Breast Imaging

Breast Imaging

Second Edition

Daniel B. Kopans, M.D.
Director of Breast Imaging
Department of Radiology
Massachusetts General Hospital
Associate Professor of Radiology
Harvard Medical School
Boston, Massachusetts

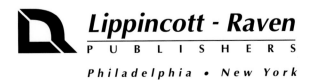

Lippincott - Raven
P U B L I S H E R S
Philadelphia • New York

Acquisitions Editor: James Ryan
Developmental Editor: Mary Beth Murphy
Manufacturing Manager: Dennis Teston
Associate Managing Editor: Kathleen Bubbeo
Production Editors: Jenn Nagaj and Elizabeth Willingham, Silverchair Science + Communications
Cover Designer: Karen Quigley
Indexer: Hope Steele
Compositor: Lisa Cunningham, Silverchair Science + Communications
Printer: Courier Westford

Printed in the United States of America

9 8 7 6 5 4 3 2 1

Library of Congress Cataloging-in-Publication Data

Kopans, Daniel B.
   Breast Imaging / Daniel B. Kopans. -- 2nd ed.
        p.   cm.
   Includes bibliographical references and index.
   ISBN 0–397–51302–X
   1. Breast--Imaging.   2. Breast--Cancer--Diagnosis.   I. Title.
   [DNLM: 1. Breast Neoplasms--diagnosis.   2. Mammography--methods.   3.
Diagnostic Imaging.   4. Technology, Radiologic.   WP 815 K83b 1997]
RC280.B8K67   1997
616.99'4490754--dc21
DNLM/DLC
for Library of Congress   97–34814
                                                                                  CIP

Care has been taken to confirm the accuracy of the information presented and to describe generally accepted practices. However, the authors, editors, and publisher are not responsible for errors or omissions or for any consequences from application of the information in this book and make no warranty, express or implied, with respect to the contents of the publication.

The authors, editors, and publisher have exerted every effort to ensure that drug selection and dosages set forth in this text are in accordance with current recommendations and practice at the time of publication. However, in view of ongoing research, changes in government regulations, and the constant flow of information relating to drug therapy and drug reactions, the reader is urged to check the package insert for each drug for any change in indications and dosage and for added warnings and precautions. This is particularly important when the recommended agent is a new or infrequently employed drug.

Some drugs and medical devices presented in this publication have Food and Drug Administration (FDA) clearance for limited use in restricted research settings. It is the responsibility of the health care provider to ascertain the FDA status of each drug or device planned for use in their clinical practice.

To the women of the world
May breast cancer soon be eliminated as a source of dread and death.

To breast cancer researchers and breast health caregivers
May our efforts soon be unnecessary.

Contents

Preface to the Second Edition ix

Preface to the First Edition xi

Acknowledgments xiii

1. Introduction 1

2. Anatomy, Histology, Physiology, and Pathology 3

3. Epidemiology, Etiology, Risk Factors, Survival, and Prevention
   of Breast Cancer 29

4. Screening for Breast Cancer 55

5. Radiation Risk 101

6. Staging Breast Cancer 107

7. Early-Stage Breast Cancer: Detection, Diagnosis, and Prognostic Indicators . . . 117

8. Mammography: Equipment and Basic Physics 135

9. Quality Assurance and Quality Control 157
   Debra Deibel

10. Mammographic Positioning 171

11. A Systematic Approach to Breast Imaging 211

12. Mammography and the Normal Breast 229

13. Analyzing the Mammogram 247

14. Benign and Probably Benign Lesions 351

15. The Mammographic Appearance of Breast Cancer 375

16. Ultrasound and Breast Evaluation 409

17. The Altered Breast: Pregnancy, Lactation, Biopsy, Mastectomy,
    Radiation, and Implants 445

18. The Male Breast 497

19. Pathologic, Mammographic, and Sonographic Correlation 511

20. Magnetic Resonance Imaging 617
    Carol A. Hulka and Daniel B. Kopans

21. Imaging-Guided Needle Placement for Biopsy and the Preoperative
    Localization of Clinically Occult Lesions 637

22. Problems and Solutions in Breast Evaluation 721

23. Palpable Abnormalities and Breast Imaging 747

24. Breast Imaging Report: Data Management, False-Negative
Mammography, and the Breast Imaging Audit. 761

25. Medical-Legal Issues and the Standard of Care 797

26. Future Advances in Breast Imaging 807

Subject Index 841

Preface to the Second Edition

This second edition of *Breast Imaging* has been delayed for several years. Unlike many new editions, most of it has been rewritten. The basic issues and observations remain the same, but the understanding of breast cancer, its development, and its diagnosis has increased since the first edition.

The delay has been primarily due to the need to stop and revisit many of the problems that appeared to have been resolved in the 1980s, but were raised once again in the 1990s. The 1993 decision by the National Cancer Institute to withdraw support for screening women ages 40 to 49 necessitated months of work to demonstrate that their arguments were inconsistent with scientific findings and their analysis incorrect. Opponents of screening began to throw one obstacle after another into the path of those supporting screening, and these obstacles had to be addressed. Once again, opposing arguments included radiation risk, the secondary "harms" (recall and biopsy) engendered by screening, and the unsupported belief that something happens abruptly to the breast and to women at the age of 50 such that screening suddenly begins to work. These arguments were developed by a fairly small group of analysts, but they were rapidly propagated by others in the lay and medical literature. The role that individuals play in these issues is impressive.

Many more individuals are now involved in imaging the breast, bringing their own agendas to the field. Most carry on the tradition of enthusiasm and dedication to the elimination of breast cancer as a major cause of death among women. With the current enthusiasm, however, has come a drift away from the importance of scientific validation. Some have adopted technologies that they believe can solve many problems, such as the lack of specificity of mammography. Their conclusions may well be true, but appropriate scientific validation should be required before a technology is adopted. It is not sufficient to merely show that a new technology can be used to evaluate the breast or breast lesions. A prospective, preferably blind, study should be required to prove efficacy.

Radiologists have been criticized in the past for our failure to validate our techniques in a prospective scientific fashion. *Breast Imaging* was written to address this criticism. Whenever scientific documentation is available, references are provided. If no data are available, then the reader should be aware that the comments are based on my experience and whatever data can be brought to bear on the subject. Although there is no doubt that some of these approaches, which are based on anecdotal evidence, will ultimately prove invalid, I have tried to provide logical arguments for adopting them.

It is hoped that the organization of *Breast Imaging* is also logical. My goal has been to provide a text that can be used by readers of varying levels of experience. I hope that it is both detailed, readable, and practical. All aspects of breast cancer detection and diagnosis originate from the anatomy, histology, and physiology of the breast. Because breast cancer cannot be prevented, and the reasons why one woman develops breast cancer and another does not remain obscure, an understanding of the epidemiology and what we know of the etiology of these malignancies form the basis of any study of the problem, and this is covered in the early chapters.

Because the only efficacious role for mammography is screening, and this has been the most contentious issue in breast care over the past 5 years, I have provided a detailed discussion of the screening issues followed by a summary of the radiation risk as a part of the "risk/benefit" equation. Because the approach to the management and treatment of breast cancer is determined by the main prognostic factor of histology, size, and nodal status, a summary of the latest staging is included in Chapter 6 as a preparation for the discussion in Chapter 7 of what constitutes early-stage breast cancer and early detection.

Because image quality is the most important technical aspect of mammography, Chapters 8 and 9 summarize the components of mammography devices and the important issues of quality control and assurance. Cancers will be missed unless the breast is properly positioned in the machine, and thus the chapter on positioning follows. Once the components are understood, the reader is provided with an organizational approach to facilitate accurate and streamlined mammographic interpretation in Chapter 11. Because the vast majority of mammograms are "normal," I have devoted a chapter to imaging the normal breast.

Chapters 13 through 15 are at the heart of the book and the subject. I have tried to provide a detailed description of an approach to analyzing mammographic findings and, based on comments from the first edition, I have added a chapter on lesions that are typically benign and require no additional evaluation. Similarly, I have tried to summarize in Chapter 15 the broad spectrum of changes that can indicate malignancy.

Ultrasound is a technology that continues to improve, and Chapter 16 has tried to take this into account. Although I still believe that if there is any doubt, tissue should be obtained for biopsy because it is so safe and simple to do so, I have tried to provide the reader with arguments that some use to defend the use of ultrasound for other than cyst solid differentiation and needle positioning. With the newer technologies, we may soon see ultrasound become a second-level screening technique.

Because of normal physiologic changes and biopsy, treatment, and cosmetic adjustments, imaging the altered breast is very common, and a chapter has been devoted to the subject.

Males rarely get breast cancer, but a small number must periodically have their breasts imaged, and I have provided a short chapter on imaging the male breast.

Most of *Breast Imaging* is organized from detection through diagnosis. Chapter 19 approaches breast abnormalities from the other direction, providing an extensive summary of the common and not so common pathologic findings in the breast and summarizing their mammographic and ultrasound features.

Magnetic resonance imaging (MRI) of the breast is gradually finding its niche. I have placed the discussion of this technology after the heart of breast imaging but before future developments, because MRI is no longer just in the future.

Interventional procedures in the breast have rapidly expanded since 1989, and Chapter 21 is quite extensive. I have tried to address all of the many ways that needles can be directed at breast lesions and used to sample or remove those lesions. Once the radiologist has all of the tools, the problem solving described in Chapter 22 becomes fairly intuitive.

Palpable abnormalities have been, until recently, the exclusive responsibility of the surgeon, but more and more radiologists have elected to become involved in the management of these lesions. I have kept this chapter separate because many may still wish to distinguish palpable lesions from imaging detected lesions, which are the responsibility of the radiologist.

Chapter 24 provides some direction for reporting breast imaging studies. The American College of Radiology has spent a great deal of time and effort developing the Breast Imaging Reporting and Data System, and this chapter follows that system.

Recognizing that ours is a litigious society and that the failure to diagnose breast cancer is the leading cause of malpractice claims, I have summarized my own perspective on the medical-legal system in Chapter 25. Unfortunately, but I believe justifiably, this is a pessimistic review. Because lawyers use the medical literature extensively in these suits, I have tried throughout this book to refrain from using terminology that can be manipulated and misconstrued by lawyers. If I have inadvertently used unjustified "imperative" language, the legitimate medical reader, as well as lawyers, should be aware that there are few, if any, absolutes in medicine, and that approaches change as our experience and understanding increase.

Exciting developments will take place in imaging the breast over the next several years, and I have concluded with a chapter suggesting where those changes will come. Digital mammography is now possible, and I expect that if there is a third edition of *Breast Imaging*, it will likely require a high-resolution display!

I have tried to make *Breast Imaging* a complete, readable, and useful text. Cases provided by the atlases that were included in the first edition have been integrated into the text to provide for more continuity. I would certainly appreciate any comments that might pertain to a third edition.

Daniel B. Kopans, M.D.

Preface to the First Edition

The development of cancer of the breast and its eventual outcome is a poorly understood, complex interaction of host as well as environmental factors. There is as yet no known way to prevent breast cancer, and once the disease is disseminated, its cure remains elusive. Data have accumulated showing that death from breast cancer can be delayed or averted by detecting and treating it earlier in its growth. Not only can mortality be diminished, but earlier detection increases therapeutic options and frequently the physical and psychological trauma of mastectomy can be avoided.

Screening is not the ultimate solution, but rather an intermediate advance until methods of prevention or therapeutic cure are discovered. The optimism that the screening trials have engendered must be tempered by the realization that, unfortunately, not all women will be saved by earlier detection. Nevertheless, at least a 30% reduction in breast cancer deaths can be achieved by screening. Recognition of this has led to a marked increase in interest in breast evaluation and mammography in particular. This book has been written not as a comprehensive and in-depth discussion of the theoretical aspects of breast imaging, but rather to provide a practical guide to imaging the breast. An attempt has been made to provide a concise overview of the major issues of breast imaging. It is hoped that this book will serve as a usable reference to guide the daily interpretation of breast imaging studies. Only modalities with demonstrated utility are discussed in detail. Experimental techniques such as transillumination, magnetic resonance imaging, and digital mammography are summarized, but should not be viewed as clinically relevant at this time.

X-ray mammography is clearly the single most important factor in early detection. Ultrasound has a limited, but useful, application in the analysis of specific lesions, while computed tomography of the breast can facilitate the positioning of guides to direct the surgeon to clinically occult lesions. These techniques and their applications are covered in detail.

Breast Imaging is deliberately organized to address the same topics from several different perspectives. The Introduction summarizes the major issues involved in breast imaging and its application for breast cancer screening. A basic review of the anatomic and histologic considerations follows in Chapter 2. The radiologist should be aware of the clinical importance of staging, and this is summarized in Chapter 3. Because the primary role of imaging is to detect breast cancer earlier, the definition of early-stage breast cancer is discussed in Chapter 4.

The bulk of the book is devoted to imaging. Redundancy is intentional because there are those who may wish to review the imaging appearance of specific pathology, or who, inversely, might desire to review the possible diagnoses for specific imaging findings.

Mammography is clearly the single most important breast imaging technique. In order to produce high-quality mammographic studies, fundamental physical factors must be appreciated, and in Chapter 5 this review precedes a discussion of the principles of patient positioning. The controversy concerning the importance of parenchymal patterns, which has filled the past decade, is addressed in the following section. An organized approach to mammographic analysis is next, and is structured from the point of view of reading the mammogram. An effort has been made to cover many of the questions that we all face in day-to-day mammographic interpretation. There are no exact answers to many of these questions, but guidelines are suggested to aid in determining which lesions require biopsy for diagnosis as well as defining findings that do not require biopsy. Further guidance is provided in a separate summary of the primary and secondary mammographic signs of malignancy.

The important distinction between detection and diagnosis is particularly stressed in Chapter 6 on ultrasonography. This modality has no efficacy for the early detection required of a screening test but does have a role in lesion analysis. The efficacious utilization of ultrasound is defined and a coordinated approach to specific problems is outlined.

Chapter 7, titled Pathologic, Mammographic, and Sonographic Correlation, catalogues the various processes that occur in the breast. These processes are grouped by anatomic and histologic criteria. Whenever possible, mammographic and sonographic examples of each are provided.

It will be apparent to the reader that there is a significant overlap in the morphology of lesions, and the nonspecific secondary signs of malignancy frequently make benign conditions indistinguishable from malignant processes. In recognition of this overlap, techniques for preoperative placement of guides to assist in biopsy of nonpalpable lesions are discussed in detail in Chapter 9. These techniques have been devised to permit early intervention and aggressive diagnosis of indeterminate lesions by permitting accurate guidance for the surgeon. Safety and accuracy are stressed in an effort to minimize the volume of tissue that must be excised so that cosmesis is preserved. The same techniques are applicable for needle placement if fine-needle aspiration cytology becomes accepted as a means to avoid benign open biopsy.

Although cancer of the breast is rare in men, a chapter has been included on the male breast, because lumps can occur, and imaging can be diagnostic.

There is great insecurity among those involved in breast imaging concerning the breast imaging report. We have evolved a straightforward, honest approach, which is summarized in Chapter 11.

Atlases of mammography and sonography are also included in this book, following Chapters 5 and 6. These are organized according to morphologic criteria found by imaging. They are included to emphasize the spectrum of characteristics that can be encountered and to provide the reader with more than one example of specific findings. It is hoped that these will be useful as an aid in day-to-day interpretation of images.

Daniel B. Kopans, M.D.

Acknowledgments

Many people have been associated with and have supported the Breast Imaging Division of the Department of Radiology at the Massachusetts General Hospital (MGH). *Breast Imaging* is a compilation of the published experience of investigators at other institutions as well as the work of those who have participated in the detection and diagnosis of breast cancer at MGH. All have contributed over many years. I apologize that some names will be inadvertently left out. I deeply appreciate the hard work and contributions to the Division of Jean Crowley, Jack Meyer, William Wood, Sheila Bucchianeri, Roberta Singer, Cynthia Puryear, Peggy McCallum, Maureen Doyle, Diane Whitmarsh, Lee Niles, Christine McGlory, Linda Johnson, Deborah Richard-Kowalski, Sandra Creaser, Jean Lamere, Jane Kelley, Sharon Mustone, Cinda Thomas, Nancy Tobin, Maria Hanley, Jayne Cormier, Dolores Dunne, Deborah Solomon, Melissa Candido, Tracy Ruvido, Lisa Dimatteo, Frances Mahoney, Miki Marino, Patricia Marotta, Susan Nugent, Donnamarie McNeil, Donna Burgess, Jackie Barrera, Joanne Merrill, Susan Cundari, Melissa Wasson, Lillian Regan, Paul Stomper, George White, Karen Lindfors, Kathleen McCarthy, Deborah Hall, Fritz Koerner, Dennis Sgroi, Gary Whitman, Priscilla Slanetz, James Thrall, Helen Mrose, and Cynthia Swann. I would also like to acknowledge all the other friends and coworkers on ACC 2 and across the country who have directly or indirectly contributed to the functioning of the Breast Imaging Division.

Debra Deibel is one of the leading experts in the United States on quality assurance and quality control and I am grateful to her for writing the chapter on those topics.

I also thank Carol Hulka, M.D., for her work in the MGH Breast Imaging Division and for permitting me to include her work in the chapter on magnetic resonance imaging.

I am particularly grateful to several colleagues. I am most grateful to Mike Moskowitz, who taught me the basics of epidemiology and the important issues in breast cancer screening. I thank Ed Sickles, who has always maintained calm in the face of intense arguments and taught me the value and importance of science. I am grateful to Steve Feig, who taught me to be thorough in analysis, and to Laszlo Tabar, who taught me the importance of technical rigor and whose work and energy are the basis of breast cancer screening. They are all good friends and major contributors to our understanding of breast cancer detection and diagnosis.

Special thanks go to Richard Moore for his creative genius and all of his help in our research efforts, as well as for developing and operating our computer systems.

I am deeply indebted to Ann Cunha, who was the Division secretary through many years of stress and difficulty and yet maintained her equanimity and humor throughout.

Finally, I wish to thank Dorothy McGrath, who has been a coanchor in the Division, a developer and editor of ideas, a creator of teaching materials, and a breast imaging educator. She has helped to raise the consciousness of technologists and radiologists throughout the country, stressing the importance of providing the best patient care possible and keeping us all in touch with the human aspects of what we do.

Breast Imaging, 2nd ed., by Daniel B. Kopans.
Lippincott–Raven Publishers, Philadelphia © 1998.

CHAPTER 1

Introduction

Although lung cancer has surpassed breast cancer as the leading cause of cancer death among American women, breast cancer remains the leading cause of *nonpreventable* cancer death. On the basis of gender alone, all women in the United States have a baseline risk of developing breast cancer of approximately 4% to 6% over the course of their lifetime. A subsegment of the population is at additional risk, giving the overall population an average risk of one chance in nine (11%) of developing breast cancer by the age of 85.

Breast cancer is one of the best studied human tumors, but it remains poorly understood. It has become fairly certain that, as with all solid tumors, breast cancer is the result of DNA alterations (damage or mutation) that lead to uncontrolled cell proliferation. Nevertheless, its actual etiology remains obscure. It is not possible to predict who will develop breast cancer. Its natural history is contested by experts. Methods to prevent it are under investigation but remain unproved, while methods to cure it are controversial and, unfortunately, not always successful. Between 30% and 40% of women who develop breast cancer die from it.

Despite the numerous large studies that have evaluated the benefit of early detection, there is no universal agreement as to who should be screened, at what age screening should begin, how often an individual should be screened, and at what age screening should be discontinued.

Our understanding of breast anatomy, histology, and pathology remains rudimentary, and basic questions remain unanswered. These range from the simplest anatomic questions, such as the distribution of ducts and their interrelation, to more complex questions, such as the possibility that there is a "stem" cell that is responsible for terminal duct differentiation and possibly the site for malignant transformation.

There is no general agreement as to whether breast cancer originates as a disease of a single cell whose progeny spread through a single duct system, or as a field phenomenon, in which multiple cells and ducts (related or separate) are simultaneously involved.

It is not known why the cells of the terminal duct appear to be the site of origin for breast cancer, and there is no basic understanding of the relationship between cancers that appear to originate from cells lining the duct and those that appear to originate from cells that line the lobule.

There are clearly lesions, such as atypical hyperplasia and lobular carcinoma in situ (lobular neoplasia), that increase the risk of developing cancer, but the relationships with invasive cancer remain obscure. Even ductal carcinoma in situ (DCIS), which has direct links to invasive cancer, remains enigmatic since it appears that not all DCIS progresses to invasive cancers.

The complexity and frustration of breast cancer are reflected in the fact that some women with microscopic, or even undetectable, breast cancer die rapidly of metastatic disease, while other women with large masses that almost replace the breast and involve axillary lymph nodes survive for many years.

Fortunately, a disease process does not have to be understood to be treated successfully. The randomized, controlled trials of screening have clearly demonstrated that the natural history of breast cancer can be interrupted if the process is detected early enough, and cure or delayed mortality can be achieved for many women. The efficacy of screening asymptomatic women has been demonstrated, particularly through the use of mammography. Mammography is the primary breast imaging technology and the only system that has been validated for screening. Nevertheless, other tests have been and will be shown to be valuable in the assessment of breast problems.

Since breast imaging was first described as a specialty within radiology (1), the field has expanded to include virtually all of the imaging technologies, including magnetic resonance imaging and nuclear medicine. The specialty attempts, using these various methods of imaging the breast, to detect and diagnose breast cancer earlier, when cure is more likely and treatment less formidable, and to assist in determining the appropriate therapy for a given lesion.

Earlier detection has permitted the more widespread use of conservation therapy with the excision of the primary lesion and radiation to reduce the likelihood of recurrence within the breast. As techniques are refined it may be possible to eliminate the tumor within the breast with little physical damage to the normal breast tissues.

Within the specialty there are numerous gaps in our knowledge. The very basic natural development of the breast as manifest by its mammographic appearance is poorly understood. Is there a "normal" breast? There has never been a study to determine whether or not there are significant changes on the mammogram that are related to the menstrual cycle. The histologic basis of all the structures seen on the mammographic image is still not clear. Why does one woman have "dense" breast tissue while another, of the same age and apparent demographic characteristics, have predominantly fat? Is one of these a normal state, while the other is an indicator of abnormality? There has been a fairly consistent suggestion that women with more radiographically dense tissues are at a slightly increased risk for cancer, but the relationships and mechanisms for this remain obscure.

Screening has been shown to be efficacious, but there are strong disagreements as to the appropriate methods of delivery of mammographic services. Is physical examination necessary? Who should perform it? How involved must the radiologist be? Is interpretation of the screening study sufficient, or must the radiologist examine and correlate the clinical examination with the mammogram? Does the psychological benefit of giving the patient an immediate report outweigh the increased detection of cancers afforded by a delayed double reading? What is the role of the radiologist in the evaluation of the palpable abnormality (2)? Additional projections (3) and spot compression views reveal more cancers on the mammogram (4), but does this actually alter management? Similarly, there is disagreement over the role of ultrasound in the evaluation of the palpable mass. The indiscriminate use of ultrasound merely adds to the expense if needle aspiration is to be undertaken to simultaneously diagnose and eliminate a palpable cyst.

Needle aspiration cytology and core needle biopsy can reduce the need for excisional biopsy for many lesions. Should lesions classified as needing short interval follow-up be aspirated or "cored" to eliminate the uncertainty for the woman, but at increased expense to the health care system? What should the threshold for intervention be when an abnormality is seen on a mammogram (5)? What should the positive predictive value be when a recommendation is made for a biopsy? What is an acceptable false negative rate?

These and many other questions remain unresolved. Most should be answered through scientific study. For some the answer is philosophical, while the economics of health care may ultimately dictate many choices (6).

The heightened awareness of the breast cancer problem has stimulated a renewed effort and increased research support to try to understand, detect, treat, and one day prevent breast cancer. The BRCA1 and BRCA2 genes, found in women with hereditary breast cancer, have been isolated. Women with an abnormal copy of the BRCA1 or BRCA2 genes face a 50% lifetime risk of developing breast cancer. Although the inheritance of a faulty BRCA1 or BRCA2 gene accounts for only 10% of all cancers, an understanding of the role of these genes in the development of breast cancer may point the direction toward more effective approaches to detection, treatment, or prevention.

There is great optimism over the potential of molecular biological research, and unraveling the molecular basis of cancers will likely lead to more effective approaches to the problem, but there have been high hopes for basic research in the past, only to end in disappointment. Clinical research is of equal importance and should be strongly supported. There is no question that mammographic screening is not the solution to the problem of breast cancer, but it is the best that is available at the present and for the foreseeable future. If properly performed, mammographic screening can reduce the death rate by at least 25% to 30% and probably more. Attention should be given to its proper performance. One of the primary messages of *Breast Imaging* is to urge the performance of high-quality mammography.

As in all medical endeavors, the practitioner should, whenever possible, use the results of scientific studies to guide clinical decisions. In the absence of science, experience must guide management. As was the goal in the first edition of *Breast Imaging,* this second edition has been written to try to provide the practitioner with the latest data available and scientific justification for the proper process whenever possible. When science is not available, it is hoped that the arguments for management decisions are logical and reasonable. Our knowledge and understanding of the breast and its characteristics and problems are constantly evolving. It is hoped that this text will provide a useful summary of the present state of knowledge and its application to breast evaluation and the breast cancer problem.

REFERENCES

1. Kopans DB, Meyer JE, Sadowsky N. Breast imaging. N Engl J Med 1984;310:960.
2. Kopans DB. Breast imaging and the "standard of care" for the "symptomatic" patient. Radiology 1993;187:608–611.
3. Meyer JE, Kopans DB. Breast physical examination by the mammographer: an aid to improved diagnostic accuracy. Appl Radiol 1983;(March/April):103–106.
4. Faulk RM, Sickles EA. Efficacy of spot compression—magnification and tangential views in mammographic evaluation of palpable masses. Radiology 1992;185:87–90.
5. Kopans DB. Mammography screening for breast cancer. Cancer 1993;72:1809–1812.
6. King MJ. Mammography screening for breast cancer [letter]. Cancer 1994;73:2003–2004.

CHAPTER 2

Anatomy, Histology, Physiology, and Pathology

As with all organ systems, an understanding of the anatomy, histology, and pathology of the breast leads to an enhanced ability to interpret imaging studies. Breast imaging primarily involves the assessment of the morphology of macroscopically visible breast structures. A basic understanding of the anatomy and histology of the breast and of the complex underlying microscopic structures in which changes take place is important for an understanding of the pathologic processes that occur and is helpful for image interpretation.

Rather than merely searching for patterns, the interpreter should try to understand the underlying processes that produce the morphologic changes visible on the various imaging studies. At times different processes may produce similar findings, but in many cases the imaging morphology reflects histologic and pathologic changes. The anatomy of the breast and the organization and distribution of the histologic elements often shape the imaging findings. Ideally the interpreter should be able to explain, using specific criteria, why a finding is judged benign or potentially malignant by being able to explain the specific characteristics of the finding that led to the particular assessment.

OVERVIEW

The breast is a modified skin gland. It develops on the chest wall between the clavicle and the sixth to eighth ribs. Breast tissue can be found as far medially as the sternum and laterally to the midaxillary line. Breast tissue frequently extends around the lateral margin of the pectoralis major muscle and may be found high in the axilla, occasionally reaching to its apex.

The skin of the breast is usually 0.5 to 2 mm in thickness. Just beneath the skin lies the superficial layer of fascia (Fig. 2-1) that, at the level of the breast, divides into superficial and deep layers. The breast develops between this split layer of fascia and is enveloped by it. The deep layer of this split fascia forms the retromammary fascia, and this lies immediately on the fascia that overlies the pectoralis major muscle providing surfaces that permit some movement of the breast on the chest wall. The fascial layers do not completely isolate the breast from the pectoralis major. Blood vessels and lymphatics penetrate the fascial layers, coursing between the muscle and the breast.

The structure of the pectoralis major muscle is important for breast imaging (Fig. 2-2). The mediolateral oblique projection is positioned so that the plane of compression is parallel to the oblique fibers of the free margin of the muscle as it extends from the ribs to the humerus. This permits maximum traction on the breast so that it can be fully positioned over the detector and comfortably compressed.

The breast is divided into incomplete compartments by varying amounts of connective tissue, described by Cooper 150 years ago and known as *Cooper's ligaments.* These planes of collagen come to peaks that attach to the skin as the retinacula cutis. The breast is primarily supported by the skin and is anchored to the chest wall medially along the sternum and superiorly toward the clavicle. It is fairly mobile inferiorly and along its lateral margins. The skin of the breast resists displacement downward but permits elevation. Displacement laterally is also resisted, but the breast is fairly easily moved medially. These movements are used to advantage in mammographic positioning (see Chapter 10).

Immediately beneath the skin is subcutaneous fat. This layer varies with individuals. In some women it is clearly separate from the parenchymal cone of the breast. In others the subcutaneous fat cannot be distinguished from fat between the glandular structures.

The nipple contains many sensory nerve endings and smooth muscle bundles. The latter perform an erectile function to facilitate nursing. The pigmented tissues of the areola contain numerous apocrine sweat glands and sebaceous glands, as well as hair follicles. The skin of the areola is thicker than the rest of the skin of the breast, tapering down toward the limbus of the areola. The small, raised nodular structures that are distributed over the areola are Morgagni's tubercles and define the openings of Montgomery's (sebaceous) glands.

The surface of the nipple itself is irregular and contains numerous crevices. The duct orifices are at the bottom of these crevices. Various investigators suggest that there are between 8 and 20 major ducts that open on the nipple. Each of these ducts and its tributaries defines a lobe or segment of the gland. Beneath the nipple openings, the major ducts dilate into their ampullary portions. These are the lactiferous sinuses. The deeper segmental ducts divide into subsegmental structures and may branch further until they form the terminal duct that enters the lobule.

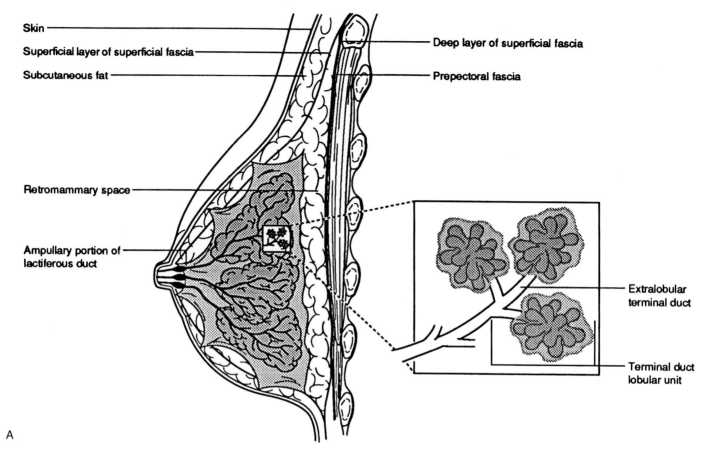

Skin
Superficial layer of superficial fascia
Subcutaneous fat
Deep layer of superficial fascia
Prepectoral fascia
Retromammary space
Ampullary portion of lactiferous duct
Extralobular terminal duct
Terminal duct lobular unit

A

FIG. 2-1. (A) This schematic representation of the basic **anatomy of the breast** can be compared to the lateral view **(B)** from a negative mode radiograph using the Xerox technique.

The lobule is defined by a final ramification of the duct into blunt ending ductules that, like the fingers of a glove, form the glandular acini and, surrounded by specialized connective tissue that is distinguishable from the stromal connective tissue, form the lobule of the breast. A terminal duct and its lobule are collectively called the terminal duct lobular unit (TDLU) (see Fig. 2-1). TDLUs can also be found as immediate branches of the major ducts and are not always at the periphery of the ductal networks.

BREAST DEVELOPMENT

The breasts have the same ectodermal origin as skin glands. They develop from the mammary ridges, which begin as ventral "streaks" in the fifth week of gestation. The mammary ridges extend longitudinally from the base of the forelimb bud (the primitive axilla) along the ventral surface of the embryo (the chest and abdomen to be) to an area medial to the base of the hindlimb bud (the primitive inguinal region). If development proceeds normally, the middle portion of the upper third of the mammary ridge persists to form the breast bud on the chest wall and eventually the tail of Spence, extending into the axilla while

the remainder of the structure disappears. Failure of portions of the ridge to involute may result in accessory breast tissue anywhere along the "milk line," extending from the axilla to the inguinal region (1,2). The axilla is the most common area in which accessory breast tissue can be found. This tissue may be in continuity with the main breast tissue (Fig. 2-3A), appear as a separate discontinuous structure (Fig. 2-3B), or it may actually form separate mounds (Fig. 2-3C). Accessory nipples are occasionally present (Fig. 2-3D).

Fibroglandular densities are frequently visible on the mammogram high in the axilla. Since breast cancer can develop anywhere that there is ductal epithelium, all of these tissues should be included and evaluated in imaging.

During the first trimester of intrauterine growth the primitive epidermal bud in the embryo begins to produce cords of epithelial cells that penetrate down into the dermis. Research indicates that there are factors that are produced in the underlying mammary mesenchyme that stimulate this growth (3). Interactions between the glandular tissues of the breast and its supporting stroma appear to continue throughout life. In the full-term fetus there is already a simple network of branching ducts, and, although lobules (the glandular elements) do not appear until adolescence, secre-

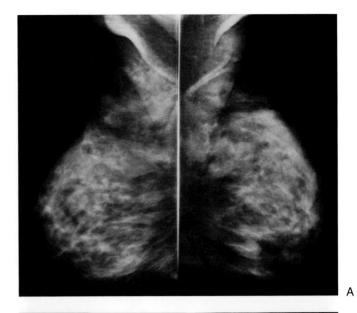

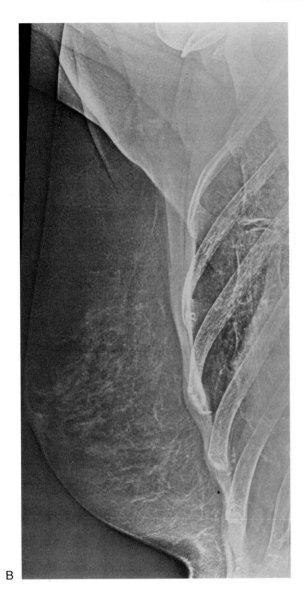

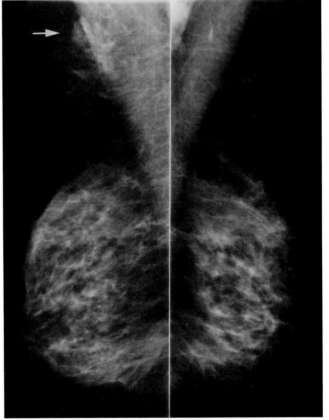

FIG. 2-3. Accessory breast tissue can form anywhere along the "milk line." Breast tissue can be found extending high into the axilla. It may be in continuity with the breast, as seen on these mediolateral mammograms **(A)**. Accessory tissue may also be separate from the main breast tissue (*arrow*), as seen on left mediolateral oblique **(B)**. *Continued.*

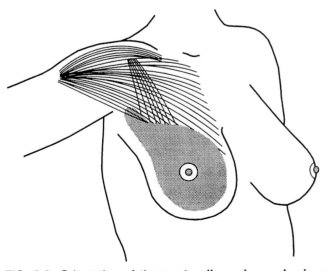

FIG. 2-2. Orientation of the **pectoralis major and minor muscles.**

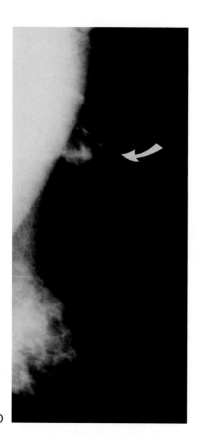
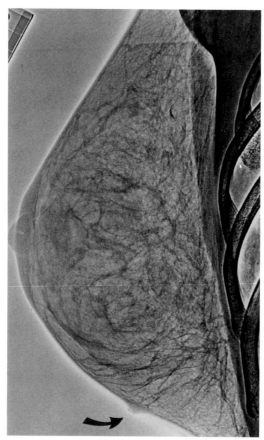

C,D

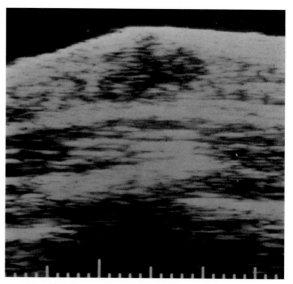

FIG. 2-3. *Continued.* Accessory tissue may even form a separate, ectopic breast, as seen in this third individual **(C)** who had a separate breast mound in her right axilla (*arrow*). Accessory nipples may be seen, as in this lateral xeromammogram where a separate nipple was visible at the bottom of the breast **(D)** (*arrow*).

tion may occur under the stimulation of maternal hormones and the newborn may have a nipple discharge.

Thelarche precedes menarche, and under hormonal stimulation the breast buds enlarge, becoming palpable discs beneath the nipple. The ducts grow back into the soft tissues, which are also stimulated to increase, and lobular development (differen-

tiation) begins. This growth may proceed asymmetrically because of the fluctuating hormonal environment and a variable sensitivity of the end-organ tissues to the stimulation.

Since the breast buds may develop asymmetrically, the detection of an asymmetric lump beneath the nipple before puberty should not be cause for concern (Fig. 2-4). Biopsy

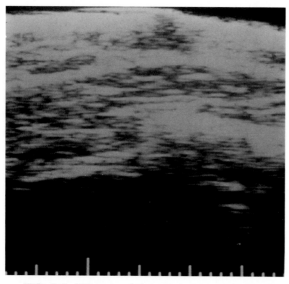

FIG. 2-4. Ultrasound demonstrates **asymmetric development of the normal breast "buds"** in a 9-year-old girl. The breast buds are the hypoechoic, triangular areas that lie beneath the nipple.

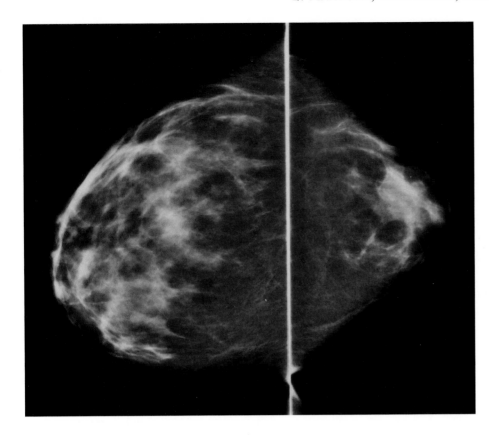

FIG. 2-5. This is a **developmental anomaly** where the left breast is much larger than the right, as seen on the craniocaudal projection.

should rarely be considered, since the inadvertent removal of the breast bud will result in failure of breast development. Only the rarest forms of breast cancer occur in pre- and pubertal females and these are usually indolent. When they do occur they are likely to grow eccentrically from the nipple, unlike the breast bud, which is centered under the nipple. Asymmetry at this stage almost always resolves in ultimate symmetrical breast development.

Although adult breasts frequently differ in size, marked asymmetry is relatively unusual (Fig. 2-5). Without skin or other changes to suggest inflammation or neoplasia, asymmetric breast size is virtually always a developmental phenomenon. There are no studies that have demonstrated any significant relationship between breast size and risk for cancer.

Probably as a result of the fluctuating hormonal environment in adolescent males, gynecomastia is fairly common during puberty. This too may be asymmetric and almost always corrects itself without the need for intervention.

Terminal Differentiation

As the breast grows, the subcutaneous adipose and connective tissues increase in volume and ductal elements proliferate, elongating and extending deeper into the subcutaneous tissues. Over a variable period of time terminal buds at the ends of the branching ducts differentiate into tufts of blunt-ending ductules that form the glandular acini of the TDLUs. The exact cells responsible for duct elongation and lobular differentiation have not been identified. Some have

speculated that there is a "stem" cell at the terminal end of the duct that is responsible for this growth. The rapid cell proliferation and DNA replication that take place in this area may account for the fact that most cancers appear to develop in the terminal duct as it enters, or along its course within the lobule. This is likely due to the fact that this is the site of most cyclic proliferation. Increased cellular proliferation increases the chance that DNA will not be copied properly and that mutations will occur.

Deng and colleagues found that there were similar genetic defects (loss of heterozygosity) in the cells of normal lobules that were adjacent to lobules containing breast cancer cells (4), while cells in lobules further away did not have the same genetic changes. This suggests that there may be a common progenitor for both the benign and malignant cells of the affected duct network. If there is a stem cell responsible for the development of the ducts and lobules, then an alteration in its DNA early in life, prior to duct elongation and terminal lobular differentiation, could be distributed into every cell in the segment. This would place the cells throughout the segment at risk for further genetic change, increasing the likelihood that one of the cells might ultimately become a cancer. This would explain the findings of Deng and his associates. It might also be the explanation for the so-called field phenomenon, in which the cells in an area of the breast have a similar abnormality while other areas of the breast are normal. This may be the explanation for diffuse adenosis, atypical hyperplasia, or even lobular carcinoma in situ.

It would be very unlikely that a carcinogen or mutagen could damage all of the cells in a segment, while sparing cells in other segments of the mature breast. However, if a stem cell were altered in the immature breast, that damage would be distributed to all of the cells of the developing segment, and only the cells of the segment would be affected. This is the likely explanation for segmentally distributed abnormalities. Our attention in preventing breast cancer is often directed toward older women. If there is a stem cell, its presence would suggest the importance of exposure to carcinogens at an early age, prior to terminal differentiation.

In mice, the period of end-bud differentiation is a time during which a carcinogen is more likely to initiate malignancy (5). A similar phenomenon may occur in humans. The breast appears to be more sensitive to radiation during this time. This maturation of the breast may take place over many years and may not be complete until the third decade of life, or it may proceed rapidly with an early first full-term pregnancy.

Additional lobular development may take place in preparation for lactation. After the cessation of lactation, many of the lobules involute. Since the breast must be complete for lactation, a full-term pregnancy likely causes rapid lobular differentiation, and it is possible that complete maturation may not occur until after a full-term pregnancy. It has been observed that women who have a first-term pregnancy by the age of 18 have a lower risk of subsequently developing cancer than women who remain nulliparous or have their first child after the age of 30. This has led to the speculation that an early full-term pregnancy offers some protection by narrowing the period of time over which differentiation takes place and, consequently, the "window of opportunity" during which a carcinogen may be most effective in causing lasting damage. If, as appears to be the case, the mature breast (differentiated terminal buds into lobules) is less susceptible to carcinogens (such as radiation), this might account for the diminished risk of breast cancer among women who bear a child early in life.

ANATOMY

In most individuals the bulk of the breast extends from the second to the seventh rib. Since breast tissues often curve

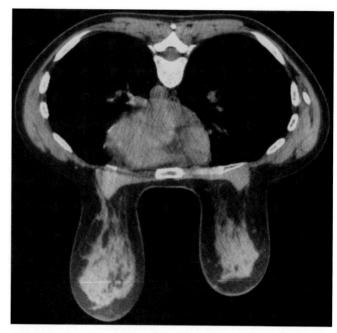

FIG. 2-6. Computed breast tomography with the breasts in the pendent position shows **breast tissue on the left adjacent to the pectoralis major muscle** extending up toward the axilla. This would be behind the pectoralis on the mediolateral oblique projection. In this individual the tissue is absent on the right after surgery for breast cancer.

around the lateral margin of the pectoralis major muscle (Fig. 2-6), the orientation of the muscle is important for optimal mammographic positioning. The pectoralis major muscle spreads like a fan across the chest wall. Portions of the pectoralis major muscle attach to the clavicle, the lateral margin of the scapula, costal cartilage, and the aponeurosis of the external oblique muscles of the abdomen. All these fibers converge on and attach to the greater tubercle of the humerus. The free fibers predominantly run obliquely over the chest from the medial portion of the thorax toward the humerus (see Fig. 2-2). The relationship of the breast to the pectoralis major muscle influences two-dimensional projectional imaging, such as mammography. Since the breast tissue is closely applied to the muscle, some of the lateral tissues can only be imaged through the muscle. As with any soft-tissue structure

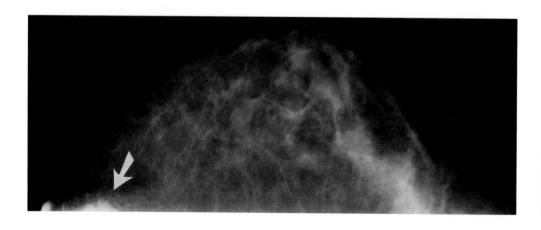

FIG. 2-7. The density seen medially (*arrow*) on this craniocaudal projection is the **pectoralis major muscle** pulled into the field of view by the compression system.

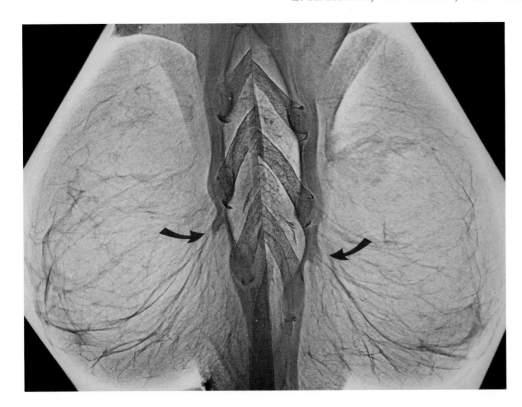

FIG. 2-8. These chest wall lateral xeromammograms show what is likely a **variation of the pectoralis major attachment** to the thoracic cage with a free margin of what is likely the inferomedial attachment (*arrows*).

overlying muscle, it is easier to project the breast into the field of view by pulling it away from the chest wall and compressing it with the plane of compression along the obliquely oriented muscle fibers of the pectoralis major muscle. In order to maximize the tissue imaged, the free portion of the muscle should be included in the field of view.

Although it has not been directly studied, it appears that there is a variable attachment of the pectoralis major muscle medially to the thoracic wall. We find that in approximately 1% of women a small tongue of muscle adjacent to the sternum is sufficiently free to be pulled into the field of view on the mammogram in the craniocaudal projection (Fig. 2-7). This is not seen on the mediolateral oblique since it is very difficult to pull this portion of the muscle into the machine in this projection, although we have seen what we believe to be a variant on a chest-wall lateral xeromammogram (Fig. 2-8). This variable portion of the muscle (Fig. 2-9) may be round, triangular, or flame-shaped and should not be mistaken for a mass.

When a flame-shaped structure that is almost completely separate from the chest wall is seen medially (Fig. 2-10A), it is likely the sternalis muscle that is being imaged (Fig. 2-10B). The sternalis muscle runs parallel to the sternum and is found in fewer than 10% of individuals. It has been speculated that it was once an extension of the rectus abdominus, but it is not connected to this or any other muscle and its origin and use is unknown. It appears to be of no functional value and can be unilateral or bilateral.

Although either pectoralis major or sternalis muscles can be imaged, care must be exercised to avoid dismissing a true medial mass as muscle since breast cancers can occur in this

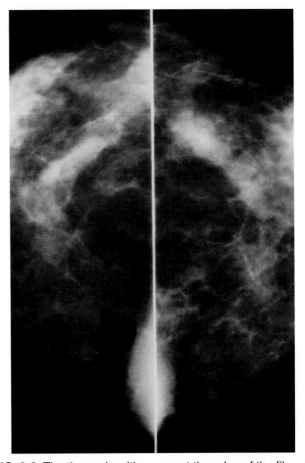

FIG. 2-9. The tissue densities seen at the edge of the film on these craniocaudal projections, medially, are the **pectoralis major muscles.**

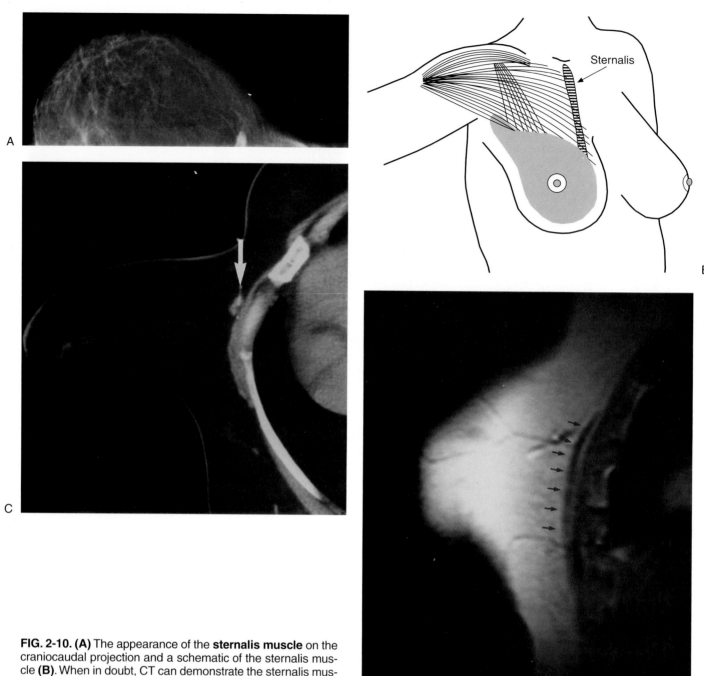

FIG. 2-10. (A) The appearance of the **sternalis muscle** on the craniocaudal projection and a schematic of the sternalis muscle **(B)**. When in doubt, CT can demonstrate the sternalis muscle. Here the patient is oblique in the scanner **(C)**. On this MRI the full course of the muscle is demonstrated **(D)** (*arrows*).

portion of the breast. If there is any doubt, CT (Fig. 2-10C), MRI (Fig. 2-10D), or ultrasound can be used to confirm or exclude a mass.

The pectoralis minor muscle lies beneath the pectoralis major muscle, extending from the third, fourth, and fifth ribs to the coracoid process of the scapula. Occasionally it can be seen on the mediolateral oblique projection as a second triangle of muscle high in the axilla above the pectoralis major muscle in the corner of the film (Fig. 2-11). This is not the latissimus dorsi muscle as some have speculated.

Vascular Supply

The lateral thoracic artery branches from the axillary artery and supplies the upper outer quadrant of the breast. The central and medial portions of the breast are supplied from perforating branches of the internal mammary artery that lies adjacent to and beneath the sternal border. Branches of the intercostal arteries provide blood to the lateral breast tissues with some blood coming from the subscapular and thoracodorsal arteries.

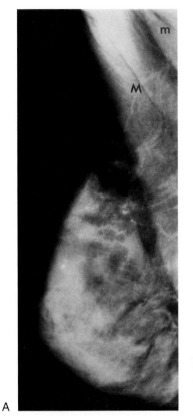

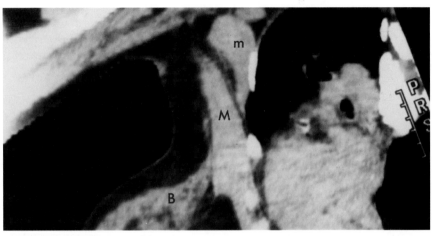

FIG. 2-11. (A) The **pectoralis major muscle** (M) is visible anterior to the **pectoralis minor muscle** (m) seen on this mediolateral oblique mammogram. The two muscles are evident on this CT reconstruction of the left breast of another patient reformatted at an oblique angle simulating the mediolateral oblique projection. The slice is through the upper outer left breast **(B)**.

Venous drainage is back through the axillary, internal mammary, and intercostal veins providing three major routes for hematogenous metastasis.

Enervation

Nerves supplying the breast originate primarily from the anterior and lateral cutaneous branches of the thoracic intercostal nerves with some enervation from the cervical plexus to the upper breast. The deep pain sensors in the breast appear to be variable. In many women, needle aspiration or needle localization with 20-gauge or smaller needles can be performed with a minimum of discomfort without the use of local anesthesia (6). To the contrary, in some women, it is extremely difficult to establish deep anesthesia. In our experience this is more likely if the breasts are extremely dense radiographically, which usually is due to fibrous connective tissue. It is merely speculation, but perhaps the nerves are more tightly tethered in these women and are not displaced from the needle path. Fibrous connective tissue may also prevent the anesthetic from reaching the nerves.

Breast pain is a fairly common symptom and is likely due to edema and swelling that occurs in many women with the normal hormone cycle. Mammography is rarely able to demonstrate the cause of breast pain. Although pain is almost always due to benign processes and breast cancer is usually painless, malignancy can occasionally cause breast pain. Focal pain and, in our experience, a drawing sensation are the types of pain that can be associated with breast cancer.

Some physicians believe that some types of breast pain are actually chest wall in origin and referred to the breast. The discomfort of costochondritis, for example, can be perceived as breast pain.

Lymphatics

The lymphatic drainage of the breast has diagnostic and therapeutic implications. Tumor can spread through the lymphatic vessels. The lymphatic system is also a route for access to the vascular system as lymph is eventually returned to the venous system through the thoracic duct and other anastomoses. Although breast cancer likely spreads primarily hematogenously, the presence of tumor in the lymphatics or in the lymph nodes indicates that the tumor has developed a metastatic potential. This increases the likelihood that tumor is elsewhere in the body.

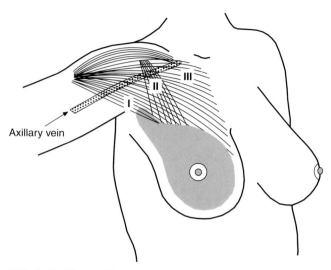

Axillary vein

FIG. 2-12. The axillary nodes are divided into three levels, as demonstrated schematically.

All breast cancers do not have the ability to metastasize. Although it is not yet possible to determine which do have the ability to spread to other organs, lymph node involvement indicates that the tumor has achieved a metastatic capability and that the disease should be considered systemic and no longer confined to the breast. Some studies suggest that spread through the lymphatics may be the primary route for access to the vascular system, although pathologists describe direct invasion of blood vessels within the breast. Lymph nodes containing tumor are usually either excised or treated with radiation to prevent recurrence, although treating the lymph nodes does not appear to influence overall survival.

The lymphatic drainage of the breast has been extensively studied. Drainage from the deeper tissues of the breast is to the surface through lymphatic channels to the skin. These then drain into a subareolar plexus and then to the axilla. There may be a small percentage of drainage to the upper abdomen and medially to the internal mammary lymphatic chain, but the primary lymphatic drainage from all parts of the breast (including the medial tissues) is to the axilla.

Although the concept of staging breast cancer is changing, the presence of tumor in the lymphatics is of important prognostic significance, and treatment may be modified based on analysis of the axillary nodes. As a consequence the axillary lymph nodes are evaluated for tumor involvement. For staging purposes (see Chapter 6) and prognostication, axillary lymph nodes are divided into three levels (Fig. 2-12). Level I lymph nodes are lateral to the lateral margin of the pectoralis major muscle and extend down into the tail of the breast. Mammography can frequently demonstrate the lowest lymph nodes in this portion of the lymphatic chain. Level II lymph nodes are beneath the pectoralis minor muscle. While the free margin of the pectoralis major muscle is retracted out of the way and preserved, the pectoralis minor muscle is transsected to

remove these lymph nodes in the modified radical mastectomy. The level III nodes are medial and superior to the pectoralis minor muscle up to the clavicle. Some data suggest that the higher the level of nodal involvement with cancer, the worse the prognosis.

Sentinel Node

As in other parts of the body, there are likely one or two lymph nodes through which the lymphatics of the breast drain first. It has been shown in patients with melanoma that technetium-99m sulfur colloid, injected at the periphery of the melanoma, will concentrate in the first lymph node that drains the area of the tumor, making it identifiable using a gamma probe (7,8). Removal and examination of this node is predictive for the presence or absence of metastatic disease, reducing the need for more complex nodal dissection and its associated morbidity and expense.

There appears to be a sentinel node for breast cancer. In a preliminary report (9), following the injection of 0.4 mCi of technetium-99m sulfur colloid mixed in 0.5 ml of saline into the tissue in a 180-degree arc around the tumor along its axillary perimeter, a probe was held over the axilla. The sentinel node was found where there were at least 30 counts in 10 seconds. The node was removed and evaluated for the presence of metastatic disease and compared to the results of the full axillary dissection. In a study of 22 women, a sentinel node was identified in 18 women who had full axillary dissections (all three levels) following radionuclide injections 1 to 9 hours before surgery. Among the 18 women, 62 radioactive and 170 nonradioactive nodes were removed. In all seven of the women who had positive nodes, the sentinel node contained tumor. In three of the patients, only this node contained tumor.

If the predictive value of the sentinel node can be validated in other trials, then the need for a full axillary dissection can be avoided. This would greatly facilitate the surgical approach to breast cancer and permit all surgery for women who elect breast preservation to be performed using only local anesthesia. This would have implications for imaging-guided needle biopsy since it would permit diagnosis, staging, and local treatment (lumpectomy) with a single operative procedure using local anesthesia.

Intramammary Lymph Nodes

Lymph nodes are found in the breast. Egan stated that whole breast dissections have revealed lymph nodes throughout the breast (10). By mammography, intramammary lymph nodes can be seen in at least 5% of normal women. They are rarely, if ever, imaged anywhere but in the lateral half of the breast and are invariably along the surface of the parenchymal cone. We have occasionally found lymphoid tissue, but not lymph nodes, elsewhere in the breast. Meyer and colleagues described three cases in which, appar-

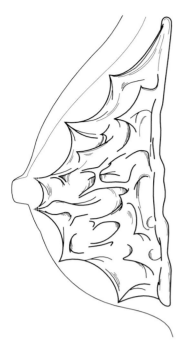

FIG. 2-13. If the glandular and fat portions of the breast are removed, what remains are **Cooper's ligaments.** This schematic depicts the fibrous connective tissues that support the ductal, glandular, and fat tissues of the breast.

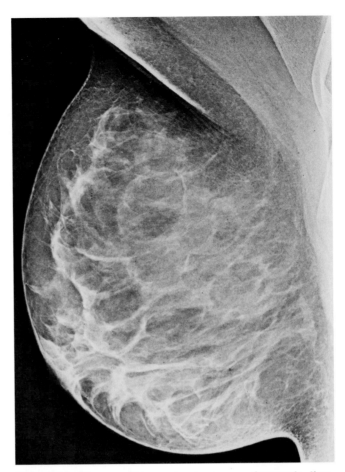

FIG. 2-14. The curvilinear structures are **Cooper's ligaments,** seen in tangent to the x-ray beam on this mediolateral xerogram.

ently complete lymph nodes were confirmed histologically in the central and medial portion of the breast (11). These, however, appear to be extremely uncommon. Virtually all intramammary nodes, visible by mammography, are in the lateral half of the breast along the margin of the breast parenchyma. They have been found as far anterior as two-thirds to three-fourths of the way to the nipple. The majority of intramammary nodes are associated with the upper outer breast tissue, although they can be found in the lower outer part of the breast or can appear to be in this area by rolling the breast when performing lateral mammograms.

Supporting Structures

The usually single layer of fascia that lies beneath the skin divides into deep and superficial layers that form an envelope within which the breast develops. The breast is given structure by the fibrous tissues that surround and course through it. Surrounded by this fascial shell the stromal, epithelial, and glandular elements of the breast are held together by an interlacing network of fibrous connective tissue. This supporting network forms planar sheets of fibrous tissue that course between the deep and superficial layers of fascia, incompletely compartmentalizing the structures of the breast. These ligaments, described by Cooper in the 1800s, form criss-crossing and overlapping structures on two-dimensional imaging and project as irregular and often spiculated shapes, frequently complicating image analysis of the breast (Figs. 2-13 and 2-14). These fibrous structures

form around and support the developing duct network as it grows back into the soft tissues of the chest.

There are two general types of connective tissue in the breast. There is usually a clear difference between the interlobular, or stromal, connective tissue described above and the specialized, loosely arranged connective tissue that surrounds and is intimately related to the terminal ducts and lobules forming the intralobular connective tissue. Together, these fibrous elements produce a cohesive structure that resists surgical dissection along tissue planes and often requires the surgeon to employ cutting techniques when operating on the breast. The fibrous connective tissues of the breast can be so tough that they make it very difficult to introduce and position needles for diagnostic aspiration or core biopsies.

There is a complex interaction between the duct network and the connective tissue elements of the breast. The percent of connective tissue decreases with increasing age in many women, while in others the percent does not seem to vary with age.

The superficial extensions of Cooper's ligaments, known as the *retinacula cutis,* attach the breast to its primary support, the skin. The deep layer of superficial fascia demarcates the back of the breast. This retromammary fascia lies

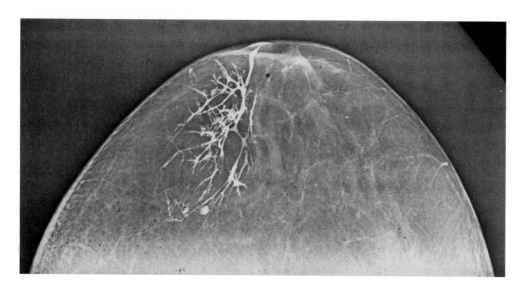

FIG. 2-15. Branches of this duct that was injected with contrast material go right to the skin of the breast.

immediately against the prepectoral fascia that overlies the pectoralis major muscle, and the relationship permits a degree of mobility for the breast to slide on the muscles of the chest wall.

Surrounding the parenchymal cone of the breast is a layer of subcutaneous fat of variable thickness. Perforated by the fibrous attachments to the skin, this fat layer does not isolate the breast, and ductal epithelium can be found directly beneath the dermis in association with the retinacula cutis. These extensions make it impossible to perform complete removal of the breast with any procedure less than a total mastectomy as ducts may extend to the skin (Fig. 2-15). To avoid devascularization and sloughing the skin, epithelial elements that can undergo malignant change are likely left behind with a subcutaneous mastectomy, making this procedure an imperfect method for eliminating the risk of breast cancer. Even a complete mastectomy cannot remove all of the ducts that attach close to the skin without devascularization and loss of the skin. It is the residual tumor extension into these ducts or the development of new cancer in these residual structures that is often the cause of recurrent breast cancer following even a modified radical mastectomy.

At the back of the breast, but within the retromammary fascia, is another layer of fat of varying volume forming the retromammary fat. The retromammary fascia slides on the prepectoral fascia permitting some mobility of the breast on the chest wall. Unfortunately, the retromammary space between the retromammary fascia and the pectoralis fascia is a "potential" space that does not completely isolate the breast. There are projections of the deep layer of fascia that traverse the retromammary space into the pectoralis major muscle, and cancer can spread through the vessels and lymphatics that penetrate to the chest wall. It was this lack of complete isolation of the breast from the pectoralis fascia that led to the surgical principles on which radical mastectomy was based.

We have shown that the majority of breast cancers develop in the parenchyma in a zone 1 cm wide that lies

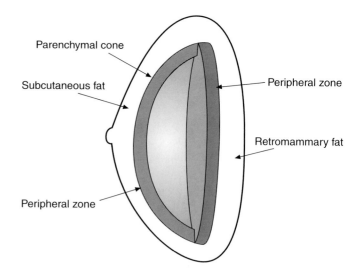

FIG. 2-16. Cancers are most commonly found at the periphery of the parenchyma. This schematic demonstrates the volume of tissue at the periphery of the parenchyma in a zone 1 cm wide that lies just beneath the subcutaneous fat and in front of the retromammary fat. More than 70% of breast cancers develop in this zone.

immediately beneath the subcutaneous fat, or anterior to the retromammary fat (Fig. 2-16). This is likely due to the fact that this is, geometrically, where most of the breast tissue is found (12). It is also possible that the majority of the TDLUs are in this zone or even, as some have speculated, that the fat acts as a reservoir for carcinogens, and, hence, the propensity for cancers to develop adjacent to these fat areas (13).

Nipple and Lactiferous Ducts

The nipple and areola contain erectile smooth muscle as well as sebaceous glands. There are hair follicles in the areola, and, on occasion, the glands or follicles may contain calcifications that rarely pose a diagnostic problem on the mammogram. Usually, eight or more lactiferous ducts have orifices originating in the nipple. Each major duct extends back into the breast in a branching network of smaller segmental and subsegmental ducts culminating in the terminal ducts and the blunt ending acini of the lobules.

Segmental Anatomy of the Breast

A major duct and its tributaries are considered a lobe, or segment of the breast. The volume and geography drained by each duct network is extremely variable (Fig. 2-17). The segmental anatomy of the breast is poorly understood. The lobes are not recognizable as histologically defined entities, since there are no boundaries separating one from another. Branches from a given duct network do not always conform to a predictable distribution. Although the major ducts tend to branch into the portion of the breast that corresponds to the quadrant of the nipple on which they open, branches can extend in unexpected directions and even branch into two different quadrants. Breast cancer appears to be a process that is confined to the cells of a single duct network. Theoretically, the removal of the entire segment (a major duct and its tributaries) should prevent recurrence. However, the segments are not evident at surgery, and, since branches of the same duct may extend into two or more quadrants (Fig. 2-18), branches of the duct and tumor may remain after resecting even an entire quadrant of the breast.

Branches from different primary ducts likely overlap and interdigitate with branches from other segmental ducts. Work by Ohtake and colleagues, in their three-dimensional studies of the ducts (14), suggests that there may be anastomoses between segmental networks, and this may be an additional way in which cancer, spreading through the duct system, involves other segments and quadrants of the breast.

The mechanism of recurrence is likely due to the fact that the duct containing the tumor is transected, and, since the pathologist evaluates only a small portion of the entire excised tissue, the extension of tumor into another part of the breast may not be appreciated. Adjuvant radiation therapy is intended to kill any residual tumor; however, if the residual tumor burden is too high, radiation may not eradicate the residual disease. Cancer that has spread into those branches and has not been eliminated by radiation is likely the source for recurrent disease. If techniques can be devised to accurately delineate a segment or eliminate the sampling

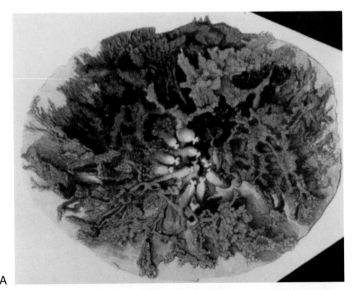

A

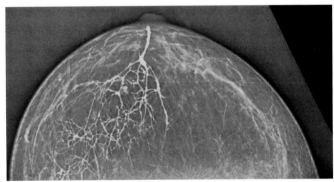

B

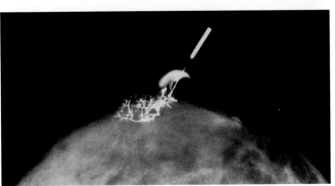

C

FIG. 2-17. **(A)** The breast is composed of lobes or segments that are defined by the major lactiferous ducts that open on the nipple. This is evident in this reproduction of the painting done by Cooper's artist following the injection of the ducts with colored paraffin. **(B)** Frequently a segment occupies a wedge of breast tissue, as seen in this duct injection imaged by xeroradiography in the craniocaudal projection. **(C) Some segments are very small,** as seen in this galactogram in the craniocaudal projection.

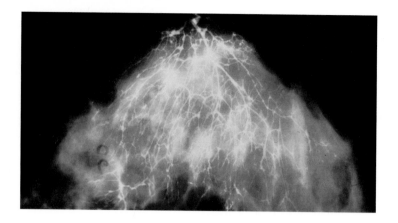

FIG. 2-18. A major duct can branch in two directions and actually involve two separate quadrants. This duct branches medially and laterally. On the craniocaudal projection the injected duct has branches that spread across the entire upper breast, so that if this patient were to have cancer and it was a segmental process a quadrant resection would likely miss branches and possible cancer that had spread within the ducts. It is likely, for this reason, that quadrant resection does not preclude recurrent cancer. (Courtesy of Norman Sadowsky, MD.)

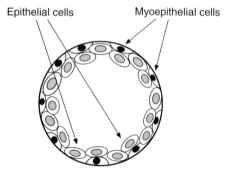

Epithelial cells   Myoepithelial cells

FIG. 2-19. Schematic of a cross section of a duct lined by epithelial cells and surrounding myoepithelial cells.

error of the pathologic tissue evaluation, therapy could be more accurately tailored.

An understanding of the development of a cancer in relationship to the duct system may have important etiologic implications. At present, it appears that most multifocal cancers are actually connected through intraductal bridges of tumor. Multiple foci likely represent areas where intraductal cancer cells have developed invasive capability.

The duct orifices are usually found at the base of multiple crypts that form the nipple surface. Immediately beneath the duct orifice in the nipple is a wider segment of the major duct known as the ampullary portion or lactiferous sinus. Beyond this point the duct begins to arborize into tapering segmental branches of varying length. Further branching may occur, forming subsegmental ducts until a terminal branch is reached. Terminal ducts and lobules may also be found branching directly from a major duct.

The ducts of the breast are lined by an inner layer of epithelial cells surrounded by a thinner, and often discontinuous appearing, layer of myoepithelial cells (Fig. 2-19). The myoepithelial cells presumably play a role in the propulsion and expression of milk during lactation. The presence of both cell types in a lesion such as a papilloma is used by the pathologist to determine that it is benign, since only epithelial cells are involved in cancer formation. Because terminal branches are not only found deep

in the breast tissue but may also form immediately off a major duct anywhere in the breast, cancers may occur immediately beneath the nipple as well as anywhere else in the breast.

Terminal Duct Lobular Unit

Branching continues until the distal duct ultimately ends in a grouping of blunt ending ductules (like the fingers of a glove) that form a collection of glandular acini defined as a lobule arrayed at the end and around a terminal duct (Fig. 2-20). A portion of the terminal duct and its ductules (acini) is surrounded by the intralobular, more loosely organized, specialized connective tissue.

The final branch from the segmental duct as it enters the lobule is termed the *extralobular terminal duct*. The portion of the terminal duct within the lobule is termed the *intralobular terminal duct*. The blunt ending tubes, or ductules, that extend like fingers into the lobule, form from 10 to 100 acini that empty into the intralobular terminal duct. Following the work done by Wellings and colleagues, histologists have termed the extralobular terminal duct and its lobule the *terminal ductal lobular unit* (15). The TDLU is the most important structure in the breast. It is the glandular unit, and it is postulated that most cancers arise in the terminal duct (Fig. 2-21) either inside or just proximal to the lobule (16). It may be significant that this is the site where the elastic tissue that surrounds the extralobular terminal duct ends, but any relationship remains to be determined. The lobule itself is usually, although not always, clearly distinguishable from the surrounding stroma and larger ducts. Its own stromal matrix (intralobular connective tissue), which some believe is derived from the dermis, contains very fine collagen fibers and reticulum and is more cellular than the extralobular connective tissue. It is also quite vascular. Although there is no demarcating membrane, the intralobular stroma stains distinctively differently from the extralobular stroma on histologic section. There are likely important chemical communications that occur between the acini and the specialized connective tissue that surround them.

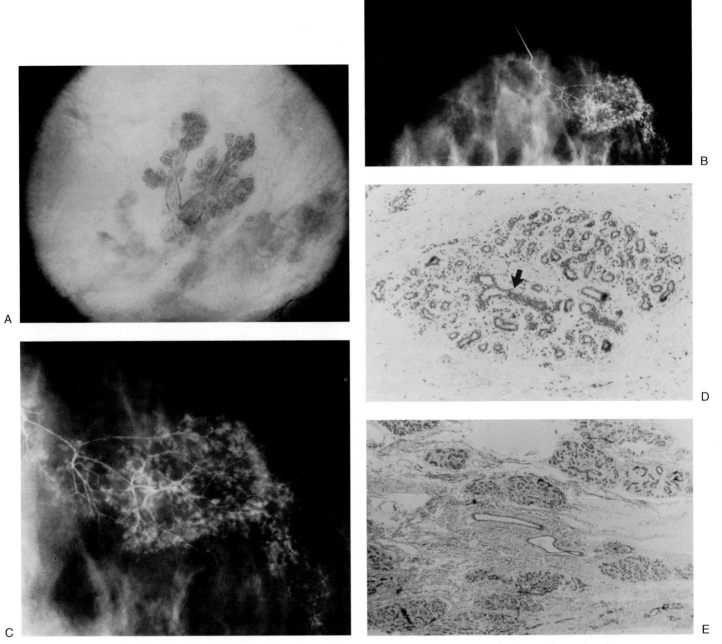

FIG. 2-20. (A) This is a thick section of tissue that has been defatted so that the three-dimensional terminal ducts and lobules are visible at 40× magnification. **(B) The appearance of TDLUs** is seen on this optically enlarged craniocaudal galactogram **(C)** in which the lobules (the small "fluffy" densities at the ends of the ducts) have filled with contrast. **(D)** This histologic section demonstrates the terminal duct and lobular acini of a TDLU. The large arrow points to the intralobular terminal duct. The TDLU is composed of the terminal duct (extralobular and intralobular portion), the ductules, or acini, of the lobule, and the specialized connective tissue that surrounds the acini and is distinct from the surrounding fat and the interlobular connective tissue. **(E)** Multiple lobules and their specialized connective tissue, as well as the interlobular, nonspecialized connective tissues, are visible in this lower magnification section.

Unlike the larger ducts, the lobule contains no elastic tissue. Although most malignant tumors in the breast are epithelial in origin, interest has been focused on the role of the contiguous, nonepithelial elements of the supporting stroma. The complex stromal-epithelial interactions and the micronutrients that bathe the terminal duct are thought by some to have a bearing on cell transformation and cancer promotion.

In addition to cancer, most of the benign lesions that develop in the breast develop in the TDLU.

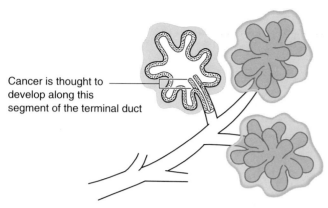

Cancer is thought to develop along this segment of the terminal duct

FIG. 2-21. Cancers are thought to arise in the intralobular portion of the terminal duct in the location suggested by this schematic.

The Normal Breast: Menstrual Variation, Lactation, and Aging Involution

Cancer is clearly the most significant pathologic process affecting the breast. Its early detection is the paramount reason for performing breast biopsies. Other abnormalities that occur in the breast are important primarily because they cause concern to the patient or physician and must be differentiated from malignancy. Of less clinical significance but potentially greater epidemiologic value has been an effort by investigators to predict which women are more likely to develop breast cancer by identifying histologic changes that may indicate a higher risk for subsequent malignancy (see Chapter 3) (17). These efforts have been complicated by difficulty distinguishing pathologic processes from the wide range of physiologic processes that occur. At a cellular level the breast is a dynamic organ that is continually changing with cyclic hormonal fluctuations. Although these primarily microscopic alterations are not visible by any presently available imaging technique, they are reflected clinically in many women by cyclic pain and swelling. Histologically the breast involutes with age, and the periodic variations are superimposed on long-term involutional changes. There is a lack of clear cut understanding of what constitutes the "normal" breast, and this has been reflected in the frequently unsatisfactory terminology that has been coined to describe various, probably physiologic, changes that occur as part of a spectrum of normal variation. Such terms as *mastopathy*, *cystic mastitis*, *dysplasia*, and the all encompassing *fibrocystic disease* are synonymous with a lack of true understanding of where normal physiology ends and true pathology begins. Autopsy studies have shown that as many as 50% of women have changes that most pathologists would characterize as fibrocystic disease (18). Similar changes were noted in reduction mammoplasty tissue and subcutaneous mastectomies performed on healthy women (19). As is discussed in the section on the normal breast, a satisfactory definition of the normal breast by imaging criteria is also lacking.

The breast is a heterogeneous organ. Further complicating breast analysis is the variable "end organ" response of its cellular constituents. This heterogeneous response can result in clinically apparent "lumps" that may merely reflect disproportionate stimulation of a volume of breast tissue, resulting in a prominence that distinguishes the particular tissue volume from the surrounding less affected tissues. The distribution of fibroglandular elements is not uniform. Neither is the distribution of fat. Islands of these various tissues may feel on clinical breast examination as thickened areas or even lumps, while by mammography the heterogeneous distribution of normal breast tissue elements may produce suspicious densities.

Fibrocystic Disease and Mammary Dysplasia

Fibrosis and cystic changes are extremely common in the breast. As noted above, at autopsy as many as 50% of women have breast elements that can be termed *fibrocystic* (20). The question that has never been satisfactorily answered is whether these changes are part of a normal spectrum or a pathologic process. The lack of uniform definitions has only added to the confusion. Any lump that is excised for whatever reason becomes, by definition, abnormal tissue. Pathologists faced with these biopsies needed to find the pathology and thus developed "wastebasket" categories. The terms *fibrocystic disease* and *mammary dysplasia* have unfortunately been used to categorize histologic variations that range from normal physiologic responses to true premalignant proliferative growth. Clinicians and radiologists optimistically trying to assure themselves that they could predict histopathology adopted these terms with little justification.

The examining fingers feel tissue inhomogeneities that are more often than not the normal variations of a heterogeneous organ. The mammogram reflects the x-ray attenuation of the tissues producing shadows that relate more to the water content of the structures than the histology. With the exception of the ultrasound diagnosis of a cyst, the calcification of an involuting fibroadenoma, or the spiculated margins of some cancers, imaging techniques are rarely able to accurately define true histology due to the overlapping appearance of many processes. The normal and the neoplastic may produce identical morphologic changes and inferring specific histology from physical examination or imaging is a statistical guess in most instances. Terms such as *fibrocystic disease* and *dysplasia* should be eliminated because they have become compromised by lack of specificity. Dupont and Page have shown that it is only the small subcategory of proliferative histologies within the category of fibrocystic disease that carries a higher risk for future malignant change (21), and within the proliferative changes it is the atypical proliferative changes that are most important.

Cysts, for example, are of no consequence unless they occur in women with a family history of breast cancer. Dupont and Page found that this combination, for unexplained reasons, increases a woman's risk 2 to 3 times. The most significant histologic risk factor among benign changes appears to be atypical epithelial hyperplasia. Women with this proliferative disorder are at five times the risk of women with no proliferative changes, and when found in women with a family history the relative risk increases to 11. Aside from these significant exceptions, no useful correlations exist between the broad category of fibrocystic disease and breast cancer risk. Furthermore, atypical hyperplasia can only be diagnosed by breast biopsy and as yet cannot be predicted by mammography although the process may produce calcifications that instigate a biopsy. The terms *fibrocystic disease* and *mammary dysplasia* cause unnecessary fear and carry an unsubstantiated prejudicial connotation. They certainly do not belong in an imaging lexicon and should probably be eliminated all together and replaced by specific histologic categories as suggested by the College of American Pathologists (17).

Cyclic Variation

The breast is a dynamic organ. Although this is not readily evident at the present level of imaging, histologic variation over the short term of the menstrual cycle is superimposed on the long-term changes of the aging process. Based on normal tissues derived from subcutaneous mastectomies and reduction mammoplasty material, Vogel and co-workers have reconstructed and detailed the monthly cellular changes occurring during the menstrual cycle (19).

During the estrogen-stimulated proliferative phase of the menstrual cycle (days 3 to 7) (Fig. 2-22), the mitotic rate in the acinar cells of the lobule increases, indicating cell proliferation in the breast as well. No secretions are seen, and the lobules are defined by a dense cellular mantle. During the follicular phase, between days 8 and 14, two distinct cell types along with more collagen are visible in the acini, while mitotic activity is diminished. The luteal phase occurs between day 15 and day 20, and the pathologist can recognize three distinctive cell types in the breast. The cells of the lobule develop vacuoles, and secretions are visible in the ducts. Vogel and associates noted loosening of the stroma within the lobule, followed by true apocrine secretion into the distended duct lumen during the secretory phase. The tissues within the lobule become edematous and there is venous congestion, which probably accounts for some of the discomfort many women experience premenstrually. Active secretion appears to end during the menstrual phase of day 28 to day 2, and then the cycle repeats itself. During the later phases there is likely apoptosis, or programmed cell death. Some have estimated that as many as two-thirds of the cells are reabsorbed in this fashion. This process ensures that a certain percentage of cells that had been formed earlier in the cycle are removed to prepare for the proliferative changes of the next hormone cycle. The role of apoptosis in breast cancer remains to be determined.

These microscopic changes have never been clearly documented at the macroscopic imaging level. Some suggest that mammography should be performed before ovulation. This is primarily to reduce the discomfort for some women when com-

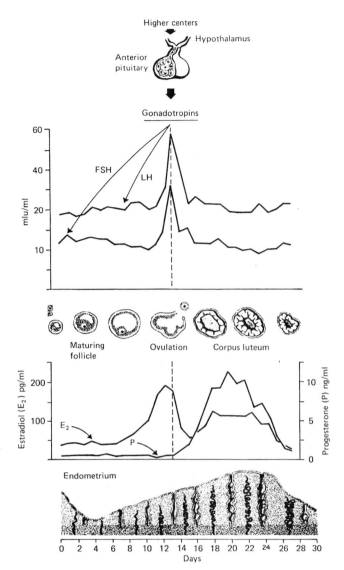

FIG. 2-22. The breast is highly sensitive to the hormone changes during the menstrual cycle. Just as with the endometrium, there is cell proliferation in the first part of the menstrual cycle. There are two cell types visible during the middle of the cycle (follicular phase), and the cells become vacuolated and secretions accumulate during the luteal phase of the cycle also associated with edema and venous congestion in the breast. The cycle begins again after apoptosis (programmed cell death) reduces the cell population at the end of the cycle. (Reprinted with permission from Scott J, DiSaia PJ, Hammond C, Spelacy WN [eds]. Danforth's Obstetrics and Gynecology [7th ed]. Philadelphia: Lippincott, 1994;30.)

pressing the edematous breast in the premenstrual phase. There are no data that determine what, if any, effect the phase of the menstrual cycle has on breast imaging and cancer detection.

Lactation

Pregnancy clearly has a profound effect on the breast. The epithelial cells begin to demonstrate changes in the first

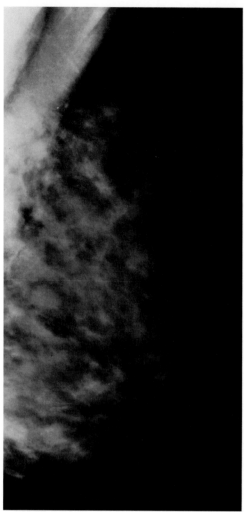

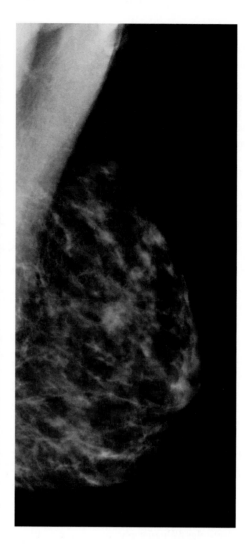

A,B

FIG. 2-23. The tissues of the **lactating breast** are often extremely and heterogeneously dense as seen on this mediolateral oblique projection **(A)**. The density often regresses after the cessation of lactation as seen in the same patient 1 year later postlactation **(B)**.

trimester. During the second trimester the lobules increase in size and there is a generalized proliferation of lobular acini, many of which begin to contain secreted material. Continued increase in the size of the lobules in the third trimester leads to replacement (crowding out) of the intralobular and interlobular connective tissue, until by the onset of lactation only thin fibrous septae separate the enlarged, secretion-distended lobules. The myoepithelial cells elongate. These are thought to be the contractile cells of the breast that aid in expressing milk. When lactation takes place, membrane-encapsulated fat globules are secreted from the epithelial cells. The membranes of these milk fat globules have been studied for their antigenic components in the search for tumor markers in nonlactating women.

When lactation ceases the breast undergoes a degree of involution, but large lobules may persist. A return to a new baseline takes approximately 3 months following the cessation of lactation. Because lactation causes a marked increase in the radiographic density of the breast (Fig. 2-23) that could obscure pathology, we recommend that routine screening mammography not be performed for at least 3 months following the cessation of lactation. True involution occurs with age.

Aging Changes and Involution

Pathologists seem in general agreement that the breast undergoes involutional changes as women age, but the timing of this involution is not clear. Over a long period of time, and apparently unrelated to ovarian activity, atrophic changes occur, but the process is not uniform throughout the breast and the timing of changes varies with individuals. The acinar lining cells of the lobules diminish, and the lobules themselves shrink in size. Connective tissue in the lobule becomes densely fibrotic or replaced by fat. Small cysts may form as the acini coalesce, but these eventually fibrose and disappear. The ductal epithelium also undergoes atrophy, and this may lead to obliteration of many of the ducts.

Intuitively, involution would be most likely associated with hormonal alterations at the time of the menopause, but at least one study questions this chronology. Aging studies, of necessity, must relate different women at varying ages since it is not possible to follow one woman over time at the microscopic level. A British investigation by Huston and coworkers (22) suggests that involution begins earlier than the generally assumed perimenopausal years. On the basis

PERCENTAGE

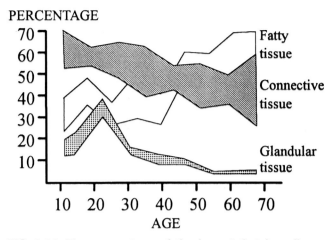

FIG. 2-24. The percentage of the breast that is collagen decreases with age, while the percentage of fat increases with age, as seen in this schematic adapted from Prechtel. (Adapted from Pretchel K. Mastopathic und altersabbangige brustdrusen verandernagen. Fortschr Med 1971;89:1312–1315.)

TABLE 2-1. *The most common benign and malignant lesions of the duct system*

Lesions of the major ducts
  Duct ectasia
  Cystic dilatation of the large duct (large duct cyst)
  Large duct papilloma
  Intraductal carcinoma extending from the terminal duct
Lesions of the minor and terminal ducts
  Hyperplasia
  Peripheral duct papillomas
  Ductal carcinoma
Lesions of the lobule
  Cyst
  Fibroadenoma
  Adenosis
  Phylloides tumor
  Lobular carcinoma
Lesions of the interlobular connective tissue
  Sarcoma

of whole breast studies, these researchers concluded that involution probably begins as early as the third or fourth decade of life and is fairly advanced by the time of menopause. This agrees with the work of Prechtel (23), cited in many pathology textbooks (24), which shows that the percent of fibroglandular tissue decreases steadily with age but that the decrease is variable among individuals with no abrupt change at any age (Fig. 2-24). In a single longitudinal study of mammographic parenchymal patterns Wolfe (25) suggested that noticeable fatty replacement occurs around the time of menopause. It is not clear how much of the observed change was technical artifact (Wolfe compared higher contrast film-screen studies of the 1960s with low contrast xeroradiographic images of the 1970s) and whether radiographically visible change actually occurs. Nor is it clear how much fatty replacement is a function of general weight gain rather than a true reflection of histologic change. Our own experience suggests that the mammographic appearance changes gradually in some but not all women and that most visible changes occur with fluctuations in the patient's weight (see Chapter 12).

The lack of a uniform definition of what constitutes the normal breast complicates determination of the abnormal. Furthermore, in all probability, host responses are important in the development of pathology. Breast evaluation is further complicated by the variable response of the end organ. This variability is suggested not only by the inhomogeneous monthly changes seen histologically, but also by the varying rate at which different parts of the breast undergo involutional change. The breast is a relatively disordered organ that lacks uniform architectural landmarks. The inhomogeneities found in varying degrees in all breasts compromise the ability of imaging studies to detect the early epithelial changes that may indicate a malignant process (see Chapter 7).

HISTOLOGY AND PATHOLOGY

Understanding the benign and malignant changes that develop in the breast is facilitated by dividing the breast into its major components and evaluating the changes that can occur in each as summarized in Table 2-1.

Relationship of Pathology to the Duct and Lobule

Benign and malignant lesions of the breast may be categorized by the level within the duct network in which they occur. Some processes are categorized as if they arose from the cells of the ducts, while others are believed to have arisen from the components of the lobules. There are few significant lesions that arise in the interlobular stroma, although fibroadenomas and phylloides tumors appear to arise from the intralobular, specialized connective tissue.

The following is a summary of the histologic and pathologic changes that can occur in the breast. For a more complete description of pathologic changes, see Chapter 19.

Lesions of the Major Ducts

Duct Ectasia

Nonspecific ectatic dilatation of the major collecting ducts can be seen by mammography and ultrasound as tubular structures beneath the nipple. Ectatic ducts may be found deeper in the breast as well. The etiology of duct ectasia has not been clearly elucidated. Periductal inflammation is either the result of duct dilatation and the extrusion of irritating materials into the surrounding stroma or the cause of duct wall weakening and dilatation. Duct ectasia is a process that generally involves the major collecting ducts.

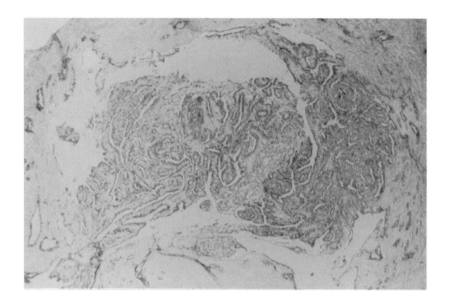

FIG. 2-25. Histologic cross section of an intraductal papilloma.

Large Duct Papilloma

Solitary benign papillomas occur in the major ducts. These are epithelial proliferations on a fibrovascular stalk (Fig. 2-25). They are usually found within a few centimeters of the nipple growing within the duct sometimes distending it. They may produce a nipple discharge that may be serous or sanguineous. Intraductal papillomas may be associated with a solitary duct enlargement. Some believe that this is due to duct obstruction. Since the dilatation is frequently both proximal and distal to the papilloma and since the normal ducts are usually blocked by keratin in the nipple orifices, obstruction is probably not the cause of the dilatation. As with cyst formation, it is likely that the papilloma causes or is associated with increased fluid secretion that is not balanced by the normal resorption mechanisms of the duct, and the fluid imbalance causes distention of the duct. Although previously the large duct papilloma was thought not to represent a breast cancer risk factor, some studies have suggested that women with solitary duct papillomas are at a small increased risk for developing breast cancer (26,27).

Paget's Disease

Paget described a form of ductal cancer that involves the large ducts. Although there is disagreement as to the exact progression of Paget's disease, these are likely ductal carcinomas that spread down the duct and out onto the nipple where characteristic Paget's cells are found in the dermis associated with an eczematoid, crusting nipple lesion. This form of ductal carcinoma often has a favorable prognosis due to its often early clinical presentation, although it may be found in conjunction with a more advanced, invasive lesion deeper in the breast.

Lesions of the Minor and Terminal Ducts

Hyperplasia

Hyperplasia likely occurs at all levels in the duct system, but the terminal duct appears to be the most significant breast structure. Wellings has postulated, and most agree, that the terminal duct is the site where most cancers develop. Hyperplasia of the epithelium in this segment is a relatively common occurrence. Several layers of otherwise normal-appearing epithelial cells form in the duct. The frequent association of hyperplasia with cysts may be the cause-and-effect relationship of a benign obliteration of the duct blocking lobular drainage and leading to cyst formation, although duct obstruction does not appear to be required for cyst formation. Gallager and Martin (28) have theorized that hyperplasia represents a nonobligatory, preliminary step toward neoplasia. Even when atypical changes develop, hyperplasia appears to represent a reversible process, but in a significant proportion of women atypical ductal epithelial hyperplasia likely progresses to intraductal carcinoma. It is likely that atypical hyperplasia is the phenotypical manifestation of genetic changes among a group of cells that place those cells closer to the changes needed for a malignancy. Since these cells likely contain several genetic alterations on the progression to malignancy, the probability of one of these cells developing all the necessary changes to become a true malignancy is greater than for normal cells.

Multiple Peripheral Papillomas

A second type of proliferation has been described in the distal ducts. Microscopic multiple papillomatous growths can be found in this region (29). Pathologists believe that these represent a different process than the solitary papillomas of the large ducts. They may represent part of a contin-

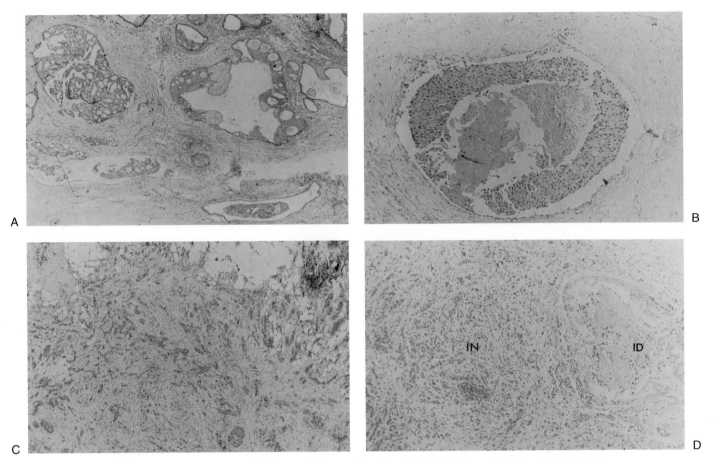

FIG. 2-26. (A) In this form of **ductal carcinoma in situ (DCIS)** ducts are filled with cells that are aligned and define cribriform spaces. **(B)** This duct is filled with so many cells that those in the center have died, probably because nutrients could not reach them. This type of comedo-intraductal cancer appears to develop invasive cells more rapidly than the better differentiated forms of DCIS. **(C)** These cancer cells have broken out of the duct and are forming a mass of **invasive or infiltrating ductal carcinoma.** The edge of the lesion is at the top of the figure. **(D)** The invasive component (IN) is on the left, while cancer continues to grow within the duct as the in situ, intraductal (ID) component in this mixed lesion.

uum of hyperplastic lesions, and it may be that multiple papillomas of this type are a premalignant change indicating a higher risk for future malignancy.

Ductal Carcinoma in Situ

The significance of ductal carcinoma in situ (DCIS) still elicits much controversy. Teleologically one would anticipate that it is the next step in a continuum that passes from hyperplasia or atypical hyperplasia to intraductal carcinoma proceeding on to frank invasion (infiltrating ductal carcinoma). Some do not believe in this progression, but there is mounting evidence that many if not all invasive cancers arise from DCIS. It is likely that some invasive cancers develop rapidly with little if any intraductal phase while some in situ cancers grow for many years within the ducts, perhaps never developing an invasive clone (see Chapter 7). It is likely, however, that breast cancer growth is a continuum that ulti-

mately results in the development of a clone of invasive cells. The duration of each step likely varies from individual to individual; in some women all the changes needed for invasion and metastasis may occur quickly, while in others there may be sufficient time at each step to interrupt the natural history of the disease. Different patterns of DCIS are emerging. The better-differentiated cribriform types (Fig. 2-26A) seem to have a slower progression to invasion, while the more poorly differentiated comedo pattern (Fig. 2-26B) seems to be more rapidly aggressive.

Invasive Ductal Carcinoma

Whether infiltrating cancer (Fig. 2-26C) develops from in situ cancer or develops directly, invasive ductal carcinoma is the most common form of invasive breast cancer and the primary lethal cancer of the breast. The cytologic features of the tumor and its growth pattern suggest an ori-

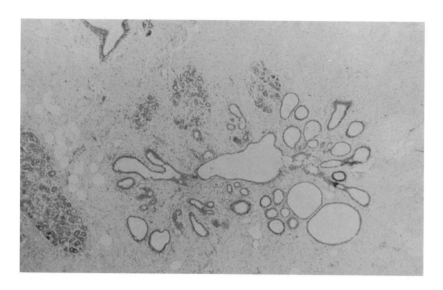

FIG. 2-27. Early microcyst formation. In this histologic section there are several normal lobules, and one whose acini are cystically dilated. This is likely the early phase in most cyst formation.

gin in the ductal epithelium. When the lesion cannot be sub-classified, it is termed *invasive ductal carcinoma NOS* (for "not otherwise specified"). Other subtypes of cancers that are thought to originate from the ductal epithelium include papillary, mucinous (or colloid), medullary, and adenoid cystic cancers. Many invasive cancers likely obliterate any residual in situ component, but as noted earlier, the in situ clones that are not destroyed by the invasive cells can continue to grow in and down the ducts, presenting invasive and in situ cancer in the same lesion (Fig. 2-26D).

Lesions of the Lobule

The most common benign lesions arise in the lobule.

Cyst

Cysts ranging from microscopic to those containing many cubic centimeters of fluid are probably the result of idio-

pathic, apocrine metaplasia of the lobular acinar epithelium. These cells appear to be hypersecretory. The increased secretion is not balanced by increased resorption, and dilatation of the lobule results (Fig. 2-27). The frequent suggestion of an associated obstructed terminal duct may be part of the process or a result of the dilating lobule causing compression of the duct.

Fibroadenoma

Fibroadenomas are the result of an idiopathic overgrowth of the specialized connective tissues surrounding the acini of the lobule. The acini are drawn out into slit-like spaces (Fig. 2-28). Subcategories of fibroadenomas have been described (intracanalicular and extracanalicular), but these do not appear to have any practical significance.

Most studies suggest that fibroadenomas carry little if any risk for the subsequent development of breast cancer. Because these lesions contain epithelium lining the stretched acini,

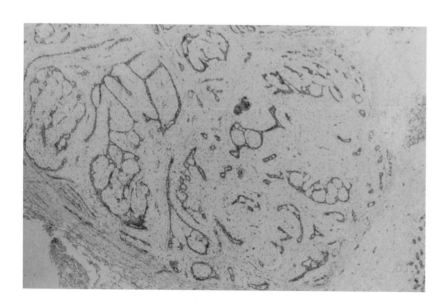

FIG. 2-28. The specialized connective tissue has overgrown, and the acini are now elongated slit-like spaces in this fibroadenoma. Normal lobules can be seen at the right edge of the picture.

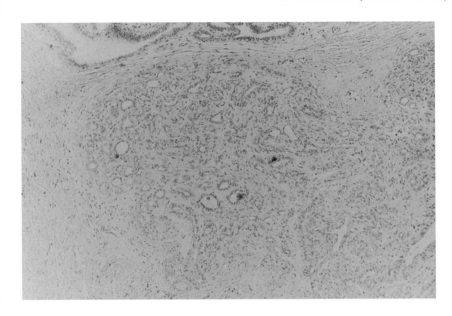

FIG. 2-29. The acini of this lobule have proliferated so that they number in the hundreds. Adenosis makes the three-dimensional lobule look like a porcupine.

cancers can arise in fibroadenomas just as they can in any breast epithelium.

One study has suggested that women with complex fibroadenomas, defined as those containing cysts, sclerosing adenosis, epithelial calcifications, or papillary apocrine changes, were at three times the risk of developing subsequent cancer than comparison groups (30). Women with adjacent proliferative disease, as well as those with fibroadenomas and a family history of breast cancer, were also at some increased risk (3.9 and 3.7 times, respectively). If Dupont and associates are correct, these risks last for many decades.

Adenosis

Adenosis is a benign proliferation of the stromal and epithelial elements of the lobule producing an increase in the number of acinar structures (Fig. 2-29). Instead of several to 100 acini, adenosis results in innumerable acini in a lobule. The individual acini are elongated. Viewed three-dimensionally, the lobule looks like a porcupine. Adenosis can be associated with a scarring process that can distort the architecture (sclerosing adenosis) and can sometimes be confused with malignant change. Calcifications are often seen in the acini.

Phylloides Tumor

The phylloides tumor is likely related to the fibroadenoma and occasionally is mistaken for it (Fig. 2-30). These are also lesions of the specialized connective tissue of the lobule. They are usually rapidly growing. Approximately 25% recur locally if not completely excised, and as many as 10% may

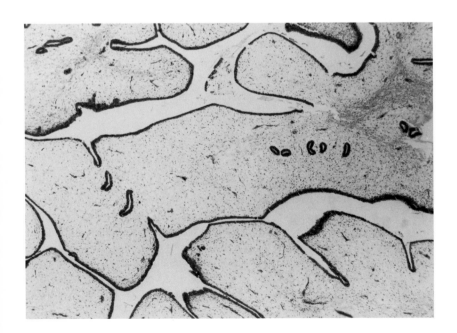

FIG. 2-30. The phylloides tumor is related to the fibroadenoma and is primarily an abnormal proliferation of the intralobular connective tissue. Note the extremely cellular stroma (numerous nucleii). The epithelium-lined spaces may be quite cystic and was the reason for the previous terminology of the cystosarcoma.

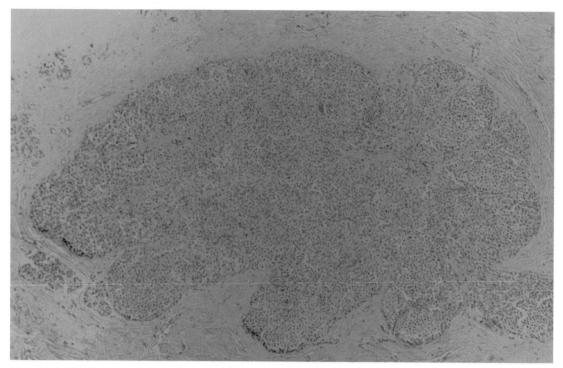

FIG. 2-31. This lobule is filled with and distended by monomorphic round cells. This is the appearance of lobular carcinoma in situ. Because this does not appear to be a direct, precursor lesion, some prefer to term this *lobular neoplasia.*

metastasize. The pathologist looks for cellular pleomorphism and invasive rather than pushing borders to suggest malignant potential. These lesions frequently have characteristics that are similar to fibrosarcomas or liposarcomas.

Lobular Carcinoma

Although most breast cancers appear to originate in the extralobular terminal ducts, there are those that appear to be derived from the epithelial cells within the lobule and are correspondingly called *lobular neoplasia* or *lobular carcinoma* (Fig. 2-31). Lobular carcinoma in situ (LCIS) is not clearly linked to invasive breast cancer, although many pathologists require the presence of LCIS to diagnose an invasive cancer as invasive lobular carcinoma. LCIS appears to be a high-risk lesion like atypical hyperplasia. It is a diffuse process usually involving large portions of breast tissue. Women with LCIS are at a higher risk for invasive breast cancer, and, unlike DCIS, the risk is bilateral. When LCIS is discovered at breast biopsy, both breasts appear to have a similar risk (15%) for the development of an invasive breast cancer within 20 to 30 years (the total risk is 30%) (31). Although invasive lobular carcinoma is not found without LCIS, women with LCIS may develop an invasive ductal cancer.

Although the pathologist finds different cytologic features and patterns of invasion that distinguish invasive lobular

from invasive ductal carcinoma, both represent cancers with equal potential for lethality.

Lesions of the Extralobular Stroma

Sarcomas

Significant lesions of the extralobular connective tissue are extremely unusual. Sarcomas such as liposarcomas and fibrosarcomas do occur, but they are very rare. Angiosarcomas can also occur and are among the most lethal of all breast tumors.

Unclassified Lesions

Radial Scar

Although a very common lesion seen histologically, the radial scar has become a more important lesion because of its visibility on mammograms and because its appearance is indistinguishable from breast cancer. Its etiology and origin are idiopathic. The lesions may be very small or several centimeters in size. Page prefers to call the larger lesions *complex sclerosing lesions.* Thought to originate at a branching point in the duct network, the lesions often demonstrate hyperplastic changes (often papillary in appearance), adeno-

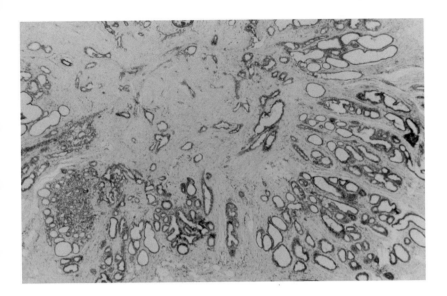

FIG. 2-32. The architecture is distorted by an idiopathic scarring process with a prominent elastic component that has been given various names, among which the term *radial scar* is the most common. This is a benign lesion whose appearance can mimic cancer.

sis, cyst formation, and a prominent fibrotic and elastic component as well as causing spiculated distortion of the tissue (Fig. 2-32). Although this is a scarring process, these lesions are unrelated to previous surgery and should not be confused with postsurgical change.

REFERENCES

1. Sloane JP. Biopsy Pathology of the Breast. New York: Wiley, 1985.
2. Haagensen CD. Diseases of the Breast. Philadelphia: Saunders, 1971.
3. Cunha GP. Role of mesenchymal-epithelial interactions in normal and abnormal development of the mammary gland and prostate. Cancer 1994;74:1030–1044.
4. Deng G, Lu Y, Zlotnikov G, et al. Loss of heterozygosity in normal tissue adjacent to breast carcinomas. Science 1996;274:2057–2059.
5. Russo J, Russo IH. Biological and molecular bases of mammary carcinogenesis. Lab Invest 1987;57:112–113.
6. Reynolds HE, Jackson VP, Musnick BS. Preoperative needle localization in the breast: utility of local anesthesia. Radiology 1993;187:503–505.
7. Alex JC, Krag DN. Gamma-probe guided localization of lymph nodes. Surg Oncol 1993;2:137–143.
8. Alex JC, Weaver DL, Fairbank JT, Krag DN. Gamma-probe guided lymph node localization in malignant melanoma. Surg Oncol 1992;2:303–308.
9. Krag DN, Weaver DL, Alex JC, Fairbank JT. Surgical resection and radiolocalization of the sentinel lymph node in breast cancer using a gamma probe. Surg Oncol 1993;2:335–340.
10. Egan RL, McSweeney MB. Intramammary lymph nodes. Cancer 1983;51;1838–1842.
11. Meyer JE, Ferraro FA, Frenna TH, et al. Mammographic appearance of normal intramammary lymph nodes in an atypical location. AJR Am J Roentgenol 1993;161:779–780.
12. Stacey-Clear A, McCarthy KA, Hall DA, et al. Observations on the location of breast cancer in women under fifty. Radiology 1993;186:677–680.
13. Falck F, Ricci A, Wolff MS, et al. Pesticides and polychlorinated biphenyl residues in human breast lipids and their relation to breast cancer. Arch Environ Health 1992;47:143–146.
14. Ohtake T, Abe R, Izoh K, et al. Intraductal extension of primary invasive breast carcinoma treated by breast conservative surgery. Cancer 1995;76:32–45.
15. Wellings SR, Jensen HM, Marcum RG. An atlas of subgross pathology of the human breast with special reference to possible precancerous lesions. J Natl Cancer Inst 1975;55:231–273.
16. Wellings SR, Jensen HM. On the origin and progression of ductal carcinoma in the human breast. J Natl Cancer Inst 1973;50:1111.
17. College of American Pathologists. Is "fibrocystic disease" of the breast precancerous? Arch Pathol Lab Med 1985;110:171–174.
18. Davis HH, Simons M, Davis JB. Cystic disease of the breast: relationship to carcinoma. Cancer 1964;17:957.
19. Vogel PM, Georgiade NG, Fetter BF, et al. The correlation of histologic changes in the human breast with the menstrual cycle. Am J Pathol 1981;104:23.
20. Love SM, Gelman RS, Silen W. Sounding board. Fibrocystic "disease" of the breast—a nondisease? New Engl J Med 1982;307:1010–1014.
21. Dupont WD, Page DL. Risk factors for breast cancer in women with proliferative breast disease. N Engl J Med 1985;312(3):146–151.
22. Huston SW, Cowen PN, Bird CC. Morphometric studies of age-related changes in normal human breast and their significance for evolution of mammary cancer. J Clin Pathol 1985;38:281.
23. Pretchel K. Mastopathic und altersabbangige brustdrusen verandernagen. Fortschr Med 1971;89:1312–1315.
24. Page DL, Anderson TJ. Diagnostic Histopathology of the Breast. New York: Churchill Livingstone, 1987.
25. Wolfe JN. Breast parenchymal patterns and their changes with age. Radiology 1976;121:545.
26. Kriger N, Hiatt RA. Risk of breast cancer after benign breast diseases: variation by histologic type, degree of stypia, age at biopsy, and length of follow-up. Am J Epidemiol 1992;135:619–631.
27. Farante G, Magni A, Campa T, et al. The risk of breast cancer subsequent to histologic diagnosis of benign intraductal papilloma: follow-up study of 339 cases. Tumori 1991;77:41–43.
28. Gallager HS, Martin JE. Early phases in the development of breast cancer. Cancer 1969;24:1170–1178.
29. Ohuchi N, Abe R, Kasai M. Possible changes of intraductal papillomas of the breast: a 3-D reconstruction study of 25 cases. Cancer 1984;54:605–611.
30. Dupont WD, Page DL, Pari FF, et al. Long-term risk of breast cancer in women with fibroadenoma. N Engl J Med 1994;331:10–15.
31. Rosen PP, Kosloff C, Lieberman PH, et al. Lobular carcinoma in situ of the breast. Am J Surg Pathol 1978;2:225–251.

Breast Imaging, 2nd ed., by Daniel B. Kopans.
Lippincott–Raven Publishers, Philadelphia © 1998.

CHAPTER 3

Epidemiology, Etiology, Risk Factors, Survival, and Prevention of Breast Cancer

EPIDEMIOLOGY: PREVALENCE AND INCIDENCE

Each year in the United States >180,000 women are diagnosed with invasive breast cancer. There are approximately 25,000 additional cases of ductal and lobular carcinoma in situ. More than 40,000 women die annually from these cancers (1). Although breast cancer has been surpassed by lung cancer as the leading cause of cancer death among women, it continues to be the leading cause of *nonpreventable* cancer death among American women. The direct causes of breast cancer remain obscure, although the mechanisms by which unrestricted cellular proliferation and metastatic spread occur are gradually being elucidated. It is still not possible to predict who will develop breast cancer, nor can we predict who will be spared, but the chromosomal abnormalities that place some women at higher risk are being discovered and may lead to a better understanding of cell control mechanisms and the sequences that lead to loss of these controls.

Lifestyle factors such as age at first full-term pregnancy relate to overall risk. There are still suggestive links between dietary factors and risk, but these may relate to breast cancer in a more indirect fashion than previously believed. The reasons for the steady increase in breast cancer incidence (see the following section) are not understood, but it is likely that a woman's exposure to her own hormones is a key factor (see Possible Reasons for an Increasing Incidence, later in this chapter). Environmental factors likely are also involved, but remain undefined.

Breast Cancer Incidence and Lifetime Risk

Incidence rates for breast cancer are compiled by the National Cancer Institute (NCI) based on detailed data collected in 10 states that participate in the Surveillance, Epidemiology, and End Results (SEER) program of the NCI. The oldest of these tumor registries was begun in Connecticut in 1940, and many of the estimates of incidence are derived from this program.

A great deal of concern has been raised over the increasing incidence (cancers diagnosed each year) of breast cancer.

This, in fact, is not a recent phenomenon. The incidence of breast cancer has been steadily rising for women at all ages since at least 1940 (2). In that year approximately 60 women per 100,000 in the population were diagnosed with breast cancer. The incidence has increased steadily by approximately 1.1% each year to approximately 75 per 100,000 in 1960, 90 per 100,000 in 1980, and 112 per 100,000 in 1987 (Fig. 3-1).

In the mid-1980s there was a sudden increase in the annual incidence over and above the steady background increase. This proved to be a temporary aberration that occurred as a result of the earlier detection of cancers as screening mammography began to be more widespread with the publication of the favorable Swedish screening results. Cancers that ordinarily would not have been detected until some time in the future were being detected earlier and added to the background, slowly increasing incidence. As more women availed themselves of screening, the apparent incidence increased. Once screening stabilizes, the incidence should return to the baseline, and this appears to be occurring.

Risks of Developing Breast Cancer

When cancer risk is discussed, it is in terms of absolute risk or relative risk. Risks are generally derived from the ratio of the incidence of breast cancer among women with the characteristic being assessed divided by the incidence in a population of women who are similar except for the characteristic being studied. For example, if the annual incidence of breast cancer in Group A is 1.5 cases per 1,000 women and in Group B the incidence is 1 case per 1,000, then the relative risk for Group A when compared to Group B is 1.5 (1.5/1). Stated another way, a relative risk of 1.5 for women in group A relative to those in group B means that women in group A are 50% more likely to develop breast cancer than women in group B. To gauge the significance of these risks one must know the characteristics of the groups being compared and the severity of the problem being evaluated. A 50% increase in risk for an uncommon problem is less significant than the same increased risk for a common disease in terms of the absolute risk and the actual numbers of people affected.

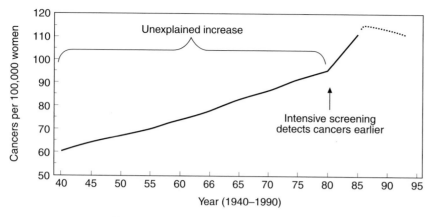

FIG. 3-1. This graph demonstrates the steady increase in breast cancer incidence since at least 1940. The data take into account the aging population. The rapid increase in the 1980s is an artifact of earlier detection that will return to the baseline increase as the number of new women being screened stabilizes. (Adapted from Miller BA, Feuer EJ, Hankey BF. Trends in invasive breast cancer incidence among American women. J Natl Cancer Inst 1991;83:678.)

The absolute risk of developing breast cancer is relative to the entire population. The relative risk is relating the risk to some special subsegment of the population. The annual rising incidence over the last 50 years has resulted in an increase in the lifetime risk, so that a 20-year-old woman who lives to age 85 has a 1 in 9 (11%) chance of developing breast cancer during that time. If she lives beyond age 85 her chances increase to 1 in 8.

Lifetime risk and annual incidence are sometimes confused. Annual risk (incidence) is the number of women diagnosed with cancer each year in a population (usually expressed as a percentage of the population). Lifetime risk is the chance that an individual will develop breast cancer during the course of her life. The cumulative risks for a 20-year-old woman at various milestones in her life have been estimated from SEER data by the NCI and are shown in Table 3-1.

The fact that a 20-year-old woman has 1 chance in 9 (11%) of developing breast cancer by age 85 has been highly publicized. Fortunately, most women are actually substan-

tially less likely to develop breast cancer. On the basis of gender alone, women in the United States have a baseline risk of 4% to 6%. A subsegment of the population is at additional risk, and these women, when combined with the general population, elevate the total average risk to 1 chance in 9 (11%) of developing breast cancer during the course of a lifetime.

Relative Risks

Other factors have been associated with increased risk. When estimates are given for these, however, the increases are compared to some baseline related to a subsegment of women. For example, the fact that women with atypical hyperplasia on breast biopsy are at higher risk than women whose biopsy revealed no proliferative changes is a relative risk among women who have been biopsied. A woman whose first degree relative (mother, sister, or daughter) had breast cancer may be at as high as 9 times the risk of the woman who is not at elevated risk, but this is not 9 times 12% (the risk for all women including those at high risk), but rather it is a relative risk of 9 times 4% to 6% (the risk for women who are not at any known elevated risk).

Incidence and Age

As noted earlier, the annual incidence of breast cancer is different from the lifetime risk. It is the number of cancers that occur in a population each year, and, as is evident in Table 3-2, the risk of developing breast cancer increases with age. Breast cancer can occur at virtually any age, and to many observers it appears that breast cancer is increasing among younger women and affecting them earlier in life. This perception is likely more a result of the increasing size of the population in the younger ages (the baby boomers). There has, however, been some shift of the incidence curves to lower ages when cohorts are evaluated by date of birth. Based on SEER data, the incidence of breast cancer for women born from 1880 to 1884 at age 50 was 95 in 100,000.

TABLE 3-1. *Risk of developing breast cancer for a 20-year-old woman*

Age	Risk
25	1/19,608
30	1/2,525
35	1/622
40	1/217
45	1/93
50	1/50
55	1/33
60	1/24
65	1/17
70	1/14
75	1/11
80	1/10
85	1/9
Lifetime	1/8

Source: Adapted from the National Cancer Institute's Surveillance, Epidemiology, and End Results Program. Statistics Review 1992. Bethesda, MD.

TABLE 3-2. *Breast cancer incidence increases with age*

Age	Cancers per 100,000 women per year
25–29	7.4
30–34	26.7
35–39	66.2
40–44	129.4
45–49	159.4
50–54	220.0
55–59	261.6
60–64	330.7
65–69	390.7
70–74	421.8
75–79	461.4
80–84	451.3
85+	411.9

Source: Based on SEER data 1984–1988 National Institutes of Health. National Cancer Institute Statistics Review 1975–1988. Bethesda, MD: National Institutes of Health; 1991. NIH Publication no. 91-2789.

A similar incidence has been found for women in their 40s in the cohort born from 1950 to 1954. The cohort with an attack rate in the youngest years appears to have been born in the 1930s (2). Reasons for these differences have not been determined.

One of the "causes" of breast cancer is aging. For most women, the development of breast cancer is likely a statistical phenomenon. The longer cells are alive, the greater the chance that DNA damage that is not fatal to the cell and that is not repaired will occur, leading to unrestricted cell growth and malignancy. The incidence of breast cancer begins to increase significantly among women in their 30s. Only 8 women per 100,000 (0.08/1,000) develop breast cancer each year while they are in their 20s, whereas >150 per 100,000 (1.5/1,000) women in their 40s are diagnosed. This rises to about 250 per 100,000 (2.5/1,000) for women in their 50s, and among women in their 60s >350 breast cancers per 100,000 (3.5/1,000) are discovered each year (3).

Because of the age distribution in the population, and as a consequence of the fact that the baby boomers are now in their 40s, the absolute number of women between the ages of 40 and 49 who developed breast cancer in 1993 was estimated to be only 8% less than for women from age 50 to age 59. In that year, there were 28,900 women between the ages of 40 and 49 diagnosed with breast cancer (16% of all the cancers diagnosed), whereas 31,500 were diagnosed among women ages 50 to 59 (17% of the cancers diagnosed) (4). It is estimated that in 1995, as a result of the large numbers of women in their 40s, there were actually more women in their 40s (33,800) than in their 50s (28,300) diagnosed with breast cancer. As the population ages, there will be an increasing percentage in the older age groups, and the total numbers of women with breast cancer will continue to increase.

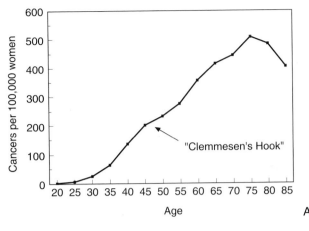

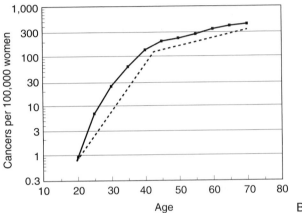

FIG. 3-2. (A) The incidence of breast cancer begins to increase around age 35, has a slight plateau around age 50 (*arrow*), and then continues to increase again at a more gradual slope, suggesting two different populations of cancer. **(B)** The change in slope can be seen when the data are graphed on a logarithmic plot. There is a rapid rise in incidence until around the age of 50 and then the rate of increase in incidence slows. (Source: Adapted from American Cancer Society. 1987–1989 SEER Incidence Rates and 1993 U.S. Census Projections. P-25, no. 1018. Atlanta: American Cancer Society.)

Are There Two Types of Breast Cancers?

The incidence of breast cancer seems to rise steadily with age until around the age of 50, where there is a slight plateau, and then begins to increase again at a more gradual rate (Fig. 3-2A). This is more apparent when the data are arranged using a semilog plot* (Fig. 3-2B). This plateau has

*Some additional data appear to support this hypothesis. In the Vancouver, British Columbia, screening trial, the breast cancer detection rate decreased between ages 45 and 55 and then increased again (5). The benefit in the Kopparberg trial reportedly decreased in the late 40s and early 50s and then increased again. In a comparison of the results from the American College of Surgeons National Cancer Database and the SEER data, the percentage of breast cancers diagnosed appeared to drop among women in their mid-40s and then rise after the mid-50s to a second peak when women are in their mid-60s (6).

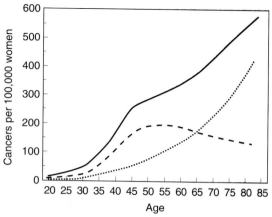

FIG. 3-3. As shown by Manson and Stallard, two overlapping curves can add to produce an overall incidence curve. This suggests the possibility of a premenopausal form of breast cancer (*dashed line*) and a postmenopausal type (*dotted line*) that add to give the solid incidence line with Clemessen's hook.

TABLE 3-3. *Age and survival from breast cancer*

Age	20-year survival (%)
<40	44
40–44	51
45–49	48
50–54	41
55–59	30
60–69	34
70–79	17

Source: Adapted from Adami HO, Malker B, Holmberg L, et al. The relationship between survival and age at diagnosis in breast cancer. N Engl J Med 1986;314:559–563.

TABLE 3-4. *Estimated cases of new breast cancers and deaths from breast cancer by age in 1997*

Age	New cases	Percent of total	Deaths	Percent of total
<30	600	0.4	100	0.2
30–34	2,500	1.4	400	0.9
35–39	6,100	3.4	900	2.1
40–44	12,400	6.9	2,300	5.2
45–49	20,200	11.2	3,400	7.7
50–54	19,200	10.7	3,800	8.7
55–59	13,800	7.7	2,700	6.2
60–64	15,000	8.3	3,000	6.8
65–69	21,600	12.0	5,300	12.1
70–74	23,600	13.1	5,600	12.8
75–79	19,900	11.0	5,700	13.0
80–84	13,800	7.7	4,900	11.2
85+	11,500	6.4	5,800	13.2

been termed *Clemmesen's hook*, and, because the rate of increase in incidence changes after this plateau, it has been used to argue that there may be two types of breast cancers—a premenopausal and a postmenopausal type. Manton and Stallard have devised a computer model by which the curve of early breast cancer, the peak rate of which occurs around age 55, when added to a late breast cancer curve that increases continually with ages over 30, forms an incidence curve that contains Clemmesen's hook (Fig. 3-3) (7).

Early Detection and Lead Time

The window of opportunity to detect breast cancers at an earlier size and stage appears to be narrower among younger women than among older women. This is reflected in the results of the Swedish two-county screening trial (8). Moskowitz's data also suggested that the lead time by which mammography can detect a cancer before it can be felt on clinical exam is shorter among younger women (9). This may indicate an actual difference in growth rate or merely a difference in the ability of mammography to detect an abnormality.

There is some evidence that this lead time for mammography is not a reflection of growth rate if, in fact, faster growing cancers are more rapidly lethal. Survival from breast cancer appears to be similar for women ages 40 to 49 when compared to women ages 50 to 59 who have the same tumor size, or histologic grade, or nodal status (10). A large study in Sweden, in fact, suggested that women diagnosed with breast cancer between the ages of 45 and 49 had the best survival (11) (Tables 3-3 and 3-4).

Although it appears that among younger women the tumor may more rapidly reach a larger size and stage and achieve the level of lethality at which it can no longer be cured, prognosis is determined by the size and stage at which the lesion is interrupted, regardless of the age of the woman. The suggestion that cancers reach the level of lethality more rapidly among younger women argues for more aggressive screening (a shorter interval between screens) for younger women (see Screening).

Possible Reasons for an Increasing Incidence

The reasons for the gradual but steady increase in breast cancer incidence over the past 50 years remain elusive and are likely multifactorial. Hormones are clearly a factor in the development of breast cancer. Pike and Henderson believe that much of the breast cancer risk can be related to a woman's exposure to her own hormones (12). They have postulated that the risk of breast cancer is directly related to the number of ovulatory cycles that a woman experiences during her lifetime.

Damage to DNA and disrupted cell regulatory mechanisms appear to be the major causes of many solid tumors including those of the breast. Irreparable damage to DNA is more likely to occur when cell proliferation is high. Active cell proliferation is highest in the breast during the midluteal phase of the ovulatory cycle (13). During the course of a normal cycle there is abundant cell proliferation followed by apoptosis—

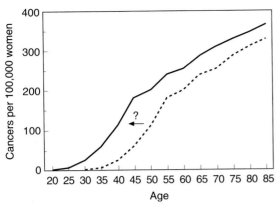

FIG. 3-4. The age of menarche has been earlier and earlier since the turn of the century. It is possible that earlier exposure to endogenous hormone cycling has shifted the incidence curve to the left (younger ages) and may account for at least some of the increase in breast cancer incidence.

"programmed" cell death (see Telomeres and Apoptosis). The more cell proliferation, the greater the likelihood that DNA replication will be compromised and abnormal copies produced. In some cells the damage may not be corrected, and, if the cell does not die, it may have acquired sufficient changes to lose proliferative control and become a full malignancy, or it may become closer to having the necessary changes such that future damage can more easily complete the transformation. The greater the number of cycles (exposure to endogenous hormones), the greater the risk for breast cancer.

Proponents of this theory suggest that the earlier onset of ovulatory cycles (early menarche) has shifted the incidence curve (that increases with age) to the left (Fig. 3-4), increasing the annual incidence for women at all ages. In societies where menarche occurs later, the incidence curve may shift to the right, into older ages, where competing causes of death might overtake the woman before breast cancer becomes a problem. Supporting this theory is the observation that early menarche (earlier exposure to cycling endogenous hormones) appears to increase the risk of breast cancer. Risk is reduced when ovulatory cycles are interrupted through early and repeated pregnancies or long periods of lactation (see Lactation). Hysterectomy with oophorectomy or early menopause reduces the risk, whereas late menopause increases the risk (14).

Early Menarche

The preceding observations suggest that it is the amount of exposure a women has to her own hormones and ovulatory cycles that may determine the likelihood that she will develop breast cancer. Additional, indirect support for this theory comes from the observations that the incidence of breast cancer is low in societies in which menarche occurs in the late teenage years. In societies and even areas of the country where the first full-term pregnancy occurs at an early age and menopause occurs earlier in life, breast cancer risk is reduced (15).

In the United States women have been maturing at increasingly younger ages, exposing the breast to endogenous estrogens and progestin cycling earlier in life (16). The average age of menarche has fallen from age 17 in the 1800s to age 12 to 13 at the present time (17). It has been postulated that nutrition is a factor in this earlier maturation, and this may be a link between dietary fat and breast cancer.

Societies that consume a high fat diet may be better nourished. Better nutrition results in earlier maturation and earlier onset of ovulation, resulting in earlier exposure to endogenous hormone cycling and the cell proliferation that appears linked to the risk of breast cancer. Similarly, the age of menopause has increased. Women are being exposed to their own hormone cycles for longer periods of time. The progressively earlier age at menarche and later age at menopause may account for some of the increased breast cancer incidence.

Late First Full-Term Pregnancy

Lifestyle changes may also account for some of the increase in incidence. Many women are delaying starting families or are not having children at all. The age of first full-term pregnancy has been increasing. A woman who has her first full-term pregnancy by age 18 has one-fourth to one-third the risk of developing breast cancer as a woman whose first full-term pregnancy is delayed until after age 30 (18).

A study by the NCI concluded that women in the northeastern United States were more likely to delay their first full-term pregnancy until later in life than women in other parts of the country and that this, along with later age at menopause, accounted for most of the excess incidence of breast cancer and breast cancer deaths that is found among women in this part of the country (15).

Lactation

There is some disagreement as to the influence of lactation on cancer risk. It seems clear that the mere fact that an individual has lactated does not influence risk. There are some data, however, that suggest that prolonged lactation helps reduce risk. If lactation is protective, it is likely not just the result of having lactated but rather is related to the duration of lactation. It has been reported that the risk of breast cancer can be cut in half when an individual lactates for a total of >10 years (19). The benefits of long duration lactation have also been suggested in a study by Newcomb and colleagues, in which the risk of breast cancer was reduced by 25% to 30% (for premenopausal women) if they lactated for a minimum of 24 months (20). Although the reduced risk may be due to alterations within the breast itself, it may be due to the cessation of ovulatory cycles that accompanies lactation supporting Pike's hypothesis.

Oral Contraceptives

Breast cancer is clearly hormonally mediated. Some have suggested that the use of oral contraceptives may be a factor in the increasing incidence, although the studies of women who have used birth control pills have produced conflicting results with no clear-cut increase in risk with their use. In a large prospective study monitored by the Harvard School of Public Health, risk of breast cancer was not increased among 118,273 nurses between the ages of 30 and 55 after 10 years of follow-up for those who used oral contraceptives versus those who did not (21). A meta-analysis reviewing the data from five prospective studies showed no evidence of increased risk, although the review of 27 case-control studies suggested a 1.73 relative risk for women who used oral contraceptives for at least 4 years prior to a first full-term pregnancy (22). Some data suggest that the use of oral contraceptives at young ages and for long periods of time may increase the risk of breast cancer before the age of 40 (23). This may be the case, but the maximum reported relative risk is 1.3 to 1.5 and, because the risk of breast cancer at these ages is very low, the absolute numbers are very small. Given that approximately 5 women out of 10,000 will develop breast cancer each year while in their 30s, a relative risk of 1.5 would increase this to $5 \times 1.5 = 7.5$. It is likely that the benefits of contraception far outweigh any breast cancer risk.

Hormone Replacement Therapy

The cardiovascular benefits and salutary effects on the prevention of osteoporosis of postmenopausal hormone replacement therapy (HRT) continue to be demonstrated. Colditz and associates have found a significant increase in the risk of breast cancer among 121,700 women in the Nurses Health Study while they were using HRT (24). The relative risk compared to women who never used HRT was approximately 1.5 for women who had used hormones for 5 to 9 years and were still using them. The addition of progestins to the estrogen replacement helps to reduce the risk of endometrial cancer, but, in their study, it did not reduce the breast cancer risk. Although there is an increased risk for breast cancer from HRT, more women die of heart disease than breast cancer, and it is likely that the benefits of HRT far outweigh the risk.

Environmental Carcinogens

Others researchers have hypothesized that environmental factors may be contributing to the increasing incidence of breast cancer with the increased exposure to environmental carcinogens. One study showed a higher concentration of DDE (dichlorodiphenyldichloroethylene), a metabolite of DDT (dichlorodiphenyltrichloroethane), in the blood of women with breast cancer (25), whereas another demonstrated higher levels of PCBs in the breast fat of women with breast cancers (26). Our own study revealed that breast cancers are more commonly found in the tissues adjacent to the subcutaneous or retromammary fat. This latter observation may merely be due to the geometry of the breast (27), but it has also been postulated that carcinogens are held in the fat, perhaps accounting for our results.

Regardless of the theories, the steadily increasing incidence has remained unexplained. The NCI review noted earlier demonstrated that the excess breast cancer incidence and mortality experienced among women in the northeastern United States compared to other parts of the country could be attributed to the later age at first full-term pregnancy and later age at menopause among these women and was probably not related to environmental factors as many have feared (15).

Surge in Incidence in the 1980s

As noted earlier, superimposed on the background of a steadily increasing incidence of breast cancer over the last 55 years was an acute upturn in the incidence curve around 1985. Although this had been hastily interpreted by some as evidence of a breast cancer epidemic, the majority of the cases contributing to the apparent rapid increase in incidence were early stage lesions and clearly attributable to the increase in mammographic screening in the middle of the 1980s.

This upturn has been carefully analyzed (28,29), and the majority of the additional increase can be explained by the detection of cancers by mammography in a given year which, without screening, would not have been detected until a year or more later. This additional increase will continue as long as new women are screened each year. Although screening accounts for much of the increased incidence, increases in women under 45 and over 65 could not be completely explained by earlier detection (30). This and the underlying steadily increasing incidence over the past 50 years remain unexplained.

ETIOLOGY

Probable Genetics of Breast Cancer

Breast cancers appear to be primarily the result of a failure of the normal regulation of cell differentiation and proliferation. Ultimately, loss of regulation is likely due to abnormalities that develop in the double helix of DNA that make up the cell's genes, which are contained in the 23 pairs of human chromosomes. Changes or mutations involving one or more gene are emerging as the direct cause of breast cancer.

DNA may be damaged by external influences such as environmental carcinogens, or by spontaneous mutation (31). If somatic cells that began life with "normal" DNA are involved, the accumulation of damage may take decades to appear, accounting for the increasing incidence of cancers with age.

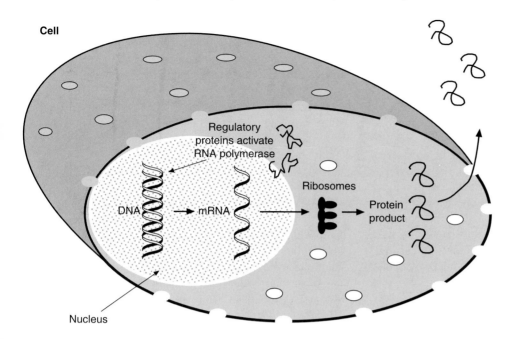

FIG. 3-5. Regulatory proteins called *transcription factors* attach to specific portions of a gene and permit the attachment and activation of RNA polymerase, which transcribes the DNA code into messenger RNA. The RNA code is subsequently used to assemble specific proteins by the cell's ribosomes.

These tumors are likely to be isolated and probably account for the majority of cancers that occur in older women. Germ cell (ova and sperm) abnormalities are the basis for the truly hereditary breast cancers and, because the abnormal inherited genes are in every cell of the body, the odds of developing a cancer earlier in life are higher. These likely account for many of the cancers that develop in younger women.

It was Knudson who postulated that women who inherit damaged DNA require less subsequent damage, and, because the inherited problem is in the germ cell, all their breast cells are primed for future change and cancer (32). Thus, women with a hereditary predisposition for breast cancer would be expected to develop breast cancer early in life (fewer subsequent events needed), and they would be more likely to develop multicentric tumors and have a higher incidence of bilaterality (33). This hypothesis is supported by the fact that the sisters and daughters of women who have bilateral premenopausal breast cancer are, indeed, more likely to develop breast cancer at an earlier age than probands.

Probably no single factor accounts for the development of all breast cancer, and it is likely that cancer induction is multifactorial. Many host and environmental associations have been reported (34), although none has been conclusively shown to be causative in humans.

Protein Synthesis

Chromosomal DNA regulates cellular functions through control of protein synthesis. In order for a protein to be created the gene in the chromosome that "expresses" it must be "turned on." Genes basically have two functioning portions, as well as long sequences that do not appear to have a function. One portion is a regulatory region that controls the transcription of the gene, and the other contains the code that ultimately determines the sequence of amino acids that will form the gene's protein product.

Transcription occurs when other proteins (transcription factors) attach to portions of the control region of the gene. This binding permits the attachment of RNA polymerase, which transcribes the coded sequence of nucleotide bases contained in the DNA of the gene (adenine, guanine, thymine, and cytosine) to produce a complimentary molecule of messenger RNA (mRNA). The mRNA passes into the cell's cytoplasm to the ribosomes. The code contained in the sequence of the mRNA is, in turn, used by the ribosomes as a template for sequencing the linkage of amino acids into proteins that are specific for the original gene (Fig. 3-5).

DNA Alterations

Breast cancer, as is likely true of most solid tumors, is the result of at least two, and probably multiple, alterations in the chromosomal DNA of a cell. This can occur as the result of spontaneous mutations that accumulate over time, endogenous processes that increase the likelihood that DNA replication, as part of normal proliferation, is compromised in some way that leads to damage, or from environmental influences such as the inhalation, ingestion, or other exposures to chemicals or radiations that damage DNA (carcinogens).

Although there are factors that have been associated with increased risk, most breast cancers occur sporadically and unpredictably and are likely the result of bad luck and cell aging. Instead of being repaired by the normal DNA repair mechanisms or instead of the cell's dying from DNA alterations, the damaged DNA becomes incorporated into the chromosome and is passed on to the cell's clones (identical offspring) at each division. If sufficient damage is accumulated in the appropriate genes, the cell loses its inhibition and is capable of unrestrained proliferation. Because DNA damage or alterations accumulate with time, it is not surprising that the incidence of breast cancer increases with age.

Genotype and Phenotype

Cells that have sustained DNA alterations may not be apparent to the pathologist. Their *genotype*, or genetic makeup, may be altered, but, because the pathologist can only see changes in the morphology of the cell or indirectly measure its nuclear or surface antigens, transformation to a malignant cell is only apparent if the cell's *phenotype* is altered. Unless the size of the cell, its shape, the appearance of its cytoplasm or nucleus become visibly altered by the change, or alterations of the antigens are demonstrable using histochemical probes, a transformed cell may not be evident.

Initiation, Promotion, and Progression

It has been postulated that there are three phases in the development of breast cancer. *Initiation* is the stage when changes have taken place in the cell that make it a cancer cell. Carcinogens are initiators. An initiator may not only transform a cell into a malignant cell, it may also cause it to replicate and grow. Alternatively, this cell may lie quiescent for a variable period of time, perhaps even many years, until, for some reason, its growth is triggered and *promotion* produces unrestrained multiplication. Promotion can be caused by some chemicals. They may greatly affect proliferation once initiation has occurred, but promoters may have no effect if the cell has not already been initiated. In other words, promoters may not *cause* a cancer, but they may trigger or support its growth. The period of promotion is also variable, but unless the cancer is destroyed, it may enter into a third phase known as *progression*, during which it spreads to other parts of the body.

By evaluating the slope of the incidence curves for cancers, epidemiologists estimate that at least two, and likely more, alterations in DNA (events) are required for malignant transformation (35). Although mechanisms have not been completely explained, there appear to be at least three major ways by which cell growth regulation is lost.

Growth Factors, Oncogenes, and Tumor Suppressor Genes

Cell proliferation and function are controlled by chromosomal DNA. As noted above, the DNA code is translated into proteins that are the true regulators of cell growth and function. Genes determine the structure, quantity, and timing of production of proteins and, thus, the properties and functions of the cell. The result is called *gene expression.*

Proper cell growth requires control of the type, amount, and timing of gene expression and protein synthesis. It is the loss of gene regulation that produces unrestricted malignant growth. There are numerous ways in which genes can be altered. The base pairs that make up the genetic code may be modified. A single point mutation resulting in the substitution of a guanine-cytosine pair for an adenine-thymine pair may have no effect (if the change is in one of the many unimportant portions of the chromosome) or may have a profound effect. The alteration may result in the substitution of the wrong amino acid in the protein that is created based on the DNA code, and this may affect the biological activity of the protein.

Translocation is another alteration in which part of a chromosome is reconstructed in a different place in the DNA chain. If this occurs in the wrong place, it may have significant effects. Genes that are switched off in their normal position may be activated when translocated.

Deletions involve the loss of portions of the genetic code. These range from the elimination of a single base pair to the loss of an entire chromosome. Once again, depending on what is lost, the result can be negligible, or devastating.

Gene amplification is the term given when, instead of having the usual two copies of each gene, one copy is duplicated multiple times. These may be joined as part of the chromosome or be extrachromosomal clumps of chromatin.

Cell function can be altered by the increased or decreased *expression* of a gene through the altered production of the protein encoded by the gene. Gene amplification can result in the overproduction of the protein product, and this can result in altered cell function. Not only can too many copies of a gene lead to overexpression, but the regulation of the transcription of the DNA into RNA into a protein may also be altered, leading to changes in the expression of the protein.

Among the molecules that are produced by the genes are a group known as *growth factors* whose purpose is to "switch on" cell growth and replication. These molecules form *ligands*, which bind to receptors in the cell or on its surface (the ligand is like a key in the receptor lock) and activate a cascade of events resulting in the activation of genes responsible for cell division.

Cells can produce growth factors that form a positive feedback through their own receptors that keep the "growth switch" turned on. This type of autoregulation is known as an *autocrine* function. The stimulation of one cell by the secretions from another is a *paracrine* effect.

Growth Factors

The protein products of the cell perform numerous functions. One category of proteins has been termed *growth factors* in that they influence cell proliferation. The overexpression of these factors has been found in many tumors. Several growth factors appear to be active in some breast cancers. The overexpression of the DNA sequences that code for these growth factors has been identified in numerous solid tumors. Among the best studied are epidermal growth factor, transforming growth factor alpha, and *HER2/neu* (also known as *erb* B2, and *int* 2).

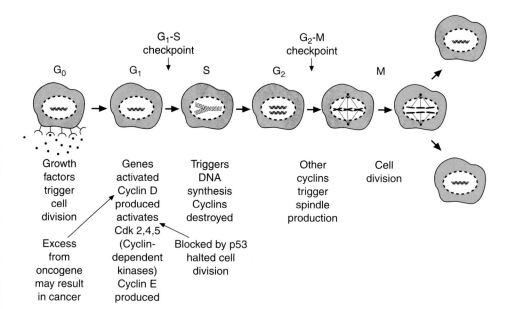

FIG. 3-6. The cell cycle has several defined stages. The resting state is termed G_0. Growth factors trigger the production of cyclins that activate cyclin-dependent kinases that trigger DNA synthesis during the S phase. When synthesis is complete, the cell is in G_2. The cycle is interrupted at checkpoints between G_1 and S and between G_2 and M, at which time mistakes may be corrected by repair mechanisms. Errors at any number of points along this sequence have been associated with breast cancers. (Adapted from Hartwell LH, Kasten MB. Cell cycle control and cancer. Science 1994;266:1821–1828.)

Cell Cycle and Cellular Differentiation

Some of the factors listed above exert their influence on portions of the cell cycle. Several basic types of cells exist. Ultimately, cells must be formed that perform their proper organ function. These cells have *differentiated*. Differentiated cells are considered to be mature. It is believed that a differentiated cell cannot become dedifferentiated and is not capable of malignant change, but the process of differentiation can be interrupted, and it is likely that it is the proliferating, undifferentiated cells that are the basis for most tumors.

Stem Cells

Because cells frequently die, they must be replaced. This is the role of the stem cell. These cells are not differentiated. In the usual course of events, when a cell dies, a stem cell divides so that two cells result. One remains a stem cell while the other becomes a differentiated replacement for the cell that died. One theory is that defective stem cells are the progenitors of cancer. Because there are likely intermediate stages between the stem cell and the differentiated cell, interruptions along the way might also lead to a variety of malignant manifestations. Deng and associates published a study in 1996 that suggests there may be a stem cell for the mammary ducts. They found that there were similar genetic defects in the cells of normal lobules that were adjacent to lobules containing breast cancer cells (36). Cells in lobules further away did not have the same genetic changes. This suggests several possibilities. If there is a stem cell responsible for the development of the ducts and lobules, then an alteration in its DNA prior to duct elongation and terminal differentiation could distribute that defect into every cell in the segment. This would place a larger number of cells at risk for further damage, increasing the likelihood that one of

the cells might develop malignant change. This would explain the findings of Deng and might be the explanation for the so-called field phenomenon. It also suggests the importance of exposure to carcinogens at an early age, before terminal differentiation. It is very unlikely that a carcinogen could damage all of the cells in a segment and not damage cells in other segments of the mature breast. However, if a stem cell were damaged in the immature breast, that damage would be distributed to the cells of the developing segment, and only the cells of the segment would be affected.

Cell Cycle

The normal cell cycle is composed of four main stages that are usually tightly controlled (Fig. 3-6). G_0 cells are in a resting state. Cells in this state can go on to become differentiated or can be triggered to divide. Growth factors secreted by other cells, or by the cell itself, activate genes that produce a family of proteins called *cyclins*. The cell enters the G_1 stage and the cyclins activate enzymes called *cyclin-dependent kinases* (CDK) that are needed for cell replication. DNA synthesis takes place during the S phase of the cell cycle and a copy of the chromosomes is formed for the new cell. This is followed by a second "resting stage" termed G_2. Other cyclins trigger the production of spindles that pull apart the two groups of chromosomes toward the centromeres into the two separate cells in the M stage of mitosis.

There are at least two checkpoints in the cell cycle, during which the process of cell division may be interrupted. Errors in DNA synthesis can be corrected during these checkpoints. Problems with the DNA template are corrected during the G_1-S checkpoint, whereas errors in the new DNA are corrected during the G_2-M checkpoint. In some tumors there appears to be a loss of these checkpoints.

Perhaps it is the loss of a checkpoint that prevents DNA repair and leads to the perpetuation of damaged chromosomes. Individuals with ataxia-telangiectasia may lack the G_1 checkpoint, and this may explain why they are so prone to radiation cell damage.

The entire sequence of the cell cycle, as well as the checkpoints, appears to be controlled by the family of molecules of the CDKs (37). These complexes of proteins direct the cell through the phases of cell division through positive and negative feedback loops. If DNA damage is present, and the CDK system is functioning normally, the process of cell division will be arrested and DNA repair effected. If the CDK system is defective, then the cell may continue to divide and the DNA may not be repaired. This can lead to genetic instability and result in cells that are even more prone to additional alterations that can ultimately lead to a malignant cell. The p53 protein appears to be involved in the regulation of the cell cycle, and this may explain why mutations of this gene are fairly commonly found in malignant lesions.

Telomeres and Apoptosis

Other genetic controls may also be affected in malignant transformation. Telomeres are DNA sequences that are found at the ends of each chromosome. They appear to be shortened each time a cell divides. When the telomere is eliminated, the cell dies through a process termed *apoptosis.* Apoptosis has been termed *programmed cell death* and is the process whereby a cell self-destructs in an orderly fashion. Unlike cellular death due to damage, the apoptotic cell is removed without any inflammatory response. There are apparently other ways in which apoptosis is triggered.

The telomere may be one way in which the organism counts the number of times a cell divides, and it may represent a mechanism to protect cells from dividing too many times, thereby increasing the risk of damage and cancer. It appears that cancers may lose this proliferation control and that their telomeres are unaffected by cell division.

Investigators have found that telomerase, a ribonucleoprotein that synthesizes telomeric DNA, is activated in cancer cells. The telomeric sequences lost with each normal cell division may actually be rebuilt by telomerase, resulting in "immortality" of the cell line. Telomerase appears to be present in germ cell lines and cancer cells but not in normal somatic cells (38).

Cell Ploidy

Normal cells have two copies of each chromosome and are termed *diploid.* They have two copies of each gene. Other areas in which cell proliferative errors can occur lie in the actual process of pulling the newly duplicated chromosomes apart into the two cells that have been created from the single parent. Spindle poles are anchoring points that develop in opposite portions of the nucleus. During mitosis filamentous structures, known as *spindles,* extend from these spindle poles to the chromosomes. When the cell divides, these spindles pull the duplicated chromosomes to their respective new cells as the cytoplasm and nucleus divide.

An error in spindle function can lead to an incomplete or abnormally large complement of chromosomes. If the cell divides properly it will have a normal diploid (two copies) complement of chromosomes. Spindle errors lead to a cell that is aneuploid (i.e., fewer than the normal number of chromosomes). An error associated with the spindle pole can lead to too many copies of a chromosome being pulled into the new, now, tetraploid cell.

Aneuploidy and tetraploidy are abnormalities of chromosome number, whereas factors that interfere with DNA replication and repair lead to abnormalities within the chromosome such as translocations, deletions, and amplification.

Genetic Repair and Damaged Repair Mechanisms

Some genetic abnormalities that have been associated with hereditary breast cancer involve genes that synthesize proteins that are involved in the repair of genetic damage (39). Damage may occur during cell division when DNA is improperly copied. Genes involved in correcting these errors are called *mismatch repair genes.* They detect and repair segments of DNA that have been incorrectly matched to noncomplimentary nucleotide sequences.

A second system is involved in more focal damage repair. This has been termed *nucleotide excision repair.* Genes involved in these processes encode for proteins that repair abnormalities that are either spontaneous or caused by exogenous factors such as chemical or radiation damage.

It is not surprising that individuals who have defective genes that encode for these repair mechanisms have a higher risk of cancer.

Oncogene Activation and Overexpression

Ultimately cell growth regulation lies in the chromosomes and the DNA code. There are likely multiple and varied pathways by which a normal cell is transformed into a malignant cell. One mechanism that can lead to unrestrained growth is the alteration of a gene that performs a normal cell function, or overexpression, of this type of gene by the overproduction of the protein product that is coded for by the gene. This class of genes, when normal, performs important regulatory functions in cell growth, but, when altered so that their normal functions are no longer regulated, they become cancer genes. The normal, or wild-type, gene of this category has been termed a *proto-oncogene.* Proto-oncogenes appear to be involved in growth control and cell differentiation.

Cell division is carefully regulated in the normal cell and is suspended when the appropriate environment signals the cell to stop dividing. Contact inhibition is one such feedback system, in which dividing cells cease to divide when they contact a neighboring cell. Differentiation into a cell appropriate for its location and function in the body also appears to be important for normal, regulated cell growth. The loss of growth regulation and the loss of cell differentiation are characteristics of malignant growth. When altered, or overexpressed, the proto-oncogenes become oncogenes.

Because these genes are so critical to cell function, only minimal damage may be needed for the cell's transformation (40). Although some oncogenes are recessive (damage to both copies is needed for malignant transformation), other oncogenes are dominant. The result of a point mutation (alteration in a single base pair), translocation (movement of part of the DNA code to an inappropriate location), rearrangement (incorrect ordering of the DNA sequence), or amplification (too many copies of the gene) can convert a proto-oncogene to an oncogene.

Oncogenes that act as dominant genes can affect a cell if a single change occurs and does not require both alleles (copies of the gene) to be altered. *Ras* is an example of an oncogene that requires only a single point mutation for its activation. Amplification of *HER2/neu* (another proto-oncogene) has been associated with breast cancers with a poorer prognosis (41), whereas other studies have suggested that activation of this oncogene is needed for in situ cancer to become invasive (42).

Suppressor Genes

A positive control on cell proliferation is exercised by tumor suppressor gene activity. Suppressor genes have normal cell regulatory functions in their normal, or wild-type, configurations. These normal functions can be altered or lost if the wild-type code is damaged, mutated, or lost. Alteration, activation, or loss of these genes can come during normal cell division, where the reconstituted DNA is incorrectly arranged, or sequences are lost in the transcription needed to copy the DNA from one cell to its progeny.

Unlike the dominant behavior of oncogenes, loss of suppressor gene activity requires that both chromosomal copies (alleles) be lost or altered. It is likely for this reason that genes that are associated with inherited susceptibility to breast cancer appear to be suppressor genes. An inherited dominant cancer gene would likely be fatal very early. In order for abnormal suppressor genes to function, both copies must be lost or altered. Thus, a woman can inherit one abnormal allele and still have normally functioning cells, but because it would only take damage to the single remaining allele, the likelihood of the cell's losing function is higher than the chance of having both damaged in a normal cell. This accounts for the increased likelihood that these women will develop cancer.

One example of a tumor suppressor gene is the gene labeled p53. This gene normally functions to inhibit unrestricted cell growth. It may also be involved in DNA repair. It is believed that when DNA is damaged, p53 is involved in temporarily stopping cell division to permit the DNA to be repaired before the abnormal DNA is copied and becomes a permanent defect passed on to the progeny and subsequent generations of the original cell. The loss of wild-type, normal p53 activity requires the inactivation or mutation of both copies of the gene for the cell to become malignant.

Carcinogens and Field Abnormalities

Carcinogens likely act by causing changes in the DNA code or sequence or by destruction of important genes. They may act on a single cell or affect a large number of cells, producing a field phenomenon where multiple cells over a large area are primed and multiple separate tumors can develop. Lobular carcinoma in situ and atypical hyperplasia may represent field changes that increase the probability of cancer because so many cells have DNA alterations that make them that much closer to being cancer cells. The fact that these represent multiple cells affected separately, rather than clones of the same parent, has been shown in cancers of the aerodigestive tract in which alterations in p53 have been found, but the mutations in the gene differ in the separate primary lesions.

Statistically, mutations causing alteration to the normal DNA are expected to occur at a relatively predictable rate. Damage to DNA can also occur as the result of external or environmental factors. Carcinogens, such as ionizing radiation, may result in significant damage to regulatory portions of the DNA code.

Many Breast Cancers Are Likely Due to Statistical Bad Luck

Mutational changes, as well as those caused by carcinogens, usually result in cell death. It is likely that many damaged cells are eliminated by the normal host mechanisms. Some chromosomal damage may be repaired by DNA repair mechanisms. However, given the number of cells and the opportunities for mutation or damage, it is statistically probable that cells with sufficient change or damage will survive and form cancers, and the likelihood of this occurring increases with age, based at least in part on the fact that the longer an organism lives, the greater the chances for the required damage or change to occur.

Superimposed on this is the potential for damage from environmental exposures, as well as problems that can occur in other cellular functions, such as those involved in DNA repair. Individuals who inherit or develop defects in repair mechanisms, such as those who are homozygotes for the ataxia-telangiectasia gene, have a reduced ability to repair DNA damage.

Breast cancer susceptibility is also likely to be related to hormones, growth factors, the individual's immune system, and other influences yet to be elucidated.

DNA Alterations and Patterns of Breast Cancer Development

Sporadic Breast Cancer

Many changes can occur in the DNA of a cell. During cell division, DNA can recombine in inappropriate sequences, altering the number and structure of the chromosomes. There may be deletions and rearrangements in the DNA sequences, breaks, alterations in the sequence of bases, and errors in the replication of the sequence during cell division. These alterations may occur in somatic cells and be confined to that cell alone producing sporadic breast cancer. This is the most common type of breast cancer and can best be described as due to bad luck. One cell has accumulated the appropriate damage, a cancer develops, and there was no way of predicting that this would occur.

Hereditary Breast Cancer

It has been estimated that approximately 90% of breast cancers are sporadic, as described above, and, therefore, unpredictable. Some women inherit an abnormal gene and are at much higher risk for the subsequent development of breast cancer. If the altered chromosomes are in a germ cell of the parent and this DNA is passed on to a child, the damage will be distributed throughout all the cells of the body. The distribution includes the white blood cells and, for this reason, when these chromosomal abnormalities are present, they can be detected through blood tests, unlike sporadic cancers.

Because a germ cell abnormality is distributed to all of the cells of the body, there are billions of cells that already have some damage. With so many cells further along in the transformation to malignancy, it takes a shorter period of time to develop any remaining changes needed for a cancer cell than for the sporadic development of cancer from cells with normal DNA. Because the cells in women who have inherited altered DNA are already closer to having acquired all the necessary DNA alterations for cancer initiation and the changes are present in all of the cells of the breast, these hereditary cancers are more likely to develop earlier in life than the sporadic cancers.

The alteration or loss of the tumor suppressor gene p53 on chromosome 17p has been identified in some women with hereditary breast cancer as well as some with sporadic cancer (43). There are some families in which these genes are passed down the generations and multiple types of cancers occur in multiple family members such as those with Li-Fraumeni syndrome. Mutation of p53 is one of the most common abnormalities found in breast cancers of all types.

BRCA1 and BRCA2

Two other heritable genes have been identified that are linked to breast cancer (see Familial and Hereditary Breast Cancer). Women who inherit (from a mother or a father) abnormalities of the BRCA1 (Breast Cancer 1) gene are at much greater risk for developing breast as well as ovarian cancer. Inheritance of abnormal BRCA2 increases only the risk of developing breast cancer (44). BRCA1 has been localized to chromosome 17q21, whereas BRCA2 is on chromosome 13q. Women with these genes have an extremely high risk of developing breast cancers over the course of their life. Initial estimates suggested that a woman who inherits BRCA1 has a 50% to 73% chance of developing breast cancer by the age of 50 and an 87% chance of developing breast cancer by the age of 70 (45). More recent estimates suggest that the lifetime risk is lower (46), but at approximately 50%, it is still extremely high.

A great deal of research has gone into determining the function of these genes. Some believe they are tumor suppressor genes. Data published in the January 24, 1997, issue of *Cell* and the April 24, 1997, edition of *Nature* suggest that the BRCA1 and BRCA2 genes code for proteins that are involved in DNA repair. This would explain why not all women with BRCA1 and BRCA2 develop breast cancer early in life. The researchers showed that embryos with two abnormal genes die in utero. A single defective allele, however, is not lethal. A woman who inherits a single allele has the defect in all the cells of her body. This greatly increases the chance that a cell will lose its second wild-type, properly functioning allele, resulting in a defect in the DNA repair mechanism of that cell. This would increase the chances for that cell to develop mutations or DNA abnormalities that would not be repaired. It is likely that many of these cells would merely die as a result, but it would greatly increase the risk that the cell would accumulate genetic changes that were not repaired and did not kill the cell and could eventually result in a malignant phenotype.

Although the discovery of breast cancer susceptibility genes has been a major achievement in the understanding of breast cancer, most breast cancers are of the sporadic type and are not related to the inheritance of a gene. Truly hereditary cancers only account for 5% to 10% of all breast cancers. Whether the changes that are being identified in the inherited forms of breast cancer will shed light on the changes that occur in sporadic cancers remains to be seen. The complexity is already apparent in that most sporadic breast cancers have normal BRCA1 and BRCA2 genes.

Clonal Nature of Breast Cancer

Breast cancers likely originate from cells derived from single clones. One clone likely overgrows another as the tumor enters the different phases of its development (Fig. 3-7). Different clones may emerge as subsequent mutations occur. The fact that many invasive cancers, presumably beginning in the ductal epithelium within the lactiferous ducts, continue to have components that remain and grow within the ducts (intraductal component) suggests that these are separate clones. The intraductal clones, unable to invade,

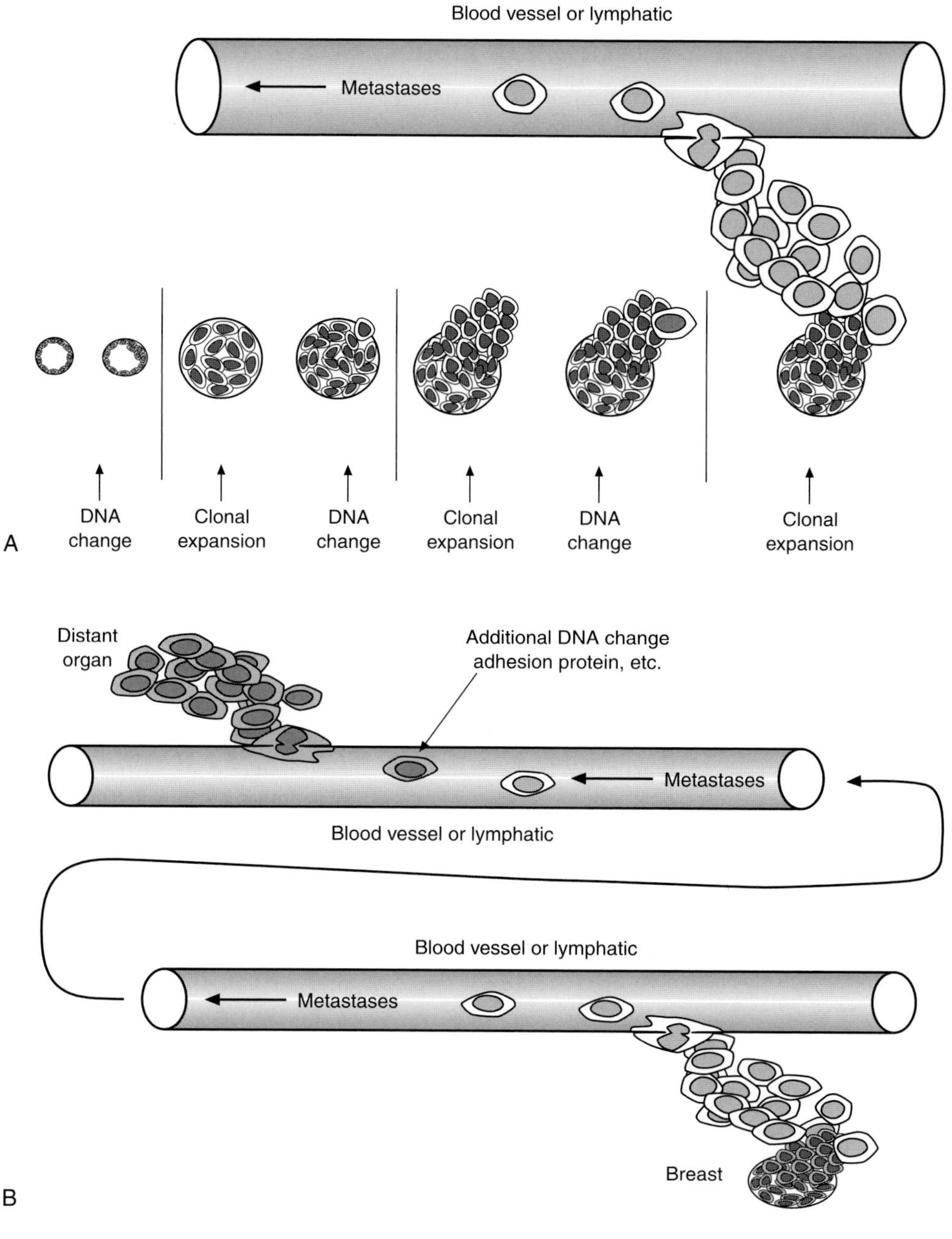

FIG. 3-7. Schematic representing the possible clonal development of breast cancers, suggesting possible stages of breast cancer progression. **(A)** One theory suggests that a cell accumulates genetic alterations that lead to its unrestricted proliferation. It may be an invasive cancer immediately, or it may only be able to grow in the duct. This clone multiplies (clonal expansion). One of the cells may develop invasive capability, which it passes to subsequent clones. The old clone may continue to grow or be overrun by the invasive clone. Genetic alterations may not be apparent to the microscopist until they are reflected in phenotypical changes to the cell and its relationships to other cells. It appears that a normal, single layer of epithelium can develop multiple cell layers (hyperplasia). When the cells appear atypical, the pathologist terms this atypical hyperplasia, and when enough phenotypical changes are visible the diagnosis is ductal carcinoma in situ. When one of these cells develops the ability to invade, its clones form invasive breast cancer. Subsequent mutations can lead to different clonal colonies. **(B)** Cells may circulate in the blood, but they must have the genetic capability to adhere to the lining of the vessel, pass through into another organ, and proliferate in that organ. Without the necessary DNA alterations, a cancer cell may not be able to successfully metastasize.

continue to grow within the duct while the invasive clone(s) infiltrate the surrounding tissue. Perhaps the fact that in situ cancer is not found in association with all invasive lesions is due to the fact that the cancer developed invasive capability early in its progression or that the in situ cancer was killed by the next clone's overgrowth (47). It is likely that intraductal clones can grow only within the ducts. The fact that in situ cancer is frequently found in association with invasive cancer supports this model of tumor growth with the in situ clones continuing to be unable to escape from the duct.

There are likely other factors that are required in breast cancer initiation, promotion, and progression. Some may act as carcinogens, whereas others are cofactors that support the development of a cancer.

Cancer Is Likely a Multistage Process

It is unlikely that only a single alteration in gene function leads to cancer. Multiple alterations are probably required to produce the various traits that characterize malignancies at various stages in their development. In lung cancer it is thought that 15 to 20 changes may be required. The development of colon cancer has been shown to represent the result of multiple hits. Vogelstein has demonstrated that the various alterations in the progressive development to a colon cancer are reflected in somatic changes in the cells and tissues that can be recognized by the pathologist (48) progressing from normal epithelium through focal proliferation to adenomas and finally carcinoma, invasion, and metastasis. Breast cancer likely follows a similar multistep process. The steps may occur over a long period, or, in some cases, it is likely that the changes occur in rapid succession or possibly even simultaneously. The fact that cancer development is a multistage process likely accounts for much of the variability in the growth and dissemination of cancers.

It is fortunate that cancer initiation likely requires multiple damaging events or hits at specific sites in the chromosomes with fairly specific alterations required for sustained cancer progression; otherwise cancer would be much more common. Because there are two copies of each gene, if the affected gene is recessive, the cell must lose its heterozygosity (become homozygotic for the specific altered gene or genes or lose it [them] completely) for cancer to result. The requirement for multiple changes reduces the probability of cancer induction in a given individual. The fact that breast cancer incidence is age related may be in part due to the statistical likelihood that, with increasing time, the chance increases that the required DNA changes will take place.

Progression of a cancer likely requires additional abnormal gene expression. The ability to invade and metastasize likely must be acquired by the cancer cell through additional mutations or damaging events. This probably explains why some cancers grow within the duct (in situ) for many years while others develop invasive ability early in their growth.

Cell proliferation is a necessary component in carcinogenesis. Without proliferation, the DNA damage is not expressed. It is possible that one effect of estrogen and progesterone is their stimulation of cell proliferation and tumor promotion. DNA damage is likely to be common, but the majority of damaged cells can either repair the damage or the damage results in cell death. Repair mechanisms are most effective when cell division is slow. Resting cells appear to be better able to repair damaged DNA. A small number of cells may survive with the damage. Among cells that are rapidly proliferating (e.g., during the menstrual cycle and during breast development) irreparable damage is more likely to occur. An abnormal p53 gene appears to be associated with reduced time in the cell cycle during which DNA damage may be repaired, increasing the likelihood that an error may be retained.

A Possible Breast Cancer Model

Proliferation

If breast cancer is like colon cancer the following sequence may occur. Some damage or mutation occurs without altering the appearance of the cell. Other changes result in noticeable changes to a cell or group of cells that alter its phenotype and are visible to the pathologist. These have become recognized as premalignant lesions (49), such as atypical hyperplasia. Subsequent damage or change to a cell in this group leads to a new clone forming in situ cancer.

Invasion

Cancer cells within the duct replicate without the normal regulation. They may proliferate without inhibition but are prevented from leaving the duct by the collagen that surrounds it forming the basement membrane. It is likely that these cells are also genetically unstable and are primed for an additional mutation or alteration. Invasion is likely the result of one of these cells developing the ability to penetrate the basement membrane. This may require the ability to secrete proteolytic enzymes, such as cathepsin D, to disrupt the basement membrane around the duct and allow invasion into the surrounding tissue. Cells with invasive capability gain access to the vascular and lymphatic systems and the opportunity to become metastatic.

Metastasis

In situ breast cancer is not lethal. Even invasive cancer that is confined to the breast is not lethal (unless it erodes a major vessel or extends directly into the lung or mediastinum). Breast cancer kills through metastatic spread and compromise of the functions of other organs. Not all breast cancers develop metastatic capability. It is well known that cancer cells are frequently shed into the blood (50) with no detrimental effect if they have not developed the ability to grow outside the breast.

For cells to be successfully metastatic, they must acquire changes beyond the unrestricted growth of a tumor. Further changes are required for cells that have gained access to the blood and lymphatic systems to be capable of exiting the vascular system and establishing metastases in other organ systems (51). It is fortunate that the process of metastatic spread is complex. To become successfully metastatic a cell must be able to escape from the duct, invade into the stroma surrounding the duct, enter the lymphatics or vascular system, avoid destruction by the immunologic system, extravasate (leave the blood), invade the new site, and proliferate in the new tissues (52). To be invasive, the tumor cells must secrete proteolytic enzymes that can dissolve the type IV collagen that forms the basement membrane that surrounds the duct. It is likely that the metastatic cancer cell must develop adhesion proteins that permit it to attach to the various structures through which it must pass. To leave the blood and invade a second organ, the cells must have the ability to adhere to the blood vessel wall and pass through the wall into the surrounding tissue (Fig. 3-7B). It is likely that these requirements prevent most of the cells that are shed into the blood from many tumors from being capable of metastatic growth. Although some cancers may have cells that achieve metastatic capability early in their development, the fact that women with cancer can be cured suggests that many cancers require time to develop the ability to spread to other organs.

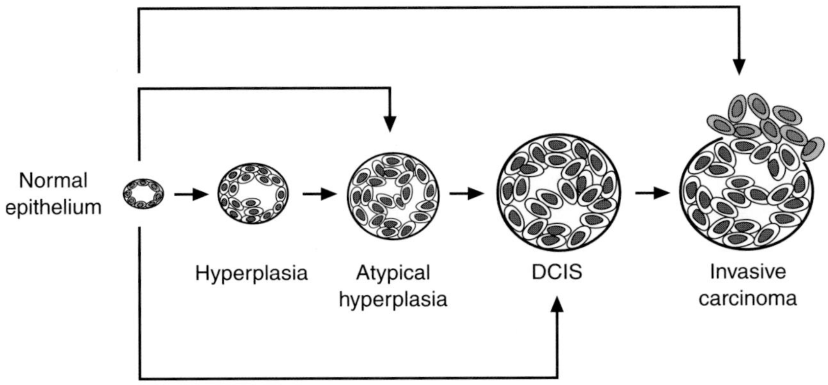

FIG. 3-8. Breast cancer may be the result of a progression from a normal epithelium through hyperplasia to atypical hyperplasia to ductal carcinoma in situ (DCIS) to invasive cancer, or perhaps from any of these stages directly to invasion. It is likely that some cancers immediately develop the ability to invade and metastasize from the first cell.

Interrupting the Natural History of Cancer

A cancer that develops over a relatively long period of time offers the opportunity of having its natural history interrupted. Earlier detection offers the ability to cure the patient before the cancer becomes successfully metastatic.

It is also likely that in some women all of these changes happen over a short period of time and that some cancers accomplish these changes early in their growth, becoming successfully metastatic before they can be detected. Perhaps, in some women, the first cell is initiated with all the necessary changes that permit its clones to be metastatic from the outset (Fig. 3-8). That some women are cured of their cancers suggests, however, that there are some cancers whose natural history can be interrupted.

Other Factors in the Development of Breast Cancer

Hormones

Clearly, hormones play a major role in breast cancer growth. In many tumors estrogen and progesterone receptors can be detected, and the growth of these lesions can be inhibited by administering competitive inhibitors of estrogen such as tamoxifen. Some investigators believe that cancer induction occurs during the breast's active growing phases in adolescence and early adulthood.

One early theory of breast cancer development invoked the effects of unopposed estrogen on cell growth. It has been shown in rats that estrogen by itself can be carcinogenic but that this effect on breast cells can be counteracted by progesterone. Luteal activity is responsible for progesterone production, and prior to the onset of complete ovulatory cycles estrogen circulates without the moderating effects of progesterone (53). Anovulatory cycles thus may subject the breast to the carcinogenic potential of unopposed estrogen. The two times in life during which unopposed estrogenic effects are most likely to occur are around the time of menarche before full ovulatory cycling and in the perimenopausal years, when luteal activity is

reduced. Ovulation may cease completely while estrogen production persists.

This hypothesized carcinogenic effect of unopposed estrogen may account for the apparent relative protective benefit from a full-term pregnancy early in life. Pregnancy not only induces differentiation of the mammary gland and the completion of the development of the terminal duct lobular unit but also appears to establish regular ovulatory cycles, reducing the time during which the breast is influenced by estrogen without the mediating influence of progesterone.

The theory that unopposed estrogen is carcinogenic is difficult to test. The effect may occur early in life, causing cell transformation, but these cells, once transformed, may remain quiescent for as many as 20 years until a subsequent event promotes one to grow as a cancer. If this hypothesis is correct, the relationship is likely to be a complex one, because studies to date only suggest a relatively small excess breast cancer in postmenopausal women using exogenous estrogen-containing hormone supplements. It is possible that the effect is greatest during proliferative cell growth when the breast is developing.

As already noted, Pike and Henderson are convinced that it is the hormones associated with the ovulatory cycle and their role in cell proliferation that account for most breast cancers. Their hypothesis is that increased cell division increases the risk of breast cancer. There is cell proliferation in the breast during both the early follicular phase as well as the premenstrual, luteal phase of the menstrual cycle, but the mitotic rate is highest during the luteal phase. They argue that it is not simply unopposed estrogen that increases the risk of breast cancers but that progesterone may play a role as well.

They postulate that it is the total number of ovulatory cycles that determines the risk due to their effects on increased cell proliferation. By this theory, late menarche and early menopause decrease the risk of breast cancer due to a reduction in the number of ovulatory cycles, moving the risk curves to later years where competing causes of death prevent cancers from becoming clinically significant during a woman's lifetime. Conversely, early menarche begins the proliferative cycles early, moving the risk curves to earlier years and hence the likelihood of cancer developing earlier in life.

The theory also accounts for the changes in risk from obesity at various stages in a woman's life as well as the effects of pregnancy and possibly lactation. Obesity, in general, is not a strong risk factor for breast cancer, but studies have shown some weak correlations. In premenopausal women, obesity does not increase the risk of breast cancer and may actually slightly reduce the risk, whereas it has the opposite association in postmenopausal women, where obesity appears to slightly increase the risk (54).

Pike postulates that premenopausal obesity increases the likelihood of anovulation and fewer cycles, whereas postmenopausal obesity increases the risk of breast cancer through the conversion by fat of the androgen androstenedione, which is secreted by the adrenal glands, to estrone, thus prolonging the exposure to endogenous estrogen. According to the theory, an early first full-term pregnancy reduces the number of ovulatory cycles early in life, displacing the breast cancer risk to later in life.

Long duration lactation (see Lactation) may have some protective effect. A study in China suggests that there was a 30% reduction in breast cancer risk for every 5 years of nursing (16). Henderson and Pike would argue that this was due to the cessation of ovulatory cycles during lactation. This theory might also explain why there is a lower risk of breast cancer among women who grow up in traditional Asian cultures compared to women in the United States. The age at menarche among Asian women is later than among Western women. In China, the average age of menarche is 17, whereas in the United States it is 12 to 13 (55). It is likely that nutrition plays a role in maturation and it is likely that it is not merely diet that directly affects breast cancer risk, but the effect that diet has on maturation, age of menarche, and, perhaps, ovulatory cycles.

Dietary Factors

As has been discussed previously, the primary mechanism for the development of breast cancer is likely chromosomal DNA alteration. The interplay of environmental (risk) factors and basic cellular mechanisms is obscure. There are dramatic geographic differences in the incidence of breast cancer that do not appear to be directly related to genetics and are not completely explained by lifestyle changes such as late first full-term pregnancy. Environmental factors may interact in an as yet undetermined fashion.

The influence of nutritional factors has been suggested both by animal models and by population studies. Japanese women, for example, have a low prevalence of breast cancer that some relate to their traditional diet, which is low in animal fat. When they change to a Western diet their breast cancer prevalence eventually approaches that of Western women (56–58). The death rate from breast cancer in other countries also appears to correlate directly with estimated fat consumption by the population, but the effects on the breast of fat in the diet are as yet not well understood.

No cause-and-effect relationship has been established, and the significance of dietary fat has been brought into question.

Willett and coworkers are following a population of 89,538 registered nurses who are participating in a long-term health study (59). Over a 4-year follow-up period, 601 cases of breast cancer were diagnosed. Detailed dietary histories were obtained, and analysis failed to show any increased risk for women whose caloric intake was 44% fat versus those with a 32% fat intake. The authors published an 8-year follow-up of this population, and there was still no relationship to breast cancer risk and total fat intake (60). Critics argue that the low end (<29% of total energy intake as fat) was not sufficiently restricted to produce a result.

Others argue, based on animal studies, that it is not merely fat but total caloric intake that relates to the risk of breast cancer. It is probable that dietary associations, if they in fact bear directly on breast cancer risk, are likely to result in complex interactions. It is possible that environmental factors work only at specific stages of breast development. It may be that dietary factors influence the growing breast but not the differentiated adult breast. It is also possible that more stringent fat restriction might have an effect, but at present it does not appear that moderate fat restriction has a demonstrable effect on breast cancer risk.

The question remains whether or not it is the diet or some other associated factors that account for this. The fact that directly measurable hereditary relationships are very uncommon suggests a complex interplay of environment and individual characteristics in the pathogenesis of breast cancer. Harris and colleagues have pointed out that these nongenetic determinants offer the possibility of developing methods of prevention (61).

RISK FACTORS: ASSOCIATION VERSUS CAUSE AND EFFECT

A number of years ago there was a headline in a Miami newspaper in which a podiatrist suggested that high-heeled shoes were related to breast cancer. He postulated that the alteration in posture and the consequent altered effects of gravity on the breast were the cause of breast cancers. The article stated that "cancer experts are not sure of the explanation," but that it was an "interesting association." Superficially, the observation seems ridiculous, but, objectively, it must be acknowledged that most individuals who wear high-heeled shoes are women and certainly most breast cancers occur among women. There is an unarguable association, but it is not likely that there is any cause and effect. This emphasizes the difficulty in assessing risk factors. Many represent interesting associations, but true cause and effect is difficult to find.

The difficulty in unraveling the various risk relationships lies in the question of cause and effect. For example, it has been shown that dietary restriction early in the lives of laboratory animals reduces the incidence of tumors (62). Dietary restriction and low body fat are related to late menarche and failure to ovulate in humans. What remains unclear is whether it is dietary restriction that is the primary association with diminished risk or if it is the reduced ovulatory activity that is protective.

Similarly, the relationship of height to elevated breast cancer risk (63) may in some way be a direct effect, or it may be that better nutrition leads to earlier menarche and it is the earlier and prolonged exposure to one's own hormones that results in the increased risk. Height may merely be an associated characteristic indicative of better nutrition.

Viruses

Viral etiologies for breast cancer have been suggested. Viruses are a potential vector for the introduction of abnormal DNA or RNA into a cell that can function as an oncogene. This could conceivably affect cell regulation. Viruses are a significant factor in the development of breast cancer in some strains of mice, but there have been no firm links in humans. Although viral particles have reportedly been isolated in human mammary tumors (64), a clear causal relationship has yet to be established.

Factors Associated with an Increased Risk of Breast Cancer

It is important to re-emphasize that factors associated with elevated risk do not necessarily define a cause-and-effect relationship. They are, for the most part, interesting associations rather than direct links. In fact, most women who develop breast cancer have no definable risks except their gender and age (65).

As mentioned previously, the composite lifetime risk of developing breast cancer for American women is now 12% (1 in 8). This overall figure includes those at all levels of risk. The baseline risk for most women in the United States is a 4% to 6% chance of developing breast cancer during their lives (66). Furthermore, figures that are given for factors associated with increased risk are often misleading. Risks are relative to some baseline, and the figures are expressed in relation to a comparison group so that the significance of the relative risk must be assessed in light of the disease incidence in the comparison group.

Further compounding the complexity of using risk factors to predict the future is that although risk factors are not directly additive, some, when found in association with one another, multiply the risk. For example, a woman with atypical proliferative change determined by a breast biopsy is four to five times more likely to develop breast cancer than a similar woman who has no proliferative changes. If she also has a family history of breast cancer, however, her relative risk jumps to 11 times the risk of the comparison women (67). The fact that these factors are not directly additive compounds the difficulty in predicting in any absolute sense an individual's true likelihood of developing breast cancer.

Because the presence of risk factors represents associations and not necessarily cause-and-effect relationships they

should be interpreted cautiously. Although women who fall into these categories are at increased risk, none of these associations has sufficient correlation to accurately predict the development of disease. Risk factors represent interesting associations, but most are of insufficient strength to have any bearing on clinical decisions. The major risk factors for breast cancer are the following:

- Female
- Age >35
- Early menarche
- Late menopause
- Nulliparity
- Late age at first full-term pregnancy (after age 30)
- Affected first-degree relative (mother, sister, or daughter)
- Previous history of breast cancer
- Biopsy proof of atypical epithelial proliferation
- Biopsy proof of lobular carcinoma in situ

All women, as a consequence of their gender, are at some risk for developing breast cancer. The presence of additional risk factors can only increase concern, and the absence of additional risk factors offers little reassurance. Risk factors are relative comparisons between populations of women with a baseline that is not zero but 4% to 6%. The absence of these associations is not protective, and no population has been identified in which there is no risk. For example, a woman who has her first full-term pregnancy by 18 years of age has a lower risk than one whose first full-term pregnancy occurs after age 30, but she may still develop breast cancer.

The majority of women do not have any apparent elevated risk other than the fact that they are female, but because this is the most significant risk, most breast cancer occurs as sporadic malignancy among women in the general population. Between 65% and 80% of breast cancer occurs in women with none of the commonly acknowledged factors that increase risk other than being female. Thus, all women must be considered at risk, and there is no population that can be safely excluded from screening.

Fortunately, most women, even those in the major risk categories (with the exception of hereditary risk), will never develop cancer of the breast. Because risk factors are generally of insufficient strength to influence most screening decisions, their value is questionable, but it is reasonable to be aware of the associations. For the few women whose mother or sister had bilateral premenopausal breast cancer and are likely to have hereditary breast cancer, earlier initiation of mammographic screening might be considered; however, advice for and management of these women are very complex.

Being Female

The single most important risk factor for breast cancer is being female. Breast cancer is almost exclusively a disease of women. It is estimated that approximately 1,000 cases (<1%) occur in males each year.

Age

Breast cancer is extremely rare through the second decade of life, and only about 0.3% of breast cancers occur in women under 30 years of age. The incidence begins to increase rapidly around age 35. This increase continues throughout life, although as noted earlier at a more gradual slope. The chance that a mass represents cancer also increases with age. A palpable abnormality in a woman over 50 years of age is eight times more likely to be malignant than one in a 35 year old (68).

In our own screening data, the positive predictive value (cancers diagnosed per biopsies recommended) for a breast biopsy recommended on the basis of an abnormal mammogram increases steadily from approximately 15% at age 40 to almost 50% by age 80. This merely reflects the prior probability of cancer at different ages (the actual cancers in the population).

Hormonal Status: Early Menarche and Late Menopause

Women who have an early menarche and a late menopause are at somewhat higher risk for breast cancer, which is probably related to the duration and type of hormonal effects on the breast (69). As mentioned previously, some have postulated that the breast may be most vulnerable to carcinogenesis during periods of unopposed estrogen stimulation. As noted above, others have suggested that it is the total exposure to estrogen and progesterone and menstrual cycling that determines breast cancer risk. These hormones stimulate cell proliferation, and it is during cell proliferation that DNA alterations occur that can lead to initiation. In a study of 63,000 Norwegian women the risk increased by 4% for every year of decrease in the age of menarche (70) between ages 16 and 13, and there was a 3.6% increase in risk for each year of delayed menopause.

Other studies have suggested somewhat higher risks associated with earlier age at menarche and later age at menopause. Moolgavkar found that a woman whose menarche was at age 10 had twice the risk of the woman whose menarche was at age 16 and that menopause at age 52 doubled the risk over menopause at age 42 (71). A similar effect was found by Trichopolous and colleagues, who found a doubling of risk between menopause at 45 and menopause at 55 (72). Hysterectomy by the mid-40s appears to reduce the risk (73). These observations suggest that the prolonged exposure of the individual to her own hormones is the likely reason for increased risk.

Family History

There are several different types of family histories of breast cancer. It is likely that most women with relatives who develop breast cancer postmenopausally are not genetically predisposed to breast cancer and that their increased risk is slight. On the other hand, a woman who has a first-degree relative (mother, sister, or daughter) with breast cancer is at a substantially increased risk of developing breast cancer herself. Estimates vary depending on the study but range from 1.5 to 2 times above the woman who has no affected first-degree relatives (74) to as high as four times the risk (75). The risk may be further increased to six times if more than one first-degree relative is affected (66). In one study the degree of risk appeared to increase if the affected mother or sister had bilateral breast cancer premenopausally (76). Such women have been reported to have approximately nine times the risk of women who have no elevated risk factors (4% to 6% lifetime risk) and have as high as a 50% (9 times 4% to 6%) lifetime risk (77). When cancers do develop in this population, they tend to occur at an earlier age than in the mother or sister. These women likely inherit damaged DNA, putting them at risk for multiple breast cancers and their development earlier in life (see Familial and Hereditary Breast Cancer). As noted earlier, a woman who inherits the BRCA1 gene has a 50% chance of developing breast cancer if she lives to age 80. Because the risk for these women is present early in life, screening of such women should probably begin 10 years earlier than the age at which the first-degree relative was diagnosed.

The relationship of a family history of breast cancer, where no genetic link is suspected, is more problematic. Women with a mother, cousin, aunt, or grandmother with postmenopausal breast cancer are at a somewhat increased risk, but this is on the order of 1.5 to 2 times the baseline risk. Although significant, this slight elevation in risk is not particularly useful in advising the woman.

Many women do not understand that the absence of a family history does not offer protection. It is important for women to know that >60% of breast cancers occur in women who have no family history of breast cancer, and that all women are at some risk regardless of their family history.

Familial and Hereditary Breast Cancer

Investigators have for many years noted that breast cancer was frequently found in several members of the same family. Claus et al. distinguish familial breast cancer from hereditary breast cancer (78). The former is defined as "two or more first degree relatives with breast cancer in the absence of hereditary breast cancer." The latter he defines as a "pattern within a particular family which shows Mendelian segregation of breast cancer." The former are probably events that happen, by the laws of probability, to cluster in a family, whereas the latter cancers are likely the result of inheritance of abnormal DNA.

DNA alterations that produce cancer initiation usually occur in somatic cells (cells from normal tissues). These sporadic cancers account for the vast majority of the breast cancers that are diagnosed at the present time. As noted earlier, there are DNA changes that increase a woman's susceptibility to breast cancer that may be passed on in the genetic material carried in the DNA of the germ cell (sperm and ova). The identification of BRCA1 and BRCA2 resulted from studies of families in which there were many relatives who developed breast cancer. In families with this genetically transmitted high susceptibility, the risk of developing breast cancer has been modeled by Hall and associates (33): By the age of 40 the risk is 37%, by age 66 the risk is 55%, and the total lifetime risk is 82%. These risks are in contrast to women who have no genetic susceptibility: 0.4% by age 40, 2.8% by age 55, and 8% over a lifetime. BRCA1 is also linked to an increased risk of ovarian cancer.

As noted earlier, these initially very high risks were likely the result of analyzing families with a high penetrance of the abnormality. More recent data suggest the risks are somewhat less, but the lifetime risk appears to be at least 50% that women with significant BRCA1 or BRCA2 mutations will develop breast cancer.

It has been known for some time that Jewish women are at increased risk for developing breast cancer. Studies of have shown that 2% of Jewish women who are of European descent (Ashkenazi) carry a deletion mutation of this gene (185delAG) that is linked to breast and ovarian cancer or a BRCA2 mutation (a deletion of thymine 617delT). These women have a 33% chance of developing breast cancer by age 50 and a 56% chance of developing breast cancer by the age of 70 (46).

A second area in chromosome 17 has also been identified as the location of a tumor suppressor gene that encodes for the protein p53. Loss or alteration of this gene also results in an increased risk for the development of breast cancer (43). This is one of the first direct links between loss of tumor suppression and the development of breast cancer.

As discussed previously, Knudson's hypothesis predicts that hereditary cancers of the breast will occur earlier in life because the inherited cells with damaged DNA have a head start and thus require fewer subsequent hits for initiation to occur.

The fact that altered or damaged germ cell DNA is incorporated in all the somatic cells of the body should result in a higher percentage of bilateral cancers. This has, in fact, been seen in women with hereditary breast cancers. This is reflected in the fact that women who have a first-degree relative with bilateral premenopausal breast cancer have nine times the baseline risk of developing breast cancer. In addition this risk occurs earlier in life.

Although there are no conclusive data available, it is considered prudent to begin screening women with genetic risk earlier than the general population. We recommend that women with a mother or sister with premenopausal breast cancer begin screening approximately 10 years earlier than the age at which the relative was diagnosed.

Familial or hereditary cancers only account for a small percentage of breast cancers that are diagnosed each year. Lynch and Lynch have estimated that, at most, 9% of breast cancers occur in the setting of the inheritance of abnormal genes (79). The discovery and cloning of these genes offers the possibility of genetic screening. However, the two

BRCA genes appear to be very large with numerous mutations. It is likely that some of these mutations do not increase breast cancer risk. Discovering which do and which do not is a formidable task, and this makes the development of a blood test all the more difficult.

Age at First Full-Term Pregnancy

Nulliparous women are at increased risk, and late parity (after age 30) further increases risk. The relationship of cancer to breast growth and maturity is suggested by the fact that women who have their first full-term pregnancy after the age of 30 years have a risk of developing breast cancer that is two times higher than women who have their first full-term pregnancy before 18 years of age (18). The risk may be even higher if the older woman has a family history of breast cancer (54). One theory is that pregnancy hastens the full development and differentiation of the terminal buds into lobular units. Without a full-term pregnancy it is likely that this process, with increased cell proliferation, may take many years. If periods of active cell division increase susceptibility to damage, shortening this period may reduce the window during which damage is more likely to occur. An early full-term pregnancy may shorten this window by completing breast development in a shorter period. As has been discussed previously, another theory suggests that the suspension of ovulatory cycles that accompany a pregnancy may push the risk curve into later years, reducing the overall risk. Women who have their first full-term pregnancy after age 35 may be at further increased risk beyond those who remain nulliparous.

History of Breast Cancer

A woman who has already had a breast cancer is at greater risk of developing a second cancer than a woman without such a history. Reports range from a 1% to 14% increase in risk, but the figure depends on the period of follow-up, because risk increases with time. If a woman survives her first cancer she has a risk of developing a second cancer that increases by about 1% each year (80) up to approximately a 15% risk.

It is important to note that the development of a second, new primary breast cancer may not alter the prognosis. Data suggest that outcome is determined by the cancer that has the worst prognosis (81). Thus, careful surveillance for the early detection of a new primary is important following treatment for breast cancer.

Benign Breast Disease and Atypical Proliferative Changes

In the past, women who have had benign breast disease were considered to be at increased risk for the future development of breast cancer. Many of these benign processes were collected under the nonspecific diagnosis of fibrocystic disease. It is unclear that true fibrocystic changes (a greater than expected abundance of fibrous tissue and the formation of cysts) represent a disease process. These breast findings are extremely common. In fact, based on autopsy data, most women have changes that can be termed *fibrocystic* (82), making this a fairly meaningless term. The lack of specificity in this term makes it impossible to accurately assess the risk for future cancer.

There are a few histologic changes that have been shown to represent a definite increased risk for the subsequent development of breast cancer. Data published by Dupont and Page suggest that the true risk lies in the small (approximately 7%) subsegment of this population in whom a biopsy diagnosis reveals proliferative changes (67). In particular atypical epithelial hyperplasia (ductal or lobular) represents a significant increased risk. Women without proliferative changes are at no significant increased risk.

Women with hyperplasia were at slight increased risk relative to the background population, but women with atypical proliferative changes followed for a median duration of 17 years were five times more likely to develop breast cancer than those with nonproliferative changes. When atypical proliferative change was found in association with a family history of breast cancer, the risk was elevated 11 times.

True cyst formation was not by itself associated with increased risk, but when present in conjunction with a family history of breast cancer a five- to six-fold risk appeared (51). Acknowledging the inaccuracies of past classifications, the College of American Pathologists has divided benign breast conditions into those with no demonstrable increased risk, those with a slight increased risk, and those with a demonstrated increased risk (Table 3-5) (83,84).

TABLE 3-5. *Histologic types of benign breast lesions and relative risk for the subsequent development of invasive breast cancer*

No increased risk
  Adenosis
  Apocrine metaplasia
  Cysts
  Duct ectasia
  Fibroadenomas (if atypical, are an increased risk)
  Fibrosis
  Hyperplasia (mild)
  Inflammation (mastitis)
  Squamous metaplasia
Slight increased risk (1.5–2.0 times)
  Hyperplasia, moderate or florid, solid or papillary
  Papilloma with fibrovascular core
  (Some studies indicate that sclerosing adenosis is a slightly increased risk)
Moderately increased risk (4–5 times)
  Atypical hyperplasia, ductal or lobular

Source: Adapted from the Cancer Committee College of American Pathologists Consensus Meeting, October 1985. Is 'fibrocystic disease' of the breast precancerous? Arch Pathol Lab Med 1986;110:171–173.

Peripheral Duct Papillomas

There is inconsistent information concerning the risks associated with the benign intraductal papilloma. It appears that the solitary papilloma that is almost always found in the large ducts of the breast has little or no importance for increased risk. However, several studies have suggested that when these lesions are multiple and found in the peripheral ducts, there is an increased risk for breast cancer (85).

Lobular Carcinoma in Situ

Lobular carcinoma in situ (LCIS), or lobular neoplasia, is an abnormal proliferation of cells in the mammary lobule that may not itself become invasive but that appears to represent a histologic indication of significant overall increased risk. Although frequently found in association with an indeterminate cluster of calcifications, LCIS is not characteristically detectable by mammography or physical examination and is usually found coincidentally when biopsy is undertaken for other reasons. The natural history of this lesion is unclear. Its importance lies in the fact that approximately 30% of women with LCIS eventually develop infiltrating carcinoma. It is of interest and importance to note that in women with this lesion the *risk for subsequent cancer is bilateral and approximately 15% for either breast over the next 20 years (for an overall 30% risk)*. Women in whom the diagnosis of LCIS is made have an increased risk of developing invasive carcinoma that is nine times the risk for most women (86).

Radiation

Ionizing radiation has been clearly shown to increase the risk of developing breast cancer. The energies from the radiation produce free radicals (charged particles) that can react with and cause damage to DNA. The type of damage caused by radiation is usually one or more breaks in one or both strands of DNA in the double helix molecule in which one or more nucleotides is eliminated (Fig. 3-9). Irreparable DNA damage is the mechanism by which radiation, as used for therapeutic purposes, kills cells (both normal and unwanted). However, some cells are only damaged and not killed by radiation, and it is these that may become malignant.

On the basis of data from women exposed to very high doses, it appears that approximately 200 rad (2 Gy) doubles a woman's risk. Not only is it impossible to predict specifically who will develop breast cancer even at these high doses, but this estimate oversimplifies a more complex relationship. Radiation risk does not appear to be absolute, but rather seems to be related to the age at which the radiation was absorbed. Older women are at considerably less risk than young girls (see Radiation Risk). The effects of low-level radiation on the breast are difficult to measure because of the large number of naturally occurring cancers and the relatively

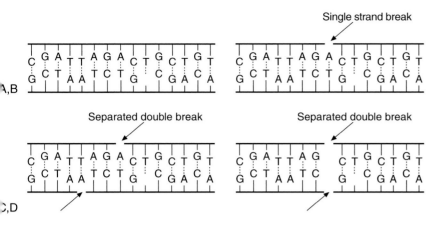

FIG. 3-9. Radiation damage is usually due to free radicals from ionization causing DNA breaks. (A) The normal double helix of DNA contains two opposite strands in which guanine is paired with cytosine and adenine is paired with thymine. Misrepair can be lethal or result in a mutation that may result in cancer. **(B)** A single strand break. **(C)** A double strand break in separate portions of the molecule. **(D)** Double stranded opposite breaks may break the DNA into two pieces.

small magnitude of the effect. Even the theoretical effects at mammographic doses do not appear to be clinically relevant.

Women who have received substantial exposure to radiation (hundreds of rads) to their breasts should be followed carefully.

Increased Breast Cancer Risk Among Women Treated for Hodgkin's Disease

Women irradiated as treatment for Hodgkin's disease are at some increased risk to subsequently develop second malignancies (87). The highest risk is for developing leukemia within the first few years after exposure. Solid tumors such as sarcomas of bone and soft tissue are less common and have a longer latency period. The increased risk for breast cancer appears to begin approximately 5 years after the radiation. The increased risk among these women for the development of breast cancer is presumably related to the scatter radiation from the mediastinal and mantle treatment portal. Dershaw and coworkers studied 27 women who had developed 29 breast malignancies after having been treated for Hodgkin's disease (88). More than 50% of the women were under 45, and 31% were under 40. Among these women, breast cancers were diagnosed between 8 and 34 years after radiation. Of the cancers, 90% (26 of 29) were visible by mammography, and 38% (11 of 26) were clinically occult and detected only by mammography. Positive nodes were found in 21%. The authors concluded that the risk of a subsequent breast cancer is fairly low but significant for women radiated in childhood or adolescence. Because mammography demonstrated 90% of the cancers, they suggest screening should begin approximately 8 years after therapy, even if the women are in their early thirties.

In a similar study, Aisenberg and colleagues followed up on 111 women irradiated for Hodgkin's disease (89). Fourteen women (13%) developed breast cancer with a median follow-up of 18 years. They estimated that women who were irradiated before the age of 20 were at the highest risk of a subsequent breast cancer (8 of 33), having 56 times the expected risk (relative risk [RR] = 56). For women who were between the ages of 20 and 29 at the time of treatment, 5 of 48 developed breast cancer (RR = 7), with only 1 of 30 women (RR = 0.9) who were >30 years old at the time of irradiation developing breast cancer. Not only does this reinforce the need for careful follow-up of these women, but it also emphasizes that the breast is susceptible to radiation carcinogenesis while it is developing (especially among teenage women), but once it has matured there does not seem to be any increased risk from radiation exposure.

Carcinogenesis and Age

The data concerning carcinogenesis raise several interesting questions. As noted above, radiation appears to be most dangerous with respect to breast cancer induction among younger women. Studies have shown that among certain rodent models, carcinogens given while their breasts are developing result in a large number of subsequent breast cancers. If the same carcinogen is given after the breasts have developed (the terminal buds have differentiated) few cancers develop (90). As noted above, among humans, a full-term pregnancy early in life has some protective effect.

All of these observations suggest that damage from a carcinogen is more likely to occur during periods of accelerated proliferation and differentiation, during which damage is more likely to go unrepaired. Proliferation and differentiation are most active while the breast is developing during adolescence and likely into the third and even fourth decades of life, with differentiation of the terminal bud and development of the terminal duct and lobule. It is likely that it is during the time of development that the breast is most susceptible to damage that may lead to cancer. The period of breast development may be a window of opportunity during which exposure to a carcinogen may be more likely to ultimately result in breast cancer.

If the period of breast development occurs over a long period, perhaps there is a larger window of opportunity for a carcinogen to cause damage. If, however, terminal differentiation and breast development occur over a short period, early in life, triggered by a full-term pregnancy in preparation for lactation, the window may be significantly narrowed and the risk of carcinogenesis commensurately reduced.

The above is theoretical but, if correct, suggests that it may be exposure to carcinogens early in life (including dietary factors) that may be most important and not exposure to the mature individual that is important.

Factors with Weak Associations

Numerous factors that appear to be associated with increased risk of breast cancer have been identified, but the relationships are weak or unconfirmed.

Exogenous Hormone Use

The low, if any, risk from the use of oral contraceptives was discussed earlier (see Oral Contraceptives). There may be some increased risk with long-term use prior to a first full-term pregnancy (use for >4 years), but there has not been any consistent risk demonstrated in numerous studies.

There are conflicting studies on the risks of HRT. Several studies suggest an increased risk while the hormones are being used but not after being used. This might suggest a promotional effect in which the hormones might support the growth of an already initiated but quiescent clone rather than a true increased risk. In one prospective study, the risk for women using hormones was increased by approximately 30% (relative risk of 1.36) when compared to nonusers, but even 10 years of use showed no increased risk once HRT was discontinued (91). Henderson summarized studies that show a 1.3 to 1.9 times risk if hormones are used for many years, but he points out that the cardiovascular and bone maintenance benefits of HRT outweigh the slightly increased breast cancer risk (6).

Obesity

Paradoxically, obesity is associated with a decreased risk in premenopausal women and a slight increased risk in older women. The reason for this is unclear, but it has been postulated that it is the conversion of androgens to estrogen (see Hormones) in the fat that accounts for the postmenopausal risk.

Lactation

Lactation has been shown in some studies to have a weak protective effect, but this may be related to the duration of lactation and could influence risk by reducing a woman's exposure to her own hormones by causing long periods of anovulation.

Alcohol Consumption

Several studies have shown an association between alcohol consumption and breast cancer risk (92). A slight increased risk has been seen with even a single drink a day (93). A meta-analysis combining results from available studies shows a consistent but low elevation of risk ranging from 1.4 to 1.7 times the risk for nonconsumers (94). No clear mechanism for this association has been identified, but at least one study has demonstrated increased levels of estrogen following alcohol consumption.

Mammographically Defined Breast Patterns and Cancer Risks

Perhaps one of the most controversial issues in breast imaging has been the significance of mammographically determined tissue patterns as indicators of risk for the subsequent development of malignancy. In his first review of these patterns, Wolfe suggested that women with a radiographically dense pattern, which he termed DY, had 37 times greater risk of developing breast cancer than women with almost all fat by mammography (Wolfe's N1 pattern) (95). Numerous studies followed in an effort to reproduce or refute this observation. Some studies supported Wolfe's contention of increased risk, albeit to a lesser degree (96–99). Other studies (100) found the risk to be higher in the P2 pattern (Wolfe later agreed). Still other studies found no increased risk (101,102). There have been studies that show that readers can agree on the classification of mammograms (103,104) and studies that show that they cannot (105). Some investigators have even studied the studies (106).

Many of these studies were not optimally designed and were flawed by biases of one kind or another. For example, none controlled for other known risk factors. Statisticians and epidemiologists have consequently disagreed on the results. The extremely high risk that Wolfe initially suggested has never been corroborated. The best analyses suggest that the radiographically dense patterns (P2-, prominent nodular densities and DY) may in fact represent a slightly higher risk. In a review of the major studies, Boyd and associates concluded, based on all the data put together, that the DY pattern carried three times the N1 risk for women under 50 years of age (106). This is approximately the same degree of risk as is carried by a woman with a mother who developed breast cancer postmenopausally.

Boyd and colleagues undertook a more rigorous review of the mammograms from the National Breast Screening Study of Canada and they concluded that the dense patterns are associated with increased breast cancer risk (106).

Because the risk for any pattern is in an absolute sense very low, the relation to cancer represents an interesting observation but is of little clinical usefulness. Given that up to 50% of breast cancers have been reported to occur in women with the low risk fatty patterns (N1 all fat and P1 15% to 25% nodular densities in predominantly fat tissue), women with such patterns cannot be excluded from screening programs. That factor, in conjunction with the fact that the vast majority of women in the so-called high-risk category will never develop cancer, makes it impossible to use

FIG. 3-10. Dense breast tissue does not preclude early detection. Clustered microcalcifications indicative of an intraductal carcinoma are evident in this close-up despite a radiographically dense breast.

these patterns to make any significant clinical decisions. Given our present level of understanding, increasing patient and physician concern on the basis of mammographic patterns is unwarranted. These patterns should be viewed as significant only from an investigational point of view; from a clinical perspective they should be used only to suggest the degree of sensitivity of the mammogram for detecting small cancers.

Age and Breast Patterns

It is a mistake to think of patterns changing at age 50. This is not the case. There is no question that older women tend to have more fat in their breasts, and mammography is better able to detect many small cancers earlier in this population, but fat replacement or deposition appears to be a progressive process that begins in some women as early as age 25 or 30. Many younger women have predominantly fat in their breasts, and a large percentage of older women have dense patterns (see The Normal Breast). Even in women with dense breast tissue, a significant number of early cancers can be found. Microcalcifications (Fig. 3-10) and areas of architectural distortion can be detected even in women who radiographically have extremely dense mammary tissues. Thus, mammographic screening in younger women should not be curtailed simply because they may have denser tissue patterns.

SURVIVAL AND BREAST CANCER

Despite the steady rise in breast cancer incidence over the last 50 years, the mortality rate has remained fairly constant. Each year approximately 25 to 30 deaths per 100,000 women in the population are attributable to breast cancer (1). The probability of surviving breast cancer varies with the age at which it is diagnosed (see Table 3-3). Contrary to popular belief, for women who are diagnosed with the disease at the same stage, younger women survive as long or even longer than older women (107), but younger women tend to be diagnosed at a later stage. In general, a woman who is in her 40s when she is diagnosed with breast cancer has a 50% chance of surviving 20 years, whereas a woman diagnosed in her 50s has only a 30% chance of surviving that long (see Table 3-3). This difference in survival may account for the delayed benefit that is derived from screening for women from ages 40 to 49. Mortality reduction for these women does not begin to appear until 5 to 7 years after screening begins (see Screening), whereas for women over 50 it begins to appear only 2 to 3 years after screening.

Until 1989 the overall death rate from breast cancer had not changed. The fact that the number of deaths per 100,000 was unchanged over 50 years while the incidence had been steadily rising could be interpreted in two ways. The overall stable death rate in the face of a steadily increasing incidence could mean that improved detection and treatment over time was saving some lives. Alternatively, however, the data could also be explained by the theory that the increasing number of cancers that were being detected were of the nonlethal variety.

In support of the improved-detection-and-treatment interpretation is the fact that between 1989 and 1992 there was an actual decrease in cancer deaths among all women except those 80 years of age and older. The NCI estimated that the decrease ranged from 3.4% among women ages 70 to 79 to 9.3% among women ages 50 to 59 (Table 3-6) (108).

Although it is difficult to attribute the reason for the decrease in death, it is in part due to earlier detection. The arguments for eliminating support for screening women under 50 are ironic because these women have taken advantage of screening, likely resulting in the decreased rate of death.

TABLE 3-6. *Decreased mortality from breast cancer 1989 to 1992*

For women ages 30–39 there was an 8.7% decrease.
For women ages 40–49 there was an 8.1% decrease.
For women ages 50–59 there was a 9.3% decrease.
For women ages 60–69 there was a 4.8% decrease.
For women ages 70–79 there was a 3.1% decrease.

PREVENTION OF BREAST CANCER

Despite the fact that the exact causes of breast cancer remain undefined, there is hope that some breast cancers can be prevented or at least delayed in their development. It has been known for many years that some breast cancers, particularly in postmenopausal women, require estrogen to support their growth. Treating women with the drug tamoxifen has been shown to increase disease-free survival in women whose cancers are estrogen receptor positive (109), and some effect has been shown even when receptor analysis suggests a negative tumor. Tamoxifen appears to compete for the estrogen receptor site and acts as a competitive inhibitor and tumorostatic agent. The fact that benefit persists after the cessation of its use suggests that it has tumoricidal properties as well.

Studies have shown that women who have had breast cancer and are placed on tamoxifen have as much as a 40% reduction in the number of cancers that develop in the contralateral breast when compared to those women with similar cancers who have not used tamoxifen (110,111). Although tamoxifen appears to oppose the estrogen effect with breast cancers, it appears to mimic the estrogen effect in terms of preserving bone density and preventing osteoporosis (112), and it also appears to have salutary cardiovascular effects (113). The only negative effect, other than producing menopausal symptoms (e.g., hot flashes) in some women, is the increased risk of endometrial cancer (114). Careful monitoring of the uterus is important for women taking tamoxifen. Tamoxifen, when given to rats, can apparently produce liver cancers (111), but this has not appeared as a problem in humans.

Based on the predominantly salutary effects of tamoxifen and the data that can be used to infer a preventive effect and likely reduction in the incidence of breast cancers, an international study was begun in 1992 to test the use of tamoxifen for the prevention of breast cancer. Women 60 and over, or high-risk younger women who have a risk profile equivalent to a 60-year-old woman's risk (Table 3-7), were recruited into a randomized controlled trial in which the study group will use tamoxifen for 2 or 5 years to determine whether such use will reduce their future risk of breast cancer.

SUMMARY AND CONCLUSION

Prevention is the ideal solution to the problem of breast cancer, but it remains an elusive goal. Without an understanding of the causes, prevention is a remote possibility. Preventive measures may also have side effects of their own that will not permit their application to the large population of women who will never develop breast cancer. A universal cure would be preferable from a public health perspective so that only women with the disease need be treated. Such a cure has also remained elusive. It is likely that for the foreseeable future early detection will remain the best hope for mortality reduction.

There is likely no single factor that explains all cancers of the breast, and the direct etiologies remain obscure. A number of factors appear to place some women at increased risk, but no woman is immune and all women have some degree of risk. The associations between specific risk factors and breast cancer are interesting and important for targeting research but are usually of little practical significance. It must be re-emphasized that all women must be considered at risk for developing breast cancer.

Risk factors define only those who may be at higher risk than the 4% to 6% baseline. No population of women has been identified that is not at risk for developing breast cancer, and screening programs must take this into account. If screening is offered only to women in high-risk groups, >65% of cancer will develop without the benefit of early detection. Until methods of prevention are defined, screening for early detection must be available to all women.

The first trials of breast cancer prevention may, possibly, open a major avenue for reducing deaths from these ubiquitous malignancies. Early detection remains the only proven method for reducing the mortality from breast cancer, and the mammographic screening of asymptomatic women remains the only efficacious method for detecting earlier stage, clinically occult breast cancer. Magnetic resonance imaging offers some hope for detecting cancers in the dense breast that are not easily detected by mammography, but the cost of the equipment and the requirement of the intravenous administration of contrast agents are limitations for wide-

TABLE 3-7. *Women eligible for the tamoxifen chemoprevention trial*

Any woman with biopsy-proven lobular carcinoma in situ (LCIS)
Age 35–39: One or more first-degree relatives with breast cancer *and* benign breast disease with at least two breast biopsies
Age 40–44: Two or more first-degree relatives with breast cancer *or* benign breast disease with at least two breast biopsies
Age 45–54: One or more first-degree relatives with breast cancer *or* benign breast disease with at least two breast biopsies
Age 55–59: One or more first-degree relatives with breast cancer *or* first live birth at age 30 or older
Age 60 and over: All are eligible

spread use. Digital mammography with dual energy subtraction or contrast enhancement may also aid in detection and the determination of the extent of malignancy. For the foreseeable future, high quality mammographic screening will be the most efficacious method for reducing the death rate from breast cancer.

REFERENCES

1. American Cancer Society. Breast Cancer: Cancer Facts and Figures. Atlanta: American Cancer Society, 1995.

2. Miller BA, Feuer EJ, Hankey BF. Trends in invasive breast cancer incidence among American women. J Natl Cancer Inst 1991;83:678. Graph.

3. National Institutes of Health. National Cancer Institute Statistics Review 1975–1988. Bethesda, MD: National Institutes of Health; 1991. NIH Publication no. 91-2789.

4. Smith RA. Epidemiology of Breast Cancer in A Categorical Course in Physics: Technical Aspects of Breast Imaging (2nd ed). Oak Brook, IL: Radiological Society of North America, 1993;21–33.

5. Burhenne HJ, Burhenne LW, Goldberg F, et al. Reply: interval breast cancers in the screening mammography program of British Columbia: analysis and classification. AJR Am J Roentgenol 1995;164:1299.

6. Mettlin CJ, Menck HR, Winchester DP, Murphy GP. A comparison of breast, colorectal, lung and prostate cancers reported to the National Cancer Data Base and Surveillance, Epidemiology, and End Results Program. Cancer 1997;79:2052–2061.

7. Manton KG, Stallard E. A two-disease model of female breast cancer: mortality in 1969 among white females in the United States. J Natl Cancer Inst 1980;64:9–16.

8. Tabar L, Faberberg G, Day NE, Holmberg L. What is the optimum interval between screening examinations? An analysis based on the latest results of the Swedish two-county breast cancer screening trial. Br J Cancer 1987;55:547–551.

9. Moskowitz M. Breast cancer: age-specific growth rates and screening strategies. Radiology 1986;161:37–41.

10. Tabar L. New Swedish breast cancer detection results for women aged 40–49. Cancer 1993;72:1437–1448.

11. Adami HO, Malker B, Holmberg L, et al. The relation between survival and age at diagnosis in breast cancer. N Engl J Med 1986;315:559–563.

12. Pike MC, Krailo MD, Henderson BE, et al. Hormonal risk factors, breast tissue age, and the age-incidence of breast cancer. Nature 1983;303:767–770.

13. Spicer DV, Ursin G, Parisky YR, et al. Changes in mammographic densities induced by a contraceptive designed to reduce breast cancer risk. J Natl Cancer Inst 1994;86:431–436.

14. Kelsey JL, Gammon MD, John EM. Reproductive factors and breast cancer. Epidemiol Rev 1993;15:36–47.

15. Sturgeon SR, Schairer C, Gail M, et al. Geographic variation in mortality from breast cancer among white women in the United States. J Natl Cancer Inst 1995;87:1846–1843.

16. Henderson BE. Endogenous and Exogenous Endocrine Factors. In Hematology and Oncology Clinics of North America: Diagnosis and Therapy of Breast Cancer. Philadelphia: Saunders 1989;3: 577–598.

17. Wyshak G, Frisch RE. Evidence for a secular trend in the age of menarche. N Engl J Med 1982;306:1033–1035.

18. MacMahon B, Cole P, Lin TM, et al. Age at first birth and breast cancer risk. Bull World Health Organ 1970;43:209–221.

19. Byers T, Graham S, Rzepka T, Marshall J. Lactation and breast cancer: evidence for a negative association in premenopausal women. Am J Epidemiol 1985;12:664–674.

20. Newcomb PA, Storer BE, Longnecker MP, et al. Lactation and a reduced risk of premenopausal breast cancer. N Engl J Med 1994;330:81–87.

21. Romieu I, Willett WC, Colditz GA, et al. Prospective study of oral contraceptive use and risk of breast cancer in women. J Natl Cancer Inst 1989;81:1313–1321.

22. Romieu I, Berlin JA, Colditz JA. Oral contraceptives and breast cancer: review and meta-analysis. Cancer 1990;66:2253–2263.

23. WHO Collaborative Study of Neoplasia and Steroid Contraceptives. Breast cancer and combined oral contraceptives: results from a multinational study. Br J Cancer 1990;61:110–119.

24. Colditz GA, Hankinson SE, Hunter DJ, et al. The use of estrogens and progestins and the risk of breast cancer in postmenopausal women. N Engl J Med 1995;332:1589–1593.

25. Wolff MS, Toniolo PG, Lee EW, et al. Blood levels of orcanochlorine residues and risk of breast cancer. J Natl Cancer Inst 1993;85:648–652.

26. Falck F, Ricci A, Wolff MS, et al. Pesticides and polychlorinated biphenyl residues in human breast lipids and their relation to breast cancer. Arch Environ Health 1992;47:143–146.

27. Stacey-Clear A, McCarthy KA, Hall DA, et al. Observations on the location of breast cancer in women under fifty. Radiology 1993;186:677–680.

28. Glass A, Hoover R. Changing incidence of breast cancer [letter]. J Natl Cancer Inst 1988;80:1076–1077.

29. Lantz PM, Remington PL, Newcomb PA. Mammography screening and increased incidence of breast cancer in Wisconsin. J Natl Cancer Inst 1991;83:1540–1546.

30. White E, Lee CY, Kristal AR. Evaluation of increase in breast cancer incidence in relation to mammography use. J Natl Cancer Inst 1990;82:1546–1552.

31. Shields PG, Harris CC. Molecular epidemiology and the genetics of environmental cancer. JAMA 1991;266:681–687.

32. Knudson AG. Hereditary cancer, oncogenes, and antioncogenes. Cancer Res 1985;45:1437–1443.

33. Hall JM, Lee MK, Newman B, et al. Linkage of early-onset familial breast cancer to chromosome 17q21. Science 1990;250:1684–1689.

34. Leis HP. Risk factors for breast cancer: an update. Breast 1981;6:21–27.

35. Stein WD. Analysis of cancer incidence data on the basis of multistage and clonal growth models. Adv Cancer Res 1991;56:161–182.

36. Deng G, Lu Y, Zlotnikov G, et al. Loss of heterozygosity in normal tissue adjacent to breast carcinomas. Science 1996;274:2057–2059.

37. Hartwell LH, Kasten MB. Cell cycle control and cancer. Science 1994;266:1821–1828.

38. Kim NW, Piatyszek MA, Prowse KR, et al. Specific association of human telomerase activity with immortal cells and cancer. Science 1994;266:2011–2015.

39. Marx J. DNA repair comes into its own. Science 1994;266:728–730.

40. Roth JA. Molecular surgery for cancer. Arch Surg 1992;127:1298–1302.

41. Kern JA, Schwark DA, Nordberg JE, et al. Studies of the HER-2/neu proto-oncogene in human breast and ovarian cancer. Science 1989;244:707–712.

42. Van Vrier M, Petrese J, Mooi W, et al. Neu-protein overexpression in breast cancer: association with comedo-type ductal carcinoma in situ and limited prognostic value in stage II breast cancer. N Engl J Med 1988;319:1239–1245.

43. Malkin D, Li FP, Strong LC, et al. Germ line p53 mutations in a familial syndrome of breast cancer, sarcomas, and other neoplasms. Science 1990;250:1233–1238.

44. Wooster R, Neuhausen SL, Mangion J, et al. Localization of a breast cancer susceptibility gene, BRCA2, to chromosome 13q12-13. Science 1994;265:2088–2090.

45. Ford D, Easton DF, Bishop DT, et al. Breast Linkage Consortium. Risk of cancer in BRCA1-mutation carriers. Lancet 1994;343:692–695.

46. Struewing JP, Hartage P, Wacholder S, et al. The risk of cancer associated with specific mutations of BRCA1 and BRCA2 among Ashkenazi Jews. N Engl J Med 1997;336:1401–1408.

47. Noguchi S, Aihara T, Koymam H, et al. Discrimination between multicentric and multifocal carcinomas of the breast through clonal analysis. Cancer 1994;74:872–877.

48. Volgelstein B, et al. Genetic Alterations Accumulate During Colorectal Tumorigenesis. In Cavenee W, Hastle N, Standbridge E (eds), Recessive Oncogenes and Tumor Suppression. Cold Spring Harbor, NY: Cold Spring Harbor Laboratory, 1989.

49. Weinberg RA. The genetic bases of cancer. Arch Surg 1990;125: 257–260.

50. Hansen E, Wolff N, Knuechel R, et al. Tumor cells in blood shed from the surgical field. Arch Surg 1995;130:387–393.

51. Hart IR, Saini A. Biology of tumour metastasis. Lancet 1992;339: 1453–1457.

52. Aznavoorian S, Murphy AN, Stetler-Stevenson, Liotta LA. Molecular aspects of tumor cell invasion and metastasis. Cancer 1993;71: 1368–1383.

53. Korenman SG. The endocrinology of breast cancer. Cancer 1980;46:874.
54. Sellers T, Kushi L, Potter DJ, et al. Effect of family history, body fat distribution and reproductive factors on the risk of postmenopausal breast cancer. N Engl J Med 1992;326:1323–1329.
55. Harris JR, Lippman ME, Veronesi U, Willett W. Breast cancer. N Engl J Med 1992;327:319–328.
56. Buell P. Changing incidence of breast cancer in Japanese-American women. J Natl Cancer Inst 1973;51:1479–1483.
57. Cole P. Major aspects of the epidemiology of breast cancer. Cancer 1980;46:865.
58. Wynder EL. Dietary factors related to breast cancer. Cancer 1980;46:899.
59. Willett WC, Stampfer MJ, Colditz GA, et al. Dietary fat and the risk of breast cancer. N Engl J Med 1987;316:22.
60. Willett WC, Hunter DJ, Meir MJ, et al. Dietary fat and fiber in relation to risk of breast cancer. An 8-year follow-up. JAMA 1992;268:2037–2044.
61. Harris JR, Lippman ME, Veronesi U, Willett W. Breast cancer. N Engl J Med 1992;327:319–328, 390–397, 473–480.
62. Welsh CW. Relationship between dietary fat and experimental mammary tumorigenesis: a review and critique. Cancer Res 1992;52:2040s–2048s.
63. Vatten LJ, Kvinnsland S. Body height and risk for breast cancer: a prospective study of 23,831 Norwegian women. Br J Cancer 1990;61:881–885.
64. Hutter RV. The influence of pathologic factors on breast cancer management. Cancer 1980;46:961.
65. Seidman H, Stellman SD, Mushinski MH. A different perspective on breast cancer risk factors: some implications of nonattributable risk. Cancer 1982;32:301.
66. Gail MH, Brinton LA, Byar DP. Projecting individualized probabilities of developing breast cancer for white females who are being examined annually. J Natl Cancer Inst 1989;81:1879–1886.
67. Dupont WD, Page DL. Risk factors for breast cancer in women with proliferative breast disease. N Engl J Med 1985;312:146.
68. Spivey GH, Perry BW, Clark VA, et al. Predicting the risk of cancer at the time of breast biopsy. Am Surg 1982;48:326–332.
69. MacMahon B, Cole P, Brown J. Etiology of human breast cancer: a review. J Natl Cancer Inst 1973;50:21.
70. Kvale G, Heuch I. Menstrual factors and breast cancer risk. Cancer 1988;62:1625–1631.
71. Moolgavkar SH, Day NE, Stevens RG. Two-stage model for carcinogenesis: epidemiology of breast cancer in females. J Natl Cancer Inst 1980;65:559–569.
72. Trichopolous D, MacMahon B, Cole P. Menopause and breast cancer risk. J Natl Cancer Inst 1972;48:605–613.
73. Lilienfield AM. The relationship of cancer of the female breast to artificial menopause and marital status. Cancer 1956;9:927–934.
74. Adami HO, Hansen J, Jung B, Rimsten A. Characteristics of familial breast cancer in Sweden: absence of relation to age and unilateral versus bilateral disease. Cancer 1981;48:1688–1695.
75. Sattin RW, Rubin GL, Webster LA. Family history and the risk of breast cancer. JAMA 1985;253:1908.
76. Anderson DE. Some characteristics of familial breast cancer. Cancer 1971;28:1500.
77. Ottman R, Pike MC, King M-C, Henderson BE. Practical guide for estimating risk for familial breast cancer. Lancet 1983;2:556–558.
78. Claus EB, Schildkraut JM, Thompson WD, Risch NJ. The genetic attributable risk of breast and ovarian cancer. Cancer 1996;77:2318–2324.
79. Lynch HT, Lynch JF. Breast cancer genetics in an oncology clinic: 328 consecutive patients. Cancer J Clin 1986;22:369–371.
80. Horn PL, Thompson WD. Risk of contralateral breast cancer: associations with histologic, clinical, and therapeutic factors. Cancer 1988;62:412–424.
81. Henderson IC. Risk factors for breast cancer development. Cancer 1993;71:2127–2140.
82. Love SM, Gelman RS, Silen WS. Fibrocystic disease of the breast: a non-disease? N Engl J Med 1982;307:1010.
83. College of American Pathologists. Is "fibrocystic disease" of the breast precancerous? Arch Pathol Lab Med 1985;110:171–174.
84. Jensen RA, Page DL, Dupont WD, Rogers LW. Invasive breast cancer risk in women with sclerosing adenosis. Cancer 1989;64:1977–1983.
85. Ohuchi N, Abe R, Kasai M. Possible changes of intraductal papillomas of the breast: a 3-D reconstruction study of 25 cases. Cancer 1984;54:605–611.
86. Rosen PP, Lieberman PH, Braun DV, et al. Lobular carcinoma in situ of the breast. Am J Surg Pathol 1978;2:225.
87. Janjan NA, Wilson JF, Gillin M, et al. Mammary carcinoma developing after radiotherapy and chemotherapy for Hodgkin's disease. Cancer 1988;61:252–254.
88. Dershaw D, Yahalom J, Petrek JA. Breast carcinoma in women previously treated for Hodgkin's disease: mammographic evaluation. Radiology 1992;184:421–423.
89. Aisenberg AC, Finklestein DM, Doppke KP, et al. High risk of breast carcinoma after irradiation of young women with Hodgkin's disease. Cancer 1997;79:1203–1210.
90. Russo J, Russo IH. Biological and molecular bases of mammary carcinogenesis. Lab Invest 1987;57:112–113.
91. Colditz GA, Stampfer MJ, Willett WC, et al. Prospective study of estrogen replacement therapy and risk of breast cancer in postmenopausal women. JAMA 1990;264:2648–2653.
92. Stampfer MJ, Colditz GA, Willett WC. Alcohol intake and risk of breast cancer. Compr Ther 1988;14:8–15.
93. Willett WC, Stampfer MJ, Colditz GA, et al. Moderate alcohol consumption and the risk of breast cancer. N Engl J Med 1988;316:1174–1179.
94. Longnecker MP, Berlin JA, Orza MJ, Chalmers TC. A meta-analysis of alcohol consumption in relation to the risk of breast cancer. JAMA 1988;260:652–656.
95. Wolfe JN. Breast patterns as an index of risk for developing breast cancer. AJR Am J Roentgenol 1976;126:1130.
96. Krook PM. Mammographic tissue patterns as risk indicators for incident cancer in a screening program: an extended analysis. AJR Am J Roentgenol 1978;131:1031.
97. Wilkinson E, Clopton C, Green R, et al. Mammographic tissue patterns and the risk of breast cancer. J Natl Cancer Inst 1977;59:1397.
98. Janzon L, Andersson I, Petersson H. Mammographic patterns as indicators of risk of breast cancer. Radiology 1982;143:417.
99. Hainline S, Meyers L, McLelland R, et al. Mammographic patterns and risk of breast cancer. AJR Am J Roentgenol 1978;130:1157.
100. Peyester RG, Kalisher L, Cole P. Mammographic tissue patterns and the prevalence of breast cancer. Radiology 1977;125:287.
101. Egan RL, McSwenney MB. Mammographic tissue patterns and risk of breast cancer. Radiology 1979;133:65.
102. Mendell L, Rosenbloom M, Naimark A. Are breast tissue patterns a risk index for breast cancer? A reappraisal. AJR Am J Roentgenol 1977;128:547.
103. Carlile T, Thompson DJ, Kopecky KJ, et al. Reproducibility and consistency in classification of breast tissue patterns. AJR Am J Roentgenol 1983;140:1.
104. Wolfe JN, Wilkie RC. Breast pattern classification and observer error. Radiology 1978;127:343.
105. Meyers LE, McLelland R, Stricker CX, et al. Reproducibility of mammographic classifications. AJR Am J Roentgenol 1983;141:445.
106. Boyd NF, O'Sullivan B, Fishell E, et al. Mammographic patterns and breast cancer risk: methodologic standards and contradictory results. J Natl Cancer Inst 1984;72:1253.
107. Adami H, Malker B, Holmberg L, et al. The relation between survival and age at diagnosis in breast cancer. N Engl J Med 1986;315:559–563.
108. Smigel K. Breast cancer death rates decline for white women. J Natl Cancer Inst 1995;87:173.
109. Early Breast Cancer Trialists' Collaborative Group. Systemic treatment of early breast cancer by hormonal, cytotoxic, or immune therapy: 133 randomized trials involving 31,000 recurrences and 24,000 deaths among 75,000 women. Lancet 1992;339:1–15, 71–84.
110. Rutqvist LE, Cedermark B, Glas U, et al. Contralateral primary tumors in breast cancer patients in a randomized trial of adjuvant tamoxifen therapy. J Natl Cancer Inst 1991;83:1299–1306.
111. Nayfield SG, Karp JE, Ford LG, et al. Potential role of tamoxifen in prevention of breast cancer. J Natl Cancer Inst 1991;83:1450–1459.
112. Fornander T, Rutqvist LE, Sjoberg HE, et al. Long-term adjuvant tamoxifen in early breast cancer: effect on bone mineral density in postmenopausal women. J Clin Oncol 1990;8:1019–1024.
113. Bagdad JD, Wolter J, Subbaiah PV, Ryan W. Effects of tamoxifen treatment on plasma lipids and lipoprotein lipid composition. J Clin Endocrinol Metab 1990;70:1132–1135.
114. Leeuwen FE, Benraadt J, Coebergh JWW, et al. Risk of endometrial cancer after tamoxifen treatment of breast cancer. Lancet 1994;343:448–452.

Breast Imaging, 2nd ed., by Daniel B. Kopans.
Lippincott–Raven Publishers, Philadelphia © 1998.

CHAPTER 4

Screening for Breast Cancer

The primary reason for performing mammography is to screen women to detect clinically occult breast cancer at a smaller size and earlier stage than it would otherwise be detected in an effort to interrupt the natural history of breast malignancies and reduce the number of women who die each year from breast cancer. Screening, however, has been extremely controversial and the debate over the efficacy of screening has dominated breast care for more than three decades. This is in part due to the fact that most physicians, and certainly most radiologists, have not had the time or training to understand the epidemiologic and statistical issues involved in the process. They understand care of the individual patient but have relied on others to analyze the screening data and draw conclusions for them. The concepts are not that difficult, and it would benefit women greatly if those involved in breast cancer detection and diagnosis had a better understanding of the issues and the results of the screening trials. It is for this reason that this chapter is extensive. It addresses many concepts that have little to do with the day-to-day care of the individual woman, but the questions are fundamental. Mammography is a screening technology. Its only real value is the earlier detection of breast cancer to reduce the death rate from these malignancies. It is, therefore, critical to determine whether screening can interrupt the growth of breast cancer before successful metastatic spread has occurred, and, if this is age related, at what age screening should begin and at what age it is no longer valuable.

RATIONALE FOR SCREENING

Not long ago it was suggested that before breast cancer could be detected it had spread from the breast to other parts of the body and become a systemic disease. Through the mechanism of randomized, controlled trials (RCTs) it is now clear that this is not the case for many women. The studies have demonstrated that the natural history of breast cancer can be interrupted and the individual can be cured, or death from breast cancer delayed, if the malignancies are detected and treated before they have successfully metastasized.

Proving this has not been a simple task. Although breast cancer is the leading cause of nonpreventable cancer death among women, it is less lethal than many other forms of cancer. Fortunately, most women who develop breast cancer do not die from it. This is partly because breast cancer is a malignancy that is directly associated with aging, and many women who develop breast cancer are of sufficient age that other illnesses frequently end their lives before they succumb to their breast cancer. Other breast cancers may never develop metastatic capability, and still others are discovered and cured before they can successfully spread. Consequently, in any study of breast cancer detection and its influence on outcome, it is very difficult to determine which cancers have actually been affected by the intervention.

Although there is no consensus, the fact that the death rate has remained fairly constant over the past 50 years while there has been a steady increase in the number of women diagnosed with invasive breast cancer since at least 1940 (see Epidemiology) suggests that some, if not a large percentage, of breast cancers are being cured. Between 1989 and 1992 there was a significant decrease in breast cancer deaths (1). It remains to be seen whether that trend will be sustained, and there is no universal agreement as to how much of the decrease is due to screening and how much is due to chemotherapy and hormonal therapy. Reinforcing the likely benefit from mammographic screening is a report from Malmö, Sweden, that the death rate from breast cancer has decreased in the city by 43% since the beginning of mammographic screening (2). The benefit was confined to the age group 45 to 65, for which screening was offered. It was suggested that therapeutic advances might account for this benefit, but these results were in contrast to an only 17% mortality reduction in the rest of Sweden (presumably exposed to the same therapeutic interventions but not to screening) over the same period.

Before large-scale screening began, most breast cancers grew large enough to be felt by the woman and her physician, yet most women did not die from their breast cancers. This suggests that there are some breast cancers that can be quite large and still have not metastasized and that treating these can cure the patient. However, although there are exceptions, it is also clear that the likelihood of cure decreases as the size of the primary cancer increases. Although there are some cancers that reach the level of incurability while still microscopic and other, very large tumors that do not result in death, studies have repeatedly shown that prognosis is directly related to the size of the cancer (3).

To reduce the death rate from breast cancers, these malignancies must be found and treated at a small size and early stage. This requires that the breast be evaluated before there are any signs or symptoms to suggest the presence of cancer. Mammography has been shown to be able to do this and to detect a large percentage of cancers before the patient or her doctor is able to feel the tumor (4).

Because there are as yet no ways of predicting who will or will not develop breast cancer, all women must be considered at risk and should be encouraged to be evaluated before there are any signs or symptoms that suggest the presence of the disease. Screening is the only way to detect cancers earlier, and this has been shown to be able to reduce the rate of death from these malignancies.

SCREENING DEFINED

Screening for breast cancer can be defined as the evaluation of a population of asymptomatic women who have no overt signs or symptoms of breast cancer, in an effort to detect unsuspected disease at a time when cure is still possible.

The primary reason for medical imaging of the breast is to screen for cancer. Just as the term suggests, screening is a filter that permits most objects to pass through while trying to sift the material to trap objects of a specific type. Screening for breast cancer tries to let most women, who do not have cancer, pass through the screen while selecting for further evaluation those women who have abnormalities that may indicate cancer. Just as a water filter may intercept beneficial minerals in an attempt to eliminate harmful contaminants, a screen for breast cancer may also find benign changes that are not immediately separable from those that are malignant. The thresholds of concern in a breast cancer screening program are similar to the pores of the filter. The tighter the pores of the filter, the more benign material is trapped along with the bad material. If the filter pores are widened to reduce the trapping of benign particles, then some of the harmful particles also pass through.

An aggressive approach to breast cancer screening traps more early breast cancers at the expense of raising concern over more lesions that prove to be benign, whereas a higher threshold for intervention reduces the number of benign lesions but permits some cancers to pass through. The differentiation of the two types of abnormalities from one another is the function of diagnosis. Finally, just as the water filter does not remove all impurities, screening for breast cancer does not detect all cancers and does not detect all cancers at a time when cure is possible.

SCREENING EFFICACY AND BENEFIT

There is no absolute definition of efficacy. In general, screening with a new technique is efficacious if the stage at which the disease is detected is reduced relative to previous methods and, more important, if the overall mortality from the disease is decreased.

Risks

The medical efficacy of screening is frequently confused with the risk versus the benefit and the cost of screening. In addition to the direct monetary and economic costs of screening, there may also be negative physical and psychological effects directly related to screening. It must be remembered that it is apparently healthy women who are being screened. Many of these women will, at one time or another, have an abnormal screen that may result in anxiety that would never have occurred in the absence of screening. Biopsies will be performed, many of which will prove to be for benign lesions. These are traumatic events that would not occur in the absence of screening. The anxiety and physical trauma that can be associated with the detection of a cancer would not have affected the woman had it not been discovered (some noninvasive cancers and other indolent lesions may never be lethal). There are subtle ancillary costs such as those to society, including the time that a woman may be away from her work or family to be screened, diagnosed, and treated.

Benefits

The principal benefit of screening is the potential to prevent the premature and often prolonged, painful death of the individual. Secondary benefits include a reduction in the trauma of treating earlier stage lesions (less surgery and exposure to chemotherapy), as well as the social benefits revolving around the importance of the individual to her family and the loss of productivity and contributions to society that arise from the premature demise of an individual woman.

There are no simple ways to compare the risks and benefits. They will be perceived differently by different women. Women should be provided with information on both the benefits and the risks so that they can decide for themselves whether to be screened.

Evidence of Benefit Versus Proof

Much of the controversy concerning who should be screened has revolved around the concepts of evidence of benefit versus proof of benefit. Evidence of benefit can come from many sources. The ability to reduce the size and stage of cancers at the time of diagnosis is evidence that there is a benefit from screening. Improved survival from screening represents evidence of a benefit. Proof, on the other hand, must eliminate lead time bias and length bias sampling and can come, therefore, only from RCTs in which two identical groups are compared (see How to Prove Screening Is Efficacious).

Even the demonstration of a reduction in breast cancer deaths among the screened women in an RCT may not be sufficient evidence of benefit because the difference may be due to chance. Most analysts do not accept proof of benefit unless the difference in the number of deaths in the screened group versus the number of control-group deaths in an RCT is statistically significant and, therefore, unlikely to be due to chance.

Statistical Significance

Even the determination of statistical significance is arbitrary because chance is always a factor, and statistical significance is chosen based on probabilities. It is generally accepted that a result is statistically significant if there is a 5% or smaller probability that the result was due to chance. Simply expressed, proof means that the results have a <5% probability of having been due merely to chance and a 95% likelihood that they represent a true relationship. This corresponds to a *p* value of 0.05 or lower in the statistical analysis.

For women aged 40 to 49 the issue of statistical significance has caused much of the disagreement in the screening debate, because evidence was available early in the debate but proof was lacking until the number of deaths grew, with the passage of time, so that the benefit became statistically significant.

Surrogate End Points

Merely showing that women whose cancers are detected earlier live longer is not sufficient to claim a true benefit. This can only be shown conclusively using RCTs in which a large group is randomly divided and one group is offered screening while the other acts as an unscreened control group. These trials are not always feasible because they are very expensive to conduct and there may be ethical and practical reasons why they cannot be performed (denial of intervention to the control group). Furthermore, if women must be followed until death, the results may not be available for many years. In the meantime, new technology may have supervened. Consequently, efforts have been made to identify other measures of benefit that directly correlate with the ultimate measure, which is the reduction of deaths from breast cancer. Analysis of the data from the RCTs of breast cancer screening has identified parameters that correlate well with decreased mortality. These include the size of the cancers, their histologic grade, and whether the axillary lymph nodes are involved or there is distant metastatic disease. These are termed *surrogate end points*. The value of surrogate end points is that they can be measured well before deaths occur. If they are directly predictive of death, then they represent useful measures.

Despite the validation of surrogate end points for breast cancer, however, there are still some researchers who do not accept these measures as being predictive and who insist that benefit can only be determined using RCTs. This has made the demonstration of efficacy more difficult. Nevertheless, the detection of cancers at a smaller size and

earlier stage has been shown to be directly related to prolongation of life (5).

Screening and Public Health

The major screening controversies have been raised as public health issues. Although some people argue to the contrary, most arguments against screening have been based on the costs. Because cost is a contentious issue, much of the recent controversy has revolved around the harms of screening. It is legitimate to ask whether the benefit for the small percentage of women whose lives may be saved by screening is worth the anxiety from false-positive studies and trauma of biopsies for what prove to be benign lesions for the many screened, healthy women who may never develop breast cancer. Furthermore, if screening is to be provided by government or insurance, the economic costs must also be considered.

Unfortunately, the public health issues have clouded the basic scientific and medical questions as to whether screening can lead to a reduction in cancer deaths for the women who participate. Despite the fact that screening has become a public health issue, screening for breast cancer is not primarily a public health concern. It differs from the usual public health problems, such as screening for tuberculosis or vaccination for contagious diseases. These should be public health concerns because the entire society benefits from their implementation. The actual benefit from screening for breast cancer is primarily important to the individual woman who is interested in reducing her risk of dying from breast cancer. It is only access to screening and the allocation of resources (who will pay the costs) that are public health concerns.

Economic and political considerations have influenced the interpretation of the scientific evidence with respect to the screening of women between the ages of 40 and 49. It is the physician's responsibility to determine the medical benefits of screening and the individual woman's right to be informed of the risks so that she can decide whether to avail herself of the potential benefit. These concepts have been frequently forgotten in public health planning, and women and their physicians have not been given all of the facts with respect to screening. Science and medical advice have been compromised in the past by efforts to reduce the cost of health care by insupportable analyses of the available data. This should be avoided in the future. Science and medicine should provide the best advice. Society will decide how to allocate resources.

Determining Efficacy

Survival Versus Mortality

Simply finding cancer earlier does not guarantee its cure. Determining whether there is a benefit from screening is not a trivial problem. It is not simply a matter of demonstrating

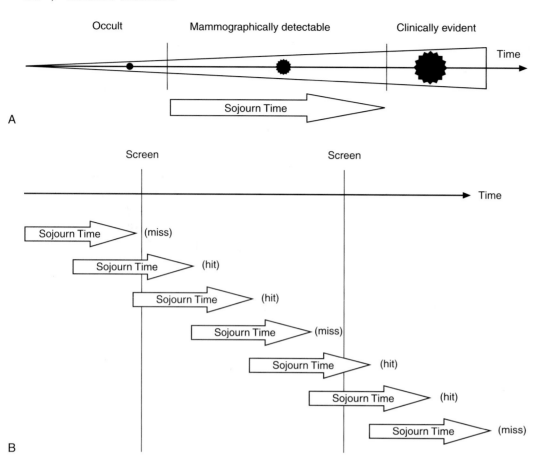

Occult   Mammographically detectable   Clinically evident

Time

Sojourn Time

A

Screen   Screen

Time

Sojourn Time   (miss)

Sojourn Time   (hit)

Sojourn Time   (hit)

Sojourn Time   (miss)

Sojourn Time   (hit)

Sojourn Time   (hit)

Sojourn Time   (miss)

B

FIG. 4-1. (A) The cancer time line. A cancer grows for a period of time during which it is undetectable. It then enters a period in its growth during which it can be detected by mammography but is clinically occult. This has been called the sojourn time. Ultimately it becomes clinically apparent. **(B) If the time between screenings is too long,** only cancers detected by chance during the sojourn period can be treated.

that women whose breast cancers are detected by screening live longer than those whose are not. There are several factors that complicate the issue and several reasons that merely looking at how long women survive with their cancers cannot be used to confidently determine the efficacy of screening.

THE CANCER TIME LINE: SCREENING INTERVAL AND THRESHOLDS FOR INTERVENTION

The success or failure of screening depends completely on the detection of breast cancer at a time when cure, or at least deferred death, is possible. Because metastatic disease is the cause of breast cancer deaths, it is not just a matter of finding cancers but rather finding them before they have successfully spread to other organs. There are conflicting pressures in this endeavor. From a medical perspective, the goal is to find as many cancers, at as early a stage, as possible. From the public health perspective, the goal is to keep the costs as low as possible. The time between screenings is of critical importance, as is the threshold for intervention. To find many cancers at a time when cure is still possible, the time between screens needs to be short and the threshold for intervention needs to be low (aggressive). Because each screen costs money, as does each intervention, the public pressure to save money on health care costs has increased

the recommended time between screenings and seeks to raise the threshold for intervention.

Sojourn Time

During some of its early growth, a breast cancer cannot be detected by any means. It then enters a preclinical period of growth when it can be detected by mammography but is not evident on clinical breast examination (CBE). Finally it becomes large enough to be clinically evident. The time that a cancer is in its preclinical phase, during which it is detectable by mammography but not yet clinically evident, has been termed the *sojourn time* (Fig. 4-1A). If screening is to find cancers earlier than they would otherwise be detected, they must be detected during this period. If the time between screenings is the same as the sojourn time or longer, only cancers that are detected by chance during their sojourn will benefit from early detection (Fig. 4-1B). The way to maximize the detection of early cancers is to make the time between screenings no more than half the sojourn time.

This can be understood by simplifying the situation. Assume that all cancers start at the same time and have the same preclinical sojourn time. If the first screen takes place before they enter the detectable phase and the second occurs after they enter the clinically apparent phase (Fig. 4-1C), it is obvious that the screen will have little value in earlier detection because by the time of the second screen they will have become clinically evi-

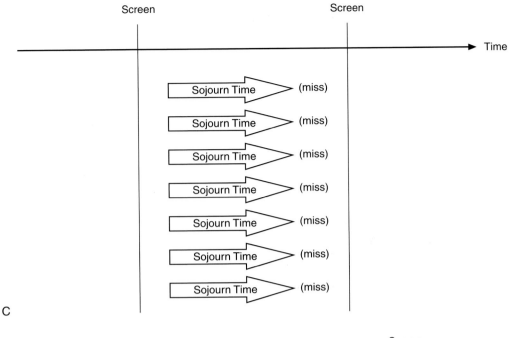

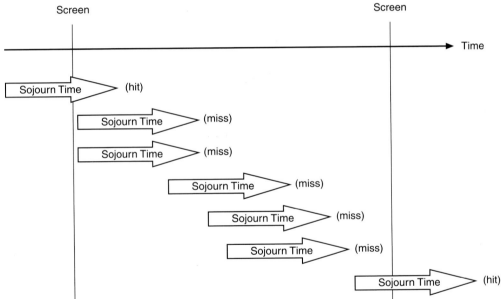

FIG. 4-1. *Continued.* **(C) If the interval between screenings is too long, there will be no benefit.** For example, if the cancers are synchronized and the first screening occurs before the start of the sojourn period and the next screening comes after the period, there will be no benefit from screening. **(D)** Even **if the cancers are not synchronized,** if the screening interval is too long the benefit is reduced.

dent. The only way to detect these synchronized cancers is to screen again before they became clinically evident.

All cancers, however, are not synchronized in their growth. Even if these cancers have the same sojourn times, which they do not, the screens fall at different places during the sojourn period (Fig. 4-1D). Some will be detected earlier by the first screen, but if the time between screens is too long most will reach clinical detectability before the next screen. To maximize the number of cancers detected during the preclinical period, the screening interval must be less than half of the sojourn time (Fig. 4-1E). Even more frequent screening may not benefit all women. If the sojourn time is very short or cancers metastasize during the sojourn

time, it may become impractical to screen with sufficient frequency to detect these cancers earlier. In fact, what is probably more important than the sojourn time is the ability to detect cancers before they successfully metastasize. For some cancers this likely occurs well before they become clinically or even mammographically detectable. This is all the more reason to screen at short intervals.

Importance of Screening Intervals and Thresholds for Intervention

To better understand the importance of screening interval and thresholds for intervention it is useful to think of cancer

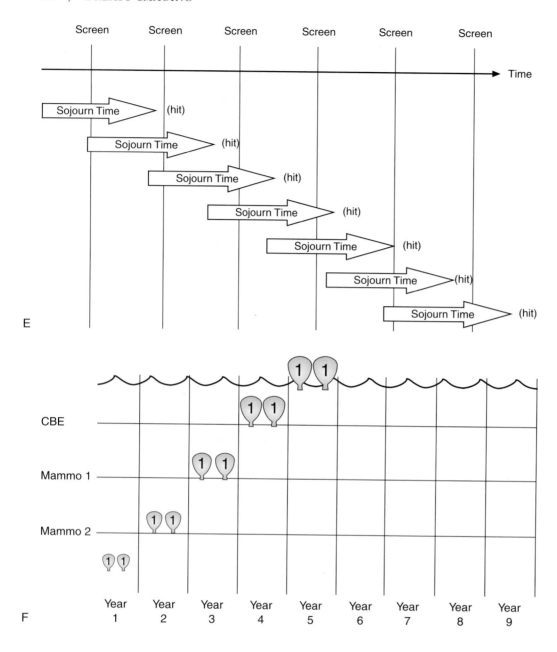

E

F

FIG. 4-1. *Continued.* **(E) The detection of cancers during the sojourn time** is maximized by screening at an interval that is no more than half the sojourn time. **(F)** Cancer is like balloons rising from the depths of the ocean increasing in size with time. (CBE, clinical breast examination.)

as a series of balloons rising from the depths of the ocean, over several years, floating at varying speed toward the surface. As the balloons rise they become larger as the pressure decreases (Fig. 4-1F). After a period of time they reach the surface, while each year new balloons begin to rise (Fig. 4-2). The time at which they reach the surface can be considered the time when the patient discovers her cancer and seeks help.

Cancer screening is similar to having a diver who descends into the water trying to find the balloons earlier, at a smaller size, before they reach the surface. The depth to which the diver can descend is similar to the sensitivity of the screen. Physical examination is like the diver who holds his breath. He can dive down to a certain depth and intercept some of the balloons earlier and at a smaller size.

For some women, this may be lifesaving. Mammography is like a diver with scuba equipment who can dive deeper and find the balloons when they are smaller. The depth to which the diver can dive is analogous to the quality of the mammography. If, for example, concern over dose leads to poor quality mammographic images, some cancers will be missed when they are very small and, as with the balloons, they will be larger by the time they are discovered. No one has yet devised a method of diving even deeper and finding them earlier or preventing them from rising in the first place.

The depth to which the diver can descend is one threshold that will determine the size at which the balloons can be detected. Because the balloons are floating to the surface at some specific rate, a certain number reach the surface each

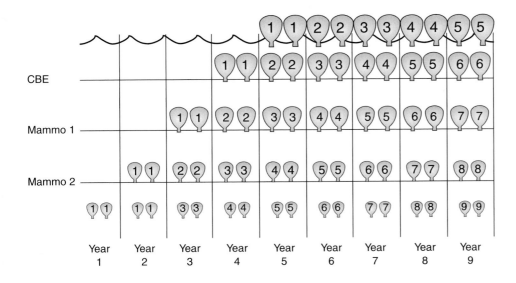

FIG. 4-2. Each year the balloons reach a new level and size while new balloons begin to rise. This is the same as cancers growing with time and new cancers developing each year. (CBE, clinical breast examination.)

Annual screen with aggressive threshold

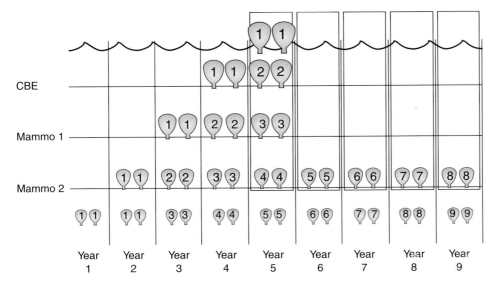

FIG. 4-3. Detection threshold. Assuming that the diver can reach to the third level, Mammo 2, then eight balloons will be found in the first year. If he dives to the same depth again a year later (1-year interval between screenings), he will find two new balloons at level Mammo 2 size, and he will find two new balloons at each successive annual dive. (CBE, clinical breast examination.)

year. This is the same as the incidence rate of cancers diagnosed in the absence of screening.

To further simplify the problem, assume that two balloons reach a new level each year and each year two of the balloons reach the surface before diving commences (see Fig. 4-2). When the dives first begin, the number of balloons that is found is determined by how deep the diver can go and how successful he is at finding the balloons. If we assume that the diver can dive deep enough to reach the third level down, we know that he is able to find eight balloons (Fig. 4-3): He will find the two balloons that reach the surface; he will eliminate two balloons that, had he not dived, would have reached the surface the following year; he will find two balloons that would not have reached the surface for 2 more years; and

he will even find the two that would not surface for another 3 years.

If he dives again the next year, the balloons that would have been found at shallower depths have already been eliminated so he will only find the two balloons that, over the course of the year, have risen from deeper and reached the depth of his dive. The first dive is analogous to the first breast cancer screen, which is called the *prevalence screen* because it finds the cancers that had been building in the population undetected. Each successive screen (dive) that finds the new cancers reaching the threshold of detection is called an *incidence screen*. The time during which the balloons could be found is the sojourn time and the number of years earlier that the balloons (or cancers) can be found by the screen is the lead

Screen every 2 years with aggressive threshold

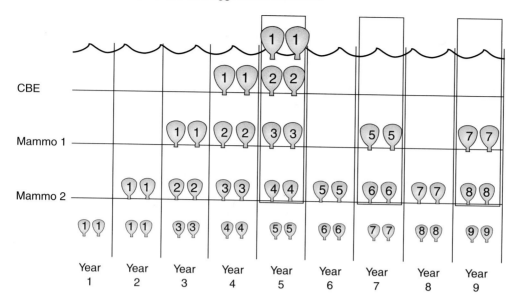

FIG. 4-4. **Increasing the interval between screenings reduces the lead time.** If the diver skips a year but still dives to the same depth, then at the next dive he will find four balloons, but two will be larger than if he had dived every year. Similarly, if there are 2 years between screenings, the cancers detected will likely be more advanced than if screening was annual. (CBE, clinical breast examination.)

time gained by screening. A simplified formula can be used to calculate how much sooner screening finds cancer by subtracting the incidence from the prevalence and dividing by the incidence. In the example of the diver, he was able to find balloons 3 years earlier than if he had waited for them to surface ([8 − 2]/[2 − 3]).

Lead time and the success of screening are influenced by the time between screens and the threshold for detection. If the diver only dived every 2 years (a longer screening interval) (Fig. 4-4), many of the balloons would have reached a larger size than if he dived every year. The lead time would be shorter, and he would find larger balloons (more advanced cancers). Similarly, if he does not dive as deep (he has a higher threshold for intervention), he will only find the larger balloons and his lead time will be shorter (Fig. 4-5). If the time between dives is too long relative to how quickly the balloons are rising, he will reach a point where he may discover many of the balloons just before or at the time they were about to reach the surface. If the time between dives is too long, he will not have added any significant lead time to their detection. He will not be finding them earlier.

One of the problems with screening is that many cancers are morphologically indistinguishable from benign lesions by imaging. Either intervention is aggressive (low threshold) to diagnose these lesions, resulting in many biopsies that result in benign histology (considered by some critics as unnecessary biopsies), or, to avoid the unnecessary biopsies, some cancers that are detected are permitted to pass through the screen (high threshold) because they have similar morphology to benign lesions. For the dive the latter is analogous to having some of the balloons in the shape of fish and trying to avoid catching fish while trying to find the balloons. The diver may fail to see these balloons, or he may let them pass to avoid catching fish. If he wishes to find as many balloons as possible, the diver may have to trap some of the fish as well.

The problem for the diver is additionally complicated in that sometimes the water is clouded and it is difficult to see the balloons, and sometimes it is so murky that it is impossible to see even the large balloons and they float by undetected until they reach the surface. This is analogous to the radiographic density of the breast where some cancers are difficult to see in dense tissue and others are completely hidden and undetectable by mammography.

In summary, the size and success at which the balloons are detected is influenced by how deep the diver can dive (the quality of the mammogram), how often the dives are made (screening interval), how clear the water is (sensitivity of mammography), and how many fish the diver is willing to catch to avoid missing the balloons (thresholds for intervention and specificity of mammography).

The detection rates at the prevalence screen can be compared to the incidence screen to provide a crude indication of lead time and a measure of how well the screening program is doing. In one of the European screening trials, the women are screened every 2 to 3 years, and each time six cancers are detected for every 1,000 women being screened. This means that the program is not advancing the detection of cancers (prevalence − incidence/incidence = [6 − 6]/6 = 0 lead time). They have essentially no lead time and are not advancing the detection of cancers. The screening program is more or less a waste of money and effort.

Screening for breast cancer is identical to the above model. The success of screening is determined by how much earlier the mammography can find cancers that are growing with time, how often women are screened, and how aggres-

Annual screen with less aggressive threshold

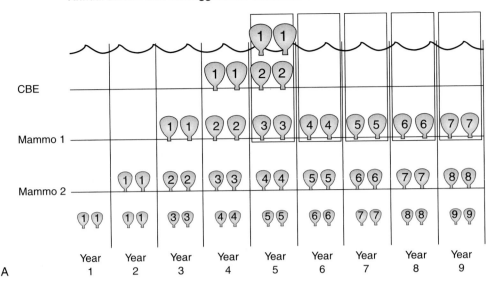

Screen every 2 years with less aggressive threshold

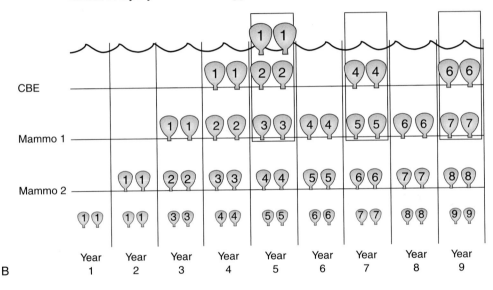

FIG. 4-5. Raising the threshold reduces the ability to detect cancers earlier. (A) If the threshold is raised (the diver does not dive as deep), fewer cancers will be detected at the first screening and those detected at the second screening a year later will be larger than if the threshold were lower. **(B) Raising the threshold and increasing the interval compromises the value of screening.** If the threshold is raised and the time between dives is lengthened, then the balloons (cancers) will be even larger at the time of detection and lead time will have been further reduced. (CBE, clinical breast examination.)

sive the radiologist is in diagnosing indeterminate lesions (the threshold for intervention).

Screening Interval and Cancer Heterogeneity

Breast cancer screening is complex as cancers do not all grow at the same rate. Another model (Fig. 4-6) is useful for understanding how the rate of growth influences the detection of cancer and the benefit from screening. The growth rates of cancers likely follow a bell-shaped, Poisson distribution. This can be simplified by dividing growth rates into three categories. A small percentage of cancers are very fast growing, another small percentage are very slow growing, and the majority are somewhere in between. The x axis of the model represents a time line. Assume that the thick horizontal line is the level of incurability. When a cancer reaches this level, it cannot be cured, and if the patient does not die from some other cause death will occur from the cancer at some later date.

The level of incurability is not the same for all cancers. It is probably determined by the time between the first transformation of a cell into a cancer cell and the development of clones of cells that are capable of successfully metastasizing. For some cancers this may be as early as the second cell if it has developed the necessary changes to become invasive and metastatic. For these cancers, even earlier detection will not save the individual. However, it is clear that for many cancers there is likely a progression from local disease (cancer confined to the breast) to the development of metastatic capability and that during this early phase the natural history can be interrupted and the patient can be cured. For most cancers the level of incurability is directly related to cancer size.

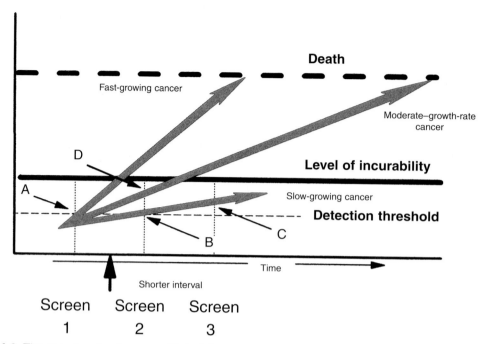

FIG. 4-6. The growth rate of cancers likely follows a bell-shaped, Poisson distribution; however, crudely there are three types of cancer. Some grow very quickly, others have a moderate growth rate, and some grow very slowly. Assume that the thick horizontal line is the level of incurability. When a cancer reaches this level, it has successfully metastasized and the patient cannot be cured. This may be the second cell that has developed the necessary changes to become invasive and metastatic, and even earlier detection will not save the individual. However, it is clear that the natural history of breast cancer can be interrupted, and the level of incurability is usually directly related to cancer size. The thin dotted line represents the detection threshold for mammography. Anything below this line cannot be detected; any cancer above the line is detectable. The vertical dashed lines represent a screening. If slow-growing cancers are evaluated, it can be seen that perhaps at the first screening they are missed because they are just below the detection threshold (*arrow*) **(A)**. They are detectable at the second screening (*arrow*) **(B)**, but even if they are missed again they are detectable at the next screening (*arrow*) **(C)** before they reach a level of incurability. In fact, some of these may never be lethal in the patient's lifetime. The fact that periodic screening is more likely to find slower-growing cancers is called length-biased sampling.

Cancers with moderate growth patterns may not be detected at the first screening (*arrow*) **(A)**, but they can be detected at the next screening (*arrow*) **(D)** before they reach the level of incurability, and it is likely that it is the detection of these cancers that has resulted in the RCTs that demonstrate decreased mortality. Cancers with rapid growth patterns may not be detected at the first screening (*arrow*) **(A)**, and, if the time between screenings is too long (screening interval), they may reach the level of incurability before the next screening. The only way to interrupt faster-growing cancers is to have a lower detection threshold or to screen more frequently (*short vertical arrow*).

The lower, horizontal, interrupted line is the detection threshold for mammography. Anything below this line cannot be detected. Any cancer above the line is detectable. The vertical dashed lines represent screening sessions. If slow-growing cancers are evaluated, it can be seen that at the first screen they may be missed because they are just at the detection threshold. They are detectable at the second screen, but even if they are missed again they are detectable at the next screen before they reach the level of incurability. In fact, some of these may never be lethal in the patient's lifetime.

Cancers with moderate growth patterns may not be detected at the first screening, but they can be detected at the next screening before they reach the level of incurability; it is likely that it is the detection of these cancers that has

resulted in the demonstration of decreased mortality in the breast cancer screening trials.

Cancers with rapid growth patterns may not be detected at the first screening, and, if the screening interval is too long, they may reach the level of lethality before the next screening. The only way to interrupt faster growing cancers is to have a lower detection threshold or to screen more frequently with a shorter interval between screenings.

Length-Biased Sampling

As the model suggests, cancers grow at varying rates and with varying degrees of virulence. Screening is performed at periodic intervals. This time between screenings is one of the factors that influences what types of cancers are diagnosed ear-

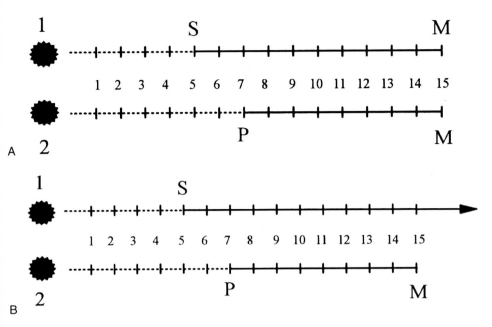

FIG. 4-7. (A) Lead-time bias can be explained by assuming there are two identical women (1 and 2) whose cancers develop at the same time and grow at the same rate. If woman 1 is screened, and her cancer is detected at point S, and woman 2 is not screened, and her cancer is not detected until it is palpable (point P), then woman 1's survival will appear to be 2 years longer than woman 2's. Although she knew about her cancer 2 years earlier than woman 2, woman 1, in this scenario, actually did not benefit because both women still died 15 years after the cancers began. This is lead-time bias. **(B)** Absolute mortality benefit. If, however, woman 1 outlived woman 2 , then there would be a benefit from screening. RCTs simulate twins by having identical populations created by the process of randomization. In RCTs, the same number of women should die each year from breast cancer. If the screened group has fewer deaths, then screening is effective because lead-time bias is avoided.

lier. Fast-growing cancers may be undetectable at one screening and grow to clinical detectability before the next screening. Periodic screening has a greater likelihood of finding slower growing cancers than rapidly growing cancers, particularly if the time between screenings is long. If only women whose cancers are detected by screening are evaluated and their cancers are slow growing, they may appear to benefit; but the conclusion is biased by the phenomenon of length-biased sampling.

Length-biased sampling suggests that women whose cancers are detected by screening frequently have more indolent disease because these are the cancers that are more easily detected. There is likely some validity to this, but there are also data that suggest that earlier detection finds cancers before a more virulent clone can develop and overgrow the other cells. If, however, screening merely selects women with nonlethal cancers, then the observation that their survival is better than women who are not screened may merely reflect this phenomenon. Length-biased sampling is one reason that evaluating the survival of women whose cancers are detected by screening and comparing them to others or to historical controls can be misleading.

Lead-Time Bias

Survival statistics (how long an individual survives with the cancer) are the most commonly used measures in cancer evaluation, but they may not provide a clear picture of the benefit of screening. Survival is a measure of the length of time between the detection of the cancer and death due to metastatic disease. By detecting a cancer earlier, survival may appear to be longer. However, this may merely be due to the fact that an individual is known to have cancer earlier in the course of the disease. The date of death may not actually be deferred, and an apparent benefit may not be real. Benefit is only real if the date of death is deferred.

This concept can be understood using the following hypothetical situation: Assume that two identical women develop identical breast cancers at exactly the same time and that the cancers will grow at the same rate. If untreated, the cancers will affect both women equally, leading to death 15 years after the tumors begin to grow (Fig. 4-7A). If one of the women were to take advantage of screening and have her cancer detected 5 years after it began growing and if she lived another 10 years, her survival from the time of diagnosis would be 10 years.

If the second woman was not screened, but waited until her malignancy grew large enough to become palpable, she might have her cancer diagnosed 7 years after it began to grow. If she were to live another 8 years before succumbing to the cancer her survival, from the time of diagnosis to the time of death, would be 8 years.

The date that a cancer begins to grow can never be determined. The only measurement that is available is the time between diagnosis and death (survival time). In the preceding example the first woman survived 10 years from diagnosis while the second woman survived only 8 years. Superficially, it would appear that the screened woman benefited from early detection, because her survival was longer. Survival analysis, however, is misleading because both women actually died 15 years after the cancer began. Their absolute mortality was actually unaffected, with no true benefit for the screened woman from screening. The apparent benefit for the first woman is due to lead-time bias. The cancer was discovered earlier in its inexorable course, and it was consequently known about for a longer period of time, but the time of death in this scenario was not altered.

Using the preceding example, a true benefit could have been established if the screened woman had actually outlived the unscreened woman (Fig. 4-7B). The unscreened woman would essentially provide a measure of the natural history of the cancer. As noted in the first scenario, if both women died at the same time (the time of diagnosis is irrelevant), regardless of the fact that one was screened, then screening would have had no benefit. If, on the other hand, the screened woman outlived the unscreened woman then, because they had both been destined to die at the same time, her deferred mortality would represent an absolute benefit from screening that was independent of lead time or any other confounding variable. Delayed mortality is proof that earlier diagnosis actually delayed her death and that there was a benefit from screening. Mortality reduction (actually delaying death), and not survival analysis, is the only accurate proof that screening is efficacious.

HOW TO PROVE SCREENING IS EFFICACIOUS

Because there is no way to identify the date that a cancer actually begins to grow, deferring death, measured as mortality reduction, is the best way to determine whether there is a true benefit from screening. The model of identical women, described above, does not exist in life. It can, however, be simulated by using the laws of probability and the structure of an RCT. By randomly dividing large populations of women and assigning one group to be screened and the other to remain as an unscreened comparison group (controls), mortality can be the end point, just as with the women in the example. If there are sufficient numbers of women involved in the study, random assignment will provide two groups that are demographically identical. The groups will be identical in all of their characteristics, such as the age distribution of the participants, their marital status, and parity. If left alone, both groups would have the same number of women develop breast cancer each year, and the same number of women would die each year from breast cancer. In effect, each woman in the screened group would have a twin in the control group. If, after screening, fewer women in the screened group die each year (because the twin in the screened group had her cancer detected before it had successfully metastasized), then an absolute benefit can be determined. Because the RCT only compares deaths each year from breast cancer and is not interested in survival, it eliminates the biases inherent in other types of analysis, including length-biased sampling and lead-time bias.

Random assignment is critical to these trials because biases can be introduced if women are selected and purposely placed in one arm of the trial or the other (selection bias). An example of obvious selection bias would come if women with palpable axillary lymph nodes were allowed to participate and were primarily assigned to one of the groups. Because these women are more likely to have advanced cancers (lymph node positive) and women with advanced cancers are more likely to die than those with lymph node negative cancers, this selection would bias the trial against the side that was given the women with the palpable nodes. This actually happened in the National Breast Screening Study of Canada (NBSS), in which more women with positive axillary lymph nodes and more women with four or more positive lymph nodes (an even worse prognosis) at the time of the NBSS nonblinded randomization were allocated to the screened group (6).

If, in an RCT, the screened women have fewer deaths per year than the unscreened control group and that difference is statistically significant (unlikely to be due to chance), then the efficacy of screening can be validated. Unless another test has a one-to-one correlation with death, most agree that the RCT, with death as the end point, is the only way that an intervention, such as screening for breast cancer, can be validated. The RCT eliminates the effects of lead-time bias and length-biased sampling. As noted earlier, some surrogate end points, such as size and stage, do appear to have a direct correlation with mortality, but these have not yet been universally accepted.

Measuring Benefit

Mortality from Breast Cancer Versus Overall Mortality from All Causes

For a benefit to be demonstrated, the control group must have women die from breast cancer while their counterparts in the screened group do not die. The effectiveness of screening is usually measured by a reduction in breast cancer deaths. Some have argued that overall mortality should be measured to see how screening affects the entire population (7). Wright and Mueller, for example, argued that, because breast cancer accounts for only 3% of all the deaths among all women each year, a 30% mortality reduction will only reduce the total deaths by 1% (8) and that screening is not worth the cost. Virtually all medical interventions can be trivialized in this fashion. Measuring mortality from all causes results in a significant dilution of the effect of screening because most women die from causes other than breast cancer. Because all eventually die and most causes of death are not preventable, a reduction in deaths from breast cancer will have little impact for the entire population but a significant impact on those whose lives are extended. To demonstrate the ability to reduce mortality from breast cancer, death from breast cancer is the appropriate measure.

Principles and Problems with Randomized, Controlled Trials

RCTs are the best method for demonstrating the efficacy of an intervention. However, the mere fact that a trial is randomized with a control group does not guarantee that its results are valid. If the trial is not properly designed and performed, its results can be misleading. RCTs can themselves be biased by faulty randomization and flawed execution. The results of the trial may apply only to the women who participated and may not relate to the general population (see Generalizability), depending on the characteristics of the population in the study.

The RCT derives its validity from the statistical power inherent in its study design and the number of participants (sample size). Because a reduction in death from breast cancer is the desired benefit, statistical proof of benefit requires that there must be enough women in the study that there will be sufficient numbers of women with cancer, and, more important, sufficient numbers of cancer deaths (called *events*) that, if there is a reduction in deaths among the screened women, the benefit (difference between the number of deaths in the screened group relative to the control subjects), will be statistically significant. If there are insufficient numbers of women in the trials or an insufficient number of events, positive results may not reach statistical validity and a true benefit may be discounted.

Some other factors that may influence an RCT include the characteristics of the population under study (age and other risk factors), how frequently the participants are screened relative to the lead time of the test (how much earlier the test can find the cancer than the care to which it is being compared), the technical quality of the screening procedure and its ability to detect breast cancer earlier, and the thresholds for intervention (see Thresholds for Intervention).

Sample Size Required to Prove a Benefit

Statistical Power

As with any intervention that does not cure every participant, the result of screening must be measured against an alternative. Most trials measure the benefit of screening versus no screening whereas some, such as the NBSS, compared mammographic screening to a single physical examination among women between the ages of 40 and 49 and to annual physical examination for women from the ages of 50 to 59. The results are compared using statistical measures (rejection of the null hypothesis) and produce a probability estimate that determines the likelihood that the results are due to chance (*P* value). The ability of a trial to provide statistically significant results is its statistical power. Because proof of benefit is measured statistically (i.e., that the benefit is statistically significant), a trial must be carefully designed so that it is large enough and properly performed so that its results are scientifically valid, and, if there is a benefit, there are sufficient numbers so that the benefit is statistically significant. As in a political poll, if there are not enough participants the results can be misleading.

To have the statistical power to demonstrate a difference between the screens and controls of a predetermined amount (e.g., a 20% improvement) the numbers of women involved in the study must be sufficient to ensure the necessary numbers of cancers, and, more important, the necessary numbers of cancer deaths so that a difference can be tested and the results will have statistical significance. The usual measure of statistical validity is that the differences between the two have a <5% probability that they are due to chance (*P* <0.05). Because the laws of probability do not permit absolutes, most studies are designed to provide an 80% chance of demonstrating the expected benefit at the 5% level of certainty. The size of the trial is influenced by the degree of certainty that is needed to accept a benefit (statistical significance). The greater the degree of certainty that is required, the larger the trial must be for any given level of benefit. A decision that requires 95% certainty needs a larger trial than one in which 90% certainty is acceptable.

The size of a trial is also influenced by the true benefit from screening. If screening were able to reduce deaths by 50%, fewer women would need to participate than would be needed to show a benefit of 25%. If insufficient numbers of women are included in a study for the amount of true benefit, the study may not reach statistical validity despite a true benefit.

The Power Calculation

Investigators use standard algorithms to estimate how large a population of women is needed to prove a benefit. This is the power calculation, and it is based on

1. The expected number of cancers that will develop in the population over the course of the trial (the prior probability of cancer in the population being studied)
2. The rate of death from breast cancer that is to be expected among these women (death rate)
3. The amount of benefit anticipated (mortality reduction)
4. The time by which that benefit is expected
5. The degree of certainty needed to accept a benefit (statistical significance)

Any alteration in these factors that involves fewer participants or fewer events can reduce the ability of the trial to have the statistical power to prove a benefit. For example, the fewer the number of deaths among control women, the more difficult it is to prove a benefit (if women do not die of breast cancer, then there is no room for a benefit from screening).

RCTs must be carefully designed to ensure that all of these factors are taken into consideration. Variations alter the statistical ability (power) to prove a benefit. Because these trials are very expensive to run, investigators try to reduce the population size as much as possible to keep down costs. This diminishes the power of the trial.

Insufficient numbers of participants, however, is one of the major weaknesses in the RCTs that have been performed. Most of the trials have had marginal power to prove a benefit from screening, and that power has been further compromised by breaking the data into even smaller numbers by retrospective subgroup analysis by age. If the number of women in the trial is too small, then the results can be misleading (9):

> if the statistical test fails to reach significance, the power of the test becomes a critical factor in reaching an inference. It is not widely appreciated that the failure to achieve statistical significance may often be related more to the low power of the trial than to an actual lack of difference between the competing therapies. Clinical trials with inadequate sample size are thus doomed to failure before they begin and serve only to confuse the issue of determining the most effective therapy for a given condition.

The controversy over screening younger women was due to the fact that some analysts ignored this basic warning and analyzed subgroups of the data from trials that had insufficient numbers of participants to permit statistically valid analyses. Inappropriate data analysis was the main reason for the screening controversy and the 1993 decision by the National Cancer Institute (NCI) to deny screening to women in their 40s.

Longer Follow-Up May Not Compensate for Inadequate Sample Size

To a certain extent, following the population for a longer period of time (woman years) may compensate for an inadequate sample size, but increasing the number of years of follow-up by increasing the length of follow-up for each woman is not as effective as increasing the total by increasing the number of women enrolled. For example, the benefit of screening is higher for 10,000 women screened each year for 5 years and followed for 5 years than for 5,000 women screened for 5 years and followed for 10 years. The first group will have had 50,000 woman years of screening, whereas the second will have had only 25,000 woman years of screening. The main advantage of longer follow-up is to permit deaths from moderate-growth tumors to occur in the control group to demonstrate the benefit for the screened group.

Selecting Populations for Study

Theoretically the main requirement for an RCT is that it compare two groups of women who are representative of the population and are apparently free of obvious cancer. If the group is divided by random assignment of individuals, the resulting test group and control group should be identical. If the numbers are large enough and allocations are truly random, then each woman in the screened group should have an identical counterpart in the control group. The same number of cancers should develop in both groups with the same number of cancer deaths expected each year in both groups. The only difference between the groups should be that one is screened and the other is not.

There are important ways that the results of an RCT, however, can be compromised, beginning with the choice of participants. Epidemiologists have clearly stated that screening trials should not include women with clinical symptoms of breast cancer (10). Because their fate is likely determined prior to their entry into the trial, women with advanced breast cancer (node-positive, incurable cancer) before the start of a trial are unlikely to benefit from screening. Furthermore, cancers that are advanced at the outset will dominate the early mortality statistics and can obscure any early benefit.

One of the major trials, the NBSS, permitted and actively encouraged women with clinical symptoms and palpable, lymph-node–positive cancers to participate in the trial. The investigators argued that they needed to include these women so that they would have sufficient numbers of women with cancer in the trial to meet their power requirement (see National Breast Screening Study). In fact, including women with clinically evident cancers increases the overall power of the trial by including more cancers and events (deaths), but it also diminishes the ability to measure the screening benefit because these women cannot be helped by screening. Using the same rationale, reduced to the absurd, the power of a trial could be increased by including women who had already died of breast cancer. This would increase the number of women with breast cancer and the number of deaths and the statistical power, but would obviously reduce any benefit from screening.

At best, inclusion of these women, if they are equally allocated to the screen and the control groups, dilutes the results. If there is not an equal distribution of advanced cancers, as occurred in the NBSS, for which screening is, *a priori,* ineffective, then the trial may be compromised and its results cast in doubt by the overweighting of inevitable deaths in the group with the excess of these cancers.

Generalizability

Screening trials must be designed with great care as errors in design can produce misleading results. Ideally, a screening trial should involve women from the same population that is expected to participate if screening is shown to be beneficial. If the population studied is not representative of the general population, then the results of the trial may not apply to the general population (generalizability). For example, women who volunteer for trials usually have a different likelihood of disease (prior probability), and, because they may have a different level of health than the average woman, they may have a different course with the same disease. The results of a trial in which women select themselves for participation by volunteering may not apply, for example, to a population of women who are referred for screening by their doctor.

The NBSS solicited volunteers to participate in the study. These women were then randomized into two groups, a screened group and a control group that was not offered mammography. Asking women to volunteer ensured that there would be a high level of compliance, but it meant that the results of the trial could only be applied to women who volunteer. This seems superficially to be a trivial point, but there are clear biases that result from studying volunteers and not the general population.

The fact that very few minority women have been included in the trials is a problem. The death rate from breast cancer for black women, particularly those younger than 40, is much higher than for white women. There are no data to determine whether these women can be helped by screening. Even older minority women may benefit more or less from screening. There are no trial data to evaluate these populations.

Trials by Invitation

The seven non-Canadian RCTs were actually not truly trials of screening, but rather of the invitation to be screened. They were population based. They targeted general population groups, randomly divided them, and then invited those allocated to the screened group in for screening. This is the proper way to allocate participants in a study. This approach more likely reflects what would occur in a general screening of the population. This screening by invitation, however, suffers from the fact that women may choose not to participate in the program. To avoid introducing selection biases, however, they must still be counted as participating. In fact, many women who are invited to be screened refuse (noncompliance). In addition, there are women allocated to the control group who undergo screening on their own, outside of the trial. Even if their lives are saved by this screening, they are still counted as unscreened controls and serve to contaminate the control group. Noncompliance and contamination cause a loss of statistical power (see Noncompliance and Contamination), and the trial must compensate for noncompliance by involving more women or be weakened by the loss of statistical power that results.

Treatment Bias

Another potential problem with the RCTs of screening is that it is difficult to determine whether women in the control group who were diagnosed with breast cancer were treated in the same way as women in the screened group. The investigators in the NBSS, in an effort to explain an excess of women with lymph-node–positive breast cancer in the screened group, revealed that the control women, cared for in community hospitals, had fewer

and less extensive axillary dissections than the screened women. If it is the case that there were treatment differences between the screened women and the control group, then it introduces a major new bias into the analysis of that trial's data.

Factors That Affect the Power and Design of Randomized, Controlled Trials

Noncompliance and Contamination

Not only have the trials not involved sufficient numbers of women, but their power has been further compromised by noncompliance and contamination. In by-invitation screening trials, some women who are invited to be screened refuse. These women are termed *noncompliers* (a woman cannot be forced to be screened). There are other women who are supposed to be unscreened controls who obtain mammograms on their own outside the study, causing contamination of the control group. Because these women are still counted with the group to which they were allocated, noncompliance and contamination dilute the effects of screening. Nevertheless, to avoid selection biases, noncompliers who die of breast cancer are still counted as having been screened, and women whose lives are saved by having their cancers detected by screening outside the trial are still counted as unscreened controls. Screening cannot affect those who are not screened, and if control women are screened, the trial merely compares screened women to screened women.

If the statistical power of the trial is to be maintained, these dilutional factors must be taken into account in designing a trial. The only way to compensate for dilution from noncompliance and contamination is to increase the number of women in the trial. The formula for increasing the number of women in the trial is the planned sample size × (1/[1 − rate of contamination − rate of noncompliance]^2). For example, if 25% of the women in the control group are expected to have mammograms on their own as contamination of the unscreened controls, the number of women needed in the trial, as originally estimated in the power calculation, must be increased by the factor 1/(1 − 0.25)^2 = 1.78. Thus, if 25% of the control women cross over and have mammograms in a trial in which 50,000 women are needed to prove a specific, anticipated benefit, the number of women in the trial must be increased by 78% to 89,000 women to retain the same power to prove a benefit. The number would have to increase to 200,000 women if, in addition, 25% of the women offered screening refused to be screened.

Despite the fact that RCTs are the only accepted method to objectively determine the efficacy of screening and have the imprimatur of science to give them validity, their results must be evaluated with a careful understanding of how they were designed and how they were executed. Significant biases have entered into these trials.

Noncompliance and contamination were significant problems in the European trials, as was noncompliance in the Health Insurance Plan (HIP) of New York trial. For example, in the HIP study only 21,000 of the 31,000 women counted as screened were actually screened. Nevertheless, all are counted as being in the screened group to avoid any biases that might occur by patient's self-selection. This dilutes the effect of the screen because, as in the Ostergotland trial in Sweden, nonattenders frequently have a higher mortality and, consequently, decrease the overall benefit from screening for the population. In the Two County trial it has been estimated that the 30% reduction in mortality for the entire screened group was actually a 40% or more reduction if only women who are actually screened are analyzed. In the Ostergotland trial, if the nonattenders are not included, the screen would have resulted in a mortality reduction rather than the lack of benefit that has been seen as a result of the deaths among women who refused screening but were still counted as having been screened.

In the Canadian trial, women were first invited to participate and were then randomized. This reduces the number of noncompliers, but, because women who volunteer for programs tend to be more health conscious and are often healthier, the results from this type of trial may not be applicable to the general population. (Other problems with the Canadian trial are discussed later in this chapter.)

There is nothing to prevent a woman assigned to a control group from obtaining a mammogram on her own, outside of the trial. This was a significant problem in the Malmö trial, in which 25% of the women who were supposed to act as controls obtained mammograms outside the screen. Among women between the ages of 45 and 54, 35% of the control women had mammography. Overall 20% of the cancers detected in the control group were detected by mammography. This obviously has a dilutional effect and significantly reduces the power to detect a benefit from a trial that is already compromised with a relatively small number of women.

The method of randomization is important. Some of the trials were randomized based on individuals. Others were randomized based on geographic location. The results of the Edinburgh trial, for example, are potentially biased as randomization was based on physician practices and there are differences in the socioeconomic status of the participants. In addition, the quality of the mammography in that trial has been considered poor.

Follow-Up

Because the actual screening in the trials is performed for a finite time, the participants must also be followed for a long enough period to permit a benefit to appear. Because breast cancers do not kill immediately and a benefit for screened women can only accrue if women in the control group die, the participants must be followed until the control women die. This may take a decade or more. For example, if ductal carcinoma is found in a screened woman, it may take 10 to 15 years for her counterpart in the control group to develop an invasive lesion and for that lesion to metastasize and be lethal. One of the problems with the trials is that the results have been analyzed too soon after the start of screening.

The length of time that the women must be followed is determined by the time period in which the benefit is expected. If, as is true for women in their 40s, the 5-year survival from breast cancers diagnosed without screening is high (11), then the women must be followed long enough for the controls to die of breast cancer so that the benefit for the screens become evident. This also influences the size of the trial. If investigators are seeking a demonstration of an early benefit, then they must screen appropriately (short interval and low threshold for intervention) and have a large number of women with rapidly growing cancers that will be lethal soon after the start of the trial. Because, for younger women, only a small number of women in the control group die rapidly from their cancers, a trial must be very large to demonstrate an early benefit. It is more likely that screening will benefit women with moderately fast-growing cancers. Because the survival for these women is also better than for older women, longer follow-up is necessary to permit the accumulation of sufficient numbers of deaths so that the benefit can be demonstrated with statistical significance.

Other Factors That Influence Randomized, Controlled Trials

Many other factors influence an RCT, including the characteristics of the population under study. If the study is designed based on an expectation that there will be a certain number of cancers developing over time and a commensurate number of deaths and the population proves to be healthier, with fewer cancers and deaths, then the trial may provide misleading results. The frequency of the screening also affects the results. If, for example, mammography can detect cancers, on average, 2 years before they would ordinarily be found, then screening every 2 years will not result in earlier detection, and there will be little or no benefit.

The technical quality of the screening and the threshold for intervention also influence the benefit. If the mammograms are of suboptimal quality for the detection of small cancers or if the radiologists decide that they must have a high percentage of biopsies where the diagnosis of cancer is made, then they, a priori, must permit small cancers to pass through the screen (12). If only single-view mammography is used then cancers will be missed (see Problems with the Other Trials).

If the detection threshold is set too high and results in little or no reduction in the size and stage of the cancers at diagnosis, then there will be no benefit from the screen (13).

Benefit Is Measured Against Death Rate Among Control Women

The survival of the unscreened control group is an important factor that has been overlooked in the analyses of the screening trials. If the background stage (control group) at which breast cancers are detected is late (more advanced cancers), then a benefit is easier to demonstrate because the prognosis for the control group is poor. This is likely the reason that the HIP study, performed in the 1960s, was successful with relatively few participants. The control women, who had only their usual health care, often presented with late stage cancer, making it easier for the screening to find cancers at an earlier stage and alter the death rate among the screened women. As health care has improved and the background stage at detection of breast cancer has improved (earlier cancers, lower stages), it becomes more difficult to lower the number of advanced stages in a screening program. Stated simply, if women do not die in the control group, there will be little benefit from screening.

Early Detection Versus Excluding the Presence of Cancer

Because screening does not detect all cancers and does not detect all cancers sufficiently early to permit cure, screening should not be thought of as a method to exclude cancer. Screening is purely a chance to detect some cancers earlier in their development at a time when intervention may be able to alter the course of the disease. Despite the fact that screening does not detect all cancers, many breast cancers can be found at an earlier stage and a significant number of women can derive life-saving benefit from the earlier detection. Along with the positive benefits of screening, however, it should be understood that, given the present state of the art, screening does not detect all cancers or save all women, and *there is still no test or combination of tests that can guarantee that a woman does not have breast cancer*. Screening is not the solution to the breast cancer problem, but until a universal cure is developed or methods of prevention are discovered, screening using mammography can save many lives. Investigation should be supported to improve on the success of mammography.

EARLY EVIDENCE OF THE BENEFITS OF SCREENING

Health Insurance Plan of New York Trial

In the early 1960s, the first RCT of screening was initiated in a health insurance program in New York. The investigators wished to determine whether screening asymptomatic women for breast cancer using CBE and mammography could lower the death rate. The HIP trial involved 62,000 women between the ages of 40 and 64 who were enrolled in the insurance plan. They were randomly divided into a screened group that was offered a CBE and mammogram every year and an equal number of women who were allocated to the control group. The study group women were then offered a screening mammogram and a physical examination each year for 4 years. The women allocated to the control group were not even informed of the study and received their usual medical care when a problem arose.

Only 65% of the women offered screening actually accepted the offer and were screened at least once. Among this group, 88% attended at least two screening sessions. As noted earlier, to avoid biasing the results, once a woman is allocated to one group or the other, she is counted as having had the intervention or as acting as an unscreened control. This is to avoid selection bias, where women who attend screening may have more favorable cancers. Thus, in the HIP trial, as well as the other RCTs, the 35% of patients who were randomized to the screened group but refused screening are included in subsequent analyses as part of the screened group, diluting the effect of the screen.

By comparing the subsequent number of deaths among the screened women with those in the control group, the investigators demonstrated that early detection could decrease the mortality from breast cancer (14).

The population size was estimated to have a 50% chance of being able to demonstrate a 20% benefit (reduction in breast cancer deaths) from screening with statistical significance should such a benefit for the screened women occur. As with most of the RCTs undertaken since HIP, this trial was designed to look for a benefit for screening women beginning at age 40. It was not designed, as has been done retrospectively, to segregate the population into those 40 to 49 years of age and those 50 and over. It was retrospective stratification that created the controversy surrounding screening.

The evaluation of the HIP populations demonstrated a mortality reduction for the screened women that began to appear approximately 3 to 5 years after the first screen (15). The data have been published with 18-year results. By that time, 163 women in the control group had died from breast cancer compared to 126 in the screened group. This 23% reduction in mortality for the screened population was statistically significant (16). Because the trial was randomized with controls, the benefit was not merely a debatable survival difference, but a true absolute mortality reduction. The HIP was the first study to show a true benefit from screening for breast cancer.

Unfortunately, it has not been possible to determine the relative contributions of mammography and physical examination to this mortality reduction. It has been estimated that 19% of the cancers detected by screening were detected by mammography alone. Furthermore, in the more modern screening trials, types of cancer in the populations shifted. There were many more advanced cancers in the HIP control groups than are now found in unscreened women in the United States. The question remained as to whether further reductions in breast cancer deaths could be accomplished by screening. In an effort to determine the benefit of mammography alone, and because mammography is more easily standardized than CBE, many of the subsequent European trials used only mammography for screening.

The benefits demonstrated in the HIP trial led to the Breast Cancer Detection Demonstration Project (BCDDP) and to the other trials of screening, the latter to corroborate the results and the former to determine if screening very large populations was feasible. The decision by the principal investigator in the HIP trial, Professor Shapiro, to analyze the data by age groups, and his conclusion that there was no benefit from screening women between the ages of 40 and 49 was the origin of the debate over the age at which screening should begin.

Breast Cancer Detection Demonstration Project

It was felt that the HIP had validated the efficacy of screening and that all that remained was to establish that large numbers of women could be screened efficiently. Consequently, the NCI, in conjunction with the American Cancer Society (ACS), undertook the world's largest screening program as a demonstration project to show that population-based screening could be performed in this country. The BCDDP, undertaken in the 1970s, evaluated >280,000 self-selected women. The program permitted any woman 35 (later raised to 40) and over to participate. The volunteers underwent physical examination and mammography in at least one of five annual screens in 29 centers across the country.

Because the study was not an RCT, the results cannot be used to prove conclusively the efficacy of screening, but important information can be deduced from the results. The BCDDP clearly demonstrated the ability of x-ray mammography to detect small, early-stage cancers (4). During the period of screening, 4,485 cancers occurred in 4,257 women within this population. The screen detected 3,557 of these cancers.

Before discussing the positive results of the project, it is important to note that >800 of the cancers that occurred were not detected by screening but appeared as interval cancers (19%). These were cancers that were diagnosed clinically within 1 year after a woman had undergone a negative screening physical examination and mammogram, but before her next screening evaluation, or within 1 year of the completion of her last screen. Given an average doubling time for breast cancer of 100 to 180 days, it is likely that these cancers were present at the time of screening but were undetected by the screen. Thus, in the BCDDP, approximately 20% of cancers were not detectable earlier by a combination of CBE and mammog-

raphy, demonstrating that even a combined screen using physical examination and mammography does not detect all breast cancers.

Benefits from Screening

The importance of mammography was demonstrated by the BCDDP. Of the cancers found at screening, >90% were detected by mammography. The ability of mammography to detect early-stage breast cancers before they become large enough to palpate was also corroborated in the BCDDP. Almost 42% of the cancers detected in the BCDDP were clinically occult and detected only by mammography.

Noninvasive intraductal carcinoma (DCIS) and invasive cancers ≤1 cm in size are favorable early-stage lesions. The presence of cancer in the axillary lymph nodes suggests a worsened prognosis. In the BCDDP, only 14% of women with small tumors (1 cm or smaller) showed evidence of axillary node involvement at diagnosis, whereas 29% of women with larger lesions had positive nodes. More than 50% of the earlier lesions were detected only by mammography, demonstrating the ability of mammography to detect breast cancer earlier in its growth.

The lack of a control group makes it difficult to use BCDDP data to directly support the benefits of screening, but the ability of mammography to detect earlier-stage, nonpalpable, clinically occult cancers was clearly demonstrated. A comparison of the mortality experience of the BCDDP population with populations monitored in the Surveillance Epidemiology and End Results program (SEER) has confirmed a survival benefit for women at all the ages studied. There was a 20-year survival among women whose cancers were diagnosed during the BCDDP of 76%. This is compared to the background survival in the SEER program of only 57% (17). The fact that survivals were the same regardless of age and that there was clear evidence of mortality reduction in the RCTs that was directly linked to survival provides inferential information that screening can benefit women regardless of age.

RANDOMIZED, CONTROLLED TRIALS OF BREAST CANCER SCREENING

Nine RCTs have been performed in Europe, Canada, and the United States since the 1960s. In these trials, women were randomly divided into two groups, one that was offered screening and the other that served as an unscreened control group. These studies have shown that there were fewer breast cancer deaths among the screened women than the controls. By demonstrating a statistically significant, absolute reduction in mortality for the screened women, the trials have shown that screening on a periodic basis can reduce breast cancer deaths. If the trials are analyzed as they were designed, this benefit has been clearly demonstrated for women who begin screening by the age of 40 (18,19).

TABLE 4-1. *The randomized, controlled trials*

Trial	Ages (yr)	Interval (mo)	Protocol	Follow-up (yr)	Invited (no.)	Controls (no.)
Health Insurance Plan	40–64	12	2-view mammogram + CBE	18	30,131	30,585
Malmö	45–69	18–24	1- or 2-view mammogram	12	20,695	20,783
Kopparberg	40–74	24–33	1-view mammogram	12	38,562	18,478
Ostergotland	40–74	24–33	1-view mammography	12	38,405	37,145
Edinburgh	45–64	24	1- or 2-view mammography alternating with CBE	10	23,226	21,904
Stockholm	40–64	28	1-view mammography	8	38,525	20,651
Gothenburg	40–59	18	2-view mammography	10	20,724	28,809
NBSS 1 (Canada)	40–49	12	2-view mammography + CBE vs. previous CBE	7	25,214	25,216
NBSS 2 (Canada)	50–59	12	2-view mammography + CBE vs. CBE	7	19,711	19,694

CBE, clinical breast examination; NBSS, National Breast Screening Study.

The basic design and results of these trials are summarized in Table 4-1.

Health Insurance Plan of New York Trial

The first RCT of screening and the prototype for subsequent trials was the HIP, which was undertaken in the 1960s. Subsequent to the HIP there have been eight additional RCTs of breast cancer screening.

Swedish Trials

After the HIP, several large-scale RCTs were undertaken in Sweden. The Swedish trials were all designed to evaluate the value of mammography alone. None incorporated CBE into their protocols (20). In an effort to reduce radiation exposure and to keep the cost of screening down, three of the five trials used only single-view, mediolateral oblique mammography.

Two County Trial (Kopparberg and Ostergotland)

The first two of the Swedish studies were designed together. Although they are actually two different trials, their data have been reported together and they are known as the Two County Trial. Women from Kopparberg and Ostergotland counties were assigned by the communities in which they lived (clusters) to be offered mammography screening or to act as unscreened controls. The randomization was by community.

In the two counties a total population of 162,981 women between the ages of 40 and 74 were available for randomization. The data concerning 134,867 women aged 40 to 74 were analyzed. The preliminary results of the Two County Trial mirrored the HIP mortality benefit by demonstrating a 30% reduction in mortality for the screened population relative to the unscreened control group—a benefit derived completely from mammographic screening (21).

Kopparberg

The Kopparberg trial began in 1977. There were 38,562 women from age 40 to 74 who were randomly assigned to the screened group, and 18,478 who were allocated to the control group. Mammography was offered to the screened women who were between the ages of 40 and 49 every 2 years and to women between the ages of 50 and 74 every 33 months. Among the women offered screening, 89% complied for at least the first screen. Single-view mammography was used.

Ostergotland

The Ostergotland trial began in 1978 as the companion trial to Kopparberg. The trial design was similar, with women ages 40 to 74 randomized by community clusters. There were 38,405 women who were offered screening, and 37,145 who were chosen to act as unscreened controls. Single-view mammography was offered every 2 years for women ages 40 to 49 and every 33 months for women ages 50 to 74, and there was 89% compliance with the first screening invitation.

It is important to recognize that in the Two County Trial women 40 to 49 years of age were screened every 2 years, and those over 50 were screened at an interval close to 3 years. A 2-year interval between screens may be too long to have much of an effect on mortality for the younger population. Another limitation of the study is that only a single mediolateral oblique view of each breast was obtained, and this practice has been shown to result in as many as 24% of cancers being missed (22,23). A third potential problem with this trial is that, after the prevalence screen, 70% of biopsies performed for mammographically detected lesions proved to be cancers. This high positive predictive value (PPV) may mean that some cancers were overlooked because they did not have sufficient characteristics to warrant biopsy, and, as a consequence, their diagnosis may have been delayed. Later in the trial, fine-needle aspiration was used, and this may account for the apparent high threshold for intervention based on the excisional biopsy rate.

For the 89% of women who complied with the first screen, the rate of stage II cancers was reduced by 25% relative to the unscreened controls, and 7 years after randomization there were 31% fewer deaths from breast cancer among those screened than in the control group. This reduction persisted for 10 years (5). Two requirements for screening efficacy were fulfilled in the Two County Trial: reduction in stage and reduction in absolute mortality.

The Two County Trial is an example of how merely reviewing statistics may not reveal the entire effect of screening. The data have been retrospectively segregated and analyzed by age. For women 40 to 49 years old in the Kopparberg trial, there was a 25% mortality reduction. This was not statistically significant because of small numbers. In the Ostergotland trial, there was no decrease in cancer deaths in the screened group compared to the controls. The reason for this is not completely clear but is almost certainly due to the fact that a large number of women who died in the screened group had refused to be screened. Almost half of the women who died of breast cancer in the Ostergotland program and were counted as having been screened had actually refused to be screened. It is required in the analysis of these trials to include these women in the screened group. Given the overall small numbers of cancer deaths, if only a few of these women had been screened and saved then the trial would show a benefit. Analysts have ignored the high cancer death rate among refusers and merely pointed to Ostergotland as an example of screening having no benefit.

Malmö

Another RCT of mammography screening began in Malmö, Sweden, in 1976 and ended in 1986 (24). Approximately 42,000 women 45 to 69 years old were randomized individually. The interval between screens for the study group was 18 to 24 months (average, 21 months). There were 20,695 women allocated to be offered screening and 20,783 randomly assigned to act as unscreened controls. For the first two screens both mediolateral oblique and craniocaudal views were obtained. If the breasts were not radiographically dense, the subsequent screens included only the single oblique view.

Compliance with screening was 70%. In the early follow-up, women ages 55 and older at entry had a 20% decrease in mortality, but because of the small numbers of participants in the trial this had not reached statistical significance. Many researchers were concerned when the early follow-up of women ages 45 to 50 showed a few more cancer deaths among the screened women than among the controls. This, however, was due to the statistical fluctuation that is expected when the number of total deaths is extremely small. By the 10-year follow-up, the benefit for women ages 45 to 49 was a 49% decrease in breast cancer deaths.

A second Malmö trial has also been performed. The details of the trial have not yet been published, but were reported at the January 1997 Consensus Development Conference in Bethesda, Maryland. An additional 17,000 women ages 45 to 48 were screened. The summary for women ages 40 to 49, provided under Proof: Statistically Significant Benefit for Women 40 to 49 Years Old, includes the combined results from the two Malmö trials.

Stockholm

The Stockholm trial began in 1981 (25). The trial randomized 38,525 women 40 to 65 years old to be offered screening and 20,651 to remain as unscreened controls. Randomization was by individual and based on a system using birth dates. Of the women invited to be screened, 82% complied with the first screen. The women were offered screening every 2 years using single-view oblique mammography. In the first screen, 53% of the cancers were palpable. Because the Two County Trial was already showing a benefit, the program was terminated early after only two screens, and, subsequently, all women have been offered screening. Stockholm has reported a 21% mortality reduction, but because of the small numbers in the trial the benefit is not statistically significant. Furthermore, having only two cycles of screening in a very small population makes it very difficult to show a benefit.

Gothenburg

The Gothenburg trial was begun in 1982. The trial randomized 52,000 women 40 to 59 years old. There were 20,724 women who were invited to be screened and 28,909 women randomized to be unscreened controls. Screening using two-view mammography was performed every 18 months, and 84% of the women invited to the first screen participated.

Edinburgh

The Edinburgh trial is complicated. Using physicians' practices for randomization, 45,130 women were divided into 23,226 in the study arm and 21,904 in the control arm. The women involved were 45 to 64 years old at the time of entry. Those in the screened group had mammography (two views) and a CBE at the prevalence (first) screen. Clinical examination only was used in years 2, 4, and 6, and CBE was combined with single-view mammography (the mediolateral oblique) in the odd years 3, 5, and 7. A relative reduction in mortality of almost 20% was reported with 7- to 9-year follow-up, but because of the small numbers of women in the trials this did not achieve statistical significance (26). That only 60% of the women complied with the offer to be screened and that the randomization by physician practice introduced socioeconomic differences has been suggested as somewhat compromising the results.

National Breast Screening Study of Canada

The NBSS had its roots in the HIP trial. The HIP study had demonstrated that the natural history of breast cancer could be interrupted and that earlier detection could reduce the number of deaths from these cancers. Although the HIP was designed to evaluate women between the ages of 40 and 64, the HIP investigators decided to try to determine if there was a subgroup of women for whom the benefit was greatest. They evaluated the data by retrospectively grouping the results by age, evaluating women from 40 to 49 years old separately from those ages 50 to 64. This was the origin of the screening controversy. What the investigators ignored was that the trial was not large enough to justify this subgroup analysis on a statistical basis. The numbers of younger women were too small to permit the benefit for the younger women to be statistically significant. Unfortunately, rather than using the analysis appropriately to suggest a new trial, the investigators suggested that there was no benefit from screening women ages 40 to 49.

Investigators in Canada recognized the possibility that there might be an age threshold for screening to be beneficial. Some also believed that the major benefit in the HIP trial came not from mammography but from the CBE. In HIP this was not unrealistic as the stage of cancers in the control group was sufficiently high that any earlier detection, even by CBE, was likely to be of benefit. With these major questions in mind, the National Cancer Institute of Canada sponsored the NBSS (27,28).

The NBSS was actually two separate studies. The first was designed to determine the efficacy of screening women 40 to 49 years old with mammography and physical examination (13), whereas the second was designed to compare the relative contributions of physical examination and mammography in the screening of asymptomatic women 50 to 59 years old (14).

The NBSS differed significantly from all of the other trials. Instead of randomizing a population and then inviting those allocated to the screening arm to be screened, the NBSS first asked for women to volunteer to participate in the trial. This approach made statistical predictions more manageable, because it increased the likelihood of compliance with at least one screen because the women agreed to participate ahead of being randomized. In the other trials women could and did refuse the invitation to be screened. Using volunteers, however, meant that the results of the trial might not apply to the general population. The other trials used a blinded randomization. The women were allocated to be screened or to act as unscreened controls before anyone running the trial had any knowledge of them as individuals.

Blinded randomization is the only way to arrive at truly random allocation. If the randomization is not blinded, there is the possibility that the allocation could be nonrandom and the trial's conclusions compromised. The NBSS made the mistake of not having a truly blinded randomization, and there is evidence that the two populations were not randomly divided.

Beginning in 1980, women volunteers were sought for the program. The NBSS thus involved self-selected women (volunteers) 40 to 59 years old who were recruited to 15 centers across Canada. The women could not have a history of breast cancer and could not have had a mammogram within 1 year of the study, but women with signs or symptoms of breast cancer were permitted to participate. This latter fact has also contributed to questions about the trial.

The fact that this trial studied volunteers had two possible effects. Volunteers tend to be more health conscious and healthier. In fact, in the report of the first 7-year follow-up data, there were many fewer deaths than expected among the trial participants, suggesting the healthy volunteer effect. The second question relates to the generalizability of the results to the population. It is unclear how the results among volunteers would apply to the general population of women.

Basic Design of the NBSS

Women 40 to 49 Years Old

For the first study, 50,430 women ages 40 to 49 were recruited to participate between 1980 and 1985. Once a woman consented to participate, she was given a thorough CBE and then assigned, on an open list, to the study or control group (it was this nonblinded randomization that has raised serious questions). The study group was offered annual mammography and physical examination, whereas women in the control group received only the initial physical examination and then were followed by mail to ascertain their subsequent health status. Both groups were instructed in breast self-examination (BSE). At the end of 7 years, there were, paradoxically, 38 breast cancer deaths among the screened women and 28 among the control group. The difference of 10 was not statistically significant, but the excess of cancer deaths in the screened group raised serious questions. Confusing the issue was the fact that 33 women who had been allocated to be screened already had lymph-node–positive breast cancer, whereas there were only 21 women with positive lymph nodes who were allocated to the control group. Of greater significance is that 19 women with advanced breast cancer (four or more positive axillary nodes) were allocated to be screened and only five allocated to the control group. These imbalances, which should not occur in a random allocation, probably had a significant effect on the results.

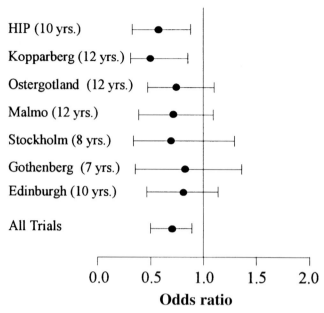

FIG. 4-8. The odds ratio of death from breast cancer for women between the ages of 40 and 74 who participated in the seven randomized, controlled trials by invitation. The dots represent point estimates (the data are analyzed at some point in time). This changes with longer follow-up. They represent the ratio of the cancer deaths relative to the number of screened women divided by the cancer deaths relative to the number of controls. If the point estimate is to the left of the line, it means that there were fewer cancer deaths among the screened women. If the dot is to the right, it means there were more cancer deaths among the screened women. The percentage of death reduction = 1 − the point estimate × 100. The bars provide the 95% confidence interval. This means that, based on the numbers of cancer deaths involved at the time the data are reviewed, the laws of probability (with 95% confidence) suggest that the true effect lies somewhere along the line. If the entire bar is to the left of the 1.0 vertical line, then the benefit is considered statistically significant ($p < 0.05$). (Adapted from Shapiro S. Screening: assessment of current studies. Cancer 1994;74:231–238.)

Women 50 to 59 Years Old

The second study in the NBSS involved women ages 50 to 59. The investigators believed that the benefit from the HIP had been due to CBE and that in that trial mammography had contributed little. They designed a trial to compare the relative contributions of mammography and CBE. The NBSS randomized the 39,476 volunteer women 50 to 59 years old into equal groups. One group was provided with mammography and CBE each year and compared to the other group that only had a CBE, but not mammography, each year. There was no unscreened control group, so the data cannot be used to determine if there was any benefit for the women in the trial from either approach to screening. At the end of 7 years from the first screen, there was no mortality difference between the two groups.

SUMMARY OF THE RESULTS

There is almost universal agreement that the RCTs of screening have demonstrated that screening is efficacious, that the natural history of breast cancer can be interrupted, and that the death rate can be reduced by periodic screening using mammography (18). In reality, because most of the trials were marginally large enough to provide statistically significant results, only the HIP trial and the combined data from the Swedish Two County Trial have sufficient numbers of women to have demonstrated a statistically significant benefit for screening (19). The other trials, with the exception of the NBSS, all show a nonsignificant benefit from screening (Fig. 4-8). The benefit from screening has been accepted based on the combination of the results from all of the trials in a meta-analysis that provides significance for the difference (10).

Many of the trials continue to be analyzed. This has been complicated by the fact that when the benefits of screening became evident many of the programs began screening their control groups. When the trials were analyzed as they were designed (not stratified by age), at 7 to 12 years of follow-up, the mortality reduction attributable to screening ranged from 3% in the NBSS for women ages 50 to 59 (Mammography and CBE compared to CBE alone) to 14% in the early Gothenburg data, 16% at Edinburgh, 18% at Ostergotland, 19% at Malmö, 20% at Stockholm, 29% in the HIP, and 32% at Kopparberg.

In an update of the seven population-based trials (Canada was not included) published in 1994, Wald and colleagues calculated a 22% mortality reduction for screening women 40 to 74 years old with a 95% confidence interval of 0.70 to 0.87 (29). Because of the small numbers of women in the trials, however, only the HIP trial and the Two County Trial are, by themselves, statistically significant.

There is no question that screening can reduce the death rate from breast cancer, with the combined data suggesting a reduction of at least 30%. This is likely a low estimate because the results are based on trials by invitation. With the exception of the Canadian trial, all of the trials first identified large populations and then randomly assigned them to the screened group or the unscreened control group. Once they were randomized, the women who were allocated to the screened group were invited to be screened. Many refused the offer. Nevertheless, to avoid selection bias, a woman who died of breast cancer and who had been offered screening is still counted with the screened group even if she had refused screening (noncompliance). Similarly, if a woman allocated to the control group had a mammogram on her own, outside of the trial, and had her life saved as a result, she is still counted as an unscreened control (contamination). Noncompliance and contamination serve to dilute the benefit from screening. The benefit, in fact, is likely considerably greater than the trials demonstrate.

Clinical Breast Examination and Breast Self-Examination as Complements to Mammography

Not all cancers are detected by mammography. Almost 9% of cancers in the BCDDP were palpable but not seen on the mammogram, and an additional 19% were found by the individual or her doctor between screenings. As many as 20% of cancers that are not evident by mammography at screening become clinically evident between annual screens. Physical examination and mammography evaluate different tissue characteristics and provide two separate, unique sources of information. The results of the physical examination should not be used to ignore mammographically detected abnormalities. Similarly, the mammogram should not be used to ignore the results of CBE. Mammography and physical examination are complementary studies, and each detects cancers not found by the other. A complete screening program should include high-quality mammography and a careful physical examination, as well as instruction for women in BSE. Just as a negative physical examination does not exclude the possibility of a mammographically detectable malignancy, a negative mammogram does not preclude the possibility of a palpable cancer.

There has been much debate over the efficacy of mammography alone. The efficacy of physical examination, alone, has never been validated scientifically. It was somewhat ironic and scientifically inconsistent when in 1993 the NCI withdrew its support for mammography screening for women between the ages of 40 and 49 but suggested that clinical examination might still be useful. Three of the trials actually included CBE and, if benefit was not accepted for mammography, then there was no support for routine CBE.

Scientific support for BSE is also lacking. The early results from a randomized, controlled study of BSE in China showed no benefit (30). This report is premature, however, with only 5 years of follow-up. Given that there are small cancers that can be detected by BSE or CBE, it is reasonable to encourage the use of both.

PROBLEMS WITH RANDOMIZED, CONTROLLED TRIALS AND ANALYSIS OF THEIR RESULTS

Screening Controversy

There is little argument that screening mammography can reduce the size and stage at detection of breast cancer (3,31) and that this can result in reduced breast cancer deaths (32). There is also little disagreement that earlier detection using screening mammography can interrupt the natural history of breast cancer for many women and that mortality can be diminished (18). Historically, controversy arose when it was decided to evaluate the results of the HIP study by dividing the women and analyzing the data for the women between the ages of 40 and 49 separately from the women between the ages of 50 and 64. This was done on the assumption that

menopause might influence the results, and age 50 was chosen as a surrogate for menopause.

It was noted that in the early years of follow-up the benefit began to appear within 2 to 3 years of the onset of screening for the older women but did not begin to appear until 5 to 7 years after the start of screening for the younger women. Because of the relatively small number of young women in the HIP, the benefit for the younger subgroup did not appear to achieve statistical significance. This was disputed in an analysis by Chu and associates (33), but many have argued that the data did not reach significance and that there was, therefore, no benefit from screening younger women. The NBSS was reportedly designed to shed more light on this question. Others felt that the trials should not be broken into subgroups and that there was sufficient other evidence of benefit, such as the results in the BCDDP, and that screening should be recommended for all women beginning by the age of 40. It was unplanned subgroup analyses of data that lacked statistical power, such as the HIP analysis, and led to the controversy.

1989 Consensus Statement

During the 1980s, medical organizations promulgated breast cancer screening guidelines that were often at variance with one another. Many of the organizations sought to reach a consensus, and in the spring of 1989 the NCI joined with the ACS, the American Medical Association, and other major medical groups and arrived at an agreement that provided women and their physicians with uniform guidelines for screening. The 1989 consensus guidelines recommended a baseline mammogram between the ages of 35 and 40, mammography and CBE every 1 to 2 years for women between the ages of 40 and 49, and annual screening for women ages 50 and over. The baseline suggestion was subsequently deleted because there were very few data that could be used to scientifically evaluate the benefit of mammography for women younger than the age of 40.

The consensus represented a political compromise. The Breast Imaging Committee of the American College of Radiology (ACR) pointed out that mammography screening of women from ages 40 to 49 on average could detect cancers about 2 years before they became clinically evident (34,35). The committee argued that screening these younger women every 2 years would mean that many cancers would be detected at about the time they would become apparent clinically, and screening at this interval or longer would likely not produce much of a benefit. Although the ACR Breast Imaging Committee voted unanimously that the guidelines should advise annual mammography for younger women, the committee was overruled based on concern that it would cause some of the organizations to withdraw from the consensus agreement. It was argued that it was best to accept a compromise to achieve a consensus and then subsequently revise the guidelines. For this reason, the optional 1 to 2 years for women ages 40 to 49 interval was adopted.

Just 3½ years later, in December 1993, the NCI withdrew its support for screening women 40 to 49 years old. The decision was made by a few individuals at the NCI who felt that the data did not justify the 1989 decision to support screening women in their 40s. They used the publication of the first results from the NBSS, published at the end of 1992, as a reason to convene a workshop in January 1993, ostensibly to review the most recent screening data. The conclusions of the workshop were preordained by the marked imbalance of presentations, weighted heavily by opponents of screening, and the fact that the summary of the workshop was written by established opponents of screening (18). The summary was published in October 1993, and the NCI presented its conclusions (that there was no benefit) to the National Cancer Advisory Board (NCAB) as it sought support for its plan to drop the guidelines for women in their 40s. The NCAB, however, having been provided with arguments in support of screening, voted nearly unanimously (13 to 1) to advise the NCI to retain support for screening women in their 40s. For the first time in its history, the director of the NCI ignored the advice of the NCAB and, in December 1993, withdrew support for mammography screening for women in their 40s. What had begun as an effort by a few people to correct what they felt had been a wrong decision in 1989 in joining the consensus, ended as an apparent political decision. The decision to drop support for screening women in their 40s and to support screening for women over the age of 50 every 1 to 2 years (also a departure from the 1989 guidelines) kept the NCI recommendations concordant with the Clinton Administration's Health Care Plan, which was announced in January 1994. The health plan had been developed during 1993 based on the advice from the NCI that it would be dropping support for screening women in their 40s. To have reversed this plan at the last minute would have dramatically affected the Administration's package. It is an unlikely coincidence that the health package only provided for screening women 50 and older every 2 years.

The NCI decision caused a great deal of confusion and was criticized because it was based on the inappropriate analysis of the data (36). The argument was perpetuated by ignoring the basic principles of statistical analysis and the analysis of data from RCTs. Studies that grouped women in their 40s and compared them to all women in the three succeeding decades of life produced a false impression that there were significant changes that occurred in screening parameters at the age of 50. The facts demonstrate, however, that there are no abrupt changes in any of the parameters of screening that occur at any age.

Why Screen Women in Their 40s?

Breast cancer is not a trivial issue for women in their 40s. More than 40% of the years of life lost to breast cancer are from women diagnosed before the age of 50 (16). Breast cancers diagnosed while women are in their 40s account for 30% of the years of life lost to these malignancies. The number of women in their 40s with breast cancer is higher than the available data suggest because, in the absence of screening, cancers that may be detectable while a woman is in her 40s are presently not diagnosed until she is in her 50s. The number of cancers diagnosed among women in their 40s will likely be even higher with appropriate mammographic screening.

Many people who oppose screening women in their 40s suggest that breast cancer is not a major problem for women at these ages. The analysis depends on the perspective. There is an important distinction between the annual breast cancer incidence (new cases per 1,000 women in the population) and the absolute numbers of cancers that develop among these women (incidence multiplied by the number of women at that age).

Breast Cancer Incidence

The incidence of cancer increases steadily with increasing age. Approximately 1.3 to 1.6 women in 1,000 are diagnosed with breast cancer each year between the ages of 40 and 49. This rises to 2.2 to 2.6 for women ages 50 to 59, and to 3.3 to 3.9 for women ages 60 to 69. Opponents of screening younger women point out that there are almost twice as many women in their 50s who develop breast cancer each year as there are in their 40s. The same analysts often ignore the fact that there are almost 1.5 times as many women diagnosed in their 60s as among those in their 50s. It is also not clear that being 1 in 1,000 is that much different from being 1 of 2 or 1 of 3 in 1,000.

Absolute Versus Relative Numbers and Biasing Data Analysis

The absolute numbers of women diagnosed with breast cancer provide a different perspective than just looking at incidence. It relates the incidence to the actual number of women at these ages at any point in time. Thus, even though the number of cancers per 1,000 is lower among younger women, if there are more women at the younger ages there could be a greater number of women with breast cancer at the younger ages. Some have trivialized the importance of breast cancer for women in their 40s by using only incidence figures. In addition, women in their 40s have been repeatedly compared to all women in four other decades of life grouped together as if the latter were a uniform group (which they are not).

Myths in Breast Cancer Detection and Diagnosis

Grouping women at different ages can be grossly misleading. For example, based on SEER estimates, in 1993 there were 28,900 women between the ages of 40 and 49

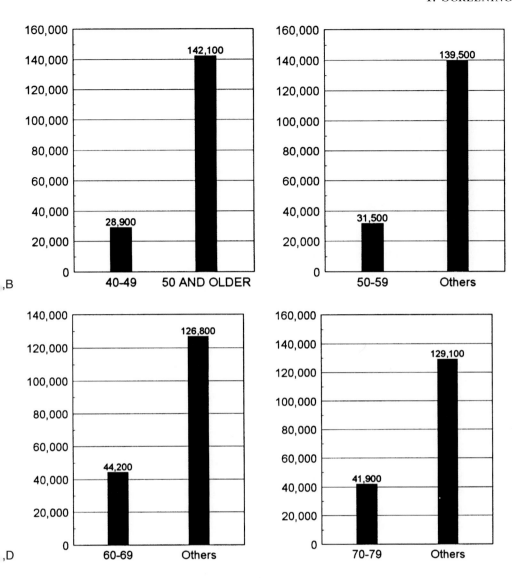

FIG. 4-9. (A) Approximately 16% of invasive breast cancers diagnosed in 1993 were diagnosed in women between the ages of 40 and 49. **(B)** Approximately 17% of invasive breast cancers diagnosed in 1993 were diagnosed in women between the ages of 50 and 59. **(C)** Approximately 25% of invasive breast cancers diagnosed in 1993 were diagnosed in women between the ages of 60 and 69. **(D)** Approximately 23% of invasive breast cancers diagnosed in 1993 were diagnosed in women between the ages of 70 and 79. *Continued.*

who were diagnosed with breast cancer. Opponents of screening pointed out that they constituted only 16% of all of the cancers diagnosed in that year. They urged that screening concentrate on the 84% of cancers that were diagnosed in all the other women (Fig. 4-9A). What this argument overlooked was that there were only 31,500 breast cancers diagnosed among women between the ages of 50 and 59 in 1993 (37). This is only 9% more than the number diagnosed among women in their 40s and constituted only 17% of all the cancers diagnosed in 1993 (Fig. 4-9B). One could argue that these women should be ignored to concentrate on the 83% of cancers that occurred in all of the other women. Age grouping can be grossly misleading. The fact is that, in 1993, no decade of life accounted for >25% of the total cancers diagnosed (Fig. 4-9C, D).

The reason that the number of cancers was so high among women in their 40s was that the baby boomers were moving through their 40s. In 1995, the ACS estimated that there

were actually more women diagnosed with breast cancer in their 40s (33,800) than in their 50s (28,300). The same was true for 1996.

By using the age of 50 as the point of analysis and comparing all women below that age with all women age 50 and older, as if they were each a uniform group, factors that change steadily with age were spuriously made to appear to change abruptly at age 50.

Age 50 Has No Biological Significance

Women and their physicians had been led to believe that something dramatic happens at the age of 50 when, in fact, it has no biological significance. The age of 50 was chosen as a surrogate for menopause because the age of actual menopause is difficult to determine. Although it was a fairly arbitrary selection, it has been imbued, by repetition, with biological significance. At one time medical oncologists thought that age

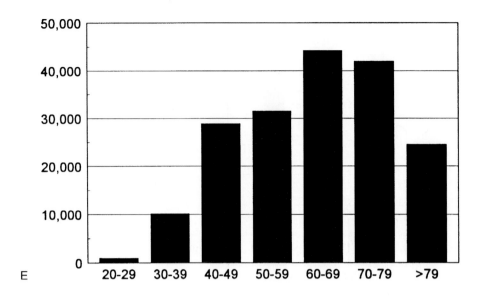

E

FIG. 4-9. *Continued.* **(E)** Totals for all age groups in 1993.

50 or menopause were major determinants in whether to use chemotherapy or hormone therapy. It is now clear that this perception was related to the way the data were grouped. Postmenopausal women can benefit from chemotherapy, and age is just one of the variables that are used to decide the best selection of therapy. Women should know that there is nothing magical that happens at the age of 50.

Age and Breast Tissue Density

One of the most repeated suggestions is that the breast is dense in women under the age of 50 and that it turns to fat and becomes more radiolucent at age 50, permitting earlier cancer diagnosis. Although a higher percentage of young women do have dense tissue, this is not a phenomenon that has an abrupt change at any age. Approximately 90% of women at the age of 30 have mammographically dense breasts. This percentage changes by approximately 1% to 2% each year and continues until approximately age 65 to 70, when 60% of women have fatty breasts. After this, the percentages appear to remain the same (see Chapter 12). There is no abrupt change in breast tissue density that occurs at any age. The misunderstanding concerning breast tissue patterns and age is, once again, a function of grouping women and using age 50 as the point of analysis. This creates the false impression that what is actually a gradually changing phenomenon changes abruptly at age 50.

There is no significant difference in the breast tissue as seen by mammography among women 40 to 49 years old compared to women 50 to 59 years old. The breasts do not turn to fat at menopause or at age 50 (38). Prechtel has shown this histologically (39), and careful analysis by age of tissue density data on mammography by Stomper (40) confirms that the percentage of women with dense breasts decreases steadily with increasing age with no abrupt alteration at age 50 or at menopause.

Age and Cancer Detection Rates

In an effort to support the arguments against screening women in their 40s, opponents of screening have used inappropriate data analysis and provided data out of context. As noted with breast tissue patterns, by comparing women 40 to 49 years old with women 50 years old and older, data that change gradually with time are made to appear to change abruptly at 50. Inappropriate grouping and comparisons have been used to trivialize the significance of breast cancer among women in their 40s.

This same type of artificial grouping was used in an article published in 1993 and used to support the NCI decision to change the guidelines. The authors assessed the prevalence of cancers in a screened population based on age. They concluded that the PPV for mammography suddenly changed at age 50 (41). The analysis of the data was skewed by the fact that women 30 to 49 years old were compared with those 50 to 70+ years old. By using the age of 50 as the point of analysis and including the extremes of what is actually only a steady and gradually increasing continuum, the results were made to appear as if there was a major change at the age of 50. They arrived at a spurious conclusion by grouping all of the younger women and comparing them to all of the older women. In doing so, they found that there were only 2 cancers per 1,000 women screened under the age of 50 and that the number appeared to jump at age 50 to 10 cancers per 1,000. In reality, a more careful examination of their data revealed that the change was more gradual. For women in their 30s the program detected 1 cancer per 1,000 women screened. This rose to 3 per 1,000 for women in their 40s, 6 per 1,000 for those in their 50s, 13 per 1,000 for women in their 60s, and 14 per 1,000 for women in their 70s. The confidence intervals overlapped for women 40 to 49 compared to those 50 to 59, showing that the difference was not even statistically significant although it is well known that the incidence of breast cancer increases steadily with increasing age. Using a different grouping it could be argued that because the detection rate for women ages 30 to 59 was only 3.3 per 1,000 and for women ages 60 to 79 it was 14 per 1,000 that screening should only concentrate on women ages 60 to 79. The conclusions are easily skewed by the way the data are grouped.

Most uninformed readers were misled by the University of California, San Francisco, School of Medicine (UCSF) analysis (41). The success of the argument was clear in a summary of the controversy written by Sox in the *Annals of Internal Medicine,* where he mistakenly concluded, based on the above review, that "the yield [of cancers] of the first mammogram was five times higher in women 50 years of age and older (10 cancers per 1,000 studies compared with 2 cancers per 1,000 studies). . . . Clearly mammography is much more efficient in detecting breast cancers in older women" (42).

Our own data confirm the fact that the number of cancers increases steadily with age (when the numbers at each specific age are counted) and that there is no abrupt change at age 50 or any other age. This trend is clearly a reflection of the prior probability of cancer that increases steadily with age, as would be expected. There is nothing magical that happens at age 50.

Age and Recall Rates, Recommendations for Breast Biopsy, and Positive Predictive Value

Opponents of screening women in their 40s have also suggested that a major change in the recall rates (abnormal mammogram), recommendations for a biopsy, and the yield of cancers from those biopsies occurs at the age of 50. In fact, the number of women recalled as the result of an abnormal mammogram is virtually the same, regardless of age. In our practice, it is approximately 6% to 8% when all screens (prevalence and incidence) are included. Sickles and coworkers have shown that the recall rates diminish after the prevalence screen (43). Their recall rate was 7% on their initial screening, and it dropped to 3% on subsequent screenings. This reflects the fact that having previous mammograms for comparison reduces the uncertainty of a borderline finding.

The percent of women for whom a biopsy is recommended is virtually the same for all women 40 to 49 years old. It ranges from 0.5% to 1.5%. Because the prevalence of breast cancer increases steadily with age, the cancers diagnosed per biopsies recommended also increases steadily with age. In our data the PPV for a biopsy for a woman 40 years old is approximately 15%, rising steadily to approximately 40% by the age of 79. The differences in PPV for mammography are merely a reflection of the steadily increasing prior probability of cancer in the population (44) and do not change abruptly at age 50 or any other age.

Much of the controversy has been manufactured. Had women and their doctors been told that age 50 was merely an arbitrary choice, then that would have been consistent with the data and discussions could have centered around the economics involved in screening. Unfortunately, the efforts were directed toward establishing age 50 as a biologically relevant age, and this is simply not true.

Other Common Myths and Lack of Logic

Unnecessary Biopsies and Scarring

Opponents of screening emphasize the harms involved. As with any test, there are false-positive screening mammograms. This is true for women of all ages. Approximately 6% to 7% of women screened for the first time are called back for immediate evaluation. This does not vary with age. The majority of these are shown to be unremarkable with a few extra mammographic views. The recall rate drops significantly if women have had previous mammograms for comparison (43).

When an abnormality is found by mammography and a biopsy is recommended, the probability of breast cancer is approximately 20% to 30%. In other words, the likelihood of a benign result is 70% to 80%. These have been termed *unnecessary* biopsies. Opponents further counsel against screening by incorrectly suggesting that biopsies lead to permanent scarring of the breast so that when a woman needs a mammogram, when she develops a mass, the mammogram will be unreadable.

These observations are not only grossly incorrect, but the logic of their application is completely inconsistent. Following a biopsy for a benign abnormality, once the breast has healed there is little if any evidence of the surgery on subsequent mammography (45), and, in the infrequent cases when changes are visible, they are rarely confusing. We undertook a prospective study of routine screening mammograms in which the radiologists were blinded to the fact that 178 women had had previous benign breast biopsies. In 170 (95%), the previous benign biopsy was not a problem for interpretation of the mammogram. For 153 of the cases (86%) there was no evidence of previous surgery on the mammogram. Among five (3%) the biopsy was evident once the history was known. In 11 cases (6%) the postsurgical change was immediately evident but was not an interpretation problem. In only eight cases (4%) old films were needed to dismiss postsurgical change. In a separate analysis, the recall rate for all women screened at the Massachusetts General Hospital from 1993 to 1996 was 6%. For women who had a previous benign breast biopsy the recall rate was 7%. A previous benign breast biopsy almost always heals with no residual abnormality visible on the mammogram.

Furthermore, the advantage of mammography is not for the woman who has a lump, but rather in the detection of clinically occult, nonpalpable cancers. By the time a cancer is large enough to feel, the chances for cure have been significantly reduced. The reason for mammography in the woman with a palpable abnormality is to screen the tissue in that breast and to screen the other breast for clinically occult breast cancer. Because mammography is not a diagnostic technique in the absolute sense and cannot be used to exclude the presence of breast cancer, its role in evaluating lumps is limited. Thus, saving mammography for when a woman has an abnormality virtually eliminates any advantage from the mammogram. The logic that mammography should be avoided until something is palpable because its use for screening leads to unnecessary biopsies is absurd.

The fact is that there is a higher percentage of unnecessary biopsies performed because an abnormality is palpated in the breast than those instigated by an abnormal mammogram. The likelihood that a palpable abnormality is cancer ranges from 5% to 30% (higher numbers are found in practices where women are referred for a second opinion and are, thus, preselected). In addition, when a cancer is palpable, it is usually larger in size and at a later stage than one detected by mammography (46). If the concern is to reduce unnecessary biopsies, then the focus of attention should first be directed toward the CBE.

Trial Designs and the Controversy over Screening 40- to 49-Year-Old Women

The design factors discussed in the section on RCTs are the key to the statistical validity. They are the reason that so much advance planning must precede the initiation of large trials. RCTs of screening are designed to answer specific questions. The power calculations are predicated on the age range of the populations to be studied to provide the necessary number of women such that, based on the prior probability (expected number) of cancers in the population, the required number will occur over the time of the trial. The calculation must, in addition, take into account the expected death rate from breast cancer to provide the required number of control group deaths, as well as to anticipate the expected reduction in deaths for the screened women over a specified period of time. Of course, these are estimates. If the death rate, for example, is higher, the number of participants can be reduced. If the death rate is lower, then the number of participants must be increased to maintain the same statistical power.

None of the seven population-based RCTs had been designed to evaluate screening benefit for 40- to 49-year-old women as a separate group. They were designed to assess a broader range of ages. For example, the HIP study was designed to evaluate the benefit of screening women 40 to 64 years old (16). The size of the population had a specified power (50%, not the usual 80%) to prove a screening benefit for this range of ages. The controversy arose because analysts tried to separately evaluate the benefit for 40- to 49-year-old women through retrospective segregation by age. Because the study was not designed for this and its power for the total population was marginal at best, there was a gross insufficiency in the number of women in the younger population. The trials, both individually and collectively, lacked the statistical power to prove a benefit in the early years of follow-up of these younger women. Although fewer women had died among the screened population relative to the controls for these ages, statisticians argued that without sufficient numbers it is not certain whether this apparent benefit was due to chance alone (33). This was, of course, circular reasoning. Because there were insufficient numbers of women to be able to have the statistical power to prove a benefit, the data should not have been analyzed as if they could be used to legitimately prove a benefit. Certainly the data should not have been used to suggest that there was no benefit. All of the trials had insufficient statistical power, individually as well as when grouped together, to be able to prove an expected benefit of approximately 25% to 30%.

Even the Canadian trial, which was purported to be designed to evaluate women between the ages of 40 and 49 separately, was actually too small to evaluate women in this age group. It lacked the statistical power to demonstrate a statistically significant mortality reduction for these women. It turns out that the design of the NBSS was based on feasibility. Because of limited resources, it was the largest trial that could be mounted. A review of the design reveals that if the NBSS design parameters had been met, which they had not, it was only large enough to permit the demonstration of a 40% or larger benefit at 5 years (47). It never had the power to show an expected benefit of 25%. The power of the NBSS was further reduced by a survival rate among the control group that was almost twice what was expected. Fewer deaths among the control women further weakened the power of the trial. In addition, 26% of the control women had mammograms. This contamination was unplanned for in the design of the NBSS. As noted earlier, to compensate for the effects of mammography in the control group (screening the controls), the NBSS would have had to involve almost 40,000 additional women in the 40- to 49-year-old group.

Retrospective Subgroup Analysis Can Eliminate the Power of the Trial

Just as the design of trials is critical for their validity, the appropriate analysis of their results is critical. The ability of a trial to demonstrate a statistically significant benefit is based on the number of cancer deaths in the screened and control groups, which is related to the number of women who develop cancer in the trial, which is related to the age of the women (and other risk factors) and the total number of women in the trial. If there are not enough women who die from breast cancer, then the trial cannot demonstrate a statistically significant benefit. The reason for the screening controversy is that analysts used data that were from trials that were not designed to answer the questions being asked. Unconscionably, they used their analyses of those data to inappropriately advise women and their physicians.

The fact is that the screening trials collectively, as well as individually, lacked the statistical power to demonstrate a mortality reduction in the early follow-up of the women under the age of 50. For a trial to have an 80% power to prove a 25% mortality reduction with statistical significance at 5 years following the first screening for women 40 to 49 years old (assuming an 80% 5-year survival among the controls), the trial would have to involve a total population of close to 500,000 women (48). This estimate was later confirmed by the International Union Against Breast Cancer (49) as well as the ACS and the NCI (50). In all the world's trials put together the total number of women who were under the age of 50 is <180,000. In other words, if all of the women in the all of the trials who were under the age of 50 were included, there were fewer than one-third the number that would be needed to demonstrate a statistically significant benefit of 25% in the early follow-up. This number was effectively further reduced by noncompliance and contamination. It should not have been surprising that the early mortality reduction among these women was not statistically significant.

By using retrospective age stratification, analysts made it impossible for the data to be statistically significant for women ages 40 to 49 in the early years of follow-up. To have then argued that the benefits that appeared did not support screening because they are not statistically significant was specious and scientifically erroneous.

The weakness of unplanned subgroup analysis can be seen in a political poll. Assume that a poll is trying to determine who will be chosen in a primary election and it takes 500 participants for the results to be statistically significant. To be safe they poll 1,000 people. The poll appears to be reasonable. The pollsters, however, then decide that it is only the Republican primary that is of interest so they look at only the results from Republican participants (a subgroup of the original poll) and they realize that only 100 Republicans participated in the poll. They certainly can look at the results, but the subgroup is too small to provide a significant sample.

The danger of subgroup analysis that lacks statistical power can be seen by reducing the subgroup still further. Most analysts agreed that screening can reduce the death rate by approximately 30% for women 50 to 69 years old. They would likely find that if the population were divided into an even smaller subgroup any mortality reduction for 57-year-old women, for example, would not be statistically significant. If, on the other hand, one accepts that subgroup analysis of data lacking statistical power is acceptable, then, reduced to the absurd, trials would require only two participants. Breaking the trials into subgroups that lack statistical power and then making medical recommendations based on that subgroup analysis is scientifically misleading and medically insupportable.

The failure to acknowledge the small numbers of women in the 40- to 49-year-old subgroup in these trials and the statistical implications of these small numbers led

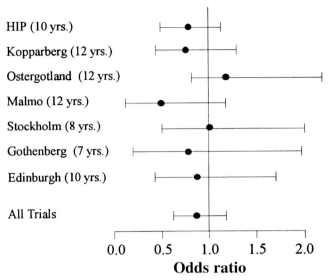

FIG. 4-10. These are similar to the data used by the NCI to dismiss the screening benefit for women 40 to 49 years old (see Fig. 4-8 for an explanation). The NBSS is not included. (Adapted from Shapiro S. Screening: assessment of current studies. Cancer 1994;74:231–238.)

to the unsupported analyses and the illegitimate use of the results of screening for these women to guide health care recommendations. A superficial review of the trials produced grossly misleading results. For example, many reviewers indicated that the trial in Malmö, Sweden, involved 42,000 women. What was usually not mentioned, however, was that <8,000 of these women were under 50 years of age (20% of the women in the trial). Approximately half of these were screened and the other half were supposedly unscreened controls, but 35% of the unscreened controls had mammograms outside of the trial. This means that the control group of women under 50 in the Malmö trial was an almost meaningless 2,400 women. This amounts to $\frac{1}{100}$ the number of women needed in a control group to prove a 25% mortality benefit at 5 years. All the other trials that had been retrospectively analyzed by age had such small numbers of 40- to 49-year-old women that even when they were combined they lacked the statistical power to prove a benefit in the early years of follow-up. Unplanned subgroup analysis that lacks statistical power is just used to define the next scientific question to be asked. It should not be used to develop medical recommendations.

The facts are that by the time of the NCI review in 1993 five of the eight trials had demonstrated a mortality reduction for women ages 40 to 49. This, however, was rejected by the NCI because the numbers of deaths involved were too small to be statistically significant. The lack of significance was clearly due to the lack of statistical power in the trials, which was reflected in the wide confidence intervals around the point estimates of the benefits (Fig. 4-10).

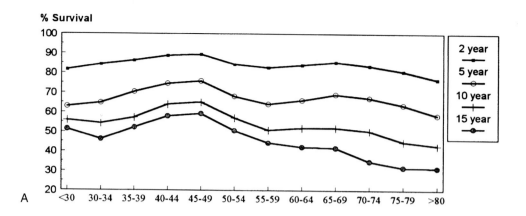

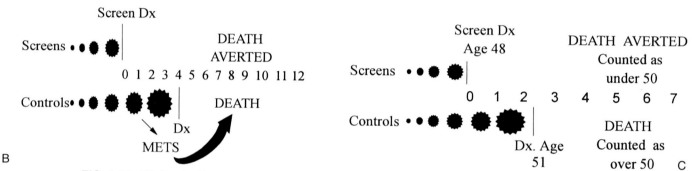

FIG. 4-11. (A) Survival by age at diagnosis. **Younger women actually live longer with breast cancer than older women,** as seen in this chart. (Adapted from Adami H, Malker B, Holmberg L, et al. The relation between survival and age at diagnosis in breast cancer. N Engl J Med 1986;315:559–563.) **(B) It is difficult to provide an early benefit from screening.** For the screened woman to demonstrate a benefit, her counterpart in the control group must develop successful metastases some time after the time that the screened woman's cancer was discovered and treated, and the control woman must then die from those metastases. This is unlikely to occur within a few years after the first screening but more likely to appear 5 or more years later and certainly not 1 to 2 years after the onset of screening. A delayed benefit makes more sense than an immediate benefit. **(C)** Data analysis should be based on the date of randomization rather than the date of diagnosis to avoid bias.

Premature Assessment of Trial Results

An additional underestimate occurred because the data were evaluated too soon after the trials began. Many of the trials were evaluated 5 years after the first screening. It may not be possible to demonstrate an early benefit if only the tumors with moderate growth are detected, and women with these cancers do not begin to die in this early follow-up period. Given the relatively favorable 5-year survival rates for breast cancer, if results are sought so soon after the start of a trial, then the numbers of women who participate must be very large to achieve statistical significance. Many of those who have analyzed the data have little experience with breast cancer patients. Health planners were looking for immediate results from the intervention. An immediate reduction in breast cancer deaths is unlikely from screening. Contrary to conventional wisdom, women under 50 actually live longer with breast cancer than do women over 50 (11) (Fig. 4-11A). In order for there to be a benefit from screening, women with breast cancer in the control group

must die. Thus, the background survival among the controls may result in a delay in the appearance of benefit for the screened women. This is likely the case in the HIP study, where the benefit for women 40 to 49 years old did not begin to appear until 5 to 7 years after screening began. A similar result has occurred in the other screening programs. In the Swedish trials, the benefit began to appear at 7 to 10 years after the first screen (20).

How Soon After the Start of Screening Should a Benefit Be Expected?

The demonstration of a benefit from screening depends on deaths in the control group. If there were no deaths in the control group, then there would be no benefit from screening. The time at which a benefit begins to appear depends on the type of cancers detected at screening whose natural history is interrupted among the screens and that progress to lethality among the controls. The RCTs, which were not optimized for screening women in their 40s, demonstrate mortality reduction that (depending on the stage at diagnosis of cancers in the control group) begins to appear 5 to 7 years after the first screening.

Early Mortality Reduction

Because a more immediate mortality reduction has been suggested among older women, some have discounted any benefit that does not appear soon after screening begins. In fact, it is difficult to explain how an immediate benefit can occur from screening (Fig. 4-11B). Breast cancer has a long natural history. Most cancers are not diagnosed until the later years of a trial (only 30% of the cancers detected in screening programs are found in the prevalence screen). Furthermore, lead times for mammographic detection range from 2 to 4 or more years before a lesion becomes clinically evident. Thus, if a cancer is detected 2 years before its counterpart in the control group, there must still be a period between the detection of the control woman's cancer and her death. It is, therefore, hard to imagine how the screened woman could have an early benefit.

The time at which a benefit appears is a reflection of how quickly the control group's cancers successfully metastasize (the screened group's cancers must be found before this occurs) and how quickly those metastases grow sufficiently to kill the control women. In order for an immediate benefit to occur, the screened woman with rapidly growing cancer must be fortuitously detected early in the trial (this is unlikely because of length-biased sampling) just prior to the successful establishment of metastatic disease (so that she will not die). Her control-group counterpart must successfully metastasize very soon after that time so that when her cancer is detected a year or more later she dies rapidly. This is a highly unlikely scenario. It is particularly difficult to explain given that among older women, where the benefit appears early, the time between screens was fairly long (2 or more years). This would increase the effect of lead-time bias and reduce the likelihood that fast growing cancers would be detected and cured. It is not scientific to reject a delayed benefit. A delayed benefit makes more sense biologically than an immediate mortality reduction, and researchers should be asking why mortality is reduced almost immediately after screening begins in women 50 and over (perhaps the primary somehow supports the metastatic growth) rather than disparaging the more biologically sound delayed benefit.

The evaluation of results too soon after the end of screening, such as appears to have occurred in the NBSS and many of the trials, also diminishes the true benefit of screening in two additional ways. It reduces the effect of benefit for cancers incident during the period of screening while emphasizing the outcome from those prevalent at initiation of screening. It also reduces the period of follow-up from the standard 5 years for incident cancers and ignores that mortality from breast cancer continues for 20 years or more.

Five years of follow-up after initial screening does not mean that 5-year survival statistics are applicable to all cancers in the studies. Because most of the cancers are not found in the first year of screening, many of the study cancers have a much smaller at-risk period. For example, if 3.2 cancers per 1,000 women are detected at the prevalence screening and, each subsequent year, 1.0 cancer is detected per 1,000 women (incidence), the measure of benefit in terms of reduced mortality at 5 years after the initial screening of 100,000 women would provide 720 cases of breast cancer in the study. However, only some of these would be subject to a full 5 years of follow-up. One hundred women with incident cancers would be detected in year 4 who would have been followed for only 1 year since diagnosis, 100 women followed for 2 years, 100 for 3 years, and 100 for 4 years. Many of their counterparts in the control group would not have even been diagnosed over the time period, and only the women with the 320 prevalent cancers would have been followed for the full 5 years of survival. Weighting the results with prevalent cancers biases the evaluation, as these are less likely to benefit from discovery than incident cancers (due to the advanced nature of many prevalent cancers). The apparent benefit of screening is reduced by mixing prevalent cases with incident cases.

As noted earlier, a delay in benefit may also occur in relationship to the interval between screenings and the growth characteristics of cancers in the population. The longer the interval between screenings, the greater the percentage of women whose cancers will grow between screenings to the level at which the tumor is incurable. Similarly, the faster the tumor growth, the more likely that short-term cancer mortality will not be affected (the tumors reach the level of incurability before they are detected). If death from cancers with moderate growth rates can be affected, evidence of a benefit is delayed because these cancers are not as rapidly lethal as the faster-growth lesions. Younger women appear to have cancers with faster growth rates (34,35,51), and this may also account for delayed benefit.

Even if the benefit is delayed for 10 years or more, it is not clear why this is not important. A benefit that occurs at 10 years is no less a benefit than one that is apparent at 5 years for these younger women. As Feig has pointed out, a woman who has her cancer diagnosed at age 45, preventing her death at age 55, actually receives a greater benefit than a women who is age 60 (she has already lived beyond age 55) who avoids dying at age 65.

Opponents' Arguments

Opponents of screening before the age of 50 have argued that, because there is a clear benefit for women older than 50 and because the benefit appears for younger women 8 to 10 years after the start of screening, the same benefit can be achieved by starting screening later. The data contradict this. The window of opportunity to delay or eliminate death from breast cancer may occur early in its growth, even though it will not become fatal for many years. There is no biological reason to believe that the cancers detected by screening in women 50 and over, that result in decreased mortality, are the same cancers that have reduced the mortality in younger women when they are detected in women in their 40s any more than it is reasonable to suggest that the benefit for women in their 50s occurred because they reached the age of 60.

An extension of this fallacious argument was used by opponents of screening to suggest that the apparent benefit for women between the ages of 40 and 49 was a consequence of their having reached the age of 50 and suddenly their cancers were cured. Not only is this biologically insupportable, but Proroc has warned that the data from RCTs should be analyzed by the age that the women were at allocation (52). Although it seems logical to analyze the results by the age at diagnosis, analyzing data by the age at diagnosis is a pseudovariable that is influenced by the study itself. Its use will bias the results against cancers detected in younger women. Because RCTs can be thought of as groups of twins, if a cancer is discovered by screening a 48 year old and her twin in the control group does not discover her cancer until she is 51 (Fig. 4-11C), the control group twin's cancer death will be attributed as a death for a cancer diagnosed after the age of 50, whereas the screened woman without a control counterpart would be attributed to a diagnosis before the age of 50 and, if she survived, would appear to have merely had a nonlethal cancer.

Despite the fact that data should not be analyzed by age at diagnosis, the HIP trial (16), Kopparberg (53), and Gothenburg (54) trials performed such analyses, and all found that the majority of the benefit was achieved for cancers diagnosed before the age of 50. Since the Gothenburg trial began screening its control group as well after the seventh year of the trial (the benefits shown in other trials made it impossible to deny screening to the controls), the investigators estimate that the majority of the benefit came from cancers detected while the women were under the age of 50. In the HIP trial, there was a 30% mortality reduction for women who began screening at ages 40 to 44. None of these women reached the age of 50 during the trial. Tabar has pointed out that in the Kopparberg trial the majority of the benefit for women between the ages of 40 and 49 was from cancers detected while they were in their 40s (53). Several of the trials suggest that the benefit is actually highest for women in their early 40s, while it diminishes for those in their late 40s and early 50s and then increases again around the age of 55. This may reflect the possibility of two breast cancer populations (see Chapter 3).

Inconsistent Use of Statistics

The opponents of screening used the lack of statistical power in the trials in a contradictory fashion. At the time that the NCI changed its guidelines, its advisors had suggested that there was not even a trend toward a benefit (18). Yet, even at that time, three of five of the Swedish trials revealed a mortality benefit ranging from 25% in Kopparberg and

27% in Gothenburg to 49% in Malmö. The Edinburgh trial had produced a 22% reduction in breast cancer mortality (55), and the HIP trial showed a 23% reduction in mortality for women 40 to 49 years old. Despite the fact that five of the eight RCTs had demonstrated a benefit, the benefit was discounted because it was not statistically significant. What was inexplicably ignored was that it would be almost impossible for a benefit to be significant in these populations because the number of women in their 40s in the trials was too small to permit statistical significance. The same reviewers, nevertheless, stated that these same trials, which were too small to be able to prove a benefit, suggested that there was no benefit from screening. What is puzzling about this conclusion is that the number of women needed in a trial to prove no benefit must be even larger than the number needed to prove a benefit.

Other Evidence That Supports Screening for Women in Their 40s

Breast cancer is still relatively uncommon, and most women still survive to die from some other problem. RCTs to study breast cancer screening must be very large to be efficacious. They are expensive to perform, and it is unlikely that a large enough, properly executed RCT will ever be undertaken. This is particularly true in light of the ethical issues involved in having an unscreened control group. Given the limitations of the RCTs that have been performed and the importance of the screening question, it is reasonable to evaluate data from other sources to assess the potential benefit of screening.

There are ample data from which a benefit can be inferred from screening women in their 40s. It has been suggested that there are differences in the cancers among women between the ages of 40 and 49 compared to those in women 50 and over. Although this may be true in terms of the lead time for detection and the screening interval, it does not appear to be true for survival. In the Swedish overview, the statistical test for heterogeneity between the two groups (younger and older women) was not significant, suggesting that there is no difference in the expected results for women at different ages.

Data from the BCDDP show that there is no significant difference between survival rates for women under age 50 and those ages 50 to 59 and no differences by age based on tumor size, grade, and stage (17,56). The Swedish Kopparberg trial confirmed that there is no difference in survival for younger women compared to older women when their cancers are collated by size, stage, and histologic grade (5). Older women have shown a statistically significant mortality reduction as a result of down-staging from screening. Mammography has been shown to down-stage tumors among younger women as well, and a mortality reduction can be expected when they are screened appropriately.

The survival of 40- to 49-year-old women with breast cancer in the BCDDP was as good or better than women 50 and over, and the percent of cancers detected by mammography for women under 50 in that study was equal to those detected by mammography alone among women 50 and over.

More modern screening programs such as that at UCSF, the program in British Columbia, and even a private practice in New Mexico, demonstrate that small, early-stage cancers can be found with proportional frequency between the two groups. In recent reviews of their data, the screening programs found that the median size for cancers in both the under-50 and 50-and-over groups was the same. The stage at diagnosis was slightly better for women under the age of 50 (31,57,58).

Ironically, at the same time that the NCI was discouraging women under the age of 50 from being screened, they announced that for women ages 40 to 49 there had been a decrease in breast cancer deaths of 8.7% from 1989 to 1992. The decrease for women ages 50 to 59 (many of these cancers were likely detected while women were in their 40s) was 9.3%. Although the NCI suggested that the decrease was due to chemotherapy, the data suggest that much of the decrease was due to screening.

Screening Women Younger Than 40

The 1989 consensus guidelines had originally included the recommendation that women between the ages of 35 and 40 have a baseline mammogram. This recommendation was quietly dropped because it had no scientific justification. None of the RCTs had included women younger than 40, and there is an absence of data. Anecdotally, we have detected nonpalpable, early-stage cancers (DCIS and invasive lesions) in younger women. The only study that sheds some statistical light on the question has been from Memorial Hospital in New York. Liberman and associates found that among 5,105 screened women between the ages of 35 and 39 biopsy was recommended in 31 (<1%). The screening detected eight cancers (five DCIS, three invasive). This rate of 1.6 per 1,000 was the same as their rate for women in their 40s (59). Just as there is no reason to believe that something magical happens at age 50, there is no reason to expect that age 40 has any mystical properties either.

NBSS: AN EXAMPLE OF HOW A LARGE TRIAL CAN BE COMPROMISED

The catalyst for the NCI's change of guidelines had been the publication of the early results of the NBSS. This was the trial that had been touted as being carefully planned and ideally designed to answer the lingering questions concerning screening. The NBSS was the only RCT that was purportedly designed at the outset to try to evaluate the efficacy of screening women in the 40- to 49-year-old age group. A superficial review of this trial fails to reveal the pronounced flaws that severely compromise the interpretation of its results.

The early data from the NBSS were used as an example of a large trial that failed to show any advantage (27), but a closer review of the trial itself reveals that it was not designed or executed properly. The power calculation (estimating the number of women needed for statistical validity) in that trial was based on a 40% reduction in mortality (47). This large a benefit, although possible, has never been suggested as likely. Assuming that the trial had met all the other statistical criteria on which it was based, which it did not, it does not have sufficient statistical power to begin with to show a benefit that is smaller than 40%.

Unfortunately, the trial did not even have the power that it was designed to have. Discounting the effects of the poor quality of the mammograms (60) on the results of the trial, other problems became apparent. The study was designed without taking into account that 26% of the women who were supposed to be unscreened controls had mammograms outside the program. In effect, this compared a group of screened women with a group of screened women. Comparing screening with screening obviously reduces the ability to prove a benefit from screening. The investigators argued that these were diagnostic mammograms. It is this failure to understand the technology that they were studying (mammography) that lies at the crux of the problems with the NBSS. The term *diagnostic mammography* is misleading to those who do not understand the technology. Mammography is not particularly useful as a diagnostic procedure. The benefit from this type of mammogram, as with all mammography, comes from screening. In the symptomatic woman the benefit still comes from screening the ipsilateral breast as well as the contralateral breast for clinically occult breast cancer. In general, mammography cannot exclude breast cancer, so its role in diagnosis is limited, but it is always able to detect unsuspected breast cancer, even in women whose clinically suspicious area proves to be benign (61). In effect, 26% of the unscreened control women in the NBSS were screened by mammography.

Proper study design requires that additional women be added to make up for the dilutional effect of contamination. To retain the power that they estimated for the trial, the investigators in the NBSS would have had to increase the number of women in the trial, under the age of 50, from 50,000 to 89,000 to make up for the contamination of 26% that occurred in the trial. Because the NBSS did not account for contamination, the trial did not have the power to detect a benefit even as large as 40%.

Poor Quality Mammography in the NBSS

Despite the fact that the most significant goal of the NBSS was to test the benefit of mammographic screening of younger women and despite concerns voiced by advisors to the program, a decision was made at the outset that the quality of the mammography was not to be of major importance. Two advisors resigned in protest. The screening centers were selected from those that had volunteered to participate. They were permitted to use whatever mammography equipment they had available. The dose for each mammogram was the overriding concern, and image quality was not a major criterion. Monitoring by physicists was primarily performed to ensure that the dose was kept low. Consequently, scatter reduction grids were not used for much of the study, resulting in image degradation.

Further affecting the quality of the mammography was the fact that there was no special training for the technologists performing the mammograms, and no special training was provided for the radiologists interpreting the studies. Thus, instead of evaluating the efficacy of high-quality mammography for screening, the designers of the trial decided to test the validity of mammographic screening as it was being generally practiced at the time the study was forming (Miller A, personal communication, 1992). In contrast, the program enlisted nurses to perform the physical examination portion of the study, and these nurses received intensive, special training (62).

As a result of concerns raised by consultants to the program and others familiar with the NBSS, the investigators organized an objective outside review of the quality of the mammograms and the results of the review were published in 1990 (62,63). Although the quality of the mammograms gradually improved, the external review clearly demonstrated that for the majority of the trial (years 1 to 4) >50% of the mammograms were judged as poor or completely unacceptable. The principal investigators had argued that the worst mammography occurred in the first 2 years of screening, when only a small number of women were screened (as the centers came on line), but their own figures demonstrated that poor image quality dominated through year 4 when all centers were active. In fact, by the fourth year, 15% of the studies were still completely unacceptable. This was not merely due to the failure to use the mediolateral oblique projection (thus underevaluating the tail of the breast where most cancers develop), as the investigators have argued; rather it is due to the overall poor quality of the images, ranging from poor positioning to poor contrast and image sharpness.

Concern about the poor quality of the images was not only voiced from critiques outside the program. The NBSS's own reference physicist stated "in my work as reference physicist to the NBSS, [I] identified many concerns regarding the quality of mammography carried out in some of the NBSS screening centers. That quality [in the NBSS] was far below state of the art, even for that time (early 1980s). Problems in the quality of mammography resulted not only from inadequate equipment in some cases, but also from inappropriate imaging technique and lack of availability of specialized training for technologists and radiologists" (64).

To the credit of the program managers, and as a result of the repeated concerns raised by advisers to the program as well as the lower sensitivity of detection found by the program's own reference radiologist (65), the quality of the mammography was improved over time. However, for a study with this importance, the quality at the outset should have been high.

Survival Among the Control Group

An additional problem with the statistical power of the NBSS was that the calculations were based on an expected mortality of 212 per 100,000 in the control group over the 5 years of the trial, when, in fact, the death rate appears to have been much lower than this figure (111 breast cancer deaths per 100,000 over 5 years), further reducing the power of the study. The control group in the NBSS enjoyed a remarkable breast cancer survival. The 5-year survival from breast cancer among women 40 to 49 years old in Canada and the United States in 1980 was 75% to 80%. The control group in the NBSS had a greater than 90% 5-year survival. Not only did this not reflect the survival in the general population, but it meant that the screened women would have to have had practically no deaths at the 7-year analysis for a statistical benefit to appear. It would appear that the women who volunteered for the NBSS did not represent Canadian women but were a selected group. Thus, the results of the trial cannot be applied to the general population. Volunteers are also likely to experience different survival characteristics than physician-referred women who constitute the majority of women being screened in the United States.

Effect of Using Untrained Radiologists

The NBSS investigators failed to train the technologists and radiologists involved in the trial. The poor training of the radiologists was reflected in the fact that the NBSS investigators found, in their own blinded review by their reference radiologist, that at least 25% of the cancers that were detected among the screened women were evident on earlier mammograms and should have been detected at least 1 year earlier than they were (65).

Randomization Process

The validity of an RCT lies in a balanced distribution of women in both groups. If neither group was screened, there should be the same amount of everything in the two groups. The same number of women should develop cancer, the same number of women should be diagnosed with advanced cancer, and the same number of women should die from breast cancer in both groups. To accomplish this, it is very important that the allocation of women to the screened group or the control group be truly random. This is the only way to achieve groups that will behave in a similar fashion. To avoid a compromise of the process of allocation, the randomization should be blind, with those doing the randomization having no information concerning the women being randomized so that there is no possibility that women could be intentionally placed in one group or the other. There is strong evidence that the random allocation process in the NBSS was, in fact, compromised and that the groups were imbalanced from the start of the trial.

The results reveal that there were more advanced cancers (axillary lymph node positive) found in the screened population in the first round of screening than in the control group. This means that, either by chance or through a flaw in the randomization process, more women with prognostically poor tumors were placed in the study group. At the time of allocation, 33 women who had positive axillary nodes at the time of entry into the trial were randomized to the screened group (30 of these cancers were palpable at the first examination), whereas only 21 were placed among the controls. The discrepancy is even greater if women with four or more nodes are evaluated. There were 19 women with these poor prognosis cancers (17 palpable at the time of allocation) that were placed in the screened group whereas only five were randomized to the control group. The difference is statistically significant. This imbalanced distribution alone would account for the failure of the trial to show any benefit for women in their 40s.

The reasons for these major imbalances are likely two design flaws in the NBSS. Because the trial was actually too small (see Statistical Power), the investigators included women with palpable abnormalities in this trial of screening. They argued that this was more realistic because, if screening is provided as a public health benefit, then women with lumps will also participate. The fact is that, without the palpable cancers that would be found among these symptomatic women, the trial would not have had enough women to meet its statistical requirements. Because these women were unlikely to benefit from screening, the inclusion of symptomatic women at best diluted the results of the trial had they been allocated equally to both trial arms. If, on the other hand, they were allocated unequally, as it appears they were, then they would have imbalanced the results.

Nonblinded Randomization

The inclusion of women with advanced cancer by itself might not have been a critical problem but for the fact that the design of the trial permitted a likely compromise of the allocation process. A key element in the design of an RCT is that the randomization process be blinded so that there is no chance for compromise of the random distributions between both groups. What has never been satisfactorily explained, and what has also been dismissed in the analyses of those opposed to screening, is that women in the NBSS had a CBE prior to randomization. By allowing women with palpable breast cancer to participate and by permitting a CBE before allocation, the randomization process could be compromised. The process was likely corrupted as the assignment to a group was made on open lists prepared ahead of time. This offered the opportunity for a nurse examiner to have a symptomatic woman placed into the screened group to ensure that she would have a mammogram, and this is the likely explanation of the imbalance of advanced and poor-prognosis cancers.

The investigators argued that the groups appeared to be randomly assigned because the major demographic features of the women appeared to be equally divided between the two groups. What they have ignored is that a shift of even 100 or more women from one group to the other would not influence the demographics of the other 24,000 women who were likely properly randomized, but it could severely affect the outcome of the trial. On the other hand, a shift of a relatively few women with advanced breast cancer would greatly affect the mortality results. The fact that there was an excess of advanced cancers and a statistically significant excess of poor prognosis cancers allocated to screening raises the possibility that the random allocation process was compromised. Regardless of the reason, this loading of the screened group guarantees that screening cannot show an early benefit in the NBSS where the results from these prevalent cancers, whose course is unlikely to be affected by screening, predominate.

The investigators have argued that the excess of advanced cancers allocated to the screened group at the start of the trial was due to the fact that screening detects more of all kinds of cancers including the advanced cancers. This is likely true. However, if the randomization process was truly random, there should eventually be the same number of all types of cancers in both groups, and the advanced cancers in the control group should rise to the surface over the course of the trial, diminishing the excess of advanced cancers in the screened group. This type of equilibration occurred in the other trials but did not occur in the NBSS. In fact the opposite happened. The excess of advanced cancers (lymph node positive) increased among the screened women relative to the controls over the course of the trial. It rose from 33 to 102 (an increase of 69 women) in the screened 40- to 49-year-old group whereas among the controls it went from only 21 to only 68 (an increase of 47). The fact that a diminution did not occur, coupled with the facts that the randomization was not blinded, that the women had a CBE before randomization, and that 90% of the poor prognosis cancers allocated to screening were palpable, suggests a probable compromise of the allocation process. As noted above, if 10 to 100 women were shifted between the two groups, the shift would not be detectable in the overall demography of the two groups. This would also account for the poorer-than-expected survival among the screened women and the better-than-expected survival among the control women that was reported by the NBSS investigators.

Although the principal investigator in the NBSS had argued that all of the other trials had had a similar experience with advanced cancers, Tarone, a biostatistician at the NCI, showed that this was, in fact, not the case, and that the excess of advanced cancers in the NBSS was the exception among the trials. He confirmed that this was an indication of a randomization failure and urged that the results of the NBSS be recalculated to eliminate the advanced cancers (6). An independent review of the randomization process was performed by MacMahon and Bailar in 1995 and 1996 (66). Unfortunately, despite the fact that the reviewers were urged to interview those responsible for the randomization, the nurses and administrative personnel were never interviewed (with anonymity and guarantees against retribution). This is the only way to determine whether the randomization was compromised, and the reviewers failed to answer the question.

Differences in Care Between the Control and Screened Groups

Not only were there major problems with the design and execution of the NBSS, but in January 1997, at the Consensus Development Conference organized by the National Institutes of Health to address the screening controversy, the principal investigator, in an effort to explain the excess of lymph-node–positive cancers, revealed that the control women were primarily treated in community centers and had fewer and less extensive axillary dissections than the screened women with cancer, who were more commonly treated in academic centers. This indicates that there were also treatment differences between the two groups and further compromises the results of the trial.

False Reassurance

Some of the trials demonstrated an excess of deaths among the screened women in the early years of follow-up. Much of this was at a time when the number of deaths was in the single digits and statistical fluctuation and chance were operative. The results of the NBSS, however, provide an important lesson for all physicians involved in breast cancer screening. Other studies, such as the HIP, have demonstrated a paradoxical phenomenon of early excess cancer deaths among women allocated to screening (although to a much smaller degree). If screening was ineffective one would anticipate the same number of deaths in both the study and control groups. Excess deaths in the study group, in the early years of follow-up, are probably an artifact of small numbers and statistical fluctuation. Persistence of an excess can only mean that diagnosis had been delayed (other hypotheses are, at best, on the scientific fringe).

Delay in diagnosis may be the result of women being falsely reassured from a negative screening study. Unfortunately, in convincing women to be screened, it is often incorrectly implied that mammography can exclude breast cancer and that a negative screening evaluation is somehow protective. It is likely that women who underwent screening and had negative results developed a false sense of security from the negative screen. Believing that a negative screen conferred a degree of protection, a woman who developed a problem in her breast during the interval between screens, assuming that the change could not be significant, would be more likely to defer immediate evaluation, or she might defer evaluation knowing that she would be screened again in the future. In contrast, her counterpart in the control group would have no similar false reassurance and would be more likely to seek immediate evaluation when she noted a breast abnormality. Thus, the screened woman would delay the diagnosis of her breast cancer and would

be more likely to present at a later stage. This problem would be amplified by poor-quality screening by converting potentially early lesions at detection into later stage and fatal cancers due to delay in diagnosis. This delay from false reassurance among screened women has been documented in a Finnish study (67).

An allocation imbalance in the NBSS can explain the fact that the excess of advanced cancers between the screens and controls did not diminish, but it cannot explain the increase in the excess during the trial. The fact that the gap widened over the course of the trial is likely due to false reassurance and delay in diagnosis among the screened women. This is the most likely explanation for the widening of the excess of advanced cancers in the NBSS. Poor-quality mammography exacerbates the problem by increasing the number of falsely reassured women and converting potentially curable cancers (by earlier detection by high-quality mammography) to incurable through the failure to detect them earlier and delayed diagnosis from false reassurance.

In the BCDDP, almost 20% of the cancers that occurred among women who had undergone both a negative physical examination and a negative mammogram were diagnosed within 1 year of the negative screen. Women undergoing screening must be aware that a negative screen does not confer protection. Mammography is used in the hope of finding a cancer earlier. It cannot be used to exclude breast cancer.

Women should understand that a change in the breast at any time, even soon after a negative screen, should be brought immediately to the doctor's attention.

Inconsistent Thresholds for Intervention

There were no agreed upon parameters for intervention in the NBSS (and apparently none in the other trials as well). If a mammogram was interpreted as positive, the case was referred to a center surgeon, who would determine whether a biopsy was indicated. This recommendation was then conveyed to the patient's nonprogram physician, who made the final decision whether to intervene. The surgeons had no agreed upon guidelines. According to Anthony Miller, the director of the NBSS, there was at least one physician who refused to biopsy lesions unless they were palpable. According to the NBSS publication, 25% of biopsies recommended from the screening mammograms were not performed, likely delaying the diagnosis of breast cancers.

Summarizing the NBSS

Perhaps the most important result of the NBSS was the demonstration that poor mammography and the poor integration of mammographic screening with diagnostic intervention reduces the effectiveness of screening. Rather than withdrawing a potentially lifesaving approach, the goal should be to provide high-quality screening and through physician education better integrate detection and diagnosis.

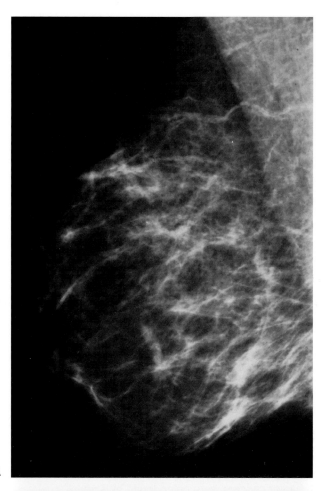

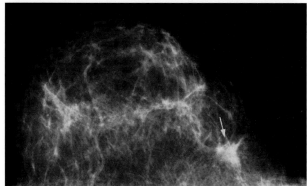

FIG. 4-12. Single-view mammography can miss almost 25% of cancers. The invasive cancer is not evident on the mediolateral oblique projection **(A)** and would be missed using single-view screening. It is only evident in the lateral left breast on the craniocaudal **(B)** projection (*arrow*).

Other Complications of the NBSS

A fact that is frequently overlooked is that the early results from the NBSS not only failed to show a benefit for screening mammography for women in their 40s, but all the screened women underwent annual physical examination as well. If this trial is used to suggest that there is no benefit from mammography, then there is no benefit from a CBE.

BSE has never been shown in an RCT to reduce mortality from breast cancer. Thus, unless one is more critical in the analysis of the NBSS, one is forced to suggest to women that they should totally ignore their breasts until the age of 50.

PROBLEMS WITH THE OTHER TRIALS

Single-View Mammography Leads to Missed Cancers

Half of the trials screened women using only a single medi-olateral oblique mammogram. This was done to reduce x-ray exposure and reduce the costs of screening. Unfortunately, single-view oblique mammography can lead to missing >24% of cancers (22,23,68) (Fig. 4-12). The exact significance of this has been debated, but it is likely that the screening trials would have further reduced mortality if two-view mammography had been performed throughout. The trials that screened these women every year and with two-view mammography demonstrated greater mortality reduction than those that screened every 2 years or with single-view mammography (57).

In addition, because it is impossible to determine if a potential abnormality is a superimposition of normal structures, based on a single projection, the recall rate is much higher if single projections are used.

Screening Intervals

The frequency of screening (time between screens) is not a trivial question. The fact that the mortality from breast cancer can be reduced proves that the natural history of breast cancer can be interrupted. This suggests that there is a period of time in the growth of many, if not all, cancers before they reach a level of lethality. The screening interval may determine the types of cancer detected and can affect how soon a benefit can be expected. Only cancers that are slow to reach the level of lethality will be detected, and the patient may derive little benefit if the time between screenings is too long. If the interval is shortened, then the tumors with moderate growth rates can be influenced, and it is likely many of these have been cured in the screening trials and account for the mortality reduction. The only way to interrupt cancers that reach the level of incurability faster is to shorten the time between screenings. If women 40 to 49 years old are to be screened, the available data suggest that it should be every year (34,35). The lead time for mammography for women from the ages of 40 to 49 is approximately 2 years. If women this age are screened every 2 years, the advantage of early detection will be diminished. Screening should be on an annual basis.

One method of determining how much earlier breast cancers are detected by mammography is to subtract the number of cancers found in each incidence screening from the number detected at the prevalence screening and divide that number by the number of cancers detected at each incidence screening. Without screening, the cancers build up in

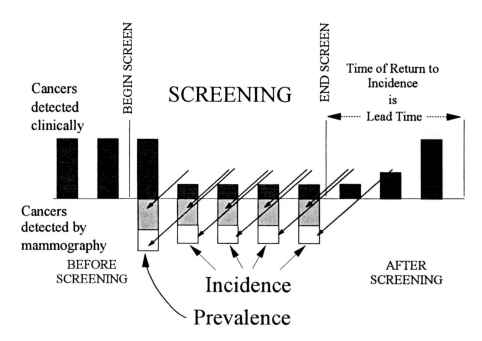

FIG. 4-13. Moskowitz estimated the lead time gained by screening by counting the number of years it took for the number of cancers surfacing in his screening population, after they stopped being screened, to be equal to the number of cancers that were found each year (incident cancers) during the screen. The bars above the horizontal line represent cancers detected by clinical examination or by the patient herself. The bars below the line represent cancers detected by mammography. At the first screening (prevalence) a large number of cancers are detected, including those that were building up in the population and those that only mammography can detect. The diagonal arrows indicate the fact that cancers detected by mammography represent cancers that are taken from the future. If they were not detected earlier, they would have come to the surface in subsequent years. When screening stops, there is initially a drop in the number of cancers surfacing. The amount of time it takes for the number surfacing each year (without mammography screening) to equal the number of cancers detected each year during screening provides an estimate of how much earlier cancers were being found by screening (lead time).

the population so that the prevalence screening includes the number of new cancers that rise to the surface each year (incident cancers) plus the cancers that have risen to the surface in previous years that could have been detected but, in the absence of screening, had collected in the population. If there are eight cancers detected per 1,000 women screened in the prevalence mammographic screen (two of which would have been detected without screening), and then two cancers are detected at each subsequent screen (incidence screen) the lead time would be $(8 − 2)/2 = 3$ years. In other words, because two cancers rise to the threshold of detectability each year (incidence) it would have taken 3 years of not screening, with two cancers each year being added to the population, to build up to the eight cancers found at the first screening.

Moskowitz reasoned that lead time can be derived by determining how long it takes for the annual detection rate to return to its baseline once screening is terminated (34). If one postulates that a new detection technique (screening) is more sensitive at finding cancer than waiting for symptoms or signs to reveal a lesion, then screening will find not only the cancers that annually rise to clinical detectability (CD) but also those occult lesions that are not yet clinically evi-

dent (O). In the first year of screening the prevalent cancers will be found. These include cancers that have been detectable for many years but were ignored, as well as those that have just reached the level of clinical detectability and cancers that are found 1 or more years earlier because of the screen. The subsequent years of screening (if the interval is within the lead-time period) will detect the incident or new cancers and will include the CDs and the Os. These two combine to produce an annual steady-state incidence during the period of screening in the population.

Screening, by detecting lesions earlier, dips into the pool of future cancers that would not have ordinarily been found until they grew to clinical detectability. Thus, when screening ceases there will be a drop in the annual incidence of cancers detected, because the screening has already eliminated many future CDs. Moskowitz found that the lead time gained by the screen is the time it takes following the cessation of screening for the incidence to return to the incidence during screening (34) (Fig. 4-13). In other words, because screening detects cancers that would not have reached clinical detectability until some future time, the time gained by the screen is equal to the time it takes for new cancers to rise from below detection thresholds, once screening stops, to

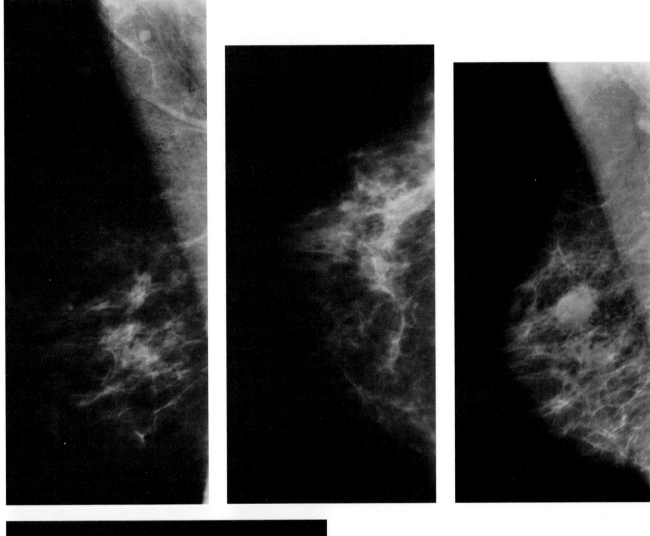

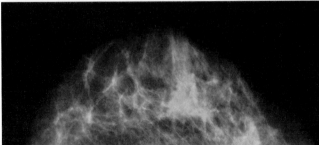

FIG. 4-14. Tumors can grow rapidly, regardless of age. In this 67-year-old woman, there was no evidence of cancer on the medial lateral oblique **(A)** and craniocaudal **(B)** projections in 1995. On the mediolateral oblique **(C)** and craniocaudal **(D)** projections 16 months later, her palpable, 1.5-cm, invasive ductal carcinoma is obvious. This cancer probably could have been intercepted earlier if Medicare had permitted screening at annual intervals. *Continued.*

replace those removed by screening and hence for the incidence to return to the annual incident steady state. The lead time gained by earlier detection is thus the amount of time it takes for the pool to be replenished to prescreening levels by the growth of new cancers in the population.

The Cincinnati BCDDP screened 10,530 women on an annual basis using physical examination and mammography. Using the preceding rationale, Moskowitz found that the lead time gained by mammographic screening of women aged 35 to 49 years was on average 2 ± 0.5 years, whereas it was 3.5 ± 0.5 years for women over 50 (34).

A similar phenomenon was seen in the Swedish Two County Trial in which Tabar and associates compared the number of cancers that rose to clinical detectability among the screened women during the interval between screenings with the number of cancers that were detected during the same period among the control women. He found that by the second year after a screening and just prior to the next screening, the screened women between the ages of 40 and 49 were being diagnosed (between screens) with 68% as many cancers as their counterparts in the control group over the same period. In other words, the lead time for mammography

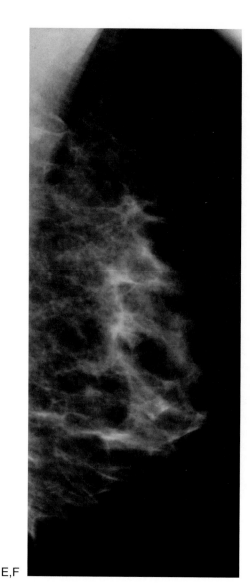
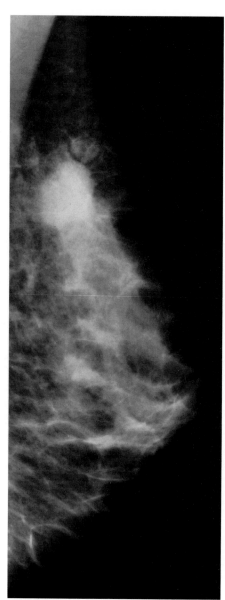

E,F

FIG. 4-14. *Continued.* In this second patient the first lateral mammogram **(E)** was unremarkable. Three months later, the 2-cm, palpable, invasive breast cancer is evident **(F)**. This cancer is so rapidly growing that even a 6-month screening interval would have been irrelevant.

among these women was about 2 years. In comparison, by the time women 50 and older were screened after almost a 3-year interval, the interval cancers among the screened women was not even up to 50% of what was occurring in the control population (35), suggesting a longer lead time for older women.

In the screening program at UCSF, the investigators found that the sensitivity of mammography (percentage of cancers detected by mammography) for women ages 40 to 49 was 87.5% if the screening interval was 7 months, 83.6% if the interval was 13 months, and 71.4% if the interval was 25 months. The numbers for women ages 50 and over were 98.5%, 93.2%, and 85.7% at the same intervals. The UCSF data indicate that screening women in their 40s every year has the same sensitivity as screening older women every 2 years.

Unfortunately, the data have only been provided with the age of 50 as the break point and the age around which the data have been analyzed. It is likely that the lead time does not suddenly increase at age 50 but that there is a progressive elongation of lead time with age, as would be expected when averages are used. For some women, regardless of age, the lead time is considerably longer, and for others it is considerably shorter (Fig. 4-14).

The Swedish data showed a mortality benefit for women over 50 screened every 2 to 3 years. This would appear to support Moskowitz's analysis predicting a longer lead time for women in this age group. Although it is likely that older women can derive benefit from screening intervals of 2 years, because these are average lead times any lengthening of the interval between screenings will likely result in a reduction in benefit. Ultimately it will be the cost of screening that determines how long the interval will be. Caution is needed. If the interval is too long and is close to the average sojourn time, money may be saved but there may be little benefit from screening.

A trial involving more than one million women to evaluate the effect of interval has been suggested and may be performed. Given the cost of such a trial and its intricacies, it is unlikely to be performed properly. It is also unlikely that the available studies will provide any additional data that can be used to convince all analysts of the appropriate intervals. However, based on the available data and the more recent favorable radiation risk assessment for women 40 and over (see Radiation Risk) it is likely that by the age of 40, women should be screened yearly. The only reason to not screen every year is economic. If cost becomes dominant then for older women—and the age at which older begins is uncertain—a cycle of screening every 18 months to 2 years may be sufficient to reduce mortality, although more frequent screening will likely offer additional benefit.

Excess Mortality in the Early Analyses of the Screening Data

As noted earlier, concerns have been raised that screening may, in fact, cause more deaths. This was based on the observation that in four of the screening trials there were, paradoxically, more cancer deaths among the screened women under the age of 50 than among the controls, in the early follow-up data. This appeared in the HIP trial, the early data from Malmö, the Ostergotland trial, and in the NBSS.

In the HIP and Malmö trials the early mortality results were based on only a few deaths among each group. Statistical fluctuation almost certainly accounts for the early excess among the screened women. That the results later reversed and the screened women have enjoyed a long-term reduction in mortality supports this analysis.

The allocation imbalance of Canadian women may make it impossible to reverse the excess deaths in that trial. As noted above, there were 14 more women with four or more positive nodes who were allocated to the screened group before screening even began. This marked disproportion of women with poor prognosis cancers more than accounts for the 10 more breast cancer deaths among the screened group in the NBSS.

In the Ostergotland trial, the excess of cancer deaths is also likely the fluctuation expected from small numbers. The lack of benefit in that trial is likely due to the fact that almost half of the cancer deaths among the screened group were among women who actually refused to be screened. The Swedish review board has concluded that, when all of the Swedish trial data are analyzed, there were, in fact, no excess cancer deaths among any of the screened groups.

IS MAMMOGRAPHY DETRIMENTAL?

Based on the incomplete analyses of the early results that suggested a possible excess of cancer deaths among the screened women, some were quick to suggest that mammography was the cause of premature death. It was suggested that the pressure from the mammogram might cause

a duct containing intraductal cancer to be disrupted permitting the cells to spill into the surrounding tissue and metastasize (69). Others have suggested that the compression might squeeze cells directly into the blood (69), whereas others cited the animal data that showed an increase in the growth of some metastatic lesions when the primary lesion is removed (70) as explaining the excess. The apparent excess was almost certainly merely due to the statistical fluctuations inherent in the small numbers of deaths at the start of the trials. The other postulated reasons cited above have no scientific basis.

Mammography requires approximately 10 to 20 pounds of compression over the surface of the breast. Even the application of the maximum compression force of 45 pounds, when distributed over the area of compression, amounts to only approximately 1 to 3 pounds per square inch (psi), depending on the size of the breast. A 250-cc breast compressed by 40 pounds experiences 3.2 psi, whereas a 750-cc breast experiences 1.4 psi (71). Squeezing the breast manually (using the fingers) can easily generate 6 psi because the force is concentrated over a very small area. Thus, the force of compression is no more likely to cause tumor spread than manual digital examination, a woman lying on her chest, or social interactions. Furthermore, although it is unlikely that compression can squeeze cells into the blood (because the veins likely close down under pressure), merely putting cancer cells in the blood does not mean that they can metastasize. Metastatic spread requires that the cells possess the biological capability to exit the blood and survive in other organ systems.

Experimental data do suggest that the growth rate of metastatic lesions may increase when the primary cancer is removed, but this appears to be a short-lived phenomenon that lasts for only a few hours (70).

Opponents of screening have only looked at the numbers generated by the trials but have not evaluated the trials and the derivation of the numbers themselves. The fact that, in virtually all major studies, mammographically detected cancers have a superior prognosis to those discovered by physical examination demonstrates that the performance of the mammogram itself has no direct detrimental effect. Our own review of women <50 years old compared those whose cancers were detected by mammography to those whose cancers were palpable. Among the women whose cancers had been detected by mammography, the 5-year survival was 95%, whereas those with palpable cancers only had a 74% 5-year survival. Among the women who died in the group with palpable cancer, only one had had a preceding mammogram (72). There is clearly no detrimental effect from the mammogram itself. In the Swedish Two County Trial the mortality from breast cancer was highest among women who were offered mammographic screening but refused (32). These women probably were compromised by their own denial, resulting in delayed diagnosis, although it could be inferred that failure to have a mammogram results in a worsened prognosis.

CLINICAL BREAST EXAMINATION

The lack of scientific analysis that has pervaded the screening controversy was clearly evident in the NCI withdrawal of support for screening women 40 to 49 years old using mammography while at the same time encouraging physicians to continue screening using CBE. Opponents of screening mammography have raised the concern that false-positive mammography leads to too much anxiety and too many unnecessary biopsies (those with benign results). False-positive CBEs cause similar anxiety and result in a higher percentage of unnecessary biopsies than mammographic screening. Spivey showed that in the best of practices 75% to 85% of biopsies instigated by CBE alone prove to be benign (73). In a review of our own patients, the PPV for mammographically instigated biopsies in an asymptomatic screening population was two to three times higher than for CBE, and in that population screening mammograms detected 10 times more of the cancers. Bassett demonstrated that, even in a surgical referral practice in which women with cancer are preselected for evaluation, the PPV for mammography was the same as for CBE whereas the stage at diagnosis for mammographically detected cancers was more favorable (46). If the desired goal is to reduce the number of unnecessary biopsies, clinical examination should be the first test to be stopped.

The lack of consistency in the NCI decision was further evident in the fact that the younger women who were screened by mammography in the HIP trial, the Edinburgh trial, and the NBSS were also screened using CBE. If these trials are used to reject mammography, then they clearly show no benefit for CBE for women between the ages of 40 and 49.

BREAST SELF-EXAMINATION

As noted earlier, the preliminary data from one of the only prospective RCTs that has assessed the efficacy of BSE has not shown a benefit. This study was among Chinese women, who have a low incidence of breast cancer to begin with, and the data were very preliminary. Because most breast cancers are still detected by the individual herself and because mammography and clinical examination in combination appear to miss 5% to 20% of cancers that occur in the interval between screens, monthly BSE would still seem to be prudent.

AT WHAT AGE DOES SCREENING BECOME INEFFECTIVE?

Although not as contentious, the decision as to what age screening should be discontinued has also been raised. There is no simple answer. None of the trials evaluated women older than age 74, and because the numbers of women older than 70 in the trials are so small, statistical power is weak. A task force that evaluated the question con-cluded that the benefits of screening for women over 65 must be balanced against the life expectancy of the individual and competing causes of death. It was concluded that whether to screen should be individualized for older women, taking into account these factors (74).

ECONOMICS AND COST BENEFIT

In 1988, Eddy and colleagues wrote that there was a benefit from screening women in their 40s but that it was expensive, and only women who were willing to pay for it should have access (75). This has clearly been the motivating perspective for health planners. However, rather than stating as bluntly as Eddy that women who could not afford to pay for screening themselves should be denied access, some health planners have avoided the issue by trying to suggest that there is no benefit. If women are to be denied access to screening because planners do not wish to allocate funds for this purpose, they should be told this directly so that the appropriate discussions can be held as to how resources are to be allocated. Health planners should cease invoking and hiding behind flawed science to suggest that there is no benefit.

Although a detailed cost-benefit analysis is beyond the scope of this text, Rosenquist and Lindfors have analyzed the cost of screening and have provided estimates of the cost per year of life saved (76). This is the standard method for comparing different interventions. It should only be used to compare screening to other health care interventions as a gauge of relative cost. They estimated that the marginal cost per year of life saved for annual mammography, beginning by age 40, through age 85, assuming a 30% decrease in mortality, was $18,600. If the same screening did not begin until age 50, the cost would be reduced to $16,800. If only women 40 to 49 years old were screened, the cost would be $26,200. Screening only women between the ages of 60 and 69 would cost $15,500, and screening only women between the ages of 80 and 85 would cost $35,000 (76). The cost per year of life saved for screening women from the age of 40 to the age of 85 is comparable to the cost per year of life saved for coronary artery bypass surgery and is less expensive than the cost of requiring seat belts, renal dialysis, cholesterol treatment, and numerous other interventions (77). Because death from breast cancer is at least five times as high as death from cancer of the cervix, screening for breast cancer is more cost-effective than cervical cancer (Pap) testing (78).

DILUTIONAL NIHILISM

Opponents of screening frequently place the intervention in the context of the entire population. This is appropriate when comparing interventions, but the distortions that this creates must be understood. By analyzing a benefit with respect to the entire population, the results of an intervention can be trivialized and made to appear not worth the effort.

This type of analysis is commonly seen in cost-benefit analyses when the intervention is said to add a number of days of life. This type of analysis that evaluates the benefit in terms of the entire population has been misunderstood by some who take the added days literally. In reality, for example, an individual who is saved from dying from breast cancer at age 40 may have 40 additional years added to her life, but cost-benefit analysis divides this result by the entire population and expresses the benefit in terms of days of life added over the entire population. This is a useful way of comparing different interventions as long as it is not misunderstood to mean that the benefit of an intervention is small.

Another example of how diluting the result can lead to trivialization of the problem can be seen in the requirement that cars have seat belts. In 1994, the National Transportation Safety Council estimated that approximately 5,200 lives are saved each year by seat belts. This can be made to appear insignificant by asking how the entire population benefits. If the benefit of 5,200 lives is diluted over all 250,000,000 Americans, seat belts benefit only 1 in 50,000. Furthermore, approximately 9 million cars are sold each year in the United States. It costs approximately $100 to install a seat belt ($400/car). Thus the cost for seat belts in new cars is $3.6 billion. If this is divided by the 5,200 lives it amounts to $700,000 for each life saved. If the individual is ignored, this same type of analysis could be used to argue that seat belts aren't worth the expense to society. Opponents of screening have used similar arguments to trivialize the benefit of screening for women 40 to 49 years old (see Economics and Cost-Benefit).

It is useful to provide a frame of reference for the screening controversy. Cervical screening is well accepted. What most people do not know is that approximately 12,000 women of all ages are diagnosed with cancer of the cervix each year, and 4,500 women of all ages die of cervical cancer annually. In 1996, approximately 33,000 women in their 40s were diagnosed with breast cancer, and almost 6,000 women died from breast cancer while in their 40s (this does not include women diagnosed in their 40s who died in their 50s or even later). There were more breast cancer deaths among women who had been diagnosed while in their 40s than cervical cancer deaths among all women.

PROOF: STATISTICALLY SIGNIFICANT BENEFIT FOR WOMEN 40 TO 49 YEARS OLD

There has been virtually no argument concerning the efficacy of screening women from the ages of 50 to 69, but despite the inappropriate data analyses many women accepted the NCI arguments against recommending screening women in their 40s. Finally, in the spring of 1996, the screening trialists met in Falun, Sweden, and updated the results from the screening trials with at least 10 years of follow-up. Despite the fact that the trials were not meant to be stratified by age, the data showed a statistically significant

benefit for screening women between the ages of 40 and 49 (53). The new director of the NCI was apprised of these updated results and urged to reconsider the NCI position. He privately acknowledged that the 1993 decision had been a mistake and agreed to review the NCI position.

Aware of the criticism that had been leveled against the NCI and the process that it had used to change the guidelines in 1993, the director sought an objective review of the data. Consequently, in January 1997, at the request of the NCI, a National Institutes of Health Consensus Development Conference (CDC) was convened to review the most recent data on screening women 40 to 49 years old. The CDC is designed as a trial with a panel selected to be the jury and an agenda that provides arguments on both sides of the issue.

The CDC panel for the screening controversy has been represented as a group of objective experts when, in fact many were not experts, having been chosen specifically because they had no previous involvement in the controversy and, hence, little understanding of the issues. Several of the panel members had significant conflicts of interest, including at least three with major NCI funding (the 1993 NCI decision was on trial). The organization of the CDC, the agenda, and the selection of panel members was strongly criticized as the conference was being prepared as being biased against screening. Although the NCI director had promised that NCI would keep hands off, the CDC was organized by the same individual who had been responsible for the 1993 workshop on the same topic that had been the springboard for the NCI guideline change. The premeeting concerns were ignored by the Office of Medical Applications of Research (the NIH group that organizes CDC) and the conference was held.

The CDC panel concluded that there was no evidence to support screening women before the age of 50. The conclusions of the panel were so at variance with the available facts that it engendered heated debate and even a Senate review. The panel issued a statement that was not only full of factually incorrect information but also did not even recognize the new data it had been asked to review. What is not generally known is that one panel member resigned in disagreement following the meeting, and two of 13 others wrote a dissenting opinion that concluded that there were data to support a recommendation to screen women in their 40s.

The data that were ignored by the CDC were subsequently presented to an ACS panel of experts that convened in March 1997 (Fig. 4-15). The data on all of the trials had an average of 12.7 years of follow-up. The trial in Gothenburg, Sweden, revealed a 44% mortality reduction that by itself was statistically significant. The strength of the benefit is reflected in the fact that 30% of the women who died in the Gothenburg trial, among the screened women, had actually refused to be screened (they are still counted as having been screened). The Malmö trial, with increased numbers, revealed a statistically significant reduction of 35%. There are only two trials for women 50 and older that are significant by themselves. When all of the Swedish trials were analyzed together, the

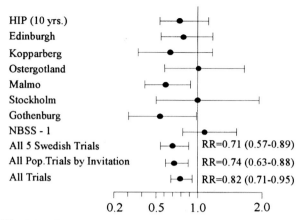

FIG. 4-15. These are the results summarizing the randomized, controlled trials for women between the ages of 40 and 49, as of March 1997, as compiled by Edward Hendrick, Ph.D., and presented to the American Cancer Society. They demonstrate a statistically significant benefit to screening (see Fig. 4-8 for details).

29% benefit was statistically significant. Adding the Edinburgh and HIP data, to combine all of the population-based trials by invitation, provided a 26% benefit that was significant. Even adding the NBSS, with its major differences from the other trials and its other major problems, the significance of a benefit remained (79). Additionally the benefit continues to increase in the trials for these younger women.

Despite having heard the same facts, the CDC panel stunned the conference participants by concluding that there was no benefit. The panel was so out of touch with the facts that its conclusions were immediately repudiated by the director of the NCI, who had been responsible for convening the meeting. The subsequent review by the ACS concluded that there was a clear benefit from screening women between the ages of 40 and 49. The ACS went even further and concluded that—based on analyses of lead time by Moskowitz (34), Tabar (35), and Kerlikowske (41), as well as the fact that the best results in the trials were from Gothenburg where women 40 to 49 years old were screened every 18 months with two-view mammography—annual mammography should be even more effective than the trial data suggest. Consequently, the ACS now recommends that women be screened annually beginning at the age of 40.

In a dramatic turnaround, the NCAB, repudiating the conclusion of the Consensus Panel, advised the NCI to recommend that women in their 40s be screened. This was immediately adopted by the NCI at the end of March 1997, and the controversy was essentially ended.

The unfortunate fact is that there is no biological significance to the age of 50. There was never any justification for using it as a cutoff. The controversy had been essentially manufactured from the inappropriate analysis and improper manipulation of data. There is a statistically significant benefit from screening women beginning by the age of 40. As noted above, the benefit is likely even greater than the trial data reveal because seven of the eight trials were by invitation and diluted by noncompliance and contamination.

SUMMARY

Screening mammography is not the ultimate solution to the problem of breast cancer. Not all lives can be saved even through earlier detection, and it is well known that mammography does not detect all breast cancers, nor are the cancers that are detected by mammography alone always curable. Until methods to prevent breast cancer are devised or a universal cure is discovered, the best opportunity women have of reducing the chance of dying from breast cancer lies in periodic screening using mammography, CBE, and monthly BSE. It is likely that screening can reduce mortality regardless of the age at which it is begun. The available data suggest that younger women should be screened more frequently. Annual screening (not the optional 1- to 2-year interval) should be recommended, certainly for women under the age of 50. The only reason to go to a longer interval for older women is to save money. In this day and age, issues of costs and benefits become mixed with medical recommendations. There are methods available that can lead to cost reduction without sacrificing screening quality, and these should be implemented before support for screening is withdrawn for economic reasons.

RECOMMENDATIONS

As recommended by the ACS, the available data suggest that there is benefit from annually screening all women beginning by the age of 40, using mammography and CBE and encouraging monthly BSE. The only reason to go to a longer time between screenings is economic (to save money). The age at which it is safe to increase the interval between screenings has not been defined. It is not likely 50.

Although there are few data that can be used to evaluate the true age at which screening becomes efficacious, there are anecdotal data to suggest that it is not unreasonable for women to begin screening in their late 30s. In the absence of data it is difficult to be firm concerning the benefit.

Below the age of 35 the risk from radiation begins to be important, and the benefit of screening becomes even less clear as a result. Although there is no study to prove efficacy, women who are at very high risk, such as those with a first-degree relative with premenopausal breast cancer (and possibly inherited BRCA1 or BRCA2 mutations), may wish to begin screening earlier (80). Although there is the unproven concern that these women may be at increased risk from radiation carcinogenesis, their background risk is sufficiently high that the benefits of early detection outweigh the slightly increased risk from the radiation. Because the risk for these women is to develop cancer even earlier than the proband, we currently suggest that these women begin screening 10 years earlier than the age at which their relative was diagnosed.

Because mammography can be expected to miss 15% of cancers, it should not be used to exclude cancer, and a clinically significant abnormality must be addressed despite a negative mammogram. Women should be reminded that a negative screening does not guarantee freedom from breast cancer and that they should bring any changes (regardless of how soon after a negative screening they occur) to their doctor's attention.

Mammography is not the ultimate solution to breast cancer. Intensive research is needed to combat these devastating malignancies, but until a safe prevention technique is devised, a better detection method developed, or a universal cure discovered, screening using mammography offers the best opportunity for reducing the death rate from breast cancer.

REFERENCES

1. Smigel K. Breast cancer death rates decline for white women. J Natl Cancer Inst 1995;87:173.
2. Garne JP, Aspergen K, Balldin G, Ranstam J. Increasing incidence of and declining mortality from breast carcinoma: trends in Malmö, Sweden. 1961–1992. Cancer 1997;79:69–74.
3. Carter CL, Allen C, Henson DE. Relation of tumor size, lymph node status, and survival in 24,740 breast cancer cases. Cancer 1989;63:181–187.
4. Baker LH. Breast cancer detection demonstration project: five-year summary report. CA Cancer J Clin 1982;32:194–225.
5. Tabar L, Duffy SW, Burhenne LW. New Swedish breast cancer detection results for women aged 40–49. Cancer 1993;72:1437–1448.
6. Tarone RE. The excess of patients with advanced breast cancers in young women screened with mammography in the Canadian National Breast Screening Study. Cancer 1995;75:997–1003.
7. Skrabanek P. Breast cancer screening with mammography. Lancet 1993;341:1531.
8. Wright C, Mueller CB. Screening mammography and public health policy: the need for perspective. Lancet 1995;348:29–32.
9. Lachin JM. Introduction to sample size determination and power analysis for clinical trials. Controlled Clin Trials 1981;2:93–113.
10. Elwood JM, Cox B, Richardson AK. The effectiveness of breast cancer screening by mammography in younger women. Online J Curr Clin Trials 1993;32.
11. Adami H, Malker B, Holmberg L, et al. The relation between survival and age at diagnosis in breast cancer. N Engl J Med 1986;315:559–563.
12. D'Orsi CJ. To follow or not to follow, that is the question. Radiology 1992;184:306.
13. Peer PG, Holland R, Jan HCL, et al. Age-specific effectiveness of Nijmegen population-based breast cancer-screening program: assessment of early indicators of screening effectiveness. J Natl Cancer Inst 1994;86:436–441.
14. Shapiro S. Evidence on screening for breast cancer from a randomized trial. Cancer 1977;39:2772–2778.
15. Shapiro S, Venet W, Venet L, Roeser R. Ten- to fourteen-year effect of screening on breast cancer mortality. J Natl Cancer Inst 1982;69:349–355.
16. Shapiro S, Venet W, Strax P, Venet L. Periodic Screening for Breast Cancer: The Health Insurance Plan Project and Its Sequelae, 1963–1986. Baltimore: Johns Hopkins University Press, 1988.
17. Smart CR, Byrne C, Smith RA, et al. Twenty-year follow-up of the breast cancers diagnosed during the Breast Cancer Detection Demonstration Project. CA Cancer J Clin 1997;47:134–149.
18. Fletcher SW, Black W, Harris R, et al. Report of the International Workshop on Screening for Breast Cancer. J Natl Cancer Inst 1993;85:1644–1656.
19. Shapiro S. Screening: assessment of current studies. Cancer 1994;74:231–238.
20. Nystrom L, Rutqvist LE, Wall S, et al. Breast cancer screening with mammography: overview of Swedish randomised trials. Lancet 1993;341:973–978.
21. Tabar L, Fagerberg CJG, Gad A, et al. Reduction in mortality from breast cancer after mass screening with mammography. Lancet 1985;1:829–832.
22. Muir BB, Kirkpatrick A, Roberts MM, Duffy SW. Oblique-view mammography: adequacy for screening. Radiology 1984;151:39–41.
23. Wald NJ, Murphy P, Major P, et al. UKCCCR multicentre randomised controlled trial of one and two view mammography in breast cancer screening. BMJ 1995;311:1189–1193.
24. Anderson I, Aspergen K, Janzon L, et al. Mammographic screening and mortality from breast cancer: the Malmö mammographic screening trial. BMJ 1988;297:943–948.
25. Frisell J, Glas U, Hellstrom L, Somell A. Randomized Mammographic Screening for Breast Cancer in Stockholm. In Breast Cancer Research and Treatment. Boston: Martinus-Nijhoff, 1986;8:45–54.
26. Roberts MM, Alexander TJ, Anderson TJ, et al. Edinburgh trial of screening for breast cancer: mortality at seven years. Lancet 1990;335:241–246.
27. Miller AB, Baines CJ, To T, Wall C. Canadian National Breast Screening Study: 1. Breast cancer detection and death rates among women aged 40–49. Can Med Assoc J 1992;147:1459–1476.
28. Miller AB, Baines CJ, To T, Wall C. Canadian National Breast Screening Study: 2. Breast cancer detection and death rates among women aged 50–59. Can Med Assoc J 1992;147:1477–1594.
29. Wald N, Chamberlin J, Hackshaw A, et al. Consensus conference on breast cancer screening: report of the evaluation committee. Oncology 1994;51:380–389.
30. Thomas DB, Dao LG, Self SG, et al. Randomized trial of breast self-examination in Shanghai: methodology and preliminary results. J Natl Cancer Inst 1997;89:355–365.
31. Clay MG, Hiskop G, Kan L, et al. Screening mammography in British Columbia 1988–1993. Am J Surg 1994;167:490–492.
32. Tabar L, Duffy SW, Krusemo UB. Detection method, tumor size and node metastases in breast cancers diagnosed during a trial of breast cancer screening. Eur J Cancer Clin Oncol 1987;23:959–962.
33. Chu KC, Smart CR, Tarone RE. Analysis of breast cancer mortality and stage distribution by age for the Health Insurance Plan clinical trial. J Natl Cancer Inst 1988;80:1125–1132.
34. Moskowitz M. Breast cancer: age-specific growth rates and screening strategies. Radiology 1986;161:37–41.
35. Tabar L, Faberberg G, Day NE, Holmberg L. What is the optimum interval between mammographic screening examinations? An analysis based on the latest results of the Swedish two-county breast screening trial. Br J Cancer 1989;55:547–551.
36. Misused Science: The National Cancer Institutes Elimination of Mammography Guidelines for Women in Their Forties. Washington, DC: House Committee on Government Operations; 1994. House Report 103-863.
37. Smith RA. Epidemiology of Breast Cancer in a Categorical Course in Physics: Technical Aspects of Breast Imaging (2nd ed). Oak Brook, IL: RSNA Publications, 1993;21–33.
38. Kopans DB. "Conventional wisdom": observation, experience, anecdote and science in breast imaging. AJR Am J Roentgenol 1994;162:299–303.
39. Prechtel K. Mastopathic und Altersabhangige Brystdrusen Verandernagen. Fortschr Med 1971;89:1312–1315.
40. Stomper PC, D'Souza DJ, DiNitto PA, Arredondo MA. Analysis of parenchymal density on mammograms in 1353 women 25–79 years old. AJR Am J Roentgenol 1996;167:1261–1265.
41. Kerlikowske K, Grady D, Barclay J, et al. Positive predictive value of screening mammography by age and family history of breast cancer. JAMA 1993;270:2444–2450.
42. Sox H. Screening mammography in women younger than 50 years of age. Ann Intern Med 1995;122:550–552.
43. Frankel SD, Sickles EA, Cupren BN, et al. Initial versus subsequent screening mammography: comparison of findings and their prognostic significance. AJR Am J Roentgenol 1995;164:1107–1109.
44. Kopans DB. The use of mammography for screening. JAMA 1994;271:982.
45. Sickles EA, Herzog KA. Mammography of the postsurgical breast. AJR Am J Roentgenol 1981;136:585–588.
46. Bassett LW, Liu TH, Giuliano AE, Gold RH. The prevalence of carcinoma in palpable vs impalpable mammographically detected lesions. AJR Am J Roentgenol 1991;157:21–24.
47. Miller AB, Howe GR, Wall C. The national study of breast cancer screening. Clin Invest Med 1981;4:227–258.
48. Kopans DB, Halperin E, Hulka CA. Statistical power in breast cancer screening trials and mortality reduction among women 40–49 with particular emphasis on the National Breast Screening Study of Canada. Cancer 1994;74:1196–1203.

49. Eckhardt S, Badellino F, Murphy GP. UICC meeting on breast-cancer screening in premenopausal women in developed countries. Int J Cancer 1994;56:1–5.

50. Eyre H, Sondik E, Smith RA. Joint meeting on the feasibility of a study of screening premenopausal women (40–49 years) for breast cancer: April 20–21, 1994. Cancer 1995;75:1391–1403.

51. Kerlikowske K, Grady D, Barclay J, et al. Likelihood ratios for modern screening mammography: risk of breast cancer based on age and mammographic interpretation. JAMA 1996;276:39–43.

52. Prorok PC, Hankey BF, Bundy BN. Concepts and problems in the evaluation of screening programs. J Chronic Dis 1981;34:159–171.

53. Tabar L, Duffy SW, Chen HH. Re: quantitative interpretation of age-specific mortality reductions from the Swedish breast cancer screening trials. J Natl Cancer Inst 1996;88:52–53.

54. Tabar L, Larson LG, Andersson I, et al. Breast cancer screening with mammography in women aged 40–49. Report of the Organizing Committee and Collaborators, Falun Meeting; 21–22 March, 1996; Falun, Sweden. Int J Cancer 1996;68:693–699.

55. Moss S, Alexander F. Presentation to the International Union Against Cancer (UICC) meeting on Breast Cancer Screening in Premenopausal Women in Developed Countries. September 29–October 1, 1993; Geneva, Switzerland.

56. Smart CR, Hartmann WH, Beahrs OH, Garfinkel L. Insights into breast cancer screening of younger women. Cancer 1993;72:1437–1448.

57. Sickles EA, Kopans DB. Deficiencies in the analysis of breast cancer screening data. J Natl Cancer Inst 1993;85:1621–1624.

58. Linvers M, Paster SB. Success of screening mammography in the private practice setting in detecting early breast cancer in women age 40–49 versus over age 50. Presented at the Society of Breast Imaging; May 10–13, 1995; Orlando, Florida.

59. Liberman L, Dershaw DD, Deutch BM, et al. Screening mammography: value in women 35–39 years old. AJR Am J Roentgenol 1993; 161:53–56.

60. Kopans DB. The Canadian screening program: a different perspective. AJR Am J Roentgenol 1990;155:748–749.

61. Kopans DB, Meyer JE, Cohen AM, Wood WC. Palpable breast masses: the importance of preoperative mammography. JAMA 1981; 246:2819–2822.

62. Miller AB, Baines CJ, Turnbull C. The role of the nurse-examiner in the National Breast Screening Study. Can J Public Health 1991;82:162–167.

63. Baines CJ, Miller AB, Kopans DB, et al. Canadian National Breast Screening Study: time-related changes in mammographic technical quality—an external review. AJR Am J Roentgenol 1990;155: 743–747.

64. Yaffe MJ. Correction: Canada study [letter]. J Natl Cancer Inst 1993;85:94.

65. Baines CJ, McFarlane DV, Miller AB. The role of the reference radiologist. Estimate of inter-observer agreement and potential delay in cancer detection in the National Breast Screening Study. Invest Radiol 1990;25:971–976.

66. Bailar J, MacMahon B. Can Med Assoc J 1996;156:193–199.

67. Joensu H, Klemi PJ, Tuominen J, et al. Breast cancer found at screening and previous detection by women themselves [letter]. Lancet 1992;339:315.

68. Andersson I, Hildell J, Muhlow A, Pettersson H. Number of projections in mammography: influence on detection of breast disease. AJR Am J Roentgenol 1978;130:349–351.

69. Watmough DJ, Quan KM. X-ray mammography and breast compression [letter]. Lancet 1992;340:122.

70. Van Dierendonck JH, Keijzer R, Cornelisse CJ, Van De Velde CJH. Surgically induced cytokinetic responses in experimental rat mammary tumor models. Cancer 1991;68:759–767.

71. Russell DG, Ziewacz JT. Pressure in a simulated breast subjected to compression forces comparable to those of mammography. Radiology 1995;194:383–387.

72. Stacey-Clear A, McCarthy KA, Hall DA, et al. Breast cancer survival among women under age 50: is mammography detrimental? Lancet 1992;340:991–994.

73. Spivey GH, Perry BW, Clark VA, et al. Predicting the risk of cancer at the time of breast biopsy. Am Surg 1982;48:326–332.

74. Kopans DB. Mammography screening for women over 65. J Gerontol 1992;47:59–62.

75. Eddy DM, Hasselblad V, McGivney W, Hendee W. The value of mammography screening in women under 50 years. JAMA 1988;259: 1512–1519.

76. Rosenquist CJ, Lindfors KK. Screening mammography in women aged 40–49 years: analysis of cost-effectiveness. Radiology 1994; 191:647–650.

77. Tengs TO, Adams M, Pliskin JS, et al. Five hundred life-saving interventions and their cost-effectiveness. Risk Anal 1995;15.

78. Mass PJ, Koning HJ, Inveld M, et al. The cost-effectiveness of breast cancer screening. Int J Cancer 1989;43:1055–1060.

79. Hendrick RE, Smith RA, Rutledge JH, Smart CR. Benefit of screening mammography in women ages 40–49: a new meta-analysis of randomized controlled trials. J Natl Cancer Institute (in press).

80. Burke W, Daly M, Garber J, et al. Recommendations for follow-up care of individuals with an inherited predisposition to cancer. JAMA 1997;277:997–1003.

Breast Imaging, 2nd ed., by Daniel B. Kopans.
Lippincott–Raven Publishers, Philadelphia © 1998.

CHAPTER 5

Radiation Risk

By 1976, the Health Insurance Plan of New York study had begun to demonstrate the benefits of screening. The Breast Cancer Detection Demonstration Project was under way when Bailar raised the concern that radiation doses required for mammography in the 1960s might induce as many cancers as might be cured from mammographic early detection (1). This pessimistic evaluation resulted in a marked reduction in the use of mammography. A reassessment of potential radiation risk was stimulated, as was research into techniques for reducing mammographic doses. Despite years of evaluation and favorable analyses, opponents of mammographic screening continue to raise questions concerning the safety of mammography.

IONIZING RADIATION AS A CARCINOGEN

Ionizing radiation is a known carcinogen. There is little question that exposure to high doses of radiation increases the risk of developing breast cancer. The likely mechanism is damage to chromosomal DNA from the free radicals that are produced when high-energy photons are absorbed in tissues. Chromosome breaks are known to occur from ionizing radiation.

The effects of radiation are not uniform, however, and depend to a great extent on the organs being irradiated. Skin and bone, for example, are relatively insensitive to radiation, whereas blood cells are fairly sensitive. The effects on the breast vary with dose and the age at which the woman is exposed. At high doses, the risk of radiation appears to be linear, with risk increasing in direct proportion to exposure. The relationship is less clear at lower doses. The few data available can support a linear relationship or a linear quadratic relationship (2) (Fig. 5-1). The linear quadratic relationship begins with a lower risk at the lower-dose exposures than the straight linear relationship and at higher doses is very similar to the straight line model.

Disagreement has resulted from the uncertainties surrounding the possible effects (or lack of effect) associated with the low doses used for modern mammography. Bailar's analysis was based on doses required to expose the high-detail, fine-grain industrial film that was used without intensifying screens in the 1960s and in the early years of mammography. Exposures at that time frequently exceeded

several rads (cGy) per image. By the time radiation risk became an issue, doses had already been significantly reduced following the introduction of the xeroradiographic technique, which reduced doses to under 2 rads (2 cGy) and eventually to under 1 rad (1 cGy). Development of lower-dose film-screen combinations has lowered exposure requirements even further, so that modern film-screen systems require well under 0.2 rads (0.2 cGy) per exposure for an average size breast.

There has never been any direct evidence that the doses required for modern mammography have any effect on the breast, particularly among women over the age of 40 in whom screening is beneficial. There is no scientific evidence that anyone ever has or ever will develop breast cancer as the result of a mammogram. All analyses of radiation carcinogenesis in the breast are based on extrapolation from populations exposed to doses that are at least two orders of magnitude higher than those required for x-ray mammography.

EVIDENCE OF INCREASED RISK OF BREAST CANCER FROM HIGH-DOSE RADIATION EXPOSURE

The evidence demonstrating the relationship of breast irradiation to excess cancer risk comes from studies of several groups of women who were exposed to moderate or large doses of radiation. The largest group included women among the more than 90,000 individuals who survived nuclear bombing but who were exposed to radiation at Hiroshima and Nagasaki (3,4). Another analysis comes from women who were treated with radiation for ankylosing spondylitis from the 1930s to the early 1950s (5). In the 1940s and 1950s approximately 600 women were treated with therapeutic doses of radiation (60 to 1,400 rads) for mastitis (6), and almost 40,000 women have been studied who underwent repeated chest fluoroscopies between 1930 and the early 1950s to monitor their pneumothorax treatment for tuberculosis (7–9). The preponderance of data from studying these women has demonstrated a subsequent increased incidence of breast cancer among those exposed to high doses of radiation. More recent studies have shown a similar risk for women irradiated for Hodgkin's disease (10–12) (see Etiology and Risk Factors in Chapter 2). These studies leave little

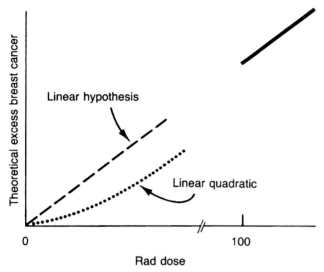

FIG. 5-1. Theoretical excess breast cancer as a result of exposure to radiation. The schematic is predicated on absolute risk assessment. The linear extrapolation from high-dose data down to mammographic levels below 1 rad is a conservative estimate. The more gradual curve of the linear quadratic is favored by many physicists.

doubt that exposure to ionizing radiation increases the risk. However, debate continues over the magnitude of the risk and its applicability for those exposed to low doses.

GENETIC ABNORMALITIES

Altered or damaged DNA appears to be the major mechanism involved in the development of breast cancers. There is some concern that women who already have, through the inheritance of damaged genes, abnormalities of DNA that predispose them to the development of malignancy may be at greater risk from carcinogens than the average individual. Some investigators have speculated that women who harbor the BRCA1 or BRCA2 gene may be at increased risk from these exposures. At this time, these concerns have not been validated. One investigator raised a great deal of concern by suggesting that those who carry the ataxia-telangiectasia gene may be at increased risk.

Ataxia-Telangiectasia Gene

A 1991 report in *The New England Journal of Medicine* suggested that women who were heterozygotes (one abnormal copy) for the ataxia-telangiectasia gene were at increased risk for radiation-induced breast cancer. This was based on a case-control study of relatives of homozygotes who had the syndrome. The authors warned that heterozygotes were estimated to make up 1% of the population, and as there is as yet no test to determine heterozygosity, they argued that all women should avoid breast radiation exposure (13). This con-

cern is an extrapolation from the fact that homozygotes are known to be extremely sensitive to radiation. They postulated that the increased risk seen in homozygotes exposed to radiation would be reflected in their heterozygote relatives.

The conclusions of this study were based on a comparison of cases with unmatched controls and a very limited sample with serious flaws. Obligate heterozygotes (blood relatives of homozygotes have one bad copy of the gene) were questioned about their exposure to diagnostic x-ray studies and the incidence of breast cancer among these women was then compared to spouses (no blood relationship), who were less likely to harbor the gene. The authors found a greater number of breast cancers among the heterozygotes and raised the warning.

Numerous letters to the editor disputed the authors' conclusions (14–18). Among the problems with the study, including the small sample size, was the lack of dosimetry. Although the authors cautioned against mammography, exposure to mammography was not even determined in the study. The majority of the exposures were from angiographic studies that exposed the breasts to less than background radiation. A major bias was the fact that the study group was older than the controls (breast cancer incidence is higher in older women). Other risk factors were not accounted for, and the reasons for undergoing x-ray studies were not solicited. The authors built their arguments on previous assumptions that they supported with their own previous work, which was similarly built on their own previous assumptions. The concerns raised by this paper are not supported scientifically and are likely incorrect. Nevertheless, as a greater understanding of the molecular biology of breast cancer develops, it may be possible to identify additional factors that predispose an individual and make her more sensitive to the many environmental carcinogens as well as radiation.

SIGNIFICANCE OF RADIATION RISK

It would be preferable to clearly demonstrate that there is no increased risk of cancer from mammographic dose levels, but this is not possible. It has been estimated that, because even the theoretical risk is so low, 100 million women would need to participate in a study to have the statistical power to confirm or disprove a significant effect on the breast at such low doses. It is impossible to perform a study that could demonstrate a true carcinogenic effect for mammographic doses below 1 rad (1 cGy), and conversely it is impossible to ever prove that a mammogram involves no risk. Compounding the difficulty in studying the effects is that even exposure to high doses does not increase the risk immediately. There is a latent period of 5 to 10 years before excess cancers begin to appear.

Not only is it impossible to predict specifically who will develop breast cancer, but the effects of low-level radiation on the breast are difficult to measure because of the relatively small magnitude of the effect and the fact that these cancers are no different morphologically or histologically from naturally occurring breast cancers.

Even at high doses, radiation exposure does not induce cancers in most women. It only increases the risk, and it is only a small number (in absolute terms) of women exposed who develop breast cancer as a result. On the basis of data from women exposed to very high doses and using an absolute risk model (the risk is the same no matter what the age at exposure), it appears that an exposure to approximately 2 Gy (200 rads) is needed to double a woman's risk. A rough estimate is that if approximately two women of 1,000 in a population develop breast cancer normally each year, exposing the breasts of all of the 1,000 women to 200 rads (approximately 1,000 times the dose of a mammogram) would increase the incidence to four cancers per year starting 5 to 10 years after the exposure. The incidence is doubled, but the absolute number is small, accounting for the difficulty in firmly establishing risk or safety.

LOW-DOSE RISK ESTIMATES AND RELATIONSHIP TO AGE AT EXPOSURE

Controversy remains about the effects of doses below the 1 rad (1 cGy) mammographic level. Some physicists favor a linear quadratic response that would suggest a lower risk than the straight linear extrapolation from the high-dose data, which is usually considered the worst-case situation (see Fig. 5-1). In 1990 the National Research Council issued a report titled Health Effects of Exposure to Low Levels of Ionizing Radiation: BEIR V (19). Based on a review of the available data, the Committee on the Biological Effects of Ionizing Radiation has calculated the potential excess breast cancer risk from radiation. They concluded that the available data showed that risk varied with the age at exposure, with risk decreasing among women exposed at older ages, and that "there is little evidence of any increased risk to women exposed after age 40."

The only study that has not demonstrated that risk decreases with age is the study of women who were treated with radiation for postpartum mastitis. It is possible that the cells of the breast tissues of these women were more susceptible to damage due to the active cell proliferation or some synergy with inflammation that the tissues were likely experiencing at the time of exposure (20).

Another way of evaluating risk is using a relative risk model. The carcinogenic potential of radiation is highest when young women are exposed and decreases with the age of the woman at the time of exposure. The expression of that risk represents a constant factor over time based on the age at exposure for the fraction of dose sustained at that age, but the excess cancers are in proportion to the incidence of the individual at the attained age. This means that successive exposures over time have incrementally diminishing relative effect as the patient ages. As noted above, the effect of radiation is also not immediate, and excess cancers do not begin to appear until 5 to 10 years after exposure (latency period). It appears that the excess of cancers that can be attributed to radiation are proportionate to the attained age of the individual. In other words, just as the natural incidence of breast cancer increases with age, the additional cancers that appear to be radiation induced also increase with age.

The BEIR V experts developed a refinement of the radiation risk model to account for these relative risks based on the age at the time of exposure and the subsequent proportionate risk as the patient ages. The model accounts for the decreasing impact of radiation exposure with age and also the age-related increasing incidence. By weighting the increased risk in relation to the age at exposure and adjusting the excess, induced cancers in proportion to the normal incidence of naturally occurring breast cancers at given, subsequent ages, one can predict the theoretical radiation-induced excess breast cancer risk over an individual's lifetime. This risk model also takes into account a latency period following exposure in which no excess cancer is expected.

Stated more simply, the relative risk factor diminishes with age, and equivalent exposures have less significance for older women. Women exposed in preadolescence and in their teens are subject to a much higher risk than women exposed to radiation in the fourth and fifth decades of life. The risk at even high-exposure doses of radiation appears to diminish significantly by the age of 40. Data from Canada, reviewing a cohort of tuberculosis patients exposed to the radiation of fluoroscopy, suggest that there may be no risk at all at any dose level for women exposed after the age of 35 to 40 years (21).

There has been one report from Sweden that suggests that some risk may persist beyond age 40 (22). The patients in that study, however, were radiated for benign conditions, and their risk may be due to the fact that they were already at higher risk (23).

Because the risk of radiation carcinogenesis for the breast decreases with the age at exposure, by the age of 35 to 40 there is probably an extremely low risk or, likely, none at all. In a large case-control study, Boice reviewed the incidence of contralateral breast cancer in women who had breast cancer in the ipsilateral breast treated with radiation (15). The ipsilateral breast received an average of 3 Gy (300 rads) of scatter radiation from the treated breast, yet there was no increased risk of contralateral cancer with more than 20 years of follow-up for women over the age of 45. Unfortunately, there were not sufficient numbers of women at younger ages to make the age of 40 the point of analysis, but with less statistical certainty, there appears to be little or no increased risk in this population (24).

The relative risks for women who are older than 40 are small, and there may, in fact, be no excess risk for women who are exposed to radiation over age 40. As stated earlier, any potential risk of radiation carcinogenesis for women over the age of 40 is so small that a randomized, controlled study would require so many women as to be impossible to perform. There are, in fact, no studies that show that exposure to mammographic levels of x-ray among women of screening age (40 and above) carries any additional risk. A reassessment of the Japanese atomic bomb data suggests that even the high-

TABLE 5-1. *Ratio of benefit to risk for women who begin annual mammographic screening by the age of 35 assuming a benefit of 5% at age 35 increasing to 25% by age 75*

Attained age	Benefit to risk ratio
40	> 400
45	352
50	66
55	47
60	37
65	38
65	33
70	29
75	27

Source: Adapted from Mettler FA, Upton AC, Kelsey CA, et al. Benefits versus risks from mammography: a critical assessment. Cancer 1996;77:903–909.

exposure risks may have been overestimated (25). In the Swedish Two County Trial of mammography screening, in which more than 100,000 women have undergone repeated mammograms since the 1970s, there has been no increase in cancer incidence associated with the screened group.

Mettler and colleagues performed a comprehensive review of the data and concluded that if there is even a 5% benefit from screening that benefit outweighs even the theoretical risk for screening women beginning at the age of 35 (26). As shown in Table 5-1, if a woman begins screening by the age of 35, the benefit-to-risk ratio remains favorable.

Decreased Radiation Risk with Age?

Given the likelihood that cancers may lie dormant for many years after initiation and that there may be many years between promotion and discovery of the tumor, it is difficult to determine when a breast cancer begins. Many breast cancers may be initiated early in a woman's life. One of the periods during which initiation is likely to occur is during breast development. During puberty and into the third and fourth decade of life, ducts are formed and terminal differentiation takes place to form the glandular tissues of the breast and the terminal duct lobular units. Active cell division occurs at a high rate during this time, and it has been shown that DNA damage or mutation is more likely to occur, and not be repaired, during periods of rapid cell division. This period then becomes a window of opportunity during which exposure to a carcinogen or spontaneous mutation is more likely to be retained and have a deleterious effect.

Evidence of the initiation of breast cancers early in life, during breast development, is found among certain types of mice. In susceptible strains, a carcinogen given during breast development results in a high percentage of breast cancers. If the same carcinogen is given after breast development is complete, breast cancer induction does not occur (27). That a similar window may exist in humans is suggested by the fact that a woman who has her first full-term pregnancy by age 18 has one-third to one-half the risk of

developing a breast cancer as a woman whose first full-term pregnancy occurs after age 30. A possible explanation for this is that a full-term pregnancy causes the rapid completion of breast development and terminal differentiation of the lobule in preparation for lactation. It is possible that the diminution in risk is due to the fact that the period of breast development, during which a carcinogen is more likely to be effective, is shortened by an early full-term pregnancy.

As a carcinogen, it is likely that radiation acts in a similar fashion. Exposure of breast tissue to radiation during active terminal differentiation may result in a higher risk of damage than exposures later in life when the lobules are beginning to involute.

The data suggest that by the time a woman is 40 years old there is probably no risk to the breast from radiation. Although there is the possibility that these events can occur at any time and the time of initiation remains uncertain, the importance of high-quality imaging should be the primary goal for mammography. If improvements in breast cancer detection can be made, they would even justify some increase in dose. Additional efforts to reduce dose should not result in reduced image quality. If image quality can be maintained, efforts to lower dose are desirable.

FILM-SCREEN MAMMOGRAPHY AND RADIATION RISK

Modern two-view film-screen mammography requires only about 0.2 to 0.3 rad (2 to 4 mGy) exposure to the breast. Using the absolute risk model, this suggests an overall theoretical risk of one in a million of inducing a carcinoma with mammography and a lower risk for women 40 and over. Hendrick has used the BEIR V calculations to predict the possible risks from screening using the relative risk model (Table 5-2). Based on the conservative estimates of BEIR V, Hendrick has calculated that performing two-view mammograms every year beginning at age 40 on through age 75 might cause 13.8 excess breast cancer deaths among a group of 100,000

TABLE 5-2. *Extrapolated estimates from the BEIR V report of possible lifetime breast cancer mortality as a result of a single mammographic study at a given age (two views of each breast) and a total of 300 mrad (3 mGy) to each breast*

Age exposed	Total potential risk of breast cancer mortality
20	2.5 per 100,000 women
25	2.3 per 100,000 women
30	2.0 per 100,000 women
35	1.7 per 100,000 women
40	1.3 per 100,000 women
45	0.9 per 100,000 women
50	0.6 per 100,000 women
55	0.3 per 100,000 women
60	0.1 per 100,000 women
65	0.02 per 100,000 women

Source: Courtesy of R. Edward Hendrick, Ph.D.

TABLE 5-3. *Extrapolated from the BEIR V report: estimates of the potential total risk of excess breast cancer death from annual mammographic study (two views of each breast) and a total of 300 mrad (3 mGy) to each breast each year**

Age exposed	Total potential risk of breast cancer mortality
20	54.1 per 100,000 women
25	41.9 per 100,000 women
30	30.9 per 100,000 women
35	21.4 per 100,000 women
40	13.8 per 100,000 women
45	8.9 per 100,000 women
50	3.9 per 100,000 women
55	1.5 per 100,000 women
60	0.4 per 100,000 women
65	0.04 per 100,000 women

*It should be noted that, over the same period of time, more than 3,000 deaths would occur as a result of naturally occurring breast cancers among women who are not screened.
Source: Courtesy of R. Edward Hendrick, Ph.D.

women (Table 5-3). It must be remembered that this is an extrapolated figure, and there will likely be no cancer deaths caused by 35 years of mammograms starting at age 40. Furthermore, over the same period more than 9,000 cancers would occur naturally (28) among 100,000 women, and at least 3,000 of these women would die of breast cancer if they were not screened. Since screening can reduce the death rate by 25% to 30%, 750 to 1,000 lives could be saved by annual mammography at the risk of possibly losing 13.8 lives due to radiation-induced cancers. This extrapolated mortality figure of 13.8 per 100,000 is probably an overestimate, if for no other reason than that screening would be expected to reduce this death rate by 25% to 30% as well, but there may be no risk from mammographic radiation among these women.

Statistical arguments are frequently not reassuring, but many of the risks of daily life that we willingly assume are as life-threatening, if not more threatening, than the theoretical (and possibly nonexistent) risk of radiogenic breast cancer at mammographic doses (Table 5-4).

TABLE 5-4. *Risks of daily living that increase the chance of dying by one chance in a million**

Breathing Boston or New York air for 2 days (air pollution)
Riding a bicycle 10 miles (accident)
Driving in a car 300 miles (accident)
Flying 1,000 miles by jet (accident)
Eating 40 tablespoons of peanut butter (aflatoxin B–induced cancer)
Being a man aged 60 in the next 20 minutes

*This is a partial list of everyday risks (adapted from Wilson Technology Review 1979 and Pochin 1978) that increase the chance of dying by one in a million, which is the risk a woman incurs from a mammogram assuming an absolute risk model. Since radiation risk is age-related, the risk of mammography for women 35 years of age and over is considerably lower and approaches zero.

Women for whom mammographic screening is likely to benefit are at very low risk, if any, for tumor induction from the radiation.

RISK TO A DEVELOPING FETUS

As with any x-ray procedure, it is generally desirable to avoid radiation to a pregnant woman. If a mammogram is requested for routine screening, we generally postpone it if there is the possibility that a patient may be pregnant, merely as a conservative precaution.

In fact, the uterus receives a minuscule amount of radiation from a two-view mammographic exposure. Any exposure would come primarily from the craniocaudal view. Since the primary beam is blocked by the cassette holder and "bucky," the transmission through it is only about 1/5,000 of the incident radiation or approximately 0.2 mR. If it is assumed that the uterus is 10 cm deep within the pelvis, the dose to the uterus would be about 1/1,000 of the entry dose (approximately 0.0002 mR).

Scattered radiation from the two views would be approximately 0.000002 mR to the uterus. All together (scatter plus primary beam) the exposure to the uterus from two views of each breast would be about 0.0004 mR. A fetus normally receives approximately 2 mR each week just from background radiation. Thus, the possible contribution from mammography is virtually zero.

If a mammogram is clinically important, there should be no hesitation. For psychological reasons, we place a lead apron around the patient's pelvis, but this is not scientifically indicated.

CONCLUSION

As with any test, risk must be weighed against potential benefit. The potential risk from radiation cannot be ignored, but this theoretical possibility must be viewed in conjunction with the reduction in breast cancer mortality shown by the randomized and controlled screening programs and other trials using mammography relative to the lack of success in reducing overall breast cancer mortality without screening. Most data demonstrate that age at exposure is the most important factor in x-ray carcinogenesis. Among women in whom the likelihood of cancer is low, and thus the benefit of early detection is low, mammography should probably be avoided unless an expected benefit for the specific individual is anticipated. Mammography is almost exclusively a screening technology, and its use should be limited to those women among whom screening has been shown to be beneficial.

The use of mammography in any woman, symptomatic or otherwise, who is under the age of 40 is anecdotal. National standards of care should be based on scientific data. Because mammography is not diagnostic in the strict definition of the term, its use to evaluate a clinically evident abnormality is limited. Its use is primarily for screening the remainder of the breast involved as well as the contralateral breast for clinically occult malignancy. The screening data have all evaluated women ages 40 and over. One study that evaluated screening women 35 to 39 years old found the same breast cancer detection rate for these women (1.6/1,000) as for women 40 to 45 years old (29), suggesting that the benefit from screening these women would likely be the same as for women between the ages of 40 and 45. Because there are no data to support screening women under the age of 35, the efficacy of mammography, even among symptomatic women, has not been proved and therefore should not be adopted as a standard of care. In the absence of proof of efficacy, each practitioner must be guided by experience as to whether or not to use mammography for evaluating a particular individual who is under the age of 35.

REFERENCES

1. Bailar JC. Mammography: a contrary view. Ann Intern Med 1976; 84:77–84.
2. Feig SA, Hendrick RE. Risk, Benefit, and Controversies in Mammographic Screening. In Haus AG, Yaffe MJ (eds), Syllabus: A Categorical Course in Physics. Technical Aspects of Breast Imaging (2nd ed). Oak Park, IL: RSNA, 1993;119–135.
3. McGregor DH, Land CE, Choi K, et al. Breast cancer incidence among atomic bomb survivors, Hiroshima and Nagasaki, 1950–1969. J Natl Cancer Inst 1977;59:799.
4. Tokunga M, Norman JE, Asano M, et al. Malignant breast tumors among atomic bomb survivors, Hiroshima and Nagasaki, 1950–1974. J Natl Cancer Inst 1979;62:1347.
5. Lewis CA, Smith PG, Stratton IM, et al. Estimated radiation doses to different organs among patients treated for ankylosing spondylitis with a single course of x-rays. Br J Radiol 1988;61:212–220.
6. Mettler FA, Hempelmann LH, Dutton AM, et al. Breast neoplasms in women treated with x-rays for acute postpartum mastitis: a pilot study. J Natl Cancer Inst 1969;43:803.
7. MacKenzie I. Breast cancer following multiple fluoroscopies. Br J Cancer 1965;19:1.
8. Myrden JA, Hiltz JE. Breast cancer following multiple fluoroscopies during artificial pneumothorax treatment of pulmonary tuberculosis. Can Med Assoc J 1969;100:1032.
9. Boice JD, Monson RB. Breast cancer following repeated fluoroscopic examinations of the chest. J Natl Cancer Inst 1977;59:823.
10. Janjan NA, Wilson JF, Gillin M, et al. Mammary carcinoma developing after radiotherapy and chemotherapy for Hodgkin's disease. Cancer 1988;61:252–254.
11. Dershaw D, Yahalom J, Petrek JA. Breast carcinoma in women previously treated for Hodgkin's disease: mammographic evaluation. Radiology 1992;184:421–423.
12. Bhatia S, Robison LL, Oberlin O, et al. Breast cancer and other second neoplasms after childhood Hodgkin's disease. N Engl J Med 1996;334:745–751.
13. Swift M, Morrell D, Massey RB, Chase CL. Incidence of cancer in 161 families affected by ataxia-telangiectasia. N Engl J Med 1991; 325:1831–1836.
14. Kuller LH, Modran B. Risk of breast cancer in ataxia-telangiectasia [letter]. N Engl J Med 1992;326:1357.
15. Boice JD. Risk of breast cancer in ataxia-telangiectasia [letter]. N Engl J Med 1992;326:1358.
16. Wagner LK. Risk of breast cancer in ataxia-telangiectasia [letter]. N Engl J Med 1992;326:1359.
17. Hall EJ, Geard CR, Brenner DJ. Risk of breast cancer in ataxia-telangiectasia [letter]. N Engl J Med 1992;326:1359.
18. Land CE. Risk of breast cancer in ataxia-telangiectasia [letter]. N Engl J Med 1992;326:1360.
19. Health Effects of Exposure to Low Levels of Ionizing Radiation: BEIR V. Washington, DC: National Academy Press, 1990.
20. Shore RE, Hildreth N, Woodard ED, et al. Breast cancer among women given x-ray therapy for acute postpartum mastitis. J Natl Cancer Inst 1986;77:689–696.
21. Miller AB, Howe GR, Sherman GJ, et al. Mortality from breast cancer after irradiation during fluoroscopic examinations in patients being treated for tuberculosis. N Engl J Med 1989;321:1285–1289.
22. Mattson A, Ruden B, Hall P, et al. Radiation-induced breast cancer: long-term follow-up of radiation therapy for benign disease. J Natl Cancer Inst 1993;85:1679–1685.
23. Kopans DB. Re: radiation induced breast cancer [letter]. J Natl Cancer Inst 1993;86:66–67.
24. Boice JD, Harvey EB, Blettner M, et al. Cancer in the contralateral breast after radiotherapy for breast cancer. N Engl J Med 1992;326: 781–785.
25. Marshall E. Study casts doubt on Hiroshima data. Science 1992; 258:394.
26. Mettler FA, Upton AC, Kelsey CA, et al. Benefits versus risks from mammography: a critical assessment. Cancer 1996;77:903–909.
27. Russo J, Tay LK, Russo IH. Differentiation of the mammary gland and susceptibility to carcinogenesis. Breast Cancer Res Treat 1982; 2:5–73.
28. Gohagan JK, Darby WP, Spitznagel EL, et al. Radiogenic breast cancer effects of mammographic screening. J Natl Cancer Inst 1986; 77:71–76.
29. Liberman L, Dershaw DD, Deutch BM, et al. Screening mammography: value in women 35–39 years old. AJR Am J Roentgenol 1993;161:53–56.

Breast Imaging, 2nd ed., by Daniel B. Kopans.
Lippincott–Raven Publishers, Philadelphia © 1998.

CHAPTER 6

Staging Breast Cancer

Although all breast cancers appear to begin in the ductal or lobular epithelium, there is a wide variation in their growth and development. It is difficult to accurately predict the course of the disease for the individual woman. There are exceptions, but for the most part these tumors grow first within the duct (see Chapter 7). As they enlarge they develop the ability, probably through mutation or further chromosonal damage, to break out of the duct and infiltrate into the periductal stroma and gain access to the lymphatics and vascular structures, ultimately spreading to axillary and other lymph nodes and to distant organs.

In an effort to better understand and treat breast cancer, efforts have been made to group lesions by the stage in this progression at which the diagnosis is made. Staging is an important but often neglected aspect of breast evaluation. Although a crude measure, it permits more accurate prognostication of the tumor's course and is a key factor in the testing of new approaches to treatment and the selection of available treatment options. By enabling the comparison of tumors with similar characteristics, staging allows detection and therapeutic interventions to be more accurately compared. Factors that affect eventual outcome have been identified, and more will be found. A fairly simple system has been devised, and radiologists should be familiar with it.

Breast cancer staging recognizes three general levels of tumor involvement loosely categorized by their growth: (1) within the breast (local), (2) the presence and character of tumor in axillary lymph nodes (regional), and (3) the status of the remainder of the body's organs in terms of metastatic spread (distant). Similarly, treatment efficacy is related to the effect of the treatment at each of these levels. Major treatment decisions depend on whether the tumor is confined to the duct (intraductal cancer [ductal carcinoma in situ]) or whether it is invasive, its size, and whether or not tumor is evident outside the breast in regional lymph nodes or other metastatic sites. The presence of tumor in the lymphatics is more an indication of the tumor's biology than anything else and establishes its capacity to exist in organs outside the breast. The significance of node involvement in treatment selection—especially the decision to employ adjuvant chemotherapy or hormonal therapy or more aggressive treatment, such as bone marrow transplantation—is the primary reason for evaluating the axillary lymph nodes. The demonstration that some women who are axillary lymph node negative may still benefit from adjuvant therapies has somewhat reduced the importance of assessing the axillary nodes (1), but most practitioners still prefer knowing the status of the axillary nodes as a measure of the tumor's aggressivity.

Staging has many uses. It may even be useful in determining whether or not axillary nodal dissection is needed. Some investigators are trying to subcategorize in situ and invasive cancers to permit more accurate prognostication. Barth and associates, in an analysis of 918 patients with T1 breast cancers (2 cm or less), found that 23% had positive axillary lymph nodes. They found, however, that lymph node positivity varied with certain factors. The strongest predictors of axillary nodal involvement were the presence of intramammary lymphatic or vascular invasion, the tumor's being palpable, and a high nuclear grade. The likelihood of positivity increased with tumor size. They found that if a tumor was nonpalpable, T1a or T1b without lymph or vascular invasion, and not high grade, the incidence of positive nodes was only 3%. If, however, the lesion was palpable, had lymph or vascular invasion, was high grade, and 1 to 2 cm in size, lymph node positivity increased to 49% (2). Women with a low or intermediate grade, nonpalpable breast cancer that is 1 cm or smaller with no lymph vessel of vascular invasion have such a low risk of nodal involvement that axillary dissection may not be required.

There are two major staging systems that have broadly similar definitions. The American Joint Committee on Cancer (AJCC) (3) and the Union Internationale Contre le Cancer (UICC) use the T, N, M classification system to define stages. The size and detectability of the primary tumor determines the T. The status of the regional lymph nodes establishes the N. The presence or absence of distant metastases determines the M.

The primary site is the breast itself along with its skin and chest wall attachments. Regional lymph nodes are those in the axilla. Although lymphatic drainage of the breast also includes the internal mammary chain as well as those along channels through the pectoralis muscles, the nodes most commonly affected and clinically accessible are those in the axilla, and it is primarily these that are studied for staging purposes. Axillary nodes have been subdivided into levels (Fig. 6-1). Level I nodes are those that are in the axilla lateral to the pectoralis major muscle. Level II lymph nodes are high in the apex of the axilla between the pectoralis major

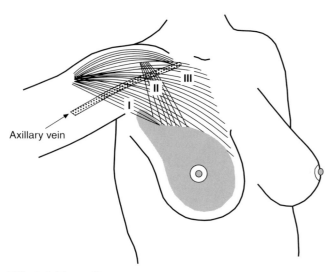

FIG. 6-1. The axillary node levels. Level I is lateral and inferior to the pectoralis major muscle. Level II is beneath the pectoralis minor muscle, and level III extends from the medial edge of the pectoralis minor to the clavicle. In general the more nodes involved and the higher the level, the poorer the prognosis.

and minor muscles, and level III nodes are infraclavicular. Tumor in supraclavicular nodes or involvement of any other lymph node group, including internal mammary nodes, is considered distant metastasis.

Cancers can be staged at the clinical level by visual inspection, palpation, and mammography with tumor confirmation by biopsy. Most treatment protocols, however, use pathologic staging. Pathologic staging includes the gross assessment of size of the excised tumor as well as histologic evaluation of the tumor, its type (if it can be classified), the grade of the cells (grade 1 is well differentiated and grade 3 is poorly differentiated) and the remainder of the breast (if a mastectomy has been performed), and the microscopic evaluation of the axillary lymph nodes removed at surgery. Studies suggest that at least 10 axillary lymph nodes should be excised from level I and perhaps level II to ensure an accurate evaluation of regional involvement (4). Despite the fact that adjuvant therapy is to be used, regardless of the node status, the presence or absence of tumor in axillary nodes is important for prognostication and future analysis of therapeutic decisions.

The actual number of involved nodes appears to directly affect prognosis. Prognostically, the absence of nodal involvement offers the greatest chance of cure, although as many as 30% of women who are lymph node negative develop recurrent breast cancer. Women with one to three nodes involved have a diminished survival expectation but do better than women with four or more involved nodes (5). Some studies indicate that infiltration of tumor from the node into the surrounding tissue is an additional adverse prognostic factor.

Women who are lymph node positive at the time of diagnosis can benefit from adjuvant chemotherapy or hormonal therapy (6). As stated above, more recent data suggest that women with large and more aggressive tumors may also benefit from adjuvant therapy even if node negative. Most of the available data are based on a rather crude analysis of lymph nodes. The node is bivalved, and several slices are shaved from each surface. The percentage of women with positive nodes increases as more thorough investigation is carried out. Staging and the conclusions based on staging will no doubt change as even more sensitive tests using immunohistochemical techniques, or even polymerase chain reaction DNA studies, are able to detect even a few cancer cells in the lymph nodes.

Although staging initially appears complex, it is based simply on the size of the tumor and the presence or absence of tumor in axillary nodes or distant sites. The stage of the tumor depends on the combinations of these factors, but basically the sequence is as follows:

Stage I cancers are less than or equal to 2 cm in diameter and have no evidence of axillary or distant metastases.
Stage II cancers are larger than 2 cm but not larger than 5 cm in diameter, or they are tumors with associated involvement of the axillary nodes but without distant metastatic spread.
Stage III cancers are tumors of any size in which the lymph nodes are fixed together in a matted axillary mass (IIIa), or tumors in which there is extension to the chest wall, or there is skin involvement, or both (IIIb).
Stage IV cancers include any tumor with associated distant metastases.

The full classification system is included in the appendix to this chapter. Mammographically detected lesions should be classified with a small m.

REFERENCES

1. Early Breast Cancer Trialists' Collaborative Group. Systemic treatment of early breast cancer by hormonal, cytotoxic, or immune therapy. Lancet 1992;339:1–15, 71–85.
2. Barth A, Craig PH, Silverstein MJ. Predictors of axillary lymph node metastases in patients with T1 breast carcinoma. Cancer 1997;79:1918–1922.
3. Fleming ID, Cooper JS, Henson DE, et al. Manual for Staging of Cancer: American Joint Committee on Cancer. Philadelphia: Lippincott–Raven, 1997:171–180.
4. Bonadonna G, Zambetti M, Valagussa P. Sequential or alternating doxorubicin and CMF regimens in breast cancer with more than three positive nodes: ten-year results. JAMA 1995;273:542–547.
5. Winchester DP, Cox JD. Standards for breast-conservation treatment. CA Cancer J Clin 1992;42:134–162.
6. Consensus Development Panel. Adjuvant chemotherapy for breast cancer: consensus conference. JAMA 1985;254:3461.

AMERICAN JOINT COMMITTEE ON CANCER CLASSIFICATION OF BREAST CANCER*

C50.0	Nipple
C50.1	Central portion breast
C50.2	Upper-inner quadrant breast

*Reprinted with permission from Fleming ID, Cooper JS, Henson DE, et al. Manual for Staging of Cancer: American Joint Committee on Cancer. Philadelphia: Lippincott–Raven, 1997;171–180.

C50.3   Lower-inner quadrant breast
C50.4   Upper-outer quadrant breast
C50.5   Lower-outer quadrant breast
C50.6   Axillary tail breast
C50.8   Overlapping lesion breast
C50.9   Breast, NOS

The following TNM definitions and stage groupings for carcinoma of the breast are the same for the American Joint Committee on Cancer (AJCC) and the Union Internationale Contre le Cancer (UICC)/TNM projects. This staging system for carcinoma of the breast applies to infiltrating (including microinvasive) and in situ carcinomas. Microscopic confirmation of the diagnosis is mandatory and the histologic type and grade of carcinoma should be recorded.

ANATOMY

Primary Site

The mammary gland, situated on the anterior chest wall, is composed of glandular tissue within a dense fibroareolar stroma. The glandular tissue consists of approximately 20 lobes, each of which terminates in a separate excretory duct in the nipple.

Regional Lymph Nodes

The breast lymphatics drain by way of three major routes: axillary, transpectoral, and internal mammary. Intramammary lymph nodes are considered with, and coded as, axillary lymph nodes for staging purposes. Metastasis to any other lymph node is considered distant (M1), including supraclavicular, cervical, or contralateral internal mammary (Fig. 6-2). The regional lymph nodes are:

1. Axillary (ipsilateral): interpectoral (Rotter's) nodes and lymph nodes along the axillary vein and its tributaries, which may be (but are not required to be) divided into the following levels:
   (i)   Level I (low-axilla): lymph nodes lateral to the lateral border of pectoralis minor muscle.
   (ii) Level II (mid-axilla): lymph nodes between the medial and lateral borders of the pectoralis minor muscle and the interpectoral (Rotter's) lymph nodes.
   (iii) Level III (apical axilla): lymph nodes medial to the medial margin of the pectoralis minor muscle including those designated as subclavicular, infraclavicular, or apical.
   Note: Intramammary lymph nodes are coded as axillary lymph nodes.
2. Internal mammary (ipsilateral): lymph nodes in the intercostal spaces along the edge of the sternum in the endothoracic fascia.

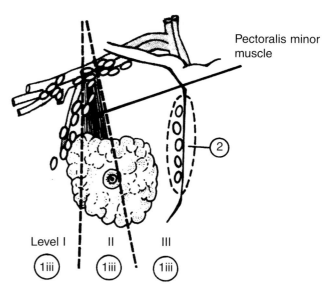

FIG. 6-2. Regional lymph nodes.

Any other lymph node metastasis is coded as a distant metastasis (M1), including supraclavicular, cervical, or contralateral internal mammary lymph nodes.

Metastatic Sites

All distant visceral sites are potential sites of metastasis. The four major sites of involvement are bone, lung, brain, and liver, but this widely metastasizing disease has been found in almost any remote site.

RULES FOR CLASSIFICATION

Clinical Staging

Clinical staging includes physical examination, with careful inspection and palpation of the skin, mammary gland, and lymph nodes (axillary, supraclavicular, and cervical); imaging; and pathologic examination of the breast or other tissues to establish the diagnosis of breast carcinoma. The extent of tissue examined pathologically for clinical staging is less than that required for pathologic staging (see Pathologic Staging). Appropriate operative findings are elements of clinical staging, including the size of the primary tumor and chest wall invasion, and the presence or absence of regional or distant metastasis.

Pathologic Staging

Pathologic staging includes all data used for clinical staging, surgical exploration and resection as well as pathologic examination of the primary carcinoma, including not less than excision of the primary carcinoma with no macroscopic tumor in any margin of resection by pathologic examination. A case can be classified pT for pathologic stage grouping if there is only microscopic, but not macroscopic, involvement at the margin. If there is tumor in the margin of resection by macroscopic examination, it is coded TX because the extent of the primary tumor cannot be assessed. If there is no clinical evidence of axillary metastasis, resection of at least the low axillary lymph nodes (level I), that is, those lymph nodes located lateral to the lateral border of the pectoralis minor muscle should be performed for pathologic (pN) classification. Such a resection will ordinarily include six or more lymph nodes. Metastatic nodules in the fat adjacent to the mammary carcinoma within the breast, without evidence of residual lymph node tissue, are classified as regional lymph node metastases (N). Pathologic stage grouping includes any of the following combinations: pT pN pM, or pT pN cM, or cT cN pM.

TNM CLASSIFICATION

Primary Tumor

The clinical measurement used for classifying the primary tumor (T) is the one judged to be most accurate for that particular case (e.g., physical examination or imaging such as a mammogram). The pathologic tumor size for classification (T) is a measurement of *only the invasive component*. For example, if there is a 4.0-cm component and a 0.3-cm invasive component, the tumor is classified T1a. The size of the primary tumor is measured for T-classification before any tissue is removed for special studies, such as for estrogen receptors.

Microinvasion of Breast Carcinoma

Microinvasion is the extension of cancer cells beyond the basement membrane into the adjacent tissues with no focus more than 0.1 cm in greatest dimension. When there are multiple foci of microinvasion, the size of only the largest focus is used to classify the microinvasion. (Do not use the sum of all the individual foci.) The presence of multiple foci of microinvasion should be noted, as it is with multiple larger invasive carcinomas.

Multiple Simultaneous Ipsilateral Primary Carcinomas

The following guidelines are used when classifying multiple simultaneous ipsilateral primary (infiltrating, macroscopically measurable) carcinomas. These criteria do not apply to one macroscopic carcinoma associated with multiple separate microscopic foci.

Breast

1. Use the largest primary carcinoma to classify T.
2. Enter into the record that this is a case of multiple simultaneous ipsilateral primary carcinomas. Such cases should be analyzed separately.

Simultaneous Bilateral Breast Carcinomas

Each carcinoma is staged as a separate primary carcinoma in a separate organ.

Inflammatory Carcinoma

Inflammatory carcinoma is a clinicopathologic entity characterized by diffuse brawny induration of the skin of the breast with an erysipeloid edge, usually without an underlying palpable mass. Radiologically there may be a detectable mass and characteristic thickening of the skin over the breast. This clinical presentation is due to tumor embolization of dermal lymphatics. The tumor of inflammatory carcinoma is classified T4d.

Paget's Disease of the Nipple

Paget's disease of the nipple without an associated tumor mass (clinical) or invasive carcinoma (pathologic) is classified Tis. Paget's disease with a demonstrable mass (clinical) or an invasive component (pathologic) is classified according to the size of the tumor mass or invasive component.

Skin of Breast

Dimpling of the skin, nipple retraction, or any other skin change except those described under T4b and T4d may occur in T1, T2, or T3 without changing the classification.

Chest Wall

Chest wall includes ribs, intercostal muscles, and serratus anterior muscle but not pectoral muscle.

DEFINITION OF TNM

Definitions for classifying the primary tumor (T) are the same for clinical and for pathologic classification. The telescoping method of classification can be applied. If the measurement is made by physical examination, the examiner will use the major headings (T1, T2, or T3). If other measurements, such as mammographic or pathologic, are used, the telescoped subsets of T1 can be used.

Primary Tumor (T)

TX	Primary tumor cannot be assessed
T0	No evidence of primary tumor
Tis	Carcinoma in situ: Intraductal carcinoma, lobular carcinoma in situ, or Paget's disease of the nipple with no tumor

T1   Tumor 2 cm or less in greatest dimension

   T1mic   Microinvasion 0.1 cm or less in greatest dimension

   T1a   Tumor more than 0.1 but not more than 0.5 cm in greatest dimension

   T1b   Tumor more than 0.5 cm but not more than 1 cm in greatest dimension

   T1c   Tumor more than 1 cm but not more than 2 cm in greatest dimension

T2   Tumor more than 2 cm but not more than 5 cm in greatest dimension

T3   Tumor more than 5 cm in greatest dimension

T4   Tumor of any size with direct extension to (a) chest wall or (b) skin, only as described below

   T4a   Extension to chest wall

   T4b   Edema (including peau d'orange) or ulceration of the skin of the breast or satellite skin nodules confined to the same breast

   T4c   Both (T4a and T4b)

   T4d   Inflammatory carcinoma (see definition of inflammatory carcinoma in the introduction)

Note: Paget's disease associated with a tumor is classified according to the size of the tumor.

Regional Lymph Nodes (N)

NX   Regional lymph nodes cannot be assessed (e.g., previously removed)

N0   No regional lymph node metastasis

N1   Metastasis to movable ipsilateral axillary lymph node(s)

N2   Metastasis to ipsilateral axillary lymph node(s) fixed to one another or to other structures

N3   Metastasis to ipsilateral internal mammary lymph node(s)

Pathologic Classification (pN)

pNX   Regional lymph nodes cannot be assessed (e.g., previously removed or not removed for pathologic study)

pN0   No regional lymph node metastasis

pN1   Metastasis to movable ipsilateral axillary lymph node(s)

  pN1a   Only micrometastasis (none larger than 0.2 cm)

  pN1b   Metastasis to lymph node(s), any larger than 0.2 cm

  pN1bi   Metastasis in 1 to 3 lymph nodes, any more than 0.2 cm and all less than 2 cm in greatest dimension

  pN1bii   Metastasis to 4 or more lymph nodes, any more than 0.2 cm and all less than 2 cm in greatest dimension

  pN1biii   Extension of tumor beyond the capsule of a lymph node metastasis less than 2 cm in greatest dimension

  pN1biv   Metastasis to a lymph node 2 cm or more in greatest dimension

pN2   Metastasis to ipsilateral axillary lymph nodes that are fixed to one another or to other structures

pN3   Metastasis to ipsilateral internal mammary lymph node(s)

Distant Metastasis (M)

MX   Distant metastasis cannot be assessed

M0   No distant metastasis

M1   Distant metastasis (includes metastasis to ipsilateral supraclavicular lymph node[s])

STAGE GROUPING

Stage 0	Tis	N0	M0
Stage I	T1*	N0	M0
Stage IIA	T0	N1	M0
	T1*	N1**	M0
	T2	N0	M0
Stage IIB	T2	N1	M0
	T3	N0	M0
Stage IIIA	T0	N2	M0
	T1	N2	M0
	T2	N2	M0
	T3	N1	M0
	T3	N2	M0
Stage IIIB	T4	Any N	M0
	Any T	N3	M0
Stage IV	Any T	Any N	M1

*T1 includes T1mic

**The prognosis of patients with N1a is similar to that of patients with pN0.

HISTOPATHOLOGIC TYPE

The histologic types are the following:

Carcinoma, NOS (not otherwise specified)
Ductal
    Intraductal (in situ)
    Invasive with predominant intraductal component
    Invasive, NOS (not otherwise specified)
    Comedo
    Inflammatory
    Medullary with lymphocytic infiltrate
    Mucinous (colloid)
    Papillary
    Scirrhous
    Tubular
    Other
Lobular
    In situ
    Invasive with predominant in situ component
    Invasive

Nipple
    Paget's disease, NOS (not otherwise specified)
    Paget's disease with intraductal carcinoma
    Paget's disease with invasive ductal carcinoma
Other
    Undifferentiated carcinoma

HISTOPATHOLOGIC GRADE (G)

GX	Grade cannot be assessed
G1	Well differentiated
G2	Moderately differentiated
G3	Poorly differentiated
G4	Undifferentiated

PROGNOSTIC FACTORS

A proliferation of prognostic factors for breast cancer is evident in that currently approximately 80 putative prognostic variables have been reported for humans with this tumor. Factors that are supported in the literature are not necessarily the final prognostic factors for breast cancer and deserve further study in an integrative model. Current therapeutic strategies for individual patients with breast cancer frequently are determined by the following prognostic variables: (1) the size (T) of the primary neoplasm (AJCC-TNM stage); (2) the presence and extent of axillary lymph node metastases; (3) pathologic stage of disease after primary therapy; and (4) the presence or absence of estrogen receptor (ER) and progesterone receptor (PR) activity (Clark et al., Tandon et al.). Figure 6-3 shows observed and relative survival rates for 50,383 patients with breast carcinoma for the years 1985–1989 classified by the AJCC staging classification.

Table 6-1 itemizes the traditional prognostic parameters for human breast carcinoma. This cancer, like other mammalian neoplasms, results from a series of genetic alterations ("hits") induced by environmental stimuli, genetic predisposition, or concurrent activity of both events.

Multiple serum biochemical markers have been included as potential prognostic indicators and have been reviewed by Stenman and Heikkinen and by Werner et al. These serum proteins include the breast mucin markers CA15-3, CA549, CAM26, CAM29, the adenocarcinoma marker carcinoembryonic antigen (CEA), cancer-associated serum antigen (CASA), mammary serum antigen (MSA), the reaction products hydroxyproline, ferritin and isoferritin (p43), tumor-associated trypsin inhibitor (TATI), the proliferation marker tissue polypeptide antigen (TPA), C-reactive protein (CRP), orosomucoid, and erythrocyte sedimentation rate (ESR) (Burke et al., 1995). The majority of these serum proteins represents a nonspecific host response to tissue damage initiated by the neoplasm. Although approved for application in clinical practice, the predominant utilization of these markers has been in investigatory studies. The indiscriminate use of these tumor-derived proteins is ill-advised, as the available research suggests that the majority of these markers lack adequate sensitivity and specificity for prediction of outcome. However, identification of elevation specific to the cancerous growth is of value when sequential testing is utilized for the purposes of quantification of tumor burden, monitoring of disease, and determination of therapeutic outcome (Burke et al.).

Table 6-2 identifies anatomic and cellular prognostic factors that have been identified and that support their application in the search for new prognostic factors. Additionally, the identification of genetic mutations and gene deletions/substitutions are an integral part of active research models that are being clinically applied internationally. Integration of oncogene protein discriminants into prognostic models that have previously shown value to predict outcome include Ha-*ras*, c-*myc*, c-*fos*, c-*erb*-B2 (*HER2/neu*), *NME1*, and *int*-2. Moreover, mutation of the tumor suppressor gene TP53 (p53) on chromosome 17p has been extensively studied and represents a common genetic mutation for multiple human neoplasms, including breast carcinogenesis. In 1993, the AJCC adopted criteria for definition of a prognostic factor that include:

   I. Statistically significant, that is, its prognostic value only rarely occurs by chance;
  II. Independent, that is, retains its prognostic value when combined with other factors; and
 III. Clinically relevant, that is, has a major impact on prognostic accuracy.

Subsequent to this adoption of definition, the College of American Pathologists (CAP) convened a multidisciplinary conference in 1994 and placed further emphasis on the sensitivity of these prognostic factors and their subsets to predict outcome when judged as relevant prognostic factors by managing physicians. Group I includes prognostic variables well supported biologically and clinically in the scientific literature. Such examples include TNM variables, histologic type, grade (histologic/nuclear), and steroid receptor activity (estrogen, progesterone). Group II was divided into two subsets of prognostic factors extensively studied both clinically and biologically. Group IIA utilized factors commonly applied in clinical trials, for example, proliferative markers such as percent S-phase fraction and Ki-67 (M1B1), and mitotic index (thymidine-labeling indices). When expanded to the biological subset, Group IIB includes prognostic factors for which biologic and clinically correlative studies had been completed; however, this subset had few outcome studies (e.g., c-*erb*-B2 [*HER2*/neu], p53, angiogenesis and vascular invasion [lymphatic/venous]). Finally, Group III represents factors that are clinically relevant and, therefore, have major implications for accuracy relative to prognosis. Group III includes some of the anatomic and cellular prognostic

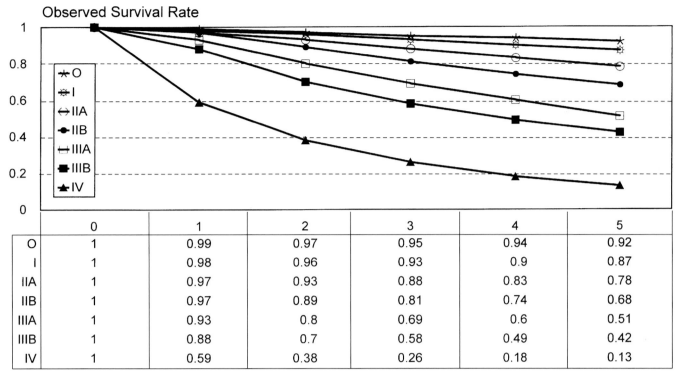

Observed Survival Rate

	0	1	2	3	4	5
O	1	0.99	0.97	0.95	0.94	0.92
I	1	0.98	0.96	0.93	0.9	0.87
IIA	1	0.97	0.93	0.88	0.83	0.78
IIB	1	0.97	0.89	0.81	0.74	0.68
IIIA	1	0.93	0.8	0.69	0.6	0.51
IIIB	1	0.88	0.7	0.58	0.49	0.42
IV	1	0.59	0.38	0.26	0.18	0.13

A   Years After Diagnosis

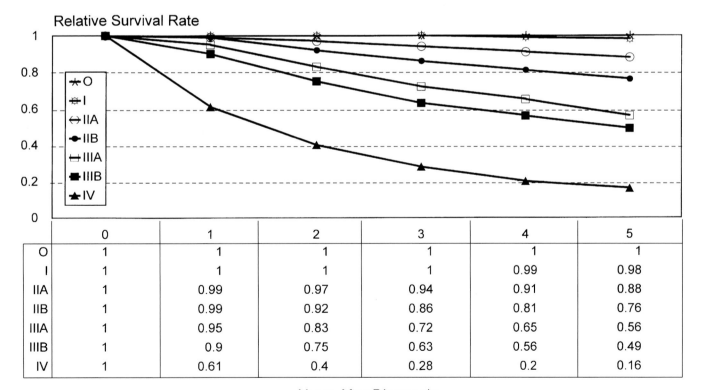

Relative Survival Rate

	0	1	2	3	4	5
O	1	1	1	1	1	1
I	1	1	1	1	0.99	0.98
IIA	1	0.99	0.97	0.94	0.91	0.88
IIB	1	0.99	0.92	0.86	0.81	0.76
IIIA	1	0.95	0.83	0.72	0.65	0.56
IIIB	1	0.9	0.75	0.63	0.56	0.49
IV	1	0.61	0.4	0.28	0.2	0.16

B   Years After Diagnosis

FIG. 6-3. Observed **(A)** and relative **(B)** survival rates for 50,383 patients with breast carcinoma classified by the current AJCC staging classification. (Data taken from the National Cancer Data Base [Commission on Cancer of the American College of Surgeons and the American Cancer Society] for the year 1989. Stage 0 includes 5,686 patients; Stage I, 21,604; Stage IIA, 10,412; Stage IIB, 5,673; Stage IIIA, 1,864; Stage IIB, 2,035; Stage IV, 3,109.)

TABLE 6-1. *Traditional prognostic parameters for human mammary carcinoma*

Tumor factors	Host factors
Lymph node status	Age
Tumor size	Menopausal status
Histologic/nuclear grade	Familial history
Lymphatic/vascular invasion	Previous neoplastic disease
Pathologic stage (TNM)	Immunosuppression
Steroid receptor status (ER/PR)	Host inflammatory response
DNA content (ploidy, S-phase)	Nutrition
EIC (in situ)	Prior chemotherapy
	Prior radiation

ER, estrogen receptor; PR, progesterone receptor; EIC, extensive intraductal component (associated with invasive carcinoma).

Source: Bland KI, Konstadoulakis MM, Vezeridid MP, Wanebo HJ. Oncogene protein coexpression: value of Ha-ras, c-myc, c-fos, and p53 as prognostic discriminants for breast carcinoma. Ann Surg 1995;221:706-720.

factors and the molecular-genetic prognostic factors that do not conform to Group I and II. With the enlarging literature relative to molecular and genetic translational research, it is highly probable that these factors will give increasing application to build prognostic models that are highly accurate for evaluation of tumor phenotype and accurately predict disease-free and overall survival outcomes when integrated with anatomic and cellular prognostic factors (Bland et al.).

BIBLIOGRAPHY

Beahrs OH, Henson DE, Hutter RVP, Myers M (eds). American Joint Committee on Cancer: Manual for Staging of Cancer (3rd ed). Philadelphia: Lippincott, 1988.

Beahrs OH, Myers M (eds). American Joint Committee on Cancer: Manual for Staging of Cancer (2nd ed). Philadelphia: Lippincott, 1983.

Bland KI, Konstadoulakis MM, Vezeridis MP, et al. Oncogene protein coexpression: value of Ha-ras, c-myc, c-fos, and p53 as prognostic discriminants for breast carcinoma. Ann Surg 1995;221:706–720.

Burke HB, Hutter RVP, Henson DE. Breast carcinoma. In Hermanek P, Gospodarowicz MK, Henson DE, et al. (eds), Prognostic Factors in Cancer, Union Internationale Centre le Cancer. New York: Springer 1995;165–176.

Clark GM, McGuire WL, Hubay CA, et al. Progesterone receptor as a prognostic factor in stage II breast cancer. N Engl J Med 1983;309:1343–1347.

Harmer MH. UICC TNM Classification of Malignant Tumors (3rd ed). Berlin: Springer, 1982.

Henson DE. Future directions for the AMCC. Cancer 1992;69 (6 suppl):1639–1644.

Henson DE, Ries L, Freedman LS, et al. Relationship among outcome, stage of disease, and histologic grade for 22,616 cases of breast cancer: the basis for a prognostic index. Cancer 1991;68:2142–2149.

Histologic Typing of Breast Tumours (2nd ed). WHO International Histological Classification of Tumours. Geneva: World Health Organization, 1981.

Hutter RVP. At last—worldwide agreement on staging of cancer. Arch Surg 1987;122:1235–1239.

Kiricuta IC. Correspondence. Eur J Surg Onc 1993;19:393–395.

Nachlas MM. Irrationality in the management of breast cancer. I. The staging system. Cancer 1991;68:681–690.

Russo J, Russo IH. The pathology of breast cancer: staging and prognostic indicators. JAMWA 1992;47:181–187.

Silverstein MJ, Poller DN, Waisman JR, et al. Prognostic classification of breast ductal carcinoma in situ. Lancet 1995;345:1154–1157.

Sobin LH, Wittekind C. UICC/TNM Classification of Malignant Tumors (5th ed). New York: Wiley, 1997.

TABLE 6-2. *Anatomic and cellular prognostic factors*

Name	Literature support	Properties
Tumor size, extent (T)	+	Pathologic more reliable than clinical
Regional lymph node involvement (N)	+	Pathologic more reliable than clinical
Metastasis (M)	+	Radiographic tests acceptable
Histology: type	+	Most breast cancer is ductal
Grade	+	Problems with uniformity of criteria
Chromatin	+	Nuclear morphology
Tumor necrosis	+	Cell degeneration and death
Mitotic counts	+	Cell activity, fixative problems, only M-phase cells
DNA ploidy	0	Conflicting results
Thymidine labeling index	+	Cell proliferation, thymidine a DNA precursor, thymidine analogue 5-bromodeoxyuridine also used, predicts recurrence
S-phase; flow cytometry	+	Cell proliferation, no standardized cutoff point
Ki-67 antibody	+	Recognizes nuclear antigen expressed only in proliferating cells
Proliferating cell nuclear antigen (PCNA)	0	Cell cycle–dependent protein that accumulates in the nucleus of replicating cells during S-phase, conflicting results
Angiogenesis[a]	+	Related to tumor angiogenesis factors
Peritumoral lymphatic vessel invasion	+	Significant for relapse-free survival but not overall survival

+, Well supported; 0, equivocal support.

[a] Factor VIII–related antigen and CD31 are vascular detection techniques for quantifying tumor angiogenesis. Basic fibroblast growth factor is an angiogenic peptide and can be measured in the urine. The degree to correlation between vascular antigens and angiogenic peptide in tumor angiogenesis is not known.

Source: Burke HB, Hutter RVP, Henson DE. Breast Carcinoma. In Hermanek P, Gospodarowicz MK, Henson DE, et al. (eds), Prognostic Factors in Cancer. Union Internationale Contre le Cancer. New York: Springer, 1995;165–176.

Sorensen ME. Managing care in breast cancer staging: routine bone scan is not indicated [abstract]. ASCO Proceedings 13:70, 1994.

Spiessl B, Beahrs OH, Hermanek P, et al. UICC/TNM Atlas: Illustrated Guide to the TNM/pTNM Classification of Malignant Tumors (3rd ed, 2nd revision). Berlin: Springer, 1992.

Stelling CB. Breast cancer staging with contrast material-enhanced MR imaging: should it change patient treatment? Radiology 1995;196:16–19.

Stenman U, Heikkinen R. Serum markers for breast cancer. Scand J Clin Lab Invest 1991;206:52–59.

Tandon AK, Clark GM, Chamness GC, et al. HER-2/neu oncogene protein and prognosis in breast cancer. J Clin Oncol 1989;7:1120–1128.

Werner M, Faser C, Silverberg M. Clinical utility and validation of emerging biochemical markers for mammary adenocarcinoma. Clin Chem 1993;39:2386–2396.

World Health Organization. ICD-O International Classification of Diseases for Oncology (2nd ed). Geneva: World Health Organization, 1990.

World Health Organization. International Histological Classification of Tumours (2nd ed). Berlin: Springer, 1988–1997.

DATA FORM FOR CANCER STAGING

Patient identification

Name _____

Address _____

Hospital or clinic number _____

Age _____ Sex _____ Race _____

Institution identification

Hospital or clinic_____

Address _____

Oncology Record

Anatomic site of cancer _____

Histologic type _____

Grade (G) _____

Date of classification _____

DEFINITIONS

Clin	Path		
		Primary Tumor (T)	
[ ]	[ ]	TX	Primary tumor cannot be assessed
[ ]	[ ]	T0	No evidence of primary tumor
[ ]	[ ]	Tis	Carcinoma in situ: intraductal carcinoma, lobular carcinoma in situ, or Paget's disease of the nipple with no tumor
[ ]	[ ]	T1	Tumor 2 cm or less in greatest dimension
		pT1mic	Microinvasion 0.1 cm or less in greatest dimension
[ ]	[ ]	T1a	Tumor more than 0.1 cm but not more than 0.5 cm in greatest dimension
[ ]	[ ]	T1b	More than 0.5 cm but not more than 1 cm in greatest dimension
[ ]	[ ]	T1c	More than 1 cm but not more than 2 cm in greatest dimension
[ ]	[ ]	T2	Tumor more than 2 cm but not more than 5 cm in greatest dimension
[ ]	[ ]	T3	Tumor more than 5 cm in greatest dimension
[ ]	[ ]	T4	Tumor of any size with direct extension to (a) chest wall or (b) skin, only as described below
[ ]	[ ]	T4a	Extension to chest wall
[ ]	[ ]	T4b	Edema (including peau d'orange) or ulceration of the skin of breast or satellite skin nodules confined to same breast
[ ]	[ ]	T4c	Both (T4a and T4b)
[ ]	[ ]	T4d	Inflammatory carcinoma

Paget's disease associated with a tumor is classified according to the size of the tumor.

Clin	Path		
		Regional Lymph Nodes (N)	
[ ]	[ ]	NX	Regional lymph nodes cannot be assessed (e.g., previously removed)
[ ]	[ ]	N0	No regional lymph node metastasis
[ ]	[ ]	N1	Spread to movable ipsilateral axillary lymph node(s)
[ ]	[ ]	N2	Spread to ipsilateral axillary lymph node(s) fixed to one another or to other structures
[ ]	[ ]	N3	Spread to ipsilateral internal mammary lymph node(s)

Clin	Path		
		Pathologic Classification (pN)	
	[ ]	pNX	Regional lymph nodes cannot be assessed (e.g., previously removed, or not removed for pathologic study)
	[ ]	pN0	No regional lymph node metastasis
	[ ]	pN1	Metastasis to movable ipsilateral axillary lymph node(s)
	[ ]	pN1a	Only micrometastasis (none larger than 0.2 cm)

Clin	Path		
	[ ]	pN1b	Metastasis to lymph nodes, any larger than 0.2 cm
	[ ]	pN1bi	Metastasis in 1 to 3 lymph nodes, any more than 0.2 cm and all less than 2 cm in greatest dimension
	[ ]	pN1bii	Metastasis to 4 or more lymph nodes, any more than 0.2 cm and all less than 2 cm in greatest dimension
	[ ]	pN1biii	Extension of tumor beyond the capsule of a lymph node metastasis less than 2 cm in greatest dimension
	[ ]	pN1biv	Metastasis to a lymph node 2 cm or more in greatest dimension
	[ ]	pN2	Metastasis to ipsilateral axillary lymph nodes that are fixed to one another or to other structures
	[ ]	pN3	Metastasis to ipsilateral internal mammary lymph node(s)

Distant Metastasis (M)

Clin	Path		
[ ]	[ ]	MX	Distant metastasis cannot be assessed
[ ]	[ ]	M0	No distant metastasis
[ ]	[ ]	M1	Distant metastasis (includes metastasis to ipsilateral supraclavicular lymph node[s])

Clin	Path	Stage grouping			
[ ]	[ ]	0	Tis	N0	M0
[ ]	[ ]	I	T1*	N0	M0
[ ]	[ ]	IIA	T0	N1	M0
			T1*	N1**	M0
			T2	N0	M0
[ ]	[ ]	IIB	T2	N1	M0
			?	N0	M0
[ ]	[ ]	IIIA	T0	N2	M0
			T1*	N2	M0
			T2	N2	M0
			T3	N1	M0
			T3	N2	M0
[ ]	[ ]	IIIB	T1	Any N	M0
			Any T	N3	M0
[ ]	[ ]	IV	Any T	Any N	M1

*T1 includes pT1mic
**The prognosis of patients with N1a is similar to that of patients with pN0.

Histopathologic Grade (G)
[ ] GX   Grade cannot be assessed
[ ] G1   Well differentiated
[ ] G2   Moderately differentiated
[ ] G3   Poorly differentiated
[ ] G4   Undifferentiated

Histopathologic Type
The histologic types are the following:
Carcinoma, NOS (not otherwise specified)
Ductal
   Intraductal (in situ)
   Invasive with predominant intraductal component
   Invasive, NOS (not otherwise specified)
   Comedo
   Inflammatory
   Medullary with lymphocytic infiltrate
   Mucinous (colloid)
   Papillary
   Scirrhous
   Tubular
   Other
Lobular
   In situ
   Invasive with predominate in situ component
   Invasive
Nipple
   Paget's disease, NOS (not otherwise specified)
   Paget's disease with intraductal carcinoma
   Paget's disease with invasive ductal carcinoma
Other
   Undifferentiated carcinoma

Staged by _____ M.D.
_____ Registrar
Date _____

Regional Lymph Nodes

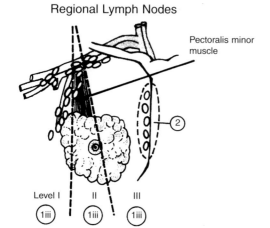

Pectoralis minor muscle

Level I   II   III
1iii   1iii   1iii

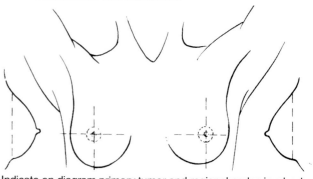

Indicate on diagram primary tumor and regional nodes involved.

Breast Imaging, 2nd ed., by Daniel B. Kopans.
Lippincott–Raven Publishers, Philadelphia © 1998.

CHAPTER 7

Early-Stage Breast Cancer: Detection, Diagnosis, and Prognostic Indicators

Despite centuries of research, there is no universal agreement over what exactly constitutes a breast cancer. Fortunately, most women who develop breast cancer do not die as a result of the malignancy. It is not clear whether this is due to earlier detection and better treatment or merely because some lesions that are classified as cancers have the potential to be lethal whereas others do not. The threat of death from some lesions, such as well-differentiated ductal carcinoma in situ (DCIS), may be extremely remote, whereas mortality from a rapidly growing, poorly differentiated invasive cancer may be more immediate. However, for any specific lesion there is no way to predict outcome with any certainty.

APPROPRIATE BIOLOGICAL MODEL FOR COMPARISON

There are two schools of thought with respect to the development of breast cancer. One school believes that breast cancer is the end result of a series of changes forming a continuum. This was first postulated by Gallagher and Martin, who based their conclusions on observations from extensive whole-breast histologic analysis (1). Their observations suggested a logical progression of epithelial transition to cancer. They demonstrated that most breast cancer originates in the intralobular terminal duct. According to their studies, normal ductal epithelium in this region can undergo reversible hyperplastic growth. In some women, the cells begin to have atypical features. They believed that atypical epithelial hyperplasia was the last reversible change that precedes the irreversible transition to carcinoma in situ, which ultimately progresses to invasive breast cancer. Once invasive, a cancer can gain access to the lymphatic and vascular systems and spread to other organs, ultimately killing the individual.

There are others, however, who believe that breast cancer is not part of a continuum but represents a duality of growth. They would argue that only invasive breast cancer is a true cancer and that it arises de novo without going through an in situ phase and that in situ breast cancer is of little consequence.

The continuum theory would compare breast cancer to cancer of the cervix, which, after a variable in situ period, becomes invasive. The dual theory likens breast cancer to cancers of the thyroid and prostate. In these organs there appear to be histologically evident cancers that remain confined locally and are not lethal and other cancers that invade rapidly and metastasize early.

Although prostate cancer has been compared to breast cancer, there are significant differences. It is likely that cancer of the prostate develops so late in life that other causes of death intervene before the prostate cancer becomes significant. In contrast, breast cancer affects women a decade or more earlier than prostate cancer affects men, and the age of onset seems to be decreasing, making it more likely that early breast cancer lesions will become significant.

The inability to accurately predict the course of a given lesion may merely indicate that the analytic tools presently available cannot distinguish between cancers with lethal potential and those that will not result in death. For this reason, most would argue that all breast cancers should be treated as if they have lethal potential.

The randomized controlled trials of screening have demonstrated that the progression of breast cancer need not lead inexorably to death. The natural history (whatever it might be) of some cancer can be interrupted and death averted through earlier detection. What remains to be determined is how best to treat the various manifestations of breast cancer to maximize the benefit while minimizing the "harm" to the individual from detection, diagnosis, and treatment.

It is well established that prognosis is directly related to (although not absolutely determined by) the size of a cancer, its histologic grade, and whether tumor cells have spread to the axillary lymph nodes (reflecting metastatic capability) (2). The detection of breast cancer "earlier" in its growth has clear advantages, and the purpose of this chapter is to review the present understanding of what constitutes "early" breast cancer. There are likely multiple paths to breast cancer. Some likely arise from a single cell and are fully capable of invasion and metastatic spread very early in their growth, if not immediately, whereas others develop in epithelium that is extensively altered and genetically unstable, with changes occurring over long periods of time and ultimately resulting in one cell accumulating all the genetic changes needed for malignant transformation.

BREAST CANCER AND ITS SUBCATEGORIES

Breast cancer is not a single disease process. It has numerous variations. Furthermore, the outcome for an individual is determined not merely by the cancer but also by the host's response to the cancer. Our ability to classify cancers remains crude. Pathologic review of the tissues using light microscopy remains the most accurate diagnostic test. Pathologists have subclassified cancers of the breast, and it is important to understand their terminology and classification.

Ductal Carcinoma (in Situ and Invasive)

A very small percentage of malignant lesions arise from the stromal elements of the breast. Ninety percent of breast cancers have cellular features that are similar to ductal epithelium and are classified as ductal cancers. When in situ (remaining confined to the duct), they are called *intraductal carcinoma*, or, more commonly, *DCIS*. When the cells have breached the basement membrane surrounding the duct and invaded the surrounding tissues they are termed *invasive* or *infiltrating ductal carcinoma*.

Because most breast cancers arise in the ducts, the earliest manifestation of breast cancer is DCIS. Because cancer that is confined to the ducts cannot spread beyond the breast and cannot be lethal, DCIS is often considered separately in cancer statistics. Some do not even consider it to be a true malignancy. The data, however, suggest that DCIS is directly related to invasive breast cancer. Virtually all invasive cancers that develop in women who have had DCIS grow in the same location as the DCIS. In many invasive cancers there are remnants of DCIS. Although all cancers may not have recognizable areas of DCIS, this lesion is almost certainly a direct precursor lesion for many, if not all, invasive cancers.

At present it is impossible to resolve disagreements over the natural history of breast cancer and the importance of in situ cancer. The diagnosis of intraductal carcinoma can only be made using biopsy. The process of making the diagnosis alters the course of the lesion, and an accurate study of its natural history is impossible. It has been shown that DCIS, if biopsied but left without definitive treatment, will progress to invasive cancer in at least 30% to 50% of women (3).

A study conducted by the National Surgical Adjuvant Breast Project (NSABP), a large multicenter collaborative group, found that women with DCIS (not further categorized) treated with excision alone had a 23% recurrence rate by 3 years, whereas those treated with excision and radiation had the recurrence reduced to 9% (4). A larger NSABP study involving only women with mammographically detected DCIS confirmed this finding. Among 818 women with DCIS randomized to be treated with lumpectomy alone

or lumpectomy and radiation therapy to 50 Gy with a mean follow-up of 43 months (range, 11 to 86 months), they found that 84.4% had no evidence of recurrence if irradiated, but there was a 20.7% recurrence rate if the patients were treated with lumpectomy alone. Of even greater concern was that 50% of the recurrences in the nonirradiated group were invasive cancers (8% overall by 4 years) and two women died of breast cancer (5).

The importance of radiation therapy has been challenged, however. Silverstein and Lagios and others have argued that if the lesions are properly evaluated and sufficient normal tissue is removed around the DCIS (DCIS is virtually always a process confined to a lobe or segment of the breast) so that the margins of the tissue are free of tumor, many low-grade lesions can be treated with excision alone (6).

The results can also be interpreted in two other ways. Those supporting the dual theory would say that, at most, <50% of intraductal cancers ever become significant, whereas the continuum proponents might suggest that if lesions are excised completely and early, their progression may be interrupted and the patient cured of the disease. Radiologists are, unfortunately, well aware of examples of lesions that were almost certainly DCIS that were overlooked or left untreated and progressed to invasive breast cancer (Fig. 7-1).

The data strongly suggest that DCIS does represent a precursor of invasive breast cancer. There has never been a reported case of "cancer calcifications" that disappeared unless they were replaced by an invasive lesion. As many point out, virtually all cancers originate in the ductal epithelium and, thus, are by definition, intraductal at the start. It is likely that if the individual lives long enough, the DCIS will progress to invasion.

Further complicating the understanding of the significance of DCIS is the fact that DCIS is not a uniform process. Pathologists have started to agree that there are distinct subtypes of intraductal cancer. They do not all agree on the classification (7), but many see a difference based on cell morphology and the architecture of the aggregated cells. Large cell tumors appear to have a different natural history than small cell cancers. Solid growth (cells abutting one another with no defined spaces within the tumor) are distinguished from those forming cribriform (sievelike) spaces. Many tumors have areas of necrosis while others have micropapillary growths.

A consensus is emerging that divides DCIS into three categories: poorly differentiated (high grade), intermediate differentiation, and well differentiated (low grade). High-grade DCIS is characterized by relatively large, pleomorphic cells with large nuclei (more than two red-cell diameters), whereas low-grade DCIS consists of monotonous, relatively small cells that are similar in morphology. The former appear to be more likely to invade early whereas the latter appear to be more indolent.

Lagios (8) was one of the first to develop a histologic grading system for DCIS that some believe can be used to predict the growth patterns of these lesions. He found that poorly differentiated DCIS, particularly of the comedo (large cell) type

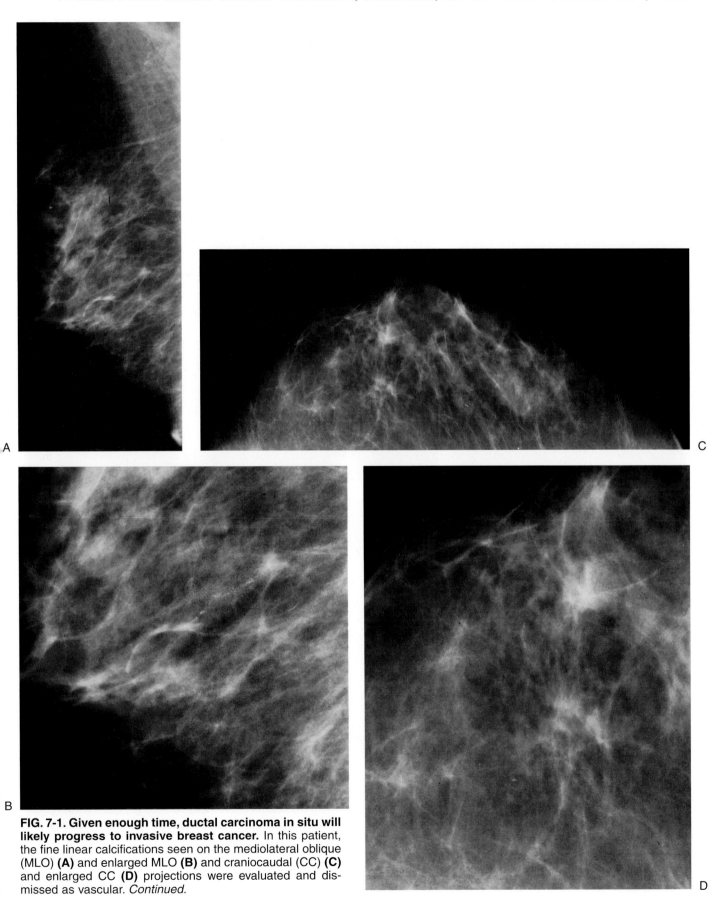

FIG. 7-1. Given enough time, ductal carcinoma in situ will likely progress to invasive breast cancer. In this patient, the fine linear calcifications seen on the mediolateral oblique (MLO) **(A)** and enlarged MLO **(B)** and craniocaudal (CC) **(C)** and enlarged CC **(D)** projections were evaluated and dismissed as vascular. *Continued.*

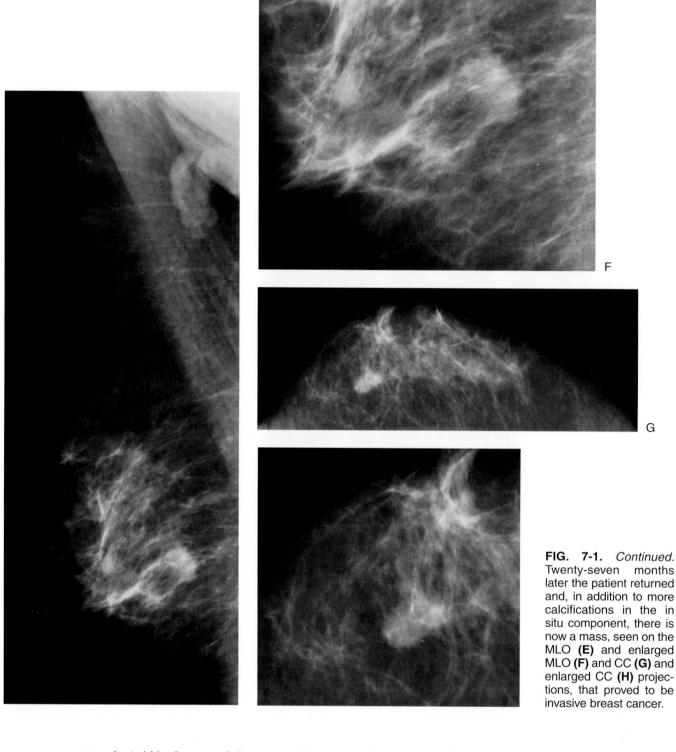

FIG. 7-1. *Continued.* Twenty-seven months later the patient returned and, in addition to more calcifications in the in situ component, there is now a mass, seen on the MLO **(E)** and enlarged MLO **(F)** and CC **(G)** and enlarged CC **(H)** projections, that proved to be invasive breast cancer.

appears to recur early (within 5 years of discovery) often with invasion. He noted that micropapillary or cribriform types progressed at a slower rate. His grading system for DCIS categorized the cytologic features of the lesions.

Initially Lagios used a classification system that was the reverse of the system used for invasive lesions. Grade I was the highest or worst grade, whereas grade IV was the lowest, indi-

cating the best prognosis. Lagios's grade I was a poorly differentiated, large cell lesion, with comedo-necrosis. Grade II was a small cell type with a cribriform pattern but with associated necrosis. Grade III was a cribriform pattern with anaplasia, and grade 4 was the small cell, micropapillary form of DCIS.

His data suggested that it might be possible to predict which lesions were likely to recur within a few years and

TABLE 7-1. *Histologic grading of ductal carcinoma in situ (DCIS)*

Cytologic differentiation
Well differentiated. Cells are uniform in size and shape (monomorphic) with evenly distributed chromatin and absent or "inconspicuous" nucleoli and rare mitoses evident.
Intermediate differentiation. Some pleomorphism. The chromatin may be slightly clumped and there are nucleoli and occasional mitoses.
Poorly differentiated. Pleomorphic cells with pleomorphic nuclei, clumped chromatin, prominent nucleoli, and frequent mitoses.
Necrosis: Necrosis is usually present in poorly differentiated DCIS, occasionally in intermediately differentiated DCIS, and usually absent in well-differentiated DCIS.
Architectural features
The polarization of the cells (orienting their long access toward a lumen) is a primary feature.
Highly polarized cells forming cribriform spaces or micropapillary protrusions into the lumen of the duct are associated with well-differentiated DCIS.
Highly polarized cells (the cells are oriented with their apices directed toward the lumen) may be present without an associated lumen and can form a solid pattern of growth. This occurs occasionally with moderately differentiated DCIS.
Less polarization (the cells are haphazardly oriented) is associated with poorly differentiated DCIS. This may form a solid pattern with or without necrosis, or pseudomicropapillary or cribriform patterns.

Source: Adapted from Holland R, Peterse JL, Millis RR, et al. Ductal carcinoma in situ: a proposal for a new classification. Semin Diagn Pathol 1994;11:167–180.

which were likely to not recur for many years, if at all (9). This could have a significant impact on therapeutic interventions. In a study of 79 women treated for DCIS by excision alone in which the tumor was <2.5 cm in its greatest extent, Lagios reported an overall recurrence rate of 10% at an average follow-up of 4 years. In this series, necrosis was an important prognostic feature. There were five out of 31 (16%) lesions of the large cell, comedo type of DCIS that recurred within 3 years of diagnosis having been treated by excision alone and an additional two of five (40%) of the small cell cribriform cancers with necrosis that also recurred. Only one of 10 (10%) of the cribriform cancers without necrosis recurred, and none of 33 micropapillary lesions had recurred after 6 years of follow-up (8).

Silverstein et al. used a similar grading system that they found predicted for local recurrence and disease-free survival. Their grade 1 lesions consisted of DCIS in which the cells had low nuclear grade with nuclei that were 1 to 1.5 red blood cells in diameter with diffuse chromatin and no visible nucleoli. Their grade 2 lesion had cells in which the nuclei were larger, 1 to 2 red-cell diameters, with coarse chromatin and occasional nucleoli. Their grade 3 (high grade) had nuclei that were greater than 2 red-blood-cell diameters with "vesicular" chromatin and one or more nucleoli (10). Using these parameters they then classified their lesions. Their group 1 consisted of lesions that had nuclear grade 1 or 2 but did not demonstrate any necrosis. Group 2 were grade 1 or 2 but with necrosis, and group 3 were the high-grade lesions. Among 238 patients, there were 31 local recurrences. Only three recurred out of the 80 lesions classified as well differentiated, group 1 (3.8%). Among the 90 women classified as group 2 (moderately well differentiated), 10 recurred (11.1%), whereas there were 18 recurrences in the 68 in group 3 (26.5%) (poorly differentiated). The 8-year actuarial disease-free survivals using the Van Nuys system were 93% for group 1, 84% for group 2, and 61% for group 3.

Holland et al. (7) have developed a similar grading scheme that is being evaluated by several groups. They divided DCIS into poorly differentiated, intermediate (or moderately differentiated), and well-differentiated lesions. Their classifications are based on cellular features as well as patterns of growth. These features include nuclear grade, architectural relationship of cells, and presence or absence of necrosis. The nuclear morphology in the cells is a primary prognostic indicator. Some of the features they suggest should be used to classify DCIS are listed in Table 7-1.

As in the other systems, their preliminary data suggest that poorly differentiated lesions recur early, with a high percentage of the recurrences being invasive cancers. Well-differentiated DCIS is slow to recur, taking 10 or more years, and invasion is less common. It has also been suggested that when an invasive cancer is poorly differentiated, any associated DCIS is also poorly differentiated, and low-grade invasive lesions tend to be associated with low-grade DCIS.

It remains to be seen whether either of these grading systems will be adopted and how they will be used in the management of DCIS. Some argue that it is only a matter of degree and that, ultimately, given sufficient time, many of these lesions, regardless of their levels of differentiation, will recur if not treated completely, and many will develop invasive capability. The importance of long-term follow-up is apparent in a review by Page et al. (11). They followed 28 patients whose previous biopsies had been incorrectly diagnosed as benign. On histologic review, the biopsied lesions were retrospectively diagnosed as low-grade cribriform DCIS. Among these 28 women, there were nine (36%) recurrences over a 25-year period. Seven of the women (25% of the total and 78% of the recurrences) developed invasive cancers within 10 years in the same quadrant of the same breast. The two other recurrences developed in subsequent years. There were even five breast cancer deaths (18%) among this group. This clearly demonstrates that even low-grade DCIS is not a totally innocuous lesion. The potential importance of DCIS is further suggested by the fact that studies such as this evaluate lesions that have been excised and some were probably completely excised. Thus, long-term follow-up of excised DCIS probably underestimates the risk from DCIS that is left alone. If a patient has a significant life expectancy, even low-grade DCIS can be an important lesion.

An Opportunity to Evaluate the Natural History of Ductal Carcinoma in Situ

Because most DCIS detected in the United States are surgically removed, the natural history of the lesion is always interrupted. The European screening trials provide an opportunity to develop a better understanding of the natural history of DCIS. In many of the trials the thresholds for intervention have been higher than those in the United States. The borderline clusters of calcifications that are excised in the United States were ignored. A review of the invasive breast cancers that were eventually diagnosed in those trials might reveal which had calcifications indicative of DCIS at an earlier screening. Unfortunately, pride (few wish to admit that they permitted cancer to pass through a screen) and the cost of such a review will likely prevent the undertaking.

Other factors will likely be discovered to help predict the natural history of DCIS. Investigators continue to elucidate the DNA sequences that are involved in the various stages of breast cancer development. The expression of several genes, such as *erb*-2 and *HER2/neu*, has already been linked to a more aggressive form of DCIS, and more details will be revealed in the future. Grading DCIS and ultimately DNA analyses may provide the patient and her physician with a better understanding of the potential virulence of these lesions.

Microscopic Invasion

As noted earlier, pure DCIS cannot be lethal. The only way that breast cancer can kill is through metastatic spread. Analysis of the significance of DCIS is further complicated because the pathologist's differentiation of in situ from invasive lesions may be inaccurate because they can only review a minute portion of the entire tumor. It would require thousands of slides to evaluate every level through a tumor to identify where it might have invaded into the stroma. This sampling error accounts for the fact that invasion may be overlooked.

Some lesions that appear confined to the ducts by light microscopy have been shown on electron microscopy to have transgressed the basement membrane into the surrounding stroma (12). This may explain why a few women with apparent intraductal carcinoma are paradoxically found to have tumor in their axillary lymph nodes when the diagnosis is made, and some actually die of metastatic breast cancer. The

likelihood of "microscopic" invasion increases with the size of the DCIS lesion. Lagios found, on careful sectioning, that if the DCIS lesion was >5.5 cm there was a 50% probability that there was microscopic invasion. For most mammographically detected DCIS, however, invasion is very rare. Only 2% of women with DCIS who have axillary dissections will be found to have tumor in their lymph nodes. For this reason, axillary node dissection is rarely indicated for DCIS.

Lobular Carcinoma

Less than 10% of cancers have cytologic features that suggest an origin in the lobular epithelium. When contained within the lobule they are designated as *lobular carcinoma in situ* (LCIS), and when they invade they are termed *invasive lobular carcinoma*. Invasive lobular carcinoma is as threatening as infiltrating ductal carcinoma.

Lobular Carcinoma in Situ

The diagnosis of LCIS causes great anxiety, and its management is perplexing. The diagnosis of this lesion is almost always coincidental. It is found periodically when a palpable mass is removed or when an abnormality detected on mammography is biopsied that proves to be benign, but the pathologist finds LCIS in the adjacent tissues.

LCIS appears to differ from DCIS in several ways. When an invasive cancer develops in association with DCIS, it grows in the same area in which the DCIS was found and is always invasive ductal carcinoma. In patients with LCIS, if invasive cancer develops, it does not always appear in the portion of the breast in which the LCIS was found (although LCIS usually involves a much larger volume of breast tissue than what is found at biopsy). Furthermore, the invasive cancer may not even develop in the same breast but rather the opposite breast, and if invasive cancer does develop, it is often invasive ductal carcinoma and not invasive lobular carcinoma. Some believe that LCIS is itself not of major consequence and prefer to reduce its significance by describing it as lobular neoplasia.

All agree, however, that LCIS is a significant indicator of increased risk for the ultimate development of invasive breast cancer. LCIS is likely one of the lesions that represents a "field phenomenon" in which large volumes of breast tissue have alterations that predispose to invasive cancer. Women with LCIS have up to a 30% risk of developing invasive carcinoma (ductal or lobular), with an equal risk (15%) that the invasive tumor will grow in either breast (13).

Because both breasts are at equal risk when LCIS is present, therapy is controversial. Most women with the disease will not develop invasive carcinoma; thus, definitive therapy is usually deferred and the breasts are followed "carefully." The probability of developing invasive carcinoma is the same for both breasts, making it difficult to recommend more aggressive therapy because both breasts must be treated equally.

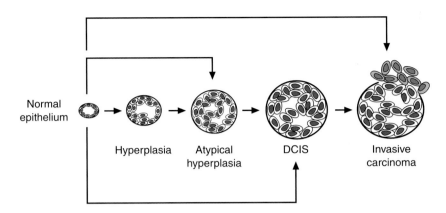

FIG. 7-2. The continuum theory suggests a stepwise progression from a normal epithelium through hyperplasia to atypical hyperplasia to ductal carcinoma in situ to invasive breast cancer. It is more likely that some cancers follow this progression, whereas others advance to invasion from any of the intermediate steps. Some cancers may be invasive with metastatic potential from the first transformed cell, whereas others replicate at each step for various lengths of time. Some intermediate changes, such as atypical hyperplasia, may represent "field" changes that occur in many cells simultaneously.

NATURAL HISTORY OF BREAST CANCER

As already noted, there is no general agreement about the natural history of breast cancer. It is generally agreed that breast cancer begins in the epithelial lining of the duct. The cells of the intralobular terminal duct are likely those responsible for most proliferation, and it is these cells that are believed to be susceptible to malignant transformation.

Cancer cells that remain confined within the duct cannot cause death. Breast cancer becomes lethal only when it develops the capability of breaking out of the duct and invading into the surrounding tissue, gaining access to the blood and lymphatic systems through which it can spread to other organs, and grow and destroy their functions. Uncertainty remains over the natural history of breast cancer and the actual steps in the progression to lethality. As with other cancers, the development and growth of these tumors is variable and likely to be influenced by individual tumor properties as well as host and environmental factors.

It is becoming increasingly apparent that cancer initiation, promotion, and progression form a multistep sequence of DNA alterations and promotional factors that eventually results in a malignant cell whose clones proliferate without restraint. The early genetic changes are presently undetectable. It is difficult to accurately relate genetic (genotypic) changes at the histologic level because many changes are probably not reflected in visible alterations in the cell's phenotype as morphologically evident changes.

The Most Likely Model

Data and experience suggest that many different paths can lead to malignancy. There undoubtedly are some cancers that develop from a single cell that, by itself, acquires all the genetic alterations needed to be an invasive cancer and whose clones are fully capable of invasion and lethal metastasis (Fig. 7-2). In other cancers, there is likely a progression that begins with some genetic alterations that may or may not be reflected in the appearance of the cell. This cell or group of cells may overproliferate with some retained controls (hyperplasia), and the process may be reversible so that a malignancy does not result. There are also cells that likely

become genetically unstable (atypical hyperplasia and in situ breast cancer). Because many of these cells may have already lost some of the usual genetic controls, the likelihood is increased that one of the group will acquire additional changes that bring it closer to a malignant phenotype.

Field Phenomena

Although it appears that many (if not most) breast cancers originate from a single cell that acquires (over a variable length of time) all the necessary DNA changes to proliferate without restraint, invade normal tissue, and spread to other organs, it also appears that some cancers arise in tissues that are "primed." This makes the ultimate change more likely. Some changes affect numerous cells such that they are not malignant but are predisposed to malignant transformation. Their genetic instability increases the risk that such a transformation will occur. In a significant number of women, a large number of cells, influenced by as yet undetermined factors, may be transformed simultaneously, each with a higher potential for subsequent transformations. When multiple cells are at risk it is described as a *field phenomenon.*

These multicell changes may be related to inherited abnormal gene sequences passed from the germ cell to all the cells in the body increasing the likelihood of subsequent cancer, but they may also be due to some environmental agent that affected many cells in a similar fashion. The mechanism for these changes remains to be elucidated.

LCIS is likely a field phenomenon in which there was not a single cell of origin but probably multiple cells that experienced a common transformation. The higher risk for women with these lesions is probably due to the greater number of cells that have a genotype that is that much closer to a true cancer phenotype.

Atypical hyperplasia may be a small focus of abnormal cells or extend over large areas. The fact that it also carries a high risk for the development of invasive cancer suggests that it, too, represents a field defect. Atypical hyperplastic tissues consist of many cells that have sustained changes (presumably in DNA or perhaps in response to growth regulation factors) that are reflected phenotypically and place the tissues closer to acquiring the necessary chromosomal alterations

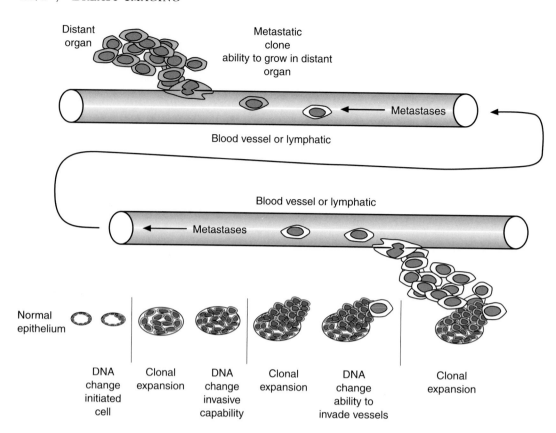

Distant organ

Metastatic clone
ability to grow in distant organ

Metastases

Blood vessel or lymphatic

Blood vessel or lymphatic

Metastases

Normal epithelium

DNA change initiated cell

Clonal expansion

DNA change invasive capability

Clonal expansion

DNA change ability to invade vessels

Clonal expansion

FIG. 7-3. Whether as a multistage process or as the direct development of an invasive lesion, a number of genetic changes most likely take place for a cell and its clones to be able to proliferate, invade, and successfully metastasize.

needed to become cancerous. The sheer number of these cells and statistical probabilities increase the likelihood of a transition of one (or more) cell to frank malignancy.

ORIGINS OF BREAST CANCER

The exact origin of breast cancer is unknown. Some have postulated that breast cancers arise from a stem cell precursor of the ductal or lobular epithelial cell, and that the various similarities to ductal or lobular elements and subclassifications of cancer represent different directions in the dedifferentiation of the cells of a particular lesion.

Although a breast stem cell has yet to be demonstrated, increasing evidence suggests that one exists. Deng et al. (14) found that there were genetic defects (loss of heterozygosity) in apparently normal cells found in normal lobules that were the same as some of the defects found in cancer cells in nearby cancer-containing lobules; cells in lobules further away did not have the same genetic changes. This finding suggests that there may be a common progenitor for both the benign and the malignant cells of the affected duct network. If there is a stem cell responsible for the development of the ducts and lobules, then an alteration in its DNA early in life, before duct elongation and terminal lobular differentiation, could be distributed into every cell in the segment. This would place the cells throughout the segment at risk for further genetic change, increasing the likelihood that one of the cells might ultimately become cancerous. This would explain

the findings of Deng et al. It might also be the explanation for the so-called field phenomenon, in which the cells in an area of the breast have a similar abnormality, but other areas of the breast are normal. This phenomenon may be the explanation for diffuse adenosis, atypical hyperplasia, or even LCIS.

It would be very unlikely that only the cells of a single segment in the mature breast could be damaged by exposure to a carcinogen or mutagen while cells in other segments were spared. If a stem cell was altered in the immature breast, however, that damage would be distributed to all of the cells of the developing segment, and only the cells of the segment would be affected. This is the likely explanation for segmentally distributed abnormalities. Efforts to prevent breast cancer are often directed toward older women. If there is a stem cell, its presence would suggest the importance of preventing exposure to carcinogens at an early age, before terminal differentiation.

The sequence of events described above and those that follow, however, are still disputed. Those who believe in a growth continuum suggest that intraductal carcinoma proliferates for a variable length of time confined within the duct. Ultimately one or more cells develop the ability to penetrate the basement membrane, and their clones invade the surrounding stroma, gaining access to the vascular and lymphatic networks and permitting metastatic spread (Fig. 7-3).

Dual theorists argue that a significant number of nonlethal cancers develop in the breast that will never affect the life of the woman. Invasive, potentially lethal cancer is interpreted as a separate distinct lesion that also develops in the epithelium but rapidly invades and metastasizes (i.e., becomes systemic and thus incurable) before it can be detected. This latter model is based on the observation that in random breast biopsies, unsuspected cancers (particularly in situ lesions) are found that never affected the life of the patient.

Autopsy studies have revealed that more cancers are found within the breast than appear to become clinically significant (15). Most autopsy studies, however, are by the nature of the population, biased. If the population is elderly, it is possible that the women died before the tumors had a chance to affect mortality. This does not prove that the same tumor, given sufficient time to grow in a younger woman, might not ultimately be lethal. In a Danish study of younger women who died from causes other than cancers, 40% of the women under age 50 years were reported to have lesions that were classified as cancer (16). This is much higher than a study in the southwestern United States where only 2.2% of women who died accidental deaths (11/500) had breast cancers at autopsy (17). In these studies, there is no independent corroboration that the lesions classified as cancer were clearly such. Other biases can enter into the analysis. In the Danish study, for example, the results were likely biased because almost half of the women were alcoholics, and alcohol has been shown to increase the risk of breast cancer.

The life expectancy of an individual most likely influences the significance of an early breast cancer. If some forms of DCIS take 10 to 15 years to evolve, DCIS in an 80-year-old woman may not have the same significance as DCIS in a 42-year-old woman.

Many Breast Cancers Arise in an in Situ Lesion

Ohuchi et al. (18), in an elegant three-dimensional pathologic analysis, demonstrated that DCIS can spread up and down the duct network and remain in situ, whereas invasive

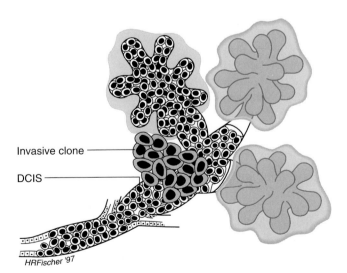

Invasive clone

DCIS

HRFischer '97

FIG. 7-4. Cells that are proliferating out of control but lack the ability to invade may continue to grow within the duct while a clone that has developed invasive capability can be growing simultaneously in the same lesion.

cancer can be found associated with a part of the process. This finding would support the continuum theory. Their data suggest that one of the already genetically unstable cells in the DCIS (19) developed an invasive clone and that this clone proliferated while the remaining in situ cells, unable to invade, continued to proliferate and spread up and down the ducts. This observation explains how DCIS and invasive breast cancer can be found in the same lesion (Fig. 7-4).

If Cancer Is Clonal, Why Is a Lesion Heterogeneous?

Invasive breast cancer likely develops from a single cell. It is the clones of this cell that form the initial tumor. There is no reason to expect, however, that once a cell becomes malignant, further DNA changes will not occur in its progeny. In fact, once a cell is genetically abnormal, the likelihood of additional changes increases. These cells are genetically unstable. The development of additional clones with different characteristics is the probable explanation for the frequent cellular heterogeneity of cancers. Eventually, the most aggressive clone likely predominates. Tabar has suggested that this predominance explains why small cancers tend to be better differentiated whereas larger cancers tend to be more poorly differentiated (20). He argues that this is an additional reason earlier detection is so important.

In situ cancer is not found within many invasive cancers for various reasons. It is possible that there are some cancers in which the first malignant cell, or one of the early in situ cells, develops all of the necessary ability (genetic changes) to invade and even metastasize. Thus, some cancers may never go through any significant in situ stage. In other cancers, it is likely that just as the invasive cancer invades and destroys normal tissue, it also destroys any in situ tumor as well, and when diagnosed, only invasive cancer is found.

Multifocal versus Multicentric Cancer

Multifocal breast cancer should be defined as multiple foci of cancer associated with one duct network, whereas multicentric cancer involves foci that are in separate lobes or segments. Multifocality is the result of cancer originating from a single cell whose clones spread up and down the duct, with the subsequent development of invasive clones forming independently at various locations. Multicentricity requires the independent transformation of two separate cells (or cell groups). Multifocality is fairly common; multicentricity is fairly unusual.

Whole breast studies by Holland et al. (21) suggest that most cancer foci are directly connected and represent contiguous spread. He found that multifocal cancers are actually part of the same lesion. Because of sampling error, the connection between the components of the lesion is not always appreciated on routine pathologic analysis. Ohtake et al. (22) used high-definition three-dimensional analysis of cancers to show that multifocal lesions are connected by ducts involved in contiguity with DCIS. True multicentricity with completely separate foci of cancer in different duct networks is extremely rare.

Molecular Biological Events

There are probably many ways that a cancer can develop (see Chapter 3). Normal control mechanisms may be lost or modified by genes that are inappropriately activated, deactivated, overexpressed, or lost completely. The activation of a proto-oncogene so that it functions as an oncogene, or the deactivation or loss of a normally functioning tumor suppressor gene, are two mechanisms that have been identified in breast cancers.

The control of the cell, regulated by the genetic code, is modulated by the proteins that are created when genes are "switched on." Feedback mechanisms act as switches, but the overexpression of a gene through the overproduction of its protein or the amplification of a gene leading to the excess generation of its product from excessive copies of the gene all contribute to loss of cell control.

Genetic Predisposition to Breast Cancer: The BRCA1 and BRCA2 Genes

Several genes have been identified that, when abnormal, predispose to the development of breast cancer. These genes were discovered because mutations of the gene were found in families that had a large number of women who developed breast cancer. Multiple diagnoses of breast cancer in the same family occur because the abnormal genes are passed in the germ cells of either the mother (ova) or father (sperm) and are the main source of inherited susceptibility to breast cancer.

The BRCA1 gene (breast cancer 1) was the first to be identified. Located on the q arm of chromosome 17, BRCA1 has a normal function, but abnormalities of the gene have been found among women in families in which breast and ovarian cancers are extremely common (23). The inheritance of the abnormal gene follows an autosomal dominant pattern, which means that women with a parent who carries a BRCA1 abnormality have a 50% chance of inheriting the gene.

Women who have an abnormal copy of BRCA1 have a 50% chance of developing breast cancer. Although the gene is primarily associated with inherited breast cancer susceptibility, women with an abnormal BRCA1 also carry an increased risk of developing ovarian cancer.

BRCA1 was the first gene discovered that was found to be abnormal and could be inherited producing susceptibility to breast cancer, but it appears that only approximately 5% of breast cancers can be attributed to an inherited BRCA1 abnormality. Another 4% to 5% are likely attributable to abnormalities of a second gene, BRCA2. Women with an abnormal BRCA2 have a high chance (50%) of developing breast cancer. This gene carries an increased risk for breast cancer but

not ovarian cancer, but it also appears to be associated with an increased risk of male breast cancer.

Clearly, having an abnormal germ cell gene in itself does not cause breast cancer (this would be incompatible with life). Genes come in two copies (alleles), and women who inherit an abnormality of BRCA1 or BRCA2 also have a normal copy of the gene. It has been shown that mouse embryos that lack either normal allele die very early in utero. Women born with one abnormal copy of a gene are further along the chain of genetic alterations that change a cell into a cancer cell. In these women it takes fewer events for a cell to develop into a malignant cell, which explains why they are at risk for breast cancer much earlier in life than an unaffected individual.

Because women who inherit an abnormal BRCA1 or BRCA2 have the gene in every cell in their bodies, the likelihood is high that one or more of those cells will accumulate other genetic changes needed for cancer to develop. This accounts for their high risk. For the same reasons, inheriting a defective gene such as BRCA1 or BRCA2 also places these women at risk earlier in life.

The functions of these two genes are being clarified. Abnormalities of the gene are apparently not common in sporadic breast cancers but only in women with the inherited susceptibility. It had been suggested that BRCA1 coded for a protein involved in DNA transcription and that it operated in the cell nucleus. Others have suggested that they have identified the protein in the cytoplasm of sporadic cancers. Some controversy existed as to the accuracy of this latter observation, but it certainly raised questions as to the true function of BRCA1 and how abnormal or absent gene function might lead to cancer. Additional information suggested that the normal BRCA1 protein inhibited cell proliferation in breast cancer cell cultures and that it was a tumor suppressor gene. In still another study, the growth of transplanted human cancers in laboratory animals was apparently inhibited when normal copies of the gene were transfected into the tumor cells

The strongest evidence suggests that BRCA1 and BRCA2 are involved in DNA repair, which also suggests that they are not directly on the path to cancer but may be involved in the mechanisms that repair DNA mutations or damage. A defect in DNA repair would permit changes to accumulate, and, if cell death did not result, the accumulation of changes would increase the likelihood of malignant transformation.

Blood Testing for Genetic Abnormalities

Because all the cells, including white cells, in women with inherited susceptibility contain the abnormal gene, blood tests can be used to screen women for the abnormality. It is estimated that 1 in 200 to 1 in 400 women carry an abnormal BRCA1 gene. Given the psychological implications of having an abnormal gene (there is even guilt among women who do not have the gene when someone else in their family is found to have it) and the medical as well as economic (insurance) implications of knowing who has an abnormal gene, the use of such screening tests will likely be limited.

Jewish Women and Risk of Abnormal BRCA1

It has long been known that Jewish women have a higher risk for breast cancer. At least part of this risk is due to the fact that approximately 1% of Ashkenazi Jewish women have inherited an abnormal BRCA1 gene (24). In a review of 418 women with early-onset breast cancer (before age 40 years) 30 women who had developed breast cancer before 30 years of age as well as 39 Jewish women with early-onset breast cancer were evaluated. Among the 30, four (13%) had chain-terminating mutations and one had a missense mutation. Two of the four Jewish women in this group had the same mutation, coded as 185delAG. Among the 39 other Jewish women, eight (25%) had this same mutation. Other mutations can occur spontaneously, but 185delAG is common among Jewish women. It has been postulated that all of these women can be traced back to a single European ancestor.

Most Breast Cancers Are Sporadic

Most breast cancers are not due to an inherited gene, and risk for them cannot be detected by a blood test. The majority of cancers appears to be due to a single cell aberration that occurs through "statistical bad luck." The longer cells are around, the greater the likelihood that one or more will develop an abnormal gene and begin unrestrained proliferation. Although many women may have cancers that also contain the same abnormal gene or genes, these are spontaneous mutations, or alterations that occur only in the changed cell and cannot be identified prospectively. Although understanding the mechanism of inherited susceptibility will lead to a greater understanding of the development of breast cancer, finding most cancers will remain the search for the proverbial needle in the haystack.

Other Genes Associated with Breast Cancer

p53 and Tumor Suppressor Genes

Some normal genes function to control cell division. These have been termed *tumor suppressor genes*. When at least one copy of these genes is present, the cell functions properly; the loss of both copies can be detected by the loss of heterozygosity in the genetic analysis of the tumor cells. The loss of a tumor suppressor gene has been found in some sporadic cancers also to be located on chromosome 17. It is a gene that codes for the p53 protein and has been found in families in which breast and other cancers are extremely common. This defective gene can also be passed between generations as an inheritance in the germ cell line, predisposing those who inherit this genetic material to cancer. Unlike BRCA1 and BRCA2, sporadic cancers (the individ-

ual has no inherited predisposition) have also been identified that have "spontaneously" developed loss of tumor suppression provide by p53.

HER2/neu (c-erb-B2)

Until fairly recently, studying breast cancer has been limited by the resolution of microscopy. Many nuclear changes are not reflected in visible alterations of the cell phenotype as seen by the pathologist until, ultimately, sufficient changes do take place that are recognized as cytologic abnormalities and eventually histologic aberration. The development of molecular biological tests permits the detection of DNA changes that are not reflected in visible cell differences under the microscope. The cytologic features of a cancer cell found in an invasive lesion may be indistinguishable from a cell found in an in situ lesion, but genetic differences have been noted in invasive lesions that are not found in in situ lesions. The activation of the oncogene *HER2/neu* (c-*erb*-B2) is one such sequence that has been identified (25). Although specific genetic abnormalities are being identified and linked to breast cancer, it is likely that multiple, as yet undefined, abnormalities must be present before a malignant phenotype becomes visible to the light microscopist.

METASTASIS

Cancer cells can be found floating in the blood of patients with breast cancer (26). Because there are cells in the blood, however, does not mean that the cancer has become metastatic. The ability to metastasize likely requires additional genetic alteration, activation, or deactivation.

Investigators have shown that to grow, a tumor must be able to stimulate the growth of a new blood supply (27). Metastatic potential increases with tumor size, which is related to tumor neovascularity. Several studies have suggested that the number of vessels at the periphery of a tumor is predictive of the likelihood of metastatic spread (28). In some series, long-term survival seems to be related to neovascularity. It is likely that the more new vessels that are formed, the worse the prognosis.

The ability of a tumor to successfully metastasize requires other genetic capabilities. Simply releasing cancer cells into the blood does not result in metastatic spread. Tumors must also be able to produce proteolytic enzymes that are necessary to disrupt the collagen that might prevent their spread (although some studies suggest that the cancer cell can induce normal tissues to produce these enzymes). Traveling through the blood, cancer cells also must be able to produce adhesion proteins that permit them to stick to vessel walls and exit from the vascular system to invade an organ (29). The metastases of many cancers to specific sites suggest that local environmental factors are also necessary for successful metastatic spread.

Breast cancer, unfortunately, is frequently successful in establishing itself in many different sites in the body. The success of screening, however, proves that it is possible to interrupt these sequential changes and successfully eliminate breast cancer before the establishment of metastatic lesions.

Does Screening Lead to the Overdiagnosis of Breast Cancer?

Some have criticized screening by arguing that it merely finds slow-growing, nonthreatening cancers. If this were so, screening would result in the diagnosis of more cancers over the long term than routine medical care. This has not been the case with long-term follow-up in the screening trials. In the Health Insurance Plan of New York (HIP) trial, earlier detection led to more cancers among the screened women in the early years of the trial, but by the seventh year (2 years after the termination of screening) the control group caught up as their cancers "rose to the surface." In the Swedish trials there has been a slight excess of cancers found, as would be expected, among the screened women. Because the control groups are now being screened, it is difficult to assess the issue of overdiagnosis, but it does not appear to be a major phenomenon.

Screening does not appear to find a greater number of cancers in an absolute sense, but it does find them earlier in their growth and reduces the stage at which the disease is found. Regardless of the true natural history of breast cancer, the fact remains that in large randomized, controlled trials, earlier diagnosis reduced the overall absolute mortality from the disease in the screened population.

The two apparently contradictory theories of breast cancer development may not be incompatible. The hypothesis suggesting two levels of tumor aggression may well represent the two ends of a spectrum. It is likely that some breast cancers develop all the necessary changes in the DNA of a cell over a short period of time with early metastatic potential, whereas others may never accumulate all the necessary changes, and it is likely that there is a spectrum of growths with intermediate potentials. Given the emerging model of progressive DNA changes leading to the development of solid tumors, a significant number of breast cancers likely develop over many years, and some progress rapidly (with the majority in between).

It is a statistical probability that some cells will acquire the appropriate mutations or chromosomal damage that permit unrestricted growth, tissue invasion capability, and metastatic potential very quickly, but other lesions will pass slowly through the various stages with clones of cells that can only grow locally, whereas others, through chromosomal change over time, develop more lethal capability. There are probably in situ cancers that never acquire the changes necessary to permit the production of enzymes needed for invasion, but on a statistical basis, the longer an in situ lesion is present, the more likely it is for one of its cells to develop the ability to break out of the duct. If this cell survives, its clonal progeny become the invasive cancer that is recognized as potentially lethal.

The significance of DCIS will remain controversial. Mastectomy is essentially a curative procedure. Because metastatic cancer cannot occur after a primary lesion has been removed, the only lesions that are not cured by mastectomy could not have been truly intraductal but had to have areas of invasion that were not apparent to the pathologist. The irony that more advanced cancers can be successfully treated by breast conservation with excision and radiation while the in situ disease is treated by mastectomy has not been lost on women and physicians. Methods to determine which of these lesions is likely to progress to invasion will help guide therapy that will increasingly focus on conservation rather than mastectomy.

Among the difficulties associated with DCIS is determining its exact extent. Many of these lesions are extremely extensive, having grown up and down the duct network. Even lesions detected by mammography alone are often more extensive than suggested by the calcifications that usually indicate their presence (30). In a study of patients with mammographically detected DCIS and apparently clear margins on pathologic analysis of the excised specimen, 40% had residual disease found upon re-excision of the surgical bed or at the time of mastectomy.

Although the pathologist should evaluate the margins of excised tissue to try to determine if the tumor comes to the margin of the excised tissue, indicating that there is residual tumor in the breast, the sampling error described above means that a duct that contains tumor and extends to the margin and into the unexcised tissue can easily be overlooked (Fig. 7-5). Some data suggest that shaving the surfaces of the excised tissue and having them analyzed separately may give a more accurate analysis of the margins. Some surgeons shave the lining of the cavity from which the specimen has been excised for the pathologist to analyze to determine if the margins are clear.

As more women with DCIS are studied and the spectrum of lesions encompassed by this terminology is better defined, therapeutic approaches will likely be modified to recognize the variety of lesions that, in the past, have all been treated as if they had the same prognosis. Until we have better methods to characterize these lesions we must rely on the results of large trials to assist in making treatment recommendations. The early studies that showed that conservation therapy (excision and radiation) was as successful in treating breast cancer as modified radical mastectomy also revealed that radiation after excision for DCIS reduced the possibility of recurrence.

What remains to be seen is the long-term survival significance. The data suggest that recurrence in the conserved breast does not compromise survival and that conservation therapy for DCIS is the correct approach. The importance of DCIS remains to be determined. It is also clear, however, that there are women with invasive cancer whose lives can be saved by detecting the lesion earlier. Any early benefit from screening is only attributable to a reduction in deaths from invasive breast cancer.

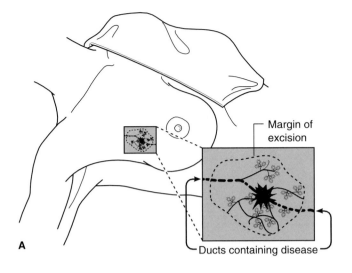

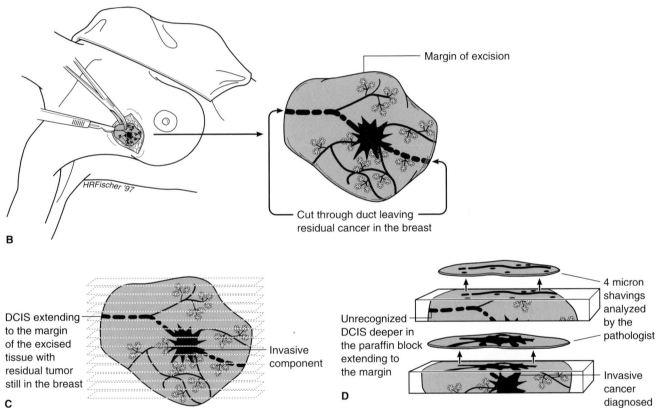

FIG. 7-5. As a consequence of the surgical excision and the way biopsy material is processed and reviewed, the pathologist may be unaware that tumor extends to the margin of the excised tissue and that there is residual tumor in the breast. The surgeon may excise a tumor without realizing that ducts containing tumor have been cut through and there is residual tumor in the breast **(A)**. The excised sample is cut into 2-mm slices **(B)** that are embedded in separate paraffin blocks **(C)**. The pathologist reviews one or two 4-μm slices that are taken from the top of each block **(D)**. If the tumor that extends to the margin is deeper in the block, it will not be seen by the pathologist and it will incorrectly appear that the tumor has been completely excised with a border of normal surrounding tissue.

GROWTH RATE OF BREAST CANCER

The fact that breast cancer is not a single disease complicates detection as well as therapy. Breast cancer doubling times range from days to several years, but the average doubling time is approximately 100 to 180 days (31,32). Although screening is an attempt to detect breast cancer early, by the time a tumor is clinically apparent (at approximately 1 cm in diameter) it has probably been growing for 5 to 10 years. Assuming the number of cells doubles every 100 days (i.e., one becomes two, two become four, four become

eight, and so on every 100 days) it would take 20 doublings for one cell to grow into 1 million cells (a mass approximately 1 mm in diameter). This lesion would have been growing for 5.5 years (20 × 100 days/365).

The mammographic detection of breast cancer that is not yet clinically evident appears to advance the time of detection by 1 to 2 years in younger women and up to 4 years for older women. Thus, *early detection* is a relative term. The size of the tumor in the breast is only important as it relates to the development of metastases. In general, the larger the tumor, the greater the likelihood that it has produced metasta-

TABLE 7-2. *Percent surviving of white women, 1974–1987*

	Year 1	Year 2	Year 3	Year 4	Year 5	Year 6	Year 7
Under 50							
1974–1978	97	91	86	81	77	73	71
1977–1980	97	91	85	80	78	73	71
1981–1987	98	92	87	82	78	75	—
50 and over							
1974–1976	94	88	83	78	74	71	68
1977–1980	94	89	84	79	75	71	68
1981–1987	96	91	86	82	78	75	—
All ages							
1974–1976	95	89	83	79	75	71	69
1977–1980	95	90	84	79	75	71	69
1981–1987	98	92	86	82	78	75	—

Source: Data from the National Cancer Institute Surveillance, Epidemiology and End-Results Program. Relative Survival Rates for Successive Numbers of Years after Diagnosis. SEER Program.

tic lesions (2). The point at which tumor cells gain access to the vascular and lymphatic system and develop the ability to successfully grow in other organs is the important factor in early detection. A life can only be saved if the primary tumor is eliminated before it has successfully metastasized.

Successful Metastases: A Speculative Model

Because the metastatic lesions are the lethal component, breast cancer can be cured if the primary lesion is eliminated before clones have spread to other organs and developed the ability to live independent of the primary lesion. The data suggest that there may be an early dependence of metastatic disease on the primary lesion. There are animal models in which metastatic lesions grow faster for a short period after the primary lesion has been removed (33). Presumably factors are elaborated into the blood by the primary lesion that reach and slow the growth of the metastatic lesions; perhaps there are other interrelations.

There has been much speculation as to the reason for the delayed benefit from screening younger women (the benefit does not appear in most trials for 7 to 10 years), but there has been little discussion and no good explanation for the almost immediate decrease in breast cancer deaths among older screened women in the screening trials (the benefit began to appear 2 to 3 years after the first screen). For an immediate benefit to appear in a screening trial, a woman in the control group must die early in the trial from breast cancer while her counterpart lives. Because periodic screening is more likely to detect the slow-growing cancers (length-biased sampling), and this phenomenon would be exaggerated by the long screening interval used in the trials, the only way that an early death could be avoided would be if metastatic disease was already established and poised to kill the control-group woman within a few years of the start of the trial but somehow regressed with the earlier detection and treatment of the screened individual. Again, this is purely speculative, but it might explain the trial results. It would imply that

metastases can be present, but not autonomous for a period of time, and reliant on the primary lesion. Until they become autonomous they are not "successful."

Regardless of the explanation, tumor cells appear to need changes that permit them to grow as metastatic lesions. They may gain access to the vascular system and the lymphatic system and even float in the blood without being able to live in other tissue environments. They develop a lethal potential only when they become successfully metastatic. For screening to be efficacious, it must result in the interruption of a cancer before this occurs. Data from the screening trials have demonstrated that *earlier* detection can accomplish this and result in a significant reduction in mortality.

SURVIVAL AND PROGNOSTIC FACTORS

Breast cancer is not uniformly fatal. In fact, because it is a series of diseases that develop with age, many women who are diagnosed with breast cancer actually die from other illness (e.g., heart disease). The majority of women with breast cancer do not die as a result of breast cancer. There appears to be a difference in the survival for younger women and older women: Contrary to common perceptions, younger women tend to live longer with breast cancer than do older women (34). The 5-year survival for women in the United States who are <50 years of age at diagnosis with invasive breast cancer is 78%, whereas for older women, it has been somewhat less (74% to 75%) (35) (Table 7-2). Survival data are influenced by the method of detection. In the screening programs, the survival for women aged 40 to 49 years was almost identical to those aged 50 to 59 years when compared by stage at detection (36,37).

Nevertheless, >30% of women who develop breast cancer will die as a result, and until recently the overall mortality has not changed for over 50 years. There may have been some progress in treating breast cancer over that time. Because the incidence has been increasing steadily over the same time, a stable mortality in face of an increasing incidence suggests some women were being cured. More recently the death rate actually appears to have decreased. This is clear evidence that earlier detection and improved therapies are having an effect. The difficulty is that breast cancer may lie dormant for many years and recur 20 to 30 years after diagnosis and kill the woman. This recurrence makes it very difficult to determine whether an individual is cured.

Treatment, either surgical or chemotherapeutic, can be disabling, which has spurred attempts to subcategorize breast cancers into groups with good prognoses and those with less favorable futures. If cancers can be accurately segregated, the treatment for favorable cancers could be less aggressive, and those with less favorable cancers could be offered more intensive therapy. Thus far, despite the optimism that is generated with the discovery of each new prognostic indicator, the major significant factors remain the size of the tumor, its histologic type and grade, the presence or absence of hormone receptors (primarily estrogen), the status of axillary nodes, and the presence or absence of distant metastatic disease.

The rates of recurrence reflect a statistical association. In general, screening can detect small cancers before they have metastasized or at a time when the tumor burden is small and can be controlled by the body's immune system. Some breast cancers are microscopic at the time of metastatic spread, however. Clearly, these lesions are "systemic" very early in their growth and detecting them will likely have little effect on the overall survival of the woman. In some cases the opposite may occur, and a small number of cancers will be relatively indolent and grow to a large size within the breast without metastasizing. Screening and earlier detection probably influence the mortality in women who have tumors that follow a growth pattern between these two extremes. There may be a period before metastasis when the tumor may be eliminated and death averted or when reducing the burden of tumor cells permits normal immunologic surveillance to prevail and eliminate the threat.

Tumor Size

Numerous studies have demonstrated a direct relationship between the diameter of an infiltrating cancer (usually measured by the pathologist) and survival (2,38,39). In the Breast Cancer Detection Demonstration Project (BCDDP), the percentage of women with positive axillary nodes increased with the size of the tumor. None of the women had positive nodes when the cancer was in situ, and if the invasive cancer was <0.3 mm, only 4% had positive lymph nodes. This increased to 10% for tumors between 0.3 and 1 cm, 22% for tumors 1 to 2 cm, 32% for tumors 2 to 3 cm, 44% for tumors 4 to 5 cm, and 50% for tumors 5 cm or more (37).

Although most staging schemes use 2 cm as the cutoff between large and small cancers (stage I), prognosis improves continuously as tumor size decreases. Rosen et al.

(40) demonstrated a significant survival difference for node-negative invasive cancers <1 cm relative to those between 1 and 2 cm (all stage I). If the tumor was <1 cm and the nodes were negative, 20% of the women had recurrence by 20 years and died. If the tumor (still node negative) was 1 to 2 cm, deaths rose to 30%.

The Swedish Two County Trial showed that if invasive cancers are <1 cm, the patients all do so well that histologic grade (which is normally an independent prognostic factor) has no influence on survival (41). Tabar and colleagues have also demonstrated that survival data parallel mortality results in that both are improved when tumors are found at a smaller size and an earlier stage (42). The biology of larger tumors appears to differ from smaller tumors.

Histologic Type and Grade

The subcategories of breast cancer have varying prognoses. Women with invasive ductal carcinomas that demonstrate varying manifestations of differentiation, such as colloid, papillary, and tubular cancers, generally have more favorable survival than those with undifferentiated invasive ductal carcinoma not otherwise specified. Typical medullary cancers also have more favorable prognoses (43). Histologic grading systems attempt to assess the mitotic activity of the cell population, the level of differentiation of the cells, their pleomorphism, and their architectural differentiation (i.e., whether they are trying to form breastlike structures, such as ducts, tubule formation, or glandular acini). Cell pleomorphism appears to be the more reliable measure.

Henson et al. found that the histologic grade of the tumor was prognostically important in an analysis of 22,616 cases of breast cancer in the Surveillance, Epidemiology, and End-Results program that monitors 9.6% of the U.S. population (Table 7-3) (44). Women whose tumors were classified stage I, grade 1 had a 99% 5-year survival and a 95% 10-year survival rate. Even if their lymph nodes contained tumor, if their tumors were <2 cm and the histologic grade was 1, their 5-year survival was 99%. Women who had tumors classified as stage II, grade 1 had the same prognosis as women whose tumors were stage I, grade 3. Both were better than those whose tumors were classified as stage I, grade 4. Histologic grade increased (worsened)

TABLE 7-3. *Five-year survival by stage*

Stage	Survival (%)
I	96
II	82
III	53
IV	18

Source: Adapted from Henson DE, Ries L, Freedman LS, Carriaga M. Relationship among outcome, stage of disease, and histologic grade for 22,616 cases of breast cancer. The basis for a prognostic index. Cancer 1991;68:2142–2149.

with tumor size. Tabar also found that the grade of the tumor appears to change as it increases in size. This may reflect progressive genetic changes as tumors age with the selection of more aggressive clones.

In an analysis of 918 patients with T1 breast cancers (2 cm or less), Barth et al. (45) found that, overall, 23% had positive axillary lymph nodes. They found that the likelihood of positivity increased with tumor size, and the strongest predictors of axillary nodal involvement were the presence of intramammary lymphatic or vascular invasion, palpability of the tumor, and high nuclear grade. They found that if a tumor was not palpable, T1a or T1b without lymphatic or vascular invasion, and was not high grade, the incidence of positive nodes was only 3%. If, however, the lesion was palpable, had lymphatic or vascular invasion, was high grade, and was 1 to 2 cm, lymph node positivity increased to 49%.

Axillary Node Involvement

Although breast cancer metastasizes hematogenously as well as through the lymphatics, the prognosis for breast cancer patients is strongly associated with the presence or absence of metastatic disease in the axillary lymph nodes at the time of diagnosis. For example, for tumors <2 cm, the 5-year survival rate diminishes from 96% in women who have no nodal involvement at the time of diagnosis to 87% in women with one to three positive nodes to 66% for women with four or more involved lymph nodes (21). Although studies suggest that even some node-negative women (with large tumors) can benefit from systemic treatment, benefit diminishes with decreasing tumor size, and axillary node assessment still provides important prognostic information. At least 10 lymph nodes must be examined for an accurate sample (46).

Lymph node positivity is not an all-or-nothing relationship. Prognosis worsens with the number of nodes involved (21). Tumor in the lymphatic system is primarily an indication of the biological potential of the tumor. When nodes are involved, the tumor has demonstrated its ability to survive outside the breast, and it must be considered "systemic"; systemic treatment with chemotherapy or hormone therapy will likely be beneficial.

Unfortunately, the absence of tumor in lymph nodes does not guarantee a cure. Approximately 30% of node-negative women develop and die from recurrent breast cancer (47). This may be an artifact of the crude method of analyzing the nodes. Merely cutting a node in half and examining histologic sections from the cut surfaces may have a large margin for error. More recent studies using multiple sectioning, immunohistochemistry, or even polymerase chain reaction to find tumor DNA have already shown higher node positivity rates than conventional sampling. The dilemma lies in the fact that all of the treatment data are based on detection techniques that find less subtle evidence of metastases.

In addition to the prognostic indicators described above, there is major interest in defining more accurate prognostic factors that can be used to better predict which women are more likely to relapse and would benefit from adjuvant therapy.

DNA Content

Flow cytometry to measure the DNA content of cancer cells has been correlated in some studies with prognosis. This method involves digestion of the tumor to prepare a suspension of its cells. After special staining, the cells flow past a laser cell counter that permits quantification of the cell population as well as a semiquantitative estimate of the DNA content of the cells. The basic measures of flow cytometry are the ploidy of the cells (the chromosomal complement) and the percent of cells in S phase (DNA synthesis). In general, cells that have an abnormal complement of DNA (aneuploid) have a poorer prognosis than those with the usual diploid complement. A cancer that has a large population of dividing cells as indicated by the percentage of cells in S phase also seems to indicate a worse prognosis (48).

Despite optimism for flow cytometry, the difficulties in standardization and the vagaries of flow analysis have not produced consistent results. Ploidy analysis is not commonly used, but the percentage of cells in S phase is used by some to estimate the growth rate of the tumor. The incorporation of radioactive thymidine into the tumor cells has been used as a measure of DNA synthetic activity. Immunohistochemical stains can be used instead. Bromodeoxyuridine is incubated with the tumor cells and then the tissue is stained, permitting the detection of cells that are actively replicating. Numbers may vary from laboratory to laboratory. Although no longer used at the Massachusetts General Hospital, the range of cells in S phase has varied from 0% to 40% with a mean of 6% and a median of 5% for invasive ductal cancers. Benign lesions rarely measure >3%. In general, the higher the percentage of cells in S phase, the greater the probability of recurrence.

Hormone Receptor Status

It is standard practice to measure the presence of hormone receptors in breast cancers (49). Many tumors have both estrogen and progesterone receptors. The presence of estrogen receptors in significant quantity is associated with a better prognosis and suggests a greater likelihood of response from hormone manipulation, such as the use of tamoxifen to block the effects of estrogen.

Oncogene Expression and Other Factors

It is becoming increasingly easier to assay tissues for the presence of a gene or its protein product. Some investigators have found that the amplification of the oncogene *HER2/neu* was associated with earlier recurrence and death. Others have been unable to confirm this (50).

Similar inconsistent results have occurred with measurements of the proteolytic enzyme cathepsin D. This may be an enzyme that helps tumors to pass through the basement membrane. Tandon et al. (51) have suggested that its presence in high concentrations was a bad prognostic sign, but others have not been able to reproduce the same results.

Epidermal growth factor and transforming growth factor alpha have been identified as other potentially useful indicators of prognosis. These appear to be important factors in hormone-independent cancers and their presence has been identified as an adverse prognostic indicator.

Tumor Angiogenesis

It is fairly apparent that cancers cannot grow beyond a volume of approximately a few millimeters without the ingrowth of blood vessels to provide nutrients. These vessels also likely provide the tumor with metastatic egress from the breast. It is not surprising that the amount of neovascularity might correlate with the biological capability of the tumor. Weidner et al. have correlated the density of the tumor vascularity surrounding the cancer with the presence of metastatic disease (28) and survival (52). The tissues were stained, immunohistochemically to detect factor VIII–related antigen (a blood vessel cell membrane factor). By evaluating the area of most "active" neovascularity, the investigators found that for every 10 vessels around the tumor counted in a 200× field, the risk of metastatic disease rose by 60%. In their test population, if there were >100 vessels in this field, all cancer recurred within 33 months, whereas <5% recurred if there were 33 or fewer microvessels in the field.

EARLY-STAGE BREAST CANCER

Gallagher and Martin initially defined the term *minimal breast cancer* to mean LCIS, DCIS, or invasive carcinoma that was no larger than 0.5 cm in diameter (1). The definition of *minimal cancer* was altered in the BCDDP to include tumors up to 1 cm in diameter, thus confusing its use.

As noted, tumor size is significant for its prognostic value. As mentioned, it has been shown repeatedly that prognosis is linked to involvement of axillary lymph nodes at the time of diagnosis, and involvement of the axilla directly correlates with the size of the cancer at the time of diagnosis. In the BCDDP, women with cancers >1 cm in diameter had a 29% likelihood of having positive nodes at the time of diagnosis, whereas only 14% of women whose cancers were <1 cm had positive nodes. The data from Evans et al. also support the importance of finding invasive cancers under 1 cm (30). In the Swedish Two County Trial of mammography screening, Tabar et al. found that women with invasive cancers <1 cm had excellent survival and that when tumors were this small, histologic grade did not effect survival and they all did uniformly well. If the tumors were >1 cm, then grade 3 tumors did worse than grade 2, which had poorer survival than women with grade 1 tumors, as would normally be expected (31).

Although Tabar et al. concluded that efforts should be made to detect cancers <1.5 cm, this was likely a practical compromise. Cancer can be detected by mammography when <1 cm. More than 50% of the invasive cancers detected by screening at the Massachusetts General Hospital are <1 cm in size. The goal of screening should be the detection of invasive breast cancer <1 cm in size.

The data support a definition of early-stage breast cancers as those that are DCIS, or invasive, but 1 cm or smaller in diameter and without evidence of axillary lymph node involvement (see Staging).

Because confused terminology makes it difficult to evaluate data, general terms such as *minimal breast cancer* should be discarded and replaced by more accurate descriptions that include size, tumor grade, lymphatic and vascular involvement, the proximity of the cancer to the excised tissue margin, and nodal status. Each of these appears to provide prognostic information, and to ensure that populations being compared are indeed comparable, these factors should be controlled.

Earlier detection, unfortunately, does not mean that a cancer is early in its development and does not guarantee a favorable result. There is also a variation in the metastatic potential of breast cancers. Some infiltrate the vascular and lymphatic system long before they are detectable by any known means. In addition, there are most certainly varying host responses to breast cancers that have not yet begun to be understood. These responses affect ultimate outcome. Even the most exacting screening program will not save all women. The mortality reduction that can be expected on the basis of the HIP and Swedish data is 25% to 40%, possibly even 50%, but not 100%. Nevertheless, screening provides an opportunity to reduce breast cancer deaths that is worthy of vigorous pursuit.

SUMMARY

The natural history of breast cancer remains largely speculative. The various stages of tumor initiation, promotion, and progression likely take place over a variable period of time. This may be very short, or occur over decades. The requirements of altered gene expression through loss, mutation, inactivation, or overexpression are probably usually chance happenings, although environmental carcinogens may play a role in some cases. Inherited genetic abnormalities may reduce the number of necessary subsequent events in others. For a cancer to be "successful," changes likely must occur in proper sequence with chance and statistical probability probably playing an important role. Some tumors may never develop the ability to grow beyond the duct, whereas others develop invasive and metastatic capability early in their growth (with the majority somewhere in between). It is likely that the natural history of tumors that develop changes over a moderately long period of time can be altered by screening and earlier detection. The effectiveness of the screen, the frequency of screening, and its ability to detect "early" breast cancer will determine how large a percentage of cancers can be affected.

REFERENCES

1. Gallager HS, Martin JE. Early phases in the development of breast cancer. CA Cancer J Clin 1969;24:1170.
2. Carter CL, Allen C, Henson DE. Relation of tumor size, lymph node status, and survival in 24,740 breast cancer cases. Cancer 1989;63:181–187.
3. Page DL, Dupont WD, Rogers LW, et al. Intraductal carcinoma of the breast—follow-up after biopsy only. CA Cancer J Clin 1982;49:751.
4. Fisher B, Redmond C, Poisson R, et al. Eight-year results of a randomized clinical trial comparing total mastectomy and lumpectomy with or without irradiation in the treatment of breast cancer. N Engl J Med 1989;320:822–828.
5. Fisher B, Costantini J, Redmond C, et al. Lumpectomy compared with lumpectomy and radiation therapy for the treatment of intraductal breast cancer. N Engl J Med 1993;328:1582–1586.
6. Silverstein M, Lagios MD. Use of predictors of recurrence to plan therapy for DCIS of the breast. Oncology 1997;11:393–410.
7. Holland R, Peterse JL, Millis RR, et al. Ductal carcinoma in situ: a proposal for a new classification. Semin Diagn Pathol 1994;11:167–180.
8. Lagios MD, Margolin FR, Westdahl PR, Rose MR. Mammographically detected duct carcinoma in situ: frequency of local recurrence following tylectomy and prognostic effect of nuclear grade on local recurrence. Cancer 1989;63:618–624.
9. Lagios MD. Duct carcinoma in situ: pathology and treatment. Surg Clin North Am 1990;70:853–871.
10. Silverstein MJ, Poller DN, Waisman JR, et al. Prognostic classification of breast ductal carcinoma-in-situ. Lancet 1995;345:1154–1157.
11. Page DL, Dupont WD, Rogers LW, et al. Continued local recurrence of carcinoma 15–25 years after a diagnosis of low grade ductal carcinoma in situ of the breast treated only by biopsy. Cancer 1995;76:1197–1200.
12. Ozzello L. Ultrastructure of intra-epithelial carcinomas of the breast. Cancer 1971;28:1508.
13. Rosen PP, Lieberman PH, Braun DV, et al. Lobular carcinoma in situ of the breast. Am J Surg Pathol 1978;2:225.
14. Deng G, Lu Y, Zlotnikov G, et al. Loss of heterozygosity in normal tissue adjacent to breast carcinomas. Science 1996;274:2057–2059.
15. Nielsen M, Jensen J, Andersen J. Precancerous and cancerous breast lesions during lifetime and at autopsy: a study of 83 women. Cancer 1984;54:612.
16. Nielsen M, Thomsen JL, Primdahl S, et al. Breast cancer and atypia among young and middle-aged women: a study of 110 medicolegal autopsies. Br J Cancer 1987;56:814–819.
17. Mettler FA, Hempelmann LH, Dutton AM, et al. Breast neoplasms in women treated with x-rays for acute postpartum mastitis: a pilot study. J Natl Cancer Inst 1969;43:803.
18. Ohuchi N, Furuta A, Mori S. Management of ductal carcinoma in situ with nipple discharge. Intraductal spreading of carcinoma is an unfavorable pathologic factor for breast-conserving surgery. Cancer 1994;74:1294–1302.
19. Visscher DW, Wallis TL, Crissman JD. Evaluation of chromosome aneuploidy in tissue sections of preinvasive breast carcinomas using interphase cytogenetics. Cancer 1996;77:315–320.
20. Tabar L, Fagerberg G, Chen H, et al. Screening for breast cancer in women aged under 50: mode of detection, incidence, fatality, and histology. J Med Screen 1993;2:94–98.
21. Holland R, Hendriks JHCL, Verbeck ALM, et al. Extent, distribution, and mammographic/histological correlations of breast ductal carcinoma in situ. Lancet 1990;335:519–522.
22. Ohtake T, Abe R, Izoh K, et al. Intraductal extension of primary invasive breast carcinoma treated by breast conservative surgery. Cancer 1995;76:32–45.
23. Weber BL, Abel KJ, Brody LC, et al. Familial breast cancer. Cancer 1994;74:1013–1020.
24. Fitzgerald MG, MacDonald DJ, Krainer M, et al. Germ-line BRCA1 mutations in Jewish and non-Jewish women with early-onset breast cancer. N Engl J Med 1996;334:143–149.
25. van de Vijver M, Peterse J, Mooi W, et al. Neu-protein overexpression in breast cancer: association with comedo-type ductal carcinoma in situ and limited prognostic value in stage II breast cancer. N Engl J Med 1988;319:1239–1245.
26. Brugger W, Bross KJ, Glatt M, et al. Mobilization of tumor cells and hematopoietic cells into peripheral blood of patients with solid tumors. Blood 1994;83:636–640.
27. Folkman J, Watson K, Ingber D, Hanahan D. Induction of angiogenesis during the transition from hyperplasia to neoplasia. Nature 1989;339:58–61.
28. Weidner N, Semple JP, Welch WR, Folkman J. Tumor angiogenesis and metastasis—correlation in invasive breast carcinoma. N Engl J Med 1991;324:1–8.
29. Hart IR, Saini A. Biology of tumour metastasis. Lancet 1992;339:1453–1461.
30. Evans A, Pinder S, Wilson R, et al. Ductal carcinoma in situ of the breast: correlation between mammographic and pathologic findings. AJR Am J Roentgenol 1994;162:1307–1311.
31. Collins VP, Loeffler RK, Tivey H. Observations on growth rates of human tumors. Cancer 1956;9:988.
32. Lundgren B. Observations on growth rate of breast carcinomas and its possible implications for lead time. Cancer 1977;40:1722.
33. Van Dierendonck JH, Keijzer R, Cornelisse CJ, Van De Velde CJH. Surgically induced cytokinetic responses in experimental rat mammary tumor models. Cancer 1991;68:759–767.
34. Adami H, Malker B, Holmberg L, et al. The relation between survival and age at diagnosis in breast cancer. N Engl J Med 1986;315:559–563.
35. National Cancer Institute Surveillance, Epidemiology and End-Results Program. Relative Survival Rates For Successive Numbers of Years After Diagnosis. SEER Program 1974–1987.
36. Tabar L. New Swedish breast cancer detection results for women aged 40–49. Cancer 1993;72:1437–1448.
37. Smart CR, Hartmann WH, Beahrs OH, Garfinkel L. Insights into breast cancer screening of younger women. Cancer 1993;72:1449–1456.
38. McGuire WL. Prognostic factors in primary breast cancer surveys 1986;5:527–536.
39. Tabar L, Duffy SW, Krusemo UB. Detection method, tumor size and node metastases in breast cancers diagnosed during a trial of breast cancer screening. Eur J Cancer Clin Oncol 1987;23:959–962.
40. Rosen PP, Groshen S, Saigo PE, et al. A long-term follow-up study of survival in stage I (T1 N0 M0) and stage II (T1 N1 M0) breast carcinoma. J Clin Oncol 1989;7:355–366.
41. Tabar L, Fagerberg G, Day N, et al. Breast cancer treatment and natural history: new insights from results of screening. Lancet 1992;339:412–414.
42. Tabar L, Gad A, Holmberg L, Ljungquist U. Significant reduction in advanced breast cancer, results of the first seven years of mammography screening in Kopparberg, Sweden. Diagn Imag Clin Med 1985;54:158–164.
43. Ridolfi R, Rosen PP, Port A, et al. Medullary carcinoma of the breast—a clinicopathological study with 10-year follow-up. Cancer 1977;40:1365–1385.
44. Henson DE, Ries L, Freedman LS, Carriaga M. Relationship among outcome, stage of disease, and histologic grade for 22,616 cases of breast cancer. the basis for a prognostic index. Cancer 1991;68:2142–2149.
45. Barth A, Craig PH, Silverstein MJ. Predictors of axillary lymph node metastases in patients with T1 breast carcinoma. Cancer 1997;79:1918–1922.
46. Fisher B, Wolmark N, Bauer M, et al. The accuracy of clinical nodal staging and limited axillary dissection as a determinant of histologic nodal status in carcinoma of the breast. Surg Gynecol Obstet 1981;152:765–772.
47. Fisher B, Bauer M, Margolese R, et al. Five-year results of a randomized clinical trial comparing total mastectomy and segmental mastectomy with or without radiation in treatment of the breast. N Engl J Med. 1985;312:665–672.
48. Johnson H, Masood S, Belluco C, et al. Prognostic factors in node-negative breast cancer. Arch Surg 1992;127:1386–1391.
49. McGuire WL, Clark GM, Dressler LG, et al. Role of steroid hormone receptors as prognostic factors in primary breast cancer. Natl Cancer Inst Monogr 1986;1:19–23.
50. McGuire WL, Tandon AK, Allred C, et al. How to use prognostic factors in axillary node–negative breast cancer patients. J Natl Cancer Inst 1990;82:1006, 1013.
51. Tandon AK, Clark GM, Chamness GC, et al. Cathepsin D and prognosis in breast cancer. N Engl J Med 1990;322:297–302.
52. Weidner N, Folkman J, Pozza F, et al. Tumor angiogenesis: a new significant and independent prognostic indicator in early-stage breast carcinoma. J Natl Cancer Inst 1992;84:1875–1887.

Breast Imaging, 2nd ed., by Daniel B. Kopans.
Lippincott–Raven Publishers, Philadelphia © 1998.

CHAPTER 8

Mammography: Equipment and Basic Physics

In 1995, the American College of Radiology (ACR) reviewed the requirements for mammography equipment and developed detailed specifications (1). The reader is referred to the ACR review for specific information, but because many of these specifications will change as technological advances are made, this chapter discusses general principles, many of which cannot change. An additional valuable reference is the syllabus for the 1993 and 1994 Categorical Course in Physics for the Radiological Society of North America on the *Technical Aspects of Breast Imaging*. Haus and Yaffe organized a review (2) that provides state-of-the-art information on the technology and equipment used for mammography for those seeking greater detail.

BASIC PRINCIPLES OF X-RAY MAMMOGRAPHY

The ultimate goal of x-ray mammography is to produce detailed images of the internal structures of the breast to permit the earlier detection of breast cancer. Because fine detail is needed, the process requires images with high spatial resolution. Because the inherent x-ray attenuation differences (tissue contrast) between normal and diseased breast tissues is so small, high-quality mammography requires the ability to enhance those differences and provide high-contrast resolution. Producing such images involves a complex interaction of many interrelated factors (Fig. 8-1).

Every component of the imaging sequence influences the resulting image and can impact the ability to detect early breast cancer. Ultimately, the image is formed by the detector, and it is the requirements of the detector that dictate the imaging parameters. Screen/film combinations, for example, require sufficient exposure to be certain that when the image is processed, the resulting picture will be optimized for viewing on a view box. This has inherent disadvantages because the characteristics of the film as a viewing medium dictate the various components of the imaging sequence and the exposure values. The development of digital mammography will alter the input requirements.

Film has a complex, sigmoid-shaped response to x-ray exposure and the light the photons stimulate in the intensifying screens. Since low levels of exposure produce little

change on the film, there is little contrast between tissues of high x-ray attenuation (the white areas of the film) because of the characteristics of the film at the "toe" of the curve. To enhance the attenuation differences and provide contrast in the high attenuation areas of the breast, greater exposure is needed to move to the portion of the Hunter and Driffield (H&D) curve (Fig. 8-2) where small changes in the amount of radiation reaching the detector lead to large changes in film blackening (higher contrast). The best contrast separation is obtained using exposures that record the x-ray attenuation on the steeply sloped linear portion of the curve where small differences in tissue contrast are amplified. At high exposures, the film density changes begin to level out (the "heel" of the curve) and contrast is no longer enhanced. The toe and heel of the film's response to light are among the limitations of film.

Direct digital acquisition of an x-ray image will not be restricted in this fashion because the image display will not be affected by the factors involved in image acquisition. Digital detectors will have, essentially, a straight line response to x-ray photons, regardless of the level of exposure. This will permit the maximum contrast separation and greater room to explore potentially even better ways to image the breast with x-rays.

Screen and Film Imaging

Haus (3) has summarized the various components of the film and screen mammographic image. He divided radiographic sharpness into contrast and blur ("unsharpness").

Contrast

There is inherent "subject contrast," which is the difference in x-ray attenuation of the various breast tissues that is determined by their thickness, density, and atomic composition. The transmission of x-rays through the tissues (penetration) is a factor of the beam quality (the energy and number of photons), which is a function of the anode/target material, the kilovoltage of the beam, and the material used to filter the beam. Contrast is also influenced by the amount of scatter reaching the film, which is influ-

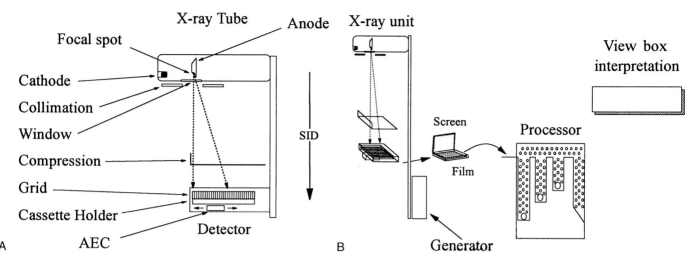

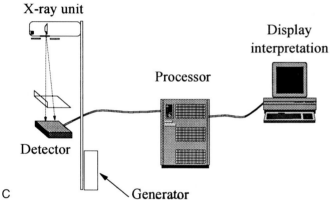

FIG. 8-1. The mammography imaging chain. Conventional mammography requires that all components of the imaging sequence be performed properly. This includes the x-ray device and its components, including the x-ray tube and its cathode, anode, focal spot, window, filtration, collimation, source-to-image distance (SID), and the compression system automatic exposure control (AEC) **(A)**; the detector and its components, including the cassette, film, and screen; or the solid-state detector, the film processor, and its components; and the interpretation system (view box or computer display). All of these components are interrelated. Alterations at any point in the sequence can influence the operation of the other elements. Even though the detector and display are different between conventional mammography **(B)** and digital mammography **(C)**, the interactions of the constituents of the system must be carefully matched and properly adjusted.

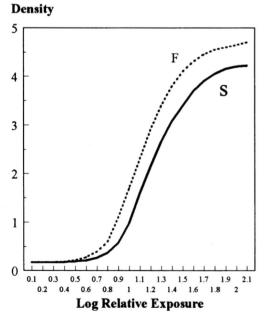

FIG. 8-2. These Hunter and Driffield (H&D) curves relate the amount of exposure to the density (blackening) of the film for a system (S) with a longer gray scale and less contrast than (F) which represents a faster film (less exposure is needed for the amount of blackening) with greater contrast (the curve rises more quickly with increasing amounts of exposure).

enced by the collimation of the beam, thinning of the breast by compression, an air gap in magnification, and a grid. The inherent tissue contrast is amplified by the contrast on the film. This is influenced by the type of film used, its processing (i.e., chemistry, temperature, time, and agitation), and factors that compromise the photographic image, including fog from improper storage, inappropriate safelights, and light leaks.

Blur

Haus breaks blur into several components beginning with actual breast motion, which can be reduced by compression to immobilize the breast and short exposure times. Next is geometric blur (geometric unsharpness), which is related to the size of the focal spot, the source-to-image distance, and the distance of the object to the detector. There is also blur related to the thickness of the phosphor of the screen that is converting the x-ray photons to light, the particle size of the phosphor, and the contact between the film and the screen.

The ability to image fine details is related to numerous factors. Anything that causes a blurring of the image can compromise the ability to find small cancers. There are several sources of blur. As with any imaging system, motion of the object being imaged or of the imaging system relative to

17.4 keV of energy with a smaller contribution from 19.7 keV. Those produced by rhodium are predominantly at 20.2 keV with a small contribution at 22.8 keV; tungsten has a characteristic emission at 59 keV (along with other very low–energy peaks). The characteristic radiations of molybdenum and rhodium are particularly valuable for screen/filming imaging since they provide an abundant source of low-energy photons that help enhance the inherently low contrast between tissue of the breast and breast cancer.

X-RAY GENERATORS

The electrical power supply of the mammographic system is among several factors that determine the x-ray output and beam quality. The generator determines the kVp and the timing involved in x-ray production. Constant potential generators produce an essentially continuous output at a single voltage level. The least efficient generators were single phase in which the kVp was reached over a period of time. Three-phase generators were an improvement, but constant potential is needed to provide more uniform photon energies. Uniform photon energy is important because it provides a "purer" x-ray output. Constant potential virtually eliminates the fluctuations (ripple) in x-ray generation that were inherent with three-phase as well as the earlier single-phase equipment. By producing an almost immediate and constant voltage and beam energy, exposure times are diminished and beam energy profiles are more uniform.

FOCAL SPOT SIZE AND GEOMETRIC CONSIDERATIONS

X-ray mammography demands high resolution to image the fine structures of masses and the morphologic characteristics of small calcifications that often indicate early-stage breast malignancy. Particles as small as 150 μm can be imaged under optimal conditions, and greater resolution is constantly being sought. The visibility of lesions is related not only to the spatial resolution of the imaging system but also to the contrast of the lesions compared to the surrounding tissue and the sharpness of the imaged structures (the opposite of blur). Resolution is determined by the size of the focal spot, by its distance from the structure within the breast to be imaged, by the distance of that structure to the detector, and ultimately by the ability of the detector to produce the image.

The focal spot is a key component of the mammographic system. The configuration of the focal spot varies with the x-ray tube. Various methods of generating x-rays from the anode are used, which result in focal spots that vary from round, to rectangular, to bipolar. The focal spot is actually an area on the anode where the electrons, accelerated from the cathode, strike the anode. In addition to the generation of x-ray photons, these impacts result in the production of heat. If the energies and time to generate photons were not limited, the heat would melt and destroy the anode. The capacity of

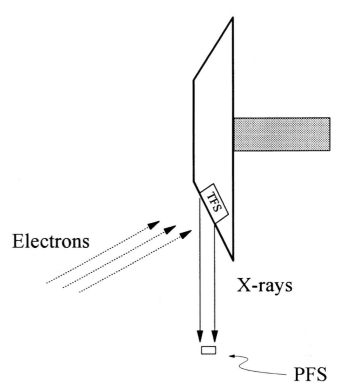

FIG. 8-4. The **anode surface is at an angle relative to the stream of electrons generated from the cathode and to the breast.** This presents a larger area from which to generate photons (TFS), but the "projected" focal spot (PFS) looks smaller on the breast, increasing spatial resolution.

the tube to dissipate this heat (heat capacity) determines its output characteristics. The design of focal spots is a compromise between the need to have a small spot size that can produce large numbers of photons over short periods of time and the need to prevent the anode from melting. Tube designs rely heavily on geometry to accomplish this.

To keep heat loading down, milliamperes up, and focal spot size small, the area on the anode that constitutes the focal spot is actually larger than the "apparent" focal spot. In addition, in most modern tubes the area struck by the electrons is constantly changed to reduce heat buildup. The latter is accomplished by rotating the anode and the former by focusing the electrons on a large area that is tilted relative to the incident beam of electrons and the breast (Fig. 8-4). In this fashion, the area over which the anode generates photons (and heat) is much larger than the apparent focal spot. This can be understood by looking from the breast back up at the anode. Depending on its location on the breast, the focal spot will appear to be quite small (toward the nipple side), and it will appear to enlarge as the perspective moves toward the chest wall (Fig. 8-5). This means that the sharpness of the image varies over different parts of the breast related to the apparent size of the focal spot and the geometric unsharpness or blur will depend on which part of the image is being considered. Unfortunately, as the apparent focal spot gets smaller away from the chest wall, there is also a drop of photon flux due to the heel effect (see below).

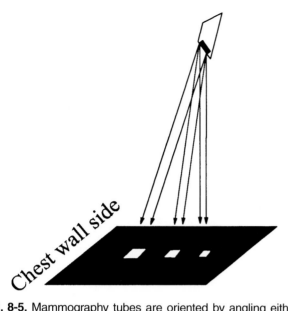

FIG. 8-5. Mammography tubes are oriented by angling either the anode or the tube so that the smallest projection of **the focal spot is at the nipple side** and gets progressively larger toward the chest wall. This schematic demonstrates how the "apparent" focal spot gets progressively smaller away from the chest wall. Because the heel effect begins to limit the photon flux as the projected spot size diminishes, the orientation of the focal spot is matched to the thinner front of the breast, which can be properly exposed with the diminished flux. The thicker chest wall side of the breast receives the most output.

"Nominal" Focal Spot Size

Geometric unsharpness would be eliminated if the focal spot were infinitely small. The closer the focal spot is to the idealized "point source," the better the possible spatial resolution of the system. Manufacturers are permitted to claim focal spot sizes that may, in reality, be considerably larger than the "nominal" figure that they quote. Dimensions of the focal spot may be 50% larger than the stated "nominal" size. For example, a nominal 0.4-mm focal spot may be as large as 0.6 mm. The actual size of the focal spot should be measured before a system is accepted.

Heel Effect

As with most factors involved in mammography, because the small focal spot is achieved by angling the anode, as the apparent focal spot size decreases, the output of the focal spot also decreases because of the heel effect. This occurs in the portion of the x-ray field in which the focal spot–to-film angle is the most obtuse. Because the angle of the exiting x-rays generated from this part of the focal spot is so steep, the apparent focal spot at this end is very small, but unfortunately, many of the photons generated at this end are reabsorbed by the anode itself. This means that the output, seen at the breast, is diminished. Tubes are oriented so that this heel falls on the thinnest anterior portion of the breast where lower flux can be tolerated.

Blur Due to Geometric Unsharpness

One form of blur in the image is due to geometric unsharpness. Although they approximate a point source, even the smallest focal spots produce geometric blurring if they are too close to the structure to be resolved, the structure is too small to be resolved, or the structure is too far away from the detector. As noted above, the blur from geometric unsharpness is the result of x-rays that are emanating from all over the focal spot. If, for example, the focal spot is rectangular, then x-rays are generated from both ends as well as the middle. The shadows cast from the x-rays generated from the ends of the focal spot are slightly different from one another, and their inexact overlap (as well as the shadows from those generated in between) causes the blur. The main shadow is not perfectly sharp but is surrounded by the penumbra (Fig. 8-6). As the name implies, geometric unsharpness is due to the geometry of the system as it relates to the size of the focal spot, the object whose shadow is being cast, and the distance of the object from the detector (Fig. 8-7). If the object is in direct contact with the detector, then there would be no blur from the geometry of the relationship. The shadow of the image would be crisp. If the object is at some distance from the film, its edges will be blurred in relation to the distance it lies away from the detector, the size of the focal spot that is generating the x-rays, and the distance of the focal spot from the object being imaged and from the detector. This is because the focal spot, although very small, has a finite size, and x-rays come from all along its surface following divergent paths. Blur from geometric unsharpness is reduced by using equipment that is designed for mammography and uses as small a focal spot as possible.

The same phenomenon can be seen when projecting a shadow onto a screen using visible light. The less focused the light source, the closer the object is to the light source, or the farther the object is from the projection screen, the greater the blurring of the shadow. This phenomenon is easily demonstrated using the light from a slide projector. If an object is held up between the light and the screen, its shadow becomes increasingly better defined as it is moved closer to the screen. As it is moved away from the screen, its margins become blurred. Similarly, the smaller the light source or the farther away the light source is from the object and the screen, the sharper the shadow of the object.

To reduce geometric unsharpness using x-rays, the focal spot must be moved as far away from the object and detector as possible, the focal spot must be as small as possible, and the object to be imaged must be pressed as close to the detector as possible. This latter requirement is one reason the breast needs to be physically compressed against the detector surface.

Haus et al. (4) has calculated that a 1-mm focal spot 28 cm from a structure can resolve 6 line-pair (lp)/mm for structures 5 cm above the recording surface. Since the size

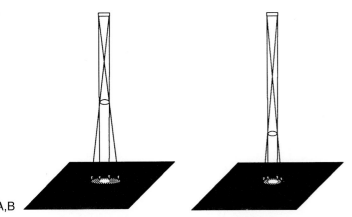

FIG. 8-6. Because the focal spot has a finite size and x-rays come from both ends as well as the middle, a secondary shadow (the penumbra) is produced **(A)** that can overlap and blur the primary shadow. This can be reduced by pressing the object (breast structures) closer to the detector, which reduces the size of the penumbra and improves the sharpness of the shadow **(B)**.

related well with the theoretic prediction that the resolution of a system is inversely related to the size of the focal spot and the distance of the structure from the detector, and directly related to the distance from the focal spot to the lesion. This relationship is summarized in the empirically derived equation

$$ALP/mm = 1.1 \times [FOD/(FS \times ODD)]$$

where ALP/mm is the approximate resolution in line pair per millimeter, 1.1 is a constant, *FOD* is the distance in centimeters from the focal spot to the object to be resolved, *FS* is the size of the focal spot in millimeters, and *ODD* is the distance in centimeters from the object to the detector.

Thus, for a specific focal spot size and a lesion a given distance from the detector, resolution increases directly with the distance of the focal spot from the object to be resolved. Doubling the distance doubles the resolution. Similarly, making the focal spot half the size will also double the resolution as long as none of the other variables is changed.

Resolution can also be increased by taking advantage of the divergence of the x-ray beam and moving the focal spot closer to the object being imaged and moving the object away from the detector. Because of beam divergence, the shadows enlarge and magnification will result (see Magnification Mammography). This will only be useful if sharpness is maintained, which requires that the focal spot size be reduced to avoid geometric blurring that increases as the distances are changed. Although the improved visibility of structures with actual radiographic magnification is primarily due to a reduction of noise (5), if the focal spot is sufficiently small, magnification will result in an absolute increase in resolution (see below).

of the penumbra relative to the main shadow cast on the film is reduced as the focal spot is moved away, this same focal spot can resolve 15 lp/mm if it is positioned 75 cm from the object to be imaged.

The resolution of a system is governed by the interaction of its components, but by holding these constant, Haus and associates used actual mammographic systems to determine the changes in resolution that occur with variation in focal spot size, in focal spot–to-object distance, and in distance of the object from the detector. The experimental findings cor-

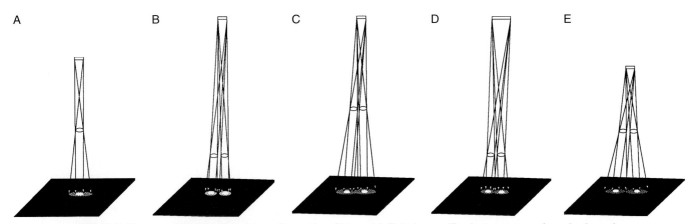

FIG. 8-7. Because the focal spot has dimension (it is not infinitely small), photons come from both ends as well as the middle. This causes an object to cast primary (umbra) and secondary (penumbra) shadows **(A)**. The capability to resolve objects and distinguish one as separate from another, such as these two round structures **(B)**, is related to many factors. The spatial resolution of a system can be reduced, causing **geometric unsharpness (blur).** Note that if the shadows (both primary and secondary) do not overlap, the two objects will be seen as separate.

Blur is increased when the secondary shadows of two adjacent structures are enlarged so that they overlap. This makes it less likely that the observer will be able to tell that the structures are, indeed, separate. This occurs when the objects are moved farther away from the detector **(C)**, the focal spot is made larger **(D)**, or the focal spot is brought closer to the objects **(E)**.

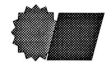

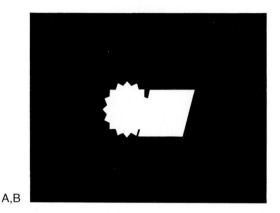
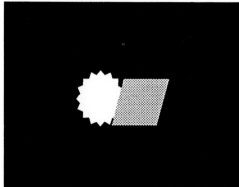

A,B

FIG. 8-8. Spatial resolution has little benefit if there is no contrast. Even though there is high spatial resolution, these two objects **(A)** appear as one on the film because there is insufficient ability to separate their slight differences in contrast. With improved contrast resolution they can be distinguished **(B)**.

Variation in Actual Spatial Resolution

The relationships discussed above assume that the detector itself can display the resolution achievable by the system, which may not be the case. Modern mammographic screen/film combinations have an inherent resolution capability of approximately 15 to 20 lp/mm. Because of the other contributions to unsharpness, however, the actual resolving power of screen/film mammography systems, operating as clinical instruments, is considerably less. Systems are required to be able to resolve approximately 13 lp/mm with the line pair bar pattern placed 1 to 2 cm from the chest wall and 4.5 cm above the film plane with the lines of the phantom oriented parallel to the anode-cathode axis. When the pattern is turned so that its lines are perpendicular to this axis, the resolution may be even lower, because most focal spots are usually more narrow than they are tall.

Improving the other elements of resolution will have little effect if the detector system is incapable of recording the improved detail. This may become a significant factor when new detectors, such as digital detectors, are devised. Spatial resolution is measured using a metal line-pair phantom that alternates metal lines with essentially empty spaces. This produces a target that has very high contrast—essentially 100% (the bars block all of the radiation and the spaces let most through).

The ability of the human eye to appreciate the resolution of a system depends not only on spatial resolution, however, but also on the contrast between the object and its surroundings. High spatial resolution is of no value if the edges that are being distinguished have the same x-ray absorption and cannot be "seen" (Fig. 8-8). The true visible spatial resolution in the breast may be considerably lower than the line-pair measurement since the differences in contrast between breast structures are considerably less than a line-pair phantom. These relationships are expressed in the modulation transfer function, which provides a better method for comparing two systems because it integrates both contrast and spatial resolution. Due to limitations in contrast, the potential for high resolution in screen/film systems is never achieved (the details are there, but because they have no contrast difference they cannot be perceived). The higher contrast resolution of digital systems may more than compensate for lower spatial resolution. This is evident when looking at the ACR phantom. Despite lower spatial resolution than screen/film systems, most digital mammographic systems can image all of the test objects in the phantom. This cannot be done with screen/film systems (Fig. 8-9).

FIG. 8-9. This image of **the ACR phantom was made using a digital detector.** Because the contrast can be exaggerated, all of the test objects are visible even the though spatial resolution is lower than that for film.

Because it is usually not uniform, the shape of the focal spot also affects resolution. It is frequently rectangular, and the output may be biphasic with greater intensity at the ends. This reduces resolving capability, because the focal spot acts as two sources rather than a point source. Efforts to reduce the size of the focal spot are complicated by the relationship between focal spot size and the amount of heat that the anode can sustain in generating x-rays, and the number of photons that can be generated per unit of time from a small surface. Reducing the size of the focal spot increases the heat loading on the tube and may preclude the use of high milliamperage (mA). This, in turn, increases the exposure time required to produce the necessary photon flux to adequately expose the detector, and longer exposures increase the chance of blur caused by patient motion.

RECIPROCITY LAW FAILURE

Until digital detectors replace film, screen/film combinations will continue to be the primary mammography detector. Another inherent property of film impacts image production. Longer exposure may result not only in blurring due to motion of the breast but also in higher dose. The relationship between x-ray exposure and film blackening is not linear. The exposure (film blackening) is generally defined as the intensity of the beam multiplied by the time ($E = I \times T$). This relationship suggests that intensity and time are reciprocal parameters. To maintain the same exposure, the equation shows that if the intensity is increased, the time of exposure can be decreased in direct proportion. The opposite would also be true. If the intensity is decreased, the time must increase. These reciprocal relationships constitute the law of reciprocity.

The failure of this relationship is called *reciprocity law failure*. This can be explained in the following way. Assume it takes 100 photons to achieve a blackening of 2 with a 1-second exposure. If the output of the tube was reduced by 50%, requiring a longer imaging time, it turns out that the law of reciprocity fails. If the output is halved, it actually takes more than just twice the exposure (dose) to achieve the same level of blackening. This is a property of the photographic process. For screen/film systems, as exposures exceed 1 second's duration, dose must be increased disproportionately to achieve the same level of film blackening. Stated another way, the light generated by a screen from a given number of photons delivered over a short period has a greater film-blackening ability than the light generated by the same total number of photons delivered over a longer period. Thus, tubes whose characteristics require longer exposures require disproportionately greater mAs (photon production) to achieve the same film blackening and image quality as a tube with higher output. The longer the exposure, the less sensitive the film emulsion to the light generated by the screen. For equivalent radiographs, a tube that requires long exposures will result in greater dose to the patient than one that produces the same output over a shorter period of time even though they produce comparable films. Most digital systems are not affected by this phenomenon.

FOCAL SPOT COMPOSITION AND FILTERS

The composition of the x-ray anode determines the x-ray spectrum that the tube can produce. This spectrum can be further refined using filters that permit photons of specific energies to pass through and block those at other energies. If the appropriate filter is chosen, the x-ray spectrum can be narrowed to a fairly small range to take advantage of better contrast from the low-energy photons.

Molybdenum Anode and Filters

The low inherent contrast of the tissue structures within the breast can be enhanced in screen/film imaging by using "softer radiation." A molybdenum anode tube takes advantage of the low-energy photons (17.9 keV and 19.5 keV) from the characteristic radiation produced by the molybdenum target and the bremsstrahlung in the 15- to 20-keV range (Fig. 8-10). The molybdenum anode, however, does not produce a completely monoenergetic, or even low-energy, beam. Some high-energy photons are also generated. By filtering the beam with a molybdenum filter, the

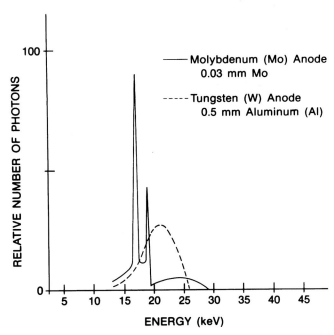

FIG. 8-10. X-ray spectrum produced by a molybdenum target anode. **Molybdenum produces more low–kiloelectron volt photons** than tungsten, which improves radiographic contrast. (Reprinted with permission from Haus AG, Cowart RW, Dodd GD, et al. A method of evaluating and minimizing geometric unsharpness for mammographic x-ray units. Radiology 1978;128:775.)

less useful photons of energies greater than 20 keV are absorbed in the filter.

Very low–energy photons are almost completely absorbed in the breast. These add to dose but do not contribute to the image. The molybdenum filter can block many of these undesirable photons as well. The combination of an anode that produces predominantly low-energy photons with a filter that permits these to pass while absorbing the very low–energy as well as high-energy photons produces an effective window, enabling the most useful photons (those that produce the greatest contrast between structures) to pass to the breast.

Other Anode and Filter Materials

Using low-energy photons helps exaggerate the contrast between breast structures, but such systems are limited by the thickness of the breast and the attenuation of its various tissues (radiographic density). Larger or denser breasts, in effect, filter the beam as it passes through and cause beam hardening (these tissues favor the transmission of predominantly high-energy photons). This diminishes overall contrast (soft x-rays are absorbed and never reach the film, whereas more energetic photons that pass through provide less information because information is related to ratio of absorbed and unabsorbed photons).

If the x-rays are too low in energy (too soft), they will be absorbed by the breast in increasing proportions, contributing to dose but not increasing the contrast because they never reach the film. To penetrate large or radiographically dense breasts, the kVp must be increased. Increasing the kVp will diminish contrast somewhat (although the actual effect has been exaggerated by some), so the increase should be tailored if possible.

One method of slightly increasing the energy of the beam is to modify the anode or the filtration to permit slightly more energetic photons to be produced and pass through. Tungsten anodes that produce a large proportion of higher energy photons can be used in screen/film imaging, but they must be specially designed using filters to reduce the large number of very high–energy photons that are generated by the tungsten anode that would significantly compromise contrast. Rhodium, palladium, or other "K-edge" filters can be used to reduce these high-keV (contrast-degrading) photons, but a tungsten anode will still produce a mammogram that has a lower contrast than a molybdenum anode, even when low kVp settings are used. (A K-edge filter is a filter composed of metals whose atoms contain K-shell electrons that will absorb x-ray photons of specific energies and slightly above and prevent those photons from passing through the filter.) Tungsten may become a more desirable anode for primary digital systems since they will not be as limited in contrast differentiation as screen/film systems (see Chapter 26). Some have suggested that silver anodes will provide the best spectrum for digital imaging.

Rhodium has been developed as an anode material as well as a filter. Because it melts at a lower temperature, however, rhodium anodes must be operated at lower mAs. The characteristic energies produced by a rhodium anode are approximately 2 keV higher than molybdenum. When this beam is filtered using a rhodium filter, this shift to slightly higher energies has some advantage over molybdenum with molybdenum filtration in radiographically dense breasts or those that are thick despite compression. In the radiographically dense or thick breast that requires 28 kVp or higher energies using molybdenum, comparable images can be obtained using rhodium (focal spot)/rhodium (filter) at 2 kVp lower than the molybdenum/molybdenum combination. Gingold et al. (6) found that 29 kVp was the crossing point above which a molybdenum target with rhodium filtration provided higher contrast and lower dose than a molybdenum/molybdenum combination, and they also found that if the exposure requires 29 kVp or higher, the rhodium/rhodium combination was even better.

Our own studies, as well as those of others, show that the main gain from rhodium, however, is in dose reduction. The image quality will be lower in contrast for rhodium/rhodium at 26 kVp than for molybdenum/molybdenum at 28 kVp, but the dose will be reduced by approximately 30% if the rhodium combination is used. Rhodium can be used to filter a molybdenum beam and will result in an intermediate dose and a slightly better image if the kVp is 29 or higher is needed for an image using molybdenum/molybdenum.

Because the filter is in the x-ray beam, its own inhomogeneities can appear on the film. Due to the distance of the filter from the film, these are usually blurred and of no consequence to the image, but if recurrent artifacts appear on the films, the filter should be evaluated for lack of uniformity.

Off-Focus Radiation

Because electrons may not be perfectly focused at the focal spot of the x-ray tube, they may strike other parts of the anode and produce photons that are off-focus. Since these act as a much larger focal spot, their presence compromises image quality. Efforts to reduce off-focus radiation improve image quality.

X-Ray Tube Window

The composition of the window through which the x-rays leave the tube is important. The glass window found on most x-ray tubes for body imaging will absorb too many of the low-energy photons that are used in mammography. Most mammography tubes, therefore, use beryllium windows to reduce the amount of filtration by the window.

Once the x-ray photons of the proper energy are generated from an appropriately small focal spot, the clarity of the image is determined by the characteristics of the system at the breast.

BREAST COMPRESSION

To provide high contrast, modern screen/film systems had to have narrow exposure latitude. This necessitated the development of x-ray systems designed specifically for mammography. With modern screen/film combinations, the breast cannot be imaged in its normal conical shape because the thin front would have to be overexposed to permit optimized imaging of the thick back of the breast; otherwise the back would end up underpenetrated if the thin front of the breast was properly exposed. One reason that breast compression is required is to even out the thickness through which the x-ray beam must pass so that a uniform exposure may be obtained. Since the dynamic range of a primary digital mammography system is so broad, exposure latitude is not as great a problem. It may be possible to perform digital mammograms with less compression than that needed for screen/film imaging. Uniform exposure, however, is not the only reason for firm compression. There are also other advantages (Table 8-1).

Importance of Breast Compression

Compression of the breast is one of the major reasons for noncompliance of women with mammography screening guidelines. The use of compression is often misunderstood. The true discomfort is difficult to measure, and many women and their physicians do not understand its great importance. Because of its narrow exposure latitude, screen/film mammography requires vigorous compression

TABLE 8-1. *Reasons for compression*

To hold the breast away from the chest wall permitting the projection of all the tissues onto the detector without the interfering noise of the other structures of the thorax

To reduce blur due to motion by physically holding the breast still

To reduce the dose needed to image the breast by reducing the thickness of the tissue through which the radiation must pass

To further reduce dose and motion because the shorter exposure time needed to image a thinned structure avoids dose increases due to reciprocity law failure when using screen/film systems with long exposure times. This also reduces the likelihood of motion.

To separate overlapping structures facilitating evaluation

To press breast structures closer to the detector to reduce blur from geometric unsharpness and improve the resolution of the system

To reduce image degrading scatter

To produce a more uniform thickness to provide more uniform exposure

of the breast to avoid underexposing the base and overexposing the thinner anterior tissues. The tissues should not be damaged, but the firmer the compression (up to a point), the better the mammogram. Firm compression, however, makes it impossible to include ribs on the mammogram. For this reason, as the breast is compressed from side to side, and again from top to bottom, it must be pulled away from the chest wall to ensure that the deep tissues are projected onto the recording system and imaged.

There are other advantages to compression in addition to making the thickness of the structures more uniform. Geometric unsharpness is diminished and resolution improved by compressing the tissues against the detector, because the closer an object is to the film, the smaller its penumbra and the sharper its shadow (see Fig. 8-7). Motion-related unsharpness is decreased because compression maintains the breast in the appropriate position. Image degradation from scatter is also reduced. Shorter exposure times are required, and thinning the structure results in reduced radiation dose. Finally, squeezing the breast between two surfaces spreads the tissues apart, separating often confusing overlapping structures on the mammogram.

Much of the concern about compression is due to unwarranted fears that it may be damaging. Aside from an occasional bruise or rare skin tear (the skin of the intertriginous inframammary fold can be friable), it is rare for compression to cause any harm.

Mammographic systems are required to be capable of producing 25 to 45 lbs of pressure. Many confuse this with the actual pressure applied to the breast. The latter is measured in pounds per square inch (psi), which relates the amount of pressure applied over the compressed surface of the breast. The psi varies with the size of the breast and the surface area of the skin that is in contact with the compression paddle and the detector. For example, if the surface of the breast that is in contact with the compression paddle is semicircular and the chest wall side measures 11 in., the area in contact with the compression device will be approximately 45 in.^{2} ($\frac{1}{2} \times$ pi $\times$ [5.5^2]) (Fig. 8-11). This means that if 45 lbs is applied over that area the pressure will amount to 1 psi (45 lbs/45 in.^{2}). If the breast is smaller, the same force will generate greater pressure, but even this is quite low. Reducing the diameter of the contact area to 7 in. doubles the pressure to 2 psi. This is actually much less than other pressures that the breast tissue may experience. It has been estimated that a clinical breast examination applies 6 psi to the breast tissues. This is considerably more than mammography, which, on average, applies only 3 psi (7). It is likely that even social interactions subject the breast to higher pressures than a mammogram (8).

The discomfort from breast compression is likely complex. There is a clear psychological component. Much of the discomfort may be due to the lack of control the individual has on the process and the mechanical, seemingly impersonal, and immodest requirements of the test. One study has shown that if women themselves are given the button that

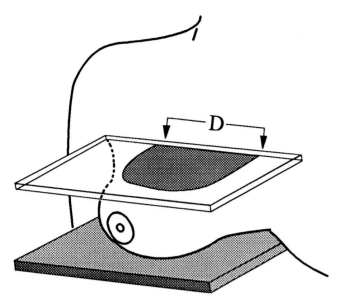

FIG. 8-11. Compression in pounds per square inch (psi). The actual pressure applied to the breast is the force applied (in pounds) divided by the area over which the force is spread, giving psi. If the breast is assumed to be a hemisphere, then psi equals one-half the area of a circle whose diameter (D) is that of the part of the breast touched by the compression paddle, divided into the number of pounds applied. This diagram depicts the surface in contact with the compression paddle and film holder. The larger the surface in contact, the lower the pressure in psi.

controls the amount of compression they often compress more tightly than the technologist.

Breast compression is important, but it should not be excessive. The technologist should be aware that once the skin of the breast is tight (taut), any additional compression will not improve the image (there is no more room for the breast to be thinned), and additional compression will only add to the discomfort. Another potential source of pain occurs if the skin is pinched in the process. The technologist should be sensitive to the patient's discomfort. If the compression is uncomfortable it is usually best to release the compression and work with the patient to alleviate the problem. It is generally easier to position the patient the second time if she has already experienced compression. The technologist should make every effort to smooth out the skin and try to ensure a comfortable procedure. If the patient is hurt or loses trust in the process, the mammograms will likely not be optimal and the patient will likely not return in the future to be screened. It may, at times, be best to desist and have the patient return in several days at a time when her breasts may be less sensitive. Compression is, however, critical for high quality imaging. Women should be educated to the importance of compression, and technologists should work with the individual to produce appropriate compression with a minimum of discomfort.

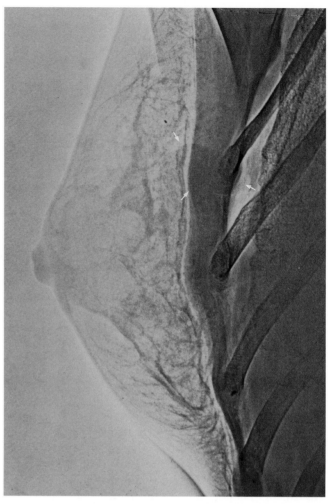

FIG. 8-12. Imaging the chest wall does not guarantee imaging all of the breast parenchyma. The arrows point to a mass that is hidden in the lateral aspect of the breast behind the curve of the thorax and the pectoralis muscles on this xeromammogram.

Possible Improvements in X-Ray Imaging and the Patient Interface

There are some modifications in standard mammography that may improve the ability to image the breast. One possible benefit would come from moving the detector away from the breast slightly (providing small amounts of magnification) around the curve of the chest wall. This would permit the deeper tissues to be imaged as was done using the xeroradiographic technique. Merely seeing the chest wall, however, does not guarantee evaluation of all of the breast tissues. Using the xeroradiographic technique, the chest wall was easily visible, but because the breast was not held firmly by the system, tissue could slip around the chest wall behind the ribs, and abnormalities could be overlooked (Fig. 8-12). Because rigid compression with close contact between the breast and screen/film detector is required, the chest wall is not imaged using screen/film combinations. Standard screen/film mam-

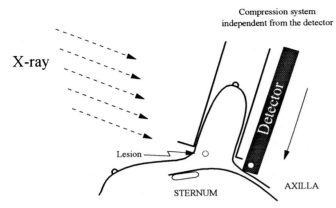

FIG. 8-13. **Separating the detector from the breast compression system** will permit the positioning of the detector slightly farther back around the curve of the chest wall. This will provide some magnification and will reduce the chance that the mammogram will not image the deep tissues. Note that the lesion is behind the compression paddles but is still projected onto the detector, which is moved farther back around the curve of the chest wall.

mographic imaging necessitates pulling the breast as much as possible away from the chest wall to project it free from the thoracic structures and onto the detector system. Some deep tissues may be missed. Separating the detector from the compression system may permit imaging the deeper tissues while preserving the advantages of rigid compression (Fig. 8-13).

Compression Paddles

For the reasons listed above, compression of the breast is needed for two-dimensional breast imaging. It was found through trial and error that compression plates should have a straight edge across the front (along the chest wall side) so that they can be brought down along the chest wall. Curved plates (and film) have been tried, but the curvature rarely conforms to the patient, and the tendency is for the corners to push the patient away from the edge of the detector.

For screen/film mammography, the edge of the compression plate along the chest wall should be molded at right angles to the plane of compression and blunted to avoid trauma to the patient. A ridge may help hold the breast tissue in the field of view and aid in pulling the breast tissue away from the chest to project it over the screen/film detector (Fig. 8-14). More gradual spoon-shaped compression plates not only fail to even out the breast thickness but have a tendency to push the back of the breast out of the field of view.

There are disadvantages to a compression paddle that is parallel to the film plane. For thicker breasts, the front of the breast may receive no compression. We have found that by keeping the chest wall side of the paddle parallel to the detector but tilting the front of the compression paddle, the tissues of the anterior breast may be better compressed and separated (Fig. 8-15). By permitting the entire paddle to rotate, thicker portions of the breast and axillary tail may be compressed

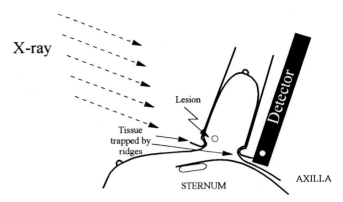

FIG. 8-14. **A ridge along the chest wall side of the compression paddle** may help hold the breast tissue in the field of view and aid in pulling the breast tissue away from the chest to project it over the screen/film detector.

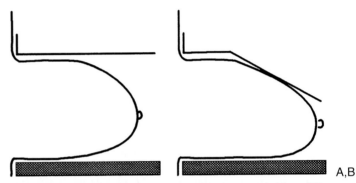

FIG. 8-15. This schematic demonstrates how **a rigid paddle** that is parallel to the detector may not compress the front of the breast **(A)**. By **tilting the front of the paddle (B)** these tissues are compressed. The effect of this type of compression is to separate the anterior structures (see Positioning in Chapter 10).

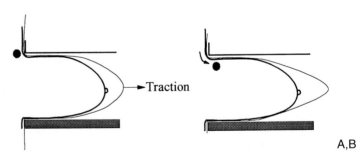

FIG. 8-16. **Traction can be applied to a partially compressed breast** if membranes are placed between the breast and the compression/detector system. This permits the breast to be pulled further into the field of view even after it is compressed. In this schematic, the breast is compressed with the membrane between the paddles and the breast **(A)**. While in compression, the breast can be pulled further into the field of view by pulling on the membranes **(B)**.

while not sacrificing compression of the thinner portions of the anterior breast. We have also developed a traction system that can aid in pulling more breast tissue into the field of view even after some compression has been applied (Fig. 8-16).

SCATTER RADIATION

The x-ray image is formed by the differential absorption of the photons passing through the breast by the tissues through which they pass. As with any shadow, the clarity of the shadow will depend on the fact that the photons that reach the detector travel in a straight line from the focal spot, through the object, to the detector. If their course is altered, the shadow becomes less distinct and sharp. Most x-ray interactions at mammographic energies involve photoelectric absorption in which an x-ray photon is completely absorbed by displacing an electron. This produces images with sharp shadows.

The other interaction between x-ray photons and tissues produces Compton scattering. In this interaction the photon transfers some of its energy to an electron. The photon continues out of the atom, but its course is altered. If this scattering is coherent (in the same direction as the original photon's course), it can contribute to the sharpness of the image. Many of these interactions, however, are not coherent, and they can cloud the image similar to the way scattered light in a room degrades the shadow of a hand cast on a white wall.

These secondary photons of scatter radiation that are generated significantly compromise image quality in mammography, reducing contrast and overall sharpness. Scatter increases with the thickness of the breast and the diameter of the field imaged. In a breast 6 cm thick, the amount of scatter reaching the recording system may equal almost half as much as that from the primary (information-containing) beam. Barnes and Berzovich (9) found that the ratio of the scatter radiation to the primary beam (S/P) might be as high as 0.86.

Scatter can be reduced by breast compression to diminish the amount of tissue traversed by the beam. Collimation to expose a smaller volume of tissue will also diminish scatter. Barnes and Berzovich also found that as the diameter of the field was reduced from 14 cm to 4 cm and the thickness of the breast from 6 cm to 3 cm, the S/P ratio decreased from 0.86 to 0.32. An air gap between the breast and the detector will also diminish the effects of scatter by spreading it over a larger area.

Despite their adverse effect on the image, scatter photons do contribute to film blackening, and when scatter is reduced by a grid, additional photons are required to produce proper exposure. This contributes to the increased dose necessitated by the use of a grid. The grid and spacer material also absorb some of the primary beam, and compensation requires a further increase in radiation dose to the patient. For screen/film mammography without a grid, 25 to 26 kVp produces the best contrast when a molybdenum target tube is used. Although most mammography grids have low attenuation carbon fiber spacers, the additional material may require an increase to 27 or 28 kVp for adequate imaging.

Various dose estimates have been recorded when grids are used. In our experience, using an oscillating grid with a 5:1 grid ratio increased the midplane dose to an average 5-cm-thick breast from 80 mrad (0.08 cGy) to 160 mrad (0.16 cGy). Others have recorded higher dose increases that relate to the type of grid, the mammography equipment used, and the size of the breast (10).

Although decreased contrast can be electronically corrected in digitally acquired images, scatter reduction will probably also improve those images, particularly for very dense or thick breasts. As an extreme example, if the attenuation of a mass permits the same photons to reach the detector as scattered photons plus normal breast tissue, there will be no contrast between the two that could be recovered electronically, and a mass may not be visible, even using a digital detector. In general, however, the scatter is distributed in a nonuniform but predictable pattern, and it is possible that an electronic filter could compensate for most of its effect and return the lost contrast. Eliminating the scattered photons, however, will still improve the visualization of breast lesions, even with a digital detector.

GRIDS

Scatter radiation causes significant degradation of screen/film images. Scatter increases with the increased compressed thickness of the breast and the radiographic density (attenuation) of the tissues. For a field of view that is 5 cm in diameter, Barnes and Berzovich (11) calculated that the ratio of scattered to primary radiation that reaches the film is as high as 0.8 for a breast that is 6 cm thick. The elimination of scatter could dramatically improve the quality of the image and the detectability of cancer.

Several types of scatter-reduction grids are available. Stationary devices attached to the film holder or inserted directly into the cassette between the breast and the film are no longer permitted. Focused grids with 80 lines per cm and a ratio of 3.5:1.0 had been shown to improve the visualization of many lesions (12), but it became evident that even these very thin grid lines compromised the image, conceivably covering significant pathology such as microcalcifications. Thus, oscillating grids are required. These devices, which have grid ratios of 4:1 to 5:1, are housed in cassette holders. The grid lines are eliminated by the motion of the grid.

Sickles (13) demonstrated that in 60% of mammograms, using a scatter-reduction grid improved image quality. In his study, the use of grids resulted in improved detection capability in 20% of women. The images that benefited most from use of the grid were of breasts that were greater than 6 cm when compressed or contained more than 50% radiographically dense tissue. Because, as yet, there are no accurate methods of predicting the radiographic density of the breast, and scatter increases with the radiographic density, the grid must either remain on at all times or a test film must be obtained. It has been our experience that most mammograms benefit from the use of a grid. Most now agree that grids improve the image most of the time, and for efficient, rapid through-put, high-quality mammography, most leave

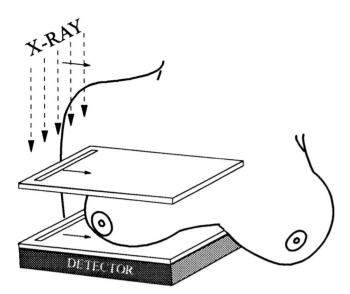

FIG. 8-17. Pre- and postbreast slit collimation. The best scatter rejection is achieved with moving slits that are aligned. The slit on the tube side of the breast prevents irradiation of the breast by primary beam that cannot get to the detector. The postbreast slit only permits directly transmitted radiation to reach the detector. The difficulty with this approach lies in the mechanics of moving the slits together and keeping the alignment as well as the demand placed on the tube.

the grid in place for all images. A doubling of the radiation dose due to the grid's interruption of the primary beam and the need to make up for these lost photons is reasonable due to the significant improvement in image quality that results and the favorable radiation risk assessment for women over 35 to 40 years of age.

New grids have been designed. A focused grid with absorbers arrayed to produce polygonal air spaces can clean up scatter in multiple directions. An early digital mammography system devised by American Science and Engineering (Cambridge, MA) had a slit that moved with the fan beam with a precollimator, preventing breast exposure to rays that were not properly aligned (Fig. 8-17). One of the new digital scanners uses a similar scatter rejecting slot.

SCREEN/FILM MAMMOGRAPHY

Major improvements have occurred since the application of the original industrial film mammography in the 1960s. This plain film (no screen) technique provided high resolution. However, since film is not very sensitive to radiation, film mammography required long exposures (increasing the likelihood of blur due to motion) and high radiation doses. Although the inherent resolution of industrial film is higher than that of screen/film combinations, the coupling of new films with rare earth screens that were more efficient in capturing x-ray photons and converting their energy to visible light led to considerable dose reduction while maintaining adequate spatial resolution.

Most modern mammography screens use variations of lanthanum and gadolinium oxysulfide to emit green light. More recently, screens that emit blue light have been developed. When combined with the appropriate film and proper processing, these systems provide high spatial resolution and contrast at acceptable dose levels. Screen/film combinations require equipment designed for mammography. In addition to the development of these detector systems, mammographic positioning and techniques have also evolved since they were first standardized by Egan (14) in the late 1950s.

Factors That Influence Image Quality

To achieve enhanced contrast resolution in an organ whose structures are inherently low in contrast, high-contrast films have been developed. The trade-off for more contrast is film with narrow exposure latitude and higher speed. Higher speed means that a lower radiation dose is needed to produce proper film blackening for optimal viewing. The dose is reduced, but higher speed means that fewer x-ray photons are needed to blacken the film (avoiding reciprocity law failure) (see Fig. 8-2). These systems have more noise (quantum mottle). If the noise is too great, fine structures and calcifications may be lost in the noise (see Fig. 8-3).

CHOOSING A SCREEN/FILM COMBINATION

The choice of screen/film combination is, for the most part, based on individual preference, as long as the combination is designed specifically for mammography and provides high resolution at low dose. Microcalcifications of 200 to 300 μm (0.2 to 0.3 mm) should be resolvable. Although there is a temptation to use fast screen/film combinations or digital detectors to reduce dose, this should not be done at the expense of image quality. There are no data that suggest that women aged 40 years and older have any significant risk from mammographic exposures. They can benefit, however, from early detection, and the ability to demonstrate small cancers is the primary benefit from mammography. The ability to detect these cancers should not be compromised by excessive noise. Within reason, image quality and not dose should be the determining factor.

Most mammography screen/film combinations use a single emulsion film and a single screen. Efforts had been made to produce dual emulsion film with two screens to increase the efficiency of photon capture, but the image quality was degraded (15).

X-Ray Film

X-ray film consists of a clear or color-tinged (dyed) backing material coated on one side with a gel that contains a uniform distribution of silver halide crystals. These crystals form grains and that contain approximately 10^9 atoms of silver. Each grain also contains an area known as the "sensi-

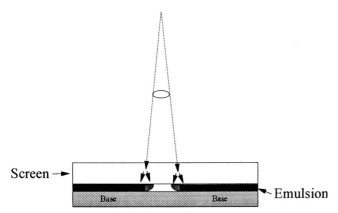

FIG. 8-18. Light spread in the detector screen can cause a blurred image. A thicker phosphor layer is more efficient in absorbing x-rays (*dotted arrows*). If the phosphor is thick, however, light generated by an x-ray photon (*solid arrows*) can spread in the phosphor as it heads to the surface. This light exposes the film and reduces the sharpness of the edges of structures. A thinner phosphor layer increases the sharpness, but it allows more x-rays to pass undetected, requiring a higher dose.

tivity spec." The crystals and the gel that contains the crystals compose the emulsion. The emulsion side of the film is placed in direct contact with the phosphor layer of the screen. The contact between the two must be tight so that the light, emitted from the screen by an x-ray's interaction with the screen phosphor, cannot spread into a wider spot. Sharpness requires that the light produce a sharp spot on the film (Fig. 8-18). If there is poor contact between the screen and film, the light will spread over a larger area, and the shadows from the tissues (absence of light exposure) will be less sharp.

The x-ray image is produced in the emulsion of the film. The silver halide grains are distributed in the gel layer. When exposed, the silver bromide of the crystal is converted by the energy transferred from the absorbed light photon into a silver ion and an electron. The silver ion is attracted to the sensitivity spec in the emulsion, forming an enlarging structure containing silver atoms. If sufficient numbers of atoms congregate, the relationship becomes stable and the grain is activated. The number of activated grains is related to the amount of exposure. Before development, the exposed film contains a "latent" image of these activated grains in which the silver atoms are grouped together, but the grouping is too small to be visible. Film development is a process that amplifies the chemical changes that are present in the latent image by converting the other silver ions in the grain to metallic silver that is black, making the image visible (see below).

Automatic Exposure Control

There is no direct correlation between radiographic density and the size, compressibility, or compressed thickness of the breast (16,17). Thus, the technologist cannot be expected to accurately predict optimal exposure values. A scout film may lead to increased radiation because of the need for repetition. Automatic exposure control (AEC) is important to reduce under- and overexposure. These are sensors that are usually under the film cassette. They measure the radiation that passes through the breast and cassette. They are calibrated such that when sufficient x-ray photons have reached the AEC, the exposure is terminated and the film will have been properly exposed. The purpose of AEC is to provide uniform and reproducible exposure and penetration of the breast tissues, regardless of their thickness or composition. It works by assessing the energy that has passed through the breast and the detector. The available systems are not perfect. Many old automatic exposure control circuits were compromised in their function by beam hardening in progressively thicker or more dense breasts. As the thickness of the breast increased or the attenuation of its tissues became greater, low-energy photons were absorbed in the breast and a greater proportion of high-energy photons reached the detector. The AEC would reach its energy peak based on these fewer, more energetic photons, and the exposure would be terminated before comparable film blackening had been achieved, producing increasingly underpenetrated images. The newer AEC systems track more accurately and should approach linearity regardless of breast thickness.

Individual variations in the distribution of breast parenchyma and the unpredictable distribution of high attenuation tissue further reduce the accuracy of automatic exposure controls, most of which are positioned along a line perpendicular to the chest wall in the center of the film holder. Given this geometry, the radiation sensor may not be optimally positioned under the densest part of the breast, which tends to extend toward the upper outer quadrant. Failure to position the AEC under the dense tissues may result in a premature termination of the exposure and an underexposed mammogram. The ability to move the AEC in the *x* as well as the *y* axis would permit greater flexibility. Systems that measure multiple areas in the breast and inform the system when the densest tissue has been properly penetrated would improve exposure control. Digital recording systems should obviate the need for AEC since the entire detector is essentially a large AEC.

In a properly exposed mammogram, the dense tissues must be penetrated so that the structures within and behind the tissue are visible. Using a screen/film combination, this is usually accomplished if the densitometric measurement of the film under the dense portions of the breast is 0.7 to 1.0 (0.8 is probably optimal). In some breasts, it may not be possible to optimally expose the full range of tissue densities, necessitating multiple exposures to optimally image all the tissues. Nevertheless, AEC eliminates significant guesswork. New circuits have been designed to improve the accuracy of these systems and for high through-put automatic exposure control is a necessity. The Mammography Quality Standards Act regulations require AEC.

A number of mammography systems use the AEC to help select the appropriate imaging factors. The exposure is begun at a low kVp setting and the AEC measures the transmitted x-rays over the first milliseconds of the exposure. If the microprocessor determines that a proper exposure cannot be completed at that kVp (the machine cannot provide enough mAs), then the kVp is automatically increased to permit completion of a properly exposed image.

FILM PROCESSING

Film will likely remain the most common form of mammographic imaging for many years to come. Processing the film is a critical part of the mammographic study. Sharp, high-contrast, artifact-free images are the goal.

The latent image that is contained in the film emulsion after exposure is not visible. If the grain of silver bromide crystals received sufficient exposure, it contains a nucleus of metallic silver atoms. The development process converts the remaining silver bromide into black metallic silver causing the entire grain to become black. The density of the blackened grains in a given area of the film gives it its "gray scale." All conventional processors transport the film through the developer, which is made up of chemicals that react with the silver halide crystals that have been activated by their exposure to x-rays and the light from the screens.

Film development is a reduction process in which electrons are provided by the developer chemistry to convert the remaining atoms of an activated silver bromide grain to metallic silver. The process of development involves multiple chemical steps. An activator in the development chemistry causes the emulsion to soften and swell so that the other chemicals can reach the silver crystals. Potassium bromide regulates the rate of development. The cluster of molecules containing silver is reduced to metallic silver through the transfer of an electron from one of the developer chemicals (typically phenidone). A second agent, hydroquinone, regenerates the electron transfer molecule so that it can reduce another silver halide molecule. The semiquinone that results from this regeneration could slow the process, but it reacts with sodium sulfite to form a hydroquinone monosulfonate salt and allows the development process to proceed and amplify the latent image. The sodium sulfite also functions as an antioxidant that maintains the stability of the hydroquinone by preventing oxygen from being dissolved in the developer solution.

The rate of the process is controlled by other chemicals, such as potassium bromide. Glutaraldehyde is added to harden the gel so that the final x-ray image resists scratching. Since there are approximately 10^9 atoms of silver in each grain, the development process amplifies the latent image information by a factor of 5×10^9 (18).

The silver halide that was not activated is not "developed." However, the developer chemicals can continue to work, gradually causing the conversion of unactivated grains to silver and "fogging" the film unless the chemical reaction is stopped. Consequently, the film is transported into the fixer chemicals where acetic acid neutralizes the development process. The unactivated silver halide dissolves in the fixer solution that also contains ammonium or sodium thiosulfate. These form with the silver halide to produce silver thiosulfate ion complexes. These are washed from the film in the wash tank. Sodium sulfite is included in the fixer as a film preservative.

The washing process is important for removing the thiosulfate from the emulsion. Over time this can react with the silver nitrate and air forming a yellow-brown stain as silver sulfate. The fixer retention test checks to ensure that only small amounts of thiosulfate remain in the emulsion.

The development process is completed in the drying chamber and the developed film is then released from the processor. Most processors move the film through these various stages using rollers. Too much or too little heat in the drying process as well as the rollers that transport the film can be sources of some film artifacts (see Chapter 9).

Based on experience, it is usually best to process film according to the manufacturer's specifications. To obtain optimized images, proper chemical concentrations are needed. Since the active chemicals are eliminated with the development process, they must be replaced. The proper replenishment rates for these chemicals are important to maintain a stable developer environment. The temperature of the chemistries also has a significant effect on the ultimate image because heating the developer speeds the chemical reactions.

When a film developer is first installed, it is important to optimize the development process. Once the parameters of development have been established to provide the radiologist with the desired film contrast and noise reduction, the processor should be maintained to ensure that those parameters remain the same and image development is stable and consistent. The procedures followed in the quality control process including sensitometric/densitometric and temperature measurements are all designed to monitor the stability of the processor functions. The radiologist should be aware that the processor quality control (QC) tests only measure the stability of the processor. The processor can be set up incorrectly and the QC will still appear consistent and in range. The processor must first be optimized before the processor QC test has any value.

Extended Processing

Tabar and Haus (19) demonstrated that by "pushing" the development process, film could be made to exhibit higher contrast, and mammograms could be obtained at lower dose. This is the origin of extended processing. The manufacturers of film built in a wide latitude for development to try to ensure that the film would not be easily fogged by overdevelopment. The usual parameters suggested for processing the film actually underdeveloped the emulsion. Tabar and Haus realized this and were the first to develop more of the activated grains by leaving the film in the developer solutions longer than was recommended. The typical amount of time that the film was in the developer chemistries in standard processing was 20 to 25 seconds. Tabar and Haus found that if they doubled this time, processing was enhanced, producing greater contrast at lower dose (more grains were developed at the same exposure). New film/screen combinations have been devised to provide similarly high-contrast images without the need for extended processing.

Processor Problems

Sprawls and Kitts (20) have summarized the problems that can occur with film processing. They cite underprocessing in particular as a major problem that results in reduced contrast and the decreased perspicuity of abnormalities. They define *optimum processing* as "the level of processing that produces the film performance characteristics (contrast and sensitivity) specified by the film manufacturer." It is reasonable for academic sites to experiment with films, screens, and processors (this is how Tabar revealed the potential for extended processing), but in general it is best for the average mammography program to use and process a film/screen combination according to the manufacturer's recommendation.

If film is underprocessed, contrast is reduced, and the film speed is diminished, requiring higher radiation dose. This can be seen using the H&D curve produced using a sensitometer to expose a film, processing it using the clinical processor, and reading the densities with a densitometer. The curve generated by this method can be compared with the curve expected by the film manufacturer. If the slope of the curve is not as steep, the contrast is lower than it should be, and if the curve is shifted to the right, a greater radiation dose is needed to achieve the same film blackening. This indicates that the processing has reduced the potential speed of the film.

Clinically the effect of underprocessing is an image that has a wide gray scale and diminished contrast. There are only two reasons for the skin line to be visible on a mammogram. The first reason is that the breast is very thin when compressed. The skin will often be evident when the breast compresses to under 3 cm. If the film is underdeveloped, the skin line will also be evident. A crude indication that the film has been underdeveloped is that the maximum density of the film will not be achieved in the areas exposed to the full beam, and the radiologist will be able to see through the darkest parts of the film not covered by the breast that should be developed to the maximum film density.

The film will be underdeveloped if the processor temperature is too low, the film does not spend sufficient time in the developer chemistry, or the developer chemistries are not sufficiently agitated to prevent a buildup of "spent" chemistry adjacent to the film emulsion that prevents fresh chemical from reaching the emulsion. Underdevelopment also results if the developer chemistry is not being replenished appropriately or the developer chemistry is diluted or contaminated.

DOSE MEASUREMENT

Despite the increasingly more favorable assessment of the risks associated with radiation (see Chapter 5), the possibility of radiation-induced malignancy continues to be an important issue in mammographic screening. Although it is likely that there is little or no risk at present levels of exposure for the screening population of women over 40 years of age (21), it is prudent to try to limit dose as long as image quality (detection capability) is not compromised.

Dose Determination

The determination of dose has generated a great deal of confusion, and many articles have been written to try to establish appropriate standards. There are several methods of measuring dose, but most agree that mean glandular dose is the most appropriate figure by which to judge exposures. Hammerstein et al. (22) argued that since it is the glandular and ductal epithelium that is at risk, the dose sustained by these components of breast tissue is the significant figure.

Because dose varies with the depth within the breast where it is measured, average glandular dose cannot be measured directly. However, direct measurements taken within phantom material have been used to create a model that enables dose in vivo to be estimated from measurable factors. These factors include the quality of the x-ray beam and its half-value layer (HVL). The HVL is a measure of the penetrating energy of the beam as determined by the thickness of aluminum needed to reduce the transmission of photons by 50%. The higher the energy, the thicker the HVL. The beam energy, the thickness of the tissue through which the beam passes (compressed thickness), and the composition (percentage of fat versus glandular tissue) of the breast all affect the dose to the breast.

An excellent review of these factors is presented in detail in a manual published by the National Council on Radiation Protection and Measurements titled *Mammography—A User's Guide* (23). This report indicates that for screen/film systems, the optimal HVL is 0.3 to 0.4 mm of aluminum. By measuring the dose at which the beam enters the breast (skin entrance dose) and knowing the energy of the beam by measuring its HVL (beam quality), dose to the breast can be estimated based on the composition of the tissues (in order to standardize dose measurements, an average breast is considered to be 50% adipose tissue and 50% glandular elements). Assuming a 4-cm-thick breast and a skin entrance exposure of 370 mrad (0.37 cGy) for screen/film systems, the average glandular dose for a beam with an HVL of 0.3 mm of aluminum is 60 mrad (0.06 cGy) (24). Adding a grid at least doubles the dose. Wu et al. (25) provide estimates of dose that are based on the energy of the beam (kVp), skin entrance dose, and the thickness of the breast.

The mean glandular dose has replaced other measures of dose. Skin entrance dose is significant only for calculating average glandular dose. Since the skin is not at risk for radiation carcinogenesis, skin entrance dose is not a useful measurement by itself. Midbreast dose is a better estimate, but it is affected by beam quality and is less accurate than average glandular dose. The average absorbed dose to the breast is a fairly good estimate (8), but it does not compensate as well as average glandular dose for variations in breast composition (26). Tables are available by which these estimates can be easily made (7), and this should be part of a quality assurance program. The ACR recommends that when using screen/film systems, the mean glandular dose to a breast that is 4.5 cm thick and composed of 50% fat and 50% glandular tissue should not exceed 0.3 rads (3 mGy) for each image. (The Mammography Quality Standards Act may change the thickness of the phantom to 4.2 cm.)

Dose Reduction

The ultimate ability to reduce radiation dose is determined by the efficiency of the detector in counting the photons reaching it. Screen/film imaging fails to record many photons passing through the breast. Rare earth screen/film combinations in common use today are more efficient in detecting x-ray photons. Physicists measure the accuracy with which a detector collects the incoming signal and converts that signal to an image. Since a signal (x-rays passing through the breast with useful information in the form of shadows) is always accompanied by noise (signals that have no useful information but can hide the primary signal), the clarity of an image is based on the ratio of the signal to the noise (signal-to-noise ratio [SNR]). Because the detector adds additional noise of its own, the measure of an efficient detector is how accurately it converts the incident signal into an interpretable image. This can be quantified by the detective quantum efficiency (DQE) of the system. This relates the accuracy and efficiency of the SNR of the signal arriving at the detector with the SNR following detection based on the following formula:

$$DQE = (SNR_{out}/SNR_{in})^2$$

Screen/film systems are quite efficient in converting incident photons into interpretable images, but they still fail to use a large percentage of the available photons. Greater efficiency in converting these photons could result in improved images or lower radiation dose.

Screen Thickness

Efficiency in detecting photons can be increased by producing a thicker medium in which to stop and record them. Most mammographic screen/film combinations use single-emulsion, single-screen combinations to preserve resolu-

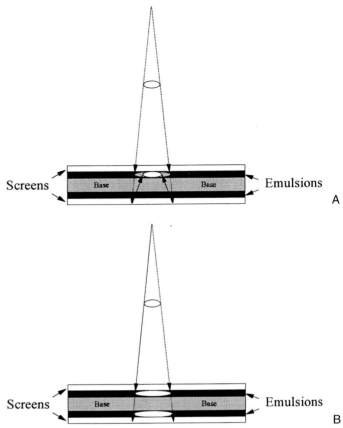

FIG. 8-19. Crossover occurs when the light from one screen crosses to the other side, exposing the other emulsion with a wide edge causing blur **(A)**. Parallax also reduces sharpness of details with dual emulsion film. The image on the tube side of the emulsion will be slightly smaller than the image on the far side and the lack of superimposition will cause blur **(B)**.

tion. Thin screens let some photons pass completely through so that they do not contribute to the image.

Thicker screens would be more efficient in absorbing these photons. However, the photon is converted to light in the screen and the light is radiated in all directions from the point of absorption. A thicker screen would permit light photons to spread over a wider area before they reached the film, so that the area of exposure would be more of a blur than a point. The thickness of the screen represents a compromise between the speed and efficiency of photon detection and the sharpness of the image. Digital detectors that use light generated by a phosphor (see Chapter 26) as the input signal have the same limitation.

Dual screen/dual emulsion systems achieve additional quantum detection efficiency and dose reduction by providing greater photon-absorbing ability. Such systems, however, risk producing blurred images from "crossover." This involves the spread of light from the screen on one side exposing the film emulsion on the other side (Fig. 8-19). Special dyes within the base of the film reduce crossover. Double emulsion films also compromise image sharpness, as the image on the far side of the film is slightly larger than the image on the near side. Parallax is created when the film is viewed, resulting in a subtle blurring of the overall image. We have found that double emulsion films can reduce the dose, but this does not compensate for the decrease in sharpness. Double emulsion films/screen systems require magnification to have resolving power that is equal to single emulsion films used for contact imaging (15).

MAGNIFICATION MAMMOGRAPHY

Magnification mammography improves the visibility of fine details and the detectability of breast lesions as Sickles has shown (27). Because of the divergence of the x-ray beam, magnification is obtained by moving the object away from the film and closer to the focal spot. The degree of magnification is calculated from this simple relationship:

$$M = FSD/FSO$$

where M is the magnification produced, FSD is the distance from the focal spot to the detector, and FSO is the distance from the focal spot to the object. For example, a structure 23.5 cm above the film will be magnified 1.5 times if the focal spot is 35 cm away from the film.

Magnification requires very small focal spots. If the focal spot is too large, geometric unsharpness will increase and blur will decrease the spatial resolution. A focal spot that measures 0.2 mm or less can resolve 17 lp/mm at 1.5-mm magnification. Since this is the approximate display resolution of screen/film combinations, focal spots this size are required for this degree of magnification. The same focal spot at two times magnification will only resolve 11 lp/mm because of the increase in geometric unsharpness that results from moving the object farther from the detector.

A conceptualization advanced by Zamenhof and Homer (28) helps explain how magnification improves spatial resolution. The detector system can be thought of as an array of resolution elements. The shadow of two closely placed structures in the breast may fall on a single resolution element in an unmagnified image (Fig. 8-20). If the objects are moved farther away from the detector, however, the divergent beam will cause the objects to be projected farther apart onto separate resolution elements, producing greater resolution.

In addition, image-degrading scatter is reduced using magnification mammography, probably because moving the breast away from the detector to achieve magnification produces an air gap, which may result in some scatter reduction from the air absorption. It is more likely, however, that the reduction is a result of the scatter photons being spread over a larger area (based on the inverse square law) and thus having a reduced impact on the image.

Although in the past magnification resulted in an absolute increase in spatial resolution compared to contact images, given the improved geometry of most modern mammographic systems, the quality of the contact image is sufficiently high that the improved image sharpness with

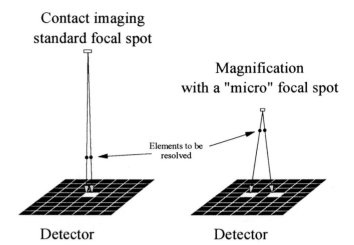

FIG. 8-20. Magnification can increase spatial resolution. Magnification can be thought of as spreading the structures over more "imaging" units, permitting the differentiation of structures and higher spatial resolution. With modern mammography systems, however, much of the gain from magnification is an increase in the ratio of signal to noise.

magnification is primarily due to the spread of the image (the signal) over a larger area. The noise remains the same so that the SNR is improved. It will likely be shown and it is our increasing belief that magnification with modern mammographic systems offers little advantage over good contact imaging unless focal spots can be made even smaller.

One disadvantage of magnification is that by bringing the focal spot closer to the breast and causing the photons exiting the breast to be spread over a larger area, increased dose is required for adequate exposure. When performing magnification mammography, the tube output is limited. Since the focal spot is smaller, the electron energy is concentrated over a smaller area. This causes an increased generation of heat that cannot be tolerated. Hence, the mA output for a magnification study drops from 100 to 150 mAs to 30 to 40 mAs or lower in most machines. This means that longer exposures are required for magnification and blur due to motion is more common. It is possible when using magnification techniques to compensate for this increased dose by using faster, double-emulsion, double-screen combinations, but the resolution gained by magnification is lost (10).

The potential to improve resolution using magnification mammography is desirable. Ideally, the mammographic detection of breast cancer could be improved if the entire breast was magnified. Unfortunately, because focal spots are made to appear small to the object by angling their surface or tilting the entire tube, magnification of large areas is not possible with present tube geometry. Tilting the anode surface is a standard approach used to improve the output of the system while maintaining an apparently small focal spot. As noted earlier, however, the small focal spot is only "seen" by a small portion of the breast tissue. As one moves away from this "sweet spot," the apparent size of the focal spot and geometric unsharpness increase.

SUMMARY

The ability to detect breast cancers earlier depends completely on high-quality imaging. Equipment should be carefully selected to provide high-quality images. The imaging sequence should be optimized and then maintained through a QC program (see Chapter 9). Until systems are devised that can mechanically position the breast, highly skilled technologists are needed to position the patient for optimized imaging (see Chapter 10). Digital mammography systems (see Chapter 26) may eliminate much of the effort needed to obtain high-quality image production, but they will introduce their own requirements, and it is likely that the intensity of effort in producing high-quality mammograms will continue for many years.

REFERENCES

1. Yaffe MJ, Hendrick RE, Feig SA, et al. Recommended specifications for mammography equipment: report of the ACR-CDC focus group on mammography equipment. Radiology 1995;197:19–26.
2. Haus AG, Yaffe MJ. A Categorical Course in Physics: Technical Aspects of Breast Imaging [syllabus]. Oak Brook, IL: Radiological Society of North America, 1992–1994.
3. Haus AG. Screen-Film Processing Systems and Quality Control in Mammography. Kodak Health Sciences Monograph based on a lecture presented at the Symposium on the Physics of Clinical Mammography Sponsored by the American College of Radiology, St. Louis. July 25–27, 1990.
4. Haus AG, Cowart RW, Dodd GD, et al. A method of evaluating and minimizing geometric unsharpness for mammographic x-ray units. Radiology 1978;128:775.
5. Niklason LT, Rosol MS, Moore RH, Kopans DB. Magnification in mammography imaging. Med Phys 1995;22:919.
6. Gingold EL, Wu X, Barnes GT. Contrast and dose with Mo-Mo, Mo-Rh, and Rh-Rh target-filter combinations in mammography. Radiology 1995;195:639–644.
7. Russell DG, Ziewacz JT. Pressure in a simulated breast subjected to compression forces comparable to those of mammography. Radiology 1995;194:383–387.
8. Kopans DB. Physical trauma and breast cancer [letter]. Lancet 1993;343:1364–1365.
9. Barnes GT, Berzovich IA. The intensity of scattered radiation in mammography. Radiology 1978;126:243.
10. Dershaw DD, Malik S. Stationary and moving grids: comparative radiation dose. AJR Am J Roentgenol 1986;147:491.
11. Barnes GT. Mammography Equipment: Compression, Scatter Control, and Automatic Exposure Control. In Categorical Course in Physics: Technical Aspects of Breast Imaging. Oak Brook, IL: Radiological Society of North America, 1993;73–82.
12. Chan HP, Frank PH, Doi K, et al. Ultra-high-density radiographic grids: a new antiscatter technique for mammography. Radiology 1985;154:807.
13. Sickles EA, Weber WN. High contrast mammography with a moving grid: assessment of clinical unity. AJR Am J Roentgenol 1986;146:1137.
14. Egan RL. Experience with mammography in a tumor institution: evaluation of 1,000 studies. Radiology 1960;75:894.
15. Oestmann JW, Kopans DB, Linetsky L, et al. Comparison of two screen film combinations in contact and magnification mammography: detectability of microcalcifications. Radiology 1988;23:657–659.
16. Swann CA, Kopans DB, McCarthy KA, et al. Mammographic density and physical assessment of the breast. AJR Am J Roentgenol 1987;148:525–526.
17. Boren WL, Hunter TB, Bjelland JC, Hunt KR. Comparison of breast consistency at palpation with breast density at mammography. Invest Radiol 1990;25:1010–1011.
18. Haus AG. Screen-Film Image Receptors and Film Processing. In A Categorical Course in Physics—Technical Aspects of Breast Imaging [syllabus]. Oak Brook, IL: Radiological Society of North America, 1993;83–99.
19. Tabar L, Haus AG. Processing of mammographic films: technical and clinical considerations. Radiology 1989;173:65–69.
20. Sprawls P, Kitts SL. Optimum processing of mammographic film. Radiographics 1996;16:349–354.
21. Mettler FA, Upton AC, Kelsey CA, et al. Benefits versus risks from mammography: a critical assessment. Cancer 1996;77:903–909.
22. Hammerstein GR, Miller DW, Masterson ME, et al. Absorbed radiation dose in mammography. Radiology 1979;130:485.
23. Feig SA, Haus AG, Jans RG, et al. Mammography—A User's Guide [NCRP Report no. 85] (Vol 85). Bethesda, MD: National Council on Radiation Protection and Measurements, 1986.
24. Shrivastava PN. Radiation dose in mammography: an energy-balance approach. Radiology 1981;140:483.
25. Wu X, Barnes GT, Tucker DM. Spectral dependence of glandular tissue dose in screen-film mammography. Radiology 1991;179:143–148.
26. Stanton L, Villanfana T, Day JL, et al. Dosage evaluation in mammography. Radiology 1984;150:577.
27. Sickles EA. Further experience with microfocal spot magnification mammography in the assessment of clustered breast microcalcifications. Radiology 1980;137:9.
28. Zamenhof RG, Homer MJ. Mammography: Part 1, physical principles. Appl Radiol 1984;Sept/Oct.

Breast Imaging, 2nd ed., by Daniel B. Kopans.
Lippincott–Raven Publishers, Philadelphia © 1998.

CHAPTER 9

Quality Assurance and Quality Control

Debra Deibel

A mammogram is among the most technically demanding of radiographic procedures. The early detection of breast cancer relies on the radiologist's ability to perceive subtle changes that are only perceptible with high-quality imaging. Appropriately designed and adjusted equipment, proper positioning to maximize tissue visualization, proper exposure, and optimal film processing are the keys to obtaining high-quality mammograms. If the information is not contained on the study, accurate interpretation is obviously impossible.

Good technique requires constant attention to detail. This begins with the selection of the equipment to be used. Although screening must be low cost to make its benefits available to all segments of the population, this does not mean low quality. The screening mammogram may be the only opportunity to interrupt the course of the disease, and, thus, the screening study must be of the highest quality. As the number of women studied increases, the savings from the purchase of inferior equipment becomes insignificant, whereas the use of such equipment may compromise the detection of early lesions. With the passage of the Mammography Quality Standards Act (MQSA) by Congress and its implementation by the Food and Drug Administration (FDA), basic quality assurance and quality control are now a matter of law.

Quality must be monitored and maintained throughout the imaging sequence. The x-ray system should be routinely monitored for tube output and beam quality with attention to resolution and contrast along with patient dose. Automatic exposure control should have a linear response and, with rare exception, should be used at all times to reduce the number of under- and over-penetrated studies. The screens in screen/film combinations should be routinely checked and cleaned to avoid artifacts that might compromise the image.

QUALITY ASSURANCE

The goal of mammography is to image all the breast tissue with high contrast and high resolution at the lowest dose with as little noise as possible to permit the detection and diagnosis of breast cancer at as small a size and early a stage as possible. If screening is to be available to all, this must be done at a reasonable cost. Quality assurance (QA) specifies the overall management program, which includes policies and procedures designed to optimize the control of the performance of the facility and its equipment. Ultimately, the physician is responsible for implementing a QA program. QA requires an entire system of monitoring that ensures that not only are the images obtained and processed properly, but that their analysis and interpretation are organized and monitored and that the information derived is accurately and effectively conveyed to the patient and her physician.

It is advantageous to use reporting systems that provide an organized structure for reporting and a standardized reporting language, such as the American College of Radiology (ACR) Breast Imaging Reporting and Data System (BIRADS). Computer systems are strongly recommended to facilitate the tracking of patients, especially those needing follow-up, to be certain that suggested measures have been taken when needed and that "the loop" has been closed. By collecting detailed statistical information such as the number of biopsies recommended and the number of cancers diagnosed, the cancer detection program can be monitored, adjusted, and improved.

QUALITY CONTROL

Quality control (QC) is the segment of the overall QA program that specifies and implements measurements of the mammographic procedure to detect any variations from the optimum so that corrective actions can be taken promptly (1). Quality maintenance through QC monitoring of the production of the image is the foundation of an early detection program. The sequence of elements that must function properly to produce a high-quality mammogram can be considered an imaging chain. A weak link or break in the chain at any point compromises the effectiveness of early detection. All components should be optimized and, once optimized, monitored to be sure that optimization is maintained.

EQUIPMENT ACCEPTANCE TESTING

A requisite for an effective QA program is to establish that all components of the imaging system are compatible and work well together. At the heart of the system is the mammography unit itself. Each site should have a medical physicist who performs a series of tests on new equipment to ensure that the equipment meets the manufacturer's specifications, the expectations of the end-user, and any mandated requirements. In addition, these acceptance tests qualify the system and provide a baseline for subsequent QC monitoring.

QC testing only ensures that the image quality is consistent with previous images without necessarily indicating the overall quality of the image. Thus, establishing an optimized baseline is the first step in a QC program. The various components and parameters of a QC program will likely vary over time as technologies evolve. The ACR publishes guides concerning these procedures (2).

ESTABLISHING THE COMPONENTS OF QUALITY IMAGING: AN OPTIMIZED BASELINE

Acceptance testing by the medical physicist, with guidance from the radiologist, should be designed to ensure the elements of image quality, patient dose, and radiation safety. The physicist should check the following:

- Mammography unit assembly evaluation (e.g., detents, locks, indicators)
- Collimation: Does the centering light field coincide with the radiation field?
- Focal spot size measurements (both large and small focal spots)
- Accuracy and reproducibility of kilovolt (peak) and timer stations
- Beam quality assessment (half-value layer) done at kilovolt (peak) used clinically
- Automatic exposure control: reproducibility, kilovolt (peak) compensation, minimum response time, backup timer verification
- Uniformity of intensifying screens
- Breast entrance exposure and average glandular dose
- Compression pressures and mechanics
- Tube leakage
- Mammography phantom image baseline
- Grid/artifact evaluation
- A processor sensitometric strip baseline

These tests are documented in both the ACR *Manual for Mammography Physicists* and in the American Association of Physicists in Medicine Report No. 29. Any problems

should initiate a call to the service engineer to take corrective action.

MAMMOGRAPHY EQUIPMENT

Detector

Screen/film combinations that are specifically designed and suited for mammography must be chosen. At the present time this involves a single intensifying screen, used as a back screen, with spatial resolution sufficient to detect microcalcifications 2 to 300 μm in size, and properly coupled with a single-emulsion film sensitive to the emission spectrum (the color of light emitted) of the intensifying screen. The cassette containing the screen and film should have very low x-ray attenuation and high durability and provide intimate contact between the film and screen. In addition, the cassette should be designed so that the edges of the film and screen are positioned tightly against the chest wall edge of the cassette to minimize the amount of breast tissue that is not imaged.

Screen/Film Contact

One cause of image blur is poor contact between the screen and the film. The cassettes should be tested by imaging a 40-mesh copper screen to ensure good screen/film contact. Areas of poor screen/film contact appear as black splotches on the resulting image. Each screen should be marked with an identification number near the left or right edge away from the chest wall. This is accomplished by affixing thin stick-on numbers that do not compromise film screen contact but prevent light from the screen from reaching the film, so that the screen number appears in white on each film. The same number should also be placed on the outside of the cassette. This numbering permits the identification of the particular cassette and its screen should a problem arise, so that artifacts related to the cassette and its screen can be rapidly resolved. Because dust causes artifacts on images and can cause poor screen/film contact, screens should be cleaned at least once a week (more frequently as needed).

Grid

The grid must be a moving grid. It must function properly and be able to continue to function even when there is firm pressure against it during breast compression. A common cause of grid artifact is poor electrical connection (Fig. 9-1).

Processing

Processing of the film is frequently the weakest link in the imaging chain. Processing involves a fairly sensitive, con-

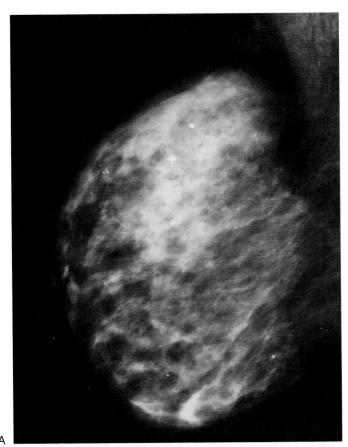
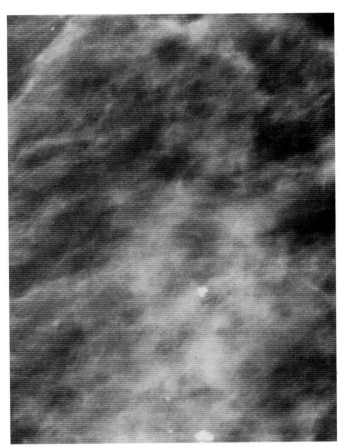

A B

FIG. 9-1. Grid lines are not immediately apparent on this mediolateral oblique projection **(A)** but are obvious on close inspection **(B)**. They can compromise the appreciation of fine details. The image should be repeated.

trolled interaction among the film, the chemicals, and the processor. It has been found that it is usually best to follow the film manufacturer's guidelines and use combinations of film, chemicals, processor cycle time, and developer temperatures that have been determined to work best. This does not mean that the individual practice cannot discover better combinations, but the recommended processing parameters have usually been carefully arrived at by the manufacturers. It is usually best to consider these components together as a complete system to obtain appropriate image quality, especially in terms of film contrast and speed.

Processor

Ideally the processor should be completely dedicated to mammography. If the processor must be used to process other kinds of film, it should be optimized for the mammography film. If the processor must be shared, it is beneficial if all single-emulsion film is directed to the mammography processor with a separate processor for double-emulsion films because the chemistry replenishment rates are determined by the amount of emulsion processed.

Daily processor maintenance includes sensitometry, monitoring of developer temperature, and cleaning of the crossover

rollers so that build-up of particulate matter or other material does not scratch or otherwise damage the film. A thorough cleaning should be performed at least monthly, and processor inspection should check for rough rollers, nonuniform transport speed, broken gears, and chemistry replenishment rates.

Control of Processing Artifacts by Proper Maintenance

If the processor is shared, bimonthly cleaning is recommended. A specially manufactured tacky transport roller cleanup film specifically designed to help clean rollers used daily may further avoid processing artifacts. Dirt and sludge from the transport rollers clings to the cleanup film, helping to keep the rollers free of dirt in the times between routine cleanings. Because the largest fluctuations in image quality have been found to be associated with processing and the processor, close attention must be paid on a daily basis.

Processor and Processing Chemistry

To maintain consistent quality, the film processor should be optimized for the type of mammographic film being used. If possible, the processor should be used only to process these films, as other films (e.g., larger sizes, double emul-

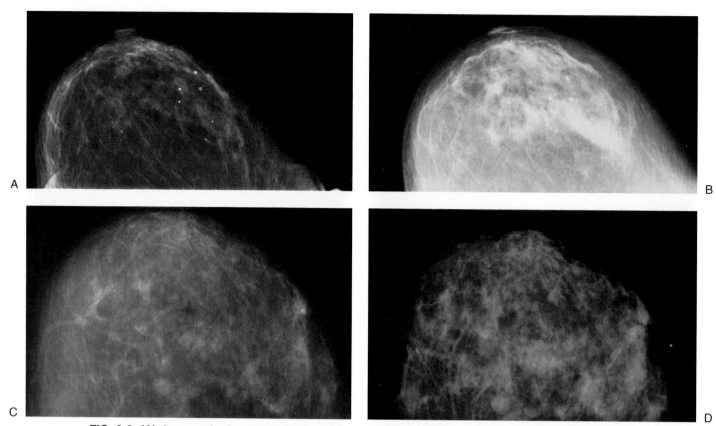

FIG. 9-2. (A) A **properly developed high-contrast** craniocaudal image using recommended developer chemistry and processing conditions. **(B)** The result of using a developer chemistry that was not recommended. The only difference between **A** and **B** is the developer chemistry. All other factors remained identical. Note that this resulted in a lower contrast image and underdeveloped film. **(C)** In another patient, contaminated chemistry and consequent underdevelopment resulted in this low-contrast craniocaudal image. **(D)** Proper development resulting in much higher contrast is evident in this image with proper processor chemistry.

sion) can affect the processing characteristics. The choice and concentration of processing chemistries is a vital part of the system. Various chemistries are rarely interchangeable. Film speed, film contrast, and base plus fog are affected by the various types and quantities of chemicals used (Fig. 9-2).

One should be cautious about the use of repackaged chemistries because there may be a tendency for these to not be as concentrated as the original chemicals from the manufacturer (4). The complex chemical reactions in film processing are beyond the scope of this discussion (see Equipment and Physics). However, several classes of chemicals are involved. The concentration of hydroquinone affects film contrast and helps determine the ultimate blackening of the film. Phenidone affects the speed of the film and the gray tones of the image. The activity of hydroquinone and phenidone are affected by the pH of the developer solution. Sulfites control oxidation and the concentration of the hydroquinone so that it is not used up too quickly. A gross measure of the concentration of these chemicals can be obtained by measuring the specific gravity of the solutions. However, only direct chemical analysis can provide absolute confirmation of the concentration of each individual component.

Chemical Replenishment Rates

As films are developed bromide is produced. Bromide is needed to control the development process but too much results in slower development. The processing parameters are dependent on a balance of bromide washing from the film and slowing development while fresh chemistry is added at the appropriate replenishment rate to maintain the desired concentrations or a seasoned chemistry. As film is processed the processing chemistries are used up and must be replenished. The proper rate of replenishment of the chemicals is necessary to maintain stable activity of the developer and fixer. The exact rate of replenishment depends on the surface area of the emulsion being processed. Because the processor cannot determine when a dual-emulsion film is being processed, these should be processed separately from single-emulsion mammographic films so that the proper chemistry replenishment rates can be maintained. Some processors track this figure directly. Usually replenishment rates are more crudely calculated using the number and size of the film processed (i.e., the total volume of film being developed per day). It is important to consult with the processor manufacturer to correctly adjust and set up the film processor to establish the appropriate replenishment rates. This will ensure the desired results and the consistency of those results.

Somewhat paradoxically, high film use per day requires lower replenishment rates per sheet of film. Very low film volume (30 to 60 films per day) is difficult to stabilize and flood replenishment is recommended. Flood replenishment requires the use of a starter solution in the replenishment tanks.

Following the initial optimization of film processing, proper replenishment is monitored and established by stable sensitometric results (film speed, film contrast, and base plus fog). The proper concentrations of these chemicals help to control artifacts and ensure that the images will not deteriorate with time.

Processing Time and Temperature

The most important time in the film processing cycle is the time that the film is immersed in the developer chemicals. This and the overall time in the processor should be chosen to optimize the sensitometric performance of the film to meet the diagnostic needs of the radiologist. Different mammography films have different processing characteristics, thus there is no best processing time or temperature that is appropriate for all mammography film.

Processing time refers to the time the film is immersed in the developer chemistry. Standard cycle processing time is considered to be approximately 21 to 32 seconds, whereas extended cycle processing time is approximately 42 to 53 seconds depending on the make and model of the processor (5). The thickness of the emulsion and the shape of the film grains determine the length of time needed for their complete development. The developer temperature is a function of film type and processing cycle time, and once again, it is usually best to follow the film manufacturer's recommendations. Developer temperature affects the film speed, film contrast, and base plus fog. No one temperature is appropriate for all films. Manufacturers have recommended immersion times and temperatures for their various products, and it is best to not deviate from these standards. As with immersion time, higher temperature, up to a point, produces higher contrast. If the temperature is too high film fog will degrade the image.

Increased film contrast may enhance perception of details in the mammogram, but the increased film speed that usually accompanies increased contrast also results in higher quantum noise in the image because fewer x-ray quanta are required to obtain a given optical density. Higher film contrast makes the noise more visible. Eventually additional processing leads to an increase of base plus fog, and the image is degraded. The goal should be high contrast with the lowest acceptable noise and an avoidance of over-processing problems.

Agitation of the Chemicals

One of the factors that is not frequently appreciated in the processing cycle is the agitation of the chemistries. Agitation is provided by roller contact and chemical recirculation pumps (6). If the film passes through with little turbulence in the chemicals, then the chemicals actually contacting the emulsion may be less potent as they are used up. Poor agitation of the various chemistries may be a significant problem in achieving the desired processing, and this should be taken into account when selecting a processor.

Wash Cycle

Washing the film after it has been developed is important for the long-term stability of the image. The removal of residual developer and fixer chemistries improves the survival of archived images. The wash water should always be filtered to remove possible contaminants and the temperature of the wash water set to the processor manufacturer's recommendation.

Drying the Film

The dryer is another key element of the processing cycle that is sometimes overlooked. Its temperature must be adjusted to be as low as possible while still providing a dry film exiting the processor. Overly dry films or films that are dried at too high a temperature can cause artifacts that interfere with the radiologist's ability to interpret the film.

Steps for Optimizing the Processor and Establishing a Baseline

The procedure for establishing processing parameters is a logical step-by-step optimization. It should begin with a thorough processor inspection by a service engineer and accomplish the following tasks:

- Drain the tanks in the processor and thoroughly clean and flush the tanks, racks, and tubing to the replenishment tanks with water.
- Drain and flush the replenisher tanks and refill with fresh chemistry mixed to proper concentration.
- Check the specific gravity with a hydrometer to provide a gross measurement of the concentration of the processor chemicals. This should agree with the desired measurement provided by the chemistry manufacturer of both the developer and fixer.
- Check the pH readings to determine whether the solutions have been properly mixed.
- Fill the fixer tank with fixer solution.
- Fill the wash tank with filtered water.
- Once again rinse the developer tank to eliminate any possibility that contaminants such as fixer have compromised the tank. Check developer tank filter.

- Fill the developer tank halfway full with developer and add the specified amount of developer starter solution to begin the seasoning of the chemistry. Add an additional amount of developer solution to fill the developer tank. To keep the pH and potassium bromide within acceptable limits, starter (from the manufacturer of the chemicals used) of a slightly higher pH is added to the fresh developer.
- Set the developer temperature control at the temperature specified by the film manufacturer for the processing cycle time being used.
- Replenishment rates should be set according to the volume of the tank and the size of films that will be used and the estimated number of films that will be processed each day.
- Wait for the processor to warm up and stabilize. The temperature should be checked with a digital thermometer that is accurate to at least ±0.5°F. (Do not use thermometers containing mercury or alcohol as they may contaminate the processor if they break.)
- Select a fresh box of film for control testing of the same type of film used for mammography. Note the emulsion number and record it.
- Using a sensitometer that is matched to the color of the light that will be emitted by the screens and produces a 21-step wedge on the control film, expose and process a sensitometric strip. This should be processed with the less exposed end being fed into the processor first, inserted on the same side of the processor feed tray each time and in the same orientation to the emulsion. It is important that these details of testing be completed precisely.
- Repeat the sensitometric strip each day at approximately the same time for 5 consecutive days. Always do this before any clinical images are processed.
- Using a densitometer, read in the center of each step of the sensitometric strip and record the densities, including an area of the processed film that has not been exposed.
- Determine the average of the densities for each step using the densities for that step from the five strips.
- Determine which step has a density closest to 2.20 and the step close to but not <0.45. The difference in densities between these two steps is designated as the density difference (DD) (often referred to as the contrast points).
- Determine the average of the densities measured from step 1 or the unexposed area of the five strips. This provides the base plus fog level (B + F).
- The numerical values of mid-density (MD), DD, and B + F are the standards that must be used when comparing future test strips in your processor using the control box of film.
- These values are recorded on a control chart and used as standards for daily processor QC.
- The control limits of MD and DD should be within ±0.10 of the optimized standards and the B + F within +0.03 of the standard. Once processing conditions (chemistry mixed to the correct concentrations as measured by specific gravity), time, temperature, and agitation have been optimized to the film manufacturer's recommendations, it should be verified that the desired film contrast is obtained.

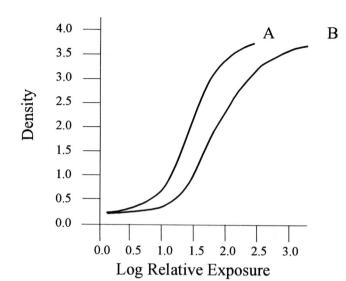

FIG. 9-3. These curves of film density plotted against the log of the relative exposure demonstrate the differences between one film with higher contrast **(A)** and another **(B)**, which has a wider gray scale.

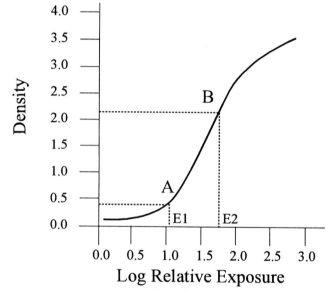

FIG. 9-4. Average gradient is calculated by finding the slope of the Hunter and Driffield curve between point A, which is the density 0.25 above the base plus fog (base plus fog is generally approximately 0.17 to 0.20) and the point on the curve that is 2.0 above the base plus fog. The formula is 1.75/(E2 – E1). In this case E2 = 1.67 and E1 = 1.09 so that the average gradient = 1.75/(1.67 – 1.09) = 3.022.

Each film has an average gradient value (film contrast), and it is important to know that value and to achieve and maintain it constantly in the processing environment.

The average gradient describes the average film contrast and is defined as the slope of a straight line between two points of specified densities. These densities are the minimum and maximum useful densities of the film along the straight-line portion of the Hunter and Driffield curve where the greatest film contrast occurs. Figure 9-3 illustrates the difference in characteristic curves of films with high and with low contrast. Using the sensitometric strip and plotting the density of all the steps is used to determine the average gradient illustrated in Fig. 9-4 (6,7).

Darkroom

The darkroom environment can be a major cause of problems. Good design and cleanliness help to control dust artifacts and ensure image quality. The darkroom should not be used as a storage room. Only the necessary processing materials should be in the darkroom. Additional objects add unwanted dust and dirt.

An adequate air supply must be provided, and the relative humidity should be maintained between 40% and 60%. Vents, which are dust accumulators, should not be located above the counters that are used for handling cassettes. One of the biggest contributors to dust and artifacts in darkrooms can be the ceiling material. The often-used acoustic ceiling tiles made of a compressed material and set into metal tracks accumulate dust and dirt that fall when the air pressure changes when the darkroom door is opened and closed. Light can also enter the darkroom through such tiles. A solid construction ceiling is strongly recommended. Sources of dust and dirt as well as light must be controlled. Food should not be allowed in the darkroom; crumbs on the screens are as bad as dust.

Care must be taken that there are no light leaks around the doors, pass boxes, or processors. Light leaks result in fog and a loss of contrast on the final image. Proper safelights, chosen to avoid the spectral sensitivity of the film being used, and correct light bulb wattage must be used. The safelight should be positioned 4 feet from the work area or the feed tray. A QC safelight test must be performed. The film in the darkroom must be kept in a clean light tight container.

Viewing Conditions and View Boxes

The display systems for reviewing and interpreting the films are often overlooked. View boxes and viewing conditions should be the same for the technologist who is critiquing his or her film for technique and the radiologist who is interpreting the study. Ideally, the view boxes used throughout the breast imaging area provide identical light conditions so that the technologist is seeing the images exactly as the radiologist will view them.

The luminance of the mammographic view box should be of a higher level than conventional view boxes. Typical view boxes have luminance levels on the order of 1,500 nit. Because of the high-contrast techniques being used, it is generally felt that mammographic view box luminance levels should be at least 3,500 nit so that the darker portions of the films can be viewed. There should be little or no ambient room light because glare compromises the ability to see contrast on the film. Masking should be available to block out extraneous light on the face of the viewing surface and around the film as this light can dramatically reduce the eye's ability to perceive low-contrast structures. The entire mammographic film not covered by the breast should be exposed and black to avoid light glare around the image. Both the technologist and the radiologist should have a high-quality magnifying lens (2× to 5×) to aid in the investigation of fine details, particularly the perception and analysis of microcalcifications.

BREAST IMAGING TEAM

High-quality mammography requires constant attention to detail. The radiologist, technologist, and physicist should work closely together to maintain image quality and the delivery of quality service. This requires that each member of the team recognize his or her importance as well as the importance of the other members.

Radiologists involved in mammography should have a firm understanding of the technology and technique. The responsible radiologist should have a solid interest in and provide oversight for the QA program. Requirements involve board certification and continuing education courses on mammography. The radiologist has the responsibility for building the entire diagnostic imaging chain and overseeing all activity to ensure that consistent, high-quality images are produced. Providing motivation and leadership to the imaging team as well as direction to the solution of problems as they are encountered are important responsibilities for the radiologist.

The radiologic technologist should be certified by the American Registry of Radiologic Technologists (ARRT) or have state licensure and must be familiar with the correct operation of the mammography equipment. It is helpful if the technologist possesses advanced-level certification from the ARRT in mammography.

The technologist must be trained, must use proper positioning to include all, or as much as possible, of the breast tissue in each required view, and must have knowledge of proper compression (see Chapter 10) and radiographic techniques. Additional requirements involve participation in continuing education courses in mammography.

The medical physicist must be certified in radiologic physics and must receive continuing education specifically in mammography physics. It is imperative that the team have a sense of cohesiveness. Once the components of the imaging system are compatible and optimized, the facility is ready to begin QA.

QUALITY ASSURANCE PROGRAM

All facilities must assign one person to be responsible for developing and documenting the QA program. This designated individual must have the authority and responsibility to complete implementation and administration of the QA pro-

TABLE 9-1. *Minimum frequencies for quality control tests*

Test	Frequency	Performed by
Processing quality control (sensitometry and temperature)	Daily before clinical images are processed and whenever processor maintenance is performed	Technologist
Darkroom cleanliness	Daily	Technologist
Screen cleanliness	At least weekly or when artifacts appear	Technologist
View boxes and viewing conditions	Weekly	Technologist
Phantom images	At least monthly	Technologist with review by radiologist and technologist
Visual checklist	Monthly	Technologist
Fixer retention	Quarterly	Technologist
Darkroom fog	Semiannually	Technologist
Screen/film contact	Semiannually	Technologist
Compression	Semiannually	Technologist
Mammographic unit assembly evaluation	Annually	Medical physicist
Collimation assessment	Annually	Medical physicist
Focal spot size measurement	Annually	Medical physicist
Beam quality assessment—half-value layer	Annually	Medical physicist
Automatic exposure control system	Annually	Medical physicist
Uniformity of screen speed	Annually	Medical physicist
Breast entrance exposure and average glandular dose	Annually	Medical physicist
Artifact evaluation	Annually	Medical physicist
View box measurement	Annually	Medical physicist

gram. The facility is responsible for providing its complete support for the program if it is to succeed. The designated individual should form a QA/QC committee composed of the radiologist, the technologist, radiation safety officer, and the medical physicist. Anyone who can make a contribution to the total QA process should be a part of the committee. The QA committee should establish specifications, guidelines, and testing procedures to fulfill obligations of compliance programs. The next step is to establish a manual to compile the necessary documentation for records. The QA manual contains

- An overview of the mammography department: responsible radiologist, technologist, and medical physicist; service technicians and contact numbers; facility license, copies of accreditation certificates, and a copy of FDA certificate
- Qualifications of the radiologists, radiological technologists, and medical physicists, including credentialing and licensing, responsibilities or job descriptions, curriculum vitae, and continuing medical education
- A list of nontechnical staff and their responsibilities or job descriptions
- New employee orientation program
- Radiation safety policy
- Dosimetry reports
- Film retention policy
- Policy and procedures for screening mammography, diagnostic mammography, positioning, special views, special procedures, copies of consent forms
- Copy of patient medical history form
- Copies of patient information
- Patient reporting and follow-up mechanisms

- Practice audit with outcome data
- Location of reference materials
- Installation manuals and service records of equipment
- Acceptance testing for all elements and baseline tests
- List of QC tests and frequencies
- List of individuals who perform QC tests
- List of acceptable control limits for each test
- Procedural description of QC tests
- List of QC equipment used to perform tests and control tests of this equipment (it is important that test equipment be monitored)
- Copies of sample charts for QC testing
- Established protocol to correct any problems noted in QC tests
- Reports of committee meetings and medical physicist annual report
- Sign-off page
- Patient complaint mechanism

QUALITY CONTROL TESTS

The minimum frequencies of QC tests for the QC mammography technologist and the medical physicist are shown in Table 9-1. The scheduling is based on the recommended minimum frequencies by the ACR in their accreditation program (2). However, it should be understood that these frequencies are the minimum, and the QC tests should be done more frequently initially to gain proficiency in performing the tests and to be able to depend on the stability of the imaging equipment. Documentation of performance, data forms, and control charts must be completed for each test for the QA

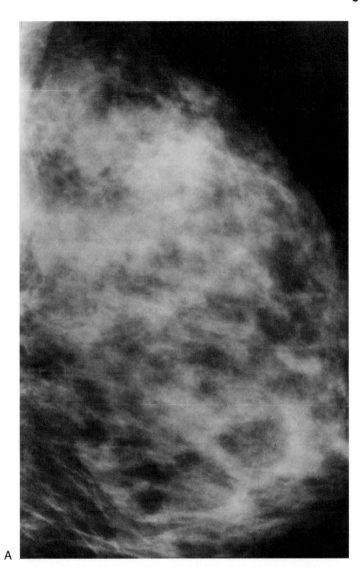

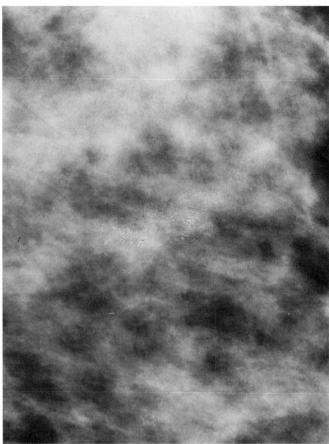

FIG. 9-5. (A) Grease on a film can simulate calcifications by blocking development. **(B)** What appear to be calcifications on this lateral mammogram are obviously a fingerprint on close inspection.

manual. It is required that the radiologist, medical physicist, and QC technologist review these data forms, control charts, and images. The QC technologist's review is continuous, the radiologist's review is quarterly, and the medical physicist's review is at least annual. At the Massachusetts General Hospital, quality is reviewed constantly and on an image-by-image basis. High-quality mammography requires a dedicated team, as it must be a constant effort. Procedure steps, required equipment, precautions, caveats, suggested performance criteria, and corrective actions are contained in the quality control manuals from the ACR Committee on Quality Assurance in Mammography (2).

Objectives for Quality Control Tests

Darkroom Cleanliness

Darkroom cleaning should be carried out at the beginning of the work period before any clinical films are handled or processed to minimize artifacts on film images. Sufficient time must be given to accomplish this task at the start of the working day. The use of daylight processors for mammography have largely eliminated the darkroom except for loading the film containers or magazines which must still be kept clean and in a clean area.

Processor Quality Control

After darkroom cleaning, before clinical images are processed and when developer temperature is at the designated level, processor QC procedures should be carried out to confirm and verify that the processor and chemical system are working according to the pre-established optimized parameters. If the density values (MD, DD, B + F) are beyond established control limits, the test should be repeated to ensure it was not a procedural error. If results remain outside control limits, the source of the problem must be determined and corrected before clinical images are processed.

Screen Cleanliness

Cleaning is performed at least weekly, or whenever dust or dirt artifacts that may degrade image quality or mimic microcalcifications are noted on images. Grease from a finger on the film can prevent its development, and the result can look like calcifications on a mammogram (Fig. 9-5).

View Box Cleanliness

The view box panels should be cleaned and visually inspected weekly for uniformity of luminance and all view box masking equipment checked for proper functioning.

Phantom Images

A radiograph is done to establish an optimized baseline to ensure image quality of the entire imaging chain. It is essential that all other components be optimized first (i.e., mammography equipment and processing). Subsequently, it

should be carried out weekly. A phantom image should be obtained after service to the mammographic equipment or whenever problems in image quality are suspected. With mobile mammography equipment, a phantom image should be done each time the unit is moved.

The phantom image is evaluated for film background density, contrast (density difference), uniformity, and the number of objects seen. The mammographic phantom approximates a 4.0- to 4.5-cm compressed breast with six different size nylon fibers which simulate fibrous structures, five groups of simulated microcalcifications, and five different size tumorlike masses (Figs. 9-6 and 9-7). Test objects within the phantom range in size from those that should be visible on any system to objects that are difficult to see even on the best mammographic systems.

ACR criteria require a minimum score that includes visibility of the four largest fibrils, the three largest simulated microcalcification groups, and the three largest tumorlike masses. The QC technologist should evaluate the phantom image and record the number of objects seen using a magnifying glass and the same viewing conditions each time. The radiologist may also wish to evaluate the phantom images. The phantom images should be compared to the baseline, and previous images should be examined for artifacts and nonuniform areas. If problems are noted, the source must be determined and corrective action taken. The medical physicist can assist in identifying the specific problem.

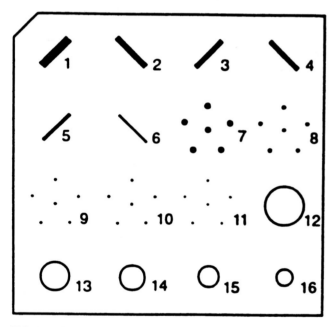

FIG. 9-6. The Radiation Measurements, Inc. (ACR), phantom contains 16 test objects seen here schematically. These include six nylon fibers of varying thickness (1 = 1.56 mm, 2 = 1.12 mm, 3 = 0.89 mm, 4 = 0.54 mm, 5 = 0.40 mm, and 6 = 0.40 mm) to simulate spicules, five groups of specs of varying sizes (7 = 0.54 mm, 8 = 0.40 mm, 9 = 0.32 mm, 10 = 0.24 mm, and 11 = 0.16 mm) to simulate calcifications, and tapered discs of varying diameter (12 = 10 mm, 13 = 7.5 mm, 14 = 6.0 mm, 15 = 5.0 mm, and 16 = 3.0 mm) whose thickness varies (12 = 2.0 mm, 13 = 1.0 mm, 14 = 0.75 mm, 15 = 0.5 mm, and 16 = 0.25 mm) to simulate masses. A flat disk is also provided to be placed on the phantom so that the density of the film under the disk can be compared to that immediately adjacent to the disk to provide a measure of the contrast range of the imaging chain. (From Radiation Measurements, Inc., Middleton, WI. With permission.)

FIG. 9-7. This is an image of the **ACR phantom** showing the various test objects that are visible using screen/film technique. At least four of the fibers, three of the simulated calcification clusters, and three of the simulated masses should be visible.

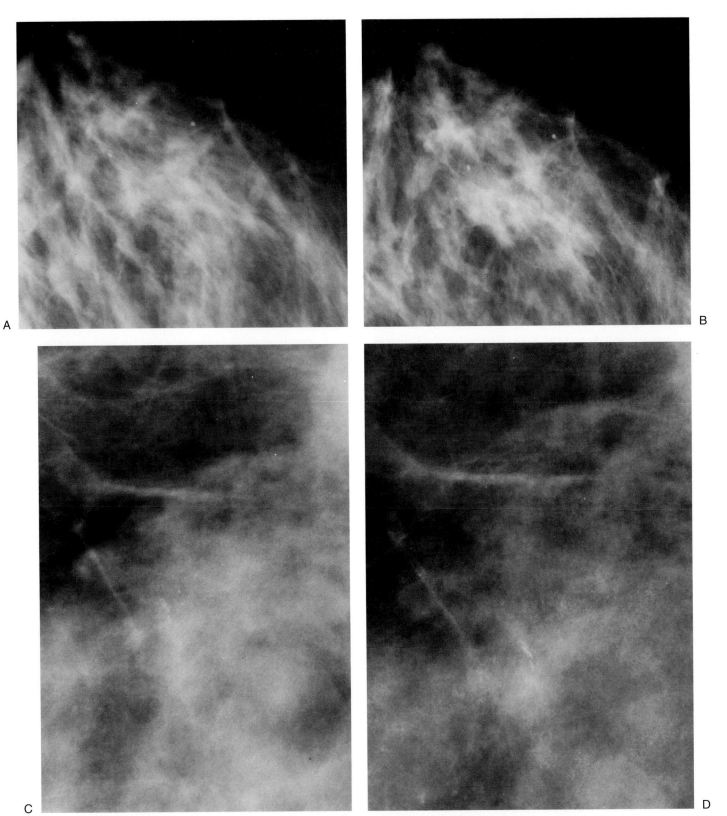

FIG. 9-8. Motion blur can be subtle. It is best seen by looking at calcifications. **(A)** Note that the benign calcifications appear blurred. **(B)** With motion eliminated the calcifications are sharply defined. **(C)** In this second case, the calcifications of ductal carcinoma in situ were barely evident due to motion blur on the magnification image. **(D)** They are much sharper on the repeat image without motion.

Visual Checklist

A visual inspection checklist for each mammographic unit and room should be based on the unit model, manufacturer, and policy.

Repeat Analysis

The number of repeated mammograms (additional patient exposure) should be tracked. There are inevitable misfires, patient motion (Fig. 9-8), and other problems that affect the images. The resulting data establish the number and cause of films that have been discarded to identify the source. The analysis helps to identify ways to improve efficiency, reduce costs, and reduce patient exposure.

Fixer Retention

Fixer retention is tested to determine the amount of residual fixer in the processed film as an indicator of how well the images will keep over time. Residual fixer indicates insufficient washing and degrades the image's stability.

Darkroom Fog

Darkroom fog is checked to prevent any unwanted film density due to fog from darkroom light leaks, poor condition of safelight filters, or film storage.

Screen/Film Contact

Screen/film contact is checked to ensure that the contact between screen and film is being maintained and not caus-

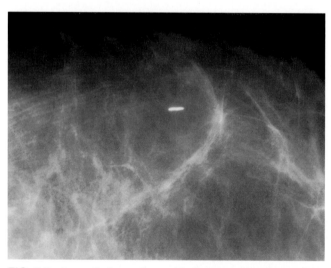

FIG. 9-9. A small piece of wood is between the film and the screen. It blocks the light from the screen so that the film under it is white. Note also that the breast structures in the area are blurred due to **poor screen/film contact.**

ing image blurring. All cassettes should be tested during acceptance testing and then at least semi-annually or when a problem of blur is suspected. The deterioration of the foam or backing on which the screens are mounted or improper cleaning can result in poor screen/film contact or blurred image quality. This can also be caused by particulate matter between the screen and film (Fig. 9-9).

Compression

The force of compression is tested to ensure adequate but not excessive force in both manual and powered modes. The medical physicist's annual tests are designed to detect problems that interfere with the image quality or increase the radiation dose to the patient. A written report of the test results should be provided to the radiologist for review and recorded in the QA manual. The medical physicist should also review the technologist's QC data and charts at an annual visit and be available to the QC technologist and radiologist.

A mammography technique chart for both phototiming and manual techniques should be completed and posted on the mammographic unit. A copy should also be placed in the QA manual. These charts should be reviewed periodically by the technologist, medical physicist, and radiologist. It may be necessary to use manual techniques to obtain appropriate film density when imaging breasts for implant views, and some phototimers do not produce acceptable densities for all kilovolts (peak) or all thicknesses of breasts.

QUALITY ASSURANCE COMPLIANCE PROGRAMS

The ACR National Mammography Accreditation Program was established in 1987 as a voluntary program. "The impetus for the program came as a result of the concerns of radiologists, other national medical organizations, the government, and the public that qualified personnel perform and interpret mammograms and that dedicated mammography equipment be used to ensure that women receive optimum mammographic examinations with the lowest possible risk" (2).

In 1992 Congress passed the MQSA. The act calls for every site performing mammography in the United States to be accredited through a nationally based, nonprofit accreditation program, such as the ACR Mammography Accreditation Program, by October 1, 1994. The FDA was given the task of monitoring all mammography facilities. The final FDA regulations will likely be completed by the end of 1997.

Many states also have state regulations for mammography. Each facility should consult its state boards to ensure compliance with both state and federal requirements.

AMERICAN COLLEGE OF RADIOLOGY ACCREDITATION

ACR accreditation requirements are likely to evolve over time. To obtain ACR accreditation for a 3-year period requires certification for each individual mammography unit. The following steps must be taken:

- An application questionnaire must be submitted to the ACR concerning qualifications of the radiologist, the medical physicist, and the radiologic technologists.
- Documentation of an established QA/QC program must be submitted.
- For each x-ray unit, a phantom image of an approved phantom must be submitted to evaluate image quality. A thermoluminescent dosimeter must be included in the field of view at the time of exposure to determine radiation dose.
- Two sets of clinical images must be submitted. These are reviewed by a panel of radiologists. The cases should consist of two fatty breasts and two dense breasts.
- The facility must submit 30 days of sensitometry and processor QC documentation.

SUMMARY

QA and QC depend on thorough preplanning of activities and proper execution of the plan. Every person involved in caring for the patient and the imaging chain has a responsibility to ensure that the result is of high quality.

REFERENCES

1. Gray JE, Winkler NT, Stears J, Frank ED. Quality Control in Diagnostic Imaging. Rockville, MD: Aspen, 1982.
2. Committee on Quality Assurance in Mammography. Quality Control Manuals. Reston, VA: American College of Radiology, 1994.
3. National Council on Radiation Protection and Measurement. Mammography: A User's Guide. Bethesda, MD: National Council on Radiation Protection and Measurement, 1986. NCRP report no. 85.
4. Kimme-Smith C, Sun H, Bassett LW, Gold RH. Effect of poor control of film processors on mammographic image quality. Radiographics 1992;12:1137–1146.
5. Haus AG. Recent Advances in Screen-Film Mammography. Radiologic Clinics of North America. Philadelphia: Saunders, 1987.
6. McKinney WE. Radiographic Processing and Quality Control. Philadelphia: Lippincott, 1988.
7. Methods for the Sensitometry of Medical and Dental X-Ray Films. Washington, DC: American National Standards Institute, 1974. ANSI PH 2.9-1974.

Breast Imaging, 2nd ed., by Daniel B. Kopans.
Lippincott–Raven Publishers, Philadelphia © 1998.

CHAPTER 10

Mammographic Positioning

One of the most critical yet difficult aspects of breast cancer detection and diagnosis is positioning the patient and properly exposing the mammogram. If the breast is not properly positioned, large volumes of breast tissue may not be imaged. Clearly, if tissues are not imaged, then the skill of the interpreter is irrelevant and cancers will be missed (Fig. 10-1). The radiologist must insist on well-positioned, properly exposed mammograms and work continuously with and support dedicated technologists whose goal is try to obtain the best images for every patient. High-quality imaging requires highly motivated technologists who recognize the importance of their work and constantly seek to improve its quality.

Imaging the anterior breast tissues is simple, but imaging the deep tissues is difficult. Given that the volume of the breast increases toward the chest wall, failure to image these tissues could exclude large areas where cancer might develop. It requires a well-trained technologist who is skilled in the proper maneuvers and a cooperative patient who is relaxed and permits the pulling and compression of the breast that is so important for high-quality imaging.

SCREENING MAMMOGRAPHY

The screening mammogram is the most important mammographic study. Although earlier detection does not guarantee cure, the screening mammogram is the only opportunity to detect a clinically occult breast cancer earlier. The fact that screening must be highly efficient and low cost, so that it can be available to as many women as possible, does not mean that the quality of the screening mammogram can be diminished. The equipment and detector system must be capable of producing excellent image quality. The technologist must strive to work with the patient to position the breast as completely over the imaging field as possible to avoid missing the deep tissues. The breast must be appropriately compressed to spread overlapping structures, and the exposure should be suitable to properly image the tissues at risk for cancer.

ROUTINE MAMMOGRAPHIC PROJECTIONS

Breast tissue can be found as far medial as the sternum, laterally to the anterior edge of the latissimus dorsi, superiorly to the clavicle and apex of the axilla, and inferiorly to just below the inframammary fold (Fig. 10-2). The mammogram is an effort to image as much of this volume as possible.

Standard Views

In general, two projections of each breast should be obtained whether the study is for screening or for a diagnostic evaluation (unless a recent two-view study is available). Two views permit an appreciation of three dimensions and an understanding of overlapping structures that may be confusing when single-view mammograms are obtained. Sickles found that single-view mammography leads to a higher rate of patient recall for additional evaluation (1). This is due to the fact that normal overlapping structures can be confusing on a single projection but are easily clarified by the second view. More important, it has been shown repeatedly that single-view mammography causes the radiologist to fail to detect 11% to 25% of cancers (2,3) (Fig. 10-3).

Two views should always be obtained as the first baseline screening examination. Some radiologists, in order to save money and radiation exposure, still argue that when the breast tissues are predominantly composed of radiolucent fat, subsequent screening studies with single-view mammograms are sufficient. Not only has this never been proved, but the cost savings is a relatively small percentage of the overall cost of screening (a sheet of film contributes $\frac{1}{25}$ of the cost of a mammogram) and the radiation exposure, relative to the benefit of early detection, is insignificant for women ages 40 and over (4). Because single-view mammography is likely to result in early cancers being missed, the effort to save money and dose will result in lives lost, and single-view screening is unlikely to be cost effective. Two-view mammography is preferred for all screening studies.

Additional Views

Additional views may be useful when a suspected abnormality is detected at screening or by clinical examination. Modified projections, coned-down spot compression, and magnification may be useful to clarify a problem (see Additional Projections).

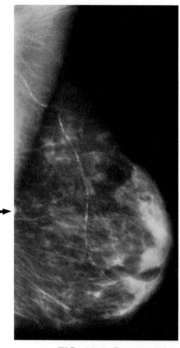
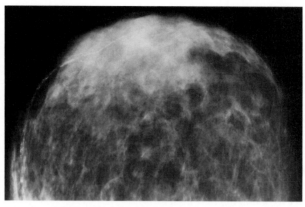
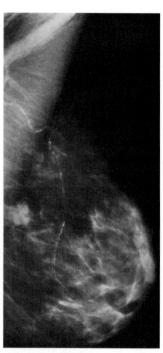

A–C

FIG. 10-1. Poor positioning can result in lost opportunity. This mediolateral oblique (MLO) projection was not well positioned and was interpreted as negative **(A)** along with the craniocaudal projection **(B)**. One year later **(C)** the breast is pulled further into the machine and the invasive ductal carcinoma is evident. It could have been detected a year earlier with better positioning. Note its front edge is barely visible at the back of the earlier MLO (*arrow* on **A**).

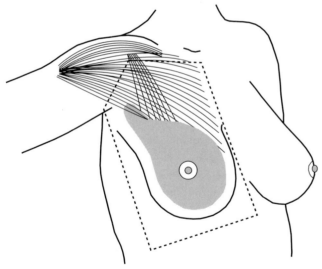

FIG. 10-2. Although the **glandular and ductal elements** of the breast are usually in the distribution shown (*dark area*), they can extend high on the chest wall up to the clavicle, high into the axilla itself, around laterally past the anterior axillary line, and down to the upper abdomen.

Positions for Mammography

Mammography can be performed with the patient seated or standing. In a screening context, when rapid through-put is desired, the standing position is preferred. The standing position also makes positioning easier if the patient has a protuberant abdomen. Most mammography systems permit imaging of women confined to wheelchairs. Recumbent imaging can be accomplished with screen/film and dedicated mammographic units for the incapacitated patient, but it is difficult. The breast must still be compressed, and a stretcher must be brought as close as possible to the detector tray so that the breast can be positioned in the unit. With some units the tray can be removed and the breast compressed directly against the film, but this usually limits the quality of the study, because the phototimer and the oscillating grid cannot be used. By padding the edges of the "bucky," the recumbent patient can be imaged, and some multipurpose chairs have also been devised to permit imaging of the recumbent patient. It is generally better, if possible, to wait for the incapacitated patient to recover so that she can be positioned in the usual fashion.

Pendent Positioning

Pendent positioning with the patient leaning forward or even prone, using gravity to assist in positioning the breast into the field of view, has advantages in some women (Fig. 10-4). With the pectoralis major muscle relaxed by having the arm hang forward, the free margin of the pectoralis falls away from the chest wall, carrying the adjacent breast tissue with it (Fig. 10-5). This can help bring the deep tissues into the imaging field.

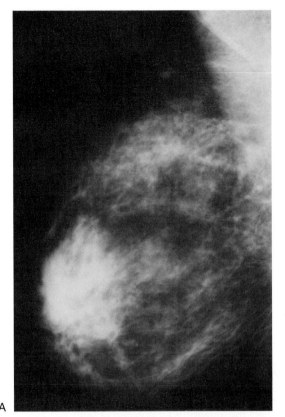
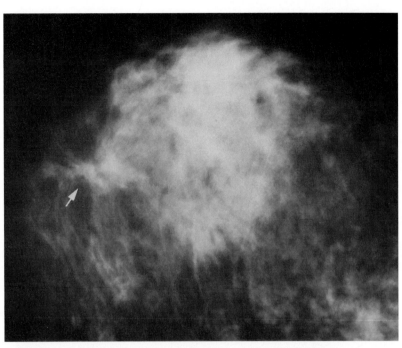

A

B

FIG. 10-3. Single-view mammography results in higher recall rates, and as much as 25% of cancers may be overlooked with a single view. The clinically occult cancer is not visible on this mediolateral oblique projection **(A)** and would have been missed had it not been for the craniocaudal projection **(B)**, on which it is clearly evident medially (*arrow*).

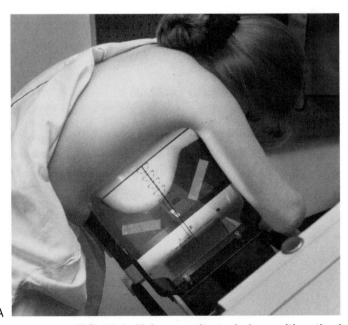
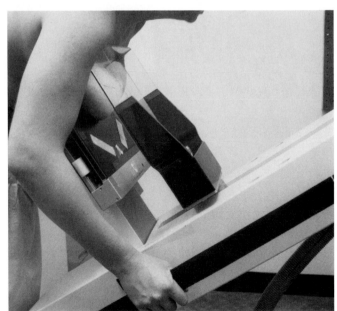

A

B

FIG. 10-4. Using gravity to help position the breast in the pendent position has some advantages. This mammography unit tilts so that the patient can lean forward and gravity can assist the technologist in positioning on the mediolateral projection **(A)** and the craniocaudal view **(B)**. Having the arms relaxed and forward relaxes the pectoralis major muscle and also facilitates positioning. *Continued.*

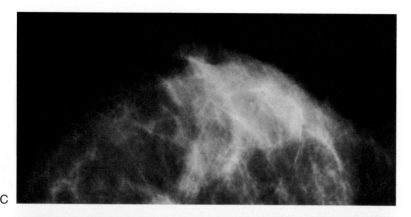

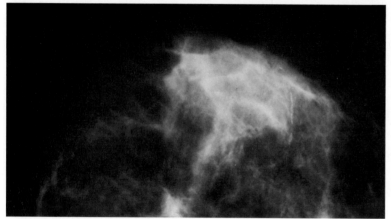

FIG. 10-4. *Continued.* **(C)** On this image obtained using conventional, upright positioning, the back of the breast is not as far into the field of view as when the patient was positioned with her breast pendent **(D)**.

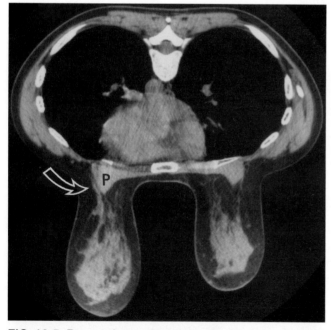

FIG. 10-5. Breast tissue lies along the lateral margin of the pectoralis major muscle. The patient in this CT scan was lying prone with her breasts pendent. Note that there is breast tissue (*arrow*) that extends along the lateral margin of the pectoralis major (P) that must be pulled into the field of view on a mammogram. The same tissue was excised from the other side when her breast cancer was excised.

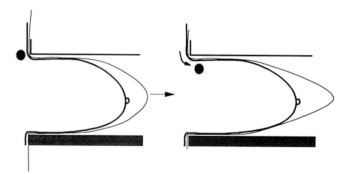

FIG. 10-6. A traction system can pull the breast (and possible lesions) further into the machine, even after some compression has been applied.

As an aid to the technologist, a membrane that lies between the compression system and the breast can be used to pull the breast further into the machine even after compression is applied (Fig. 10-6). This too can help ensure that the deep tissues are included in the imaging (see Chapter 26).

Need for Compression

As long as fine detail is needed on breast images, it is likely that the breast will always need to be compressed. Compression holds the breast away from the chest wall to permit transmission imaging without obscuration by the structures of the thorax. It prevents motion, spreads the overlapping strictures of the breast, reduces scatter by reducing the thickness of the tissue, permits more uniform exposure by converting the cone shape of the breast into a rectangular solid, reduces the dose required for proper exposure, and, by pushing the tissues close to the detector, reduces geometric blur.

Proper Compression

Insufficient compression permits tissue to slip out from the field of view. Too much compression does nothing to improve the image and only results in discomfort and even pain for the patient. Among the goals of compression is to thin the breast as much as possible and spread the structures. The determining factor is the elasticity of the breast, and, in particular, the elasticity of its envelope, the skin. As compression is increased, the breast tissues push out perpendicular to the compression planes and against the exposed skin. Once the exposed skin is tight, additional pressure only pushes the tissues against an unstretchable envelope and does not improve the image, but causes pain. Thus, the compression should be applied until the skin becomes taut (or the patient asks that it be stopped).

Pain and Compression

Contrary to popular belief, women who are polled with regard to mammographic compression acknowledge that most of the time there is little or no discomfort from mammography (5). If the breast is sore to begin with, compressing it will likely exacerbate the discomfort. Unless an immediate study is needed, mammography can be delayed until the breasts are not uncomfortable.

Mammography should not be painful. If it is, it may mean that skin is being pinched and the technologist should stop and release the compression. Much of the discomfort is due to the anxiety and loss of control associated with the procedure. Technologists should recognize this and be as supportive as possible. Each step of the process should be explained, and the patient should be warned when pressure is to be applied. If the patient expresses pain, compression should be stopped. If the positioning is unsatisfactory, compression should be released, the technologist should try to determine what was causing the discomfort, the procedure should be discussed again with the patient, and then the technologist should try to reposition so that it is more comfortable.

There is clearly a psychological aspect to the discomfort associated with breast compression. Although mammography systems are expected to be able to generate 25 to 45 lb of force, pressure is related to the surface area over which the force is applied. This is expressed in pounds per square inch (psi). Because even the smallest breasts have surface areas that are over 10 in.², the actual pressure on the breast is quite low. For example, if the surface of the breast that is in contact with the

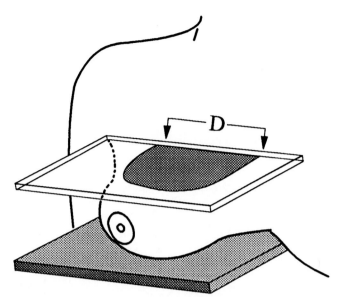

FIG. 10-7. The amount of pressure applied to the breast is the number of pounds applied divided by the area of the compression paddle's contact with the breast (*shaded area*), which equals pounds per square inch.

compression paddle is semicircular (Fig. 10-7), and the chest wall side is 11 inches across, the area in contact with the compression device is approximately half the area of a circle that is 11 inches in diameter (5.5 inches in radius). This is approximately 45 square inches ($\frac{1}{2} \times$ pi $\times 5.5^2$). This means that if 45 pounds is applied over that area the pressure amounts to 1 psi (45 lb/45 in.²). If the breast is smaller, the same force amounts to greater pressure, but even reducing the diameter to 7 inches only increases the pressure to 3 psi. In our experience the amount of force rarely exceeds 20 lb. It has been shown that the average (depending on breast size) pressure generated from mammographic compression amounts to approximately 3 psi. This is the equivalent of applying 45 lb to a breast whose skin area, in contact with the compression paddles, is 15 in.², suggesting a diameter at the chest wall that is a little less than 7 inches. These numbers may not have much meaning until it is realized that the pressure from a mammogram is actually much less than the 6 psi that can be generated by the examining fingers of a clinical breast examination (CBE) (6). A mammogram likely delivers less pressure to the breast tissues than social interactions.

Lack of control is also a component of the discomfort. Many women who control the compression button actually satisfactorily compress themselves with less reported discomfort than if the technologist compresses them (7).

Mediolateral Oblique Projection

The single most useful mammographic projection of the breast is the mediolateral oblique (MLO) image. Ideal MLO positioning should permit the breast to be imaged from high in the axilla down to and including the inframammary fold (Fig.

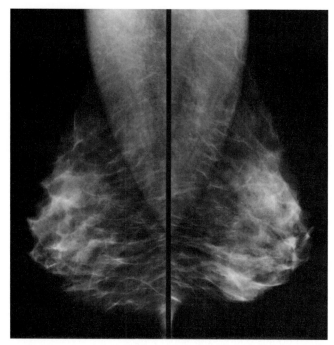

FIG. 10-8. A well-positioned mediolateral oblique mammogram should include tissue from high and deep in the axilla down to the opened, inframammary fold with the front of the breast pulled up and out from the chest wall.

10-8). The term *oblique* is used differently than in other areas of radiology. It does not apply to the patient, but rather to the plane of breast compression. Breast tissue often is found lateral to and curving around the free, lateral margin of the pectoralis major muscle as it courses toward the humerus (see Fig.

10-5). Although there is no direct attachment of the breast to the pectoralis, there are penetrating blood vessels and lymphatics that go from the breast into the muscle, and the adherence of the retromammary fascia to the prepectoral fascia makes it very difficult to pull the breast away from the muscle.

Just as it is easier to pull the skin of the arm away from the muscle by pinching it parallel to the muscle fibers, it is easier to pull the breast away from the chest wall by pulling it and compressing it along a plane that is parallel to the angle of the pectoralis muscle fibers. This also reduces the discomfort from compression. Usually the most lateral and superior portions of the breast and its tail must be imaged through the pectoralis major and, for these reasons, the muscle should be included in the MLO image.

Proper positioning is accomplished by determining the angle of the free margin of the pectoralis major muscle while the patient's humerus is slightly raised, keeping the muscle relaxed (Fig. 10-9). The gantry should be rotated so that the plane of the detector parallels the muscle as it passes obliquely across the chest. This has been shown to be the best way to permit the breast to be pulled away from the chest wall and to permit the maximum amount of tissue to be brought into the field of view. This angle, which varies from individual to individual, permits the necessary compression of the tissues of the breast with the least amount of discomfort.

It is important that the patient be instructed to relax her shoulders as much as possible to avoid tension in the pectoralis muscles, because this reduces the amount of tissue that can be imaged. The arm, however, should never be elevated higher than the shoulder, and every effort should be made to avoid tightening the chest muscles, which tends to pull the breast out of the field of view. The best mammo-

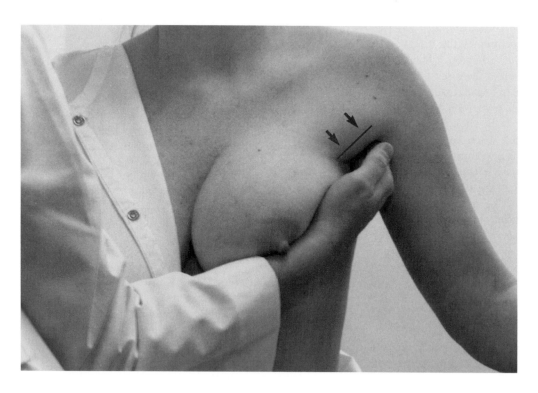

FIG. 10-9. The technologist's fingers are behind the free margin of the pectoralis major muscle. It is the angle of the muscle (*line* and *arrows*) that determines the angle to which the gantry is rotated.

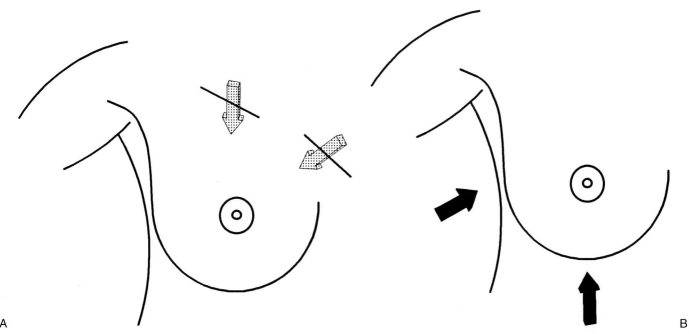

FIG. 10-10. (A) The medial and superior margins of the breast are fixed and immovable (*patterned arrows*). The mobility of the lateral and inferior margins **(B)** (*solid arrows*) is used to properly position the breast.

grams are obtained when a woman can actively relax the pectoralis major muscle.

The breast is positioned by taking advantage of its movable margins. One of the goals of positioning is to press the breast and its structures as close to the detector as possible to reduce blur from geometric unsharpness. Because it is firmly attached to the chest wall medially along the sternum and superiorly below the clavicle, the breast cannot be moved laterally or inferiorly on the chest wall, but it can be elevated and moved medially (Fig. 10-10). In positioning for the MLO the technologist raises the breast and pulls it forward and medially, trying to gather all the deep lateral tissues. She guides the patient into the machine so that the corner of the cassette is high and deep in the axilla, positioning the edge of the cassette against the ribs to keep the breast from sliding back laterally.

The patient is then rolled slowly toward the cassette holder, so that the edge of the cassette keeps the breast from slipping out of the field of view, and the detector pushes and holds the breast medially, preventing it from slipping back laterally and out of the field of view. As the compression paddle is brought across the sternum and against the breast, the technologist removes her hand. As this is done, the technologist should continue to hold the breast and slide her hand up and out to ensure that the breast continues to be held medially, is pulled forward away from the chest wall, and is pulled up so that the structures are spread (up and out). The patient should be as far into the machine as possible to image the tissues from high in the axilla and the upper outer quadrant of the breast down to the inframammary fold (IMF). The breast should be pulled up and out (Fig. 10-11)

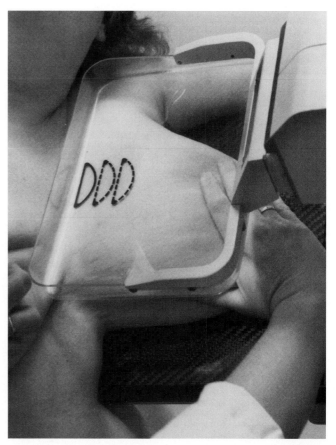

FIG. 10-11. The breast should be pulled up and away from the chest wall as the compression is being applied to open the inframammary fold.

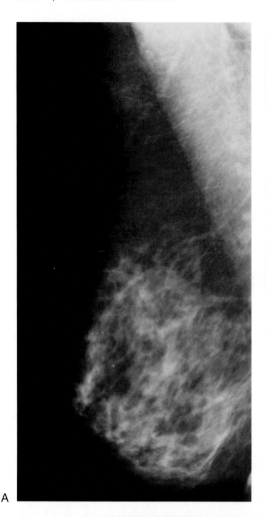

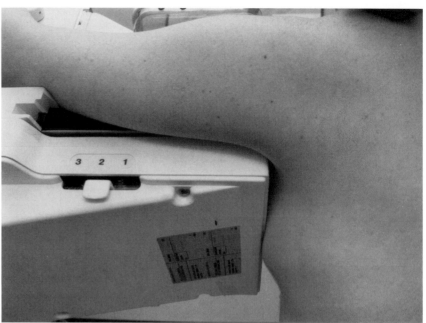

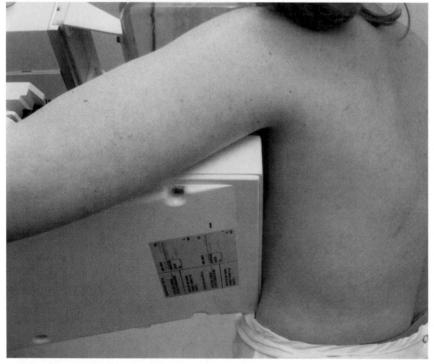

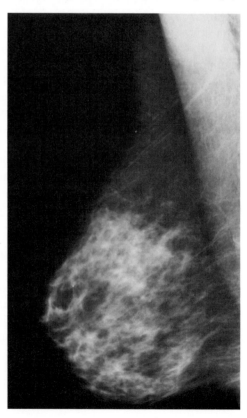

A

B

C

D

FIG. 10-12. The breast should be pulled up and away from the chest wall. In this mediolateral oblique projection the breast is drooping and the inframammary fold is not even on the film **(A)**. This can occur because the patient has been allowed to pull out of the compression, as seen from behind **(B)**, and the bottom of the breast has slipped out. By pulling the breast up and away from the chest wall and being sure that the detector is as close against the chest wall as possible **(C)**, the inframammary crease is visible and open **(D)**.

so that the IMF is open and there is no overlap between the bottom of the breast and the upper abdomen (Fig. 10-12). The open IMF should be visible at the bottom edge of the film (Fig. 10-13).

If the corner of the detector has been properly placed high in the axilla, then the compression paddle, which is aligned with the detector, encounters the breast high and deep along its superomedial margin (Fig. 10-14). During positioning the technologist must hold the breast to maintain its position and smooth the skin to eliminate any folds. Because the breast is anchored medially, the compression paddle cannot push these tissues any distance. If the breast is not properly held medially, then the tethering of the breast along the sternum pulls the medial tissues out of the field of view as the paddle slides over the anchored tissues (Fig. 10-15).

By moving the breast as far medially (toward the sternum) as possible, the skin over the medial breast is relaxed, and the compression paddle does not have to move as far to compress the breast. This reduces, but does not eliminate, the possibility that a lesion in the medial breast will slip out

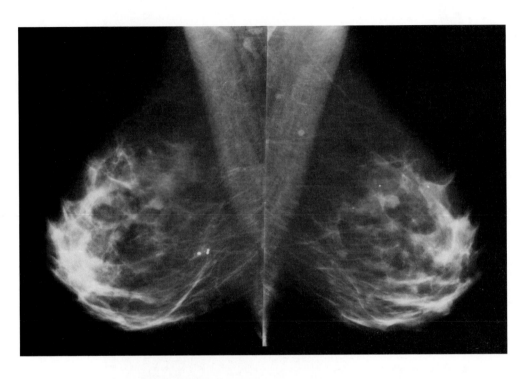

FIG. 10-13. On well-positioned mammograms the inframammary folds are open with no overlap of the breast and upper abdomen.

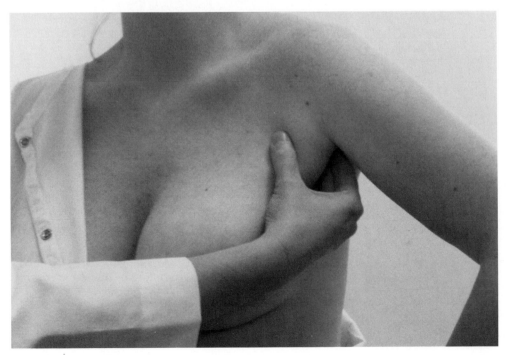

FIG. 10-14. The corner of the detector should ideally be placed high in the axilla, as shown in this picture where the technologist has placed her fingers. The compression paddle will be at the level of the technologist's thumb.

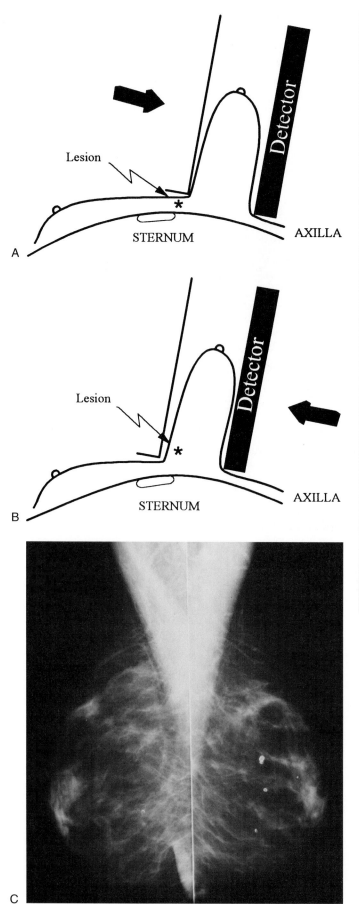

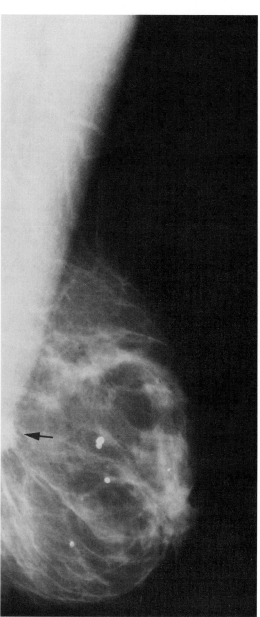

FIG. 10-15. (A) This schematic is a perspective looking down from above. If a lesion is in the medial portion of the breast it may be pulled out from the field of view if the breast is moved laterally during compression (*arrow*). The breast should be moved medially **(B)** (*arrow*) to avoid requiring the compression paddle to move too far laterally. **Medial lesions can be pulled out of the field of view from under the compression because the breast is tethered medially.** No abnormality is evident on these bilateral mediolateral oblique projections **(C)**. A repeat image on the same day of the right breast demonstrates an invasive cancer **(D)**. The medial tissues had been pulled from the field of view on the first study.

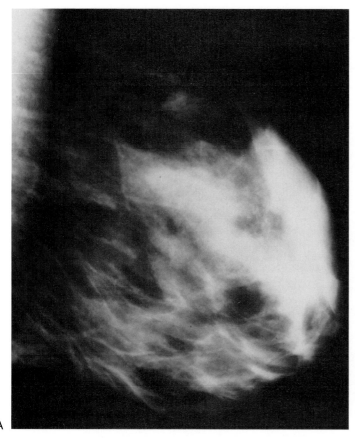

A

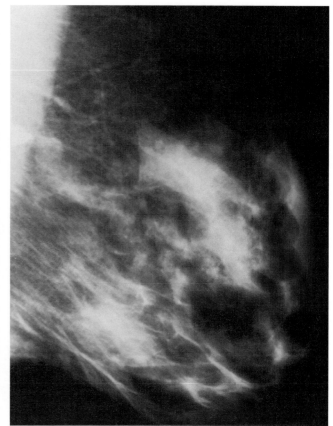

D

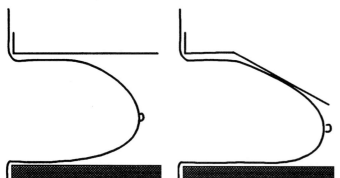

B,C

FIG. 10-16. The tilt paddle is able to compress the anterior breast tissues. This mediolateral oblique projection was performed with a standard compression paddle. The front of the breast is not compressed, and the structures overlap **(A)**. Using standard, flat compression the back of the breast is compressed, but the front is frequently not **(B)**. The tilt paddle first holds and compresses the back of the breast, and then it tilts to compress the front **(C)**. The result is better overall compression and separation of the anterior structures **(D)**.

from under the compression paddle and not be imaged (see Fig. 10-15C). The technologist should try to be sure that the breast is as far into the machine as possible.

Tilting Compression Paddles to Follow the Contour of the Breast

On occasion the axillary tissues are very thick. They may be even thicker than the breast itself so that even with firm compression the lower breast is not optimally compressed. Furthermore, it is common to find that the compression paddle compresses the back of the breast, but the thinner, front tissues are not even touched by the paddle and the structures are not spread. We have designed a tilting compression paddle that can correct this problem (see

Chapter 26). It not only rotates to compensate for thicker tissues in the upper outer portion of the breast, but it tilts so that the anterior, subareolar tissues are compressed (Fig. 10-16).

If a tilt paddle is not available, the technologist should image the high deep tissues separately (Fig. 10-17A) and then repeat the view of the front of the breast with better compression if necessary (Fig. 10-17B). Similarly, if the breast is too large for the cassette, it should be imaged as a mosaic, using several overlapping views.

Gauging Proper Mediolateral Positioning

A properly positioned MLO study shows tissues extending from the axillary tail to the upper abdominal wall (Fig.

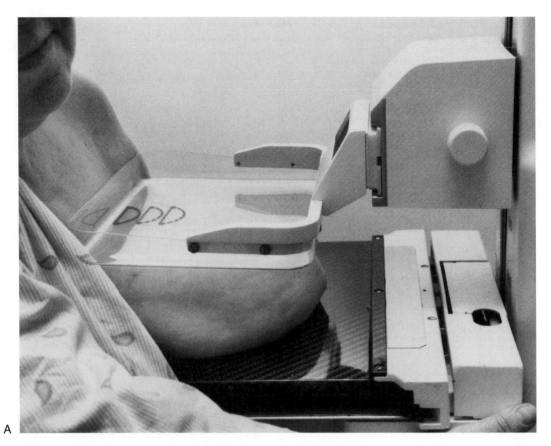

A

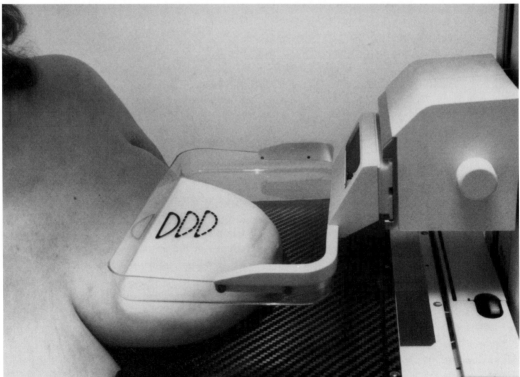

B

FIG. 10-17. In a patient with a large breast or when the deep tissues prevent compression of the anterior breast, two images may be needed. In this patient the anterior breast is not well compressed **(A)**. Having obtained a good image of the deep tissues, a second image was obtained of only the front of the breast **(B)** to provide better compression to the anterior tissues.

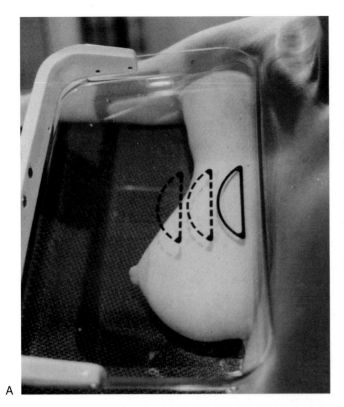

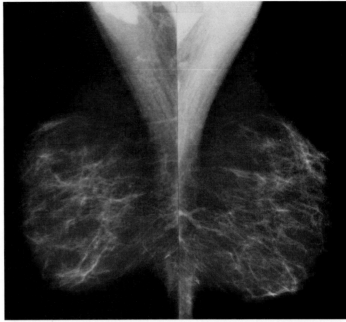

FIG. 10-18. A well-positioned mediolateral oblique projection images the tissues from high in the axilla to just below the inframammary fold **(A)**. The mammogram **(B)** should ideally appear as in this 36-year-old woman (note that not all young women have dense tissues).

10-18). If the breast is not well positioned, cancers can be missed. The pectoralis muscle should be visible extending obliquely in the upper half of the image. It should be very wide at the top and taper as it crosses the upper breast. Studies have suggested that breast tissue is maximally imaged when the pectoralis muscle is visible down to the axis of the nipple.

Technologists should make every effort to include as much breast as possible in the compression to avoid missing deep lesions. The degree of gantry rotation for the oblique view may vary depending on the patient's body habitus, and technologists should adjust the machine to the geometry of the particular individual. The goal is to project as much tissue as possible onto the detector. The way to accomplish this may vary among women. Any obliquity that accomplishes this is satisfactory as long as both breasts are imaged symmetrically.

As the only constant reference point, the nipple should ideally be projected in tangent to the x-ray beam on all images. This also reduces the chance of confusing the nipple as a mass or a true subareolar mass being mistaken as the nipple. If positioning the nipple in profile reduces the amount of breast tissue imaged, then the technologist should ignore trying to image the nipple in profile in favor of projecting the maximum amount of tissue onto the film. When the nipple is not in tangent, it can be mistaken for a mass (Fig. 10-19A). If there is any question of a subareolar abnormality, an additional view of the front of the breast, with the nipple in profile, can be obtained (Fig. 10-19B).

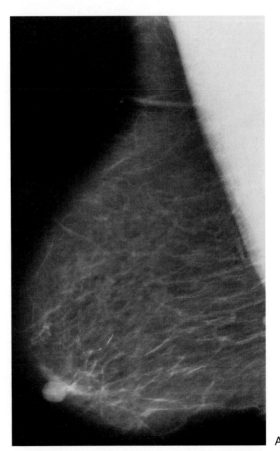

FIG. 10-19. If the nipple is not in profile it can be mistaken for a mass. On this projection there appears to be a subareolar mass **(A)**. *Continued.*

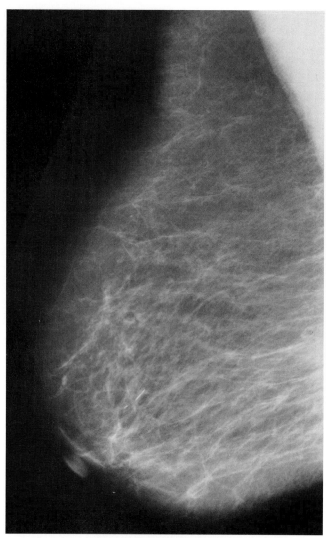

B

FIG. 10-19. *Continued.* The "mass" proved to be the nipple when the patient was repositioned with the nipple in profile **(B)**.

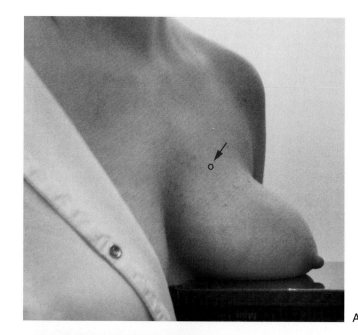

A

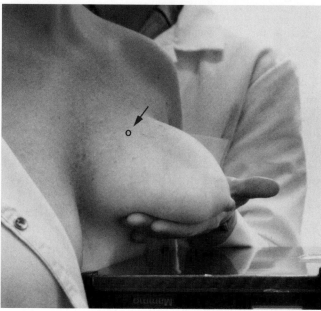

B

FIG. 10-20. Just placing the breast on the detector **(A)** may result in deep tissues, particularly at the top of the breast (*arrow* and "O" on skin), being pulled out of the field of view by tethering at the top of the breast as the compression paddle traverses the upper chest. Elevating the breast **(B)** relaxes the upper skin, and a lesion is less likely to be excluded from the field of view. The detector is then raised to this level. *Continued.*

Craniocaudal Projection

The second view that should be routinely obtained is the craniocaudal (CC) projection. Compression is usually applied from the top of the breast (although some units permit compression from the bottom up) with the detector system under the caudal surface. The gantry is positioned with the beam perpendicular to the floor.

Whenever possible, the nipple should be projected in profile, although, as with the MLO projection, maximizing the tissues imaged takes precedence over imaging the nipple in profile. In the standard CC view, the axis of the nipple is perpendicular to the edge of the detector. Optimal CC positioning is achieved by having the technologist elevate the breast by gathering the tissues from below and pulling the breast up and away from the chest wall. The skin and tissues at the top of the breast are fixed, but the lower breast and its attachment at the IMF are movable and can be ele-

vated, relaxing the skin of the upper breast. If the breast is simply placed on the detector (Fig. 10-20), the compression paddle may not be able to keep the deep tissues in the field of view. Elevation of the IMF permits more breast tissue to be pulled into the field of view as well as better and more comfortable compression.

The technologist should raise the breast with a flat palm underneath so that the IMF is raised as high as it will move

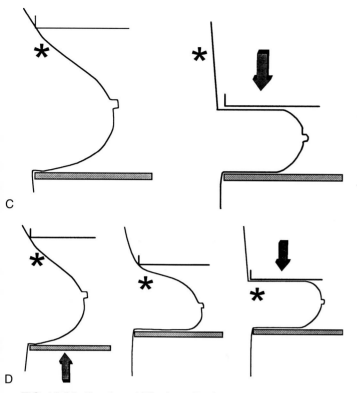

C

D

FIG. 10-20. *Continued.* The benefit of elevating the breast can be seen schematically. Failure to raise the breast can result in the lesion not being imaged **(C)**. Elevation permits more of the upper breast to be included in the field of view **(D)**.

(Fig. 10-21). The detector should be raised to this level so that when the breast is placed on the detector the bottom of the breast is as high as possible, while avoiding raising it so high that attachments at the bottom of the breast pull breast tissues close to the chest wall out of the field of view. Elevating the breast relaxes the upper tissues so that when compression is applied, the attachments at the top of the breast do not pull high, deep lesions out of the field of view (see Fig. 10-20). The patient should be guided into the machine so that the edge of the cassette is against the ribs, pushing up slightly from beneath the breast. The breast is then pulled into the machine with two hands (Fig. 10-22).

Because the medial tissues may inadvertently be pulled out of the field of view on the MLO by normal tethering along the sternum, many radiologists suggest that special attention be paid to these tissues on the CC projection. As the patient moves against the film holder for the CC projection, the opposite pendent breast may bump against the holder and prevent the patient from pressing as close into the detector as possible. To prevent this, the opposite breast should be placed up on the detector so that the patient can move into the field of view as deeply as possible (Fig. 10-23). Care should be taken to be certain that the medial tissues are imaged. Since breast cancer is most commonly found in the lateral breast, however, these tissues should not be neglected, and the technologist should draw the lateral tissues into the field of view as the compression is applied (Fig. 10-24).

Since the skin of the upper breast cannot be stretched, the technologist should carefully guide the compression paddle over the clavicle. It is a good idea to gently pull some of the skin up and over the clavicle before lowering the compression so that as the paddle is brought down the skin can be released,

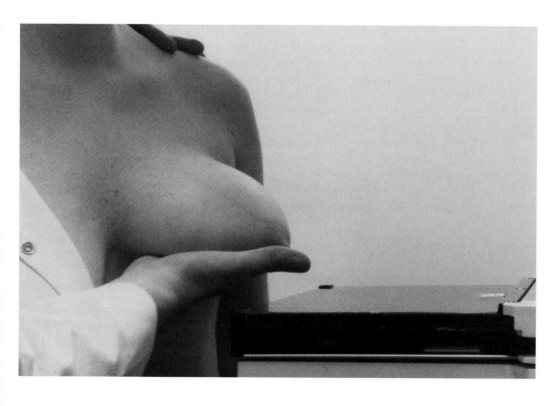

FIG. 10-21. The technologist should elevate the breast with a flat palm as high as it can be moved to relax the upper breast tissues. The detector should be elevated to this level.

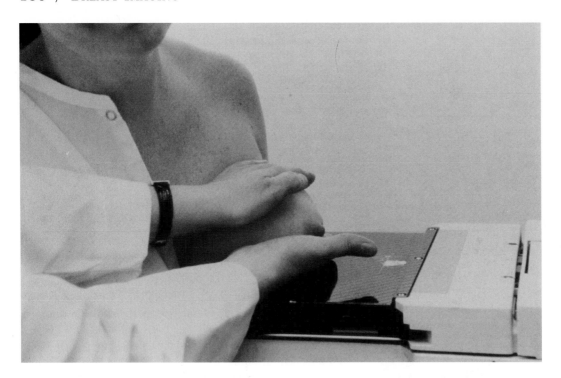

FIG. 10-22. The breast is pulled into the machine using two hands.

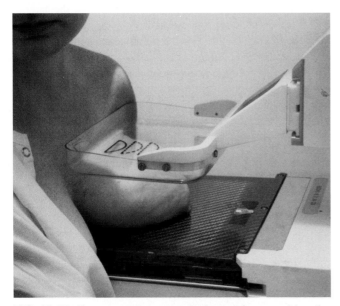

FIG. 10-23. To prevent the opposite breast from pushing the patient away from the detector, the breast is placed up on the detector as seen on this craniocaudal position.

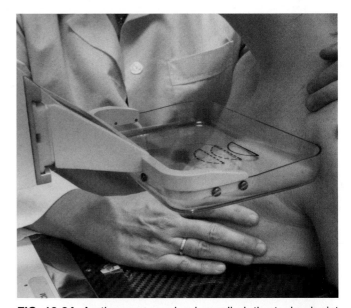

FIG. 10-24. As the compression is applied, the technologist should try to **pull the lateral tissues into the field of view** as demonstrated here.

preventing uncomfortable stretching. The compression is brought down from above along the chest wall to push the tissues against the detector. If the breast has been maximally elevated, then the compression must travel only a short distance to compress the tissues, and it is unlikely that a lesion in the upper breast will be pulled out from under the compression by tethering of the upper breast. Breast tissues are to some extent elastic, but there is a limit, and as the compression is brought down, a lesion high in the breast may be pulled out of the field of view by normal superior attachments. If a lesion high in the

breast is suspected, undercompression can be used on subsequent imaging to evaluate these tissues.

Quality Control

The properly positioned CC view should complement the MLO. Ideally the nipple should be perpendicular to the edge of the film. A small portion of the opposite breast should be visible on the mammogram, indicating that it was draped on the detector and that there is the likelihood that the medial

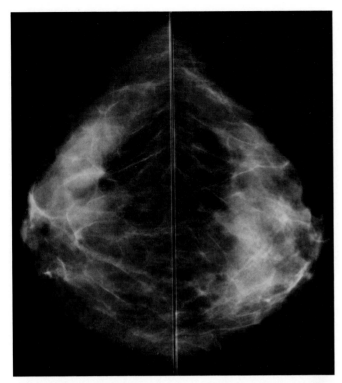

FIG. 10-25. Ideally there **should be fat between the edge of the film and the parenchyma on a well-positioned craniocaudal (CC) projection.** These are the CC projections of the patient in Figure 10-8.

breast tissues have been included on the image. The lateral tissues should have been pulled into the field of view so that, if possible, there is fat visible behind the lateral portion of the fibroglandular tissues (Fig. 10-25).

Maximizing the tissue imaged on the CC view is usually compromised by the shape of the thorax blocking the positioning of the detector. Generally, more breast tissue can be projected on the MLO view than on the CC view because of the slope and curve of the chest wall. Although the technologist should strive to image all of the breast tissues by ensuring that the medial (sternal) tissues are included on the CC projection, there is the possibility that some of the lateral tissues will not be included in the field of view. If the images suggest that there is likely glandular tissue extending laterally off the film, rotating the patient so that the lateral tissues lie on the detector (CC exaggerated laterally) can provide a better evaluation of the lateral tissues (Fig. 10-26). In a screening setting technologists should be trained to automatically obtain these additional views if the lateral tissues extend beyond the standard CC projection.

As with the MLO, the opposite breast should be positioned symmetrically in the craniocaudal projection so that the mammograms can be viewed as mirror images.

Properly Positioned Projections

The properly positioned MLO should include as much breast tissue as possible. The image should include the free margin of the pectoralis major muscle to ensure that the patient is as far over the detector as possible and that the tail

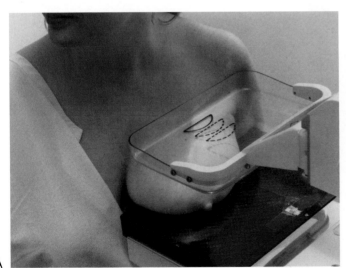

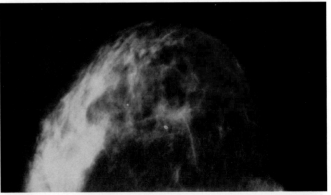

B

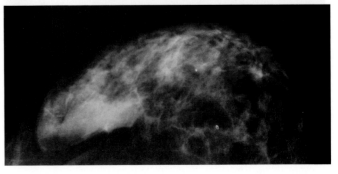

C

FIG. 10-26. A craniocaudal (CC) projection exaggerated laterally is used to image the tissues that wrap around the chest wall. As seen here **(A)** the patient is turned medially to permit these tissues to be positioned over the detector (note that the nipple is no longer perpendicular to the edge of the film). On this CC projection **(B)** the lateral tissues are not completely imaged and are off the edge of the film. The CC exaggerated laterally **(C)** images these tissues.

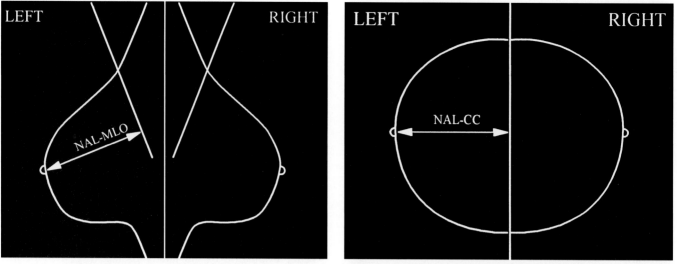

FIG. 10-27. (A) Schematic indicating the visualization of the pectoralis major on the mediolateral oblique (MLO) down to the level of the nipple axis line (NAL) on the MLO. **(B)** The corresponding line from the nipple to the back of the film on the craniocaudal should be no more than 1 cm shorter than the NAL on the MLO. If it is shorter, there is likely breast tissue that is not being projected onto the detector.

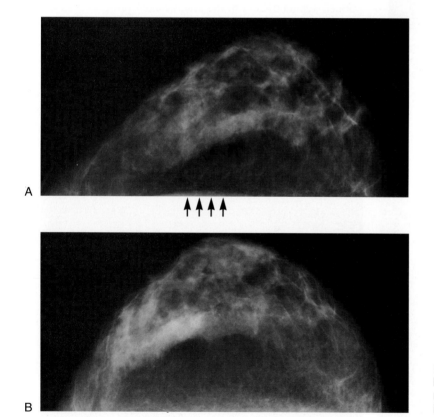

FIG. 10-28. Although there is pectoralis muscle visible (*arrows*) on this craniocaudal (CC) projection **(A)**, more breast can be pulled into the machine as seen in this second CC projection **(B)**.

of the breast is imaged. Ideally, the IMF should be on the image, and the breast tissues pulled up and out to spread the structures and open the IMF so that the bottom of the breast and the upper abdomen do not overlap. Although the individual's habitus or condition may interfere with optimal positioning, usually the pectoralis major muscle should be visible down to the axis of the nipple on the MLO view (Fig. 10-27).

The CC view should image as much of the breast as possible although the geometry of the breast and chest wall frequently means that less tissue is imaged than on the MLO. It has been suggested that the distance from just under the nipple to the chest wall edge of the film on the CC projection (NSL-CC) should be no more than 1 cm shorter than the distance back from the nipple, in the axis of the nipple

(NAL-MLO) to the pectoralis major muscle in the MLO (see Fig. 10-27). Stated another way, NAL-MLO minus NAL-CC should be less than or equal to 1 cm.

It has been estimated that the pectoralis major muscle should be visible on approximately 30% of CC views. Seeing the pectoralis major muscle is likely a result of a relaxed patient permitting the muscle to bulge forward. It does not necessarily indicate that more breast tissue is imaged (Fig. 10-28).

MAMMOGRAPHY AID TO POSITIONING (MAP)

Louise Miller, one of the leading mammography technologists in the United States, has devised a mammography aid to positioning (MAP) that is a visual aid to help in training technologists to understand the relationships of the breast to the underlying muscles of the chest wall and how they relate to the various components of the mammographic image.

The MAP is made by drawing on the skin of a volunteer the area of the chest wall that can contain breast tissue and is thus at risk to harbor a malignancy (Fig. 10-29). This is the area that the technologist is trying to include on the mammogram. By also drawing the anticipated location and course of the fibers of the underlying pectoralis major muscle, the relationship of these structures, as seen on the mammogram, is visually apparent. If the patient is properly positioned for the MLO, it is clear on the MAP that the free margin of the pectoralis major can be imaged down to the level of the nipple (Fig. 10-30). When the MLO is properly positioned, all of the muscle that is free from attachment is in the field of view, permitting inclusion of the tissue along its posterolateral surface.

Because the corner of the compression paddle is aligned with the corner of the film holder, if the muscle is not wide at the top of the mammogram, this indicates that the axillary corner was not positioned deep in the axilla, as is also clearly evident on the MAP (Fig. 10-31). Using the MAP it can be demonstrated that, if the pectoralis muscle appears to

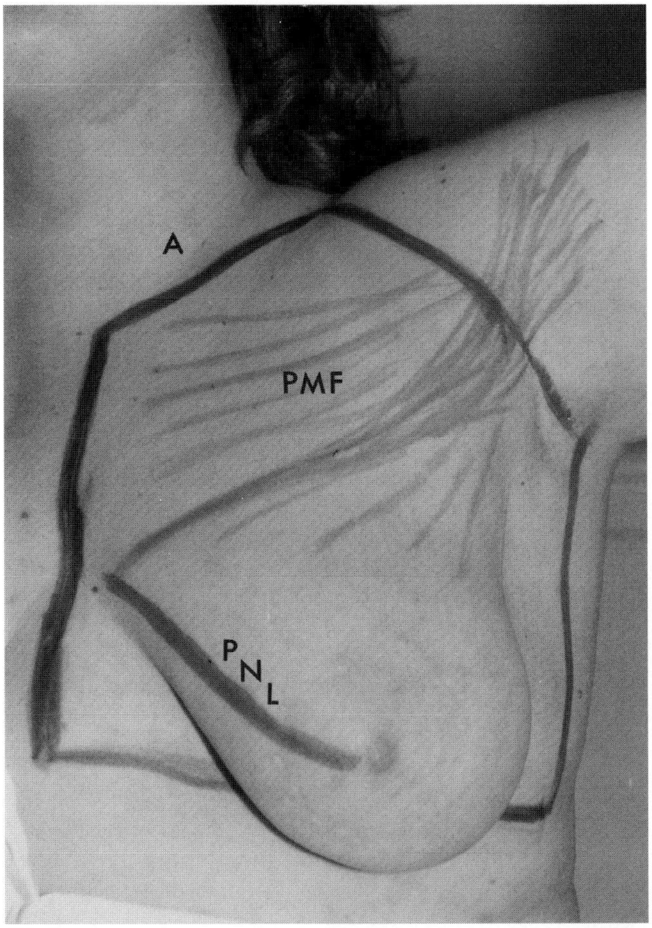

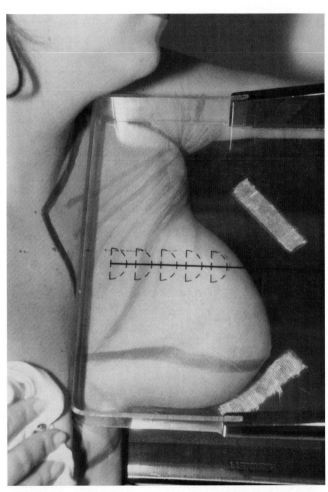

FIG. 10-29. The area of potential breast tissue (*dark outer line A*), as well as the expected course of the pectoralis major muscle fibers labeled PMF, is outlined on this volunteer. The posterior nipple line (PNL) is drawn on medially so that the technologist can appreciate how it relates to the pectoralis major in the mediolateral oblique projection.

FIG. 10-30. Using the MAP, the technologist-in-training can visually appreciate the relationship of the breast and pectoralis major muscle as they appear on the mammogram. The relationship of the posterior nipple line to the pectoralis muscle is also apparent.

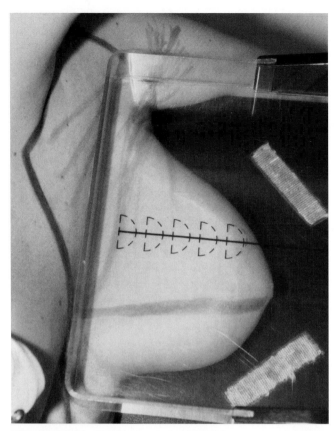

FIG. 10-31. The MAP allows the technologist to understand what has happened when the mediolateral oblique presents only a narrow margin of pectoralis muscle. This occurs because the detector is not positioned deep enough into the axilla. If the pectoralis appears thin and vertical in its orientation, the breast has not been properly positioned.

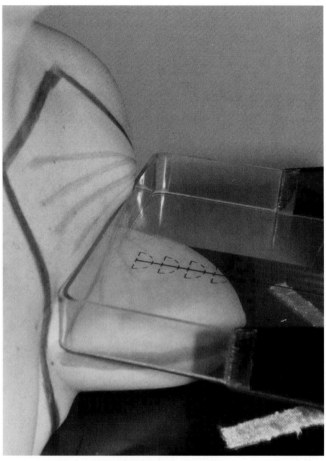

FIG. 10-33. The MAP clearly shows how the pectoralis major muscle can be pulled into the field of view on the craniocaudal projection.

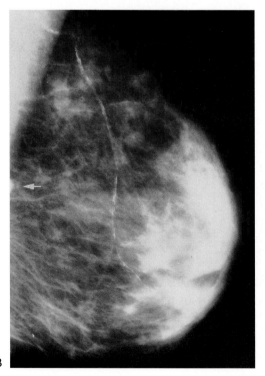
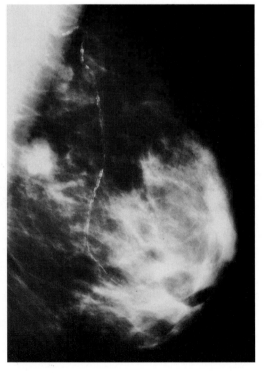

A,B

FIG. 10-32. This right mediolateral oblique **(A)** was poorly positioned and a small cancer, visible in retrospect (*arrow*), was missed. A year later the patient returned, and with better positioning (still not optimal) the larger cancer is now obvious **(B)**.

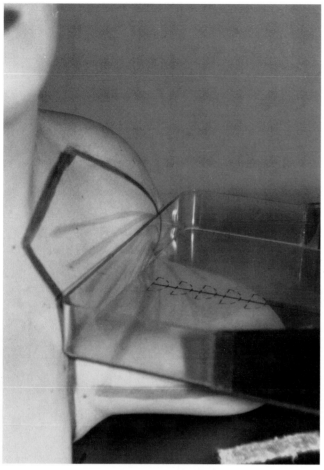

FIG. 10-34. Even the periodic medial bulge of the muscle on the craniocaudal projection is evident using the MAP.

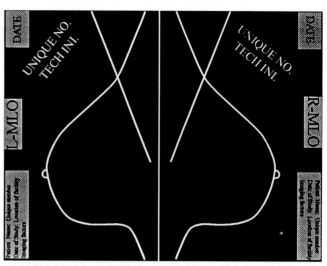

FIG. 10-35. Films should be labeled with an identifying code that is unique for the patient, the date of the study, the projection, and the name and location of the facility, as well as the technologist's initials. Imaging factors recorded on the image may also be useful.

be vertically oriented, the patient is not properly positioned and deep tissues may not be imaged. Poor positioning can lead to deep cancers being overlooked (Fig. 10-32).

The MAP can also be used to evaluate the CC projection. If the patient is relaxed, the pectoralis major muscle can be drawn into the field of view (Fig. 10-33). It is even possible to see how a bulge in the sternal insertion of the pectoralis may be imaged (Fig. 10-34).

IDENTIFICATION MARKERS

In addition to identifying the patient, proper labeling is important to avoid right-left and medial-lateral confusion. Efforts should be made to avoid label clutter, but a right and a left marker should be visible on all images (Fig. 10-35). An indication of the projection should be attached to the film. Some technologists prefer to place radiopaque markers that indicate the projection of the image. We prefer stickers that wrap over the edge of the film (readable from either side of the film) so that the projection is easily identified without hav-

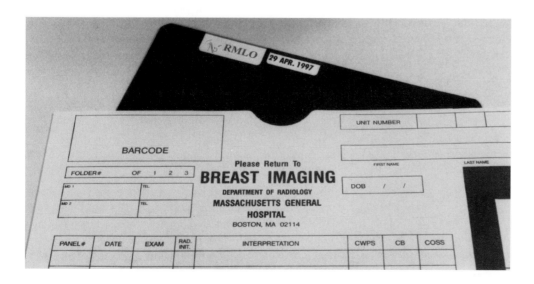

FIG. 10-36. An example of **edge stickers.** These facilitate retrieval of particular images by the projection and the date of the study without having to hold each image up to the light.

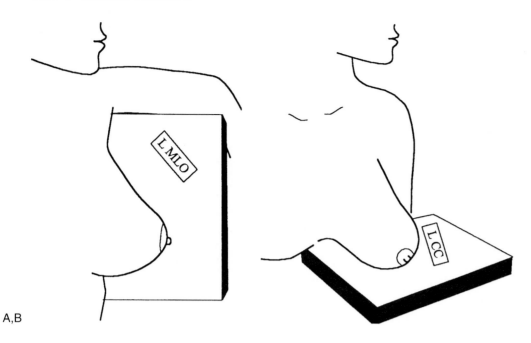

A,B

FIG. 10-37. Radiopaque markers should be in the axillary portion of the images as seen on the mediolateral oblique **(A)** and craniocaudal **(B)** projections.

ing to hold the film up to the light and can be more easily retrieved from a file jacket. Similarly, color-coded date stickers that wrap over the edge permit sorting through a folder to retrieve specific films without having to hold each one up to the light (Fig. 10-36). Ideally, the film should be blackened to its edges so that when the mammogram is being viewed there is no extraneous light that might compromise viewing.

By convention, radiopaque identification markers should be placed along the upper axillary portion of the breasts in the lateral views and along the axillary side of the breast in the CC projections (Fig. 10-37). When supplemental views are obtained, they should be labeled in a similar fashion and the projection should be indicated.

Each film should contain a unique number that identifies the patient. The date of the study, as well as an indication of the projection, should be on the film. The name of the facility should be on each image, along with its address, so the film can be returned to the appropriate facility should it be loaned out for review and become separated from its film folder. As with all plain x-ray imaging, the technologist's initials should be on the film so that she can provide information about the imaging and patient should the radiologist need additional information.

Placing a number sticker directly on the screen of each cassette blocks light and appears on every mammogram. In this way, if there is a problem caused by the screen, the screen can be identified. We also place a radiopaque marker on the detector of each mammography unit so that it can be identified on each image to aid in trouble-shooting imaging problems.

PHYSICAL EXAMINATION

Although mammography is the most valuable method of screening for breast cancer, there are some cancers (even

some small ones) that are palpable but not visible on the mammogram. Although physical examination as the only method of screening has not been well studied, it is likely that some lives can be saved by detecting cancers earlier based only on the CBE. It is advisable that patients referred by a physician for screening should have been examined by that physician. If a center accepts self-referred patients, they should be examined at the screening center. Otherwise, they should be informed that the mammogram is only part of a complete screen and advised to seek a CBE if they do not wish to have one provided by the center. To be performed properly, a CBE should be done systematically (8). Examiners should be properly trained and monitored, just as those who perform mammograms are trained and monitored.

Although interested x-ray technologists can be trained to perform CBE, this should not be a requirement. Their primary responsibility should be to obtain high-quality mammographic images.

Radiologists certainly can perform CBEs, but this should not be a requirement. The radiologist's responsibility is to supervise the performance of high-quality mammographic imaging and provide reasonable interpretation of the images (see Chapter 25). Any physician who takes responsibility for performing a CBE should recognize that it takes 5 to 15 minutes to perform a thorough one. Any faster likely means that the examination was not thorough.

Correlative Clinical Breast Examination

Individual radiologists may wish to perform, or have their technologists perform, focused CBEs to identify the area of concern for which a patient is referred for imaging. Ostensibly, this is to ensure that an area that is clinically suspicious is included on the mammogram. There are several fallacies associated with this approach. The idea was originally promulgated at a time when mammographic positioning was poor and large volumes of breast tissue were frequently not included on the standard projections (see below) (9). With modern positioning it is rare that an area of clinical concern is not imaged on the standard views. A second problem is that there is no guarantee that an area found by a technologist (or even the radiologist), in a cursory examination, will actually correspond to the area of concern to the referring physician. Finally, there are no data that show that this actually results in earlier diagnosis of cancer, and no data that show that mortality is affected by such an examination. Individuals may decide that they wish to perform such examinations, but until the procedure is taught in a structured fashion and certification similar to that for mammography is required, CBE of any kind should not be considered part of the standard of care for mammography. Radiologists should be aware, however, that their CBE or that performed by their technologists carries potentially significant medical/legal consequences that should be considered (see Chapter 25).

MAMMOGRAPHY FOR THE INDIVIDUAL WITH A SIGN OR SYMPTOM THAT COULD INDICATE BREAST CANCER

There has been considerable debate concerning the appropriate evaluation of women who are sent for mammography because they have a clinically evident abnormality (10). The mammogram actually has little value in the evaluation of a palpable abnormality because, even if the mammographic evaluation is negative, the clinical finding must be pursued to a satisfactory conclusion.

In the past we and others have suggested that a focused clinical examination by the radiologist or technologist of the area in question should be correlated with the mammogram. In an early study we found that by tailoring the mammogram to a clinically evident abnormality found by the radiologist's focused examination, we were able to image an additional group of breast cancers that were not evident on the primary mammographic views (9). Our study, however, was done during an era when positioning was not taught well and was often far from optimal. It was not unusual for large volumes of tissue to be excluded on the two basic projections. By focusing the technologist on a specific area, tissues that had been excluded were imaged, and the cancers that they contained became evident.

Modern mammography is performed in a far more rigorous fashion and the images are of much higher quality than the mammography of the late 1970s and early 1980s. Routine positioning is far more successful in evaluating the majority of the breast tissues than in the past. It is much less likely that tissues containing a lesion will be omitted from the standard contact images. Thus, the focused or correlative clinical examination has less (if any) validity.

Sickles has demonstrated that spot compression of clinically suspicious areas will demonstrate a few additional cancers (11), but these were lesions that were clinically suspicious to begin with, and there are no data that show that the additional images actually influenced the care of the patients.

Spot Compression of a Palpable Finding

Although there are no data that prove that spot compression of a palpable finding leads to earlier diagnosis and there are no data that this influences mortality, a number of lecturers in breast imaging stress the need to perform spot compression of palpable abnormalities. Sickles' data, noted above, employed magnification with spot compression, and his results suggested that magnification permits better visualization of some palpable findings than the conventional two-view images. His data, however, do not separate the benefit of magnification from the spot compression. We find that magnification, because of long exposures, may be too susceptible to motion when evaluating an area of clinical concern. Consequently, we perform spot-compression views without magnification.

Without the referring physician present, it is impossible to know the precise area that raised the referring physician's concern. Consequently, the technologist asks the patient to point out the problem. A marker is placed over the area indicated by the patient, and then the technologist obtains a spot-compression view to try to better image any lesion that is in the area. The goal of the spot-compression view is to try to push the edge of a mass, should one actually be present and not visible on the standard views, against the subcutaneous fat in an effort to better image its margin. The technique that we use was described by Wende Logan. The technologist places a radiopaque marker over the area indicated by the patient and draws an imaginary line between the nipple and the lesion (Figs. 10-38A, B). The gantry is rotated so that the plane of the detector is parallel to this line (Fig. 10-38C). The breast is placed on the detector and rotated so that the marker is in tangent to the x-ray beam (Fig. 10-38D), and the spot-compression paddle is used to compress the area of concern indicated by the patient (Figs. 10-38E, F). The geometry is such that this provides the best opportunity to push the margin of a lesion (should there be a lesion) against the fat for better contrast and visualization of its margin.

Our practice is to perform spot-compression imaging of any clinically suspicious area if the patient can point it out to the technologist. Because there is no scientific support for this maneuver, its use is anecdotal and should not be considered a standard of care. Because what the technologist or radiologist feels on CBE may differ from what concerned the referring physician, we focus on whatever area the patient suggests was the area of concern. We have seen only a few rare cases where spot-compression views of an

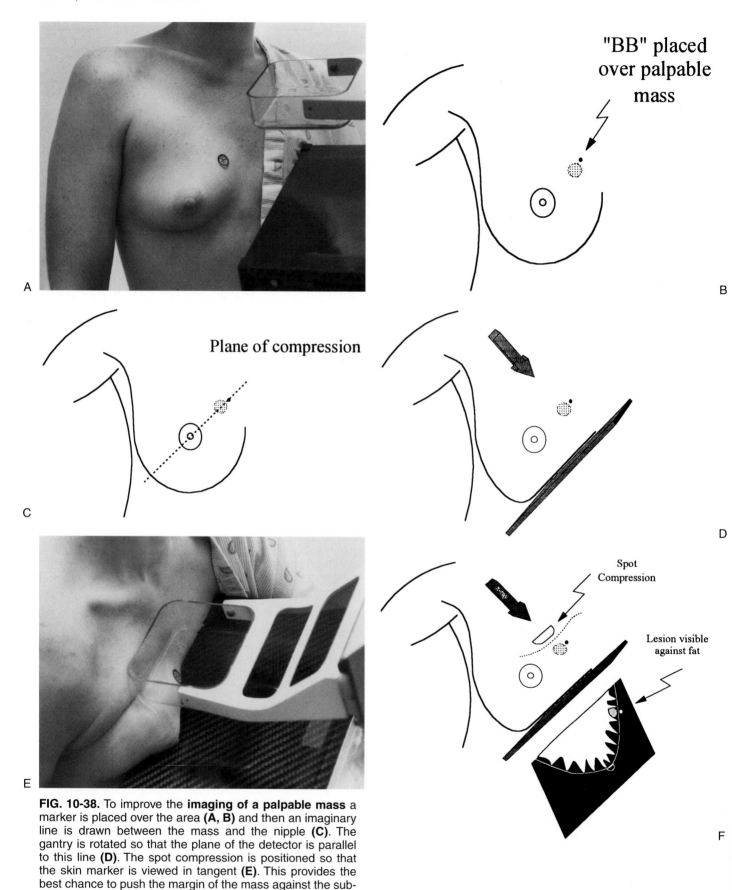

FIG. 10-38. To improve the **imaging of a palpable mass** a marker is placed over the area **(A, B)** and then an imaginary line is drawn between the mass and the nipple **(C)**. The gantry is rotated so that the plane of the detector is parallel to this line **(D)**. The spot compression is positioned so that the skin marker is viewed in tangent **(E)**. This provides the best chance to push the margin of the mass against the subcutaneous fat so that it may be better seen **(F)**.

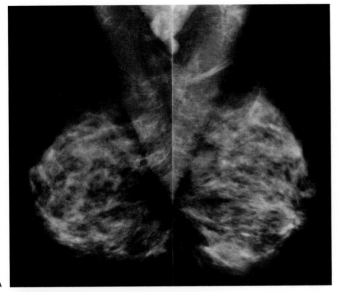

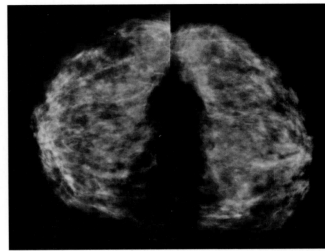

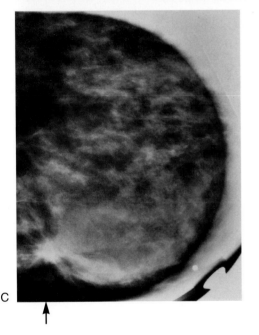

FIG. 10-39. Spot compression of a palpable area rarely alters management of a clinically evident problem. In this case the preliminary mediolateral oblique **(A)** and craniocaudal **(B)** mammograms were unremarkable, but the patient and her doctor had felt a nonspecific area of thickening in the lower right breast. A spot compression view **(C)** of the area indicated by the patient revealed an irregular, spiculated mass that proved to be an 8-mm invasive breast cancer.

area of clinical concern, as indicated by the patient, have actually revealed an unsuspected cancer (Fig. 10-39). It has been our experience that when a lesion is palpable and has malignant features by mammography, the clinical concern is usually sufficient that the area would be biopsied even if the mammogram had been unremarkable. There is no documentation that spot compression of a palpable abnormality has a major role in altering management, and there has been no cost-benefit analysis of the extra imaging required. In an informal poll of registrants at our postgraduate courses, <5% perform spot-compression imaging of palpable areas. Spot compression of a palpable finding should not be considered a standard of care, although in our practice we believe it is, on rare occasions, useful and worthwhile.

ADDITIONAL PROJECTIONS: EXAGGERATED VIEWS

Because of the curve and slope of the thorax and the geometry of the breast, there will likely always be tissues that are not projected onto the detector. This is especially true of the deep tissues and, in particular, the upper inner quadrant where the tissues are fixed and difficult to pull into the field of view. Once the standard projections have been obtained, however, there is no limit to the maneuvers and other projections that can be used to answer specific questions. The x-ray beam can be directed from any angle (Fig. 10-40), the patient can be turned to permit imaging of specific portions of the breast, and the breast itself can be rolled from side to side and forward and back to permit the x-ray beam to pass through different tissues at different

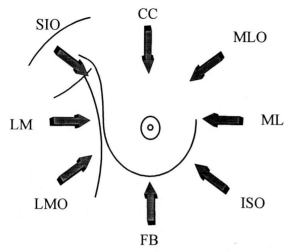

FIG. 10-40. The gantry can be rotated so that the beam comes from any direction. (CC, craniocaudal; MLO, mediolateral oblique; ML, mediolateral; ISO, inferosuperior oblique; FB, from below; LMO, lateromedial oblique; LM, lateromedial; SIO, superoinferior oblique.)

angles (see Chapter 22). Just as the radiologist performing fluoroscopy moves the patient and uses the compression paddle to sort out the various overlapping structures in the abdomen, the breast can be moved and spot compression applied to sort through the various overlapping structures of the breast.

Imaging the Lateral Breast Tissues

XCCL (Exaggerated Craniocaudal View Laterally)

If a lesion is suspected in the lateral half of the breast, the patient may be rotated in the CC projection so that the lateral half of the breast is positioned over the detector, permitting more complete projection of these tissues onto the recording system (Fig. 10-41).

Axillary Tail View

The axillary tail (AT) view is a projection that is used to isolate the axillary tail and any lesion within the tail of the breast. In the past this was termed the "Cleopatra view" (12), because the patient was positioned in a semireclining posture to permit positioning the cassette and compression

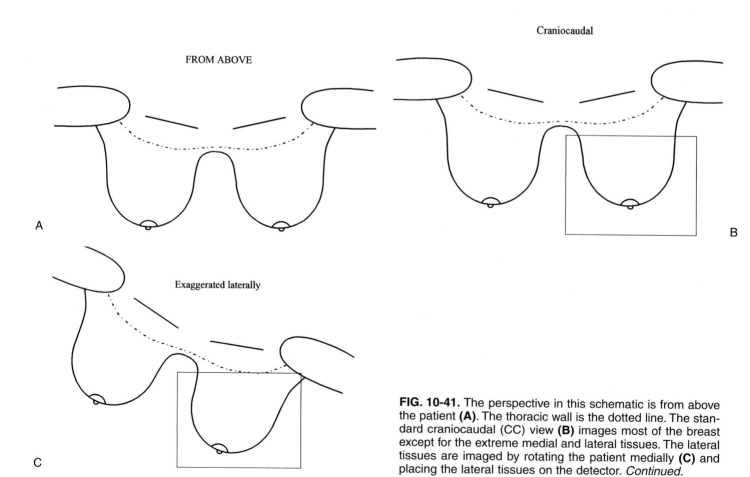

FIG. 10-41. The perspective in this schematic is from above the patient **(A)**. The thoracic wall is the dotted line. The standard craniocaudal (CC) view **(B)** images most of the breast except for the extreme medial and lateral tissues. The lateral tissues are imaged by rotating the patient medially **(C)** and placing the lateral tissues on the detector. *Continued.*

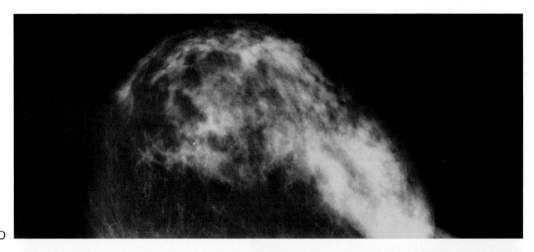

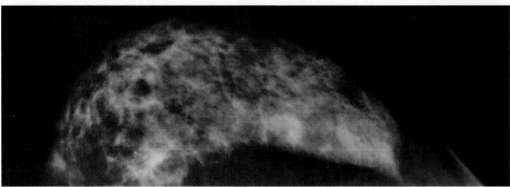

FIG. 10-41. *Continued.* In this patient the **standard CC projection** of the left breast failed to adequately image the lateral tissues **(D)**. A **CC exaggerated laterally** was used to image these tissues **(E)**.

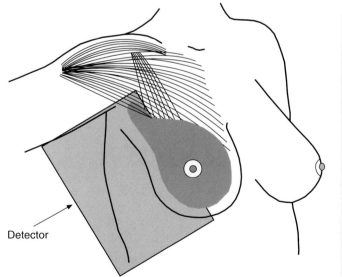

Detector

A

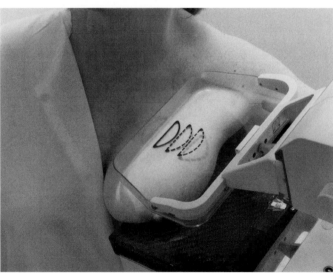

B

FIG. 10-42. If an abnormality is suspected in the axillary tail of the breast, these tissues can be isolated on the mammogram using the axillary tail (AT) view, which projects only the lateral tissues, which extend up into the axilla, onto the detector **(A)**. Many mammographers make the mistake of including central and even medial tissues on this image as if it were a poorly positioned mediolateral oblique. This is an example of an incorrectly positioned AT view **(B)**. *Continued.*

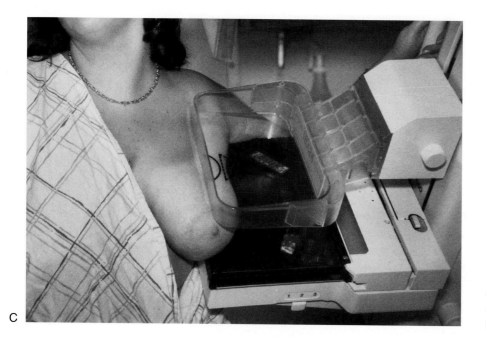

C

FIG. 10-42. *Continued*. Note that central tissues are being included. The AT view should isolate the axillary tail, as in this picture **(C)**.

system along the tail of the breast. This same projection of the tail of the breast is now more easily accomplished with modern mammographic equipment and does not require the patient to contort into an uncomfortable position because the gantry can be rotated to parallel the tail of the breast.

This view is used primarily to confirm the location of a lesion. It is therefore important to include only the tail of the breast in the AT projection. A common mistake is to merely repeat an MLO projection, which includes tissues from medial to lateral and does not isolate the tail of the breast. The AT view is positioned in a more anteroposterior direction, placing the edge of the detector along the edge of the

chest wall so that only the lateral (no central or medial) tissues are included in the field of view and only the tail of the breast is under the compression (Fig. 10-42).

Imaging the Medial Tissues

Cleavage View

Because standard CC imaging tries to include all of the medial tissues, additional imaging of these tissues is rarely needed. If, however, a medial lesion is suspected, the patient is placed in the CC projection but rotated so that more

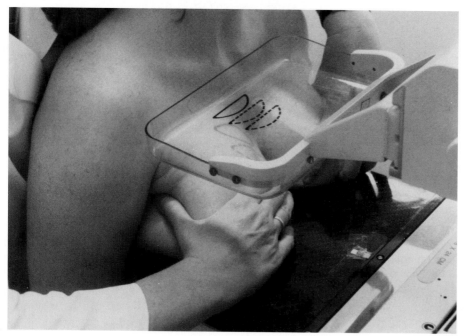

A

FIG. 10-43. **The cleavage view is used to image the tissues in the medial breast.** The patient is moved so that both breasts are on the detector with the medial portion of the side in question covering the automatic exposure control **(A)**. *Continued.*

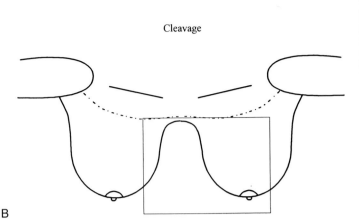

Cleavage

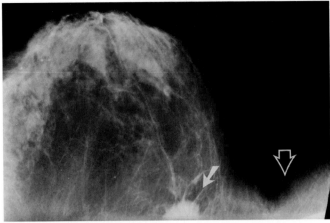

B   C

FIG. 10-43. *Continued.* Both breasts are included in the compression **(B)**. Medial lesions, like this invasive breast cancer **(C)**, can be imaged in this fashion.

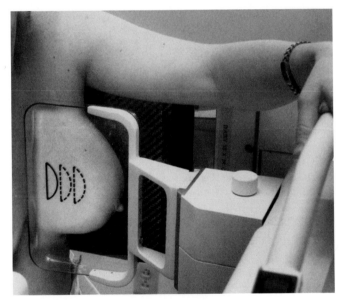

FIG. 10-44. The **straight lateral view** is positioned with the x-ray beam parallel to the floor.

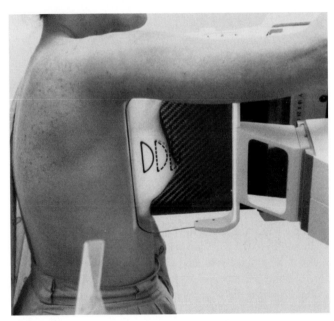

FIG. 10-45. The **lateromedial projection** is used to image medial lesions, triangulate possible abnormalities, and (with magnification) determine if calcifications are benign milk of calcium. Here the patient is positioned for the lateromedial projection.

medial breast tissue is projected onto the cassette (Fig. 10-43). This cleavage view is the best way to project the tissues that are close to the sternum over the detector. Both breasts are placed on the cassette so that the tissues overlying the sternum are in the field of view. It is frequently helpful if the technologist positions herself behind the patient and reaches around on both sides, grasping the breasts and simultaneously pushing them together and pulling them away from the chest wall and onto the detector. The technologist can use her body to gently push the patient into the machine while compression is applied. It is important to be certain to offset the breasts so that the side in question covers the automatic exposure control so that the image will be properly exposed. If the automatic exposure control (AEC) is under the space between the breasts, there will be only air in the x-

ray path, and the AEC will terminate the exposure too soon and the image will be underexposed.

Straight (90-Degree) Mediolateral Projection

The straight lateral projection is the third most useful projection. If a lesion is seen in the MLO but is not visible in the CC, the straight lateral projection can be used to determine if the lesion is real and for triangulation (see Chapter 22). When evaluating calcifications, the straight lateral magnification view is used to determine if the calcifications are

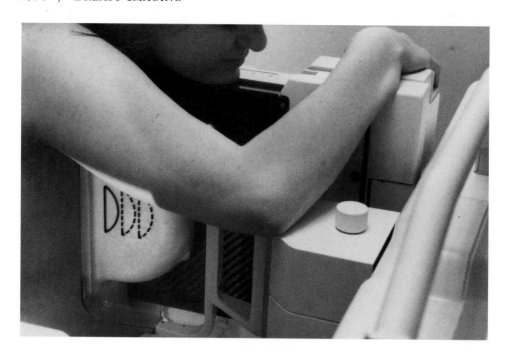

FIG. 10-46. The **lateromedial projection** is obtained by placing the detector against the sternum. Having the patient relax her arm and place her chin on the detector permits the breast to be pulled into the machine, as shown here.

benign milk of calcium precipitated and collected in the dependent portion of benign cysts.

Orthogonal views (obtained at 90 degrees to one another) provide the best understanding of the three-dimensional relationships of breast structures. Thus, if a lesion that requires intervention is detected, a straight lateral view that is the 90-degree complement of the CC view is often useful.

The straight lateral view is positioned in the same way as the MLO view, except that the compression is not parallel to the course of the pectoralis major muscle, but rather the x-ray beam is parallel to the floor with the compression at right angles to the CC view (Fig. 10-44). Every effort should be made to project as much tissue as possible onto the detector, but the MLO view generally permits more complete evaluation than the straight mediolateral view.

Lateromedial Projections

It should come as no surprise that basic x-ray principles apply to mammography. Since the resolution of very small details is critical, blur caused by geometric unsharpness can be a significant problem (see Physics in Chapter 8). This is particularly true if large focal spots are used with short source-to-object distances or there is a long object-to-detector distance. Blur can be reduced by shortening the distance between the lesion and the detector by bringing the lesion closer to the recording system. Thus, if a lesion is present in the medial tissues of the breast, the image will be sharper if a lateromedial projection is used (Fig. 10-45). This places the detector along the medial aspect of the breast with the x-ray beam and compression coming from

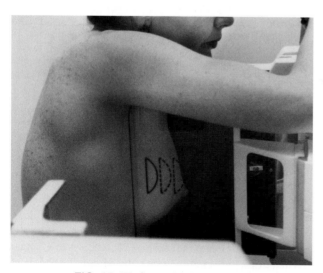
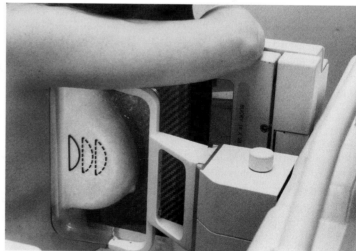

FIG. 10-47. Once the breast is positioned, the arm is gently raised out of the field of view.

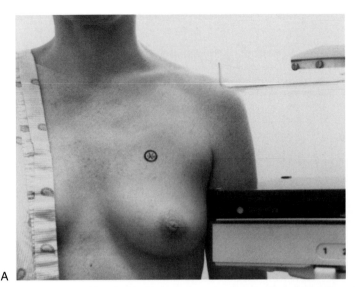
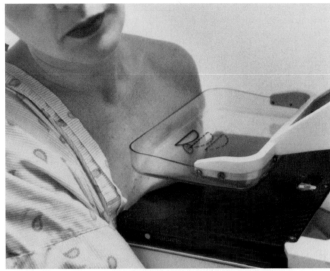

A   B

FIG. 10-48. If there is a lesion in the upper breast, isolating that area using a "lumpogram" may be helpful. Here the marker is placed over the possible lesion **(A)**, and then just the tissues containing the lesion are compressed **(B)**.

the lateral surface. This position may even occasionally project more tissue than the mediolateral position, but in general the mediolateral projection is favored as the standard view.

The patient is positioned so that the detector is on the sternum, or even slightly offset to the opposite side of the sternum. The patient leans against the detector. Some technologists find it helpful if she rests her chin on the detector (Fig. 10-46). This permits the technologist to push the breast across the chest toward the detector (Fig. 10-47). Because lesions that are close to the detector are more sharply imaged, the lateromedial projection provides a sharper image of a lesion in the medial breast tissues.

Imaging the Tissues of the Upper Breast

On occasion a lesion is seen high in the breast. On routine CC compression these tissues may be pulled out of the field due to tethering of the upper breast skin as the breast is compressed. The upper part of the breast may be studied by modifying the CC compression. The lower part of the breast is ignored, and only the area in question is compressed and projected onto the detector in the "lumpogram" described by Sickles (Fig. 10-48).

Caudocranial Projection

In most systems the gantry can be rotated 180 degrees to permit the detector to be placed against the top of the breast, closer to an upper lesion, and a caudocranial projection can be obtained. This takes advantage of the free margin of the breast, and elevating it toward the detector helps to prevent the upper tissues from coming out of the field of view. Frequently, because of the slope of the chest wall, the cau-

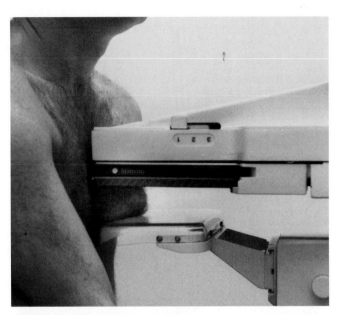

FIG. 10-49. The **caudocranial projection** is useful for kyphotic women and those with small breasts. Here it is used to image a man.

docranial projection gets farther back in the upper breast than the CC projection (Fig. 10-49).

POSITIONING THE MALE BREAST

The male breast is positioned in the same way as the small female breast. The MLO is used to image from the lateral projection (Fig. 10-50). The CC projection can be done as a craniocaudal projection or as a caudocranial view (see Fig. 10-49). Other projections may be helpful in men as they are for women (Fig. 10-51).

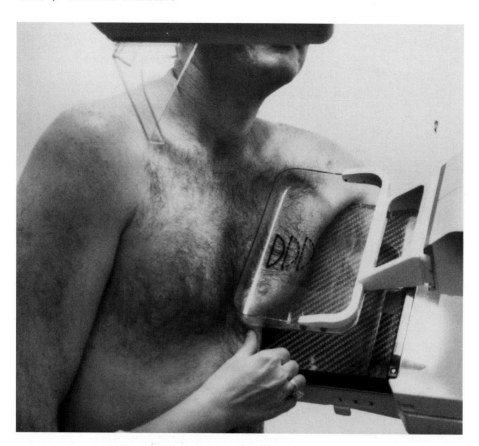

FIG. 10-50. The **mediolateral oblique projection in a man** is positioned exactly as it is for the woman, as seen here.

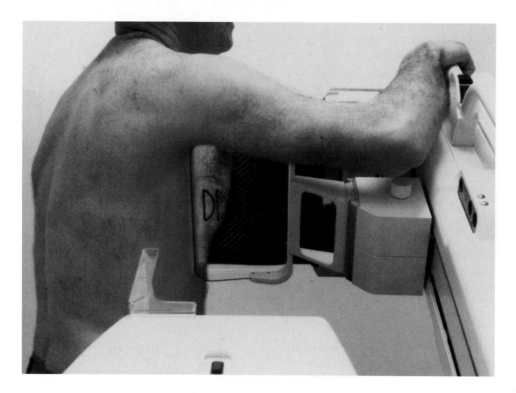

FIG. 10-51. A man is positioned for a lateromedial projection.

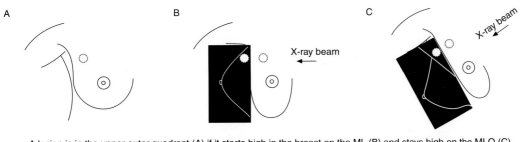

A lesion is in the upper outer quadrant (A) if it starts high in the breast on the ML (B) and stays high on the MLO (C).

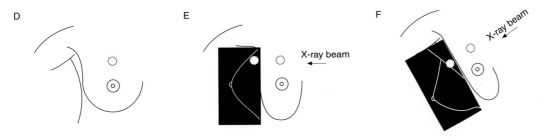

A lesion is at 12:00 (D) if it starts high on the ML (E) and moves down a short distance on the MLO (F).

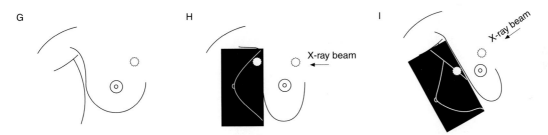

A lesion is in the upper inner quadrant (G) if it starts high on the ML (H) and moves a longer distance down on the MLO (I).

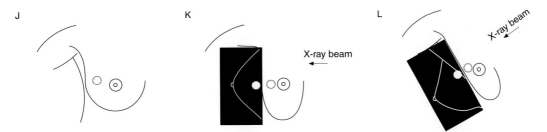

A lesion is in the midlateral aspect of the breast (J) if it starts in the middle of the breast on the ML (K) and moves up a short distance on the MLO (L).

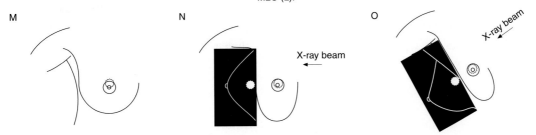

A lesion is in the center of the breast (M) if it starts in the middle of the breast on the ML (N) and in the middle on the MLO (O).

FIG. 10-52. The **location of a lesion** can be predicted by its movement between the straight lateral and the mediolateral oblique projections. *Continued.*

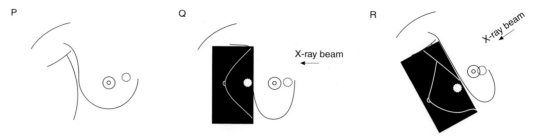

A lesion is in the midmedial breast (P) if it starts in the middle of the breast on the ML (Q) and moves down on the MLO (R).

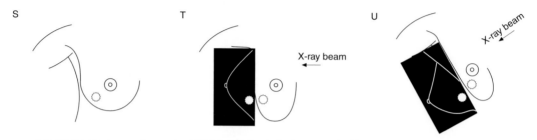

A lesion is in the lower outer quadrant (S) if it starts low in the breast on the ML (T) and it moves up on the MLO (U).

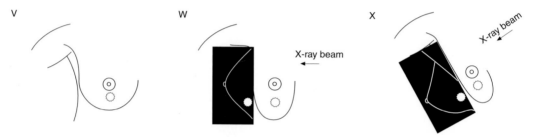

A lesion is in the 6:00 region of the breast (V) if it starts low in the breast on the ML (W) and moves up a short distance on the MLO (X).

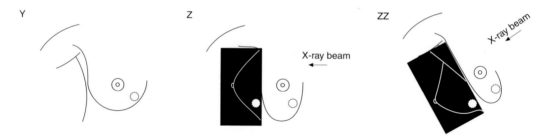

A lesion is in the lower inner breast (Y) if it starts low in the breast on the ML (Z) and stays low on the MLO (ZZ).

FIG. 10-52. *Continued.*

TRIANGULATION TRICKS

Techniques to triangulate lesions in the breast are described in detail in Chapter 22. Several basic concepts are presented in this section.

On occasion a lesion is seen in the CC projection that is not clearly identifiable in the lateral view. Creative positioning can be helpful. Some problems of localization can be solved by using the simple concept that a lesion moves in the direction that the tissue in which it lies is moved. Additional information about location can be derived by observing the shift of the lesion relative to other structures that accompanies slight repositioning or changes in tube angulation (13,14).

In general, if a lesion is seen only in one projection, it is best to return to the projection on which it was seen, modify the projection, and observe its shift in relationship to the background structures as an indication of its location.

Parallax and Lesions Seen Only in the Mediolateral Oblique Projection

Parallax can also be used to define the location of a lesion within the breast by comparing its shift relative to the nipple and other breast structures between the MLO and straight lateral views. When a lesion is seen in the MLO projection but is not evident in the CC projection, a straight lateral mammogram frequently demonstrates the finding (assuming it is real). Because the gantry rotates from the straight lateral through the oblique projection to get to the CC, Sickles has shown that placing the images on a view box with the nipples in line, the top of the breasts in the lateral projections at the top of the view box, and the lateral portion of the CC projection also at the top, with the images lined up so that the mediolateral (ML) is first, followed by the MLO, followed by the CC (from the straight lateral through the oblique to get to the

CC), a line through the lesion on the ML through the lesion on the MLO, points to its location on the CC.

Using this approach and working from the ML through the MLO to determine where a lesion is likely to be in the breast (Fig. 10-52)

1. If a lesion starts high in the breast on the ML and stays high on the MLO, then it is lateral on the CC.

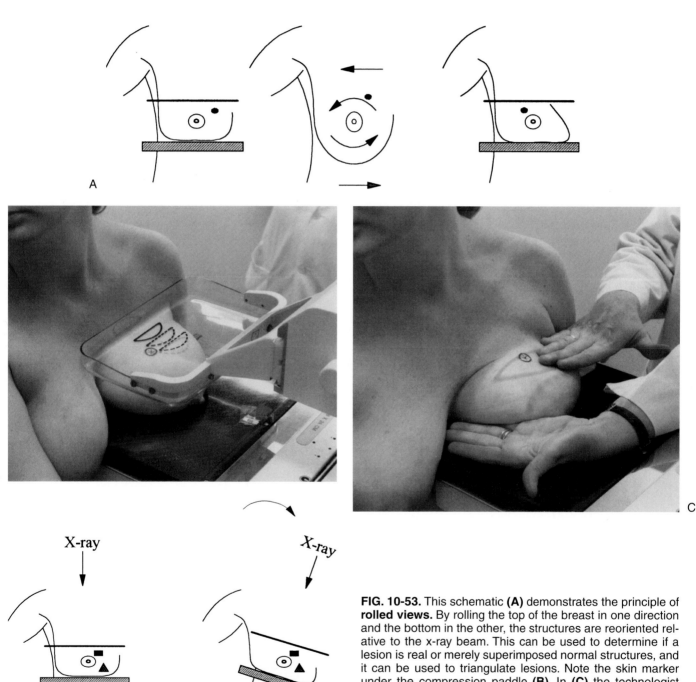

FIG. 10-53. This schematic **(A)** demonstrates the principle of **rolled views.** By rolling the top of the breast in one direction and the bottom in the other, the structures are reoriented relative to the x-ray beam. This can be used to determine if a lesion is real or merely superimposed normal structures, and it can be used to triangulate lesions. Note the skin marker under the compression paddle **(B)**. In **(C)** the technologist has rolled the top of the breast laterally and the bottom medially. The marker, on the top of the breast, moves laterally. By recompressing with the breast in this new position, the location of structures can be determined. The same effect can be achieved by angling the gantry and recompressing **(D)**.

2. If a lesion starts high on the ML and moves down a short distance on the MLO, it is central on the CC.
3. If a lesion starts high on the ML and moves rapidly down on the MLO, then it is medial on the CC.
4. If a lesion starts in the middle of the breast on the ML and moves up on the MLO, then it is lateral on the CC.
5. If a lesion starts in the middle of the breast on the ML and moves down on the MLO, it is medial on the CC.
6. If a lesion starts in the middle of the breast on the ML and stays in the middle on the MLO, then it is in the center on the CC.
7. If a lesion starts low in the breast on the ML and stays low on the MLO, then it is medial on the CC.
8. If a lesion starts low in the breast on the ML and moves up a short distance on the MLO, then it is central on the CC.

9. If a lesion starts low in the breast on the ML and it moves rapidly up on the MLO, then it is lateral on the CC.

Rolled Views and Lesions Seen Only in the Craniocaudal Projection

Determining the location of a lesion seen only in the CC view can be facilitated by rolling the breast (as under a fluoroscope) and obtaining a second projection. The technologist places one hand on top of the breast and the other beneath the breast and rolls the top in one direction and the bottom in the other with the nipple as the axis of rotation (Fig. 10-53). The breast is then recompressed holding the new tissue orientation. By knowing which way the top and bottom were rolled,

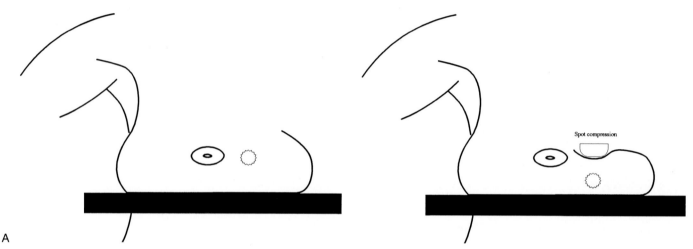

A   B

FIG. 10-54. Spot compression reduces blur by pushing the tissue **(A)** closer to the detector **(B)**, reducing geometric unsharpness.

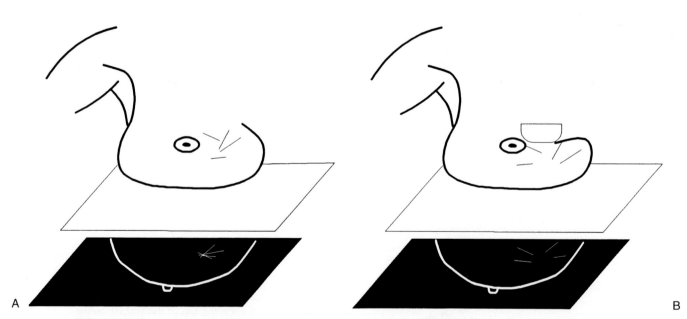

A   B

FIG. 10-55. Spot compression can separate overlapping structures. The structures in **A** are in different parts of the breast but appear as a single structure on the mammogram. Spot compression can spread them apart, proving that there is no significant lesion **(B)**.

and observing the movement of the lesion between the two images the location of the lesion can be determined.

Similar parallax can be achieved by angling the tube/compression system by 15 to 20 degrees to reorient the projection of the structures relative to one another. The apparent movement of the lesion between the nonrotated and rotated views can reveal whether it is in the top, middle, or bottom of the breast. This information can then be used to determine its location in the lateral projection.

The same technique can also be used to determine whether a lesion is real. Benign overlapping structures that are superimposed on one projection, causing a worrisome shadow, can be separated and eliminated as a cause for concern by reorienting the relationships of internal tissues in this way.

FINDINGS ON THE SKIN AND SKIN LESIONS

Structures in or on the skin may be projected as intramammary lesions because of the basic spherical geometry of the breast. It is not the pigment of a lesion that causes it to be imaged on a mammogram. Nevi are rarely visible. Skin lesions are usually only visible when they are firm and raised and retain an air to soft tissue interface when the breast is compressed. The most common skin lesion that projects on the mammogram is the seborrheic keratosis. Markers placed on these lesions can confirm their dermal location (see Chapter 13).

Calcium deposits in the skin can be more problematic. When they lack the classic lucent-centered appearance of benign dermal deposits, they can simulate intramammary clustered microcalcifications. Tangential views of the skin will confirm their dermal location. The process can be facilitated by using mark-

ers placed on the region of interest and obtaining tangential views to the marker. This is described in Chapter 22.

SPOT COMPRESSION OF NONPALPABLE LESIONS

When the entire breast is compressed, it is compressed only as much as its least compressible part. By substituting a small compression paddle, pressure can be applied over a smaller area (more pounds per square inch) to a smaller volume. Spot compression is useful for spreading overlapping structures and can push a lesion closer to the detector, reducing geometric unsharpness and blur (Fig. 10-54). One of the major uses of spot compression is the demonstration that structures that appeared on the original image to represent significant architecture actually represent a benign overlap of unrelated structures, forming what Sickles has termed a *summation shadow* (Fig. 10-55).

Some technologists prefer to "cone" down when performing spot compression. By collimating the x-ray beam, scatter can be reduced. However, the technologist must be careful to be certain that the lesion does not get squeezed out from under the compression paddle like a watermelon seed, giving the false impression that the lesion is not real. To avoid this we leave the cones open when spot compression is applied so that the field outside the compressed area is visible, reducing the likelihood of this occurrence. There is still the problem that the lesion may be squeezed out the back (chest wall side) of the compression. This can be reduced by using a compression device on a movable arm so that the edge of the paddle need not align with the back of the detector.

It is not always easy to position the spot-compression device directly over the area to be evaluated. Although a

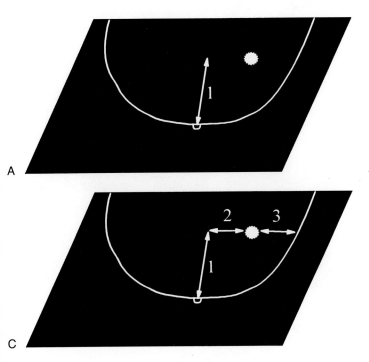

A

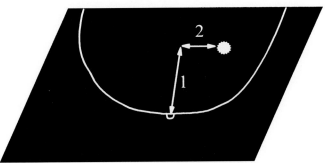

B

C

FIG. 10-56. To accurately position the spot compression device, measurements are taken from the film that include **(A)** the distance back to the lesion in the axis of the nipple, **(B)** then the distance to the lesion, and **(C)** then the distance from the lesion over to the skin. *Continued.*

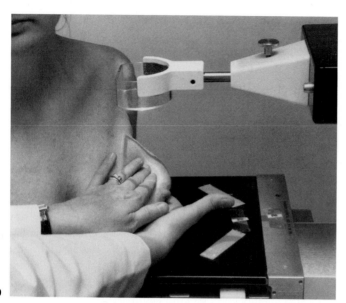

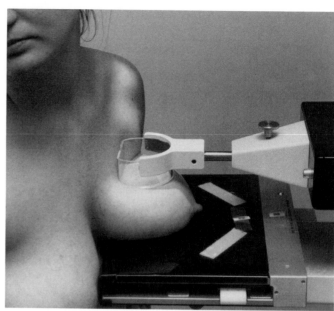

D

E

FIG. 10-56. *Continued.* These measurements are then transferred to the breast in simulated compression **(D)**, and the compression is applied at their intersection **(E)**.

ruler can be used, this may upset the patient (some technologists have found that a ruler suggests an abnormality to the patient). Most technologists use their fingers as a measuring tool. They measure the number of finger widths back from the nipple (Fig. 10-56A) in its axis and then the number over to the lesion (Fig. 10-56B). Some mammographers suggest

getting a third measurement from the lesion to the skin to better triangulate the target (Fig. 10-56C). These measurements are transposed from the mammogram to the patient as her breast is held against the detector in simulated compression, the way the film from which the measurements had been derived (so that the measurements are more accurate)

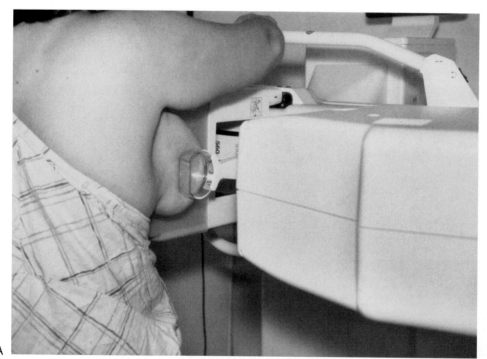

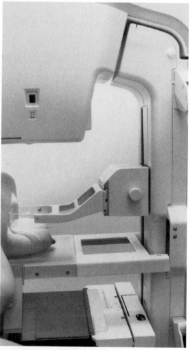

A

B

FIG. 10-57. Magnification reduces the effect of noise. As shown here, the breast is elevated from the detector and moved closer to the focal spot on the mediolateral **(A)** and craniocaudal **(B)** projections. Because of beam divergence the image is magnified. Using the spot compression device can reduce obscuration from the overlapping of tissues.

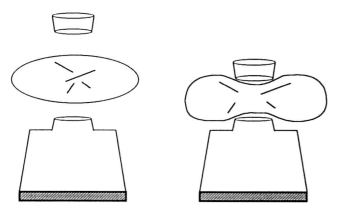

FIG. 10-58. This schematic demonstrates **dual spot** magnification.

was obtained (Fig. 10-56D). The spot-compression paddle is then used (Fig. 10-56E).

MAGNIFICATION

When an appropriately small focal spot is used (actual measurement of 0.2 mm for 1.5 magnification or a smaller focal spot for higher magnification), direct magnification mammography can improve resolution because of the divergence of the x-ray beam and the projection of information onto a larger area of the recording system. Although from a scientific point of view magnification improves spatial resolution, in fact, as a consequence of the actual focal spots involved, improved mammographic imaging is due to a reduction in scatter-related image degradation and a reduction in noise. The latter is less obtrusive because the signal (the lesion) is enlarged while the noise is spread over a larger area, improving the signal-to-noise ratio.

Sickles has shown that magnification improves the visibility not only of calcifications but of masses as well (15). Magnification does require higher dose to the patient and should be used selectively as a problem-solving technique to determine the following:

- Is a lesion real?
- Do microcalcifications represent benign collections (vascular, fat necrosis, secretory)?
- Are there more calcifications than can be seen on the contact study, and is biopsy indicated?

- Are calcifications part of a diffuse process not evident on the contact study and more likely to be benign?
- Will the analysis of the margins of a mass aid in lesion management?
- What is the extent of the cancer?

Magnification is performed by moving the focal spot closer to the breast and moving the breast farther away from the detector (Fig. 10-57). Magnification mammography can be performed in all mammographic projections. The entire, although somewhat reduced, field can be magnified. Many mammographers prefer to cone down to further reduce scatter when obtaining magnification images. Probably the sharpest images are obtained using coned-down, top-and-bottom spot-compression and magnification imaging (Fig. 10-58).

REFERENCES

1. Sickles EA, Weber WN, Galvin HB, et al. Baseline screening mammography: one vs. two views per breast. AJR Am J Roentgenol 1986;147: 1149–1153.
2. Muir BB, Kirkpatrick A, Roberts MM, Duffy SW. Oblique-view mammography: adequacy for screening. Radiology 1984;151:39–41.
3. Wald NJ, Murphy P, Major P, et al. UKCCCR Multicentre randomised controlled trial of one and two view mammography in breast cancer screening. BMJ 1995;311:1189–1193.
4. Mettler FA, Upton AC, Kelsey CA, et al. Benefits versus risks from mammography: a critical assessment. Cancer 1996;77:903–909.
5. Stomper PC, Kopans DB, Sadowsky NL, et al. Is mammography painful? A multicenter patient survey. Arch Intern Med 1988;148:521–524.
6. Russell DG, Ziewacz JT. Pressure in a simulated breast subjected to compression forces comparable to those of mammography. Radiology 1995;194:383–387.
7. Kornguth PJ, Rimer BK, Conaway MR, et al. Impact of patient-controlled compression on the mammography experience. Radiology 1993;186:99–102.
8. Miller AB, Baines CJ, Turnbull C. The role of the nurse-examiner in the National Breast Screening Study. Can J Public Health 1991;82: 162–167.
9. Meyer JE, Kopans DB. Breast physical examination by the mammographer: an aid to improved diagnostic accuracy. Appl Radiol 1983; 103–106.
10. Kopans DB. Breast imaging and the "standard of care" for the "symptomatic" patient. Radiology 1993;187:608–611.
11. Faulk RM, Sickles EA. Efficacy of spot compression—magnification and tangential views in mammographic evaluation of palpable masses. Radiology 1992;185:87–90.
12. Goodrich WA. The Cleopatra view in xeromammography: a semireclining position for the tail of the breast. Radiology 1978;128:811.
13. Swann CA, Kopans DB, McCarthy KA, et al. Localization of occult breast lesions: practical solutions to problems of triangulation. Radiology 1987;163:577–579.
14. Sickles EA. Practical solutions to common mammographic problems: tailoring the examination. AJR Am J Roentgenol 1988;151:31–39.
15. Sickles EA, Doi K, Genant HK. Magnification film mammography: image quality and clinical studies. Radiology 1977;125:69–76.

Breast Imaging, 2nd ed., by Daniel B. Kopans.
Lippincott–Raven Publishers, Philadelphia © 1998.

CHAPTER 11

A Systematic Approach to Breast Imaging

BASIC PRINCIPLES: DETECTION VERSUS DIAGNOSIS

To use breast imaging technologies appropriately, one must understand the difference between detection and diagnosis. *Detection* is the ability to find unsuspected anomalies among which a significant number will prove to be malignant. *Diagnosis* is the ability to characterize a detected anomaly as benign or malignant. A useful detection technique may have no value for diagnostic evaluation, and conversely, a diagnostic test may be of little use until an anomaly has been detected.

Screening and Threshold Sensitivity

Screening is an evaluation to detect unsuspected disease. There are various levels of screening. For a woman who has a lump detected on clinical examination, the uninvolved areas of breast tissue can be screened for breast cancer. An individual, asymptomatic woman can be screened, as can large populations.

The term *screening* is derived from the process of filtering or sifting. A screen over a window is used to filter out bugs while letting air through. It is common to use a screen to sift a material such as soil to remove rocks. To accomplish this a screen is used with openings that are chosen to allow the desired size particles to pass through while holding back the undesirable particles. The size of the openings will determine the size of the rocks that will be trapped and prevented from passing through the screen. If the soil clumps are similar to small rocks, then openings that are too small will trap good soil as well as the unwanted rocks. If the openings are made larger, more soil will pass through, but rocks will also be allowed to pass through the screen.

The size of the openings in a sifter can be compared to the threshold sensitivity of a breast cancer screening program. The thresholds that are used by the radiologist to raise concern over a lesion are like the openings in the sifter. Just as with the stones and soil, the lower the radiologist's threshold, the more cancers will be detected, but the higher the percentage of benign lesions (soil) that will be trapped by the screen. If the threshold for intervention is raised (the openings enlarged) fewer benign lesions will be investigated (false positives), but more cancers will be missed (1,2) as false negatives (see Positive Predictive Value).

If screening is to be successful, cancers must be found at a smaller size and earlier stage than they would be without screening. Ultimately, screening for breast cancer is only efficacious if mortality can be deferred or prevented.

Detection must precede diagnosis, and detection of breast cancer at an earlier stage is the most important function of an imaging technique. Mammography is an excellent detection technique, but it is not diagnostic unless the lesion has the typical characteristics of a malignant process, characteristic benign calcifications, or is an encapsulated fat-containing lesion defining a benign mass. If intervention is to be undertaken earlier, many benign lesions will require biopsy because they frequently cannot otherwise be distinguished from cancer. Until preventive measures can be discovered or improvements in therapy developed, reductions in mortality from breast cancer will only come with improvements in detection capability.

Improvements in diagnostic capability will benefit women by reducing the number of biopsies of benign lesions that must be performed. Ultrasound is an example of a useful diagnostic test in its capacity to determine that a mass is a cyst. However, the fact that it is useful to further characterize a lesion once it has been detected has no bearing on its ability to detect a lesion de novo. Diagnostic studies are only of use once the lesion has been detected. Because breast biopsy (needle or excisional) is a relatively safe procedure with very low morbidity, a noninvasive diagnostic test must be extremely accurate in separating benign from malignant lesions if, by using it, a biopsy is to be avoided.

X-ray mammography is currently the only imaging modality with proved efficacy for screening and the earlier detection of breast cancer. Based on the increasing prevalence of breast cancer with age, the concomitant decreasing radiation risk with increasing age, and the evidence of mortality reduction, it is reasonable for screening to begin for women by age 40. An annual mammographic study in conjunction with a careful physical examination should be coupled with reinforcement of the potential benefits of breast self-examination.

Providing Low-Cost, High-Quality Screening

Efforts should be made to reduce the cost of mammographic screening so that all women can be tested, but image quality must not be sacrificed. Low-cost screening does not imply low-quality mammography. Because the screening study is the earliest opportunity for detection, it should use the highest quality mammography. Well-trained technologists are required to position the breast properly, and experienced radiologists are needed to interpret the studies.

In an effort to reduce the expense of screening and make it available to all segments of the population, efficiency must be improved while maintaining quality. The screening session is the time at which the full benefit of mammography is realized, and mammographic imaging at screening must be optimized. Although the psychological aspects of breast cancer detection and diagnosis are quite unique, the mammography screening study is identical to cervical cancer screening using the Papanicolaou test. The study is either negative, requires close follow-up, requires recall of the patient for additional evaluation, or is sufficiently suspicious to require a biopsy.

Educating Women on Approaches to Screening

Unfortunately, the media have promoted the idea that the screening mammogram should be reviewed immediately by the radiologist and a report should be immediately available to the screened woman. Given the relatively slow progression of most breast cancers, there is no biological reason to rush the interpretation of the mammogram. It is more important to avoid overlooking an early breast cancer than it is to provide an immediate report. Because of the fears associated with breast cancer, there is great psychological pressure on the screened woman. Unfortunately, in an effort to promote screening, women have been led to believe that a negative mammogram is reassurance that they do not have breast cancer. This is the unjustified reason for the pressure for immediate interpretation.

The reality is that a negative mammogram does not ensure that a woman does not have breast cancer. In fact, as many as 20% of cancers that become clinically evident over the course of 1 year will not have been seen on a mammogram at the start of that year (3). Mammography has little if any efficacy for excluding cancer, and a negative mammogram provides little reassurance. Its value is its ability to demonstrate many cancers at an earlier stage, not its ability to exclude cancer. Having a radiologist on site during the screening phase will reduce the necessity to recall patients with questionable abnormalities, but it will significantly increase the cost of screening, and rushing the review of the mammogram to provide an immediate report could result in early cancers being overlooked.

Accuracy and Cost-Effectiveness of On-Site Reading

Most well-trained radiologists can read 40 to 50 mammograms in a 2-hour "batch-reading" session if those studies are organized on an alternator along with previous available examinations so that film handling by the radiologist is minimized. If the interpreting radiologist is experienced, between 93% and 96% of the studies will be read as negative, and 4% to 7% percent of women screened will be recalled for additional study. Having a radiologist on site

reading the same cases, as they are performed, and discussing the mostly negative (93% to 96%) results with the patient would save the 4% to 7% recalls, but it would mean that the same number of cases would take 8 hours of radiologist time. This inefficient approach is not cost-effective.

Batch reading is not only more efficient, it also permits more than one review, which facilitates double reading at little added expense with a demonstrated benefit in detection. In our own practice, we found that our detection of clinically occult malignancy increased by over 7% by just having a second radiologist quickly review the batch and look for abnormalities that were overlooked by the primary reader (see Perception and Double Reading).

If a radiologist is asked to consult on each study as it is taken, he or she will be involved for a full 8-hour day to interpret the same number of studies. The cost will have to be increased to account for this inefficient use of radiologist time as well as the delay in patient through-put created by such a system. Double reading in such an "on-line" system will lead to further increase in cost.

It is more cost-effective to separate the screening component from the diagnostic or lesion evaluation function of breast imaging. The less frequently used, often more expensive modalities, such as ultrasound- and imaging-guided biopsy technologies, are more efficiently used when grouped centrally. Multiple, highly efficient peripheral screening sites should ultimately be linked to a central comprehensive evaluation center to expedite the analysis of any abnormality found at screening. The comprehensive center will permit the rapid evaluation of a woman with any type of breast problem in a cost-effective manner. The separate screening centers need only produce high-quality contact mammographic studies and clinical breast examinations by trained examiners if the patients do not have a referring physician to perform the clinical study. Magnification mammography, ultrasound, computed tomography (CT), magnetic resonance imaging (MRI), fine-needle aspiration cytology, core needle biopsy, localization, and excisional biopsy capabilities can be concentrated in a centralized breast evaluation center fed by multiple screening sites. The evaluation center should also be used to assess women with clinically evident signs or symptoms of breast cancer and can facilitate the multidisciplinary care of women diagnosed with breast cancer. Organizing breast cancer detection and diagnosis as separate functions is likely to be more cost-effective in the long run.

The negative implication of this approach is that 4% to 7% of women may be asked to return for additional study after an abnormal screening test with their attendant increased anxiety and some additional cost. The number of recalls decreases with repetitive screening (4). The breast, by mammography, is quite stable from year to year, and it is only changes, with their higher likelihood of malignancy, that elicit recall among women who are repetitively screened. Women and physicians must be educated to understand these issues so that costs may be kept down, permitting high-quality screening to be available to all women.

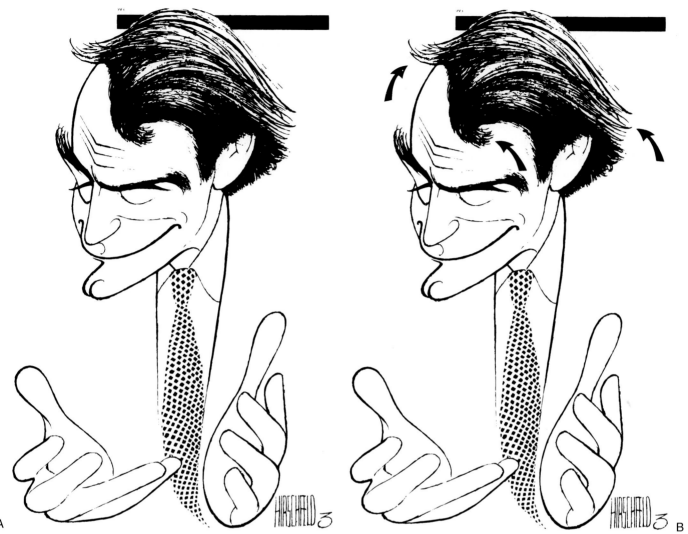

FIG. 11-1. The perception problem. In this drawing by Hirschfeld entitled *Charlie Rose* **(A)**, the artist has included his daughter's name, Nina, into the drawing three times. (Copyright Al Hirschfeld. Drawing reproduced by special arrangement with Hirschfeld's exclusive representative, The Margo Feiden Galleries Ltd., New York.) The difficulty of the visual search for "Ninas" is similar to the radiologist's search for abnormalities on a mammogram. The Ninas are all defined by strands of hair **(B)** at the edges (*arrows*). The difference is that the radiologist is not provided with a description of the abnormality, and is not informed as to which, out of the thousands of images being reviewed, contains the abnormality.

Perception and Double Reading

Double reading is strongly recommended. It is a psychovisual fact that all observers (even the most experienced) fail to perceive significant abnormalities. This has been demonstrated in other types of image interpretation, and mammographic interpretation is no exception. Studies have shown that skilled observers fail to detect pulmonary abnormalities that are visible in retrospect (5), and even experts will fail to perceive significant bowel lesions on barium enemas and fractures on bone films.

This phenomenon is clearly demonstrated in daily life in the common occurrence of searching for a known object such as car keys. The harder one searches, the more frustrated one may become. However, another observer might easily point out that the keys are lying on a table in clear view. The reason for the failure to perceive by the first observer is unclear but common to all. The failure to see a cancer, which, in retrospect, may even be obvious, is not negligence but appears to be an immutable psychovisual threshold of the human visual process.

Failure to Detect a Cancer

The fact that a radiologist is not negligent for not having seen a cancer when it is visible in retrospect is not always clear to those outside of radiology. It is helpful to explain the problem by using a more commonly understood comparison. The caricatures drawn by the artist Hirschfeld are a good example. The artist periodically includes his daughter's name (Nina) in his work (Fig. 11-1). He facilitates the search for the name by indicating the number of times her name is incorporated in his drawings and he writes this beside his signature. The visual search for "Ninas" is similar to the radiologist's search for cancers. The difference lies in the fact that the radiologist is not provided with any indication as to which images contain the abnormality or its definition. Compounding the difficulty is that there will only be two to 10 cancers found among every 1,000 women screened. This means that the radiologist must review 4,000 images (two of each breast) to find the small number that contain a visible cancer. It is virtually inevitable that cancers will be missed, despite careful image review.

Most observers fail to see different lesions on mammography. Fortunately, just as the second observer easily saw the keys on the table, the failure to perceive a cancer can be reduced by having a study reviewed by a second reader (double reading). Using a double-reading system, Bird (6) had a 5% improvement in cancer detection. Tabar et al. (7) and Thurfjell et al. (8) found that double reading increased the detection rate of breast cancer by 15%.

Although there are benefits from double reading, it is not clear that it should be the standard of care. Double reading can lead to an increase in the number of false-positive results. Unless it is practiced in an efficient manner, double reading will increase the cost of screening, and increased cost may force a reduction in access for many women. To keep costs to a minimum, efficient interpretation with a minimum of added effort is required.

Double reading, with little or no increased cost, can be accomplished if screening is provided in a rapid throughput, high-quality setting, with the film interpretation deferred and performed by batch reading.

Massachusetts General Hospital System

As noted above, in our own study at Massachusetts General Hospital a second reader increased the detection rate of malignancy by 7%. Our system involves mounting the screening studies on an alternator. The main reader reviews the studies methodically and uses the previous studies as well as the history to render an interpretation using short codes into a computer beside the multiviewer. Subsequently, when given the completion command, the computer can easily translate the codes into a full written report. When uninterrupted, it takes the main reader 1 to 2 hours to review approximately 30 to 40 studies (this can be faster if computer interactions are kept to a minimum). The main reader circles any suspicious areas with a wax marker. Once the main reader's review is complete, the quick reader reviews the cases, trying to find significant abnormalities that the main reader may have overlooked. The quick reader can review the same cases very rapidly because the quick reader has no paperwork to do and does not even interact with the computer unless a problem is found.

The quick reader's review can be completed in 10 to 15 minutes or less. If the quick reader finds an abnormality that was overlooked by the main reader, the computer code is changed, and the quick reader becomes the interpreter and is responsible for that case. When the quick review is complete, the computer is directed to finalize the reports and they are sent to the referring physicians with a copy in lay terms to the patient.

In our prospective study of 5,899 women screened by mammography, a total of 39 malignant lesions were detected (6 to 7 per 1,000 women screened). The main reader detected 36 of the 39 while an additional three were detected by the quick reader. The quick reader missed eight cancers that were detected by the main reader. These data show that if a single reader is used, methodical review is needed (slow is better than fast), but it is preferable to have a second observer because this rapid review can improve the detection rate of breast cancer at minimal cost.

Diagnostic Mammography

Although the term *diagnostic mammography* has come into general use, it is really a misnomer. The greatest benefit from mammography is derived from its use as a screening test in the evaluation of asymptomatic women. Capable of detecting breast cancers 1.5 to 4.0 or more years earlier than they might ordinarily be found (9,10), mammographic detection at a smaller size and earlier stage has been shown to interrupt the natural history and lethal progression of the disease and result in reduced or delayed mortality (7,11). Mammography can be of some diagnostic value and can be used to heighten the concerns raised by clinical examination when there is concordance between the mammogram and physical examination and both are suspicious, but it cannot be used to reliably differentiate benign from malignant processes and cannot be used to exclude cancer.

In the symptomatic patient, mammography occasionally provides a useful check on a suspicious clinical finding. There is the theoretical possibility that a palpable lesion may not be of sufficient concern on clinical examination to prompt a biopsy by itself. If the mammogram demonstrates a suspicious finding, it might prompt earlier intervention. There are anecdotal cases of this happening, but it has never been documented in a prospective scientific fashion, and, in our experience, is very rare.

Cancer, even when palpable, can be missed at biopsy. The simultaneous demonstration of a mammographically suspicious lesion can be used to reduce a possible delay in diagnosis when, for whatever reasons, the biopsy of a suspicious mass produces benign results (12). If the mammogram suggests a highly suspicious lesion (Fig. 11-2) and the biopsy fails to confirm malignancy, the mammogram should be repeated as soon as possible to confirm that the suspicious abnormality has indeed been removed or to permit rebiopsy if necessary.

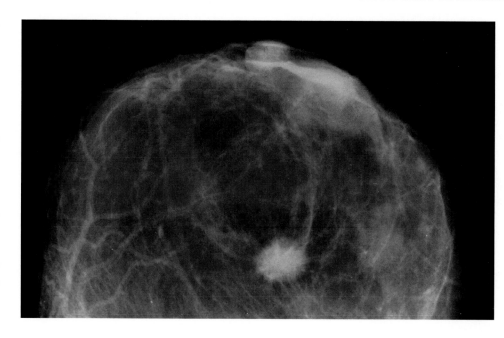

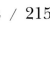

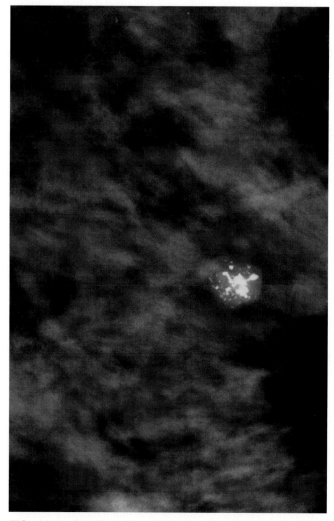

FIG. 11-2. A spiculated mass is almost always cancerous. If the biopsy of this palpable, very dense, spiculated mass comes back benign, the diagnosis should be questioned and a repeat mammogram should be obtained to try to ensure that the mammographically suspicious lesion was actually removed at surgery.

Mammography can, on occasion, be used to avoid the biopsy of a benign mass. The demonstration of a calcifying fibroadenoma (Fig. 11-3) or an encapsulated lesion containing fat, such as a lipoma (Fig. 11-4), oil cyst, or hamartoma, is sufficiently diagnostic that biopsy can be avoided. However, given the importance of early breast cancer diagnosis, the relatively low morbidity from a tissue diagnosis, and the fact that mammography does not reveal all cancers and that some cancers have benign characteristics on mammography, it is usually unsafe to rely on a mammogram to exclude the possibility of cancer.

As many as 60% of palpable abnormalities are not visible on the mammogram (13). Even with tangential, spot-compression views, palpable cancers may not be defined on the mammogram. Ultimately, just as a mammographically detected abnormality must be resolved satisfactorily, a clinically detected abnormality must be resolved satisfactorily. In reality, among women in whom malignancy is clinically suspected, mammography is used primarily to screen the remainder of the breast in question as well as the contralateral breast for clinically unsuspected cancer (14).

The major benefit from mammography is the ability to detect clinically occult, nonpalpable anomalies in the breast. Many of these prove to be malignant, but others with similar morphologies prove to be benign. Because mammography and physical examination provide information based on different tissue characteristics (15,16), concerns raised by one can rarely be negated by lack of corroboration from the other and, as has been often reiterated, a negative mammogram should not result in delayed intervention when a clinically suspicious lesion is present. Similarly, a negative physical examination should not delay diagnosis in the breast containing a mammographically suspicious abnormality.

FIG. 11-3. Calcified fibroadenoma. A calcifying, involuting fibroadenoma requires no additional evaluation even if palpable.

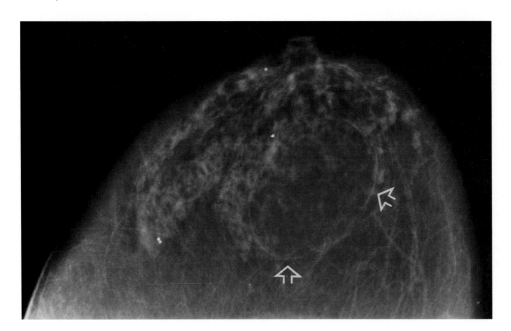

FIG. 11-4. Lipoma. This radiolucent, encapsulated lesion (*arrows*) is a benign lipoma and requires no further evaluation even if palpable.

Although mammography can demonstrate a few additional cancers when special views are used to image clinically suspicious tissues (6,17), some cancers can be obscured or overlooked on routine screening mammography and physical examination remains an important component of screening.

SCREENING TERMINOLOGY

Many of the measures of a screening program involve statistical concepts. The following is a short summary of several important terms.

1. *Prevalence* is the number of cancers in a population at a given point in time. If there has been no screening there will be a number of cancers that will be growing undetected in the population. When screening begins, the cancers that have been building in the population (over many years) will be found as well as the cancers that could only be detected for the first time in the population in that year (the incident cancers). Thus, in the first year of screening (prevalence year) there should be more cancers detected than in subsequent years (incident years).

2. *Incidence* is the number of cancers that are diagnosed each year subsequent to a prevalence screen. It is a measure of the number of cancers that rise to the level of detectability for the threshold of detection that is in effect at the time and over the time period (usually 1 year). The number of incident cancers depends on the ability of the screen to detect small cancers and the growth rate of the cancers in the population.

3. *Lead time* is a measure of how much earlier a screening method can detect cancer over a comparison method (e.g., usual medical care). The lead time can be gauged by subtracting the number of cancers found at the incidence screen from the number found at the prevalence screen and dividing the result by the number found at the incidence screen. In other words,

$$\text{Lead time} = \frac{(\text{Prevalence} - \text{incidence})}{\text{Incidence}},$$

or the number of years earlier that a cancer can be detected by the new threshold = [(old cancers that could have been detected years earlier plus the new cancers detectable for the first time this year) – (the new cancers detectable for the first time this year)] / the new cancers detectable each subsequent year at the new threshold.

For example, assume the prevalence screen detects six cancers per 1,000 women, and the incidence screen detects two cancers per 1,000 women. The lead time for the screen is (6 – 2)/2 = 2 years. Put another way, the lead time is a measure of how many incidence years (as measured by the screen) of growth occur before a lesion is detected in a prevalence screen.

4. *Prior probability of cancer* is how many cancers are expected to occur in a given population over a period of time. This is a measure of the expected prevalence and incidence of cancer in a population. For example, because cancer is more common among older women, the prior probability of cancer is higher among older women than among younger women.

5. *Positive predictive value* (PPV) is a measure of the discriminating power of the method being analyzed. It is defined as

$$\frac{\text{Number of true cancers}}{\text{Number of tests called positive for cancer}}$$

This may be used to measure the discriminating power of the mammogram as a measure of what percentage is read as abnormal and needs additional imaging, or as a measure of the aggressivity of intervention when biopsies are recommended. For the latter,

$$\text{PPV for biopsy recommended} = \frac{\text{Number of cancers diagnosed}}{\substack{\text{Number of lesions} \\ \text{recommended for biopsy}}}$$

6. *True-positive results* are the lesions that are called cancer and prove to be cancer.

7. *False-positive results* are lesions that are called cancer that prove to be benign.

8. *False-negative results* are mammograms or lesions that are called negative or benign but prove to be cancer.

9. *True-negative results* are mammograms or lesions that are called negative and prove to be negative.

10. *Interval cancers* are cases where no cancer is detected at screening but a lesion is diagnosed before the next screen. The interval is usually 1 or 2 years.

11. *Sensitivity* is a measure of the test's capability of finding cancers that are in the population. It is calculated by dividing the number of cancers correctly diagnosed by the screen by the total number of cancers that are actually present in the population:

$$\text{Sensitivity} = \frac{\text{True positives}}{(\text{True positives} + \text{false negatives})}$$

Sensitivity decreases as false negatives increase.

12. *Specificity* is a measure of how successful a screen is at saying that cancer is not present when it really is not present. It is calculated by dividing the number of cases correctly called negative by the number of cases that actually are negative for cancer.

$$\text{Specificity} = \frac{\text{True negatives}}{(\text{True negatives} + \text{false positives})}$$

Specificity diminishes as false positives increase.

Gauging the Success of a Screening Program

The most important measures of a successful screening program are the number of cancers found each year in the population being screened relative to the prior probability of cancer in that population, the percentage of cancers detected by the screen as this relates to the number of cancers that could be detected during the interval (sensitivity), the size of the invasive cancers, the percentage of invasive cancers less than 1 cm in diameter (measured by the pathologist), the types (histology and grade) of cancers found, the percentage with positive axillary nodes, the percentage with distant metastatic spread, the percentage with ductal carcinoma in situ (DCIS), and the ability to predict which woman does not have breast cancer (specificity). The following are goals for successful screening:

1. In the first year of screening (prevalence), depending on the age ranges and other risk factors of the women being screened, six to 10 cancers per 1,000 women screened should be detected.

2. In subsequent screens (incidence) of the same women, between two and three cancers can be expected per 1,000 women.

3. The goal is to maximize the detection of small invasive cancers. A successful screening program should try to detect 40% to 50% of invasive cancers when they are 1 cm or smaller in diameter. Some suggest 1.5 cm should be the goal (17), but the former is possible if intervention is aggressive.

4. Twenty percent to 30% of the cancers should be DCIS (lobular carcinoma in situ is not counted as a malignant lesion). Statistics should be kept that include DCIS and also those that measure only invasive cancers.

5. The rate of node positivity will be higher in the prevalence year (because undiagnosed cancers have been building up in the population before screening begins), but should drop below 20% as the program progresses.

In addition to these, the sensitivity, specificity, and the PPV of an abnormality detected by screening and the PPV of a lesion that is biopsied are useful for gauging the success of a program.

Positive Predictive Value

PPV is meaningless without some qualification. If one wishes to measure the number of women recalled for additional evaluation, the PPV is applied to the interpretation of the screening mammogram. Most measure the PPV as a recommendation for a biopsy. This is a measure of the thresholds being used for intervention in a program (the aggressivity of the screening program). PPV is only meaningful in the context of the number of early cancers diagnosed.

There is significant variation in PPV between radiology groups practicing mammography. This underscores the variation in populations being screened, the approach to interpretation, and the thresholds for intervention. Much of this variation is due to the threshold sensitivity of various groups. Some require a higher probability of cancer before biopsy is undertaken, whereas others will have a lower threshold (18). In many European countries, thresholds are determined by cost. Borderline lesions may be allowed to pass through the screen to keep costs down (19)—one reason that some programs do not detect a high percentage of early cancers.

Given the variability in the presentation of breast cancer and its frequent morphologic similarity with benign lesions, in the future, the best approach to interpretation will likely involve the estimation of the probability of malignancy for a given type of lesion. This will evolve along with a better understanding of and correlation between the morphology of breast cancers seen mammographically and their histologic characteristics. The implementation of adjunctive techniques, such as fine-needle aspiration cytology or core biopsy, will be useful for modifying probabilities. Ultimately, predictive values will be determined by "acceptable" false-negative rates (20).

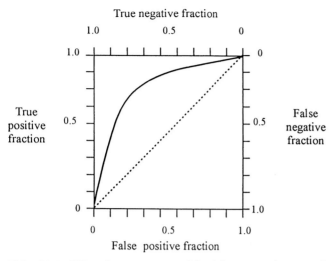

FIG. 11-5. What is an acceptable false-negative rate? This receiver operating characteristic curve (the dotted line represents random chance) graphically demonstrates that for operators who have the same powers of observation (they operate on the same curve), the only way to reduce the false-positive rate is to increase the false-negative rate by having a higher threshold for intervention and permitting cancers to pass through the screen.

Receiver Operating Characteristic Analysis

Most experienced readers recognize the same features of lesions on mammograms. They operate on the same receiver operating characteristic (ROC) curve, which is a plot that relates true positives and false positives (Fig. 11-5). This means that although they recognize the same findings on mammograms, they interpret the significance of those findings differently and have different thresholds for concern. For example, one radiologist may feel that all solid masses need to be biopsied. For circumscribed masses, this may mean that only 5% prove to be cancer. Another radiologist may believe that it is not reasonable to biopsy 100 women to find five cancers. They both see the same things on the mammograms, but the first radiologist, with a lower threshold for intervention, will find more early cancers than the second. This, however, will be at the expense of more false-positive interpretations. The second radiologist will have fewer false positives, but will let more cancers and more false negatives pass through the screen. If the observers have comparable perception skills, they are operating on the same ROC curve. The only way that the false-positive rate can be reduced is for the false-negative rate (missed cancers) to rise (21). Similarly, if the goal is to reduce the false-negative rate, then the false-positive rate must rise. The exact level of operation that is correct is philosophical and ultimately dictated by cost (economic and human).

It can be argued that the fundamental purpose of screening is mortality reduction, which is contingent on detecting as many cancers as possible at an earlier stage. Efforts to reduce the false-positive rate should not do so at the expense of increased false negatives.

STANDARDIZED REPORTING AND OUTCOME MONITORING

Reporting and data management are described in Chapter 24. Groups involved in breast cancer detection and diagnosis should try to standardize their reporting. This will reduce confusion for the referring physician and improve the communication of information. The American College of Radiology (ACR) Breast Imaging Reporting and Data System (BIRADS) was devised for just that purpose (see Chapter 24). Part of the system includes the recommendation to monitor the results of each radiologist as well as the overall screening program so that weaknesses can be corrected and the program improved. Hopefully groups will eventually be able to pool data and help refine diagnosis on a national scale.

By monitoring their own results, individuals and groups can develop probabilities based not only on national data but also on their own experience, which will have greater significance in their own particular populations. Standardization will not only help the individual group compare itself to other groups in the country, but if similar data are gathered by all groups, the effect of screening can be monitored nationally. It may even be possible to improve screening guidelines by analyzing such data, and perhaps discover new information that will have an impact on diagnosis and therapy.

Use an Organized Approach

Mammography and its interpretation should not be haphazard. The entire sequence from image production through interpretation, communication of results, and follow-up to determine outcome should be organized to try to ensure a high probability of detecting breast cancers earlier. Parameters for intervention should be carefully thought out so that image interpretation follows specific guidelines. Interpretation should not be a random process but rather based on supportable principles. If specific thresholds are used, outcome monitoring can help adjust thresholds based on fact rather than whim.

Thresholds for Intervention

Several studies have shown that there is a benefit from the detection of invasive breast cancers before they become >1 cm in size. Although there is no biological reason to suggest that there are absolute prognostic thresholds, there is a clear survival advantage for women whose cancers are 1 cm or smaller. Rosen et al. (22) followed up women over a period of 20 years. Among those with negative axillary nodes and stage I cancers, women whose invasive cancers were 1 cm or smaller enjoyed longer survival than those whose cancers were 1.1 to 2.0 cm. Tabar et al. had similar results (23).

Histologic grade measures the differentiation of cellular features. Well-differentiated cells look similar to normal breast cells, whereas poorly differentiated cells are markedly different. For most cancers, those composed of poorly differentiated cells have a worse prognosis than better differentiated cancers. Tabar found that for invasive cancers <1 cm, the usual association of higher grade with poorer prognosis did not hold, whereas it was predictive for a worse prognosis for cancers >1 cm (23). According to the Swedish data, women whose cancers were diagnosed when <1 cm uniformly do well, regardless of the histologic grade of the tumor (23). This observation along with the survival analyses would suggest that the goal should be to diagnose invasive breast cancer before it gets >1 cm and thresholds should be set accordingly.

A Systematic Approach

The ability to detect breast cancers earlier requires high-quality imaging, proper film processing, systematic review of the images, reasoned interpretation, the ability to solve problems raised by the imaging, and the ability to guide the diagnostic removal of cells or tissue for diagnosis. The interpreter should participate in all aspects of this process. It is very important that quality control be supervised by the interpreter(s) of the images so that any image degradation can be detected and corrected as quickly as possible.

Errors can be reduced by following a carefully structured approach to the process. The detection and diagnosis of breast cancer can be divided into five very specific tasks:

1. Detection—Find it.
2. Verification—Is it real?
3. Triangulation—Where is it?
4. Identification—What is it?
5. Management—What should be done about it?

Detection

Having obtained high-quality images, the interpreter should have a systematic approach to the images.

Separating Screening from Diagnosis

There are >50 million women >40 years of age in the United States. The cost of screening must be kept to a minimum so that women at all economic levels may be screened. The system of detection and diagnosis should be organized so that high quality is maintained while providing highly efficient service. We have found that the Swedish model permits high quality with efficiency, and the screening service is separated from the problem-evaluation service. Asymptomatic women who only require screening have their mammograms in a screening center designed for high quality and efficiency. It is exclusively designed for mammography. The technologists are dedicated and strive to obtain the highest quality studies possible.

The screening study is the only opportunity to detect a cancer in its preclinical stage. Thus, screening mammograms must be the best possible. Equipment capable of producing high-quality images should be used, and the technologists should be the most proficient. It has been shown that single-view mammography may result in the failure to detect 5% to 20% of breast cancers (24,25). Thus, certainly the initial screening study should be a two-view examination. If the breast is predominantly composed of fat, it might be possible to use single-view oblique laterals for subsequent screens although this approach has never been validated scientifically. We prefer to obtain two views at each screen.

Systematic Review of the Images

As with most imaging studies, abnormalities on mammography are generally readily apparent to the trained reader. However, a systematic approach to image analysis is important to appreciate subtle changes and reduce false-negative interpretations due to observer error. Individuals will develop their own routine, and as long as the basic conventions are maintained, there is no one "correct" sequence.

Image interpretation, however, should not be arbitrary. The radiologist should adhere to a system to avoid common mistakes such as right/left confusion or failure to understand the three-dimensional location of an abnormality. Image interpretation should not be based on subjective opinion but on the analysis of specific morphologic criteria. Thresholds for various levels of intervention should be defined and not subject to daily fluctuations. Image interpretation should be as consistent as possible. Without an organized approach, improvements are more difficult.

Exposure and Viewing Conditions

The type of view box used is an individual preference, but the details of the image must be readily visible. Modern film/screen combinations and exposures result in high-contrast images with maximum film densities as high as four or more on densitometric measurement.

The skin line is often not visible without a bright light, but the assessment of the skin is rarely important. Bright overall illumination is needed to assess the dark portions of the film. Haus (26) has found that five experts in mammography use illumination that, on average, is twice as bright as conventional view box illumination at the level of 3,500 nits.

Alternators with films loaded for batch interpretation are more efficient in the screening setting. Extraneous light should be reduced, and masking around the images is preferable to reduce peripheral glare that can compromise the eye's ability to see contrasting structures.

When previous films are available, comparison should be made. Ideally, the observer should compare the current study with prior studies that are two or more years old, because a subtle abnormality may only be apparent as a progressive change over a long period of time, and may be difficult to appreciate over the short interval.

A bright light is helpful to assess changes at the edge of the parenchyma in the dark portions of the film under the

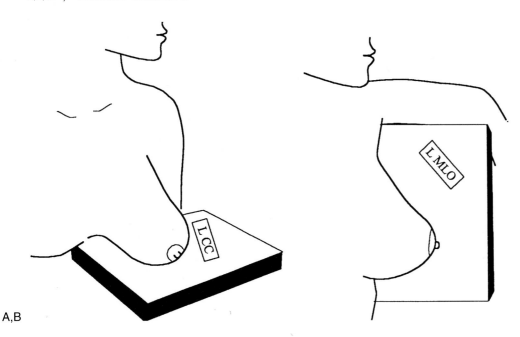

FIG. 11-6. Location for opaque markers. Schematic showing the location of radiopaque markers on the craniocaudal projection **(A)** and the lateral projection **(B)**.

subcutaneous fat. Analysis of the skin rarely contributes information that is not already clinically evident because skin changes associated with cancer are usually late changes and appreciated on clinical evaluation.

Virtually all abnormalities are visible to the unaided eye, but use of a magnifying lens will frequently facilitate the analysis of small structures and is a valuable aid for the detection of microcalcifications. A lens or other system that permits 2× to 5× magnification is useful. We have also found that a reducing or minifying lens that compresses the image can aid in the appreciation of broad areas of asymmetry.

Positioning the Films for Viewing

The breasts are best viewed as symmetric organs. By convention, mammograms should be labeled with radiopaque markers on the axillary side of the craniocaudal views (Fig. 11-6A) and along the upper axillary side of the breast on the lateral views (Fig. 11-6B). Markers should be in this location no matter how the image is obtained so that the medial, lateral, top, and bottom sides of the breast can be identified. The film should have a unique identifying number for the patient permanently attached as well as the date of the study, and identification

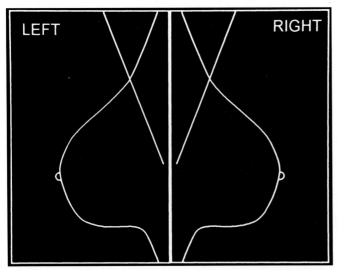

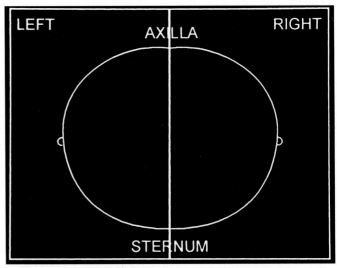

FIG. 11-7. Viewing mirror images aids mammographic interpretation. Asymmetries can be appreciated by placing the lateral views **(A)** back to back and the craniocaudal views so that corresponding portions of the breast are viewed as mirror images **(B)**.

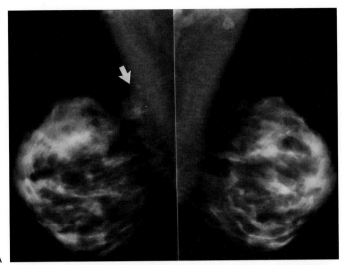
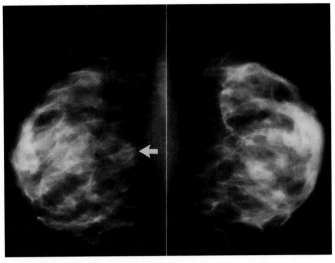

A

B

FIG. 11-8. Viewing mirror images facilitates perception. The focal asymmetry (*arrows*) on the mediolateral oblique (**A**) and craniocaudal (**B**) projections proved to be an island of breast tissue.

of the facility performing the study. Compression thickness, pressure, milliamperes, and kilovolt peak information are potentially useful data to include on the image. The availability of these data may help select techniques for future imaging of the individual. The ACR recommends the use of permanent flash card information on the films. We have found permanent stickers to be more reliable and readable using reflected light. All mammograms should also be labeled with left and right markers, and the mammographic projection should be recorded on the study (27).

The positioning of mammograms on a view box is a matter of individual preference, but it should be organized, and mistakes will be avoided if the same system is consistently followed. It is less confusing if images are mounted the same way each time. The x-ray convention is to position the images on the view box as if the observer is facing the patient with the left breast on the observer's right and the patient's right breast on the observer's left. Because we prefer to have the nonreflective emulsion side of the single-emulsion film facing the observer to avoid any extraneous light reflecting from the films, we position the mammograms opposite to this convention with the left breast on the observer's left, and the right on the observer's right.

We prefer to position the films as mirror images, with the chest wall side of the breasts against one another and with the labels at the top of the images. The chest wall side of the lateral projection is placed against the chest wall side of the opposite breast (Fig. 11-7A). The same mirror image orientation is used to position the craniocaudal views, but the films are rotated so that the axillary portions are opposite as are the sternal portions (Fig. 11-7B). The reader then knows that the upper halves of the lateral projections and the axillary halves of the breasts in the

craniocaudal projections are always at the top, with the sternal sides of the craniocaudal views at the bottom. Viewing the breasts as mirror images aids the appreciation of asymmetry.

Image Interpretation

With mammograms, as with other x-ray imaging, finding lesions is based on observing disruption of the normal patterns. There is a marked variation in the patterns of the internal structures of the breast, and only experience can give a broad familiarity with the normal spectrum.

Area for area, the breasts are remarkably symmetric. If the mammograms are obtained using symmetric positioning, the architecture and distribution of density should be mirror images (Fig. 11-8). The images should be compared area for area: The subareolar regions should look similar, the upper right breast should be the mirror image of the upper left, and so on. Tabar and Dean (28) suggest masking all but small mirror-image sections of the mammogram, when learning, to help appreciate asymmetric areas.

Large areas of asymmetry are more easily appreciated by viewing the back-to-back images from a distance or through a reducing lens to compress the scale and bring the entire image into foveal vision. The reader should assess asymmetric density differences and asymmetric architectural differences on two projections to determine if they are three-dimensionally real. Changes from previous studies, if they are available, should be sought.

This global evaluation is followed by a close-up individual review of each image, looking for abnormal densities, areas of architectural distortion, and microcalcifications. Finally, a magnifying lens should be used to search each image for small lesions and microcalcifications.

The detection of breast cancer involves the screening of tissues thought to be normal. This usually involves the evaluation of asymptomatic women in an effort to detect clinically occult abnormalities that have a significant probability of malignancy. It also applies to symptomatic women in whom the asymptomatic portions of the ipsilateral breast are screened as well as the contralateral breast.

An anomaly detected at screening may be of sufficient concern to instigate immediate intervention, or if borderline in appearance, it may require additional evaluation to resolve it as inconsequential or requiring tissue diagnosis. This latter process has been termed *diagnostic mammography*. It is more appropriately called *breast lesion evaluation* or, as Sickles has termed it, *problem solving*. This also applies to the symptomatic woman for whom imaging techniques may be applied to the area of concern raised by the clinical breast examination. The value of mammography is limited in this latter application, and once again, is more valuable in screening the clinically unremarkable tissues.

Develop a Reasoned Approach

The radiologist should develop an approach to detection and diagnosis in which each step and decision can be supported. In the screening setting the radiologist may prefer to delay a final assessment until additional evaluation is undertaken, but the process should be considered incomplete until the evaluation has taken place. At that time, a final assessment should be rendered. Final assessments should adhere to the ACR BIRADS (see Chapter 24).

Ideally, significant abnormalities should be fully characterized by their shape, margin characteristics, size, x-ray attenuation, location in the breast, and effect on the surrounding structures if they are masses; if calcifications are detected, they should be characterized according to their location, size, number, morphology, distribution, and heterogeneity.

The initial assessment should determine whether the finding can be characterized as benign without the need for further evaluation. Ideally, guidelines should be established so that interpretation is consistent, concise, and clearly represented to the referring physician or patient. Thresholds for various levels of intervention should be followed and used consistently. In the screening setting, a computerized reporting system is quite useful. Computerized reports enforce consistent terminology that is more easily understood by the referring physician and requires the radiologist to provide consistent analysis. The radiologist should avoid relying on intuition concerning the significance of a finding but should have carefully thought-out reasons for interpretive conclusions.

Because screening in the United States is not centrally controlled, it is important for individual practitioners to monitor their own results to ensure that they are detecting earlier stage lesions. If guidelines are followed and defined thresholds are used, monitoring permits the modification of thresholds for intervention and can minimize the number of women who require interventional procedures for what prove to be benign processes. The organization of mammographic interpretation is facilitated by the fact that the detection and diagnosis of breast cancer is virtually the only significant process of consequence in the breast; other processes in the breast are only important if they interfere with breast cancer detection.

Verification

Before raising concern when a potential abnormality is detected, the radiologist must be convinced that a finding at screening is truly a three-dimensional reality. Methods for affirming the presence of a lesion as well as triangulating its location are described in detail in Chapter 22.

Lesions seen in only one projection must be confirmed as significant before suggesting any intervention. Normal breast structures may overlap on the projected two-dimensional image and form "summation shadows" that mimic a significant abnormality. Overlapping structures can be differentiated from true breast lesions by various techniques. This differentiation can usually be made on the initial screen by comparing the two standard projections. Failure to demonstrate an abnormality on two views is usually sufficient to determine whether an observation represents a real lesion or superimposed tissues. If there is any question, multiple haphazard additional views are to be discouraged. The confirmation and search for corroboration of an abnormality should be carefully tailored to minimize x-ray exposure for the patient.

Return to the View on Which an Abnormality Is Suggested

In general it is more useful to return to the projection in which the abnormality is seen and modify that projection to alter the direction of the x-ray beam as it passes through the tissues. If the suspicious finding is distorted architecture, spot compression is used to better separate structures and eliminate confusing overlap. Alteration of the angle of the incident x-ray beam relative to the tissues may accomplish the same thing. Angling the gantry and reimaging will produce a different projection of the various tissue elements on the detector. This can also be accomplished by rolling the breast and recompressing to reorient the tissue relationships relative to the beam (29,30).

Magnification Reduces Noise and Improves Sharpness

The improvement in sharpness through direct mammographic magnification can be used to better determine the true nature of an abnormality as well as improve the visualization of its morphologic characteristics. The latter may be important for lesion analysis.

Triangulation

Once an abnormality has been confirmed and determined to be potentially significant, its three-dimensional location in the breast must be determined. The radiologist should avoid a recommendation for intervention unless there is an accurate idea of the true location of the lesion within the breast. Abnormalities suggested in only one projection must be corroborated by other views or by other imaging techniques such as ultrasound or CT. Maneuvers such as rolled views that can be used to establish the existence of a lesion can also be used to establish its location within the breast so that a needle can be accurately introduced into it. Evaluation of the apparent motion of a lesion against the background of the breast tissue through parallax shift can also be used to determine its location (see Chapter 22).

The radiologist must be certain that the lesion is in fact within the breast. Because the majority of the skin surface projects over the breast on two-view imaging, skin lesions and calcifications can be mistaken for intramammary abnormalities. Placing markers on cutaneous structures to confirm that they represent the shadow on the mammogram is fairly straightforward. Using the localization grid to place a marker on skin calcifications to permit tangential imaging for confirmation is described in Chapter 22.

Raised skin lesions, or skin lesions with irregular surfaces that trap radiopaque powders and ointments can project onto a mammogram and be mistaken as being within the breast (flat pigmented lesions usually are not visible). Any question is easily resolved by placing a marker on the skin lesion and imaging the marker en face and also with a tangential x-ray beam. Skin calcifications may be shown by placing a marker on the surface in which the calcifications are likely to be located and then imaging the marker in tangent. This will confirm their dermal location (31).

Rolled Views

If an intramammary lesion is seen on only the craniocaudal projection, rolled views can determine in which third of the breast the lesion lies. Simple fluoroscopic principles are applied. If the lesion moves in the direction that the top of the breast is rolled, the lesion is in the top of the breast. If it moves with the bottom then that is its location. If it remains relatively stable, it is likely in the center. Orthogonal views can then be obtained concentrating on the third of the breast in which a lesion lies to confirm its location.

Straight Lateral Projection

If a lesion is seen only on the oblique view then a straight lateral projection should be obtained. The shift of the lesion

relative to the projection of the breast tissues can be used to determine its location in the breast (29). We have also used ultrasound and CT for the accurate triangulation and localization of true intramammary lesions when modified projections are inconclusive (32,33).

Assessment

Once the lesion has been confirmed as real, and its location in the breast has been confirmed (skin lesions excluded), lesion analysis should proceed. The first decision to be made is whether the lesion is morphologically benign. A finding that is benign by mammographic criteria needs no further evaluation.

Mammographic interpretation should not rely on intuition. The interpreter should have specific reasons for deciding that a lesion is benign. Magnification views for improved morphologic characterization and lesion definition and ultrasound for cyst/solid differentiation are the primary noninvasive methods of lesion analysis.

Morphologic analysis coupled with the location of the lesion can be used to avoid arousing concern over the common intramammary lymph node. A round, lobulated, circumscribed, or reniform lesion in the outer periphery of the breast makes it virtually certain that the finding represents a benign intramammary lymph node and requires no additional concern (Fig. 11-9). Lucent-centered, spherical calcifications (Fig. 11-10) are almost always due to benign processes, including the calcification of accumulated debris in and around the ducts, fat necrosis, and skin calcifications. Calcifications that have a diameter >0.5 mm and form continuous rod-shaped deposits several millimeters long are due to the calcification of debris within the duct that is unrelated to a malignant process.

Magnification in conjunction with a horizontal-beam lateral projection can demonstrate the crescentic, concave-up, dependent collection of precipitated "milk of calcium" in benign cysts. Densely calcified fibroadenomas need not arouse alarm, and radiolucent encapsulated masses, such as lipomas, oil cysts, galactoceles, and the mixed-density hamartoma, are always benign.

An apparent focal cluster of calcifications on contact imaging may be shown on magnification imaging to merely represent a more prominent group in tissues that actually contain numerous similar, round, amorphous, scattered calcifications, reducing the likelihood of malignancy. Lucent centers may also be revealed by the higher resolution of magnification, and biopsy can be avoided.

Only a circumscribed lesion with sharp margins does not require open biopsy and can be followed (20). Some prefer to use magnification images to evaluate margins. We have found that it is extremely rare for a sharply defined, circumscribed mass on modern mammograms to become ill defined on magnification, and we may recommend short-interval follow-up based on the contact screening images.

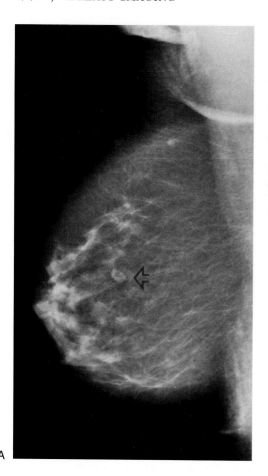

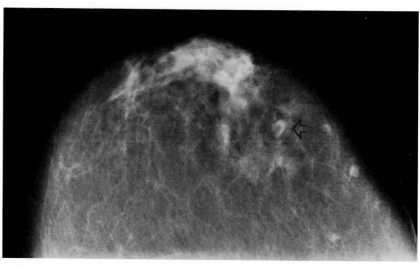

A

B

FIG. 11-9. Intramammary lymph nodes. This mass (*arrows*) and the other smaller masses have the typical appearance and location of benign intramammary lymph nodes on the mediolateral oblique **(A)** and craniocaudal **(B)** projections, and no further evaluation is needed.

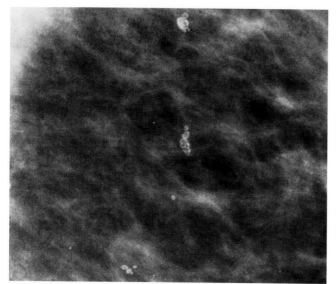

FIG. 11-10. Lucent-centered calcifications are due to benign processes. These are typical skin deposits.

Ultrasound as an Adjunctive Study

For lesions close to 1 cm or larger, ultrasound can differentiate a cyst from a solid lesion. A cyst should have sharp anterior and posterior walls with no internal echoes and have enhanced through-transmission by ultrasound (Fig. 11-11). The assessment of a solid lesion as seen by ultrasound is purely a statistical probability because benign and malignant solid lesions can have similar ultrasound morphology; however, most fibroadenomas are ovoid on ultrasound and cancers are frequently more spherical or triangular.

Management

Thresholds for intervention should be defined and applied consistently. Criteria that prompt a biopsy may differ between radiologists, but the criteria used should be supported by data. The available data (see Chapter 16) suggest that the best opportunity for cure for infiltrating breast cancer is to discover them when they are <1 cm in diameter (22,23). Any spiculated lesion that is not due to previous surgery, even one that is stable over time, is highly suspi-

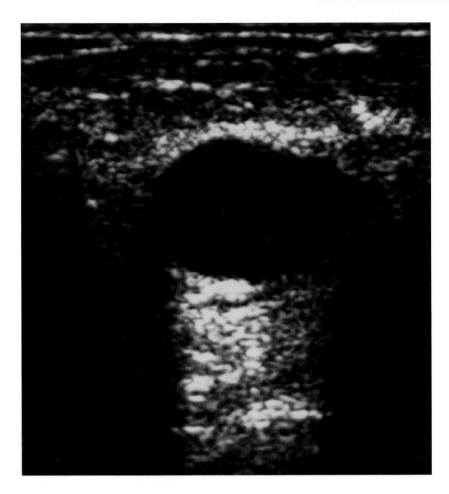

FIG. 11-11. A cyst on ultrasound. By ultrasound a cyst should have well-defined margins, sharp anterior and posterior walls, and no internal echoes, and there should be enhanced through-transmission of sound.

cious, and these are only rarely benign. Any suggestion of an ill-defined, infiltrative margin should probably prompt intervention. Calcifications that do not have clearly benign morphologies warrant careful evaluation. Those that are typical of intraductal cancer forming in necrotic cancer cells in the duct filled by breast cancer should be biopsied. Five or more indeterminate, irregularly shaped calcifications <0.5 mm in a 1-ml volume of tissue should be viewed with a high degree of suspicion.

The ACR has developed the BIRADS (see Chapter 24). This provides five assessment categories for mammography reporting.

1. Negative mammogram
2. Benign finding—negative mammogram
3. Probably benign finding—short-interval follow-up is recommended
4. Suspicious abnormality—biopsy should be considered
5. High probability of malignancy

In the screening setting, the patient may need to be recalled for additional evaluation before she fits into one of the above categories, but each mammographic assessment should ultimately fit into one of the above categories.

Negative Mammogram

If the mammogram is negative, no further x-ray analysis is needed. This does not mean that further assessment is not required. If the patient has a clinically evident abnormality, clinical decisions must be made. The fact that the mammogram is negative does not alter this, just as a negative physical examination does not alter the need to pursue a lesion that is suspicious by mammography.

Benign Finding

The primary determination that must be made is whether the lesion is benign. If a finding has clearly benign morphologic characteristics, there is no need for further analysis or intervention.

High Probability of Malignancy

Lesions that have a high probability of malignancy require intervention. This generally means a tissue (or cytologic) analysis.

Indeterminate Lesion

Ultimately, when a lesion is confirmed and has a finite probability of malignancy but its histology remains uncertain based on morphologic analysis, a recommendation for further analysis should be made. This may be merely short-interval follow-up in the case of a lesion that has a minimal probability of malignancy (2% or less) or the recommendation to obtain tissue for more suspicious lesions. Recommendations should be made according to established guidelines such as those described above, and the consequences of the recommendation should be monitored so that modifications in the guidelines can be based on data and not anecdotal evidence.

In general, if the lesion is circumscribed and meets the size criterion for investigation, ultrasound- or imaging-guided aspiration is recommended to establish the cystic or solid composition of the lesion. The accuracy of fine-needle aspiration cytology, or core needle biopsy remains uncertain. Ideally, because there is some operator dependence for these procedures, the accuracy should be established for each radiology group (34). If biopsy is not used to diagnose solid lesions that have reached the threshold, women with those lesions should be followed very carefully to ensure that false-negative results are corrected expeditiously (35).

If the results of a needle biopsy are discordant with the expected diagnosis, rebiopsy or excisional biopsy should be performed. For example, if the lesion is a spiculated mass and the report states "fibrocystic tissue," there is a high likelihood that the needle missed the target, and excisional biopsy should be performed. On the other hand, if the lesion is round or ovoid with sharply defined margins, and the needle biopsy material is interpreted as a fibroadenoma, the results are congruent, and reliance on the needle biopsy is justified. Several studies have demonstrated that if the histology of a core needle biopsy is read as atypical hyperplasia (a high-risk but benign lesion), excisional biopsy is warranted because many prove to be breast cancer at excision (36).

From Probably Benign to Suspicious: Biopsy Should Be Considered

The lesions that fall in between *clearly benign* and *high probability of malignancy* constitute the most difficult, and there is no unanimity among experts as to their appropriate management. These lesions range from those with ill-defined margins to those with clustered calcifications with heterogeneous morphology. Some of these lesions will be classified as probably benign whereas others will be grouped with suspicious lesions for which a biopsy should be considered.

There is general agreement that the category of *short-interval follow-up* should include only lesions that are probably benign and have a very low probability of malignancy.

The stability of a lesion over time is not necessarily reassuring by itself. Breast cancer can be stable (37). The principle of short-interval follow-up is one that applies to lesions that have a very low probability of malignancy to begin with and have an additional level of certainty added by their stability. Probabilities are multiplicative. Cancer can be stable over several years, although this is rare. Stability for a worrisome lesion is, therefore, not reassuring. Stability for a lesion that is unlikely to be cancer to begin with, however, multiplies a low probability by a low probability, resulting in a reassuring, extremely low probability.

Suspicious: Biopsy Should Be Considered

There are no absolute criteria for prompting biopsy because imaging probabilities must be assessed in light of individual patient factors such as age, quality of life, risk from intervention, and so forth. Due to the true uncertainties of lesion analysis, however, the referring physician, whenever possible, should be given probabilities that can be presented to the patient so that together they can make an educated decision concerning the desirability of intervention or close follow-up. For example, some women might wish to avoid surgery and select short-interval follow-up for a lesion with a 2% to 5% probability of malignancy whereas another woman might elect surgery for a 1% chance of cancer. If needle biopsy or open biopsy is elected, the radiologist and surgeon should be able to offer the patient a safe, accurate procedure that has a high likelihood of arriving at the correct diagnosis with as little cosmetic damage and morbidity as possible (see Chapter 21).

Needle Positioning

The most accurate needle positioning methods involve holding the breast in the compression system of the mammographic unit and inserting a needle into the lesion for needle biopsy, or a needle or wire guide through or alongside the lesion parallel to the chest wall to guide an excisional biopsy (38). Accurate positioning can also be accomplished for selected lesions using ultrasound, CT, and MRI. Accurate positioning for needle biopsy is critical if the results are to be accurate. Accurate guide placement for excision is needed to permit a small amount of tissue to be removed to accurately determine the histology of the lesion in question (39). Specimen radiography with compression should be performed on all nonpalpable, excised lesions, and radiography of core samples should be used to determine that tissue containing calcifications has been sampled.

If the lesion proves to be malignant and contains mammographically visible calcifications, postsurgical mammography with magnification may be helpful to assess the extent of the lesion and the possibility of residual cancer by defining residual calcifications. It is recommended that for breast conservation, all gross cancer should be removed and the margins of the excised tissue be free of tumor (clear margins), which indicates that the gross tumor has been removed. This appears to minimize the likelihood of recurrence after radiation, although overall survival does not appear to be affected.

Short-Interval Follow-Up

The value of short-interval follow-up (a time period less than the recommended annual screening interval) is still debated. Some would argue that if the lesion is of insufficient concern to prompt immediate biopsy, there is little or no advantage in short-interval follow-up, and unnecessary concerns are raised and cost increased.

There are few prospective, objective data on short-interval follow-up (39). Even the timing of the short interval has no truly scientific basis. Most schemes rely on analysis of the expected doubling times of breast cancer. Our own experience suggests that whatever the interval, it should not interfere with annual screening. We have adopted a six-month short interval and recommend monitoring at this interval for a total of 2 years. Sickles has suggested a six-month initial short interval and then directed annual follow-up for a total of 3 years (35).

In our screening program, approximately 2% to 4% of women screened have findings that are placed in our short-interval follow-up. Although cancers can be stable for more than two years (36) it has been our experience that these almost always have suspicious characteristics on the initial study. It is very rare for a lesion that is classified as probably benign, but ultimately shown to be malignant, to also be stable for two years.

A lesion that has an extremely low probability that remains stable over two years almost guarantees benignity. Because the number of these lesions is so small, it is almost impossible to arrive at statistically significant conclusions about follow-up intervals. Moskowitz has pointed out that age may play a role and he suggested that, in women under 50 years, the interval should be shortened to 3 months due to the apparently faster growing tumors in this age group, but this remains purely speculative (personal communication).

It must be emphasized that a lesion that is classified as probably benign should have a very low probability of malignancy. For example, short-interval follow-up should not be used to evaluate suspicious lesions seen in only one projection. If a lesion is suspicious, an expeditious determination of its histology should be undertaken. If this is not possible, referral to another center may permit earlier intervention.

If a lesion has suspicious morphology, stability is much less reassuring. A spiculated lesion of any size is suspect regardless of its stability. Prospective studies are needed to develop policies based on data rather than supposition, but until these are available it is likely that a lesion that is stable over a 2-year period, and has probably benign characteristics to begin with, is very unlikely to be malignant.

Communication of Breast Imaging Results

The communication of results of breast imaging studies has been problematic (40). The written report may not be sufficient. It is suggested that an abnormal screening examination that requires additional evaluation and significant findings that suggest a finite probability of malignancy should be communicated in writing and through direct telephone communication to the referring physician's office. Many states require that the patient be informed directly.

We have found that in addition to written and verbal communication of the need for prompt evaluation, errors can be reduced by maintaining a file of patients who fit into the categories requiring immediate attention. This file is reviewed on a periodic basis to ensure that appropriate follow-up has occurred. Computerization can facilitate this process and automatically generate follow-up lists and letters if appropriate intervention has not occurred.

THE AUDIT

As with all of medicine, mammography and breast imaging are continuously evolving. New observations will continue to be made. A good screening program should track the results of abnormalities that are discovered (see Chapter 24) (this is mandated in most states and required under the Food and Drug Administration guidelines). By learning what an abnormality proved to be, the radiologist and group will improve their image interpretation and can modify their approaches to better detect and diagnose early breast cancer.

SUMMARY

The ability to detect early breast cancer requires the following:

1. Optimized imaging using (a) dedicated mammographic equipment, (b) highly skilled technologists to properly position the breast to maximize the visualized tissue, (c) proper processing of the image to enhance soft-tissue contrast and preserve high resolution, and (d) a quality control program to guarantee that these elements remain constant.

2. Interpretation should use (a) a systematic review by a trained radiologist with comparison to previous studies whenever possible; (b) defined parameters and thresholds for interpretation; (c) the appropriate communication of a finding to the referring physician or a structure to provide follow-up for the self-referred patient; and (d) a system of follow-up, at least for abnormal studies, to try to ensure that concerns are appropriately transmitted and to assess the results of the applied thresholds.

By developing a reasoned, consistent policy, a breast imaging group can provide concise accurate reports based on interpretations that are not arbitrary but carefully thought out. By monitoring the results of their activities, accuracy will be improved.

REFERENCES

1. Elmore JG, Wells CK, Lee CH, Feinstein AR. Variability in radiologists' interpretations of mammograms. N Engl J Med 1994;331:1493–1499.
2. Kopans DB. The accuracy of mammographic interpretation. N Engl J Med 1994;331:1521–1522.
3. Baker LH. Breast cancer detection demonstration project: five-year summary report. CA Cancer J Clin 1982;32:194–225.
4. Frankel SD, Sickles EA, Cupren BN, et al. Initial versus subsequent screening mammography: comparison of findings and their prognostic significance. AJR Am J Roentgenol 1995;164:1107–1109.
5. Austin JHM, Romney BM, Goldsmith LS. Missed bronchogenic carcinoma: radiographic findings in 27 patients with a potentially resectable lesion evident in retrospect. Radiology 1992;182:115–122.
6. Bird RE. Professional quality assurance for mammographic screening programs. Radiology 1990;177:587.
7. Tabar L, Fagerberg G, Duffy S, et al. Update of the Swedish two-county program of mammographic screening for breast cancer. Radiol Clin North Am 1992;30:187–210.
8. Thurfjell EL, Lernevall KA, Taube AAS. Benefit of independent double reading in population-based mammography screening program. Radiology 1994;191:241–244.
9. Moskowitz M. Breast cancer: age-specific growth rates and screening strategies. Radiology 1986;161:37–41.
10. Tabar L, Fagerberg G, Day NE, Holmberg L. What is the optimum interval between mammographic screening examinations? An analysis based on the latest results of the Swedish two-county breast screening trial. Br J Cancer 1989;55:547–551.
11. Tabar L, Duff SW, Krusemo UB. Detection method, tumor size and node metastases in breast cancers diagnosed during a trial of breast cancer screening. Eur J Cancer Clin Oncol 1987;23:959–962.
12. Meyer JE, Kopans DB. Analysis of mammographically obvious breast carcinomas with benign results on initial biopsy. Surg Gynecol Obstet 1981;153:570–572.
13. Faulk RM, Sickles EA. Efficacy of spot compression—magnification and tangential views in mammographic evaluation of palpable masses. Radiology 1992;185:87–90.
14. Kopans DB, Meyer JE, Cohen AM, Wood WC. Palpable breast masses: the importance of preoperative mammography. JAMA 1981; 246:2819–2822.
15. Swann CA, Kopans DB, McCarthy KA, et al. Mammographic density and physical assessment of the breast. AJR Am J Roentgenol 1987; 148:525–526.
16. Boren WL, Hunter TB, Bjelland JC, Hunt KR. Comparison of breast consistency at palpation with breast density at mammography. Invest Radiol 1990;25:1010–1011.
17. Meyer JE, Kopans DB. Breast physical examination by the mammographer; an aid to improved diagnostic accuracy. Appl Radiol 1983;103–106.
18. Van Dijck JAAM, Verbeek ALM, Hendriks JHCL, Holland R. The current detectability of breast cancer in a mammographic screening program. Cancer 1993;72:1933–1938.
19. Kopans DB. Mammography screening for breast cancer. Cancer 1993;72:1809–1812.
20. Brenner RJ, Sickles EA. Acceptability of periodic follow-up as an alternative to biopsy for mammographically detected lesions interpreted as probably benign. Radiology 1989;171:645–646.
21. D'Orsi CJ. To follow or not to follow, that is the question. Radiology 1992;184:306.
22. Rosen PP, Groshen S, Saigo PE, et al. A long-term follow-up study of survival in stage I (T1 N0 M0) and stage II (T1 N1 M0) breast carcinoma. J Clin Oncol 1989;7:355–366.
23. Tabar L, Fagerberg G, Day N, et al. Breast cancer treatment and natural history: new insights from results of screening. Lancet 1992;339: 412–414.
24. Muir BB, Kirkpatrick A, Roberts MM, Duffy SW. Oblique-view mammography: adequacy for screening. Radiology 1984;151:39–41.
25. Wald NJ, Murphy P, Major P, et al. UKCCCR multicentre randomised controlled trial of one and two view mammography in breast cancer screening. BMJ 1995;311:1189–1193.
26. Hendrick RE, Committee on Quality Assurance in Mammography. American College of Radiology Mammography Quality Control Manuals (rev ed). Reston, VA: American College of Radiology, 1994.
27. Bassett LW, Hirbawi IA, DeBruhl N, Hayes MK. Mammographic positioning: evaluation from the viewbox. Radiology 1993;188: 803–806.
28. Tabar L, Dean P. Teaching Atlas of Mammography. New York: Thieme, 1985.
29. Swann CA, Kopans DB, McCarthy KA, et al. Localization of occult breast lesions: practical solutions to problems of triangulation. Radiology 1987;163:577–579.
30. Sickles EA. Practical solutions to common mammographic problems: tailoring the examination. AJR Am J Roentgenol 1988;151:31–39.
31. Kopans DB. Breast Imaging. Philadelphia: Lippincott, 1989;331–334.
32. Kopans DB, Meyer JE. Computed tomography guided localization of clinically occult breast carcinoma—the "N" skin guide. Radiology 1982;145:211–212.
33. Kopans DB, Meyer JE, Lindfors KK, Bucchianeri SS. Breast sonography to guide aspiration of cysts and preoperative localization of occult breast lesions. AJR Am J Roentgenol 1984;143:489–492.
34. Kopans DB. Fine-needle aspiration of clinically occult breast lesions. Radiology 1989;170:313–314.
35. Sickles EA. Periodic mammographic follow-up of probably benign lesions: results of 3,184 consecutive cases. Radiology 1981;179: 463–468.
36. Gisvold JJ, Goeliner JR, Grant CS. Breast biopsy: a comparative study of stereotaxically guided core and excisional techniques. AJR Am J Roentgenol 1994;162:815–820.
37. Meyer JE, Kopans DB. Stability of a mammographic mass: a false sense of security. AJR Am J Roentgenol 1981;137:595–598.
38. Kopans DB, Meyer JE, Lindfors KK, McCarthy KA. Spring-hook-wire breast lesion localizer: use with rigid compression mammographic systems. Radiology 1985;157:505–507.
39. Gallagher WJ, Cardenosa G, Rubens JR, et al. Minimal-volume excision of nonpalpable breast lesions. AJR Am J Roentgenol 1989;153: 957–961.
40. Robertson C, Kopans DB. Communication problems after mammographic screening. Radiology 1989;172:443–444.

Breast Imaging, 2nd ed., by Daniel B. Kopans.
Lippincott–Raven Publishers, Philadelphia © 1998.

CHAPTER **12**

Mammography and the Normal Breast

The primary role of mammography is to screen asymptomatic women in the hope of detecting breast cancer at a smaller size and earlier stage than the woman's own surveillance or her doctor's routine examination might ordinarily achieve. Smaller size and earlier stage at diagnosis have been shown to reduce or delay mortality from breast cancer (1–4). Mammography is also used to evaluate women with palpable abnormalities, but the fact that mammographic morphologic criteria are frequently not specific limits its utility as a diagnostic technique. Mammography is best thought of primarily as a screening test. Management of a clinically apparent lesion must ultimately be determined by the clinical assessment. In the symptomatic woman, because mammography cannot be used to exclude breast cancer and the mammographic findings are frequently not specific, it should be used primarily to survey the remainder of the ipsilateral breast and screen the contralateral breast to detect clinically occult cancer (5).

DETECTION VERSUS DIAGNOSIS

In 1979, Moskowitz (6) emphasized the difference between detection (screening) and diagnosis. Mammography is primarily useful for detecting abnormalities, including many early-stage and curable cancers. It is less valuable for diagnosis to determine whether a lesion that has been detected is benign or malignant. The distinction has become increasingly important as we enter a period in which large populations are being screened for breast cancer. If the benefits of screening are to be available to all women, the cost of mammography must be reduced. Image quality, however, must be maximized. This can be accomplished by developing efficient screening programs. As has been shown in Europe as well as in the United States (7), costs can be reduced by separating screening (*detection*) from the evaluation of women who have a clinically evident problem or a problem detected by mammographic screening (*diagnosis*).

To determine what is abnormal, it is important to understand the normal breast. There is a wide variation in "normal," and a familiarity with the range is required for accurate imaging interpretation.

GENERAL PRINCIPLES

The Normal Breast

In view of the enormous amount of work that has been done in an effort to understand the breast and the development of breast cancer, it is surprising that the normal breast has never been clearly defined. This is likely due to the fact that since breast cancer is really the only significant abnormality that occurs in the breast, it is really only the changes that appear to predispose to breast cancer that are considered significant. There is a large range of histologic findings that occur in women who never develop breast cancer, but where normal ends and abnormal begins is not obvious, and past classifications have been found to be inaccurate. For example, it was relatively recently that the term *fibrocystic disease* was discarded in favor of more accurate subcategorization of the changes that had been formerly grouped under this term. This change in terminology occurred when it was recognized that most of the changes that had been grouped in this nonspecific classification were of no particular significance and were so common that it would be difficult to classify them as a disease (8).

Compounding the difficulty of defining normal is the wide variation among individuals. It is also difficult to obtain significant amounts of histologic information concerning the normal breast at different ages because normal breasts are rarely available for histologic evaluation. The preponderance of data comes from autopsy series, which tend to be biased toward an older population of women or from those with significant diseases. Other data are derived from mastectomy material and breast biopsies, which are, by definition, abnormal tissue. Furthermore, because it is not possible to histologically follow the actual development, monthly changes, and long-term evolution of the mammary tissues in a single individual, most studies can only look at a cohort of women at one point in time. Inferences must be made by comparing histopathology from different women at varying ages, and these are influenced by such factors as reproductive history and the use of exogenous hormones. Consequently, an accurate definition of what constitutes normality is difficult.

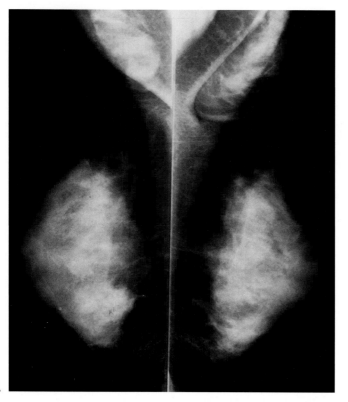

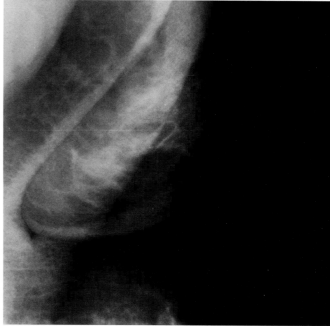

A

B

FIG. 12-1. **(A)** Accessory breast tissue is seen high in the axilla on these mediolateral oblique projections. **(B)** The appearance of this tissue is identical to normal breast tissue on a photographic enlargement of the right axillary tail.

The Mammogram and the Menstrual Cycle

Although the physiologic changes of the menstrual cycle can be dramatic, they have never been scientifically evaluated with reference to mammography. The effects of the menstrual cycle on the mammogram have been fictionalized, but little has been clearly documented. Clinically there are fairly significant, cyclic changes that occur in the breast that vary with the individual. Histologic evaluation has documented significant, periodic cellular changes (9). Some magnetic resonance data have demonstrated increased contrast enhancement during the premenstrual phase of the menstrual cycle (10), but correlates have never been documented and there are no data suggesting that any visible changes are evident on the mammogram.

The Normal Mammogram

There is an extremely wide variation in the mammographic appearance of the breast, and it is likely that all these variants are normal. In all likelihood, most breast cancers form in normal breast tissue with a single cell developing the malignant genotype (and ultimately the malignant phenotype) that is transferred to its clones. Despite the difficulty in determining with any precision what is normal and what is abnormal, there are likely some abnormal breast tissues. The higher, and often bilateral, risk of breast cancer, associated with atypical ductal or atypical lobular hyperplasia and lobular carcinoma in situ (LCIS), suggests that these precursor lesions may represent field abnormalities where a large number of cells are in some way primed, increasing the likelihood that one cell or a group of cells will become overtly malignant. Because of this increased risk, it is reasonable to consider these abnormal breast tissue, but they have never been demonstrated as different mammographically. Although there appears to be some increased risk associated with the dense breast patterns, there are as yet no accurate indicators that are visible by mammography that can predict where, or even in whom, a cancer will grow. There are as yet no mammographically defined indications of the presence of either atypical hyperplasia or LCIS.

The presence of these high-risk lesions does seem to have some associations. For example, LCIS usually occurs in women whose breasts are radiographically dense. It is unclear whether this is due to the age at which LCIS is usually found (most often in the premenopausal woman) or a true relationship to breast density. Stomper et al. (11) have noted, and our data agree, that atypical hyperplasia is often found by biopsies instigated by mammographically detected calcifications. They found that as a consequence, mammography was able to define more women with atypical hyperplasia than could biopsies due to clinically evident abnormalities. We have found a similar association with calcifications adjacent to LCIS. Although these associations are interesting, their significance and practical use remain unclear.

DEVELOPMENTAL VARIATIONS

The breasts usually develop in a fairly symmetric fashion. Although small areas of tissue are not identical in both breasts, the general distribution of tissues is symmetric, and tissues should be evaluated to search for asymmetries. Although the breasts generally develop simultaneously, occasionally one will begin to develop before the other. As a consequence, the asymmetric development of one breast before the other in the preadolescent or adolescent female may be thought, by an inexperienced examiner, to represent a mass on clinical examination. Surgery should be avoided since removal of the breast bud will result in the subsequent failure of breast development. There are occasional masses that develop in the adolescent breast, but these are uncom-

mon and are usually eccentric from the nipple. Since breast cancer is extremely rare among young women and the odds are extremely high that a true mass is benign, observation rather than intervention is reasonable if there is any question.

Accessory and Ectopic Breast Tissue

Fairly striking developmental variations in breast tissue are occasionally seen. Breast tissue may be present anywhere along the "milk line," which, in the embryo, extends from the axilla to the groin (see Chapter 2). Ectopic breast tissue (discontinuous with the gland and in an uncommon location) is fairly unusual because all but the thoracic portion of the mammary ridge is usually resorbed during fetal development. Accessory breast tissue (extending from the main gland) is fairly common, appearing high in the axilla, either unilaterally or on both sides (Fig. 12-1). On rare occasions, an accessory nipple may be imaged (Fig. 12-2) or a complete accessory breast. These variations are important because wherever there is ductal epithelium, it is possible for breast cancer to develop. Since the most common location of accessory tissue is in the axilla, the properly positioned mammogram should attempt to image as much tissue as possible in this area.

Asymmetric Breasts

Once development is complete, there is usually only a minor difference in the sizes of the two breasts. On occasion, however, one breast may develop noticeably larger than the other (Fig. 12-3). The exact reason for this has never been determined, but it is likely due to differential end-organ response to hormones and growth factors. Other than the psychological difficulty that this may induce, there is no reason

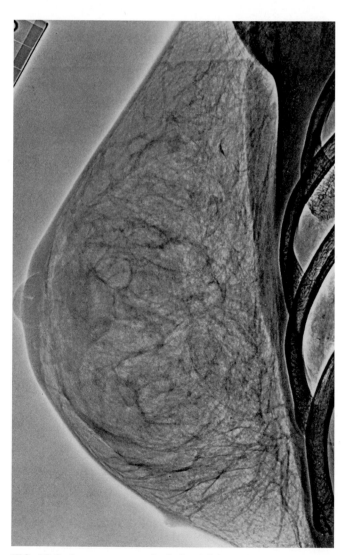

FIG. 12-2. An accessory nipple is visible at the bottom of the breast on this lateral xerogram.

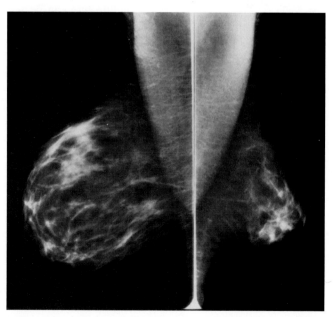

FIG. 12-3. Both breasts are normal even though the left breast developed to be considerably larger than the right.

to believe that it is of any particular consequence. Rapid asymmetric enlargement during adolescence can sometimes be caused by the growth of a giant fibroadenoma. Phylloides tumors can also grow rapidly and result in breast enlargement. Very large cysts may occupy large volumes of the breast, but these usually do not occur until a woman is in her 30s.

It is rare that cancer will cause a significant enlargement of one breast without any other evidence of malignancy, such as a mass, skin thickening, or erythema. Similarly, non-neoplastic inflammation will almost always result in pain or erythema. Noticeably asymmetric breasts with no other associated abnormality are almost always a developmental phenomenon.

Breast Size and Cancer Risk

Although one might expect that a greater volume of tissue might mean a greater risk of malignancy, there does not appear to be any relationship between breast size and cancer development. No good studies of the relationship of risk to size are available, in part, due to difficulty in measuring size. Using bra size as a crude measure of breast size, we found that the percentage of women who were diagnosed with breast cancer was approximately the same for each size.

Breast Composition

The composition of the breasts is also extremely variable. Adipose tissue comprises a large portion of many breasts and is radiolucent. The radiographically visible densities include to varying degrees ducts, lobular elements, and fibrous connective tissue structures. Ducts can frequently be seen as thin linear structures (usually 1 mm or less in diameter) radiating back from the nipple and crisscrossing the tissues. Lobules and the intralobular connective tissue project as vague "fluffy" densities whose architecture can be seen following the injection of contrast material (Fig. 12-4 A–C). The ducts and lobules are often hidden within the connective tissue (Fig. 12-4 D–G).

There are two different types of connective tissue in the breast. The specialized intralobular connective tissues contribute to the visibility of the lobule. The major component of radiographic density on the mammogram is due to the extralobular connective tissues, which are likely responsible for most of the gross variations in density. Studies have suggested that women whose breasts are radiographically dense are at greater risk for breast cancer. The debate over this has continued for over 20 years. There does appear to be some increased risk for women with dense patterns, but it is of no practical significance, and none of the many variations can truly be labeled as abnormal.

Breast Variation with Age

The conventional teaching has been that the breast, its ducts present at birth, develops during adolescence with

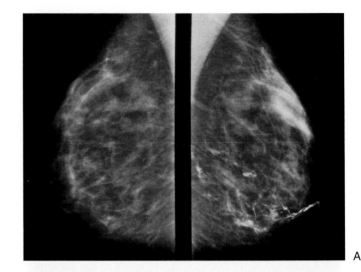

A

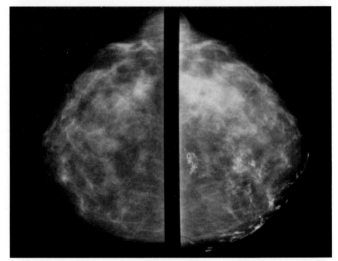

B

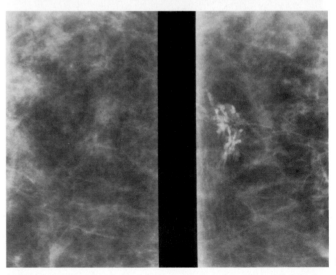

C

FIG. 12-4. Ducts are fine linear structures, whereas lobules produce ill-defined densities. These structures are seen on the pre-contrast injection (on the left) and post-contrast injection (on the right), lateral **(A)**, and craniocaudal projections **(B)**. The terminal ductules (acini) appear like fingers of a glove on this close-up view from the craniocaudal projection of the pre- and postinjection images **(C)**. *Continued.*

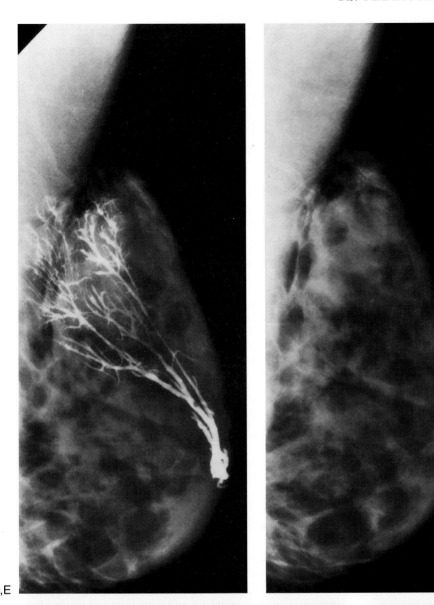

D,E

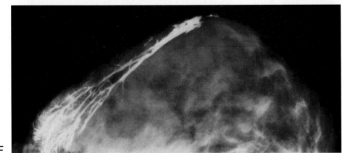

F

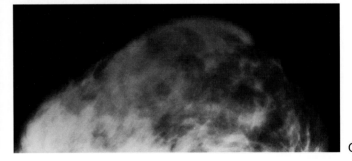

G

FIG. 12-4. *Continued.* The ducts are clearly visible when injected with contrast **(D, F)**, but are normally silhouetted by the intra- and extralobular connective tissues **(E, G)**.

growth into the mid-20s, and "maturation" (end-bud differentiation into lobules) with the first full-term gestation. Conventional teaching further holds that the breast undergoes involution after menopause with diminution in epithelial, stromal, and lobular elements and an increase in fat content. This "conventional wisdom" is actually not accurate. At

least one autopsy series suggests that, in fact, involution significantly precedes menopause in many women and can begin as early as the third decade of life (12).

Mammography offers the opportunity to study the breast over time at a macroscopic level. In 1976, Wolfe (13) published a review of cases of women who had had mammo-

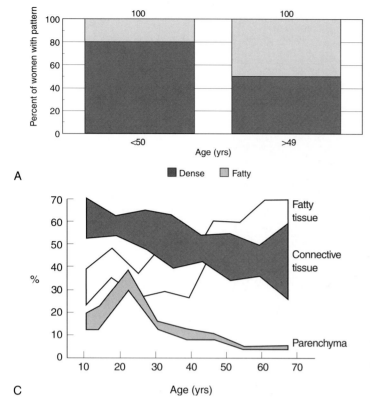

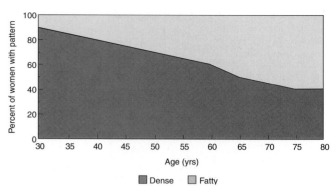

A

B

Dense   Fatty

C

FIG. 12-5. (A) This graph demonstrates the percentages of women with dense breast tissues and those with fatty patterns. By making age 50 years the point of analysis, it appears that the tissue patterns change at age 50. If the same data are viewed as percentages at each age **(B)**, it becomes apparent that there is no dramatic change at age 50 but rather change that occurs in some women at different ages and never occurs among others. These data from the Massachusetts General Hospital screening program almost duplicate the histologic analysis by Prechtel **(C)**. This histologic analysis of the change in the proportions of the tissue components of the breast demonstrate the same findings as are noted mammographically. There is a gradual decrease in the connective tissue and glandular components and a similar gradual increase in the adipose components with no abrupt change at any age. (Adapted from Prechtel K. Mastopathic und Altersabbangige Brustdrusen Berandernagen. Fortschr Med 1971;89:1312–1315.) *Continued.*

grams over a 5- to 10-year period. He suggested that among some women in this group who had dense mammary tissues, involutional changes with fatty replacement were apparent on the mammograms. The conclusions, however, must be challenged. The images displayed in the article suggest that Wolfe was comparing parenchymal patterns obtained with the plain film techniques of the 1960s that used low kilovolt peak (kVp) and produced high-contrast images, with the flatter, lower-contrast, xerographic images obtained at higher kVp in the 1970s. This comparison, coupled with the conventional teaching of fatty involution, may have biased his results. Other studies have shown that the percentage of younger women who have radiographically dense breasts is higher than that among older women, but this is far from universal, and there are many women in their 20s who have fat as the predominant tissue and many women in their 80s who have extremely dense breast tissues.

In our experience with women who have had mammograms over a period of 10 years or more, we have rarely seen a significant change in the radiographic density of the breast unless there has been a significant increase or decrease in body weight. In fact, it is likely that obesity is one of the most significant influences on parenchymal density because the breast is one area where fat deposition and resorption are very common. Body habitus and percent body fat were not controlled for in Wolfe's work.

Based on the involutional changes that have been fairly well documented at the microscopic level, one would expect changes in the radiographic appearance of the breast over time, but these have not been convincingly shown in longitudinal studies, and may be too subtle to be obvious on mammography. We can only extrapolate from horizontal studies in which older women tend to have a greater proportion of fat in the breast than younger women. Progression from one radiographic pattern to another, in any large population of women, has never been objectively demonstrated.

Breast Density and Age

The failure to understand the changes that take place in the breast with increasing age has led many to continue to believe that there is dramatic change in the mammogram at 50 years. This is an artifact of data analysis. Much of the confusion is due to analyses that group women into those younger than a certain age (usually 50 years) and those older than that age. By analyzing the data in this fashion, with a single age as the point of analysis, differences that occur steadily with age can be made to appear to occur at that age. If the point of analysis is age 50 years, any changes with age will appear to occur at that age (Fig. 12-5A). If the data are analyzed properly com-

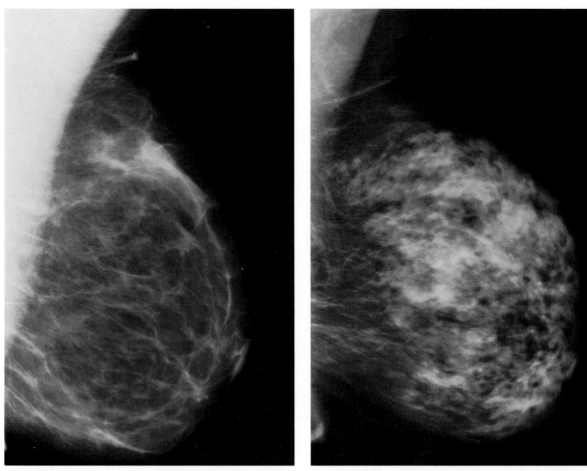

D   E

FIG. 12-5. *Continued.* Young age does not always mean dense and older age does not always mean fatty. **(D)** This 22-year-old woman has a tissue pattern that is almost entirely fat. **(E)** This 79-year-old woman has a very dense tissue pattern (she was not using hormones).

paring ratios at each age, a different picture emerges (Fig. 12-5B). Women with dense patterns do not change their patterns at age 50 or at any other single point in life. There is no question that a high percentage of women have dense breast tissue at 30 years (approximately 90% dense versus 10% fatty), but this ratio does not change abruptly. It decreases steadily at approximately 1% to 2% per year so that by 40 years the ratio is 80/20. By 50 years, it is 70/30, and the 50/50 ratio occurs at approximately 65 years.

Stomper et al. (14) found similar gradual changes with no abrupt change at any age. They also noted that women with fewer than two pregnancies tended to be more likely to have dense breasts. In addition, they found that benign calcifications were very common on normal mammograms. They were present on 8% of the mammograms performed for women ages 25 to 29 years and increased to 86% of the mammograms performed on women ages 76 to 79 years.

There is no major change that occurs at 50 years or at menopause. This same, gradual decrease in dense tissues

(connective tissue and glandular elements) that is evident by mammography has also been noted histologically by Prechtel (15) (Fig. 12-5C), whose data show a gradual change in percentages with age that almost directly reflects mammographic pattern changes with age. Prechtel's analysis also shows no abrupt change at 50 years or at menopause.

Although a higher percentage of younger women have dense tissue patterns, the breast tissues of many young women are almost all fat. It is not uncommon for women in their 20s to have almost all fat tissue patterns (Fig. 12-5D). Similarly, it is not uncommon for women in their 70s and 80s to have very dense patterns (Fig. 12-5E). Decrease in breast tissue density is rarely dramatic and is usually subtle. The trabecular densities become thinner, and the percentage of fat gradually increases in some women. It is extremely rare, in our experience, for the breast tissues to suddenly change.

The most frequent association with significant change in density is weight gain or loss. The breast is a repository

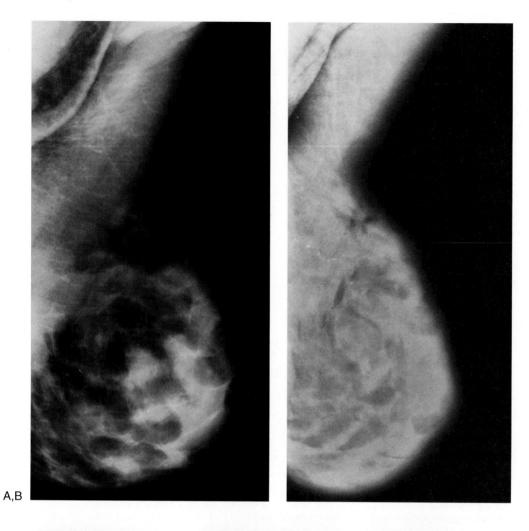

A,B

FIG. 12-6. The change in pattern from dense tissue mixed with fat **(A)**, to a very dense pattern **(B)** was the result of a 20-lb weight loss in this 43-year-old woman.

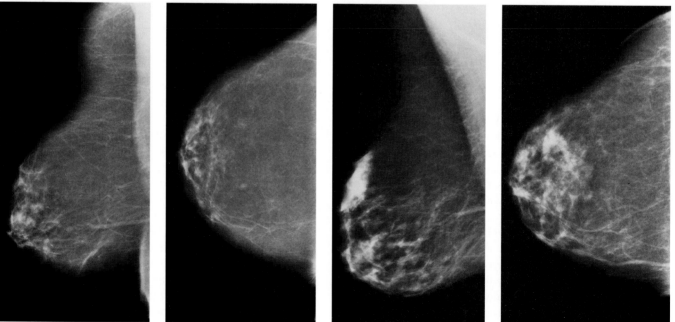

A–D

FIG. 12-7. This 53-year-old-woman had a pattern of predominantly fat on the mediolateral oblique (MLO) **(A)** and craniocaudal (CC) **(B)** projections. Her breasts resisted compression. At 57 years she had lost a significant amount of weight, and the fibroglandular tissues were less separated by fat, producing areas of greater tissue density even though her breasts were more compressible on the MLO **(C)** and CC **(D)**.

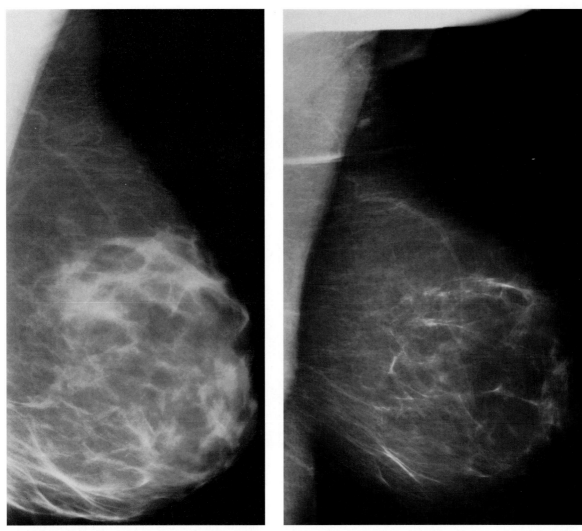

FIG. 12-8. From age 35 years **(A)** to age 37 years **(B)** the patient gained 45 pounds. The breasts became less compressible, and the dense structures were spread farther apart by fat. In addition, there was likely some resorption of fibrous and glandular tissues.

for fat, and weight gain and loss may be visible in the tissue density of the breast. The most dramatic changes in breast patterns are usually related to changes in weight (Fig. 12-6).

Clinical Assessment Does Not Predict Radiographic Density

Many have mistakenly confused the physical firmness of the breast tissues with their radiographic density (x-ray attenuation), incorrectly believing that firm breast tissue is radiographically dense. This is not the case. Studies have shown that the radiographic density of the breast cannot be predicted based on size, firmness (measured by the forces needed for compression), or compressed breast thickness (16,17). Contrary to conventional wisdom,

breasts with a higher fat composition often require greater compression forces (18) and are frequently firmer. In fact, it has been our anecdotal experience that the breasts that are the most difficult to compress frequently have a pattern that is almost all fat. A possible explanation is that in some individuals, if the skin cannot stretch and excess amounts of fat are deposited in the breast, the breast will become less compressible (Figs. 12-7 and 12-8).

It is clear that there is a general trend toward less dense breast tissue (a higher percentage of fat) with increasing age, but this is likely a combination of genetics (19), body habitus, and weight. An increase in fat content in the breast appears to be possible at virtually any age (Fig. 12-9). The actual role and interaction of hormones remain to be elucidated.

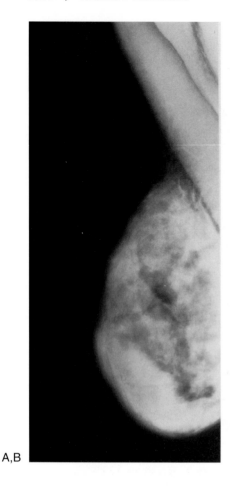 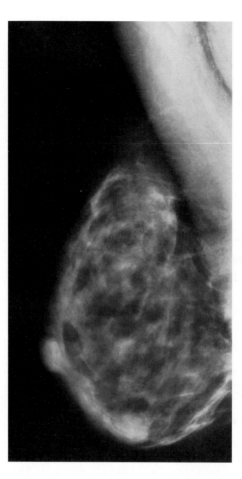

A,B

FIG. 12-9. This individual, aged 36 years, had extremely dense breast tissue **(A)**. By 39 years, she had gained a considerable amount of weight, and her breast tissues had a much higher proportion of fat **(B)**.

BREAST TISSUE (PARENCHYMAL) PATTERNS

Initial studies of the patterns of breast tissues seen by mammography were performed by Wolfe (20). His results suggested that women with dense tissues were at elevated risk for breast cancer. Although the dense tissues projected on the mammogram are primarily the shadows of the stromal elements as well as the parenchyma (the functioning glandular elements), the overall appearance of these tissues has been called the *parenchymal pattern*. There has been a great deal of misunderstanding concerning these patterns as they appear on the mammogram.

Although the system of dividing the patterns into four major types, first devised by Wolfe, is now widely used, it is clearly an oversimplification. There is a continuum that produces a broad spectrum of patterns, and indeed it is still unclear which patterns represent the normal breast or which, if any, are abnormal.

In 1967 Wolfe developed a classification of mammographic patterns by dividing breasts into four categories (20). Although the patterns are no longer classified using his labels, the general observations have remained. They have been adapted by the American College of Radiology (ACR) in the ACR Breast Imaging Reporting and Data System (BIRADS) as patterns 1 through 4. Wolfe labeled a breast

that was almost completely radiolucent because of a high proportion of fat as the N1 or normal breast (Fig. 12-10A). This was an arbitrary decision. Fewer than 50% of women have an N1 pattern, depending on the age of the population studied. Many cancers are found in N1 women. One might therefore question the validity of implying that this pattern is normal and the others abnormal.

Wolfe's second category included breasts that were predominantly fat by radiography but in which between 15% and 25% of the parenchyma demonstrated serpentine, beaded, or nodular densities. He believed that these densities corresponded to prominent ducts visible because of periductal collagenosis, although this has never been shown conclusively to be the case. Wolfe termed this the *P1 pattern* (Fig. 12-10B). When these beaded and nodular densities increased to occupy more than 25% of the parenchymal cone of the breast, the parenchyma was classified as having a P2 or prominent duct pattern (Fig. 12-10C). In fact, although these "nodular densities" often are ductal structures, Wellings and Wolfe (21) later showed that many of them may be related to the lobules and not the ducts, and this was confirmed in a later study that showed that the nodular densities are frequently due to intralobular proliferation.

Wolfe's fourth pattern classified the breast that was radiographically dense with relatively homogeneous sheets of

-D

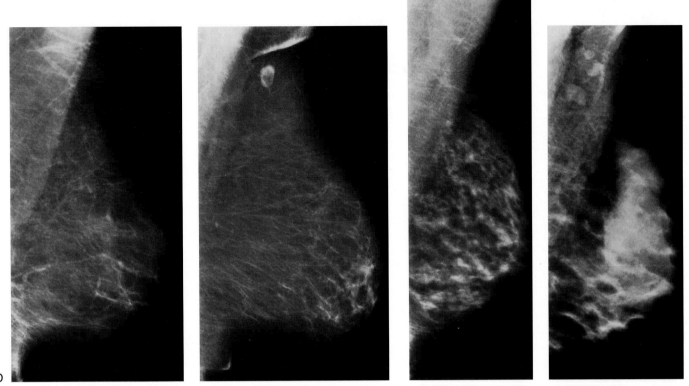

FIG. 12-10. (A) Wolfe's N1 type breast (now the American College of Radiology [ACR] pattern 1). Almost all of the tissue appears to be fat. **(B)** Wolfe's P1 type breast (now ACR pattern 2) with predominantly fat, but some (up to 25%) visible fibroglandular density. **(C)** Wolfe's P2 pattern (now ACR pattern 3), is heterogeneously dense with a large percentage (>25%) of the volume as visible fibroglandular tissue. **(D)** The most dense patterns were called DY by Wolfe (now ACR pattern 4). These are extremely dense and predominantly due to large percentages of fibrous connective tissue.

density occupying more than 25% of the volume of the parenchymal cone. He labeled this the *DY pattern*, insisting that it represented mammary dysplasia (Fig. 12-10D). This is a nonspecific term that has little true meaning, but it confused some into thinking that this was an abnormal state. In most series, approximately 25% to 30% of women fall into this category, and it would be unusual for this large number of women to have abnormal breasts. Wellings and Wolfe (21) showed that this diffuse density is usually due to the common finding of stromal fibrosis. Fibrous tissue is a major constituent of the breast and is probably the major component of radiographically visible densities.

In fact, the true histologic correlates of Wolfe's parenchymal patterns have never been clearly elucidated. The few histologic studies that have been undertaken (18,22) were influenced by the fact that the tissue sampled was from breast biopsies, which are, once again, by definition, abnormal. Thus, any extrapolation to the breast in general and the population as a whole is biased. In a study we performed in conjunction with the Harvard School of Public Health, we found that nodular densities on the mammogram actually represented the lobules of the breast and when prominent,

were frequently associated with intralobular hyperplasia (23). This study, too, was limited only to biopsy material.

As with any other x-ray analysis that relies predominantly on patterns of density and morphology, the underlying histology of these patterns is likely varied. The so-called prominent duct pattern is probably a conglomerate of histologies representing lobular as well as ductal structures. The diffuse densities in the breast in all probability relate to nonspecific fibrosis, a phenomenon that is extremely common in younger women. To suggest that this represents an abnormal state of "dysplasia" incorrectly oversimplifies and prejudices analysis when so many women have this pattern.

Tissue Patterns and Breast Cancer Risk

In 1979 Wolfe (24) suggested that the tissue pattern of the breast, as seen by mammography, might predict risk for developing breast cancer. He thought that the most dense patterns carried a much higher risk than did breasts that were predominantly fat. This report was followed by numerous studies, some supporting and some refuting the hypothesis. Although the actual level of risk varied enormously in

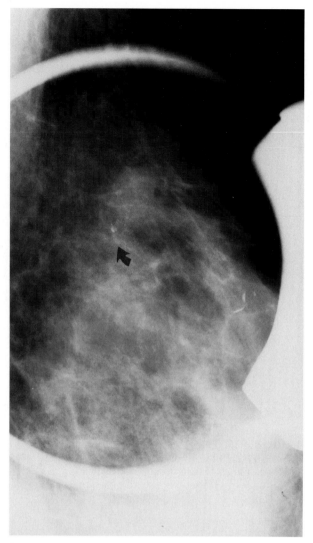

FIG. 12-11. As with many cancers, this one is at the periphery of the parenchymal cone.

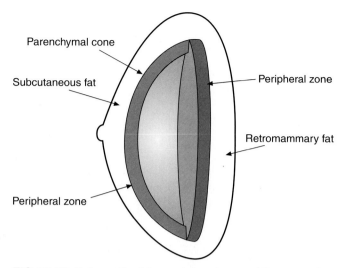

FIG. 12-12. Schematic of the peripheral zone of the parenchymal cone of the breast. More than 70% of cancers develop in this zone that is 1 cm deep beneath the subcutaneous fat and in front of the retromammary fat. This is likely because more than 50% of the breast tissue (by geometry) is in this zone.

the studies, there appeared to be a slightly increased risk for women with dense breast tissue. The most convincing data are from a review of the mammograms from the National Breast Screening Study of Canada. In that screening program, Boyd et al. (25) found that the risk for developing breast cancer was five times greater for women with dense breast tissue when compared to those with fatty tissue. The results seem to hold up even when the potential for masking is accounted for. Since cancers appear to occur in women with every tissue pattern, tissue density is not useful for deciding screening interval (unless intervals of less than 1 year are considered). The associations do raise interesting questions about the determinants of tissue patterns and how they might be related to risk.

Given that significant numbers of cancers occur in women in each pattern group, it is likely that there is a range of normal and that risk for any individual woman will never be determined from macroscopically visible factors, because most cancers are likely sporadic and develop in nor-

mal tissue. Nevertheless, some interesting associations between the dense mammographic patterns and the risk for developing breast cancer have been suggested, and work continues to try to determine these associations. It is possible that the gene or genes that are involved in breast tissue density are also related to cancer susceptibility.

Location of Breast Cancers

Many cancers develop at the periphery of the parenchyma beneath the interface between the subcutaneous fat or retromammary fat and the parenchymal cone of the breast (26) (Fig. 12-11). This is likely a probabilistic relationship because, based on plane geometry, in most breasts, more than 50% of the tissue lies in a 1-cm zone at the periphery of the glandular structures (Fig. 12-12). Since more than 70% of breast cancers detected by mammography alone lie in this zone, questions arise concerning other possible reasons. If carcinogens are held in breast fat, their proximity to the terminal ducts in these zones may play a role. Nevertheless, the radiologist should pay close attention to this zone.

Increasing Breast Tissue Density

It is unusual for the normal breast to increase in density, radiographically, over time. The most common reason for this is weight loss, with a crowding of the trabecular structures as fat is resorbed from the breast. The most dramatic changes in pattern are frequently due to weight changes as discussed in the section on Breast Variation with Age.

A second reason for increasing density in the breast is hormone replacement therapy (HRT). The use of exogenous estrogen can cause the radiographic density of the breast tis-

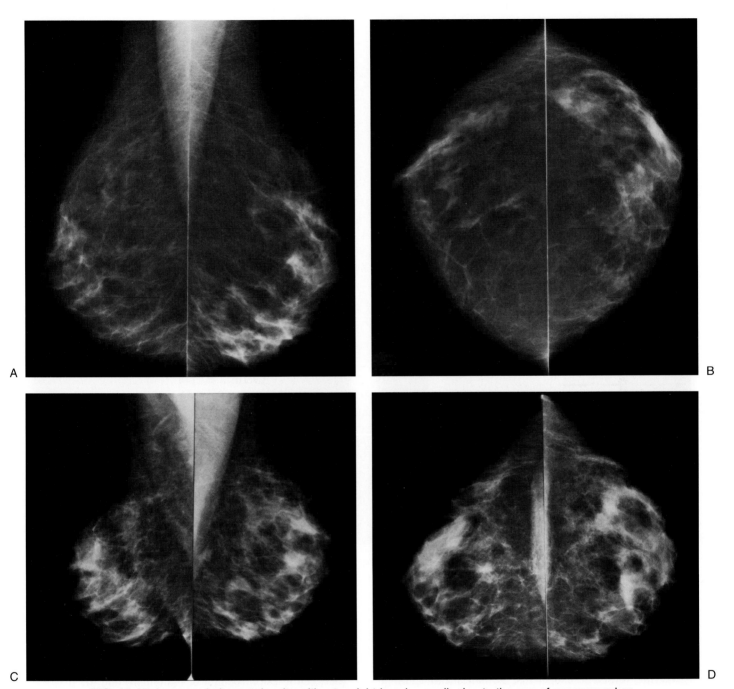

FIG. 12-13. Increase in breast density without weight loss is usually due to the use of exogenous hormones. This patient had premature menopause at 35 years and this mammogram at 38 years **(A, B)**. She was on hormone replacement therapy when this second mammogram was taken at 44 years, revealing increased parenchymal density **(C, D)**.

sues to increase in some women. A great deal of concern has been raised that HRT will cause increased density and mask breast cancers. This has not been the case in our practice. Although some studies with limited numbers of women have suggested that 17% to 27% of women will develop denser patterns with HRT (27–29), it has been our experience in evaluating more than 200 women that this happens less than 5% of the time, and for most women, there is no

increase in breast tissue density with the use of HRT. The differences in the study results may be due to the types, doses, and combinations of hormones used, but it does not seem to represent a major problem.

When exogenous hormones do cause changes, they may result in diffuse increases in tissue density (Fig. 12-13). The effect may be dramatic (Fig. 12-14). Although uncommon, we have also seen cysts develop in women on HRT. The

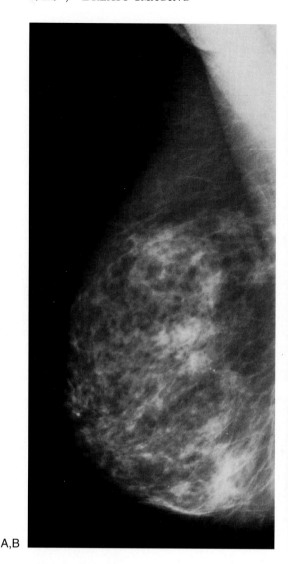
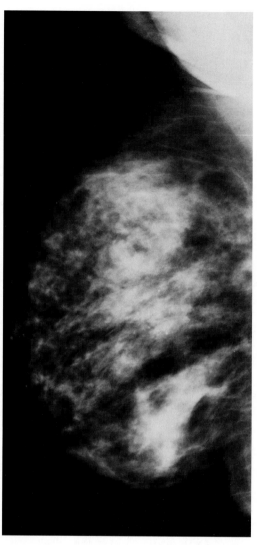

A,B

FIG. 12-14. This fairly striking increase in density from age 63 years **(A)** to age 65 years **(B)** is attributed to hormone replacement therapy.

development of a solitary density would be difficult to attribute to HRT, but if HRT is suspected, it might be reasonable to withdraw HRT for three months and evaluate any regression of the density. Clearly if the new density has malignant features, delay in diagnosis is not advised.

Varying forms of exogenous hormones can cause an increase in tissue density. Estrogen in vaginal creams is readily absorbed through the mucosa and can produce changes in the breast. The use of such creams should be noted in the history.

THE RADIOGRAPHICALLY DENSE BREAST

There has been much concern about the radiographically dense breast. It has never been accurately defined. We have used the term to indicate the mammographic appearance of a breast in which there is sufficient x-ray attenuation from normal breast structures that the ability of mammography to detect small cancers may be reduced because cancers may

be masked by the highly attenuating surrounding tissue. This is the same as the silhouette phenomenon that causes loss of the heart border with the silhouette sign in chest radiography. If tissues of the same x-ray attenuation abut one another and there is no discernible contrast difference between a lesion (benign or malignant) and the tissue surrounding it, the border will be invisible on the x-ray imaging. Tumor masses may be impossible to distinguish from normal connective tissues unless there is some distortion of the architecture or the there is deposition of calcium.

Many have failed to understand the significance of the radiographically dense breast. It is different from the breast that feels firm on physical examination. Intuitively one would expect small, firm breasts to be radiographically dense and large and soft breasts to be radiolucent. As noted earlier in the section called "Clinical Assessment Does Not Predict Radiographic Density," the size, consistency, and compressibility of the breast are unrelated to its radiographic density. Radiographic density is different from physical firmness. Two studies have now demonstrated that there is no relationship between the physical examination and tactile qualities of breast tissue and the radiographic appearance of those tissues. Physical parameters such as size, compressed thickness, and resistance to compression do not correlate with radiographic density (14,15).

The highest attenuators in the breast that are not calcium are the fibrous structures, which tend to be the extralobular connective tissues. These may be found in firm as well as soft breasts. One study suggests that it is breasts with high fat content (radiolucent) that are frequently the firmest, requiring higher pressures for compression during mammography (16).

As one would expect, density does correlate somewhat with body fat, but there are no accurate correlations that permit the prediction of radiographic density from physical parameters. Height and weight are perhaps the best predictors of radiographic density (30). Because the breast is a repository for fat, tall, thin women tend to have dense patterns, and short, heavy women tend to have lucent patterns, but even this is not a perfect correlation. This has practical implications in that technologists cannot be expected to be able to predict radiographic density, and photo-timing is required for optimal mammographic exposure control.

The only way to determine radiographic density and tissue patterns is from the mammogram itself. The lack of correlation between the characteristics of breast tissue on the clinical breast examination and those found on the mammogram explains the importance of the clinical breast examination as a part of screening. The two studies measure different tissue characteristics. The mammogram measures the density of the atomic groupings in the breast tissue, whereas the physical examination measures the resiliency and elasticity of the molecules formed by these atoms and forming the tissues. The mammographic measurement of tissue characteristics are different from those measured in the clinical breast examination. This accounts for why they are complementary studies, and each finds cancers that are not evident by the other.

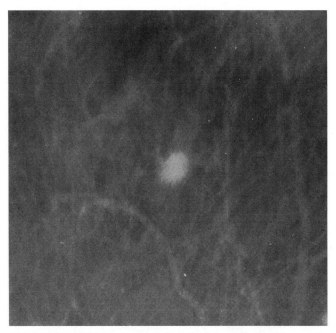

FIG. 12-15. This 6-mm invasive ductal carcinoma is easily visible because it is surrounded by fat tissue.

Cancer Detection and the Dense Breast

An understanding of breast tissue patterns as they apply to the sensitivity of mammographic detection of breast malignancy is important. The greater the amount of fat within the breast, the easier it is to recognize a water-density tumor (Fig. 12-15). As in any other x-ray study, the margins of a water-density cancer will be obscured or invisible when they are contiguous with normal tissue of equivalent x-ray attenuation (Fig. 12-16). In breasts in which the parenchyma is nonuniform, the x-ray attenuation will vary in a nonuniform way, making it difficult to detect a small cancer whose margins are similarly nonuniform. In the breast that is heterogeneously dense or extremely dense, the sensitivity of mammography, not only for

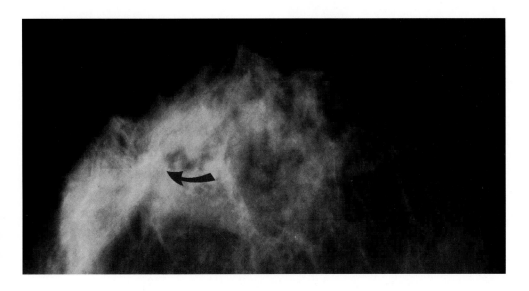

FIG. 12-16. This cancer is obscured by the dense tissues of the breast and was evident on the mammogram only because it distorted the architecture (*arrow*).

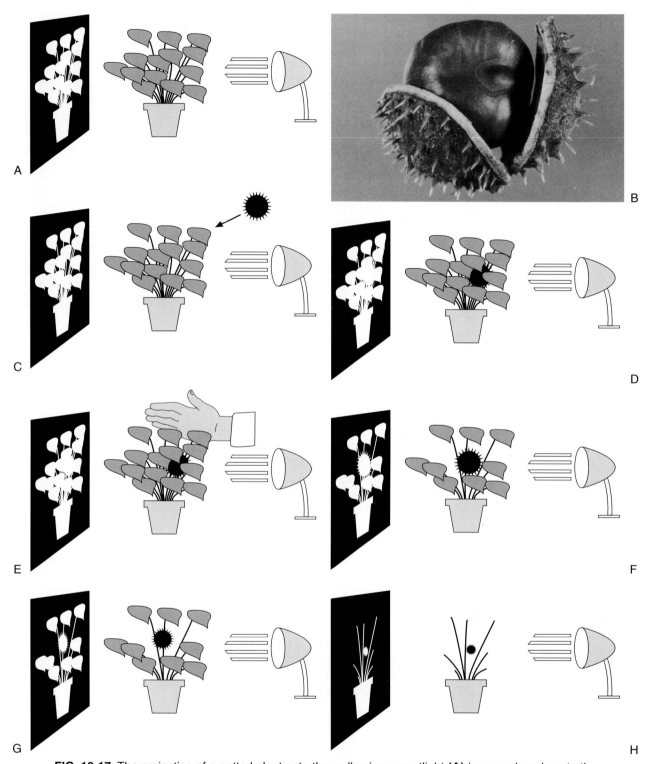

FIG. 12-17. The projection of a potted plant onto the wall using a spotlight **(A)** is a good analogy to the breast and cancer detection by clinical breast examination and mammography. Assume that a chestnut, with its prickly shell **(B)**, is placed in among the branches and leaves of the plant **(C)**. If the leaves are densely packed, the nut—even a very large one—may not be visible **(D)**, yet fingers pressed against it can easily feel it **(E)**. If the plant has fewer leaves, analogous to the breast with less fibrous tissue, then the nut becomes more visible **(F)**. If there are few leaves, then even a very small nut is visible **(G)**, and if an extremely small nut is nestled between the rigid stems of the plant, the nut may be easily visible, but not palpable because it is protected by the stems **(H)**.

the early detection of malignancy, but also for large cancers is somewhat diminished because of the difficulty of finding ill-defined cancers within the inhomogeneous background.

The fact that mammography can detect very small cancers but can also miss some very large cancers is confusing to clinicians and the public. Figure 12-17 is useful for explaining how mammography can detect many very small cancers, but some large palpable cancers can still be difficult to image.

The dense breast is not the only reason for overlooking cancers. It is of some interest that among cancers overlooked in the screening study in Nijmegen, the Netherlands (31), many cancers were overlooked in women with predominantly fatty breast tissue. Detecting small cancers in the dense breast is more difficult, but early-stage breast cancer can be detected by mammography among these women. In a review of 118 women with breast cancer detected by mammography alone (32), among women under the age of 50 years, we found that 70% were detected in women with radiographically dense breast tissue and these were at a smaller size and earlier stage than among women with palpable cancers. Even though a higher proportion of younger women have dense tissues, recent data from modern mammography screening programs show that mammography can detect early cancers among women aged 40 to 49 years at the same proportion as for women aged 50 to 59 years (33,34). The dense breast does reduce the sensitivity of mammography somewhat, but should not deter screening among these women and is not the sole cause for overlooking breast cancers.

Although disputed (35), it may be the masking of cancers by dense tissues that accounts for some of the apparent increase in risk attributed to tissue patterns. Cancers in women with the more lucent (fatty) patterns may have been found earlier and removed from the population before the data acquisition in which the excess risk appeared.

Acknowledging the fact that parenchymal densities may mask small cancers, the ACR BIRADS has adopted a similar system to that proposed by Wolfe, dividing breast patterns into four major groups (see Chapter 24):

1. Predominantly fat
2. Fat with some fibroglandular densities
3. Heterogeneously dense
4. Extremely dense

These are not used to suggest any particular risk for breast cancer but to alert the clinician that when the dense patterns are present, the sensitivity of mammography may be diminished (36). It is important to understand that although the dense patterns may reduce the sensitivity of mammography, early cancers may still be detected mammographically. Mammographic screening is still valuable in women with dense breast tissue.

CONCLUSION

A familiarity with the wide variation found on normal mammograms will assist the radiologist in determining when a finding is abnormal. Each step of the process—from obtaining the mammogram to its interpretation and communication of the results to the patient's physician—should be performed systematically, with an effort toward high quality and efficiency. Once an abnormality is appreciated, analysis should proceed in a systematic manner. Before recommending additional evaluation, the radiologist should determine how the next study will alter the course of management. Tests should not be ordered haphazardly, but with reason and specific goals in mind.

REFERENCES

1. Shapiro S, Venet W, Strax P, Venet L. Periodic Screening for Breast Cancer: The Health Insurance Plan Project and its Sequelae, 1963–1986. Baltimore: Johns Hopkins University Press, 1988.
2. Tabar L, Gad A, Holmberg LH, et al. Reduction in mortality from breast cancer after mass screening with mammography. Lancet 1985; 13:829–832.
3. Morrison AS, Brisson J, Khalid N. Breast cancer incidence and mortality in the breast cancer detection demonstration project. J Natl Cancer Inst 1988;80(19):17–24.
4. Tabar L, Gad A, Holmberg L, Ljungquist U. Significant reduction in advanced breast cancer, results of the first seven years of mammography screening in Kopparberg, Sweden. Diagn Imaging Clin Med 1985;54:158–164.
5. Kopans DB, Meyer JE, Cohen AM, Wood WC. Palpable breast masses: the importance of preoperative mammography. JAMA 1981;246:2819–2822.
6. Moskowitz M. Screening is not diagnosis. Radiology 1979;133:265–268.
7. Bird RE, McLelland R. How to initiate and operate a low-cost screening mammography center. Radiology 1986;161:43–47.
8. Love SM, Gelman RS, Silen W. Fibrocystic "disease" of the breast—a non-disease? N Engl J Med 1982;307:1010–1014.
9. Vogel P, Georgiade NG, Fetter BF, et al. The correlation of histologic changes in the human breast with the menstrual cycle. Am J Pathol 1981;104:23–34.
10. Harms SE, Flamig DP, Hesley KL, et al. Fat-suppressed three-dimensional MR imaging of the breast. Radiographics 1993;13:247–267.
11. Stomper PC, Cholewinski SP, Penetrante RB, et al. Atypical hyperplasia: frequency and mammographic and pathologic relationships in excisional biopsies guided with mammography and clinical examination. Radiology 1993;189:667–671.
12. Huston SW, Cowen PN, Bird CC. Morphometric studies of age related changes in normal human breast and their significance for evolution of mammary cancer. J Clin Pathol 1985;38:281–287.
13. Wolfe JN. Breast parenchymal patterns and their changes with age. Radiology 1976;121:545–552.
14. Stomper PC, D'Souza DJ, DiNitto PA, Arredondo MA. Analysis of parenchymal density on mammograms in 1,353 women 25–79 years old. AJR Am J Roentgenol 1996;167:1261–1265.
15. Prechtel K. Mastopathic und Altersabbangige Brustdrusen Verandernagen. Fortschr Med 1971;89:1312–1315.
16. Swann CA, Kopans DB, McCarthy KA, et al. Mammographic density and physical assessment of the breast. AJR Am J Roentgenol 1987; 148:525–526.
17. Boren WL, Hunter TB, Bjelland JC, Hunt KR. Comparison of breast consistency at palpation with breast density at mammography. Invest Radiol 1990;25:1010–1011.
18. Russell DG, Ziewacz J. Experimental investigation of tissue pressures that are developed within a breast compressed during mammography. Presented at the 79th Scientific Assembly and Annual Meeting of the Radiological Society of North America. Chicago, November 28–December 3, 1993.
19. Pankow JS, Vachon CM, Kuni CC, et al. Genetic analysis of mammographic breast density in adult women: evidence of a gene effect. J Natl Cancer Inst 1997;89:549–556.
20. Wolfe JN. A study of breast parenchyma by mammography in the normal woman and those with benign and malignant disease of the breast. Radiology 1967;89:201.

21. Wellings SR, Wolfe JN. Correlative studies of the histological and radiographic appearance of the breast parenchyma. Radiology 1978;129:299.
22. Fisher ER, Palekar A, Kim WS, et al. The histopathology of mammographic patterns. Am J Clin Pathol 1977;421:29.
23. Brisson J, Morrison AS, Burstein N, et al. Mammographic parenchymal patterns and histologic characteristics of breast tissue. Breast Disease 1989;1:253–260.
24. Wolfe JN. Breast patterns as an index of risk for developing breast cancer. AJR Am J Roentgenol 1976;126:1130–1139.
25. Boyd NF, Byng JW, Fishell EK, et al. Quantitative classification of mammographic densities and breast cancer risk: results from the Canadian National Breast Screening Study. J Natl Cancer Inst 1995;87:670–675.
26. Stacey-Clear A, McCarthy KA, Hall DA, et al. Observations on the location of breast cancer in women under fifty. Radiology 1993;186:677–680.
27. Berkowitz JE, Gatewood OMB, Goldblum LE, Gayler BW. Hormonal replacement therapy: mammographic manifestations. Radiology 1990;174:199–201.
28. Stomper PC, Van Voorhis BJ, Ravnikar VA, Meyer JE. Mammographic changes associated with postmenopausal hormone replacement therapy: a longitudinal study. Radiology 1990;174:487–490.
29. McNicholas MMJ, Heneghan JP, Milner MH, et al. Pain and increased mammographic density in women receiving hormone replacement therapy: a prospective study. AJR Am J Roentgenol 1994;163:311–315.
30. Brisson J, Morrison AS, Kopans DB, et al. Height, weight, mammographic features of breast tissue, and breast cancer risk. Am J Epidemiol 1984;119:371–381.
31. Peer PG, Holland R, Jan HCL, et al. Age-specific effectiveness of Nijmegen population-based breast cancer screening program: assessment of early indicators of screening effectiveness. J Natl Cancer Inst 1994;86:436–441.
32. Stacey-Clear A, McCarthy KA, Hall DA, et al. Breast cancer survival among women under age 50: is mammography detrimental? Lancet 1992;340:991–994.
33. Sickles EA, Kopans DB. Deficiencies in the analysis of breast cancer screening data. J Natl Cancer Inst 1993;85:1621–1624.
34. Clay MG, Hiskop G, Kan L, et al. Screening mammography in British Columbia 1988–1993. Am J Surg 1994;167:490–492.
35. Boyd NF, O'Sullivan B, Campbell JE, et al. Mammographic patterns and bias in breast cancer detection. Radiology 1982;143:671.
36. Bird RE, Wallace TW, Yankaskas BC. Analysis of cancers missed at screening mammography. Radiology 1992;184:613–617.

Breast Imaging, 2nd ed., by Daniel B. Kopans.
Lippincott–Raven Publishers, Philadelphia © 1998.

CHAPTER 13

Analyzing the Mammogram

By far the most important function of mammography is the earlier detection of breast cancer. The performance and acquisition of high-quality mammography is the key to the ability to accomplish this task. No amount of interpretive expertise can correct for the fact that the lesion is not imaged due to poor positioning, is hidden by underpenetrated tissue, or is overlooked because the image is blurred. Similarly, no observer is perfect, and all observers are subject to periodic failure to perceive a lesion that is visible in retrospect. Double reading should be encouraged, but it must be accomplished efficiently so that there is no significant increase in cost. Double reading reduces the false-positive rate, but if women are denied access to screening because of increased cost the benefit of double reading is lost. A systematic approach to the entire process improves efficiency (see Chapter 11), maintains quality, and helps to diagnose breast cancers earlier.

BATCH AND DOUBLE READING

Interpreting screening studies in batches can reduce the cost by maximizing the radiologist's productivity. The disadvantage of the patient's not having an immediate report is more than offset by the reduced expense and the added advantage that reading mammograms on an alternator permits double reading. As has been shown in the interpretation of chest x-rays, there is a psychovisual phenomenon that guarantees that all radiologists will periodically fail to perceive significant abnormalities (1). Mammographic interpretation is no exception. Because different readers overlook different findings, having more than one reader interpret a mammogram reduces the error rate. Interpreting mammograms on an alternator permits multiple reviewers with little increase in cost. In our own experience, double reading in this fashion increased our breast cancer detection rate by 7%. Bird found that a second reviewer increased the cancer detection rate by 5% (2), and Tabar has reported as high as a 15% improvement in cancer detection with double reading (3). This increased yield from double reading has also been documented by Thurfjell and colleagues (4).

DETECTION, DIAGNOSIS, AND DIAGNOSTIC ACCURACY

Mammography is invaluable in the detection of anomalies in the breast, but it is less suited for the differentiation of those anomalies into benign or malignant diagnostic categories. As breast imaging techniques have evolved, a better understanding of the underlying histopathologic changes that account for some of the mammographic findings has developed. Nevertheless, the problem remains that the diagnosis (in the true sense of the word) of many lesions, based on imaging criteria, often defies the high levels of certainty required if a tissue diagnosis is to be avoided. In view of the important consequences of early breast cancer detection and the high level of safety in obtaining a tissue diagnosis, the accuracy of a noninvasive diagnostic study should approach 100%.

Despite uncertainties, criteria have been established to assist in diagnosis. Before the instigation of an invasive procedure it is important to analyze and categorize anomalies in the breast so that appropriate action can be taken. Mammography and appropriate diagnostic techniques, such as ultrasound for differentiating cysts from solids, should be used to maximize the diagnosis of early cancers and reduce the need to biopsy benign lesions whenever possible.

FILM REVIEW

The acquisition and interpretation of mammograms should be undertaken in an organized and structured fashion (see Chapter 11). High-quality mammography is required, and the images should be viewed in an appropriate environment with reduced ambient light and good viewing conditions. Films should be reviewed using a consistent viewing scheme. The radiologist should systematically search the images for masses, calcifications, areas of asymmetry, architectural distortion, and changes from previous studies when they are available. Interpretive decisions should be based on established thresholds for intervention, and the interpreter should have reproducible and consistent reasons for interpretive decisions.

VIEW BOX ANALYSIS

The View Box

The viewing conditions for mammography are important. Although ideal viewing conditions have never been scientifically determined, there are general principles that apply. When reviewing modern, high-contrast films with a high maximum film density, bright backlighting is desirable. In general, the light output of a mammography view box should probably be twice as bright as a standard lightbox. Although there have never been any truly scientific studies of the appropriate light output, Haus found that five experts use view boxes with approximately 3,500 nits (candela/m^2) of light output to view high-contrast images (5).

Because extraneous light reduces the eyes' ability to perceive low-contrast objects, the images should be masked. Masking ensures that glare from around the images, which can dramatically interfere with visualization of details on the mammogram, is eliminated as much as possible. Ambient light also compromises viewing, and reading rooms should have low light levels. The view boxes used by the technologists should be matched to those used by the radiologists so that properly exposed mammograms appear the same, facilitating quality control.

Positioning Films on the View Boxes

The films should be positioned in a standard and consistent fashion on the view box. They should be placed the same way each time to minimize left-right confusion. Most reviewers find that it is preferable to match the mediolateral oblique (MLO) images from each breast and place them back to back as mirror images and to position the craniocaudal (CC) views base to base as mirror images with the lateral (axillary) portions of both at the top. Although the convention is to place the mammograms as if the patient were facing the viewer,

many reviewers prefer to have the dull emulsion side up to minimize reflection from the nonemulsion surface. This places the left breast on the left and the right on the right.

If there are two banks of view boxes, we place the new films on the bottom row with older films above (Fig. 13-1), although the specific arrangement of the films is up to the preference of the interpreter. Because subtle changes may not be apparent from one year to the next, we routinely compare films from two or more years earlier with the present study.

Quality Control at the View Box

Checking the Positioning

The images should first be evaluated with respect to quality. The breasts should ideally have been positioned sym-

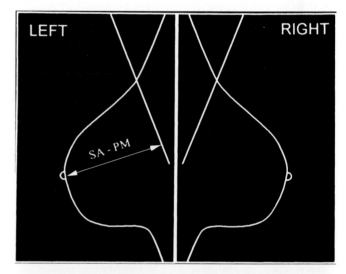

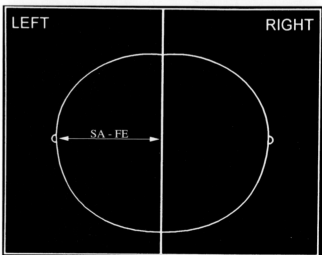

FIG. 13-2. Schematic showing the posterior nipple line in the two standard projections. The distance from the subareolar region (SA) to pectoralis major (PM) on the mediolateral oblique should be no more than 1 cm longer than the distance SA to the film edge (FE) on the craniocaudal view.

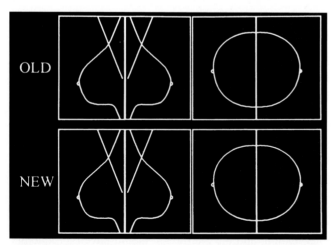

FIG. 13-1. To avoid confusion, the **films should be arranged the same way each time.**

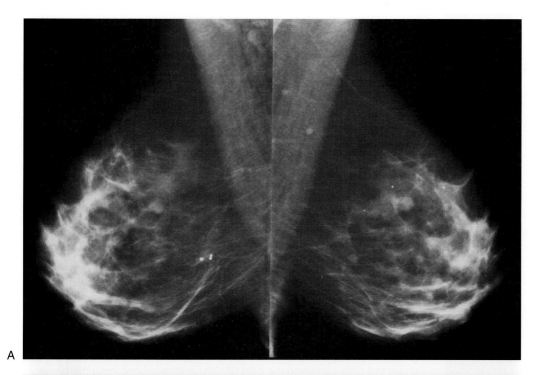

A

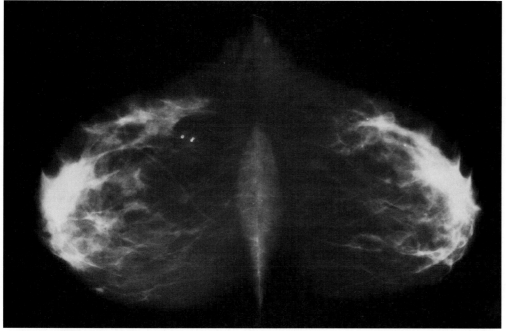

B

FIG. 13-3. The breasts should be symmetrically positioned with the breast pulled up and out to open the inframammary fold, as on these mediolateral oblique **(A)** projections. The pectoralis major muscle is visible on approximately 30% of craniocaudal projections, as it is here **(B)**. *Continued.*

metrically for the exposures. The technologist should have tried to maximize the amount of tissue projected onto the detector. The nipple should be in profile, if possible. This is not an absolute requirement: If, to position the breast to maximally visualize the breast tissues, the nipple goes out of profile, the visualization of the tissues takes precedence. If there is a question of a subareolar mass versus the nipple, an additional view of the subareolar tissues with the nipple in profile will clear up any confusion.

Eklund and Cardenosa have described measurements that provide some indication that the maximum tissue to be

imaged is on the films (6). Habitus and patient infirmities may preclude optimal positioning, but there are some goals for which to strive. On most mammograms, the pectoralis major muscle should be visible down to the level of the axis of the nipple on the MLO projection (see Chapter 10), and the distance from immediately beneath the nipple to the edge of the film on the CC view should usually be within 1 cm of the distance from under the nipple to the pectoralis major on the MLO (Fig. 13-2) (7). The breasts should be pulled upward and out, not drooping, and the trabecular structures should be separated by firm compression. Ideally

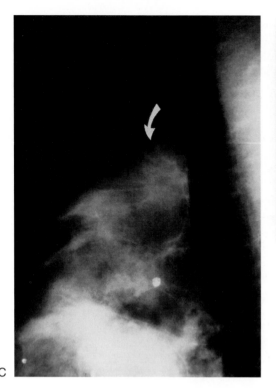

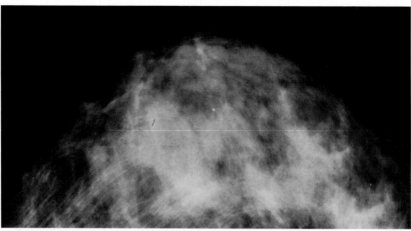

C

D

FIG. 13-3. *Continued.* **Proper penetration is important.** The cancer (*arrow*) on this mediolateral oblique projection **(C)** would not have been seen had the tissue not been properly penetrated.

The curvilinear lines that project over the medial portion of the left breast on this craniocaudal projection **(D)** are due to the **patient's hair** slipping under the tube cone into the field of view and projecting onto the breast.

the junction with the upper abdomen should be visible with the inframammary fold open and no overlap of breast and upper abdomen (Fig. 13-3A). On approximately 30% of the CC projections, the pectoralis major muscle should be visible at the back of the breast (Fig. 13-3B).

Penetration

To see lesions in dense fibroglandular tissue, the x-ray beam should be sufficiently energetic to penetrate these tissues. Although it has never been documented scientifically, many radiologists believe that the dense portions of the breast should be penetrated so that they measure approximately 0.8 or higher on a densitometer. This is a level at which structures can be seen through the dense (white) portions of the mammograms (Fig. 13-3C).

Blur

There are many causes of blur or unsharpness on an image. Blur due to motion of the breast during the exposure is often difficult to appreciate. Most breasts have at least one calcification, and observation of the sharpness or lack of sharpness of calcifications may indicate a motion problem.

Tissue Inclusion

Given the geometry of the breast and chest wall it is likely that some breast tissues will be missed no matter

how well the patient is positioned. Nevertheless, the goal of every mammogram should be to image as much tissue as possible with high spatial and contrast resolution. The criteria described above are optimal. Individual patients vary, and it is usually not possible to accomplish ideal positioning in every projection for all women. For example, visualization of the pectoralis major muscle on the CC view is expected in only 30% of mammograms. Although it is rare that all of the positioning criteria are met, the technologist should strive to accomplish optimal positioning with each exposure.

Artifacts

Although it is almost impossible to eliminate all artifacts, efforts should be made to reduce them to a minimum. The screens should be cleaned at least once a week to eliminate dust that can block the light from the screen from reaching the film and cause bright specks that simulate microcalcifications. Scratches on the screen or on the film can cause pseudolesions or distract from seeing real lesions. Unusual artifacts usually have a simple explanation (Fig. 13-3D).

MAMMOGRAPHIC INTERPRETATION

The observer should avoid the urge to immediately view mammograms "up close." It is preferable to sit back and view the images from a distance, bringing foveal vision to bear on the entire image. Some observers find the use of a minifying lens beneficial to reduce the size of the images. This aids in appreciating areas of asymmetry.

The images should then be viewed from a distance of 1 to 1½ feet to begin evaluating some of the tissue details. Finally, the observer should evaluate the mammograms so as to view the subtle details. Although all structures visible on the mammogram can be seen with the unaided eye, a magnifying glass is helpful to make small detail more obvious.

The images should be systematically reviewed with particular attention to the deep tissues, especially near the inframammary fold and high in the axilla (tumors are often overlooked here). Because most cancers develop at the interface between the edge of the parenchyma and the subcutaneous and retromammary fat (8), these tissues should be evaluated for architectural distortion, masses, or calcifications.

Calcifications

There is a tendency to concentrate on looking for calcifications because they are such specific, high-contrast structures. The interpreter should realize that, although significant calcifications are important to find and often represent early intraductal cancer, it is the small invasive cancers that are most important to find before they become 1 cm in size. Invasive cancers are potentially lethal, and prognosis is improved if they can be treated while they are ≤1 cm in size (9,10). The analysis should include a search for small masses and areas of architectural distortion.

Review of Old Films

If old films are available, comparison is important to search for any changes. If the patient has been studied previously at another center, she should be urged to obtain and bring her old films with her at the time of her examination. If she does not bring these films, an effort should be made to obtain them if the present study suggests an abnormality. If the present study is unremarkable, obtaining outside films adds little advantage. Bassett and associates, in a review of 1,432 cases in which 87% had previous films, found that clinical management was altered in 35 of the 1,093 cases where the previous films were located. Of the seven biopsies that were performed as a result, two cases of cancer that would have been missed without the previous mammograms were diagnosed. The two cancers were detected because of changes between mammograms from their own facility. Their estimated cost for obtaining the 134 outside studies, of the 274 that they requested, amounted to $12.52 per study (postage and labor) with an average delay of 43 days before the outside studies arrived. The outside studies resulted in the avoidance of six workups and one biopsy (11).

Although it is preferable to have all previous studies, given the difficult logistics of obtaining outside studies, the delays involved, the cost, and the marginal benefit (as well as the frequency with which loaned films are lost), we confine our efforts to obtaining outside films when there is a management need for them. As noted, we request that all women obtain their outside studies and bring them in to their appointment, but if the mammogram is negative we do not routinely seek outside films.

Neodensities

Fortunately, the mammographic appearance of the breast is fairly stable from year to year. Changes such as the development of new masses (neodensities) or new calcifications should be analyzed to determine their significance. It is a good idea to compare studies that are at least 2 years apart because changes may not be as apparent from one year to the next (Fig. 13-4).

In general a new focal abnormality warrants careful review and often requires ultrasound (for cyst/solid differentiation) or tissue evaluation (needle biopsy or open biopsy) as needed to make a diagnosis. The development of multiple (three or more) similar findings in noncontiguous areas usually represents a benign change, almost always cysts.

ANALYZING LESIONS DETECTED BY MAMMOGRAPHY

See also Chapters 14 and 23.

Problems can be avoided if the interpreter follows a simple approach to the images (see Chapter 11): (1) Find it. (2) Is it real? (3) Where is it? (4) What is it? (5) What should be done about it?

Find It

The major effort in screening is to detect cancer earlier. Breast cancer usually presents as one or a combination of the following (see Chapter 15):

- Neodensity or new calcifications
- Mass
- Calcifications: focal or segmental
- Asymmetry: focal or more diffuse asymmetric density
- Architectural distortion
- Skin changes
- Trabecular changes
- Nipple changes
- Axillary nodal abnormalities

The mammograms should be reviewed to detect areas that have changed or developed since previous studies (neodensities or new calcifications), as well as masses, calcifications, architectural distortion, focal asymmetry, and areas of diffuse asymmetry. Any suspicious finding should be assessed to determine whether it is real and to determine its location and significance and what the next step should be in its management (see Chapters 11 and 24).

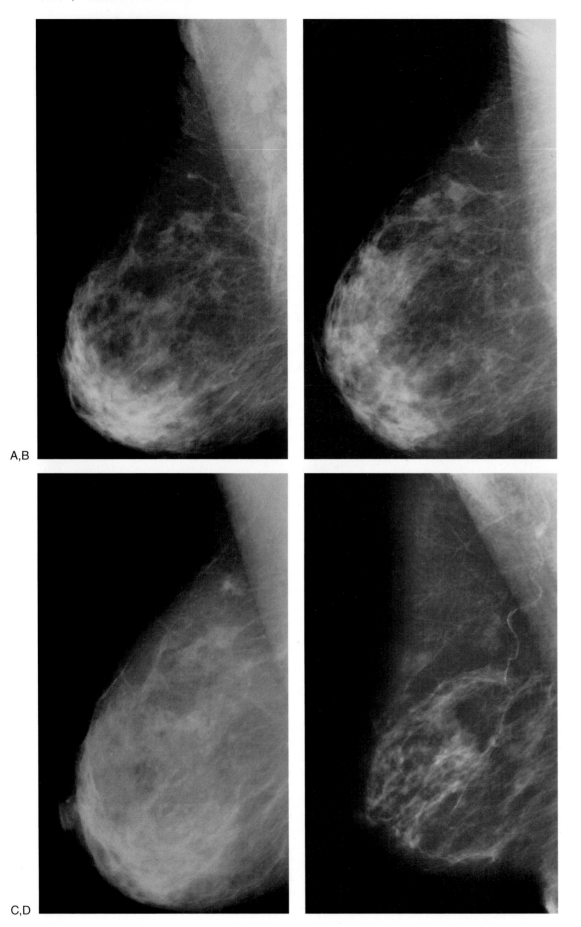

A,B

C,D

FIG. 13-4. If possible the present study should be compared to a comparable study from 2 or more years earlier. (A), (B) For example, the changes between these two studies, obtained 1 year apart, are subtle and difficult to appreciate, as are the changes between B and (C). C was obtained 1 year after B. The small cancer at the top of the breast is best appreciated by comparing A and C. In a second patient, subtle progressive changes are evident as the invasive lobular and ductal cancer grows slowly from 1990 until it is obvious in 1994. The subtle changes that occurred from year to year are more apparent if the progressive studies are compared to the first year. The first mediolateral oblique is from 1990 (D), the second is from 1991 (E), the third from 1992 (F), and the last from when the patient returned following a 2-year interval in 1994 (G), at which time the cancer is obvious. The corresponding craniocaudal projections are 1990 (H), 1991 (I), 1992 (J), and 1994 (K).

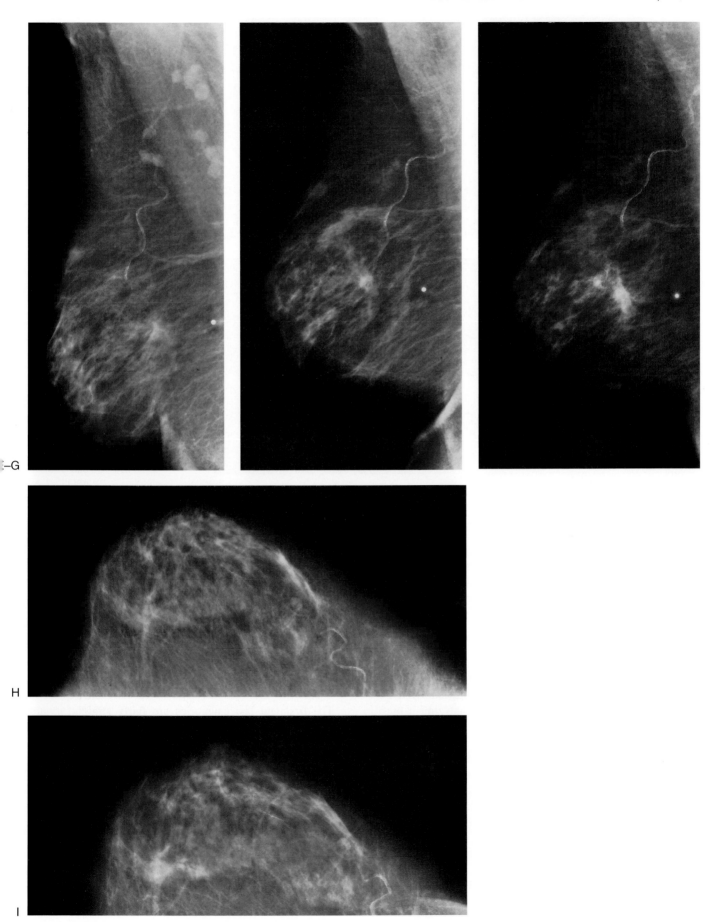

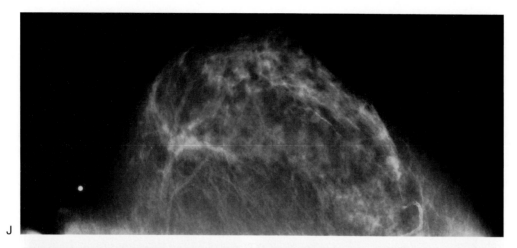

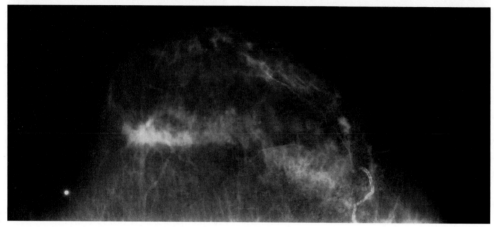

Is It Real? If So, Where Is It?

Many anomalies that are detected prove to be pseudo-lesions and are merely overlapping normal structures. Either using the standard screening images, or additional views, the radiologist should determine first if a finding is real, and second where it is, three-dimensionally, in the breast.

What Should Be Done About It?

Much of what is detected by mammography proves to be benign. Once an anomaly has been detected and shown to be three-dimensionally real, the first step in analyzing it is to try to determine if it can be categorized as a benign finding. If its morphology clearly indicates a normal structure or a benign process, further evaluation is unnecessary (see Chapter 14). If it is not clearly benign, analysis should proceed.

The interpreter should have specific reasons for rendering a specific interpretation. Thresholds for intervention and guidelines should be defined so that analysis is not based on subjective assessment but on objective criteria. For example, it is not sufficient to say "I think these are benign calcifications." One should be able to explain why they are categorized as such (e.g., they are smooth, round, >1 mm, and have lucent centers). These are benign characteristics that support the interpretation.

The observer should assign an assessment that meets one of the five categories that conform to the Breast Imaging Reporting and Data System (BIRADS).

1. The mammogram is negative with no abnormality seen.
2. There is a benign finding.
3. There is a finding that is probably benign, but short-interval follow-up is suggested because stability over a period of time will provide additional reassurance.
4. Indeterminate: There is a finite probability of malignancy, and biopsy should be considered.
5. There is a very high probability of malignancy.

The first and last categories are fairly straightforward. Benign changes require no further evaluation. Changes suggesting malignancy require intervention.

USE OF MAGNIFICATION MAMMOGRAPHY

There are no data other than anecdotal that many of the high-probability lesions found on the screening contact mammograms require additional evaluation other than a tissue diagnosis. Some interpreters suggest that, in cases in which conservation therapy (lumpectomy and radiation therapy) is to be used, additional evaluation of high-probability lesions should involve magnification views in an attempt to better define the extent of a lesion (multifocality) (12) or to search for multicentricity. Although magnification does improve the visibility of structures, it is rare, with modern mammographic techniques, to find additional abnormalities on the magnification images that were unsuspected on the conventional contact study. Consequently, that magnification may not be routinely needed.

It is likely that if whole breast magnification could be accomplished, more early cancers would be detected, but although magnification mammography is valuable for improving mammographic sharpness its value in evaluating targeted areas of the breast has to some extent been exaggerated. Because magnification results in decreased noise, the margins of masses are better seen and the morphology of calcifications is sometimes clearer. We assume that this improved sharpness has a benefit, but there have been no prospective film/screen studies to establish the need for magnification in most cases.

WHEN IS ADDITIONAL EVALUATION WARRANTED?

There has been a certain bandwagon effect of educators stressing the need to work up a finding as mindless exercise rather than having specific reasons for additional evaluation leading to documented benefit. As with any medical test, when suggesting or performing additional evaluation, the radiologist should ask two questions:

1. How is the next test going to alter the care of the patient?
2. How will the results of the next test benefit the patient?

Whether choosing extra views, magnification, or ultrasound, the radiologist should be able to answer these questions with specific reasons for the workup. If there is no benefit for the patient, then the additional test is of no value.

Searching for Multifocality

When a tumor has been excised, the mammographic demonstration of calcifications adjacent to the tumor bed can suggest the presence of residual cancer. Dershaw and associates (13) studied a group of 43 women whose breast cancers had associated microcalcifications that were mammographically visible. In addition to their primary excision, these women underwent re-excision of the cancer site for suspected residual disease. The investigators found that residual calcifications on the mammogram, consistent with those evident on the preoperative magnification mammograms, correctly predicted residual intraductal cancer (ductal carcinoma in situ [DCIS]) tumor in 20 of 29 women. In 31% of the women, these calcifications were due to benign processes and constituted false positives. Among the 13 women in whom no residual calcifications were seen, four were found to have residual tumor for a false-negative rate of 31%, demonstrating once again that mammography cannot be used to exclude residual cancer.

Significance of Residual Calcifications

If cancer is present, magnification may demonstrate additional calcifications that are indicative of tumor in ducts. It has been postulated that these should all be resected in an effort to excise all gross tumor and reduce the likelihood of failure. The prediction of recurrences within the breast, however, have all been related to pathologically evident tumor at the resection margin. The significance of residual calcifications by mammography can only be postulated. Although excision of all visible calcifications might seem to make sense, there are in fact only indirect data that suggest that this influences recurrence rates in the breast. There are no data that show that overall mortality is affected if all the mammographically evident calcifications are not resected.

The data do indicate that residual calcifications following excision of a cancer that had associated calcifications strongly suggest residual disease. The benefit of excising these calcifications has been derived by combining several observations. The issue revolves around the ability of radiation to destroy remaining cancer cells after surgical removal of the bulk of the tumor. Because radiation kills in a logarithmic fashion, with each treatment killing a percentage of the tumor that remains, the goal of surgery is to eliminate as many tumor cells as possible so that the radiation can eliminate any remnants. Some invasive breast cancers are associated with a large component of tumor that extends through the ducts. This has been termed *extensive intraductal component* (EIC). Some data suggest that women with cancers and EIC who are treated with adjuvant radiation therapy have a higher risk of recurrence of cancer in the breast (14). This is likely the result of excessive residual tumor burden and not any inherent resistance of intraductal cancer to radiation.

By extrapolation it has been suggested that, because EIC predicts for higher local recurrence and residual calcifications indicate residual intraductal carcinoma, residual calcifications that are not excised might predict for a higher recurrence rate. This has not been confirmed directly. Although most therapy is directed at eradicating all tumor from the breast, it is not apparent that this influences the ultimate prognosis, and the necessity of removing all calcifications associated with a cancer remains, intuitively, a good idea, although scientifically unproved. We nonetheless recommend that all tissue containing malignant-appearing calcifications be removed.

FINDINGS THAT MAY STIMULATE ADDITIONAL EVALUATION

Indeterminate Lesions

If the morphologic features of a finding cannot be characterized as indicating a benign, or probably benign, process, then the lesion is indeterminate. Within the indeterminate category of findings on mammography, there is a broad spectrum of possibilities. Probabilities range from lesions

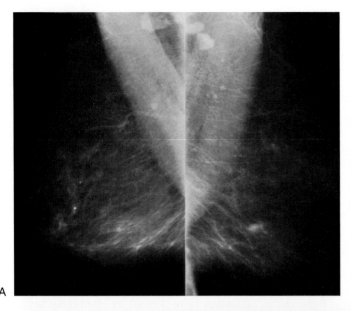

A

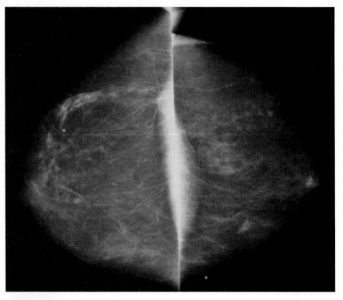

B

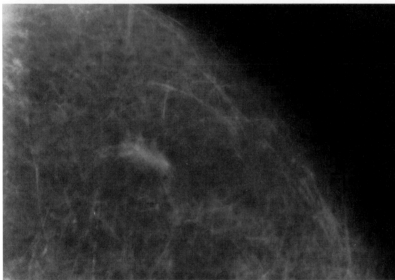

C

FIG. 13-5. Three-dimensionally real, focal asymmetries should be evaluated. (A) There is a focal asymmetry in the right breast toward the bottom on the right mediolateral oblique and medial on the craniocaudal (CC) view **(B)**. On the magnification mammogram, in the CC projection, the spiculated margin of this invasive ductal carcinoma is evident **(C)**.

with <5% likelihood of malignancy to those with >50% probability. Additional evaluation using special views, especially magnification, may be useful to better refine the morphologic characteristics of the lesion. It is possible with sufficient data to develop probabilities for a specific type of lesion. As data accumulate, practices with sufficient experience can provide to a patient and her physician probabilities that are sufficiently accurate that the patient and her physician can make a more informed decision as to whether to follow a lesion or to excise it.

Focal Mammographic Abnormalities

Asymmetry

Normally the breasts are fairly symmetric on a mammogram. Asymmetry may be indicative of a significant process; each mammogram should be assessed for the presence of asymmetries.

Focal Asymmetric Density versus Asymmetric Breast Tissue

Many asymmetries are visible by mammography. A three-dimensional, real, focal asymmetry may represent a mass that could be significant, whereas asymmetric breast tissue is a normal variation.

Mammographic interpretation includes the search for asymmetries. The breasts should be compared as symmetric organs. One may be larger than the other, but the internal structures are usually quite symmetric over broad areas of analysis. There are typically small areas that are not mirror images, but the distribution of tissues is usually fairly symmetric. When asymmetric areas are present, the observer must determine whether these are true asymmetries or merely the

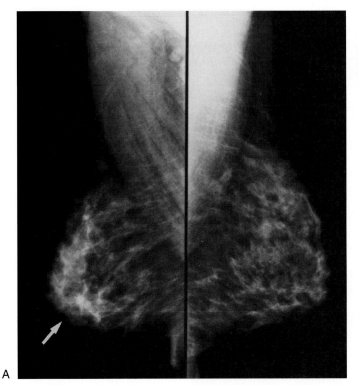

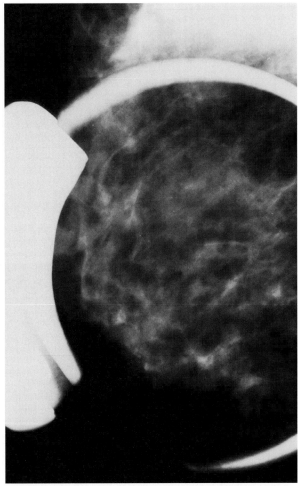

A

B

FIG. 13-6. What appears to be a spiculated area seen only on the mediolateral oblique projection **(A)** (*arrow*) proved to be a **superimposition of normal structures** when the area was compressed with the spot compression device **(B)**. *Continued.*

result of differences in positioning or compression. True asymmetries are three-dimensionally real and present in both projections (Fig. 13-5). Overlapping tissue structures that form summation shadows and normal tissue variations are the most common form of unimportant asymmetries (Fig. 13-6).

If an asymmetric density is three-dimensionally real, then the observer must decide whether or not the asymmetry is due to focal, benign asymmetric breast tissue or a true focal asymmetry that could represent a significant mass. The former is a normal variant as discussed in the next section; the latter requires further evaluation. Usually the distinction is easily made by "dissecting" the components of the finding on the mammogram that comprise the asymmetric volume and concluding that it is composed of unrelated, superimposed structures. Spot compression mammography, rolled views, or changing the angle of the x-ray beam may help spread or reorient tissue structures to determine whether or not a mass is present (see Chapter 22).

Focal Asymmetric Density

The perception of a focal asymmetric density is usually an initial assessment. It is the first impression that draws the observer's eye. It may, in fact, be a mass, but until it is cate-

gorized more completely it is perceived because its mirror image counterpart is lacking in the other breast.

A focal asymmetric density must first be distinguished from asymmetric breast tissue. The asymmetric density that should be considered suspicious is usually smaller than asymmetric breast tissue, and the density is concentrated toward its center. Unlike asymmetric normal tissue, the suspicious asymmetric density appears to be forming a mass with a dense central zone with density tapering toward its periphery (Fig. 13-7). The finding becomes more suspicious when it is present in two projections and when the density is not diffuse, but rather concentrated around a point in the breast (Fig. 13-8). A focal asymmetric density is a three-dimensional structure with definable margins that either fade into the surrounding tissue or are obscured by them.

Once the observer's attention is directed toward asymmetric density, on closer inspection it may become apparent that it actually represents a suspicious mass. Spot compression may help separate overlying structures, pressing the tissue closer to the film to better define the margins of the lesion. Magnification mammography may show that the margins of an asymmetry are irregular or spiculated. A focal asymmetric density that is, three-dimensionally, more

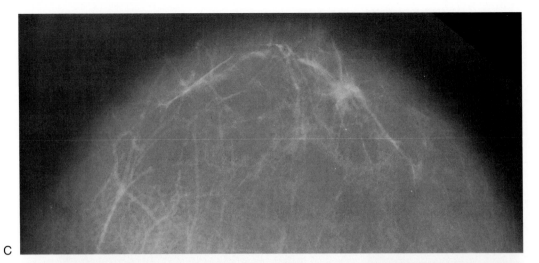

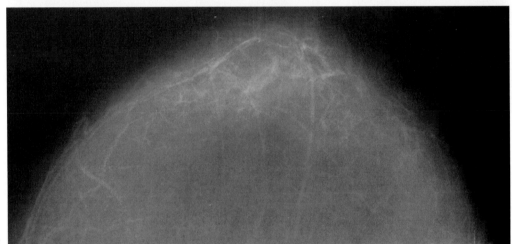

FIG. 13-6. *Continued.* In this second patient there appears to be a spiculated lesion lateral to the nipple on the craniocaudal projection **(C)**, but when the breast was rolled slightly to reorient the structures **(D)**, it is clear that the original "lesion" was due to **superimposed, normal structures.**

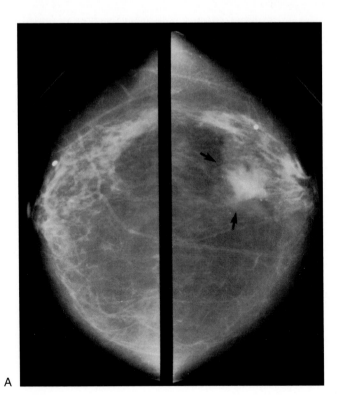

FIG. 13-7. **Breast cancer that presents as asymmetry usually presents with the density concentrated centrally in the asymmetry.** (A) This cancer is first perceived as a focal asymmetric density on the craniocaudal projection with the density concentrated centrally (*arrows*) and fading toward the periphery of the tissue volume. **A focal asymmetry should draw the observer's attention.** *Continued.*

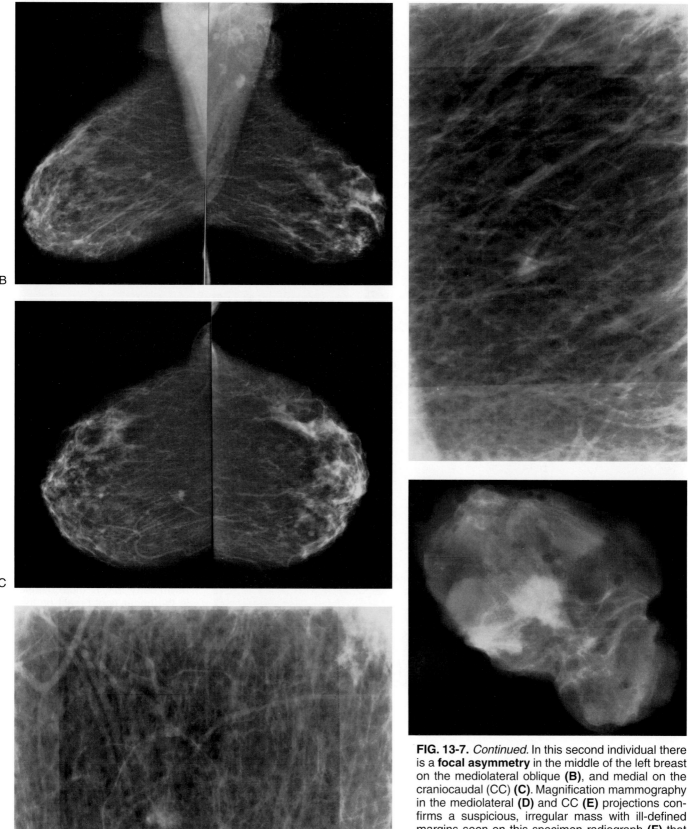

FIG. 13-7. *Continued.* In this second individual there is a **focal asymmetry** in the middle of the left breast on the mediolateral oblique **(B)**, and medial on the craniocaudal (CC) **(C)**. Magnification mammography in the mediolateral **(D)** and CC **(E)** projections confirms a suspicious, irregular mass with ill-defined margins seen on this specimen radiograph **(F)** that proved to be an invasive ductal carcinoma with associated ductal carcinoma in situ at biopsy.

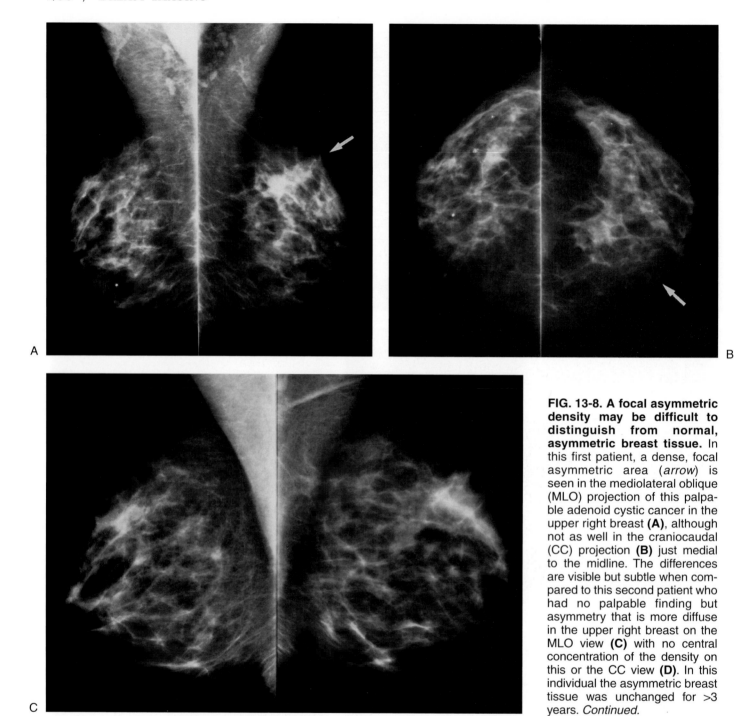

FIG. 13-8. **A focal asymmetric density may be difficult to distinguish from normal, asymmetric breast tissue.** In this first patient, a dense, focal asymmetric area (*arrow*) is seen in the mediolateral oblique (MLO) projection of this palpable adenoid cystic cancer in the upper right breast **(A)**, although not as well in the craniocaudal (CC) projection **(B)** just medial to the midline. The differences are visible but subtle when compared to this second patient who had no palpable finding but asymmetry that is more diffuse in the upper right breast on the MLO view **(C)** with no central concentration of the density on this or the CC view **(D)**. In this individual the asymmetric breast tissue was unchanged for >3 years. *Continued.*

attenuating than the normal breast tissue and that does not merely represent a superimposition of structures should be considered suspicious and warrants biopsy.

Asymmetric Breast Tissue

Breast tissue asymmetry can be the result of either a greater volume of fibroglandular tissue on one side or greater density to the tissue relative to the mirror image area in the other breast. Asymmetric breast tissue should be distinguished from a focal asymmetric density. The latter may prove to be a true mass, whereas the former is merely a normal variation.

Asymmetric breast tissue is a term that should be reserved for broad areas of greater parenchymal volume or greater radiographic density of the tissue that do not form a mass but that are distinctly different from the corresponding contralateral volume of tissue. By definition, in asymmetric breast tissue, the architecture of the breast is maintained, the underlying tra-

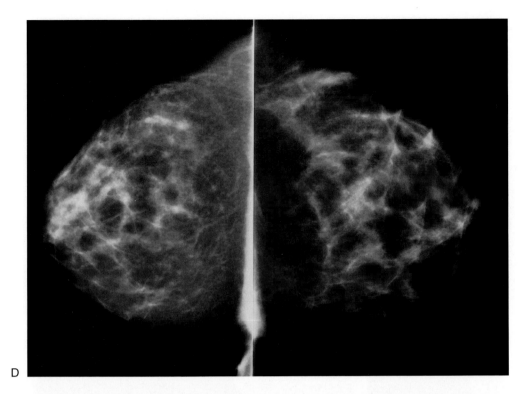

D

FIG. 13-8. *Continued.*

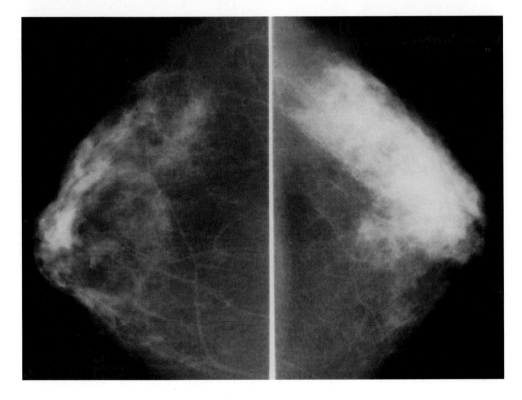

FIG. 13-9. Benign, asymmetric breast tissue, as seen in the lateral right breast on these craniocaudal projections, **has no architectural distortion, no suggestion of mass formation, and no significant calcifications. If there is no corresponding palpable asymmetry and it has not appeared over time, the asymmetric tissue represents a normal developmental variant.**

becular pattern is preserved, and there is no architectural distortion. There is no mass formation, and there are no significant calcifications associated with the asymmetric tissue.

It is important to recognize that benign asymmetric breast tissue is a developmental variant. It should not develop between successive mammograms in mature women. Tissue volumes that increase in density and cannot be accounted for by differences in imaging technique and positioning or attributed to weight loss or hormone replacement therapy should raise suspicion. Invasive lobular carcinoma is notorious for causing a diffuse, asymmetric increase in density over time with little mass formation or architectural change.

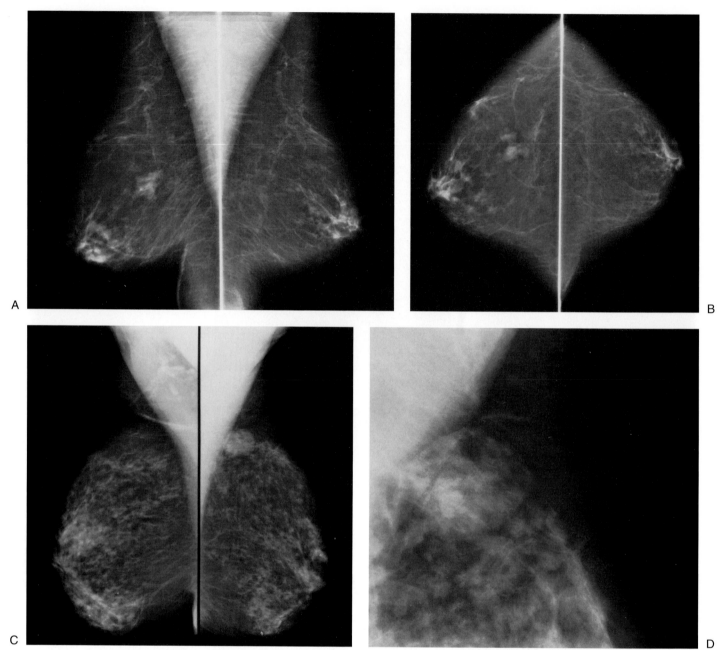

FIG. 13-10. A benign, focal asymmetric density. The focal asymmetric density visible in the center of the left breast on the mediolateral oblique (MLO) **(A)** and craniocaudal **(B)** projections was stable for 3 years and is a benign asymmetry. In this second patient, the asymmetric tissue has a rounded contour on the MLO projection **(C)**, but there is no real mass on the magnification image **(D)**. This density had been present since the patient's first mammogram 9 years earlier and is another, but unusual, manifestation of asymmetric breast tissue.

Although structures in front of and behind the area can on occasion confuse the image and make it appear as if the lesion contains fat, normal asymmetric breast tissue can frequently be distinguished from a mass if fat is seen distributed through the volume. Breast cancer rarely contains fat.

The morphology of asymmetric breast tissue is similar to that of the contralateral breast, except that there is greater tissue volume or the tissue has greater radiographic density on the involved side (Fig. 13-9). Simple, benign asymmetric breast tissue rarely has definable margins, but rather fades at the edges, and it does not have an easily defined, radiodense center. There should be no suggestion of an underlying mass or architectural distortion. If significant (not clearly benign) calcifications are present, the entity is no longer a simple asymmetry and may require further evaluation (biopsy). Benign, asymmetric breast tissue may occasionally occupy a small volume and merely be an island of normal breast tissue (Fig. 13-10).

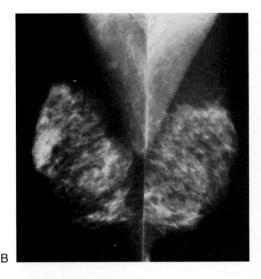

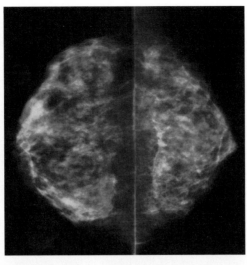

FIG. 13-11. Normal asymmetric breast tissue appears as greater tissue density in one breast compared to its mirror image volume in the other breast. There is greater tissue density in the superolateral subareolar region in this 56-year-old woman, as seen on the mediolateral oblique **(A)** and craniocaudal **(B)** projections. This had not changed in more than 3 years.

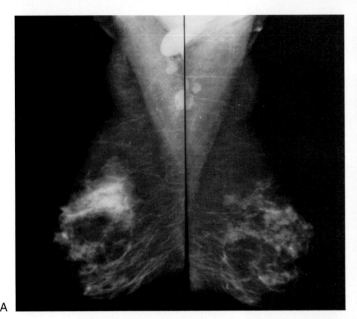

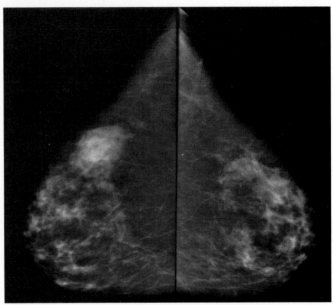

A

B

FIG. 13-12. There is a greater volume of breast tissue seen in the left breast on the mediolateral oblique **(A)** and craniocaudal **(B)** projections. This **asymmetric breast tissue** was unchanged over 3 years. (Note: The large axillary nodes are incidental. One was biopsied and proved to be a benign reactive lymph node.)

Asymmetric breast tissue had been implicated in the past as a secondary sign of malignancy based on incomplete or retrospective analyses. In a review of women whose mammograms had been read as negative but who proved to have cancer (palpable lesions), some had asymmetric tissue that corresponded to the location of the lesion (15). Asymmetric density was thus implicated.

Unfortunately, this type of analysis ignored the denominator of the equation: How many women have asymmetric density, but *do not have breast cancer*? Using similarly flawed reasoning, Wolfe suggested that asymmetrically prominent ducts were an indication of cancer (16), but he too had no denominator for the phenomenon and, because he only reported a few cases, they likely had been clinically evident for the biopsy to have been done. In an effort to

understand the true value of asymmetric tissue or tissue density as an indication of malignancy, we undertook a prospective evaluation. In a study of 8,408 women, 221 (3%) were found to have prominent asymmetric breast tissue (asymmetric volume or density) (17). The asymmetries included greater tissue density in one quadrant compared to its mirror image in the other breast (Fig. 13-11), a greater volume of radiographically dense tissue on one side versus the other (Fig. 13-12), or what appeared to be more prominent ducts on one side relative to the other (Fig. 13-13). Among these women, 20 had corresponding palpable asymmetries and underwent excisional biopsies. Of the 20, two women were diagnosed with invasive breast cancer and a third with lymphoma of the breast. The other 17 women who were biopsied had benign histologies. The 201 with asymmetric breast

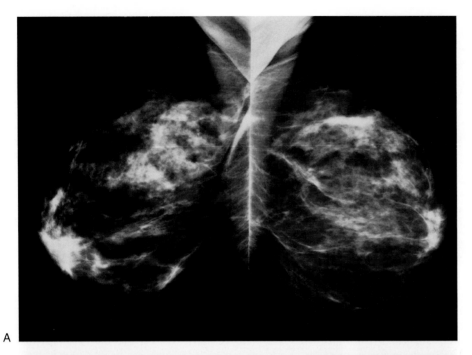

A

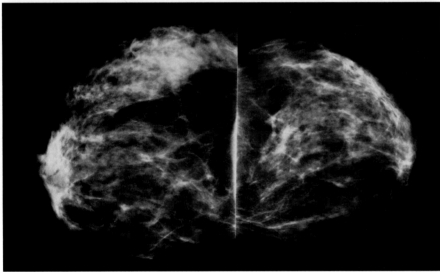

B

FIG. 13-13. Normal asymmetric tissue density presenting as prominent ducts. The nodular-appearing densities are more prominent in the upper outer left breast as seen on the mediolateral oblique **(A)** and craniocaudal **(B)** projections. In fact, these are likely lobules, but they have been termed prominent ducts. The appearance has remained unchanged for 5 years in this 67-year-old woman.

tissue with no palpable findings were followed up 36 to 42 months after the mammogram, and none had been diagnosed with breast cancer.

Despite the fact that the tissues are often prominently asymmetric by mammography, this asymmetry is not usually evident by clinical examination. We and others have shown that clinical breast examination (CBE) evaluates different tissue parameters than mammography (18,19). The mammogram measures the concentration and "Z" of the atoms making up the tissues, whereas clinical examination measures the elastic properties of the molecules formed by the atoms. Our study indicated that asymmetric breast tissue on the mammogram was significant only when it was also palpable, and biopsy of simple asymmetric breast tissue is recommended only when there is a corresponding palpable asymmetry.

Because our study failed to reveal any cancer among the women with nonpalpable asymmetric breast tissue with >3 years of follow-up, there is no reason to evaluate these women at any increased frequency. The use of ultrasound has never been shown to add any clinically useful information in this situation as long as there is no reason to suspect a mass in these tissues.

Thus, asymmetric breast tissue, with no evidence of mass formation, no architectural distortion, and no significant calcifications, that has not developed over time, is a normal variant and needs no additional evaluation or follow-up, unless it is palpable.

Asymmetric breast tissue is most common in the upper outer quadrant. Virtually all of these asymmetries are normal variations due either to developmental asymmetry or, per-

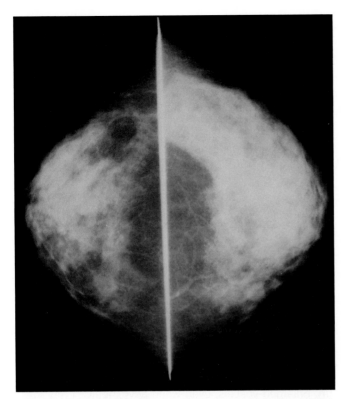

FIG. 13-14. Iatrogenically created asymmetric breast tissue. The asymmetric tissue density seen on the craniocaudal view of the right breast is the result of surgical removal of tissue from the left breast.

haps, to differential end-organ response to hormonal stimuli. Asymmetric breast tissue may be iatrogenically created with decreased density on the contralateral side secondary to the surgical removal of breast tissue (Fig. 13-14).

Asymmetrically dense breast tissue can be associated with breast cancer, but when cancer is found in tissue with the above characteristics it is virtually always clinically evident (Fig. 13-15) or the mammographic appearance does not meet the true definition of asymmetric breast tissue (no associated mass, no architectural distortion, and no calcifications). If the attenuation of asymmetric tissue increases over time, the insidious growth of invasive lobular carcinoma should be suspected (20).

Asymmetric Vasculature

The vessels of the breast are generally symmetric in size and distribution. They may become engorged because of either distal obstruction or increased flow due to hyperemia (Fig. 13-16). A dilated vessel can be a normal variant or accompany inflammation as well as neoplasia (Fig. 13-17). An asymmetrically large vein that is >1.5 times the size of its contralateral counterpart may be a subtle indication of an abnormality. We have found this to be an extremely uncommon finding, because it is more likely to be associated with later stage cancers, and it is becoming increasingly rare to see these tumors. Asymmetric vessels are generally either a normal variation or secondary to differences in mammo-

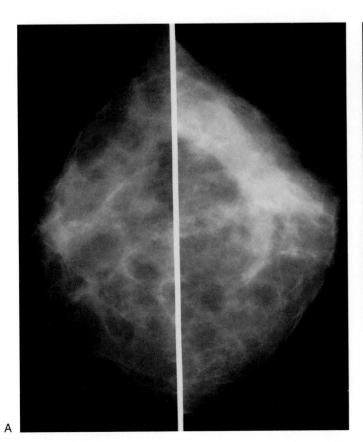

A

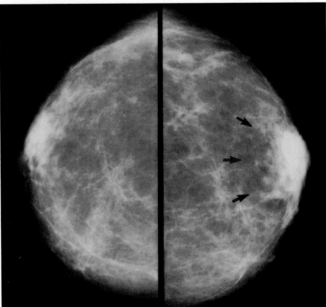

B

FIG. 13-15. Asymmetrically dense breast tissue and cancer. Asymmetrically dense breast tissue can be associated with malignancy. The asymmetrically dense breast tissue in the lateral aspect of the right breast on these craniocaudal (CC) projections was palpable, and biopsy revealed an invasive ductal carcinoma **(A)**. Invasive ductal carcinoma was also found where these palpable, asymmetrically prominent ducts (*arrows*) are seen in the subareolar region of the right breast on these CC projections **(B)**.

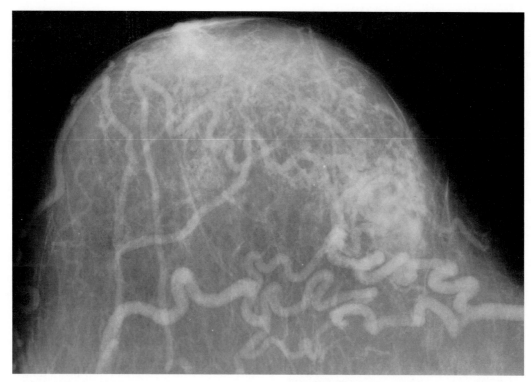

FIG. 13-16. Asymmetric vasculature is usually benign. Enlarged vessels, even when asymmetric, are usually not due to malignancy. The large veins on this craniocaudal projection were due to the patient's congestive heart failure.

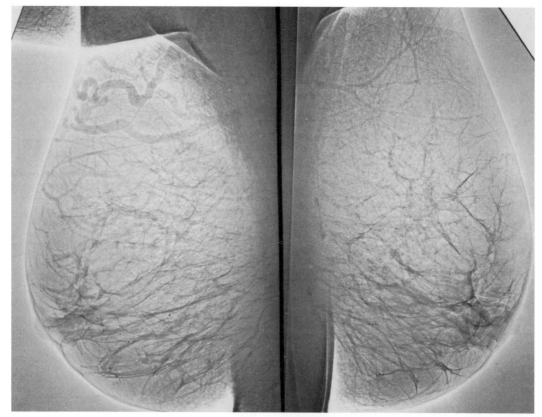

FIG. 13-17. Asymmetric vasculature is rarely associated with cancer. Asymmetrically dilated vessels associated with breast cancer are so uncommon that we have only seen two cases. The enlarged vessel on the left was associated with a palpable breast cancer in the left axilla on these lateral xerograms.

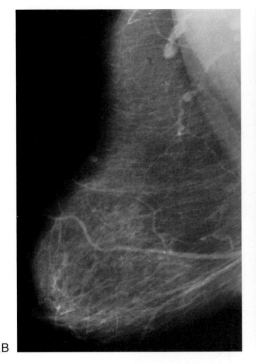

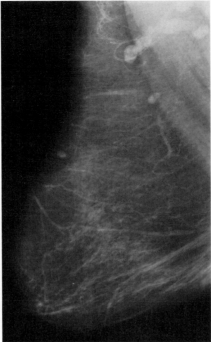

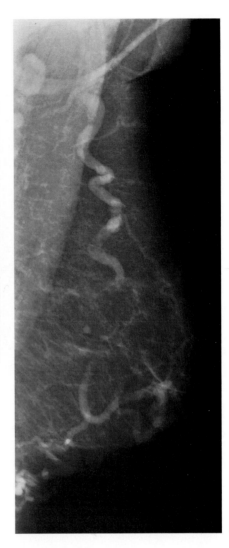

A,B

C

FIG. 13-18. The vessel seen on this mediolateral oblique (MLO) **(A)** is more prominent than the one on the MLO taken a year later **(B)** due to better compression on the second MLO.

The vessel in this second patient **(C)** is prominent due to **collateral flow secondary to thyroid cancer causing obstruction in the superior mediastinum.**

graphic compression (Fig. 13-18A, B), although on occasion an obstruction in the axilla or mediastinum can cause dilatation through collateral flow (Fig. 13-18C).

ANALYZING MASSES

As with any significant finding, masses should be described (see Chapter 24) as to their location, size (the largest diameter of the mass; spicules are not counted), shape, margin characteristics, x-ray attenuation (if significant), and effect on the surrounding architecture. Any associated findings (architectural distortion, associated calcifications, trabecular changes, skin thickening or retraction) should also be reported. The ACR-BIRADS lexicon and approach to reporting should be followed.

Location

Although the caution may seem trivial, the interpreter must first determine that a lesion is, in fact, within the breast. As a consequence of the basic spherical shape of the breast and the geometry of compression, only thin strips of the skin surface are imaged in tangent and the vast majority of the skin surface is projected over breast tissue. As with calcifications, some masses that project on the mammogram are actually benign skin lesions (Fig. 13-19). The radiologist should be alert to the fact that the presence of a skin lesion does not preclude the possibility of an intramammary lesion. If there is any question, a marker can be placed on the skin lesion to identify it for the radiologist.

The term *mole marker* has been coined to describe a metallic (radiopaque) marker that is placed on a skin lesion so that its location can be confirmed on the mammogram. In fact, moles or nevi are rarely visible on the mammogram. The pigment of a lesion does not make it radiopaque. Only raised skin lesions, such as seborrheic keratoses (Fig. 13-20) and attenuating lesions such as sebaceous cysts (Fig. 13-21), can project as intramammary processes. These are visible because they have an air–soft tissue interface or are more attenuating than the underlying breast tissue. Placing a small metallic marker that will appear on top of them on the mam-

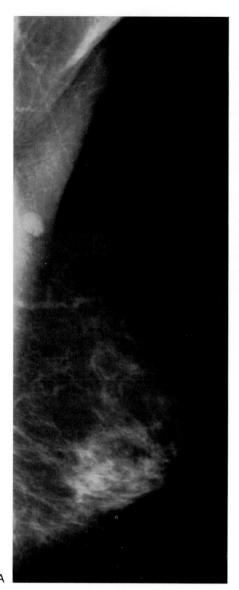

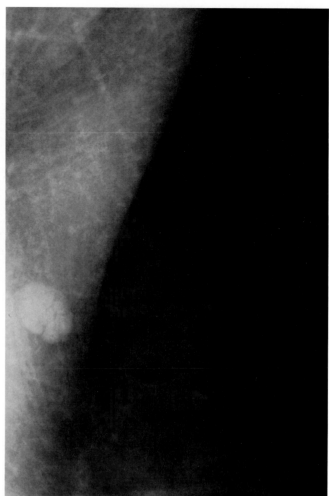

FIG. 13-19. Skin lesion projecting over the breast. On this mediolateral oblique, there is a mass that projects over the axillary tail of the breast **(A)**. The fact that it is a benign, seborrheic keratosis on the skin is apparent on closer inspection, where its verruciform features are evident **(B)**.

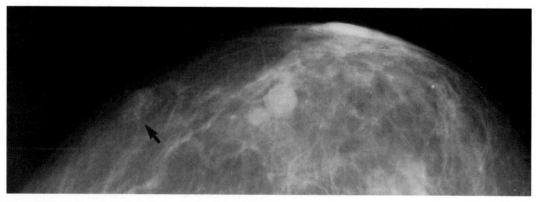

FIG. 13-20. This **seborrheic keratosis** on the skin is raised and has an air interface. This makes it visible on the craniocaudal view projected over the breast.

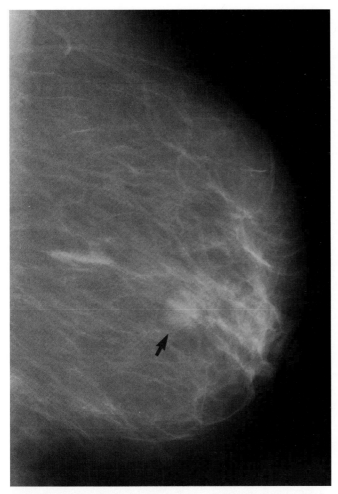

FIG. 13-21. In addition to being more attenuating than the fat of the breast, this **epidermal inclusion cyst** (*arrow*) is slightly raised and is visible on the mediolateral mammogram.

mogram will confirm the etiology of the density on the mammogram, eliminating any concern (Fig. 13-22).

Seborrheic keratoses typically have a verrucous appearance, with air trapped in their interstices, making them easily distinguishable from intramammary lesions (Fig. 13-23). On occasion they can trap powders, and these can mimic clustered microcalcifications.

Because some skin lesions have irregular margins, careful correlation should be made—cancers have been mistakenly dismissed when a skin lesion was depicted on the patient diagram as overlying the same area as the cancer. Pigmented lesions (moles) are not visible on the mammogram and do not need to be marked unless they are raised above the skin. If there is any question, markers should be placed on the skin lesion or the lesion should be placed in tangent and re-examined.

Location of Breast Cancer

Breast cancer can occur anywhere in the breast or, indeed, wherever breast tissue is found. Cancer can develop anywhere along the milk line where the embryologic structure was not resorbed. We have seen primary breast cancer high in the midaxillary line, as well as in an island of breast tissue in the anterior abdominal wall (Fig. 13-24). Breast cancer has been described in other rests of breast tissue (21).

Statistically, the most common location for breast cancer is the upper outer quadrant of the breast. Estimates vary. In a survey conducted by the American College of Surgeons, cancers were found at the listed frequencies in the following locations (22):

Upper outer = 36%
Upper inner = 9%

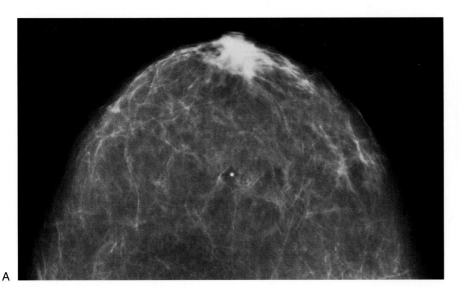

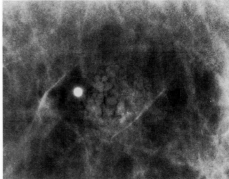

FIG. 13-22. Use of a marker on a skin lesion. A metallic marker was placed by the technologist on the raised skin lesion evident on the breast. It is visible on the craniocaudal mammogram **(A)** adjacent to a density projecting over the center of the breast. Closer inspection **(B)** demonstrates the classic, verruciform appearance of the seborrheic keratosis.

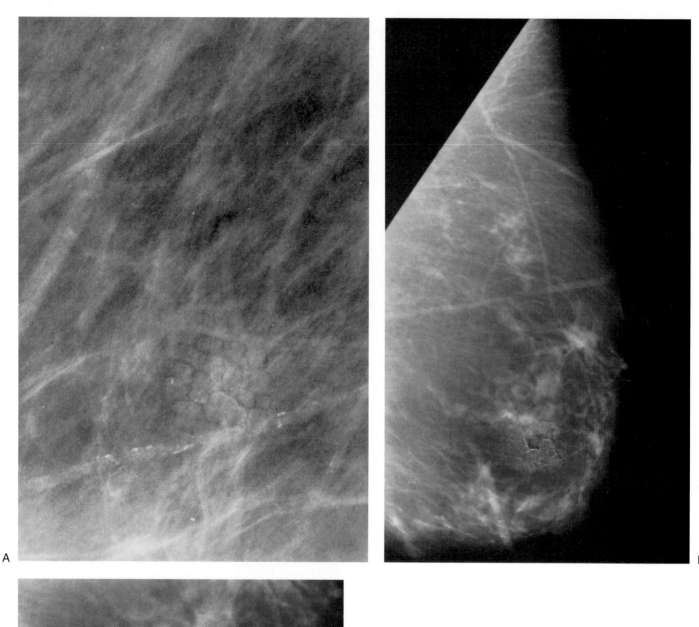

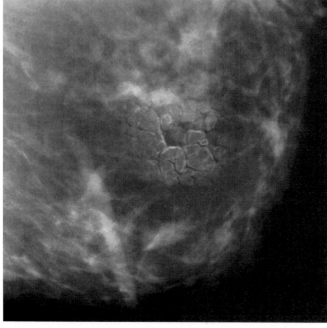

FIG. 13-23. (A) A **benign seborrheic keratosis** is more evident on this lateral projection **(B)** due to powder or ointment emphasizing its typical verruciform surface, which is seen close up **(C)**.

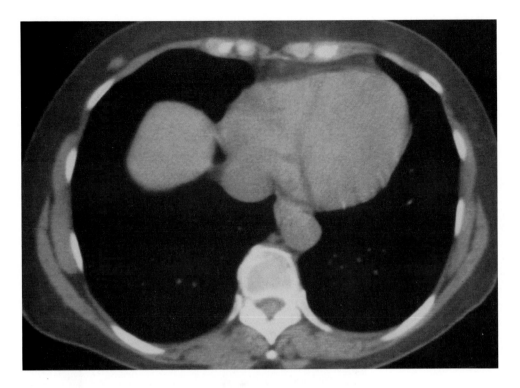

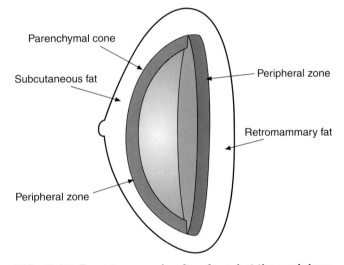

FIG. 13-24. Cancer can develop in rests of breast tissue. Primary breast cancer can be found anywhere along the milk line. This palpable cancer, visible on this CT scan of the upper abdomen in the anterior abdominal wall on the right side, apparently developed in a rest of breast tissue that had not resorbed during embryologic development. The patient had presented with metastatic disease in an axillary lymph node.

Lower outer = 6%
Nipple or subareolar = 7%
Lower inner = 5%
Axillary tail = 1%
Overlapping quadrants = 17%
Not reported = 18%

Although the numbers differ somewhat, the distribution was similar in Sickles' review of mammographically detected cancers (23):

Upper outer = 52%
Upper inner = 15%
Retroareolar = 14%
Lower outer = 11%
Lower inner = 8%

FIG. 13-25. Breast cancer is often found at the periphery of the gland. This schematic depicts a zone 1 cm wide beneath the subcutaneous fat and anterior to the retromammary fat. More than 70% of breast cancers develop in this zone. For most women, depending on the size of the breast, more than 50% of the parenchyma is in this zone.

Peripheral Zone Beneath the Fat

Our own analysis suggests that most breast cancers develop at the periphery of the glandular tissue, just beneath the subcutaneous fat or anterior to the retromammary fat. The radiologist should carefully evaluate the breast parenchyma in a zone 1 cm wide, immediately beneath the subcutaneous fat and anterior to the retromammary fat. Among women under the age of 50, >70% of breast cancers were found in this peripheral zone (8). This is likely true among older women as well. Although other reasons for this observation cannot be excluded, such as the possibility that carcinogens may collect in the fat subjecting the underlying lobules to damage (24), the most likely reason is that, on a geometric basis, this volume of tissue accounts for >50% of

the breast parenchyma (depending on the size of the breast) (Fig. 13-25).

Mammographic Blind Spots

On the MLO projection the most common location to fail to image a lesion is the medial area because this part of the breast is further away from the film and more likely to slip

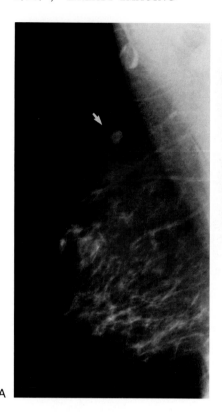

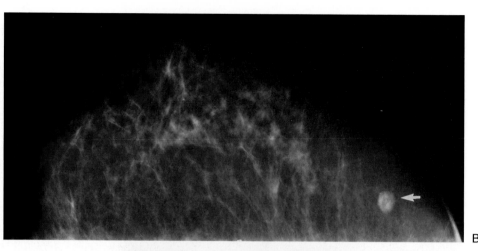

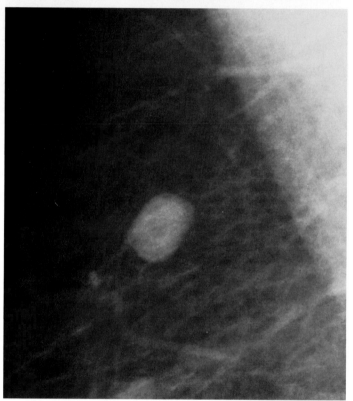

A

B

C

FIG. 13-26. Typical intramammary lymph node. This is the typical location and appearance of an intramammary lymph node (*arrows*) projecting over the upper outer aspect of the breast, as seen on the mediolateral oblique (MLO) **(A)** and the craniocaudal **(B)** projections. On close inspection **(C)** the typical lucent hilum is visible on the MLO image. No further evaluation is needed.

out from under the compression plate. The CC views can be positioned to be certain to include these tissues. The problem of positioning is complicated by the fact that, in our experience, cancers are occasionally missed in the fibroglandular tissues in the lateral portion of the breast that extends off the edge of the film in the CC view. An exaggerated CC view to image these tissues may be valuable.

The tissues of the upper breast may slip out from under the compression paddle on the CC projection if the breast is not elevated to relax the skin. This is frequently the reason that a lesion is seen deep in the breast on the lateral projection and not on the CC view.

Cancer may be found anywhere there are epithelial elements. Although it is uncommon, cancer can occur in the

subcutaneous fat. Ducts can be found in the subcutaneous fat following along the retinacula cutis to the skin, and cancer can occur here as well.

Location of Benign Lesions

Most breast lesions, both benign and malignant, can be found anywhere in the breast. When the morphology of a mass suggests an intramammary lymph node, location can guarantee the diagnosis. Intramammary lymph nodes are extremely common findings and are recognizably visible in approximately 5% of all mammograms. Typically, they are reniform or multilobulated masses that are <1 cm in size and have a lucent notch (Fig. 13-26). The vast majority of intra-

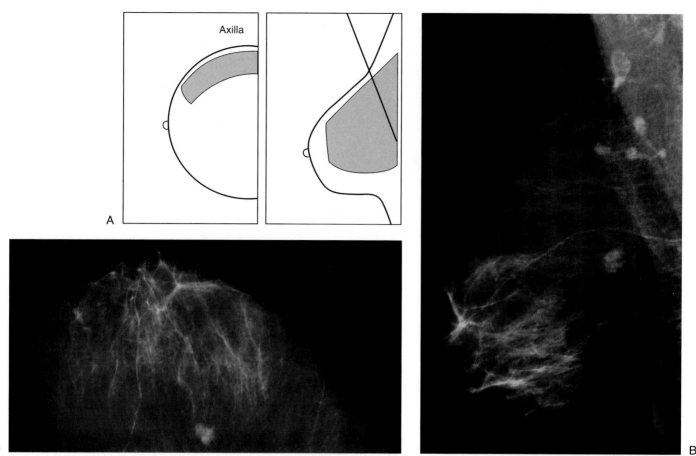

FIG. 13-27. (A) This schematic depicts the **usual location of intramammary nodes** in the lateral portions of the breast on the craniocaudal (CC) and mediolateral oblique (MLO) projections (*shaded areas*). This **rare, central intramammary lymph node** is the only case that we have seen, in more than 150,000 mammograms, of an intramammary lymph node that was centrally located in the breast on the MLO **(B)** and CC **(C)** projections. It proved to be a benign reactive node at histologic analysis.

mammary lymph nodes occur at the edge of the breast tissue in the outer portions of the breast. Although pathologists have described lymph nodes in all parts of the breast, the only part of the breast in which intramammary nodes are routinely seen on mammography (Fig. 13-27) is the outer quadrants. They are usually above the mid-plane but may be in the lower outer quadrant. They may be found as far as two-thirds to three-fourths of the way from the chest wall to the nipple. They are usually so characteristic in appearance that they do not require further investigation (see Chapter 14).

On rare occasions, intramammary lymph nodes have been described on mammograms in locations other than the lateral tissues. Meyer and colleagues reported two cases of lesions that were in the medial part of the breast that were histologically reported as lymph nodes (25). We have seen lymphoid tissue in other parts of the breast and a single case of an intramammary node anterior to the pectoralis major muscle in the center of the breast (Fig. 13-27B, C). Assuming that the Meyer cases are truly lymph nodes, nodes in this location should be extremely uncommon as only two were found among their thousands of breast biopsies.

The diagnosis of an intramammary lymph node should not be considered when a mass is seen in any other section of the breast unless the lesion has a clearly defined lucent hilum. If an upper outer quadrant lesion does not have the characteristics of a benign intramammary node, including a lucent hilar notch and smooth, and sharply defined margins, then suspicion should be aroused. Not all upper outer quadrant masses are benign lymph nodes, and this is the most common location for cancer (Fig. 13-28). If the morphology is not clear, magnification mammography may better demonstrate the shape and margins.

Because they are usually malleable and conform to the confines of the duct, benign large duct, intraductal papillomas are rarely visible by mammography unless they calcify or cause a cystic dilatation of the duct. Large duct papillomas are almost invariably found in the subareolar region within several centimeters of the nipple. Unfortunately, breast cancers can also occur in this area so that location cannot be used as a differential point.

Cysts and fibroadenomas can be found anywhere there are lobules, and lobules can be found everywhere in the

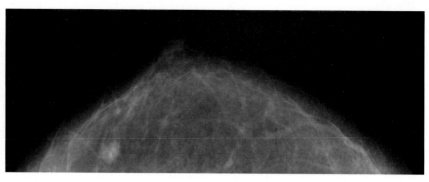

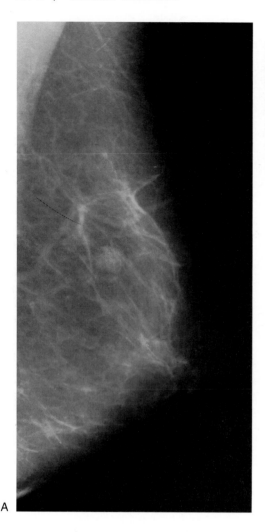

FIG. 13-28. Not all upper outer quadrant masses are benign lymph nodes. The density seen on the mediolateral oblique **(A)** and the craniocaudal **(B)** projections is in the typical location of an intramammary lymph node, but it proved to be an invasive breast cancer. If there is any doubt, magnification mammograms help to evaluate the margins of the lesion.

breast. The location of a lesion in the breast, by itself, has no differential value.

Determining the location of a lesion is important should further evaluation or a biopsy be necessary. Its coordinates should be clearly stated to guide the clinician. BIRADS, to assist the clinician, suggests that the location of a lesion be provided based on the face of a clock. Translating the mammographic location to the clinical location is a bit of a problem because the breast is distorted for the mammogram, but a conversion can be made. The radiologist should translate the location with care because, for example, 2:00 in the left breast is in the upper outer quadrant, while it is in the upper inner quadrant in the right breast (Fig. 13-29). The depth of the lesion is defined as anterior, middle, or posterior (see Chapter 24).

If further evaluation or intervention is required for a particular lesion, its location should be defined three-dimensionally by imaging (see Chapter 22). The triangulation of a lesion is usually easily accomplished by orthogonal x-ray imaging. Altering the projection can aid when triangulation is difficult. Ultrasound and computed tomography are also useful.

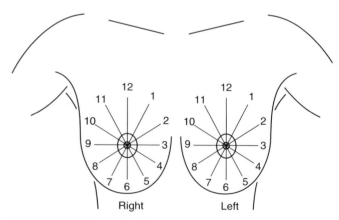

FIG. 13-29. Schematic of the "clock face" method of defining location within the breast.

Size

Any lesion, regardless of size, should be suspected if it has morphologic criteria that suggest possible malignancy. The size of a cancer at the time of diagnosis is, however, an important prognostic indicator (26). Although the traditional

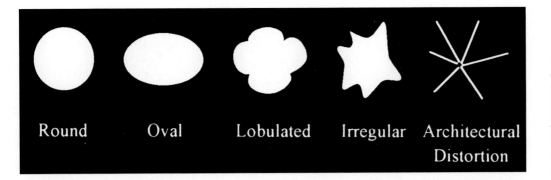

FIG. 13-30. Mass shape, as defined by the American College of Radiology Breast Imaging Reporting and Data System, can be divided into five shapes—round, oval, lobulated, irregular, and (though not strictly a mass) architectural distortion.

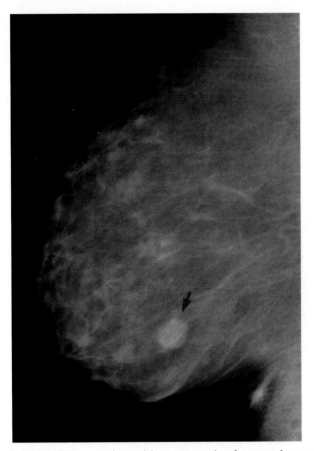

FIG. 13-31. This **cyst** (*arrow*) is an example of a **round** mass.

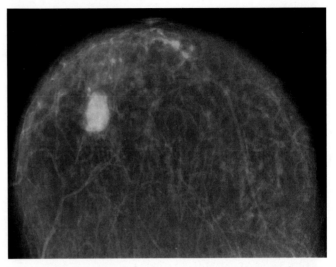

FIG. 13-32. This **hematoma** is an example of an **oval** mass.

staging of breast cancer uses 2 cm as the cutoff for stage I infiltrating cancers, even within stage I lesions there is a significant difference in prognosis that improves with the diminishing diameter of the tumor (9).

Many years ago Gallagher and Martin demonstrated the benefit of finding infiltrating cancers 5 mm or smaller (27). This is a desirable goal but difficult to achieve even with mammography. A number of studies have looked at 1 cm as a threshold and have shown that finding infiltrating cancers ≤1 cm has a survival benefit that is almost as high as a 5-mm threshold (28–30). The detection of invasive cancers at 1 cm or smaller is an achievable goal. In our prac-

tice, >50% of the invasive cancers detected by screening are ≤1 cm in diameter.

Shape

The shapes of masses (Fig. 13-30) can be divided into round (Fig. 13-31), oval (Fig. 13-32), lobulated (Fig. 13-33), irregular (Fig. 13-34), and architectural distortion (Fig. 13-35). The probability of malignancy increases as a lesion becomes more irregular in shape. An area of architectural distortion (particularly if spiculated) that is not associated with a mass in an area where there has been no prior surgery frequently is due to an underlying malignancy.

Margins

The interface between a lesion and the surrounding tissue (Fig. 13-36) is one of the most important factors in determining the significance of a mass. Circumscribed masses whose margins form a sharp, abrupt transition with the surrounding tissue are almost always benign (Fig. 13-37). Because some lesions with ill-defined margins appear to be

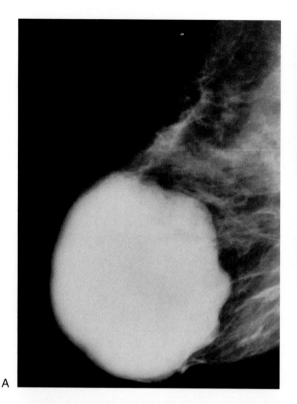

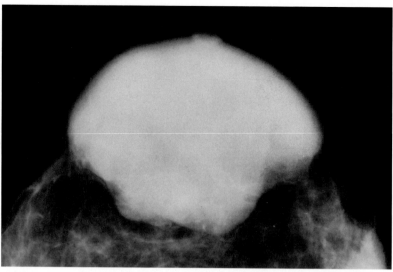

A

FIG. 13-33. This **giant fibroadenoma** in the lateral **(A)** and craniocaudal **(B)** projections is an example of a **lobulated** mass.

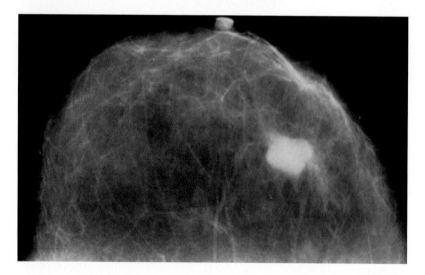

FIG. 13-34. This **invasive cancer** is an example of an **irregular** mass.

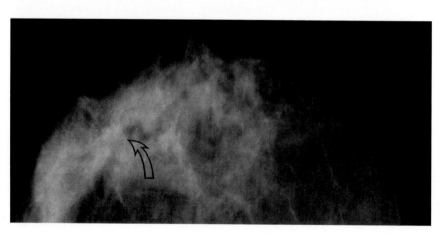

FIG. 13-35. The **architectural distortion** (*arrow*) on this craniocaudal projection was the only mammographic indication of the invasive cancer in the lateral right breast.

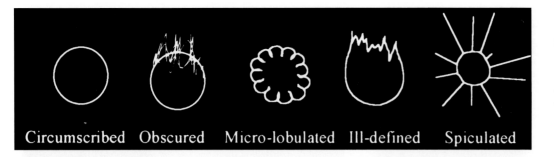

Circumscribed Obscured Micro-lobulated Ill-defined Spiculated

FIG. 13-36. A mass can have one of five margins. The American College of Radiology Breast Imaging Reporting and Data System defines these, as represented by this schematic—circumscribed, obscured, microlobulated, ill defined, and spiculated.

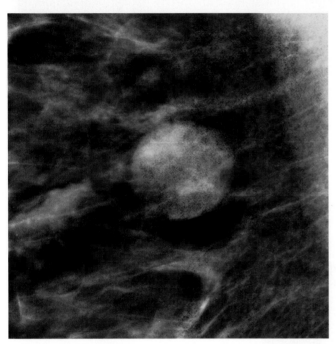

FIG. 13-37. This **cyst** is an example of a lesion with a **circumscribed margin.**

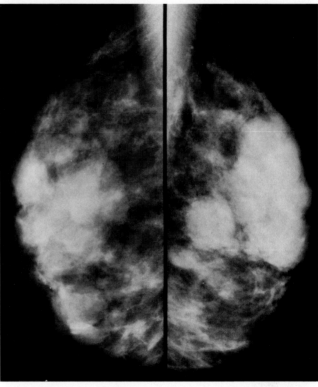

FIG. 13-38. The **multiple cysts** in these lateral mammograms are circumscribed masses, but they have margins that are **obscured** by the normal surrounding tissues.

circumscribed at low resolution, it may be valuable to obtain magnification images whose reduced noise and improved sharpness can increase the confidence of circumscription or reveal a less well-defined margin that should increase concern.

An obscured margin (Fig. 13-38) occurs when the normal surrounding tissue hides the true edge of the lesion. The interpreter must decide whether a lesion's margin is obscured or truly ill-defined due to infiltration. The latter raises the level of concern.

The microlobulated margin (Fig. 13-39) reflects the irregular surface that can be produced by a breast cancer (although fibroadenomas and cysts can have a microlobulated margin). The irregular protrusions that form at a tumor's edge can form short undulations at the surface of the lesion when seen on the mammogram. These are distinguished from a lobulated mass whose undulations are large. Microlobulations are only a few millimeters across.

The vast majority of breast cancers have an irregular interface as they invade the surrounding tissue. This pro-

duces the truly ill-defined margin (Fig. 13-40) that should raise concern. The probability of malignancy is high in lesions with ill-defined margins, although benign masses, including cysts and fibroadenomas, can appear to have ill-defined margins due to abutting normal tissues or, in the case of cysts, pericystic inflammation.

The classic breast cancer has a spiculated margin (Fig. 13-41) due to fibrous projections extending from the main tumor mass. The exact etiology of spiculation is unclear. Some have postulated that it is normal tissue being drawn toward the malignancy in a cicatrizing process. Careful microscopic analysis of these projections reveals associated cancer cells, and the spiculations are likely a reaction to this infiltration. By convention, the diameter of a cancer is measured across the tumor mass and excludes the spicules.

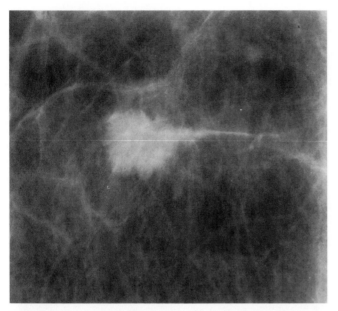

FIG. 13-39. This **invasive cancer** has a **microlobulated** margin.

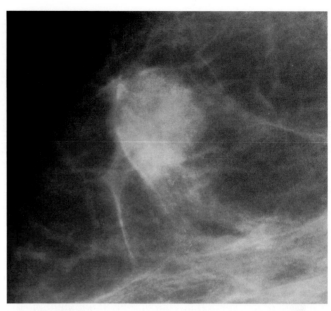

FIG. 13-40. This **invasive cancer** has an **ill-defined** margin.

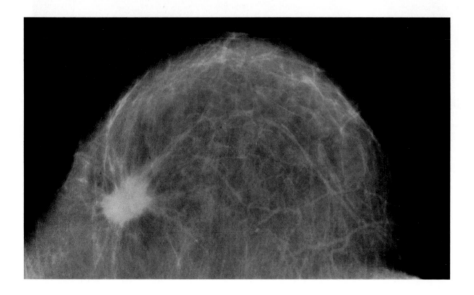

FIG. 13-41. An **invasive cancer** with a **spiculated** margin.

Postsurgical and Post-Treatment Change

Spiculated masses or areas of architectural distortion that appear spiculated should always be biopsied unless the distortion can be directly attributed to previous surgery. The analysis of breast lesions is thus aided by having some historical information. Knowledge of previous surgery, the site of the incision, and, in particular, the site from which tissue was removed is important for the interpretation of masses as well as calcifications. The site of tissue removal is important as the skin incision may be remote from this volume, and the distorted architecture after surgery is generally at the site of tissue removal.

If a benign diagnosis is made by biopsy, the breast usually heals with little or no distortion visible on subsequent mammography. Architectural distortion is not uncommon during the first year after any form of breast surgery, but this should resolve in almost all cases within 12 to 18 months (31). Some have argued that screening should be discouraged because it leads to breast biopsies and biopsies scar the breast, compromising the interpretation of future mammograms. This is not the case. Once healing is complete, postsurgical changes after a benign biopsy are rarely evident on a mammogram, and it is even more unusual for any changes to create difficulty in mammographic interpretation.

Irradiation for breast cancer may delay healing and may result in permanent scarring that is visible by mammography (see Chapter 17). This may be a problem in the early follow-up period. We generally obtain a new baseline mammogram 6 months after the completion of radiation. It is not unusual to see an area of spiculated architectural distortion in the excision site

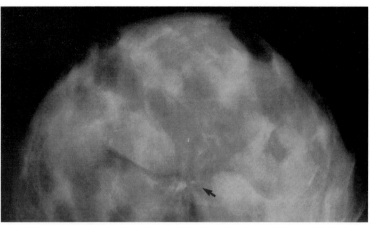

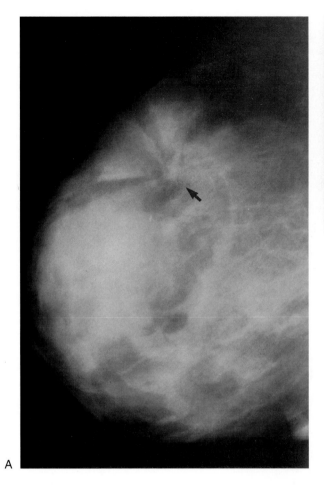

A

B

FIG. 13-42. This **spiculated architectural distortion** (*arrow*) on the lateral **(A)** and craniocaudal **(B)** mammograms proved to be an idiopathic radial scar.

at that time. If the margins of resection were clear when the cancer was removed, the likelihood of recurrent cancer is very low. If there are no other changes that suggest recurrent disease, we generally recommend annual screening. If there is a lingering question these women may be placed in a short interval follow-up program of mammography every 6 months for 2 years. Post-treatment change should remain stable or improve over that time, and at the end of the 2 years the patient can return to annual screening. For most cancer patients, the post-treatment change is clear, and the short interval follow-up is not needed.

Postsurgical fat necrosis in either the irradiated or nonirradiated breast can produce calcifications that can at times be confusing (32) (see Chapter 17).

Benign sclerosing duct hyperplasia (radial scar) may produce spicules visible by mammography (Fig. 13-42). The likelihood of the diagnosis can be suggested from morphologic criteria (long spicules without a central mass with fat trapped within), but a biopsy is still required to safely make the diagnosis (33).

TYPES OF MASSES

Circumscribed Masses (Round, Oval, or Lobulated)

Perhaps one of the most controversial subjects in mammography is the management of the solitary circumscribed mass. Statistically, a lesion that is round, oval, or lobulated with sharply defined borders that suggest a sharp separation of the margin of the lesion from the surrounding tissues has a very high likelihood of being benign. Unfortunately, as with all signs, this does not always indicate a benign lesion. There are a small number of cancers that are round, oval, or lobulated with circumscribed margins.

Although it had been taught that circumscribed cancers were usually the more indolent medullary subtype, in fact, medullary cancers often have an indistinct margin. The most common cancer that grows as a circumscribed mass is infiltrating ductal carcinoma NOS (not otherwise specified). Lymphoma, colloid carcinoma, and papillary carcinoma can on occasion appear as round, smoothly marginated lesions. Papillary cancers are frequently intracystic, and the cyst accounts for the smoothness of the margin.

Halo Sign

A dark, thin (1 mm or smaller) line can frequently be seen surrounding circumscribed masses. This halo of apparent radiolucency is actually an optical illusion. This Mach effect (34) is due to the retina's integration of the abrupt transition of the interface between structures that causes the cones of the retina, which are adjacent to the projection of the edge

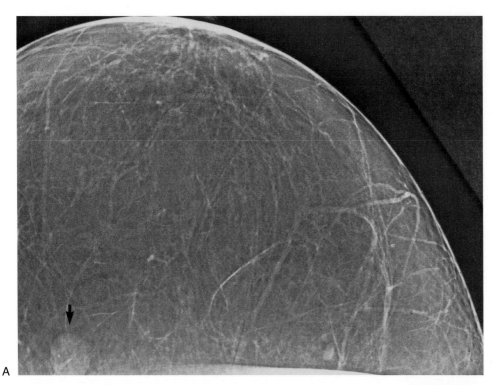

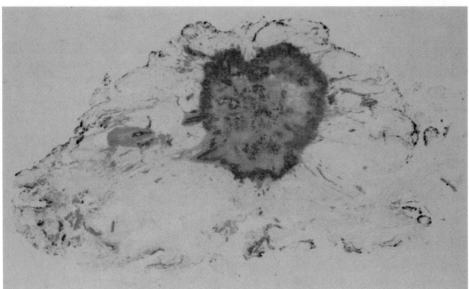

FIG. 13-43. The mass in the medial left breast on this craniocaudal xerogram **(A)** appears to be well circumscribed and has a **surrounding halo.** A photomicrograph **(B)** of the **invasive cancer** that was excised reveals that the lesion's margin is actually ill defined. This ill definition was not evident at the level of resolution of the contact mammogram.

of the mass on the retina, to be suppressed. This fools the visual system into believing that there is a dark band adjacent to the edge of the mass. Densitometry shows that there is no actual decrease in density. This can also be demonstrated by covering the mass, which causes the halo to disappear. An associated halo had been considered by some radiologists to be pathognomonic of a benign process, but sharply marginated malignant lesions can also produce halos (34). The apparent sharpness of the edge can vary with the resolution of the image. A sharp edge on contact mammography may be shown to be ill defined on magnification.

A lesion with a halo that appears to be smoothly marginated at the macroscopic level of a mammogram (Fig. 13-43A) may have an infiltrative margin when viewed at the microscopic level (Fig. 13-43B).

Probability of Cancer When a Mass Is Sharply Circumscribed

Most investigators have found that the probability of malignancy for round or oval masses with circumscribed margins is approximately 2% (35). Sickles (36) and Varas and colleagues (37) have also shown that circumscribed masses have a <5% probability of malignancy if there is no evidence of infiltration on magnification mammography. In our own practice, 5% of circumscribed masses excised after needle localization are malignant. The differences likely lie in the fact that we eliminate most cysts by ultrasound or aspiration, and they are not included in our statistic. Because the probability of malignancy is so low for these lesions, most agree that it is reasonable to follow them at short interval if they are found on a first mammogram and intervene only if they enlarge or demonstrate any other significant changes.

Significance of Size

Size does not predict malignancy. It has been suggested that the size of a circumscribed lesion could be used to guide intervention in the belief that the larger the lesion, the greater the likelihood that it is malignant. There is no scientific support for this approach. In a review of data from his screening program, Sickles found no significant increase in risk with increasing size for solitary circumscribed lesions (38). In his review, the increasing age of the patient had a weak association with the risk that one of these masses was malignant, and our own data agree with this, reflecting the prior probability of cancer in the population. It is likely that those who perceive a difference associated with size have also included palpable lesions, whereas Sickles reviewed predominantly nonpalpable lesions found at screening. It is also important to note that the lesions that Sickles described had sharply defined margins on magnification imaging. Any suggestion of infiltration or spiculation should prompt early intervention regardless of the size of the lesion. A circumscribed mass that was not present previously but develops should be investigated.

Prognostic Importance of Size

Although not a useful criterion for the diagnosis of cancer, size is a factor when the lesion proves to be cancer. If intervention (tissue diagnosis) is ever to be undertaken for a newly discovered circumscribed mass, it should be done while the prognosis, should it be a cancer, is most favorable. As noted previously, Rosen's data from Sloan-Kettering (9) and Tabar's data from Sweden (10) demonstrate an apparent worsening in prognosis when cancers are >1 cm among women with generally favorable lymph node–negative (stage I) cancer. The size of a cancer is also directly related to the probability of involvement of the axillary nodes (27) and thus to prognosis (see Chapter 6). It is likely that there is a continuum and no abrupt threshold, but cancer >1 cm is twice as likely to have spread to the axillary nodes as a lesion 1 cm or less in diameter. Although 1 cm may be an artificial figure, there are data indicating its importance. Maximizing the diagnosis of cancers when they are ≤1 cm is a desirable goal.

When to Intervene

Using this rationale, the data suggest that if a solitary circumscribed lesion seen on the first mammogram is ever to be primarily evaluated, it should be while it is 1 cm or smaller. If it is not primarily evaluated, a protocol for follow-up should be devised that offers the opportunity to expeditiously detect a change that would indicate that the lesion is malignant and prompt early intervention.

Although the standard of care supports following well-circumscribed round or oval lesions (39), our own approach has been more aggressive. To diagnose invasive breast cancers before they reach 1 cm in diameter, we arbitrarily set a threshold of 8 mm for intervention for solitary circumscribed masses seen on a first mammogram. This was not chosen because of a belief that the likelihood of malignancy increases with size but was based on the data demonstrating the advantages of diagnosing cancers while they are <1 cm in diameter. In our practice, any solitary circumscribed lesion that is 8 mm or larger is investigated by ultrasound (for cyst/solid differentiation), needle aspiration (for cyst/solid differentiation), or excisional biopsy (if solid), assuming that there are no previous films demonstrating its stability. Fine-needle aspiration or core needle biopsy, if accurate, may be used to avoid excisional biopsy, particularly if the diagnosis is clearly a fibroadenoma. Among our own screen-detected cancers diagnosed since 1978, >50% of the infiltrating lesions have been under 1 cm.

This approach applies only to solitary circumscribed masses. There should be no size threshold for spiculated or ill-defined masses, and a biopsy should be recommended at any size for these other lesions, but for the "most likely benign" circumscribed mass, our threshold for investigation (ultrasound, aspiration, or biopsy) may be considered for newly discovered solitary lesions approaching 1 cm.

Isolated small (<8 mm), round, smoothly marginated densities occur so frequently that it is impractical to evaluate them. It is reasonable to merely follow these at 6 month intervals if primary evaluation reveals no suspicious morphology. This is particularly true when many similar densities are scattered throughout the breast. Multiple rounded densities with sharp margins that do not distort the normal breast architecture almost invariably represent a benign process.

LESIONS THAT ARE ROUND, OVAL, OR LOBULATED WITH CIRCUMSCRIBED MARGINS

Fibroadenoma

The most common sharply marginated mass among women in their teens, 20s, and early 30s is the fibroadenoma. Radiographically, a fibroadenoma is, for all practical purposes, indistinguishable from a cyst or even a well-circumscribed carcinoma. However, in general it has

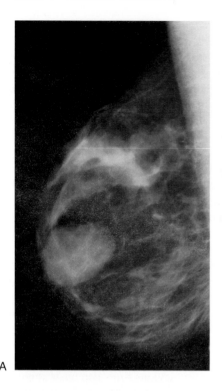

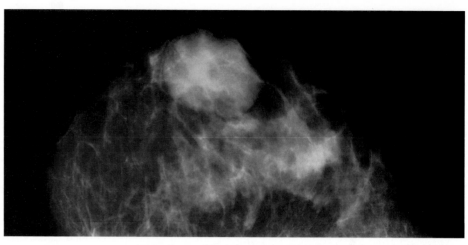

FIG. 13-44. On mediolateral oblique **(A)** and craniocaudal **(B)** projections, **fibroadenomas,** such as this mass in the subareolar region of the left breast, **usually have sharply defined margins** that are on occasion somewhat flattened. They tend to be oriented with their longer axis in the direction of the ducts, but these are not diagnostic features.

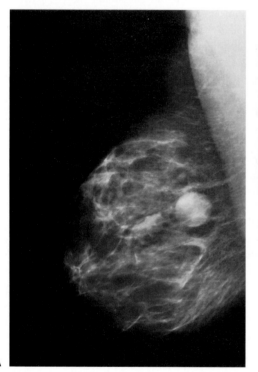

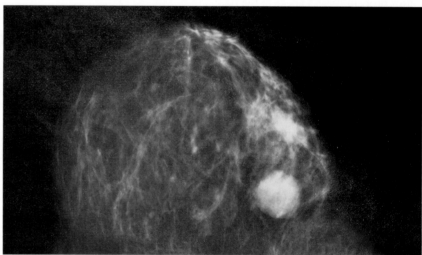

FIG. 13-45. Cysts rarely distort the surrounding tissue. This round, well-circumscribed mass on the mediolateral oblique **(A)** and craniocaudal **(B)** projections proved to be a cyst.

sharply defined margins that may be slightly more angular (Fig. 13-44) than the usually round or ovoid cyst. Like other benign lesions they usually do not distort the breast architecture but rather fit in it. When the typical large calcifications are present within the fibroadenoma, the diagnosis can be made without a biopsy (see Calcifications).

Cysts

Cysts are probably the most common masses found in the breast. They are rare before the age of 30 and begin to be frequently diagnosed beginning in the fourth decade of life. Although more common in premenopausal women, they can be found in women of all ages and are not that unusual in postmenopausal women. As described in the section on pathology, they most likely represent dilatation of the terminal ducts within the lobules that is the result of an imbalance between secretion and resorption. Macrocysts (visible by mammography) are usually multiple and bilateral (see Fig. 13-38). They also rarely distort the architecture of the breast, appearing rather as round densities within it (Fig. 13-45).

Cysts may be clearly defined. They more commonly have margins that are partially obscured by the surrounding parenchyma (Fig. 13-46). At times their margins are not visible on the mammogram, causing only focal increased density. Portions of their margins may be seen as bulging, rounded contours within the dense background of the breast (Fig. 13-47).

There is no unanimity in the appropriate management of cysts. It is best to separate those that are detected only by mammography from those that are palpable. This is likely an artificial distinction, but the clinician should have a say in the management of a palpable cyst, whereas the lesion found only on mammography should be managed by the radiologist.

Ultrasound is a safe, easy, and accurate way of evaluating lesions to determine if they are cysts or solid. Most clinicians agree that if a lesion meets all the criteria for the ultrasound diagnosis of a cyst (round or oval, sharply defined, with no

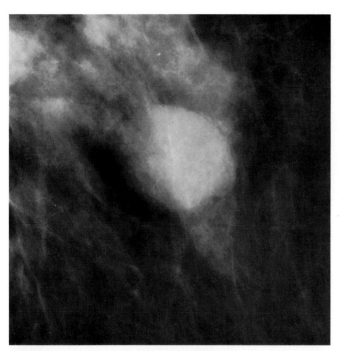

FIG. 13-46. Cysts frequently are partially obscured. This mass has a partially obscured margin but was found to be a benign cyst under imaging-guided aspiration.

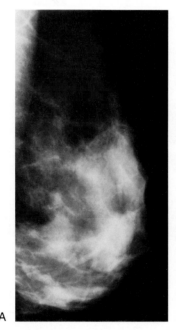

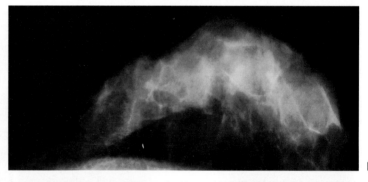

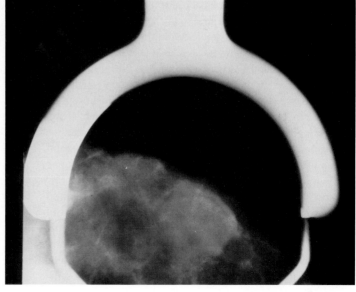

FIG. 13-47. Aspiration can make the diagnosis of a cyst. There is a palpable mass in the anteromedial tissues of the right breast on the mediolateral oblique **(A)** and craniocaudal **(B)** projections. Its anterior margin is sharply defined on the spot compression view **(C)**, but the surrounding tissues obscure its posterior margin. *Continued.*

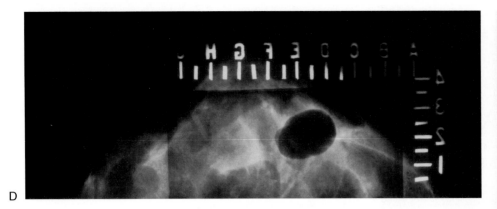

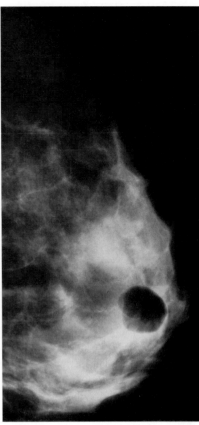

FIG. 13-47. *Continued.* Ultrasound was indeterminate; at the request of the referring physician, the mass was aspirated and air introduced, as seen on the craniocaudal **(D)** and lateral **(E)** projections, which confirm a benign cyst.

internal echoes and with enhanced through transmission of sound) (Fig. 13-48), the diagnosis is virtually ensured (40).

For palpable lesions that are thought to be cysts, the approach may be different. Some surgeons argue that a palpable cyst may hide something beneath, and they aspirate palpable masses despite the ultrasound diagnosis of a cyst, although the data supporting this approach are obscure. Furthermore, many palpable cysts are painful, and the presence of a lump causes anxiety for some women. Aspiration is the fastest, and often least expensive, way to both diagnose and eliminate a palpable cyst. Although many advocate the use of ultrasound to evaluate palpable masses, the routine ultrasound evaluation of palpable masses is not cost effective if the clinician is going to aspirate the mass despite the ultrasound diagnosis of a cyst.

The nonpalpable lesion detected only by mammography is the responsibility of the radiologist. The ultrasound demonstration of a cyst is sufficient, and no further evaluation is necessary if the imaging criteria are present. If there is any question, then imaging-guided aspiration using mammographic or ultrasound guidance can be diagnostic while simultaneously eliminating the mass. Although not required, the introduction of a small amount of air (less than the amount of fluid removed) following the fluid aspiration may be of value. It has been suggested that this might reduce the likelihood that

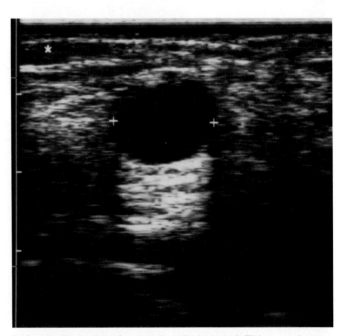

FIG. 13-48. A classic cyst by ultrasound. This round mass has **sharply defined anterior and posterior margins with no internal echoes. There is enhanced through-transmission of sound.** These features **define a simple, benign breast cyst and no further intervention is required.**

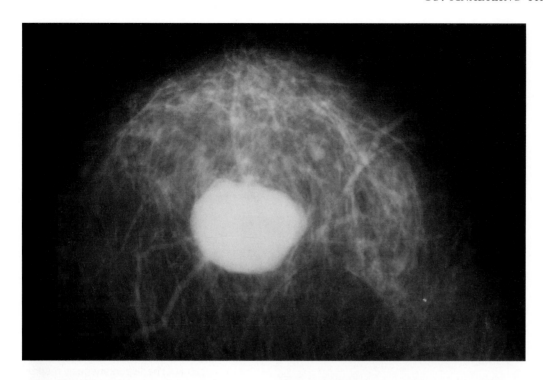

FIG. 13-49. Intracystic cancer can bleed. This mass, seen on the cranio-caudal projection, was high in x-ray attenuation due to hemorrhage from intracystic cancer.

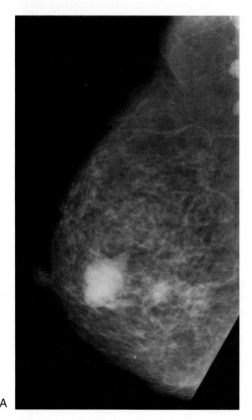

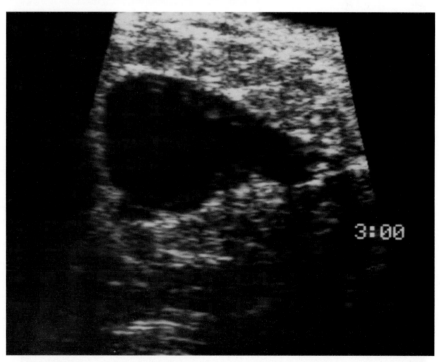

A

B

FIG. 13-50. Cancers associated with a cyst are extremely unusual. The lobulated mass, seen on this straight lateral projection (A), is complex on ultrasound (B), with a thickened wall. Cancer was found abutting the cyst and growing into it.

the fluid would reaccumulate, although this is probably not the case. If patients are followed for several years, as many as 40% of cysts refill despite the introduction of air. Nevertheless, the appearance of a smooth thin wall on pneumocystography is reassuring and helps confirm that the aspirated lesion was the same as the abnormality visible on the mammogram.

We have never demonstrated an intracystic cancer with a pneumocystogram, although other radiologists have demonstrated this lesion. Intracystic breast cancer is extremely rare. It has been our experience that the few intracystic cancers that do occur present as palpable cysts that have high x-ray attenuation due to blood from internal hemorrhage (Fig. 13-49).

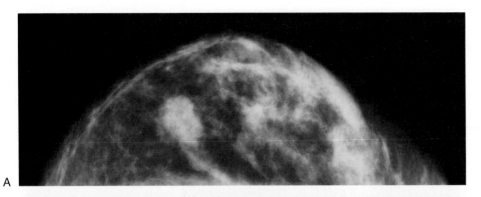

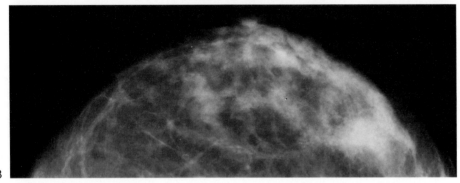

FIG. 13-51. Cysts may resolve spontaneously. The cyst in the medial left breast seen on this craniocaudal projection **(A)** had spontaneously resorbed on a follow-up study 3 months later **(B)**.

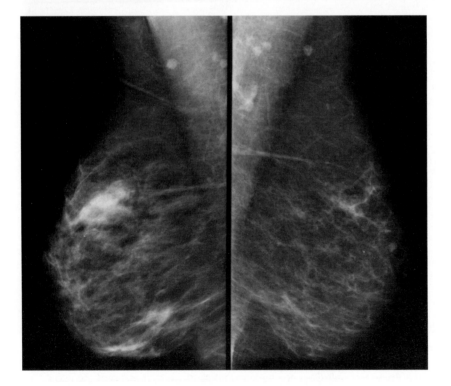

FIG. 13-52. An unusual effect of hormone replacement therapy is an increase in tissue density. The mediolateral oblique (MLO) on the right was imaged before the use of estrogen. The MLO on the left is of the same breast with the image reversed. It was obtained 2 years after the right image. The increased tissue densities are due to the institution of hormone replacement using estrogen.

Although it is likely that nonpalpable, intracystic cancers will be found as the use of screening increases, the probability is low. For this reason we do not recommend reaspiration if a cyst recurs as long as the following criteria are met. If a nonpalpable cyst is aspirated and completely emptied with no suspicious residua and the fluid is unremarkable to visual inspection (clear, yellow, green, or brown), we no longer recommend reaspiration if it recurs unless there are other reasons to empty it once again. This differs from many surgeons who reaspirate recurrent palpable cysts and surgically excise them if they continue to recur. The rationale for this approach is not clear, nor is it universally accepted. There are no data that suggest that the recurrence of a nonpalpable cyst has any significance.

Breast cyst fluid is virtually never clear. At best it is turbid yellow or green. Because intracystic cancer is extremely rare and cytology may be negative even when cancer is present, many discard cyst fluid without submitting it to cytologic analysis, unless the fluid represents old blood. If the aspiration reveals old blood (thick maroon material), the aspiration should be terminated (so that the lesion remains visible) and biopsy is indicated.

On rare occasions we have found cancers abutting a solitary cyst (Fig. 13-50). Although the relationship is not clear, it is possible that the cancer may be the cause of duct obstruction, leading to a solitary cyst (see Chapter 16). Signs of malignancy, as well as other lesions with suspicious morphology, should not be overlooked simply because cysts have been identified in the breast.

Cysts may spontaneously resolve (Fig. 13-51) or persist over many years. Although they are most common before menopause, cysts can occur in postmenopausal women. Exogenous hormone therapy can lead to the postmenopausal development of cysts along with increased fibroglandular density (Fig. 13-52). Although in some small series these effects have been reported to occur as often as 27% (41) of the time, in our experience, in an unpublished review of 100 women, the percentage was closer to 5% of women using such hormonal supplementation.

Abscess

Most infections of the breast are treated before they form an abscess. Furthermore, most breast abscesses occur in young women and are often associated with nursing. Consequently, it is rare that a mammogram is indicated in a woman with an abscess, and most are treated clinically. On the rare occasions when we have been asked to image these, we have found that they run the spectrum of findings. They may be round and well circumscribed or irregular and ill defined or only evident by skin and trabecular thickening. Even ultrasound cannot always differentiate an abscess from a cyst or other abnormality; aspiration is generally needed to make the diagnosis.

Intraductal Papilloma

Intraductal papillomas usually extend within the lumen of the duct and are not evident on conventional mammograms. On occasion they form visible masses that may be circumscribed. If the duct is cystically dilated around the papilloma, they may appear as cysts (Fig. 13-53). They rarely present as lobulated masses within several centimeters of the nipple.

Focal Fibrosis

The breast is a fairly dynamic organ and appears to readily produce and resorb collagen. On occasion focal areas of fibrosis occur and may appear as isolated islands of density (42). The

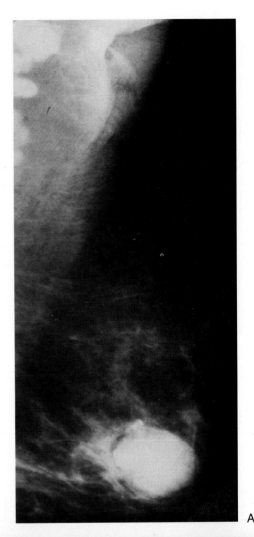

A

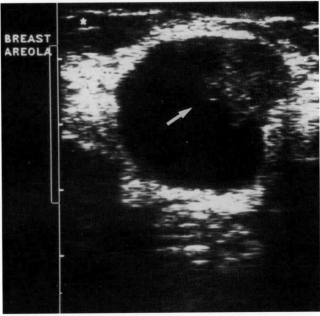

B

FIG. 13-53. Intracystic papilloma. This circumscribed mass **(A)** in the subareolar region is a cyst that contains **(B)** an intracystic mass (*arrow*) that proved to be a benign papilloma. The cyst is actually a cystically dilated duct.

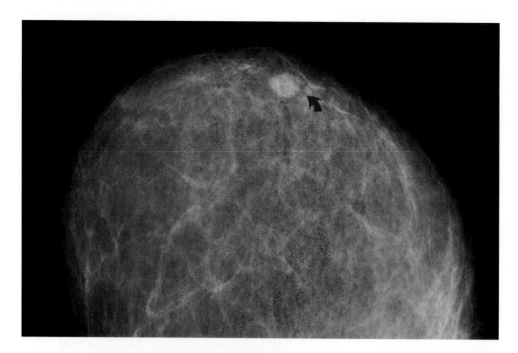

FIG. 13-54. The sharply circumscribed lesion in the subareolar region proved to be a **focal area of fibrosis.**

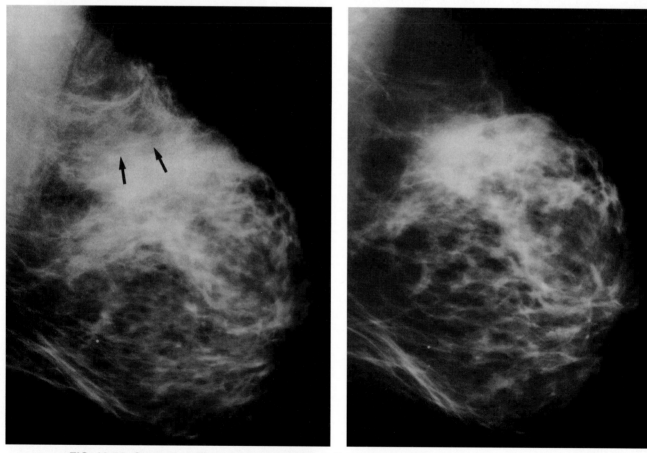

A

B

FIG. 13-55. Contusion. This individual sustained direct trauma to the upper outer right breast. Trabecular thickening **(A)** (*arrows*), presumably due to blood and edema dissecting along tissue planes, is evident. Several months later **(B)** the blood and fluid have resolved, the bruise is no longer evident, and the trabecular pattern has returned to being thin and fine.

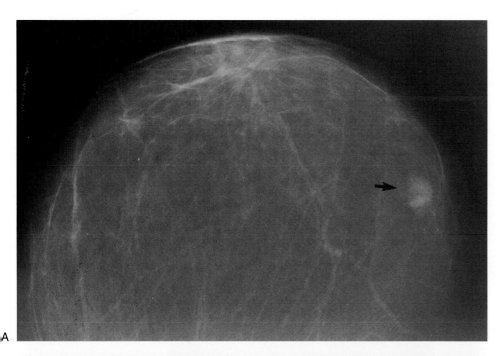

A

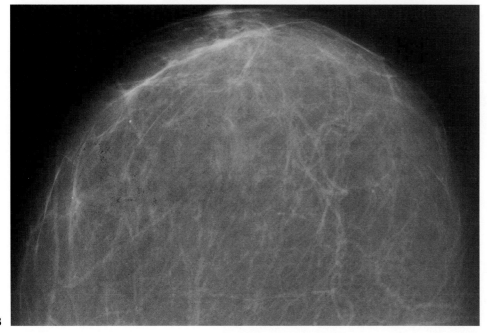

B

FIG. 13-56. Hematoma. (A) A smoothly lobulated circumscribed mass in the lateral left breast (*arrow*) where the patient had sustained a direct blow. **(B)** Several weeks after the injury the hematoma has resolved.

margins of such fibrotic islands are sometimes smooth and well demarcated (Fig. 13-54), but usually they are more difficult to evaluate because they fade gradually into the surrounding tissues. Coned-down spot compression may help eliminate concern by showing undisrupted architecture through the density.

More recently some of these lesions have been recategorized as *pseudoangiomatous stromal hyperplasia* (43,44). These are benign lesions that may resemble focal fibrosis or fibroadenomas on imaging. The lesions have clefts that are lined by fibroblasts (spindle cells) that give the appearance of small vessels (hence the name). They have no known malignant potential.

Hematoma versus Contusion

Trauma to the breast can cause a hard mass or thickening that is obvious on physical examination. Radiographically, a contusion may appear as very subtle diffuse infiltration of tissues by blood or edema. Producing only mild architectural changes with some thickening of the breast trabeculations (Fig. 13-55), a contusion rarely produces a radiographically visible mass.

If, on the other hand, trauma results in a true focal collection of blood, a fairly well-circumscribed lesion may be seen (Fig. 13-56). Hematomas are not uncommon after surgery

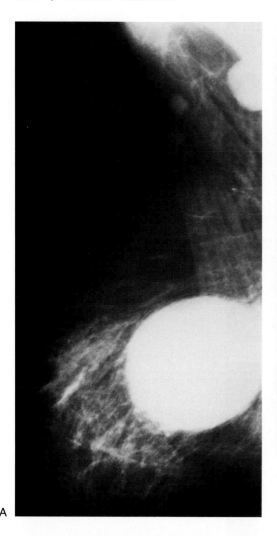

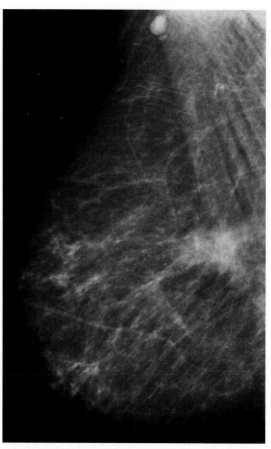

A

B

FIG. 13-57. (A) This **postoperative hematoma** (the high attenuation is due to the presence of blood) was present 9 days after an excisional biopsy for ductal carcinoma in situ. The axillary nodes are reactive. Nine months later **(B)** the hematoma has resolved with minor, residual postsurgical change.

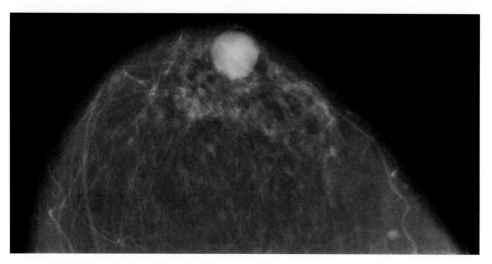

FIG. 13-58. This **phylloides tumor** increased from 2.5 to 3.5 cm in <6 months in this 74-year-old woman who initially refused surgery.

(Fig. 13-57A). They should resolve spontaneously within several weeks (Fig. 13-57B), but it is not uncommon for architectural change to persist for up to a year after a breast biopsy with benign results (31) and longer if the breast has been irradiated for cancer. Usually there are no long-term sequelae of trauma to the breast, and permanent architectural distortion is fairly unusual.

On rare occasions, architectural distortion and scarring may persist, forming a worrisome spiculated density. Alternatively, trauma may result in one of the several forms of fat necrosis,

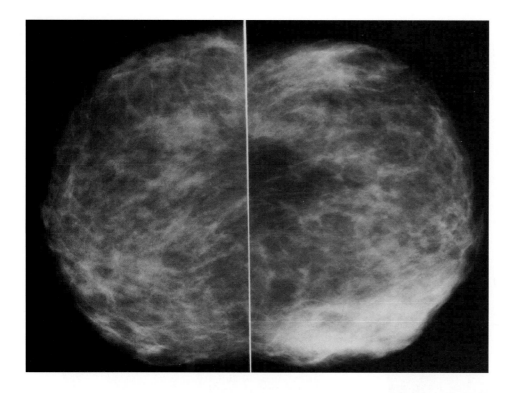

FIG. 13-59. The area of diffuse asymmetric increased density in the medial right breast proved to be **lymphoma.**

such as the encapsulated, gelatinized fat of the post-traumatic oil cyst with the typical lucent appearance (see Chapter 14).

Phylloides Tumor

Phylloides tumor is a rare lesion that used to be more common. It usually forms a slightly lobulated density with sharply defined margins and is often rapidly growing (Fig. 13-58). Usually the tumor is benign, but approximately 15% are malignant and are locally invasive, recurrent, or metastatic beyond the breast (see Chapter 2). Although their natural history is difficult to determine, this lesion is probably a variant of the fibroadenoma. It is radiographically indistinguishable from the so-called giant fibroadenoma that can be seen in adolescent women and women in their 20s (see Fig. 13-33).

Lymphoma

Malignant lymphoma of the breast can have varying morphologic characteristics, from diffuse increased density (Fig. 13-59) to a sharply marginated lesion (Fig. 13-60). Primary lymphoma of the breast is a relatively rare phenomenon, and lymphoma is usually evident elsewhere in the body when detected in the breast.

Circumscribed Breast Cancer

Unfortunately, as many as 7% of malignant lesions can be well circumscribed (Fig. 13-61). It was commonly believed that

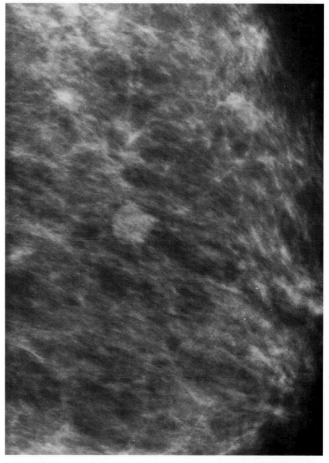

FIG. 13-60. Lymphoma is often well circumscribed. This solitary circumscribed mass proved to be primary lymphoma of the breast.

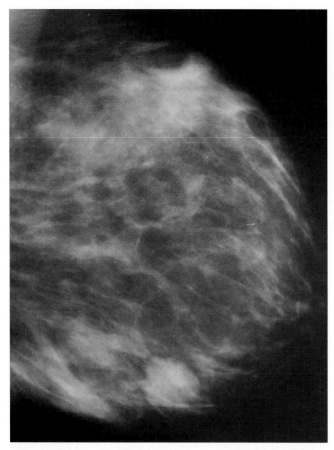

FIG. 13-61. The **circumscribed** mass with obscured margins in the lower right breast proved to be **infiltrating ductal carcinoma.**

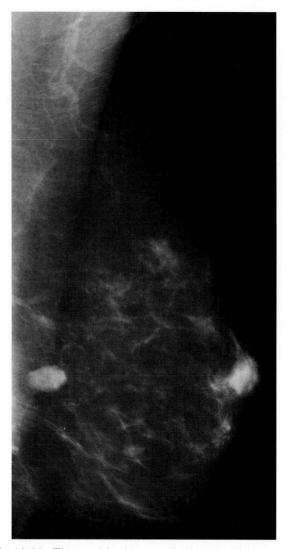

FIG. 13-62. The ovoid, circumscribed mass deep on the mediolateral oblique projection is **lymphoma, metastatic to the breast.** There is another less well-defined focus in the subareolar tissue.

circumscribed cancers are usually of the medullary type and have a more favorable prognosis, but in fact "garden variety" infiltrating ductal carcinoma (NOS) is more commonly the diagnosis when the margins of a cancer are sharply marginated on the mammogram (45). Although it has been suggested that circumscribed margins indicate that a cancer is slow growing, circumscribed borders do not guarantee indolence.

Usually a well-circumscribed malignant lesion has some part of its margin that is ill defined, suggesting infiltration. As with many other descriptors, this appearance can also occur with benign processes. The overlap of normal tissue structures can cause sharply defined margins to appear ill defined. Coned-down spot compression may help in the evaluation of these densities.

Metastatic Disease to the Breast

Lesions metastatic to the breast from another primary malignancy are frequently round and fairly well marginated. When multiple round densities are seen—particularly when they occur unilaterally—the question of a metastatic process should be considered (Fig. 13-62). Although it is not common, virtually any other malignancy can be metastatic to the

breast. When metastatic disease is found in the breast, the primary cancer is usually already known.

The most common lesion to metastasize to the breast is melanoma (Fig. 13-63), followed by lymphoma and lung cancer. We have also seen ovarian cancer and renal cell carcinoma spread to the breast (Fig. 13-64). Metastatic lesions are usually multiple. Although metastatic lesions may be ill defined, they are frequently distinguished from primary breast malignancy by their often well-defined margins.

Unusual Circumscribed Masses

There are other extremely rare lesions that may be circumscribed (see Chapter 19). These include such unusual lesions as sarcomas, malignant fibrous histiocytomas, and myoid hamartomas. None has distinguishing features by imaging.

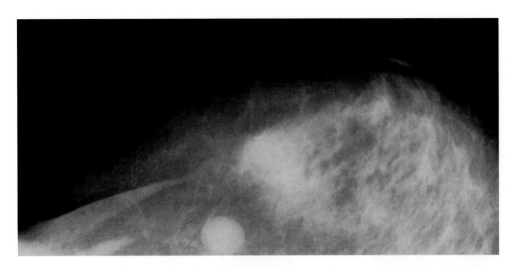

FIG. 13-63. The circumscribed mass in the lateral right breast is **melanoma that is metastatic to the breast.**

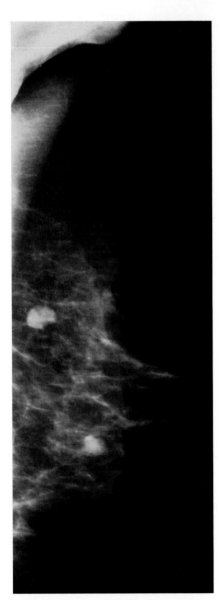

FIG. 13-64. These circumscribed lesions seen on the mediolateral oblique projection are **metastatic ovarian cancer** in a 61-year-old woman.

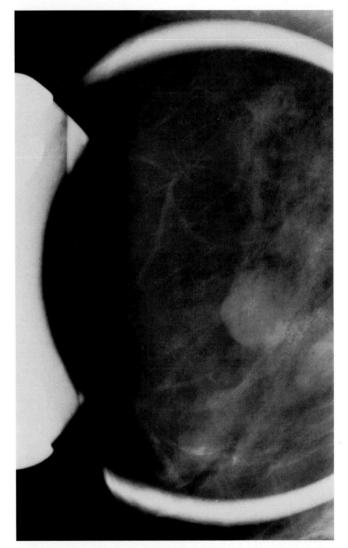

FIG. 13-65. This nonpalpable mass in a 54-year-old woman has a circumscribed anterior margin, as shown on a magnification lateral mammogram. The posterior margin is either obscured or ill defined. Ultrasound proved that the lesion was a **benign cyst,** and no further evaluation was needed.

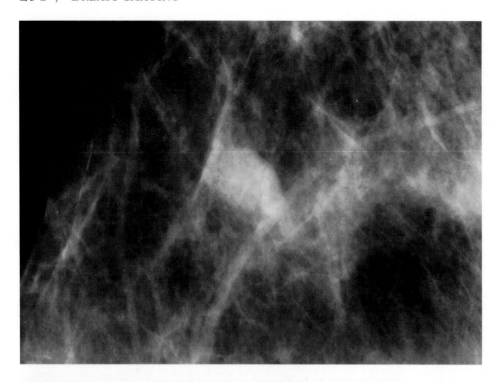

FIG. 13-66. This nonpalpable mass in a 42-year-old woman has an obscured inferior and deep margin. Ultrasound showed a solid mass, and biopsy revealed a **benign fibroadenoma**.

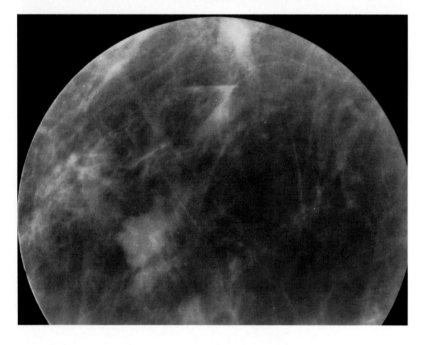

FIG. 13-67. A mass with a **microlobulated** margin should arouse suspicion. This 8-mm mass has a microlobulated margin and proved to be ductal carcinoma in situ.

LESIONS WITH OBSCURED MARGINS

Differentiating a well-circumscribed margin that is obscured from normal surrounding tissue from a lesion whose margin is ill defined because it is infiltrating into the normal tissue is one of the major problems in diagnosis. If high-resolution tomography can be developed, the differentiation of benign from malignant masses will be greatly facilitated. A margin that is obscured may look ill defined simply because the tissues in front and in back of the lesion are superimposed, and the con-

glomerate shadow obscures the margin. Many lesions, benign as well as malignant, develop in lobules that are immersed in normal extralobular fibrous-connective tissue. Their margins are immediately contiguous to this tissue with its similar x-ray attenuation, making it impossible to determine where the lesion ends and the fibrous tissue begins. It is not unusual for cysts (Fig. 13-65), as well as fibroadenomas (Fig. 13-66), to have obscured margins, and this often results in the need for ultrasound to differentiate a cyst from a solid mass or a tissue diagnosis if the lesion is solid. Pericystic inflammation (perhaps from leaked cyst contents) can also blur the margins of these benign lesions. Ultrasound is useful to avoid more aggressive intervention for a benign cyst.

LESIONS WITH MICROLOBULATED MARGINS

Many well-circumscribed lesions within the breast have a degree of lobulation. Fibroadenomas, for example, are usually not perfectly round and smooth, but have undulating lobulated margins. The more lobulated the lesion (lobulations per surface area) and the smaller the undulations, however, the more likely it is to be malignant. When the lobulations are multiple and only several millimeters in size, the degree of suspicion should be increased. Some have described this microlobulation as knobby. The ACR BIRADS prefers the term *microlobulated* margin. This morphologic characteristic is a strong indication of cancer (Fig. 13-67) but once again not pathognomonic because benign masses can have similar margins (Fig. 13-68).

LESIONS WITH ILL-DEFINED MARGINS: BREAST CANCER AND EVERYTHING ELSE

Breast Cancer

The ill definition of a margin is an important characteristic of breast cancer. Most invasive breast cancers have ill-defined margins as a result of tumor infiltration into the surrounding tissue and the irregular fibrosis that frequently accompanies the tumor (Fig. 13-69). Most ill-defined masses should be investigated, although many benign lesions can have ill-defined margins.

Cysts and Fibroadenomas

Virtually every benign lesion of the breast can also be found with margins that radiographically appear ill defined. This is true of cysts (see Fig. 13-51), whose margins may

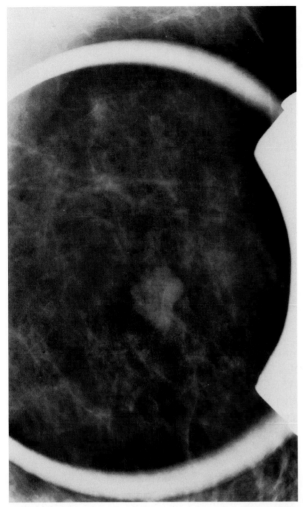

FIG. 13-68. Benign masses can have microlobulated margins. This mass, on magnification mammography, proved to be a benign cyst.

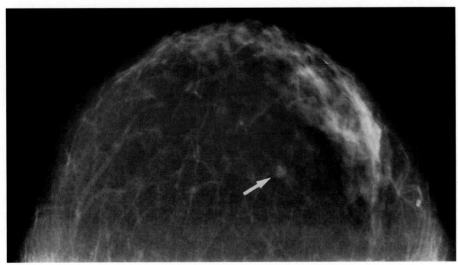

FIG. 13-69. The 7-mm **ill-defined** mass **(A)** in the midlateral aspect of the left breast on the craniocaudal projection remains ill defined on the magnification image **(B)** and represents a **nonpalpable infiltrating ductal cancer.**

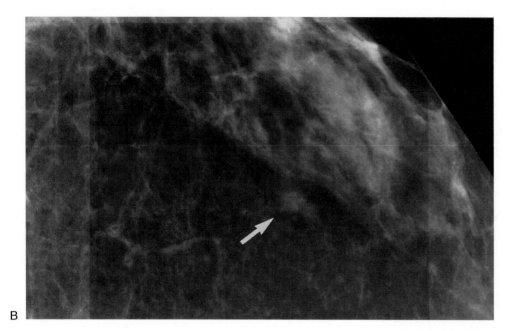

B

FIG. 13-69. *Continued.*

appear ill defined due to pericystic inflammation or pericystic fibrosis. Fibroadenomas can appear to have ill-defined margins (Fig. 13-70). Many benign lesions appear to have ill-defined margins because they blend seamlessly into normal breast tissue and their margins are actually obscured. A solid mass with ill-defined margins should be biopsied.

Contusion versus Hematoma

Contusion or hematoma from blunt trauma to the breast may produce a hard mass, but this is generally more apparent on physical examination than on the mammogram. Nevertheless, a bruise can produce an ill-defined lesion.

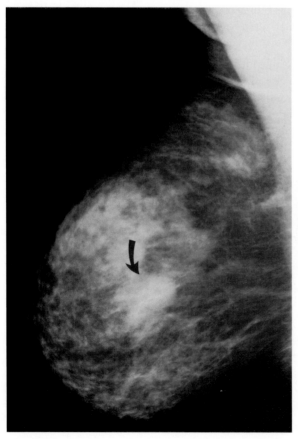

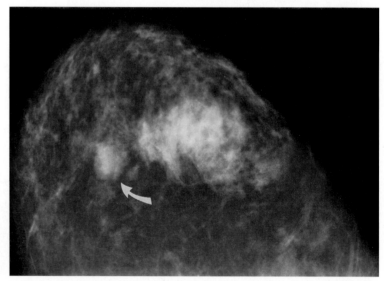

A

FIG. 13-70. Fibroadenomas can appear to have ill-defined margins, especially if they are not surrounded by fat. The ill-defined mass (*arrow*) on the mediolateral oblique **(A)** and craniocaudal **(B)** projections in this 51-year-old woman proved to be a fibroadenoma.

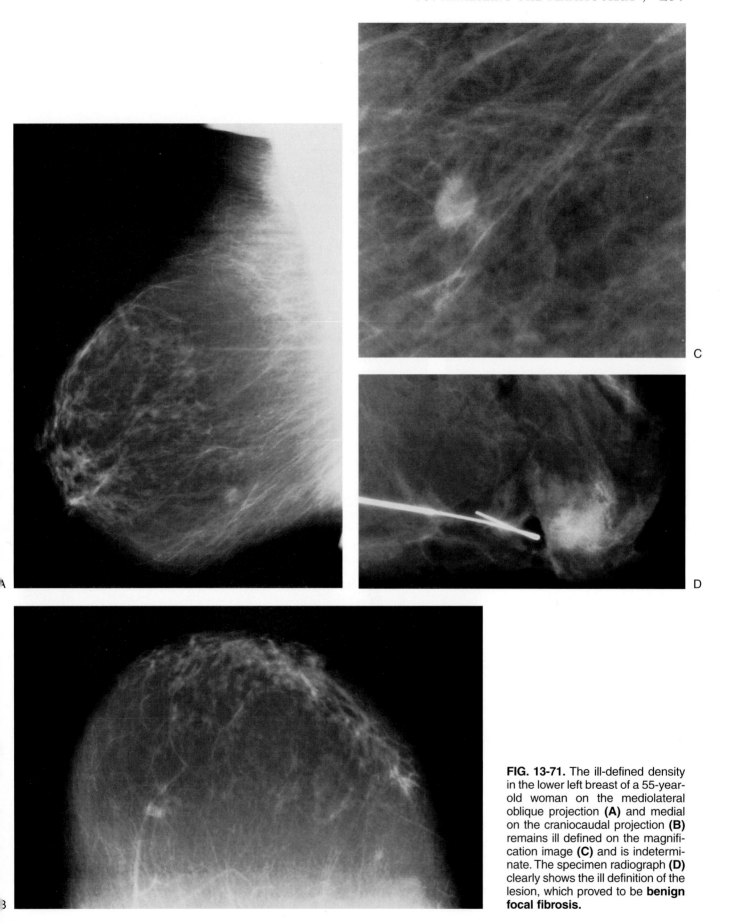

FIG. 13-71. The ill-defined density in the lower left breast of a 55-year-old woman on the mediolateral oblique projection **(A)** and medial on the craniocaudal projection **(B)** remains ill defined on the magnification image **(C)** and is indeterminate. The specimen radiograph **(D)** clearly shows the ill definition of the lesion, which proved to be **benign focal fibrosis.**

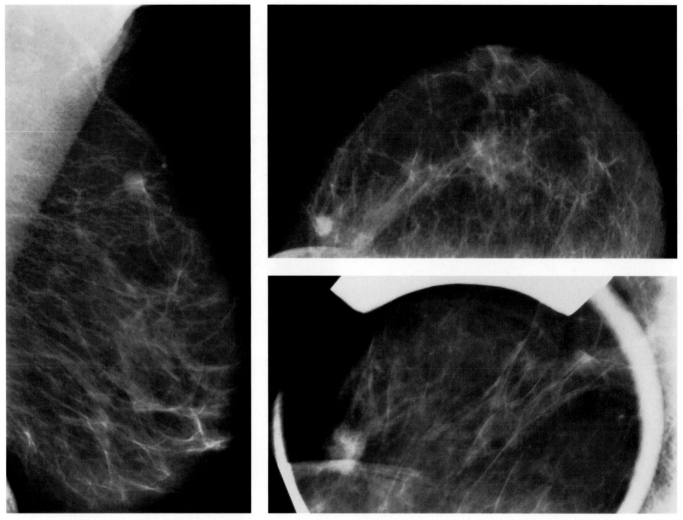

FIG. 13-72. Magnification can help evaluate the margins of a lesion. Based on the mediolateral oblique **(A)** projection the density in the upper breast could easily be an intramammary lymph node. The craniocaudal (CC) **(B)** projection is more worrisome, and the CC magnification view **(C)** defines a spiculated ill-defined mass that proved to be invasive breast cancer.

Extravasated blood generally dissects along the fibrous planes of the breast, producing trabecular thickening, but it can collect and appear as a mass radiographically.

Focal Fibrosis

Focal fibrosis frequently has ill-defined margins and is indistinguishable by mammography from a malignant process (Fig. 13-71).

Infection

Infection in the breast, including true abscess formation, is usually not clearly demonstrated mammographically; most are treated medically without the need for a mammogram. As with a hematoma, thickening of the trabecular pattern and architectural distortion in a nonspecific pattern is more likely.

EVALUATION OF ILL-DEFINED MASSES

Ultrasound can be useful to evaluate ill-defined lesions to determine if a cyst is present. Spot compression may aid in spreading overlapping structures, and magnification may improve the visualization of the lesion's margins (Fig. 13-72). In general, however, solitary lesions with ill-defined margins that are not cysts or islands of normal breast tissue should be biopsied.

ARCHITECTURAL DISTORTION

Breast cancer does not always produce a mammographically visible mass. It may produce only an area of architectural distortion. In general, the flow of structures within the breast is directed toward the nipple along duct lines. This pattern is superimposed on the crescentic planes of Cooper's

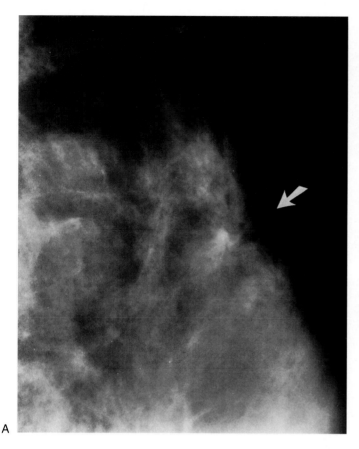

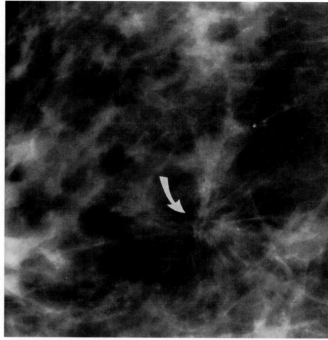

FIG. 13-73. Architectural distortion. The edge of the parenchyma is pulled in (*arrow*) due to an invasive cancer **(A)**. In this second individual **(B)** the cancer was apparent as a small area of spiculated architectural distortion (*arrow*).

ligaments, which form arcing curvilinear densities that criss-cross the breast to insert on the undersurface of the skin, producing concave scalloped surfaces at the edge of the mammary parenchyma. Disturbances in this normally symmetric flow—especially the pulling in of structures toward a point eccentric to the nipple—should be carefully evaluated (Fig. 13-73). Distorted architecture should be regarded with a high degree of suspicion and, if three-dimensionally real and not due to previous surgery, biopsy is indicated.

There are also benign causes of architectural distortion. The most common is apparent distortion due to the super-imposition of normal structures. Additional views, especially spot compression and rolled views (see Chapter 10), will resolve apparent distortions due to the superimposition of normal structures.

Postsurgical Change

Postsurgical scarring (Fig. 13-74) and fat necrosis are the most common nonmalignant causes of architectural distortion, although it is surprisingly uncommon for the breast to form a permanent radiographically noticeable scar (even if there is palpable scarring). Persistent postsurgical scar is rare and should resolve within 1 year to 18 months after surgery for a benign process (see Chapter 17). If it has not resolved,

the pathology of the biopsy should be reviewed to be sure that a high-risk lesion such as atypical hyperplasia was not present, possibly indicating the edge of a malignancy that was missed at surgery. Unless architectural distortion clearly coincides with a region of previous surgery, it should be investigated. The observer should remember that the tissue that was excised may lie at a distance from the surgical skin incision.

Radial Scar

Idiopathic tethering of the surrounding tissue is seen with an uncommon entity that has been variously termed a *radial scar*, *indurative mastopathy*, *sclerosing duct hyperplasia*, or *elastosis*, among other terms (Fig. 13-75). Frequently, dense radiating lines that are usually very long (≥1 cm) without a central mass are interspersed with trapped fat, forming lucent zones near the center of the area. These morphologic characteristics may suggest the diagnosis, but the lesion still should be biopsied because some cancers can have the same appearance. Because this benign lesion cannot be definitely distinguished from cancer by mammography and can sometimes fool even the pathologist by its gross appearance, excisional biopsy should be performed to make a definitive diagnosis. Core needle biopsy is probably not sufficient for the diagnosis of these lesions.

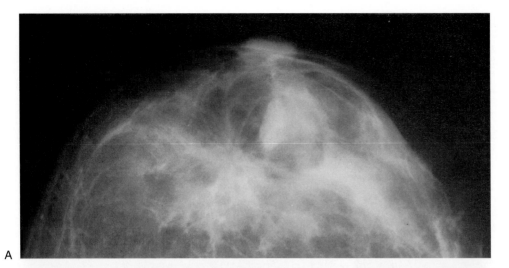

A

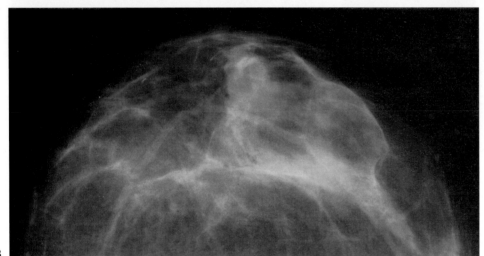

B

FIG. 13-74. Postsurgical change is a cause of architectural distortion. In this individual there was spiculated architectural distortion several months after the removal of a benign lesion (A). One year after the surgery (B) the distortion is gone and there is no mammographic evidence of the previous surgery.

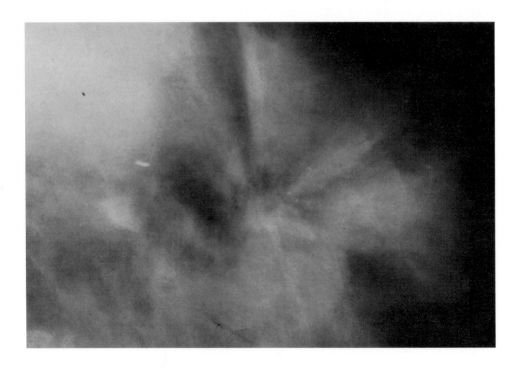

FIG. 13-75. The only way to make the diagnosis of a radial scar is through a surgical excision. This spiculated architectural distortion proved to be a benign radial scar.

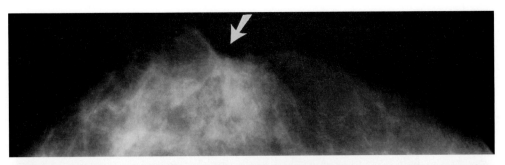

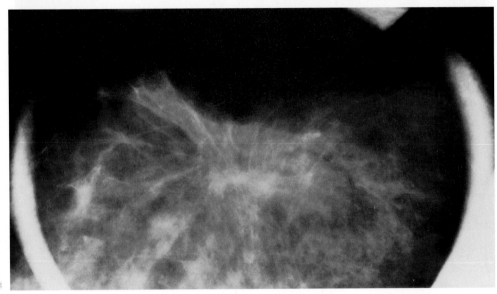

FIG. 13-76. The edge sign. The normally convex or scalloped edge of the parenchyma is pulled in **(A)** (*arrow*). A spot magnification image **(B)** reveals the spiculated invasive cancer that is the cause.

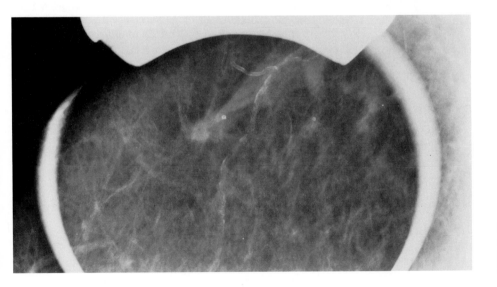

FIG. 13-77. A spiculated mass is almost always cancer. This 8-mm spiculated lesion was a nonpalpable, **invasive ductal carcinoma.**

Distorted Parenchymal Edge

The most common type of architectural distortion is spiculated distortion without a visible mass. This usually occurs in heterogeneously dense breast tissue. Because cancers are most common at the interface between the parenchyma and the subcutaneous and retromammary fat, spiculated distortion is fre-

quently found at the edge of the parenchymal cone (Fig. 13-76). The underlying mass is not apparent, and the observer's eye is drawn to the desmoplastic reaction that subtly distorts the architecture.

When a tumor occurs at the edge of the mammary parenchyma, either beneath the subcutaneous fat or adjacent to the retromammary fat, it can distort the edge of the

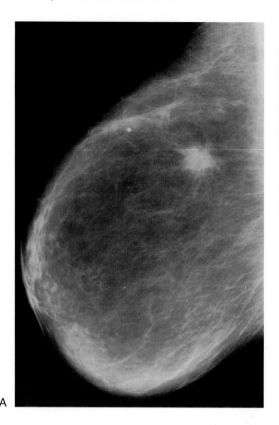

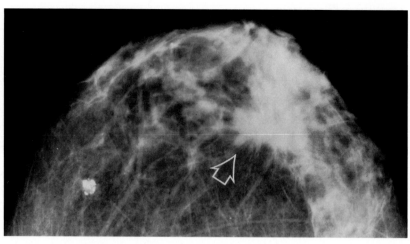

FIG. 13-78. The spicules are fibrous structures likely induced by the spreading cancer cells. If carefully evaluated there would likely be cancer cells along the fibrous spicules of this palpable invasive ductal carcinoma **(A).** In this second individual **(B)** the cancer is hidden by the dense tissue in the lateral portion of the breast and only the spicules (*arrow*) extending into the retromammary fat are visible.

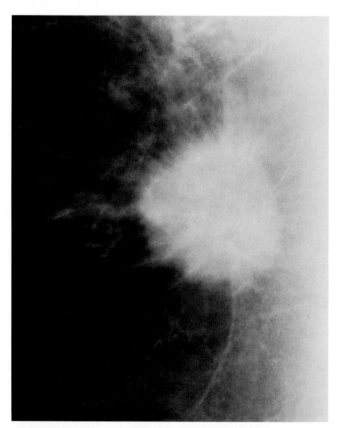

FIG. 13-79. This **invasive cancer,** seen photographically enlarged, has very short spicules, giving it a **brush border** appearance.

parenchyma. This architectural distortion may manifest itself as an actual pulling in, thickening, or merely as a flattening or straightening of the edge. Tethering of the edge of the parenchymal cone in one breast may be recognized by comparison with the corresponding mirror-image tissue of the opposite side.

The normal insertions of Cooper's ligaments in the skin produce a scalloped, concave margin to the parenchyma. A flattening, bulge, or convexity seen along the edge of the parenchyma may also indicate a possible cancer. A convexity is more likely due to a cyst or fibroadenoma. Nevertheless, it may still require investigation.

LESIONS WITH SPICULATED MARGINS (CANCER, POSTSURGICAL CHANGE OR SCARRING, AND UNCOMMON LESIONS)

A spiculated margin is one of the most significant findings on mammography. Although not a feature of all cancers it is one of the most typical features of many.

Breast Cancer

The presence of spiculations or a more diffuse irregular appearance (Fig. 13-77) is almost pathognomonic of breast cancer. These radially oriented filamentous structures represent fibrosis interspersed with tumor extending into the tissue surrounding the cancer (Fig. 13-78A). The desmoplasia

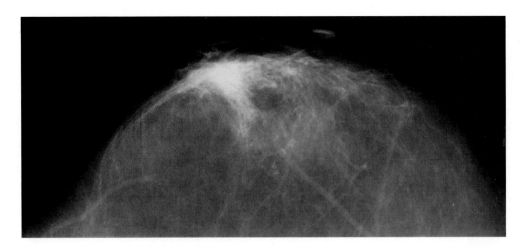

FIG. 13-80. The spiculated density in the subareolar area following a biopsy with benign results is **postsurgical change** that may persist for several weeks to even several months but usually resolves.

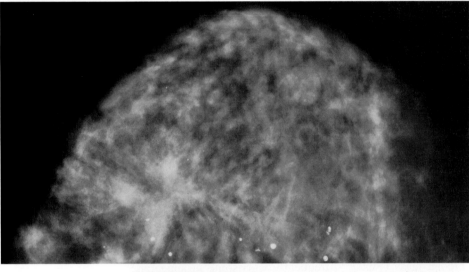

A

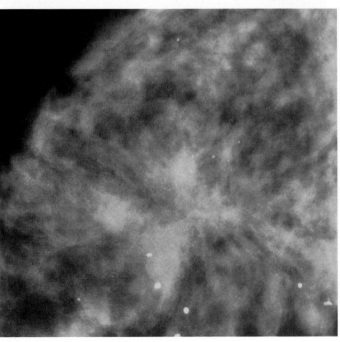

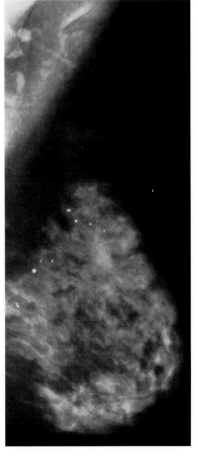

FIG. 13-81. Rarely, a postsurgical scar becomes a fixed spiculated change. This woman had a benign biopsy 6 years earlier, accounting for the architectural distortion seen on the craniocaudal projection **(A)** and photographically enlarged **(B)**. One distinguishing feature, in addition to the fact that the distortion was stable for 6 years, is that the change is barely visible in the mediolateral oblique **(C)** projection.

B,C

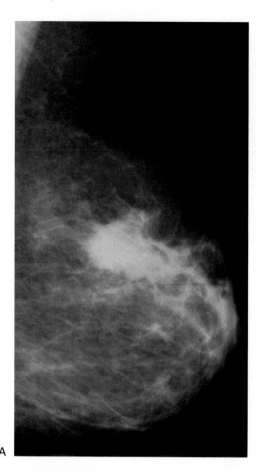

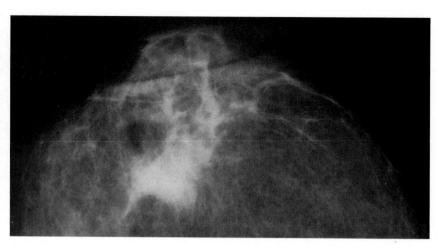

FIG. 13-82. Postsurgical change in the period immediately after a biopsy may be dramatic if a hematoma has formed, as in this patient who has a large, irregular, spiculated mass in the lateral **(A)** and craniocaudal **(B)** projections.

distorts the tissue surrounding a cancer. When a cancer with spiculation develops in a background of dense breast tissue its mass may be obscured, but a subtle "sunburst" pattern can be noted. These are the desmoplastic spicules of the lesion radiating from the underlying hidden mass (Fig. 13-78B). Occasionally spiculations appear to represent only fibrosis, but this is probably a sampling error, and tumor cells are usually found in association with this process. The spicules may extend over several centimeters or be only a few millimeters in size, producing a "brush" border (Fig. 13-79). When spicules are present the diagnosis of cancer is virtually certain.

Postsurgical Change and Scar

Architectural distortion and increased density may persist for many months after surgery; given sufficient time, the breast usually heals without radiographically visible scarring unless a large amount of tissue has been removed or there have been postoperative complications. In the early postoperative period (weeks to several months) spiculated architectural distortion is not unusual (Fig. 13-80). Sometimes, particularly if there is a hematoma, a large, spiculated mass is seen after surgery for a benign lesion. This usually is reabsorbed, and the breast heals without an obvious residual. On occasion, however, even a small

biopsy may result in a persistent ill-defined or spiculated residual scar (Fig. 13-81).

Postsurgical change is usually easily diagnosed. Postsurgical change is frequently a planar phenomenon and is frequently worrisome in appearance in only one projection. It may not even be evident in an orthogonal view (see Fig. 13-81). Cancer is usually evident and worrisome in the two projections. On occasion a mammogram is obtained soon after a surgical biopsy and distorted architecture is found. It can be reasoned that, if the biopsy had revealed a benign lesion, and the suspicious lesion had been excised, that the distorted architecture is unlikely to be due to an occult cancer. It is rare for breast cancer to occur in a region of a previous biopsy, although this may happen either by coincidence or because a sampling error caused the cancer to be missed at the previous excision. Significant growth of tumor, however, is unlikely within 1 year of surgery. Consequently, the rapid development of a malignant mass missed by the biopsy is unlikely. Healing may require many months to more than a year, and a new mass detected by physical examination or mammography soon after surgery is in all probability related to the surgery (Fig. 13-82).

In such cases, follow-up rather than rebiopsy is reasonable. It is not unusual for the biopsy site to appear spiculated soon after the biopsy and for this appearance to persist for as long as 6 months to a year after surgery for a benign lesion. If the breast has also been irradiated for cancer, the distorted architecture can remain for 18 to 24 months or longer, due to the delayed healing caused by the radiation. These changes usually resolve ultimately, leaving little evidence of the previous biopsy, but in some women fat necrosis may lead to calcium deposition or a persistent scar.

A spiculated area or architectural distortion seen on a mammogram that is done more than a year after surgery should be carefully correlated with the previous surgical site (from which the tissue was actually removed). It must be remembered that the skin incision may be at a distance from the area biopsied, which can complicate analysis. If there is any question, biopsy is prudent. Postsurgical change should stabilize or improve (resolve) with time. The appearance of distortion where none had been present previously or an increase in density or distortion over time should engender a high degree of suspicion.

Uncommon Spiculated Lesions

There are rare benign lesions, such as extra-abdominal desmoid tumors, granular cell tumors, and radial scars with elastosis, that can mimic the classic appearance of breast cancer. Desmoid and granular cell tumors are extremely uncommon (see Chapter 19).

False-Negative Biopsy

The likelihood of cancer is so great that if a lesion with spiculated margins is biopsied and the results are benign, skepticism should prevail. It should be demonstrated that the lesion has, in fact, been removed either by specimen radiography for nonpalpable lesions or by repeating the mammogram at the earliest possible time for these as well as lesions that were palpable (46). It is possible that the cancer was missed at biopsy. Furthermore, especially for nonpalpable lesions, if a large tissue sample has been obtained it must be carefully evaluated histologically at several levels because the actual tumor may occupy only a small portion of the tissue sample and could be missed with routine pathologic sampling.

Radial Scars

Radial scars are being diagnosed with increasing frequency. None of these lesions can be safely diagnosed without a biopsy. The radial scar is an idiopathic lesion. It is a scarring process characterized by lobules trapped in elastic tissue with ducts containing epithelial hyperplasia radiating from the center. Papillomatosis and adenosis are frequently present. Radiographically, as noted previously, it can appear as spiculated architectural distortion that is indistinguishable from breast cancer. It may even have the appearance of a spiculated mass (Fig. 13-83). Although the diagnosis can be suggested by the long spicules with little or no central mass, these lesions must be excised to avoid overlooking a malignancy.

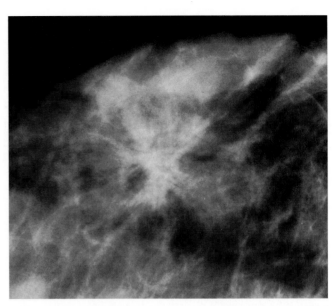

FIG. 13-83. Radial scars may appear as spiculated masses. This spiculated mass was palpable in a 27-year-old woman and proved to be a radial scar when excised.

NEODENSITY

The breast, at the level of resolution of mammography, is a fairly stable organ. Among many women however, it begins to involute long before menopause (see Chapter 12). If there are any changes, fibrous connective tissue and glandular elements are replaced by fat as the individual ages. Even when exogenous hormones are used, the parenchymal densities of the breast remain relatively stable over time. New masses, focal areas of increased density, new calcifications, or architectural changes require careful evaluation.

Thickening of the trabeculations of an area may indicate a significant process (see Chapter 15). Subtle changes may take place over several years. It would be ideal to compare the present examination with all previous studies, but this may compromise efficient review. A comparison study should probably be from at least 2 years prior to the present examination to reduce the likelihood of overlooking a subtle change.

Cysts are the most common masses that appear over time. They are frequently multiple and bilateral. The greatest problem with cysts is that a significant abnormality may be more difficult to appreciate because the tissues are obscured by the cysts. As with other possible abnormalities, spot compression and varying the projection may help to determine if there is a superimposed problem. Ultrasound is helpful in distinguishing cysts from solid lesions, but ultrasound should be targeted to a specific area and not used to survey the breast. Future investigations may prove that ultrasound can be used to survey breast tissue and find occult cancers, but the data do not yet support this application.

Fibroadenomas can enlarge over time. Because these lesions likely develop with the breast, it is rare for them to

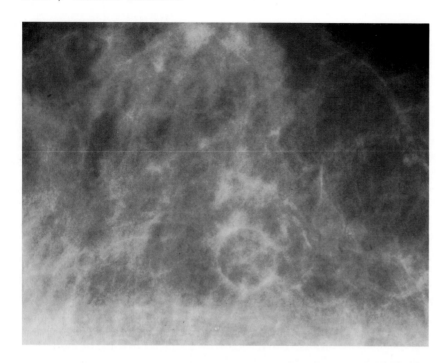

FIG. 13-84. The post-traumatic oil cyst is a form of fat necrosis. The oil cyst is oval or, as in this case, round with low-attenuation, gelatinized fat within a capsule.

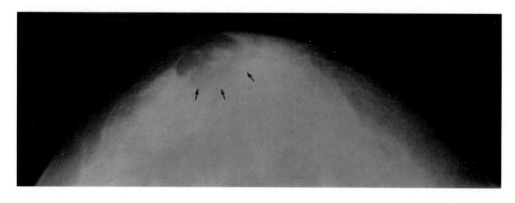

FIG. 13-85. Lipomas can be palpable. This lipoma (*arrows*) was excised, despite the fact that the mammogram was diagnostic.

appear in an area that was clear on previous mammograms. A new, solid mass should be viewed with suspicion.

X-RAY ATTENUATION

The x-ray attenuation of a lesion is a useful measure of its significance. The absolute attenuation of a breast lesion cannot be determined from two-dimensional imaging, but relative comparisons can be made.

Low-Attenuation Lesions

Most benign lesions are isodense or slightly denser than an equal volume of normal fibroglandular tissue. Breast cancers are frequently more highly attenuating. This remains a subjective analysis (particularly when there is little or no fibroglandular tissue for comparison) and is not an absolute diagnostic criterion. There are benign lesions that are highly

attenuating, and there are malignant lesions that are lower in x-ray attenuation.

Encapsulated Fat-Containing Lesions

Encapsulated fat-containing lesions are benign and radiolucent. Although moderately uncommon, they are important because encapsulated lesions that contain fat are never malignant. Radiolucent lesions are always benign, and the diagnosis can be made from the mammogram. Lesions that truly contain fat (not just appear to have fat or to trap fat) are never malignant. Lucent lesions include the post-traumatic oil cyst (Fig. 13-84), lipoma (Fig. 13-85), and the extremely rare galactocele, all of which have a similar appearance. All have a capsule whose inner wall is visible in contrast to the high-fat material making up the lesion. The oil cyst is a form of fat necrosis that contains gelatinized fat defined by a thin capsule. Its appearance is characteristic. Lipomas and high–fat content galactoceles present no diagnostic dilemma and are always benign.

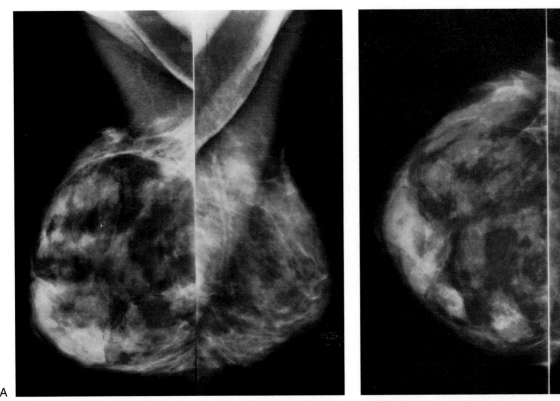

FIG. 13-86. The large mass that is displacing the normal architecture in the left breast on the mediolateral oblique **(A)** and craniocaudal **(B)** projections in this 39-year-old woman is encapsulated tissue of mixed density. This is typical of a benign hamartoma.

Encapsulated lesions of mixed density, such as the hamartoma (Fig. 13-86), that contain fat are never malignant and can be characterized directly from the mammogram as benign processes. These benign lesions truly contain fat. The interpreter is cautioned that some lesions, as a consequence of tissue projecting behind and in front of them, may appear to contain fat when in fact they do not.

Breast Cancer

Most breast cancers have a higher x-ray attenuation than an equal volume of fibroglandular tissue (Fig. 13-87A). This is likely due to the dense fibrosis associated with these lesions and perhaps the fact that they are less compressible than normal or benign tissues. There are many cancers that are isodense, and occasionally some, such as colloid can-

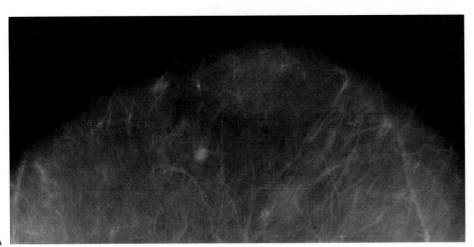

FIG. 13-87. (A) Breast cancer is usually highly attenuating. Despite its very small size, this invasive breast cancer is extremely attenuating. *Continued.*

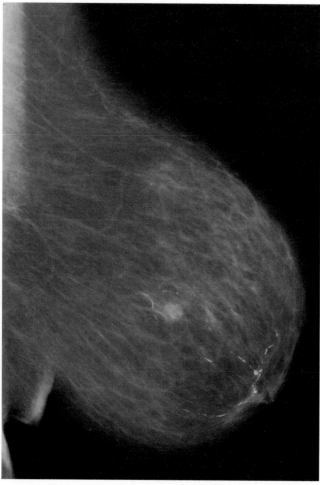

B

FIG. 13-87. *Continued.* **(B) Breast cancer is not always dense.** This invasive cancer is not particularly dense for its size.

cers, may be less attenuating than an equal volume of breast tissue; this characteristic, therefore, does not have a perfect correlation (Fig. 13-87B). Benign lesions can also have higher attenuation. Bleeding into a cyst can result in a highly attenuating mass. Because intracystic bleeding can indicate an intracystic mass, highly attenuating cysts should be carefully evaluated (Fig. 13-88).

OTHER LESIONS

Solitary Dilated Duct

On rare occasions, a solitary duct or network may appear dilated and form a tubular or branching structure (Fig. 13-89). A solitary dilated duct has been described as an indicator of cancer. This, however, is an extremely unusual event, and the reported cases are anecdotal. The usual cause of solitary duct dilatation is idiopathic duct ectasia.

An intraductal papilloma can cause duct dilatation. The mechanism is not clear. It has been suggested that the papilloma obstructs the duct and the buildup of fluid causes the duct to dilate. This does not make physiologic sense. It would imply that the ducts usually secrete fluid to be blocked. If this were the only mechanism, then fluid would normally have to drain from the nipple such that the drainage could be blocked by the papilloma. This is not the case, because nipple discharge is unusual. Furthermore, the ducts are generally blocked by keratin plugs in the nipple orifices. If it was blockage of normal secretions, then this would lead to diffuse ductal dilatation in most women.

In our experience, when a single dilated duct harbors an intraductal papilloma, the tumor is usually distal in the duct

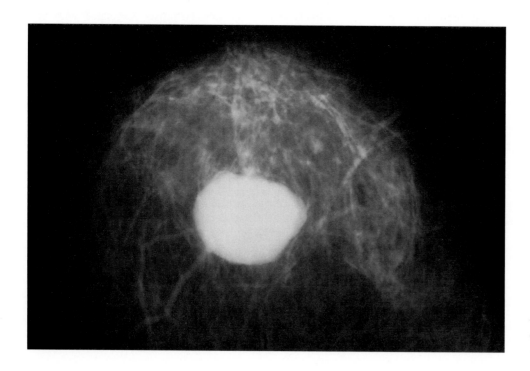

FIG. 13-88. The high attenuation of this mass was primarily due to **hemorrhage from an intracystic cancer.**

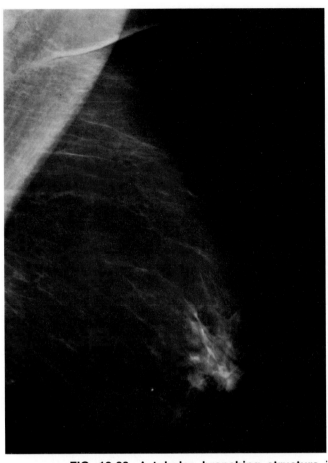

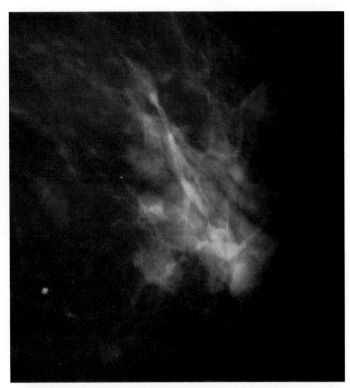

A   B

FIG. 13-89. A tubular, branching structure is seen on the mediolateral oblique (MLO) **(A)** and enlarged MLO **(B)** images. *Continued.*

(relative to the lobule) but is rarely obstructing it. This suggests that the papilloma itself probably is the cause of, or related to, increased secretion that is not balanced by resorption, leading to dilatation of the widest portion of the duct according to Laplace's law (47).

When a dilated duct is found in association with cancer, the dilated duct is almost always accompanied by a discharge, or other signs, such as calcifications or an associated mass, are present. Because a solitary dilated duct is so rarely caused by cancer, if there are no associated signs or symptoms and there are no previous mammograms to determine the chronicity of the finding, these patients are placed in a short-interval follow-up program with mammography at 6-month intervals. If there is no change after 2 years, we return the patient to annual screening. Cancer in this setting is so rare that short-interval follow-up for these women may ultimately prove to be unnecessary.

Because duct dilatation is probably not due to obstruction, cancers as well as benign lesions associated with solitary dilated ducts are, in fact, usually not at the nipple but further back in the duct. If biopsy is undertaken, it may be necessary to excise the deep segments of the duct. If the dilatation is associated with a discharge, galactography may help to evaluate the deeper duct segments. There have been several

anecdotal cases of cannulating ducts that are not discharging and injecting contrast to define filling defects, or of using ultrasound to guide injection directly into a dilated duct.

STABILITY OVER TIME

For most lesions, stability over time is an indication that a mass is benign. However, the shape and margins of the lesion must be taken into account. If a mass is round or ovoid, or even lobulated with circumscribed margins, the likelihood of malignancy is probably 5% or less. If it is then found to be stable over a 2-year period (our arbitrarily chosen interval), then the likelihood of malignancy is even less because cancers are rarely stable (low probability multiplied by low probability). Stability for indeterminate or suspicious lesions, however, is much less reassuring. Although unusual, we have seen spiculated or ill-defined masses and areas of architectural distortion (Fig. 13-90) that were cancers but were stable for as long as 5 years (48). Lesions should only be classified as "probably benign" when they have benign morphology and the expectation is that they will not change over the period of follow-up. Lesions that are probably benign can be reasonably followed at short intervals to assess

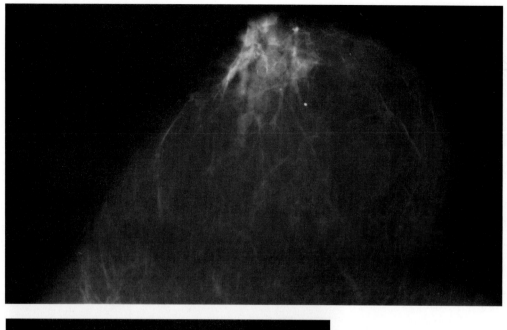

C

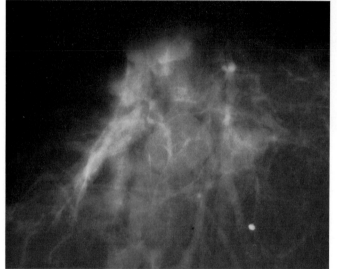

D

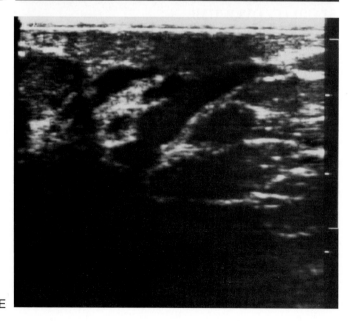

E

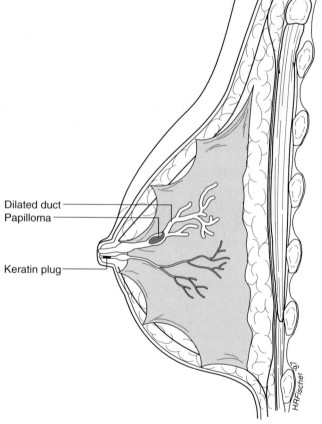

Dilated duct
Papilloma

Keratin plug

F

FIG. 13-89. *Continued.* The structure is also shown on the craniocaudal (CC) **(C)** and enlarged CC **(D)** images. On ultrasound **(E)**, the structure is shown to be fluid-filled dilated ducts due to **ectasia.**

Intraductal papillomas are generally found near the nipple. **(F)** As depicted in this schematic, if ductal dilatation is present it is generally on both sides of the papilloma, suggesting that the dilatation is not an obstructive phenomenon. Most normal ducts are effectively obstructed by a keratin plug in the nipple orifice.

—C

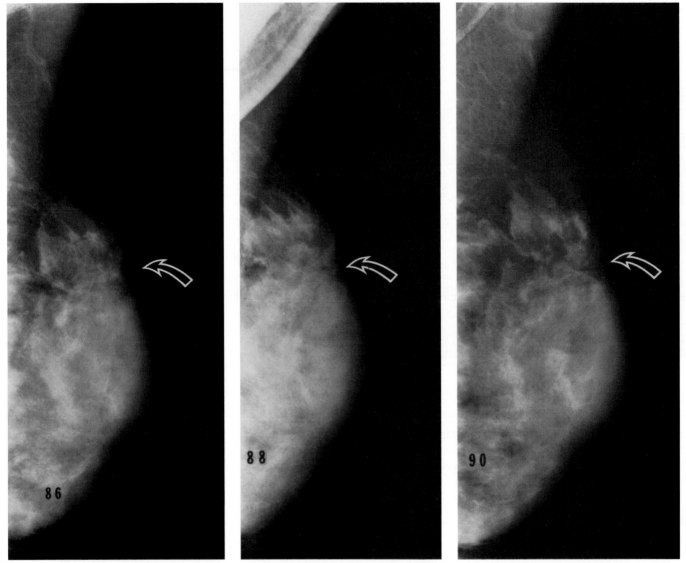

FIG. 13-90. Cancer can be stable for as long as 5 years. Architectural distortion (*arrow*) was unchanged from 1986 **(A)** to 1988 **(B)** to 1990 **(C)**, yet it proved to be invasive ductal carcinoma at biopsy in 1990.

their stability (39). Biopsy should be undertaken for any lesion that has worrisome morphology, despite its stability.

RULE OF MULTIPLICITY

Because most breast cancers are solitary and distinctive in appearance, the presence of three or more findings that have similar morphologic characteristics usually means they are due to benign processes. This is particularly true if the findings are in multiple areas of the breast and especially if the similar findings are bilateral. Cysts are frequently multiple. Fibroadenomas may also be multiple. The rule of multiplicity for masses generally applies to those that are round or ovoid with circumscribed or obscured margins. Clearly multiple spiculated masses should not be considered benign.

Multiple Rounded Densities

Multiple rounded densities, defined as three or more rounded densities in a breast (Fig. 13-91), are not very common. In a screening population of approximately 23,000 women, multiple rounded densities were found on the first screen in 120 women (0.5%). When these are of relatively low x-ray attenuation (density), they most likely represent cysts. We have adopted a practical approach to such lesions. Due to the multiplicity of these structures, biopsy is impractical and would result in unacceptable morbidity to the patient. With the exception of metastatic disease to the breast and the generally obvious multifocal cancer (dense, ill-defined, or spiculated lesions), multiple rounded densities are invariably benign. Unless one of the densities distinguishes itself with a different, suspicious morphology and prompts a biopsy, a recommenda-

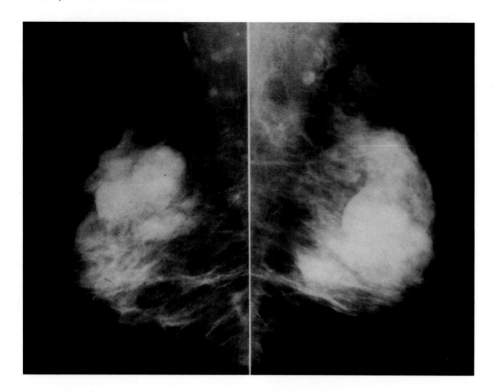

FIG. 13-91. The **multiple rounded densities** seen bilaterally on these mediolateral oblique mammograms are all likely cysts.

tion for a 6-month follow-up is made. Invariably there is no change. We now avoid ultrasound because it may demonstrate hypoechoic areas and areas of shadowing that never prove to be malignant and are only confusing. Ultrasound may be helpful if there is a specific, focal area of concern.

Multiple Vague Densities

At times the observer is confronted with a mammogram where there are numerous (three or more) vague, ill-defined densities, any one of which, if solitary, might elicit additional evaluation. These likely represent islands of breast tissue (lobules and connective tissue), and if there are no other reasons to suspect malignancy many observers would dismiss them as normal mammograms. We place these in our short-interval follow-up program, but this is overly cautious.

SIGNS THAT WARRANT BIOPSY ONLY WHEN PHYSICAL EXAMINATION PROVIDES SUPPORTING EVIDENCE

Although intuitively it might seem appropriate that CBE should be correlated with the mammogram, this is rarely critical for making management decisions. The two methods of breast evaluation actually measure different tissue characteristics, and the results are often discordant. Cancers detected by mammography are frequently not palpable, and some cancers that are palpable are not evident on the mammogram. It is well established that, if either test raises sus-

picion, that suspicion should be acted on regardless of the results of the other test. A complete screening program should probably include CBE, but the so-called correlative CBE has no documented practical value.

Asymmetric Dense Breast Tissue

The only situation in which the correlation of the CBE with the mammogram may assist management is when asymmetric breast tissue is evident on the mammogram. A review of false-negative mammograms in women with palpable cancers occasionally reveals an asymmetric increase in the density of the breast tissue in the region of the cancer without other suspicious changes (15). As a result, although nonspecific and common in normal women, asymmetric breast tissue density can be associated malignancy. More important, however, the converse is not true: Asymmetric breast tissue density is *unlikely* to be due to breast cancer if the density is not forming a mass, the architecture is preserved, and there are no microcalcifications associated with the asymmetry (see Asymmetric Breast Tissue, earlier).

At least 3% of normal women have significantly asymmetric breast tissue that appears as increased volume or density relative to the same projection of the contralateral breast. This usually merely reflects normal asymmetric development (Fig. 13-92). In some women it no doubt represents the variable end-organ response of breast tissue to hormonal factors, with one part of the breast being more sensitive to hormone stimulation. However, in a woman who has a palpable thickening that is of some concern on physi-

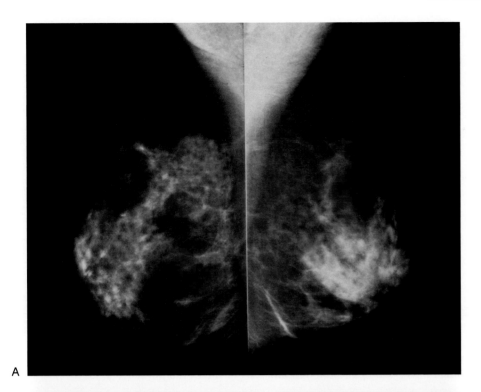

A

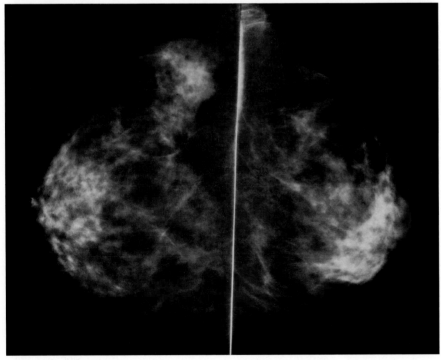

B

FIG. 13-92. Asymmetric breast tissue is usually a normal variation. The asymmetric breast tissue in the upper (as seen on the mediolateral oblique projections) **(A)** and outer (as seen on the craniocaudal projections) **(B)** left breast was stable for >4 years, as was the asymmetric tissue density in the anterior, lower inner right breast.

cal examination, the presence of corresponding asymmetric dense breast tissue on mammography should increase the level of concern and prompt a biopsy (Fig. 13-93).

Some palpable cancers do not produce a lesion with mammographically demonstrable margins, nor do they produce calcium deposits. The only visible finding may merely be an increase in radiographic density in a volume of breast tissue. Thus, when asymmetric tissue is palpable, malig-

nancy becomes a concern. Normal, asymmetric breast tissue is usually not palpable, and asymmetrically dense tissue, without the margins of a mass or other secondary signs of malignancy, is not by itself an indication for biopsy.

Asymmetric dense breast tissue must not be confused with a focal asymmetric density (Fig. 13-94). The latter is part of the spectrum of lesions with ill-defined margins. A focal asymmetric density almost always has a shape centered on a point

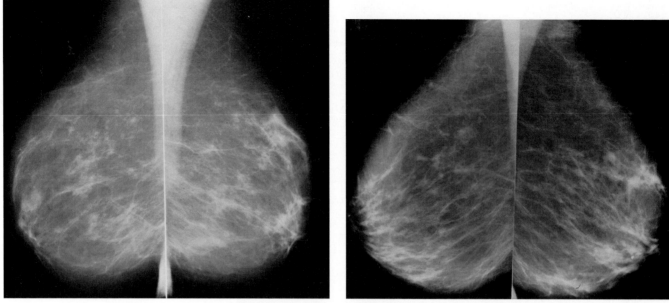

FIG. 13-93. Significant asymmetric breast tissue is palpable. In this patient **(A)** there is asymmetry in the anterior upper right breast that was not palpable and is a normal variation. In this second patient **(B)** a similar asymmetry was **palpable,** and biopsy revealed invasive ductal carcinoma.

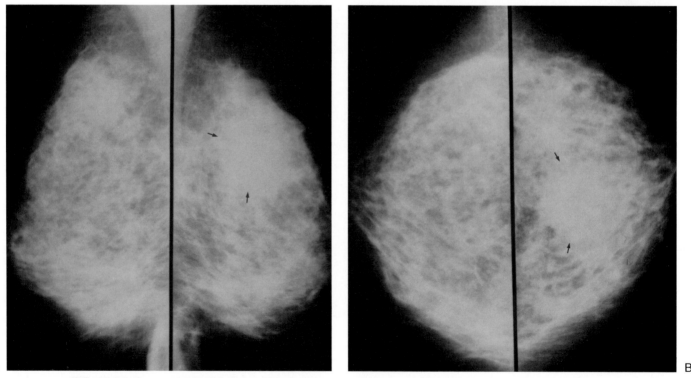

FIG. 13-94. Asymmetrically dense tissue is not always a normal variation. In this case the asymmetry is centrally dense in the lateral **(A)** and craniocaudal **(B)** projections with the density decreasing toward the periphery. This is trying to form a mass, and biopsy revealed invasive breast cancer.

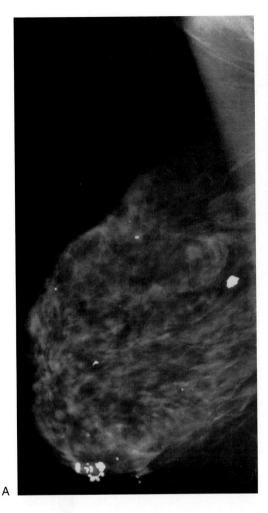

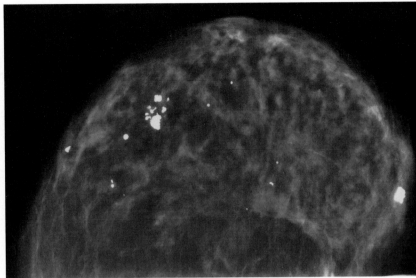

FIG. 13-95. The **large calcifying masses** in this 70-year-old woman on the mediolateral oblique **(A)** and craniocaudal **(B)** projections are typical of calcifying, **involuting fibroadenomas.** The appearance is so characteristic that there is no need for a tissue analysis.

and is most dense at the center. Asymmetric breast tissue is almost always benign and requires no additional investigation if there is no corresponding, palpable asymmetry. A focal asymmetric density, on the other hand, should be suspect and frequently requires additional evaluation such as magnification imaging to determine whether or not it is significant.

When assessing asymmetric density, the observer should remember that the asymmetry may be due to increased density on the ipsilateral side or to decreased tissue on the contralateral side. For example, in a woman who has had a previous biopsy, asymmetry may be due to the removal of tissue on the contralateral side rather than increased density ipsilaterally.

CALCIFICATIONS

Masses with Associated Calcifications

The etiology of a mass can frequently be inferred by associated calcifications. A mass that contains large (>1 mm) calcifications with a popcorn appearance is diagnostic for an involuting fibroadenoma (Fig. 13-95) or, less commonly, a papilloma. Fine curvilinear calcifications that delineate the wall of a round or oval mass almost always indicate a benign

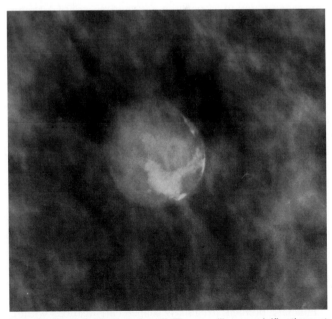

FIG. 13-96. **Calcified cyst wall.** The curvilinear calcifications at the surface of this round mass permit the diagnosis of a cyst.

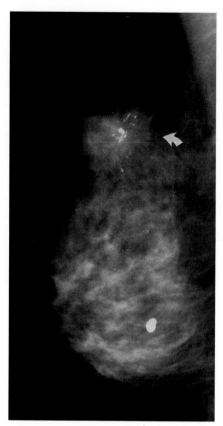

FIG. 13-97. Pleomorphic calcifications in a mass. These calcifications are in the intraductal component of a cancer (*arrow*) that has both invasive and intraductal portions.

cyst (Fig. 13-96). Pleomorphic calcifications that are <0.5 mm, when found in association with a mass, are of concern just as they would be if no mass were present (Fig. 13-97). When due to cancer, these calcifications almost invariably occur in the intraductal component of a mixed lesion (invasive cancer with an associated intraductal cancer). Some intraductal cancers have tissue reaction outside the duct without apparent invasion (49), or the duct may become dilated with the growing intraductal cancer such that a mass may still represent intraductal disease without invasion. This is, however, relatively uncommon, and a mass usually indicates an invasive lesion. Some cancers can have large calcifications associated with them, probably as a result of their engulfing some neighboring benign deposits. As with calcifications that are not associated with a mass, calcifications associated with a mass should be judged by the most worrisome, and if there is a question biopsy should be considered.

Calcifications in Cancer

Punctate, pointed, irregularly shaped calcifications within a mass that are heterogeneous in size and morphology or fine, linear, branching deposits filling the narrowed duct lumen are strong indicators of cancer (Fig. 13-98). Usually when calcifications of this type are present within a lesion,

A

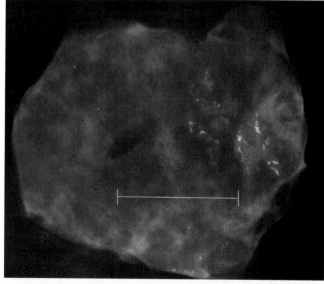

B

FIG. 13-98. (A) Pleomorphic calcifications in an irregular, ill-defined mass are almost diagnostic for a malignant process, as in this invasive and intraductal cancer. The fine linear branching calcifications of poorly differentiated comedocarcinoma (ductal carcinoma in situ) are well seen in this specimen radiograph (B) in which the marker represents 1 cm. Mammography can demonstrate calcifications in the breast that are as small as 150 μm.

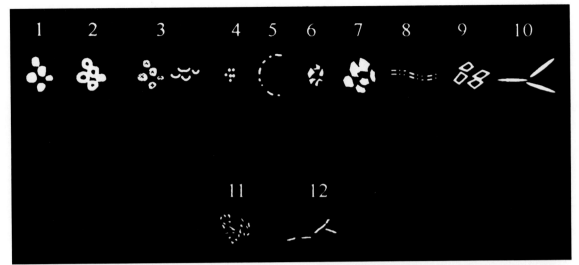

FIG. 13-99. This schematic represents many of the **types of calcifications** that can be seen by mammography. (1) Calcified debris in ducts; (2) dense, lucent-centered calcifications in fat necrosis; (3) precipitated calcifications in small cysts (milk of calcium); (4) concretions in small, cystically dilated lobules; (5) rim calcifications in the wall of a cyst; (6) early deposits in an involuting fibroadenoma; (7) large deposits in an involuting fibroadenoma; (8) vascular calcifications; (9) skin calcifications; (10) calcified rods in secretory disease; (11) pleomorphic deposits in intraductal cancer; (12) fine linear calcifications found in comedocarcinoma.

the irregularity of the mass itself is sufficient to arouse significant concern. Although it used to be stated that up to 50% of malignant masses contained calcifications, the percentage is lower now that lesions are being discovered at an earlier stage. The presence of calcifications within lesions that already exhibit morphologic signs of malignancy merely increases the likelihood of cancer.

In large cancers, necrosis can produce calcifications, but fortunately these large cancers are becoming less common, and, as noted previously, calcifications associated with an invasive cancer are almost always due to an intraductal component. The presence of a large number of calcifications may signal the presence of an EIC. In some series, EIC has predicted a greater risk of recurrence for women whose breast cancer is treated by lumpectomy and radiation. It is likely that invasive cancers with an EIC are characterized by tumor extending undetected along the ducts beyond the margin of resection such that the volume of residual tumor is sufficiently great to escape complete elimination by radiation. This results in a greater chance of recurrence.

Analyzing Calcifications Without an Associated Mass

Calcium deposits are extremely common in the breast. Stomper and associates reported that they found benign calcifications on 8% of the mammograms performed for women between the ages of 25 and 29 with a steady increase to 86% of the mammograms performed on women between the ages of 76 and 79 (50). It has been our experience that most women have one or more calcifications visible on x-ray. Calcifications are seen even more extensively and more frequently by microscopy.

Breast cancer is just one of the many mostly benign processes that result in calcium deposition. Some are produced by active cell secretion, whereas others form in necrotic cellular debris. They may be a response to inflammation, trauma, radiation, or foreign bodies. Calcifications are found within the ducts, alongside and around the ducts, in the lobular acini, in vascular structures, in the interlobular stroma, in fat, and in the skin. Depending on their etiology and location they may be punctate, branching, linear, spherical (shell-like), fine, coarse, cylindrical, smooth, jagged, regular in size and shape, or heterogeneous (Fig. 13-99).

Although they are termed *calcium deposits*, their exact composition remains uncertain. They have been analyzed by Galkins and associates, and in fact many may not contain just calcium (51). The exact reason for this is unclear. Spectral analysis of calcifications revealed other elements, including unexpected heavy metals such as iron. Should higher "Z" material be present it may some day be possible to do in vivo spectral analysis to aid in diagnosis. More likely, the higher attenuation of these materials may permit x-ray dual energy subtraction to highlight the particles associated with cancer, leading to earlier detection (see Chapter 26).

The morphology and distribution of breast calcifications can often indicate their etiology (Figs. 13-100 through 13-103). Certain patterns are never associated with malignancy (see Chapter 14). Some calcifications form in the extralobular stroma, but most occur in the lobules and ducts. When lobular they are virtually always benign and usually in cystically dilated acini. Intraductal cancers may clog the duct, and central portions of the tumor may die from lack of oxygen and nutrients diffusing in from the periductal vascu-

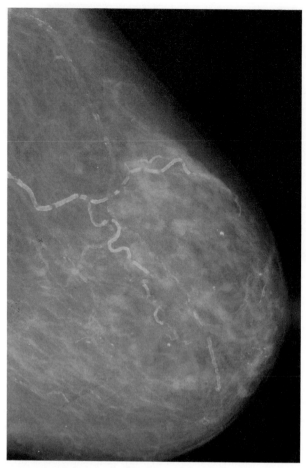

FIG. 13-100. **Vascular calcifications** usually have a typical appearance and should cause no concern.

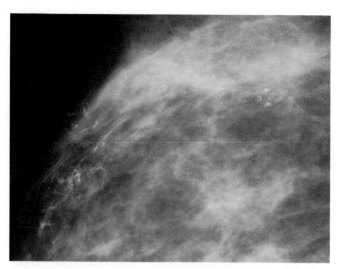

FIG. 13-102. **Pleomorphic calcifications in a segmental distribution** are always of concern, as in this poorly differentiated comedocarcinoma.

lature. The necrotic (comedo) cells may calcify, producing a characteristic fine linear pattern that branches with the duct. Difficulty in diagnosis arises when the calcifications form small clustered particles. These frequently cannot be differentiated from benign collections.

As with masses, if the morphologic characteristics of calcifications indicate a benign process, then no further analysis is needed (see Chapter 14). Most calcifications have characteristically benign morphology, but certain shapes and patterns should prompt a biopsy. A careful search for the clustered

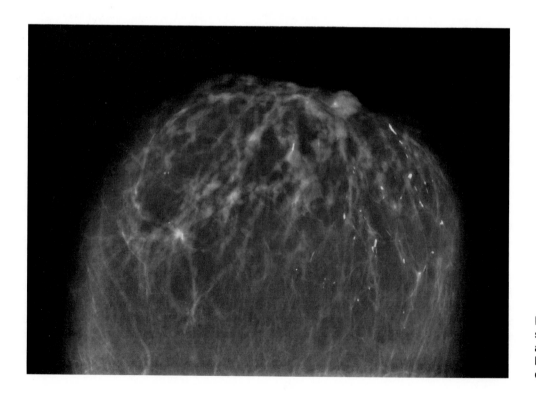

FIG. 13-101. **Linear, solid, rod-shaped calcifications** virtually always represent a **benign process**, such as these due to secretory deposits.

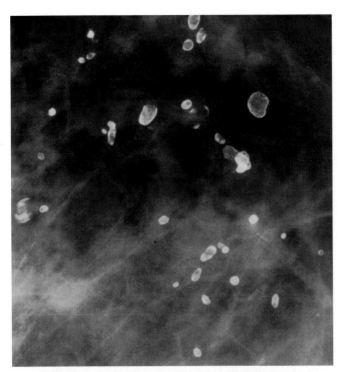

FIG. 13-103. Large (>1 mm) lucent-centered calcifications are always due to a benign process, such as these that likely represent fat necrosis or calcified debris.

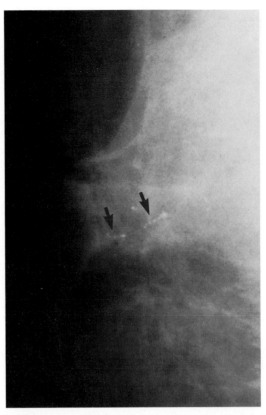

FIG. 13-104. These calcifications (*arrows*) were due to **intraductal carcinoma** extending into the nipple in a patient with **Paget's disease.**

microcalcifications that may herald an early-stage cancer should be done on all mammograms. The fact that some cancers produce radiographically visible calcium deposits early in their growth can be considered fortuitous. Although the pathologist sees microscopic deposits in many breast cancers, many produce no radiographically detectable calcifications.

When visible on the mammogram, calcifications can be seen by the unaided eye, but a magnifying glass is indispensable to aid in finding them. Magnification mammography, by reducing the effect of noise, improves the clarity in viewing and analyzing these particles. Irregular, heterogeneous deposits that lack benign morphology, grouped in isolation without an associated mass in a small volume of breast tissue and greater than four in number should be viewed with suspicion. In 20% of cases, these groups represent cancer (52).

The recognition that certain patterns of calcium deposition are associated with malignant processes has made possible the early detection of many cancers. The detection of these clustered microcalcifications associated with cancer is unique to mammography and one of its most important functions. No other imaging technique can find these tiny deposits, which when found in isolation may herald the presence of a highly curable intraductal cancer or early infiltrating lesion.

Unfortunately, benign and malignant processes can produce similar patterns of calcium deposition and frequently cannot be differentiated. Biopsy is often required for diagnosis. Analysis of the location, size, morphology, number, distribution, and any associated findings of the deposits can, however, eliminate many from suspicion.

The initial assessment of calcifications is made to determine if they conform to well-established benign morphologies. Calcifications with benign morphologies require no further investigation. If the characteristics of the calcifications are such that they cannot be reliably classified as due to benign processes, then additional evaluation is indicated.

Magnification mammography is the primary technique used to further analyze calcifications. A clearer appreciation of the morphology and distribution of the calcifications is afforded by magnification, and this is used to ultimately decide, using objective criteria, whether or not a biopsy to establish a firm diagnosis is needed.

Location

The major determination is whether or not calcifications are truly intramammary or are in the skin. This may seem trivial, yet numerous women have undergone truly unnecessary surgery to try to remove calcifications that were benign skin deposits (53). It is not difficult to appreciate the fact that most skin calcifications project over the breast in two views, because only thin portions of the skin are actually seen in tangent on the two-view mammogram. Tangential views of the skin containing the calcifications will confirm the location of these particles (see Chapter 22).

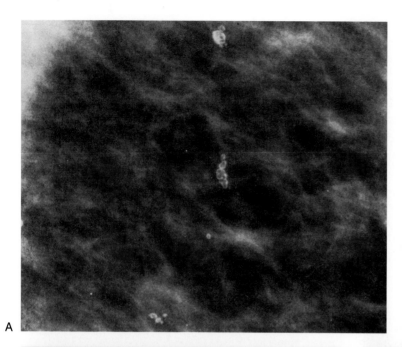

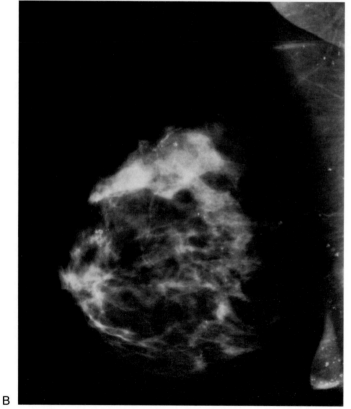

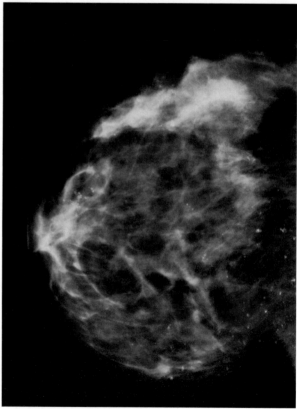

FIG. 13-105. **(A) Calcifications that have lucent centers and geographic shapes** are almost always benign skin calcifications, as seen here enlarged many times.

Skin calcifications are most commonly found along the sternal borders of the breast, as seen here on the mediolateral oblique **(B)** and craniocaudal **(C)** projections in this second individual. This is likely due to the high concentration of hair follicles here.

Calcifications of the Nipple and Skin

Calcifications of the nipple occur infrequently. On occasion, the clinically evident extension of intraductal carcinoma onto the surface of the nipple, known as *Paget's disease,* can produce microcalcifications extending along the duct network in a single-file pattern (Fig. 13-104). Vir-

tually all other calcifications of the nipple represent benign processes and are rare.

Calcifications in the skin, however, are extremely common. As already mentioned, they usually have a typical appearance, often having central lucencies with a spherical or polygonal shape (Fig. 13-105A), and are frequently scattered widely over the breast, especially along the sternal side

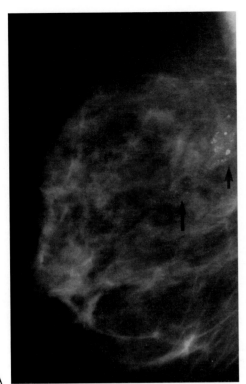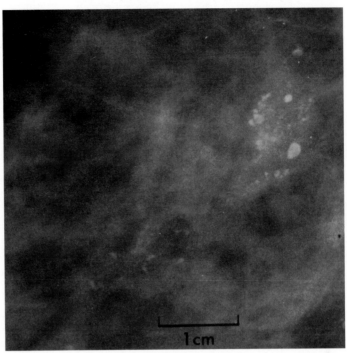

FIG. 13-106. Calcifications should be judged by those with the worst morphology. There are large, benign calcifications **(A)** with lucent centers in this segmental grouping (*short arrow*), but the other very small, pleomorphic calcifications (*long arrow*) are due to intraductal carcinoma. These are seen to better advantage on this enlarged image **(B)**.

(Fig. 13-105B, C). On occasion they may be mistaken for intramammary deposits, but this can be resolved using tangential views.

Size

The calcifications associated with breast cancer (as well as those from benign process) are often truly microscopic, and the pathologist sees many more than are radiographically visible. These calcifications rarely form in the tumor when it has infiltrated beyond the duct but more frequently form in the necrotic cancer cells that frequently die in the central portions of a duct that is stuffed with and distended by malignant cells.

Within a given group of calcifications, size may vary from barely perceptible to large coarse deposits. Calcifications up to 2.0 mm in diameter may still be considered suspicious microcalcifications, but there are invariably other smaller calcifications. The calcifications that are associated with cancer are usually ≤0.5 mm in size.

Calcifications as small as 0.2 and 0.3 mm are visible on mammography. In general, the smaller the particles the greater the suspicion although small deposits can be formed by adenosis and fibrocystic processes. When all the calcifications are >2 mm, a benign process is likely. The significance of a cluster, however, relates to the smallest calcifications in the group, not the largest (Fig. 13-106), and although calcifications associated with cancer may be large, the smaller, more suspicious calcifications are invariably present. The observer is reminded that the presence of typical benign calcifications does not preclude the possibility of a coincident, malignant process. A lesion should be evaluated according to its worst characteristics.

Number

The use of a threshold number to categorize suspicious groupings of calcifications has caused much debate. Because one or more mammographically visible calcifications are present in virtually every breast, and because clustering of calcifications is often an indication of a malignant process, the question must be posed: What constitutes a significant cluster?

The answer depends on the pattern of deposits, which is defined by their individual morphology and distribution relative to one another. In addition, it is very clear that few if any cancers have been discovered because of a single calcification. In our experience and that of others, it is rare (if ever) that two, three, or four calcifications have been the only indication of a cancer. The number five in a cubic centimeter has been derived from general experience (on contact, nonmagnified images). In a large series, Egan and

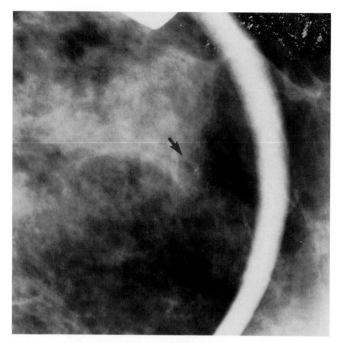

FIG. 13-107. It was the **clustering** five calcifications in 1 cc of tissue, as seen on this magnification view, that led to the diagnosis of **ductal carcinoma in situ** in this 55-year-old woman.

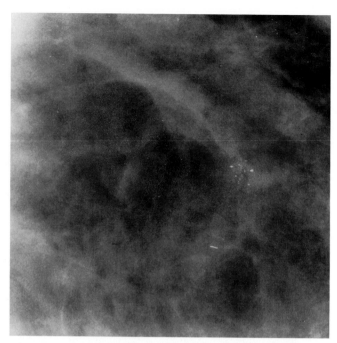

FIG. 13-108. The **variation in size and shape** of these very small calcifications led to their biopsy and the diagnosis of **ductal carcinoma in situ.**

associates found that, among 115 patients biopsied for microcalcifications alone, all lesions diagnosed as cancer had at least five visible flecks of calcium in a 0.5 × 0.5–cm field. The probability of malignancy was zero when there were fewer than five calcific particles (54).

Once the cluster has been defined, then it can be analyzed. It is likely that no absolute minimum threshold exists. No doubt some cancers contain fewer than five calcifications, but this is exceedingly rare. We have found that the risk of malignancy increases considerably when there are five or more isolated calcifications (not part of a diffuse process) visible in a volume of approximately 1 cc. Using this as a threshold (and excluding calcifications with benign morphology), 20% to 25% of the clusters can be expected to indicate cancer.

This threshold should not be considered absolute. If fewer calcifications are visible, but their morphology is of sufficient concern, then biopsy should be undertaken. These percentages apply only to women who have isolated microcalcifications without a visible tumor mass. The risk of malignancy increases if other secondary signs of malignancy are present. The number of calcifications, along with their size, morphology, and distribution, must be evaluated. This is clearly an observational phenomenon and not a fact of nature.

There are undoubtedly rare cancers that indicate their presence by forming fewer than five calcifications, but on a statistical basis the probability of malignancy increases with the number of calcifications. It is the clustering of small heterogeneous calcifications in isolation in a small volume of tissue that should raise concern about the possibility of breast cancer (Fig. 13-107). Many who use the term *cluster* fail to define it but merely assume its recognition. To avoid

raising concern over the large numbers of women who have one, two, three, or even four particles closely grouped on their mammogram that are invariably the result of a benign process, the threshold of five is useful and reasonable.

Morphology

The morphologic characteristics of calcifications are the most important elements in their analysis. The shapes of the particles and heterogeneity of the shapes and sizes are frequently valuable in determining the likely cause of the deposits. A better understanding of the microscopic histologic and pathologic environment in which calcifications form also helps in understanding the morphologic changes seen on mammography (55). Calcifications that can be categorized as due to benign processes need no further evaluation.

Calcifications that vary in size (most <0.5 mm) and shape are a cause for concern (Fig. 13-108). Calcifications due to breast cancer are either due to cellular secretion or the calcification of necrotic cancer cells.

Virtually all calcifications that form in breast cancers (including invasive lesions) form in the intraductal portion of the cancer. Although the multiplying cells can expand the duct, the necrosis usually occurs irregularly in the center of the duct. One study suggests that this occurs when the tumor diameter enlarges beyond 180 μm (56). The cells in the center become hypoxic as their distance from their blood supply increases and eventually the center of the tumor becomes necrotic. Because this is an irregular process at the center of the intraductal cancer, the calcifications formed are very small, irregular, and haphazard.

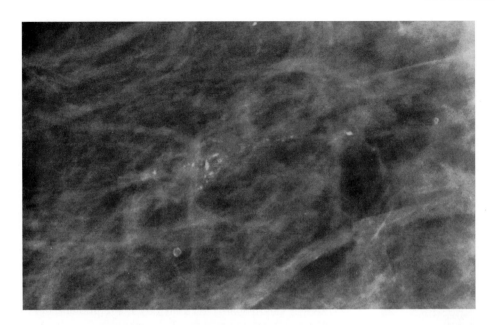

FIG. 13-109. The **fine linear branching pattern of calcifications** in this craniocaudal projection is due to **ductal carcinoma in situ** of the comedo type.

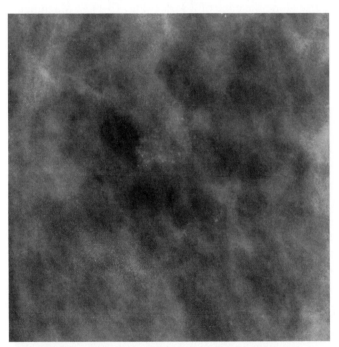

FIG. 13-110. These clustered, punctate calcifications are nonspecific but were forming in the **cribriform** spaces of low-grade **ductal carcinoma in situ**.

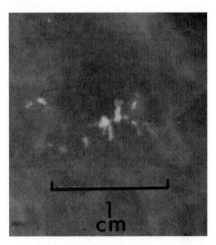

FIG. 13-111. **Ductal carcinoma in situ** usually forms calcifications that are heterogeneous in size and shape, as in this cluster.

Although these calcifications have been termed *casting*, they are actually the result of irregular patterns of tissue necrosis within cancer in a duct and are not molded by it. Their distribution, however, is guided by the course of the duct, giving a very distinctive linear, branching (Fig. 13-109) pattern. This pattern of calcium distribution is due to comedonecrosis. In other cancers it is likely that the secretion of calcification into the cribriform spaces generated by some cancers accounts for the less characteristic patterns of calcium deposition (Fig. 13-110). Suspicion should be aroused when

a group of calcifications is very heterogeneous. Calcifications associated with breast cancer are usually extremely variable in shape as well as size. The morphology of calcifications is very important in assessing their significance. Those associated with cancer are usually irregular, with pointed angular shapes (Fig. 13-111). This heterogeneity is reminiscent of fragments of broken glass. Although there are exceptions, the calcifications associated with cancer are rarely round or smooth. Calcifications associated with cancer have been variously described as having comma shapes with pointed projections and irregular surfaces. Delicate linear deposits <0.5 mm in diameter that may be branching and associated with punctate calcifications in a dot-dash pattern are almost always due to a malignant process (Fig. 13-112). The more criteria the calcifications fulfill, the greater the probability of cancer, although Sickles has shown that most calcifications associated with malignancy do not appear in a typical form (57).

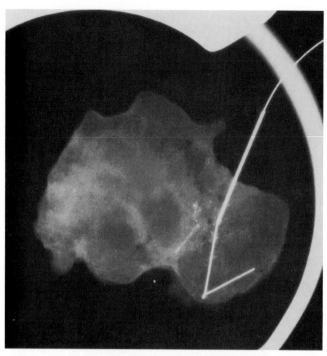

FIG. 13-112. The **"dot-dash" pattern of interrupted calcifications** due to **ductal carcinoma in situ** is clearly visible in this specimen radiograph.

Calcifications Typically Associated with Benign Processes

Lucent-Centered Skin Calcifications

Calcifications that have lucent centers are always due to benign processes (they are only coincidentally found in association with cancer) and need no further analysis. The simplest to evaluate and dismiss are skin calcifications with their typical lucent-centered, often geometrically shaped morphology (see Fig. 13-105). If there is any question, magnification views and tangential views of the skin at the location of the calcifications can be definitive (see Chapter 22).

Vascular Calcifications

Vascular calcifications are generally not a problem, having the usual appearance of parallel, serpentine deposits that course along the edge of a vessel (Fig. 13-112). Magnification mammography can be helpful in evaluating borderline deposits to confirm their etiology.

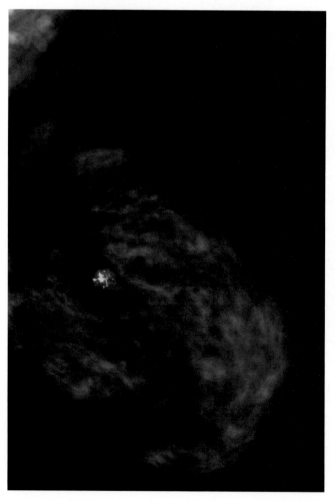

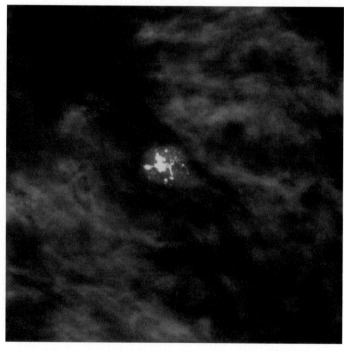

FIG. 13-113. Calcifications that look like popcorn are typical of an **involuting fibroadenoma,** as seen on the mediolateral oblique (MLO) **(A)** and MLO photographically enlarged **(B)** and on the craniocaudal (CC) **(C)** projection and CC photographically enlarged **(D)** in this 43-year-old woman. *Continued.*

Coarse Deposits

Coarse or popcorn-like calcifications are typical of involuting fibroadenomas (Fig. 13-113) and need not elicit concern. The timing and causes of involution are not clear. Although many observers have suggested that loss of hormonal support at menopause is the cause, premenopausal women can have calcifying fibroadenomas.

Rod-Shaped Calcifications

Large (>0.5 mm across) rod-like calcifications that only occasionally branch and are solid or have lucent centers are the kinds of calcifications found in secretory disease (Fig. 13-114). These calcifications form in debris that collects in the duct lumen or causes an inflammatory reaction around a duct. The latter can result in lucent-centered rods (Fig. 13-115). These benign calcifications are frequently bilateral.

Round (Acinar) Calcifications

Other calcifications that are typically associated with benign processes include smooth, round calcifications 0.5 mm or larger. These deposits are probably concretions formed in the acini of microcystically dilated lobules

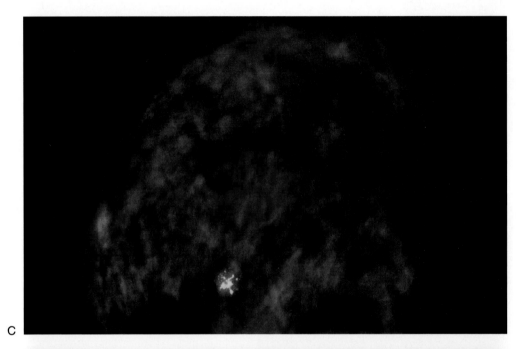

C

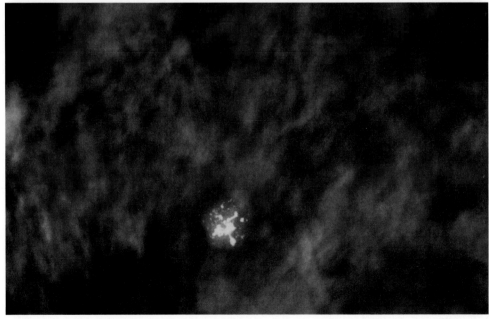

D

FIG. 13-113. *Continued.*

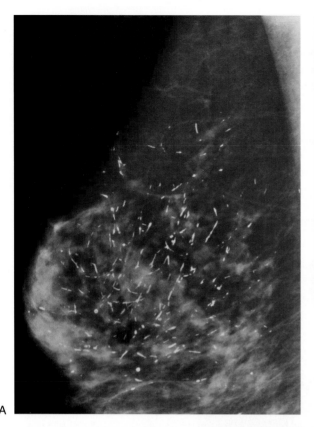

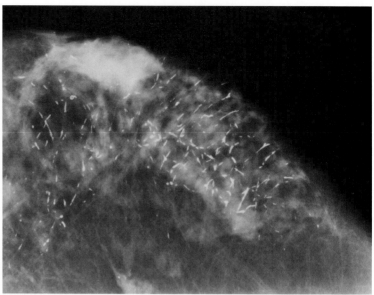

A

B

FIG. 13-114. Solid rod-shaped calcifications are typical of the calcification of benign intraductal cellular material in **secretory disease,** seen here in an 83-year-old woman on the lateral **(A)** and craniocaudal **(B)** projections.

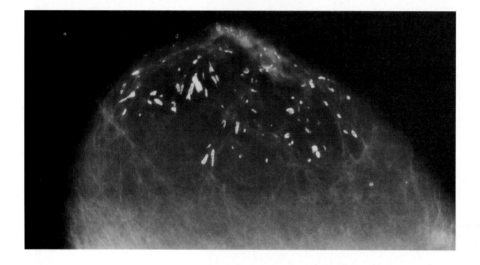

FIG. 13-115. Secretory calcifications can be tubular with lucent centers, as in a number of these calcifications seen on this craniocaudal projection. This is presumably secondary to periductal inflammation.

(Fig. 13-116). When extensive, they may be found in the fibrous, extralobular stroma. It is likely that these latter calcifications are formed in the "burned-out" remnants of atrophic lobules.

Other Spherical Lucent-Centered Calcifications

Spherical or lucent-centered calcifications can be found, coincidentally, in association with breast cancer, but they are invariably the result of benign processes (Fig. 13-117). They may form in debris collected in a duct or in small areas of

fat necrosis. Because these calcifications probably do not appear suddenly completely formed, if a cluster appears to be forming in a spherical pattern, it is reasonable to follow them at short intervals to monitor their coalescence rather than to intervene immediately (Fig. 13-117 B–E).

Rim Calcifications

Rim or eggshell calcifications are very thin, benign calcifications that appear as calcium deposited on the surface of a sphere. These deposits are usually under one mil-

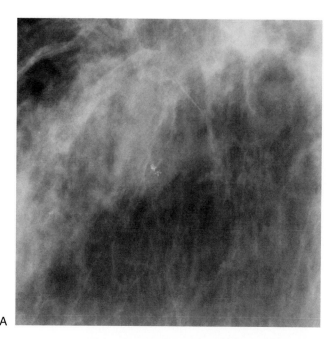

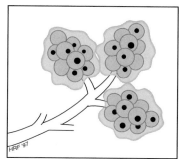

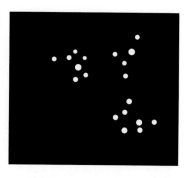

FIG. 13-116. (A) Acinar calcifications. These small, round, regular, tightly grouped calcifications are likely in a microcystically dilated lobule. **(B)** This schematic suggests the development of acinar calcifications.

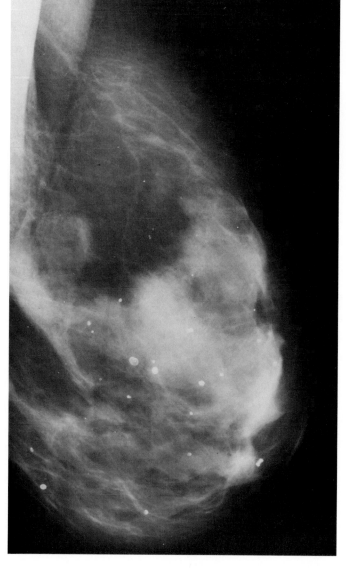

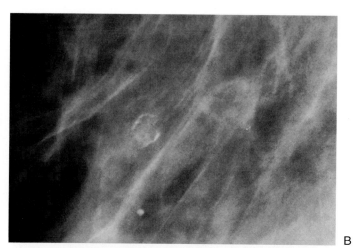

FIG. 13-117. Lucent-centered calcifications are due to benign processes (A). In this second case, the calcifications on the mediolateral oblique **(B)** and craniocaudal **(C)** magnification views were forming in a spherical distribution. *Continued.*

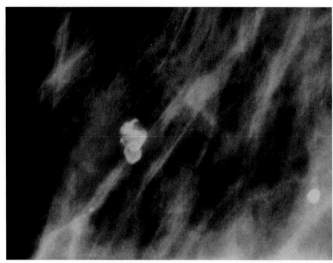

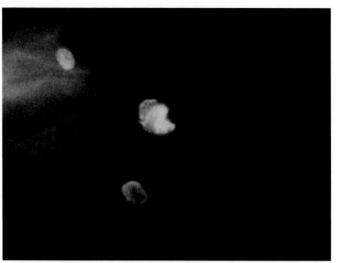

D

E

FIG. 13-117. *Continued.* They were followed and ultimately formed an obvious spherical deposit **(D, E)**, likely due to fat necrosis (note that others have also formed in the interim).

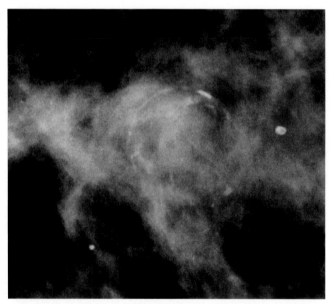

FIG. 13-118. Thin rim calcifications usually delineate the wall of a cyst. In this case the outline of a 1-cm cyst is visible in dense tissue because of the calcium that is forming in its wall.

limeter in thickness when viewed on edge. Although fat necrosis can produce these thin deposits, fat necrosis usually results in thicker calcium deposition. Calcifications in the wall of cysts are the most common rim calcifications (Fig. 13-118).

Calcifications Whose Morphology Varies Between Projections

Because they represent solid particles, most calcifications have a similar appearance when viewed on orthogonal projections. Calcium that has precipitated in cysts is influenced by gravity and has a different morphology in the CC projection than on the lateral view. Calcifications that appear round and amorphous on the CC projection and are curvilinear or linear in the lateral projection are almost always due to milk of calcium. On the CC image the x-ray beam passes through a thin layer of the powdery particles, and they often appear as indistinct and fuzzy, round, amorphous deposits because they form in a pool in the dependent portion of the cyst. The same deposits appear as sharply defined, semilunar, crescent-shaped, curvilinear (concave up), or linear calcifications in the horizontal beam lateral because the photons pass through a thicker layer of calcium that is precipitated in and defines the dependent portion of a cyst (Fig. 13-119).

Milk of calcium is felt by virtually all experts to be formed by a benign process. There is a slight suggestion that milk of calcium may represent a risk factor for breast cancer. Sickles reviewed >200 cases of mammographically evident milk of calcium (58). Although he did not comment on the fact that 8 of the 200 (or 40 of 1,000) cases had an associated malignancy, this is more than four times the expected prevalence of breast cancer in the normal population (at most 10 cancers would be expected among 1,000 women in a prevalence screen). It is likely that these women had other reasons for this higher prevalence of malignancy, but we have a low threshold for biopsying clusters of these calcifications if they are not clearly milk of calcium.

Calcifications that form in the wall of a cyst may have a similar appearance, as would concretions in cysts that have solidified in the same orientation as free-flowing milk of calcium. It would be extremely unusual for the calcifications of breast cancer to form this pattern.

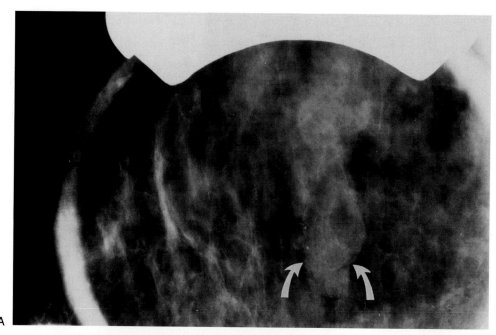

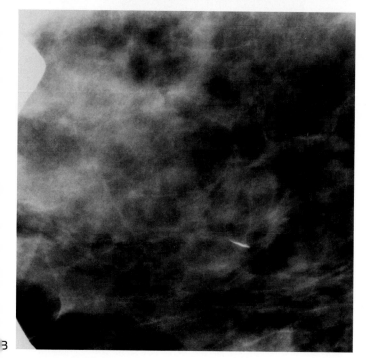

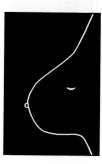

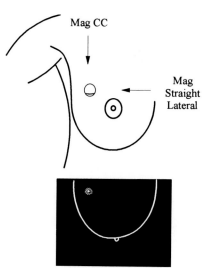

FIG. 13-119. Milk of calcium layers in cysts. (A) In this individual the cyst is barely visible (*arrows*) on the craniocaudal (CC) projection because the beam is passing through a very thin layer of calcium. On the magnification straight lateral projection **(B)**, the layering calcium delineates the curved bottom of the cyst. This phenomenon is depicted by this schematic **(C)** as the milk of calcium forms a "puddle" of calcium in the dependent portion of a cyst. When viewed from above in the CC projection, the density of the calcium decreases from the center, producing an amorphous appearance. In the lateral projection the calcifications form a crescent-shaped concave shadow.

Suture Calcifications

Suture calcifications probably represent calcium deposited on the gut matrix of suture material (59). These are relatively common in the postirradiated breast, and, on occasion, when extensive surgery (such as reduction mammoplasty) has been performed. They are probably the result of delayed resorption of the resorbable suture material that permits the calcium to form. They are typically linear or tubular in appearance and knots are frequently visible (Fig. 13-120).

Large Irregular, Dystrophic Calcifications

Large (>0.5 mm), irregular calcifications may have no apparent underlying cause and are termed *dystrophic*. Dystrophic calcifications usually form in the irradiated breast or in the breast after trauma (perhaps due to fat necrosis). Although irregular in shape, they are usually >0.5 mm in size (Fig. 13-121). They may have lucent centers. Benign, dystrophic calcifications frequently have an appearance that resembles crushed lava (Fig. 13-121 D–G).

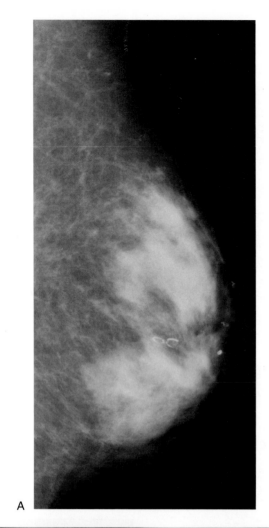

A

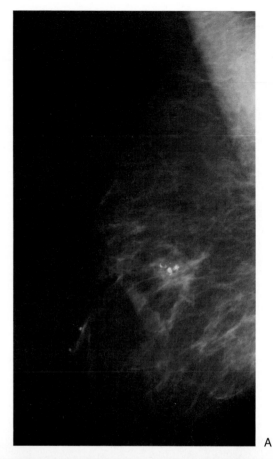

A

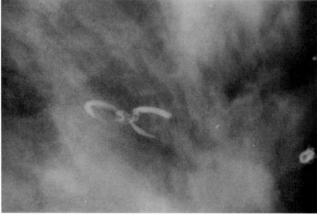

B

FIG. 13-120. Calcified sutures likely occur when there is delayed resorption of the organic material. In this case even the knots and loops calcified following radiation for breast cancer, as seen on the lateral **(A)** and photographically enlarged **(B)** images.

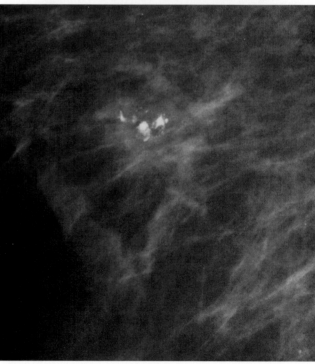

B

FIG. 13-121. These calcifications, seen on the mediolateral oblique (MLO) **(A)** and the enlarged MLO **(B)** and craniocaudal **(C)**, developed in a 57-year-old woman 5 years after excision and radiation for an invasive breast cancer. Because of the small size of several, they were excised revealing fibrosis, radiation change, and benign **dystrophic calcifications.** *Continued.*

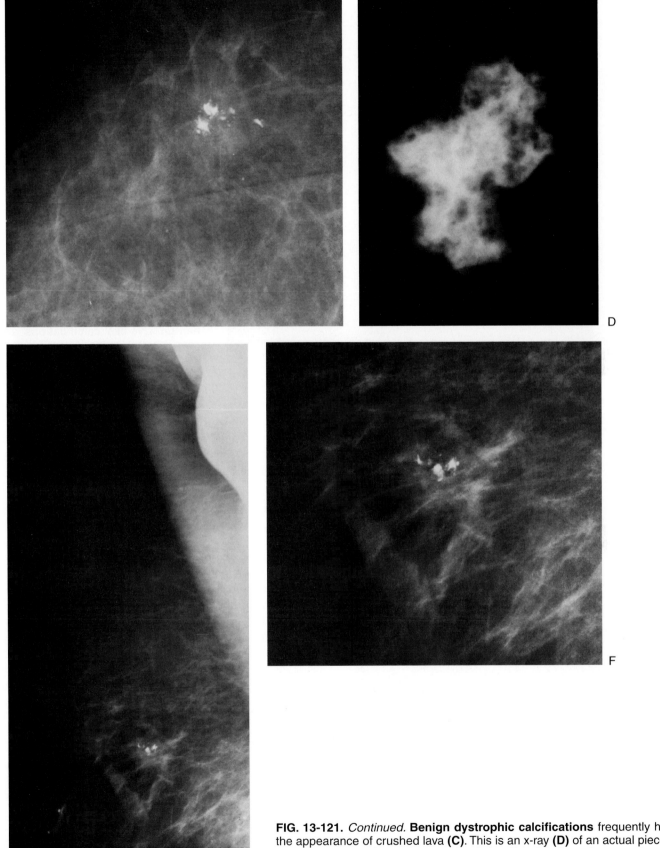

FIG. 13-121. *Continued.* **Benign dystrophic calcifications** frequently have the appearance of crushed lava **(C)**. This is an x-ray **(D)** of an actual piece of lava. Note that in this patient previously irradiated for breast cancer the dystrophic calcifications seen on the mediolateral oblique **(E)** and enlarged **(F)** projection resemble the lava. *Continued.*

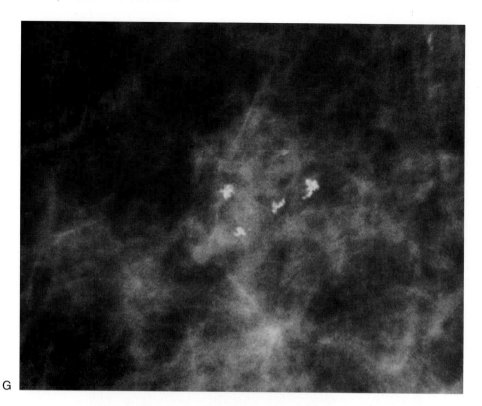

FIG. 13-121. *Continued.* Similar **benign lava-like calcifications** are seen on this magnification view in another patient **(G).**

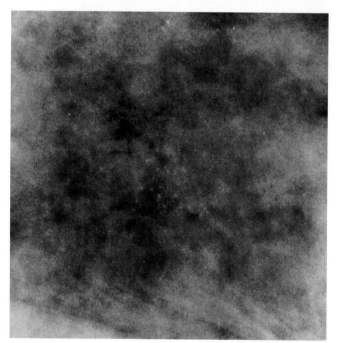

FIG. 13-122. These are **punctate calcifications** formed in microcysts.

Punctate Calcifications

Punctate calcifications are round or oval and very small (<0.5 mm) but very sharply defined, pinpoint deposits (Fig. 13-122). Very round, regular, punctate calcifications are rarely associated with breast cancer, but if they include or are associated with calcifications whose shapes are not round or smooth but heterogeneous, they should be viewed with suspicion. Punctate calcifications are frequently found in the fibrous stroma with no apparent etiology. They may have formed in the remnants of burned-out lobules.

Morphologies That Should Arouse Immediate Concern: Indistinct, Amorphous Calcifications

Indistinct or amorphous particles that do not layer in the horizontal beam lateral images are of intermediate concern. They are round or flake-shaped calcifications that are sufficiently small or hazy in appearance that a more specific morphologic classification cannot be determined (Fig. 13-123). Although they do not layer in the dependent portions, many of these are likely deposits in small cysts. Adenosis may also cause these calcifications, and if highly magnified innumerable extremely small particles may be found to be the cause of what appears to be a larger single particle. Occasionally breast cancer can produce these types of calcifications.

Morphologies That Suggest a High Probability of Malignancy

Pleomorphic or Heterogeneous Calcifications

Pleomorphic or heterogeneous calcifications, sometimes called *granular*, are neither typically benign nor typically malignant, but calcifications that are irregular and vary in

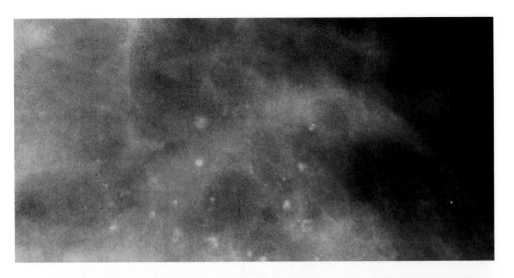

FIG. 13-123. Amorphous calcifications are basically round but have fuzzy edges. These proved to be small cysts.

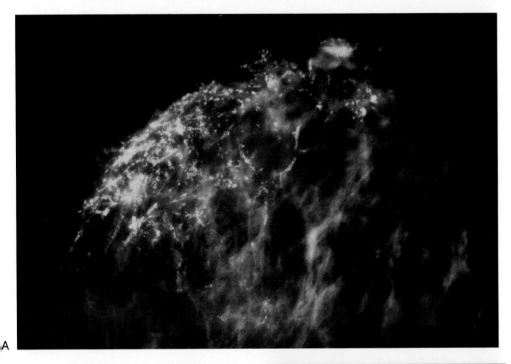

A

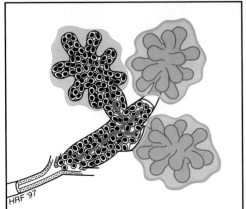

B

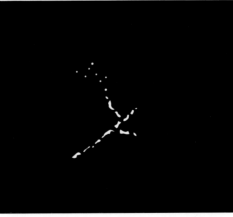

FIG. 13-124. These calcifications **(A)** are formed in the typical fine **linear branching pattern of comedocarcinoma.** The schematic **(B)** demonstrates how the cancer cells in the center of a duct filled with tumor can necrose and calcify. Since the pattern of necrosis is irregular, the pattern of calcification is irregular although the general distribution suggests that the calcifications are forming in the ducts.

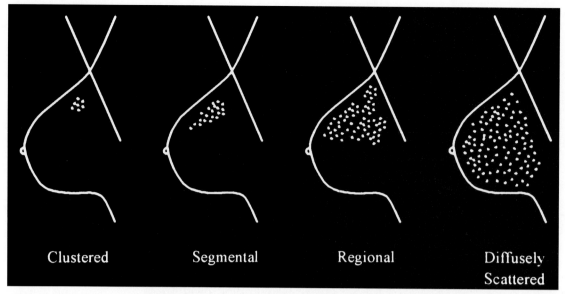

Clustered   Segmental   Regional   Diffusely Scattered

FIG. 13-125. This schematic depicts the four **patterns of calcium distribution.** Beginning from the left is the clustered grouping, followed by segmentally distributed, then regional, and diffusely scattered.

size and shape and are <0.5 mm in diameter should be viewed with a high degree of suspicion.

Fine Linear or Branching Calcifications

Fine linear or branching calcifications are thin, irregular calcifications that appear linear but when carefully evaluated actually are discontinuous irregular particles that form in a linear pattern and are <1 mm in width. Their appearance is explained by the irregular calcifications of necrotic tumor in the lumen of a duct that is irregularly involved by breast cancer (Fig. 13-124). They almost invariably are due to comedo-carcinoma.

Distribution of Calcifications

The distribution of calcifications (Fig. 13-125) is often a clue to their etiology and importance. The ACR BIRADS defines four distribution patterns:

1. Clustered
2. Segmental
3. Regional
4. Diffusely scattered

An isolated focal collection of heterogeneous calcifications must be carefully assessed. On the other hand, the parallel distribution of vascular calcifications along vessels makes it unlikely that they will be confused with malignant deposits.

Diffusely scattered, lucent-centered calcifications generally represent secretory deposits, fat necrosis, or skin deposits. In general, diffuse calcifications randomly distributed across large volumes of breast tissue are caused by benign processes. This is especially true when each is fairly uniform in shape although varying in size. Round, amorphous, scattered calcifications are

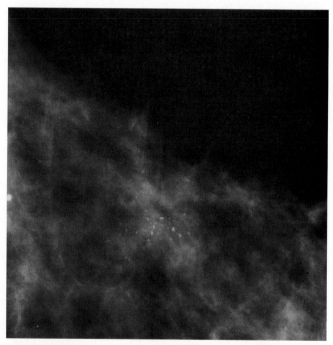

FIG. 13-126. Clustered calcifications. Five or more calcifications in a cubic centimeter of tissue constitutes a cluster. These are small and pleomorphic and proved to be due to **ductal carcinoma in situ** found at routine screening in a 51-year-old woman.

generally seen in benign conditions, and when bilateral the confidence that they represent a benign process is increased.

Clustered Calcifications

Many calcifications form in nonspecific patterns. These are the types of calcifications that are the most difficult to accurately analyze and are the cause of most benign biopsies. Heterogeneous calcifications whose pattern of distribution can only be termed *clustered* and cannot be accurately placed in benign categories may be caused by adenosis, peripheral duct papillomas, atypical hyperplasia, and other benign breast conditions. Unfortunately, cancer can also produce these clusters of calcifications and biopsy is needed to establish an accurate diagnosis (Fig. 13-126).

Segmentally Distributed Calcifications

This distribution is thought to represent calcifications within a single duct network of a lobe or segment. A lobe or segment of the breast is defined by the major duct opening on the nipple and its branches spreading into the breast, terminating in its lobules (see Chapter 2). The data suggest that breast cancer is a process that initially is confined to a single duct network. True multicentric cancer (multiple duct networks involved) is unusual, whereas multifocality (cancer at multiple sites within one duct network) is relatively common (60).

Calcifications whose distribution suggests a duct network are of concern. Extensive intraductal carcinoma can produce innumerable calcifications throughout large portions of the breast, and on rare occasions this can occur bilaterally. These are usually readily distinguishable from benign conditions because of the markedly heterogeneous morphology of the deposits: irregular shapes, sizes, and angulation of

surfaces that typify suspicious particles (Fig. 13-127A, B), whereas benign conditions usually produce round and regular calcifications (Fig. 13-127 C–E).

A large number of calcifications that are relatively confined to a volume or segment of the breast must be distinguished from diffuse, randomly distributed calcifications. The latter are almost always associated with a benign process, whereas the former must be carefully evaluated. Rarely, an entire duct network may be diffusely filled with cancer with calcification over a large volume of tissue. When segmentally distributed calcifications are caused by cancer they generally indicate diffuse intraductal tumor (with or without invasion), and the pathologist frequently sees the comedo, poorly differentiated variety (see Chapter 2). The segmental distribution of calcifications is an important analytic observation, and biopsy is usually indicated.

Regional and Diffusely Scattered Calcifications

Calcifications that appear randomly distributed throughout large volumes of breast tissue or throughout the entire breast are almost always benign. Although breast cancer can be extensive, this is very unusual and diffusely scattered calcifications are almost always due to benign processes. These should be distinguished from calcifications that are extensive but still occupy only a segment of the breast. The latter should be considered highly suspicious and should be biopsied. Diffuse calcifications must be randomly distributed throughout the breast to be dis-

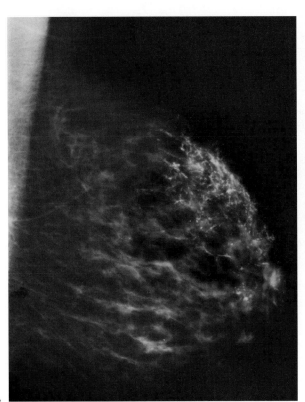

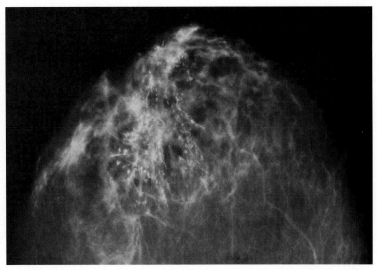

FIG. 13-127. Segmentally distributed calcifications are those that form in a single-duct network. When they are heterogeneous and irregular, they are usually due to **ductal carcinoma in situ,** as seen on the mediolateral oblique **(A)** and craniocaudal **(B)** projections of this patient with comedocarcinoma. *Continued.*

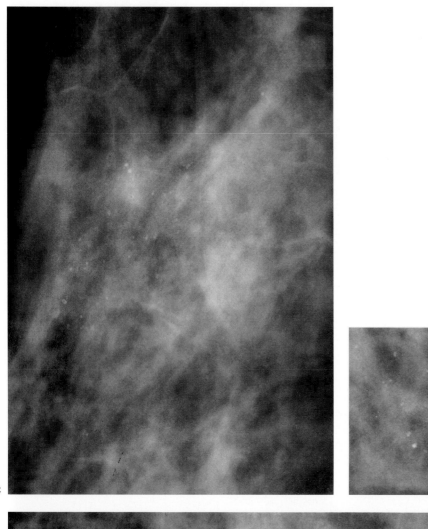

C

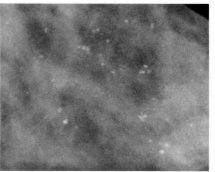

E

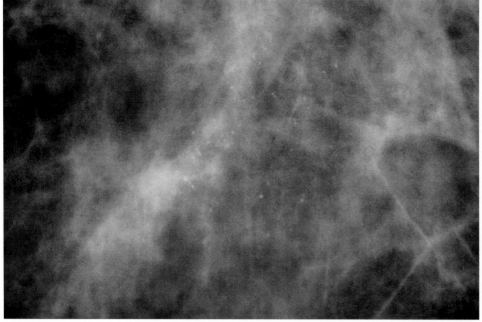

D

FIG. 13-127. *Continued.* **Segmentally distributed calcifications may be due to benign processes.** Occasionally segmentally distributed, round, regular calcifications can be seen in benign stromal fibrosis, as on these mediolateral oblique **(C)** and craniocaudal **(D)** projections and on this specimen radiograph **(E)**.

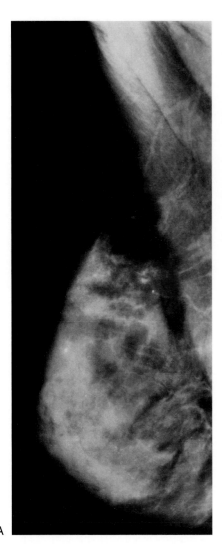

A

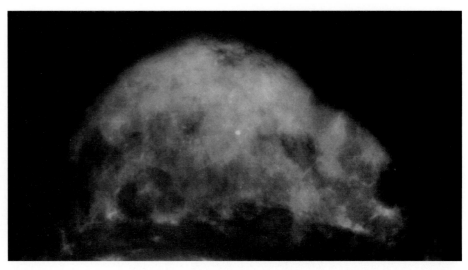

B

FIG. 13-128. Diffusely scattered, amorphous calcifications are due to benign processes. The more one looks, the more calcifications become apparent throughout the mediolateral oblique **(A)** and craniocaudal **(B)** projections. These had been stable for 4 years in this 50-year-old woman.

missed as benign. Despite the fact that they are usually benign, diffuse microdeposits may be difficult to assess. The observer must first recognize that a diffuse pattern is present. Several of the calcifications may be more prominent than others, and it might initially appear that one is dealing with a focal cluster. On close inspection, occasionally with the assistance of magnification views, the multiplicity and widespread distribution of the calcifications become evident. Even randomly distributed calcifications may have several areas where a number of particles are close together. If their morphology is the same as the others they should not raise concern.

Multiple amorphous, relatively round, monotonously similar calcifications that likely form in cystically dilated lobular acini are benign. When these are distributed throughout the breast and bilaterally, they are of no concern (Fig. 13-128); however, an isolated group of calcifications, within a diffuse pattern, that has malignant characteristics should be biopsied.

Secretory calcifications may also produce a diffuse pattern of calcium deposition. They are thick rod-shaped or spherical deposits oriented along duct lines. Unlike calcifications associated with cancer, they rarely have branch points and are usually bilateral. One should always remember that several processes can coexist simultaneously, and the observer should be careful to search among the diffuse calcifications for an isolated group that is different and may represent a focus of malignancy.

Multiple Groups of Calcifications

It is fairly common for multiple clusters of calcifications that are morphologically similar to appear. Many of these are fibroadenomas whose mass is not visible. Others likely represent debris in the ducts or deposits in cystically dilated acini. As with masses, if there are three or more groups of widely separated clusters with similar morphology, the likelihood of breast cancer is very low (Fig. 13-129) (the rule of multiplicity). In our practice, if no group is any more worrisome than the others, the mammogram is repeated at 6-month intervals over 2 years to assess the stability of the finding and no intervention is indicated.

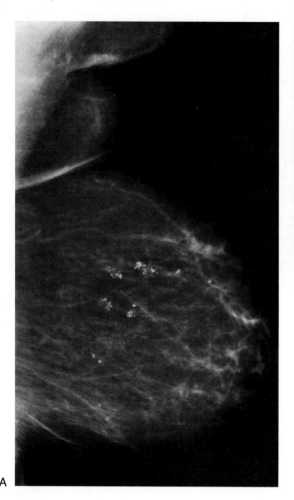

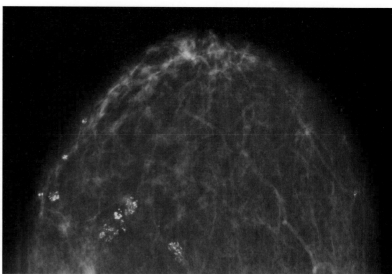

FIG. 13-129. Multiple groups of calcifications are usually due to benign processes. These have been stable for 9 years on the mediolateral **(A)** and craniocaudal **(B)** projections in this 74-year-old woman.

Stability of Calcifications

The majority of calcifications found in the breast are due to benign processes. These are easily separated from other deposits. Large calcifications or those with lucent centers can be ignored and do not require additional evaluation (except for extremely rare lesions such as osteogenic sarcoma). Sickles defined calcifications that formed clusters of very round deposits as almost always benign and demonstrated that they can be followed with repeat mammograms over short intervals (36) because they have a low (<1%) probability of malignancy. In his review, interval change prompted biopsy among some of these patients with only 11% of these proving to be due to cancer. As with masses, the classification "probably benign" to begin with and stability for 2 years markedly increases the probability that calcifications are due to a benign process.

As with masses, however, stability of indeterminate or suspicious calcifications should be less reassuring. Lev-Toaff and colleagues reviewed 1,882 cases in which calcifications without a mass proved to be caused by breast cancer. For 105 of these women there were old studies for comparison. In 26 of these cases (25%) the calcifications, which were ultimately biopsied, proved to be cancer despite having been stable for 8 to 63 months (mean, 25 months). Thus, for indeterminate or suspicious calcifications stability is not a reliable indication of a benign process (61). It is somewhat reassuring that, in their study, calcifications that were stable were rarely associated with invasive breast cancer (12%), whereas 29 of the 79 women with increasing calcifications (37%) were associated with invasive cancer. It is of interest that all of the calcifications were partially or completely in the cancers. Some had calcifications in both benign and malignant tissues.

The authors only reviewed lesions that proved to be cancer. Their observations do not alter the legitimacy of short interval follow-up for calcifications that are probably benign. Our policy has been to obtain mammograms every 6 months for 2 years for calcifications that are probably benign. If they are stable over this period, we believe that return to annual screening is reasonable. If calcifications have worrisome morphology, stability is not reliable.

ASSOCIATED FINDINGS: SKIN, NIPPLE, AND TRABECULAR CHANGES AND AXILLARY ADENOPATHY

Other features involved in the assessment of a mammographic abnormality include skin and nipple changes, axillary abnormalities, and associated calcifications. Skin and nipple changes and axillary adenopathy are generally evident clinically. The mammogram should be performed to emphasize the analysis of the breast tissues. High-contrast mammograms maximize the perception of breast cancer, and images should be obtained to permit assessment of the breast parenchyma with imaging of the skin and nipples secondary in importance.

Some radiologists wish to see the skin on mammograms. This is a habit left over from when more cancers were found at an advanced stage in which the skin was frequently involved. There is an additional fallacy in the desire to evaluate the skin because only small portions of the skin are visible in tangent on a mammogram. If the radiologist wishes to assess the skin, this is best accomplished by examining the patient.

Skin Changes

The skin forms the outer envelope of the breast. The epidermis is in direct continuity with the ductal epithelium as it descends from the surface of the nipple through the duct orifices and becomes the ductal epithelium. Some observers believe that this is the route of spread for duct carcinoma out onto the nipple in the form of Paget's disease.

The skin generally forms a smooth convex surface, surrounding the mammary parenchyma and separated from it by a variable layer of subcutaneous fat. Away from the areola, normal skin is approximately 0.5 to 2.0 mm in thickness. On rare occasions normal skin thickness may be up to 3 mm, but when this occurs an underlying abnormality should be considered. The skin of the areola varies in thickness between individuals, as does the nipple. In some individuals the nipple is flush with the areola, whereas in others it is extremely prominent.

The breast itself is attached to the skin by the extensions of Cooper's ligaments, known as the *retinacula cutis*. The breast is supported by the skin through these attachments. The normal skin overlying the breast measures up to 2 mm in thickness, although it normally thickens to form the areola. Breast cancer may involve any of these structures through contiguous spread, extension through the duct network, or through the lymphatics.

Although the interpretation of mammograms should include an evaluation of the skin, if it is visible, skin changes associated with malignancy generally occur late in the disease process and frequently are apparent clinically. On occasion, a cicatrizing tumor deep within the breast can cause skin retraction through the tethering of Cooper's ligaments and the retinacula cutis, but in general cancers that cause skin retraction are close beneath the dimpling and are usually superficial lesions (Fig. 13-130). Because the mammogram only provides tangential evaluation of small strips of the skin, skin retraction is usually more evident on the clinical examination (as a puckering or dimpling of the skin) than by mammogra-

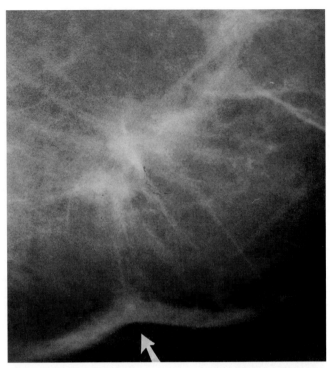

FIG. 13-130. Skin retraction. The desmoplastic reaction to this superficial cancer caused skin dimpling and local thickening (*arrow*), as seen in tangent.

phy, and its presence on the mammogram is usually merely corroborative rather than the key to interpreting a mammogram.

Visualization of the skin on a mammogram is not a primary concern, and mammographic exposures should be determined by the breast tissues and not the skin. When retraction caused by a cancer is evident clinically, the tumor mass is generally visible mammographically. If no underlying lesion is evident, the retraction is likely to be due to posttraumatic scarring.

Skin Thickening

Thickening of the skin can have many causes, and its mammographic appearance is nonspecific. Skin thickening can be focal or diffuse, unilateral or bilateral. Skin thickening can occur as a result of tumor invasion (local) (Fig. 13-130); tumor in the dermal lymphatics (Fig. 13-131); or lymphatic congestion through obstruction of the lymphatic drainage within the breast, in the axilla (regional), centrally in the mediastinum (central); or even congestive heart failure (Fig. 13-132).

Focal skin changes are better seen by clinical examination than mammography because they go unnoticed by the latter unless imaged tangentially. Ultrasound can demonstrate skin thickening directly (62), but despite some reports that suggest the cause of skin thickening can be inferred by ultrasound, this is usually not of practical importance.

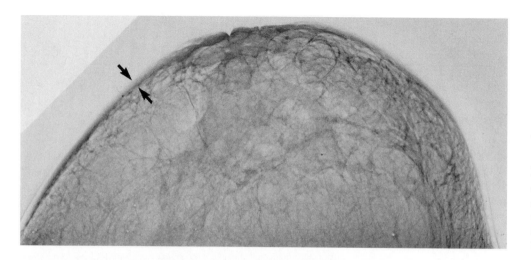

FIG. 13-131. Diffuse skin thickening can be due to inflammatory cancer. The skin is not well seen on film/screen mammography. Diffuse skin thickening is visible on this xerogram of a woman with inflammatory breast cancer, although the diagnosis is made clinically.

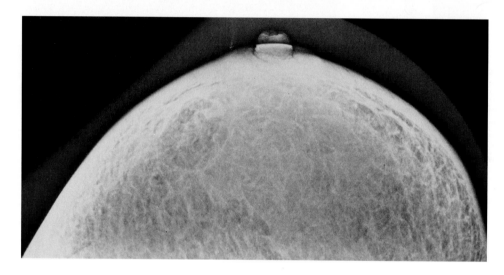

FIG. 13-132. Congestive heart failure can cause skin thickening, as seen on this negative-mode craniocaudal xerogram.

Benign inflammation can also cause skin thickening. Such thickening can be seen in patients with an aseptic mastitis as well as those with mastitis that has a bacterial etiology.

The major differential diagnosis for skin changes includes direct involvement by a malignancy, infection, nonspecific inflammation, primary skin processes such as psoriasis, lymphatic obstruction (local, regional, and central), vascular obstruction (congestive heart failure, vena cava superior syndrome, and anasarca), and systemic diseases with skin involvement (e.g., scleroderma, dermatomyositis, congenital absence of the lymphatics).

Focal Skin Thickening

Focal skin thickening is rare. It is also rare when a focal area of skin thickening is apparent on the mammogram, because skin thickening is only apparent when the skin is seen in tangent, and only a small portion of the skin is seen in tangent on a mammogram. Infection or postsurgical scarring are the most likely causes of focal thickening, and these are usually clinically obvious. Generalized edema may produce what appears to be focal thickening of the dependent, usually inferior, skin of the breast.

Diffuse Skin Thickening

Diffuse skin thickening is more common than focal. Because the lymphatic drainage of the skin is continuous with the lymphatics that pass through the breast, lymphatic congestion of the skin may be associated with a subtle or pronounced thickening of the trabecular pattern of the breast defined by Cooper's ligaments. Skin and trabecular thickening are most often due either to benign inflammation, inflammation after radiation treatment, direct dermal lymphatic involvement by tumor cells, or secondary edema due to lymphatic obstruction from tumor cells (see Chapter 19). When tumor cells obstruct the dermal lymphatics, diffuse thickening that is indistinguishable from the other causes of skin thickening occurs.

Irradiation of the breast is another common cause of diffuse skin thickening. The response to radiation varies, but in most women there is a self-limited swelling due to edema

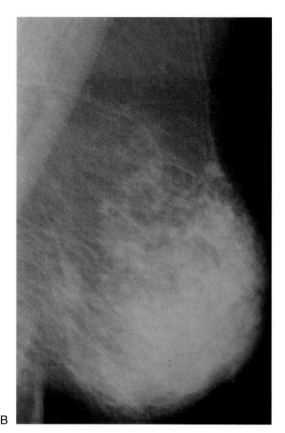
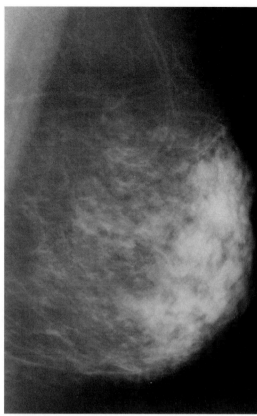

FIG. 13-133. Benign thickening. (A) The skin and trabecular thickening was caused by a non-neoplastic **inflammation. (B)** The condition resolved spontaneously.

A,B

that manifests as radiographically visible skin and trabecular thickening (see Chapter 17). This may resolve or become a fixed fibrotic change.

Skin Thickening Secondary to Dermatologic Problems, Congestive Heart Failure, Vascular Compromise, and Absent Lymphatics

Thickening can have other less common causes. Occasionally, dermatologic problems such as psoriasis produce skin thickening. This etiology should be considered, especially when the thickening is bilateral. Another uncommon cause of bilateral skin thickening is congestive heart failure (see Fig. 13-132). Any process that obstructs venous return to the heart, such as mediastinal tumor (superior vena caval obstruction), can cause skin and trabecular thickening in the breast. We have seen one case of Milroy's disease with a congenital absence of the lymphatics that produced thickened skin.

Skin Thickening and Breast Cancer

Skin Thickening Due to Inflammatory Cancer. Thickened skin invariably accompanies inflammatory carcinoma, a highly aggressive manifestation of breast cancer with poor prognosis, in which tumor is found permeating the dermal lymphatics (although this infiltration is not always present even when the skin is thickened). By itself, however, the thickened skin is a nonspecific finding, and the diagnosis of inflammatory carcinoma is based on the clinical findings with erythema and increased skin temperature over one-third of the breast surface. The thickened skin accentuates the pores and has the classic appearance that suggests the skin of an orange *(peau d'orange)*. Radiographically nonspecific skin thickening is seen, and almost invariably the overall trabecular pattern of the breast appears thickened due to congestion in the intramammary lymphatics. On occasion an underlying tumor mass that is not detectable on clinical examination is visible mammographically.

Skin Thickening Due to Neglected Cancer. At times it is difficult to differentiate true inflammatory cancer from a neglected carcinoma that has ultimately spread to involve the skin. Inflammatory cancer tends to have a much shorter clinical course in which the cancer becomes evident over several days, weeks, or a few months, than a neglected carcinoma. Neglected cancers have a history that goes back over many months or even years, during which time the individual has either denied the presence of a problem or has chosen to ignore it.

Skin Thickening Due to Advanced Cancer. Diffuse skin thickening associated with noninflammatory cancer is a late change indicating advanced disease. It is often accompanied by generalized thickening of the trabecular structures coursing through the breast. The radiographic appearance is nonspecific and may merely reflect edema. When the thickening is due to direct tumor invasion of the dermal lymphatics, it is a poor prognostic sign.

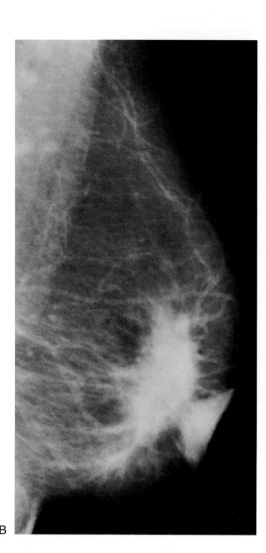

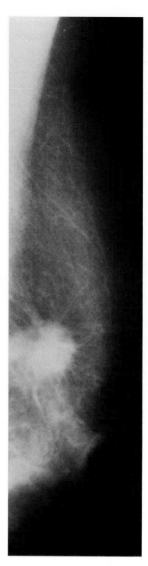

A,B

FIG. 13-134. Nipple areolar retraction. (A) The nipple areolar complex is pulled in by the obvious, large, invasive cancer lying beneath. **(B)** In this second patient the large cancer deep in the breast is causing the nipple to be retracted.

Trabecular Thickening and Distortion

Cooper's ligaments and the lactiferous ducts produce a fine trabecular pattern of curvilinear septations coursing through the breast. Extensions of Cooper's ligaments pass through the subcutaneous fat and insert in the skin as the retinacula cutis, giving a scalloped, concave appearance to the edge of the parenchymal cone. Both benign and malignant processes can result in thickening of these structures. Although the parenchyma appears to be separated from the skin by the layer of fat, epithelial elements, in which cancer can form, may be found immediately beneath the skin, making it impossible, for example, to remove the entire tissue at risk by performing a subcutaneous mastectomy. The ducts have a network of lymphatics that surround them.

There are many causes of edema of the breast, including infection and inflammation, and these may produce trabecular, as well as skin, thickening (Fig. 13-133). Rarely, skin and trabecular thickening can stem from unusual causes of lymphatic impedance, such as axillary nodal obstruction, or from central causes, such as superior vena caval obstruction or even congestive heart failure.

Skin and Nipple Retraction

Although skin and nipple changes occasionally are helpful in analyzing the mammogram, when visible mammographically skin and nipple retraction are generally late changes and are evident clinically. The best way to evaluate the skin and the nipple is to directly examine the patient. Although on occasion the mammographic compression makes nipple retraction more evident, the mammogram should be exposed to enhance the visibility of internal structures and is not made to evaluate the skin and nipple.

As a secondary sign of malignancy, nipple retraction is generally associated with large cancers (Fig. 13-134) that are evident on the mammogram; it is rarely the most significant indication of malignancy. Although malignant lesions

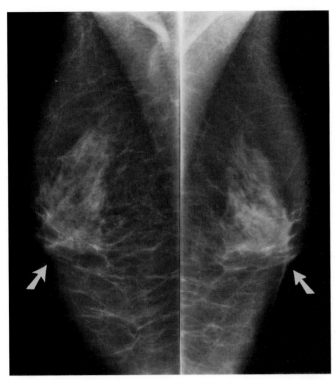

FIG. 13-135. Areolar tethering. In some women the lower edge of the areola is normally tethered and appears pulled in (*arrows*), as seen in these lateral projections.

may produce mammographically visible alterations in the nipple and skin, a palpable lesion is frequently evident.

Retraction or inversion of the nipple is usually the result of a benign idiopathic process and may be bilateral or unilateral. Benign changes invariably occur over a long period of time. When nipple inversion happens over a short interval (several months), a malignant etiology should be sought. Because of the contraction of fibrous structures, cancer may cause the nipple to deviate in the direction of the tumor (see Chapter 15).

In some women, particularly on a poorly compressed mammogram, there is some normal tethering from Cooper's ligaments in the 6 o'clock subareolar region that may suggest skin retraction (Fig. 13-135). This is usually symmetric, and no underlying mass is seen. This phenomenon is not commonly seen on mammograms obtained with vigorous rigid compression systems.

Skin or nipple retraction may result from benign scarring, usually in a postsurgical setting along the skin incision. Fat necrosis has also been reported as a benign cause of skin retraction.

Nipple and Nipple Discharge

Evaluation of the nipple, as the skin, is generally better accomplished by visual inspection. Paget's disease is thought by many to be a process in which intraductal cancer grows along the duct and out onto the nipple (a few

pathologists believe some cases may originate de novo in the nipple). Paget's disease is not detectable by mammography unless there is an associated underlying mass, architectural distortion, or calcifications. Unusual primary lesions of the nipple can be imaged if they cause distortion of the nipple or produce calcifications (see Adenoma of the Nipple, in Chapter 19).

Nipple Discharge

Nipple discharge is a fairly common occurrence. Discharges may be unilateral, bilateral, from a single duct, or from multiple ducts. The discharge may be clear, milky, yellow, green, brown, or bloody. In general, bilateral discharges are due to a central hormonal cause, such as elevated prolactin levels. Primary breast malignancy is rarely the cause of a bilateral discharge. Most unilateral, multiduct discharges are due to benign processes. It is unusual, although not impossible, for a malignancy to cause a unilateral, multiduct discharge. In general, if breast cancer is the cause of a discharge, it is a unilateral, solitary duct discharge. Nevertheless, most unilateral, solitary duct discharges are still due to benign causes.

The association of breast cancer with a discharge varies depending on the reported series. The incidence has been reported to be as high as 17% (63). In one series only 7% of the discharges were due to malignancy (64). These results were similar to a second series of 72 discharges evaluated by ductography in which 7% were due to cancer (65).

Contrary to conventional wisdom, a discharge due to breast cancer does not have to be bloody. In Urban's series, 50% of the discharges due to cancer were serous, and 50% were bloody. Furthermore, there is no unanimity as to which type of discharge requires further investigation. Given sufficient stimulation to the nipple areolar complex, a discharge may be elicited from many breasts. Some believe that only the spontaneous discharge is important.

Unilateral Solitary Duct Discharge

The most common cause of a unilateral, single-duct discharge is a large-duct papilloma. These are benign hyperplastic growths with a fibrovascular core. They have no known predisposition toward malignancy and usually occur within a few centimeters of the nipple in the large ducts. The discharge from a papilloma may be serous or sanguineous. Benign duct ectasia may also produce duct discharge, and even an apparently normal duct may discharge.

Management of Duct Discharge

There is no agreed-on management for duct discharge. In general, bilateral discharges are investigated for a central etiology such as a pituitary problem. Cytologic analysis (Pap smear) of discharged material may help if positive, although not all discharges caused by cancer are cytologically positive. Mammography should be obtained to determine if there is any abnormality detectable by mammography to account for the discharge. In our experience it is rare that the standard mammogram reveals the underlying problem. Magnification mammography has been advocated to evaluate the subareolar tissues, but there has been no documentation that this has any clinical efficacy.

It is usually a clinical decision as to how vigorously to pursue a duct discharge. If the clinical concern is high, many surgeons perform a dissection of the involved duct. The clinical assessment will try to delineate a "trigger point." This is the point where pressure by the examiner can produce the discharge. Surgical intervention is achieved by eliciting the discharge in the operating room. The surgeon places a sialogram-type probe in the orifice of the discharging duct and with a circumareolar incision exposes the subareolar ducts. With the probe in place, the problem duct is identified and the surgeon proceeds to dissect the branching network as it extends back into the breast. If the discharge is bloody, the involved ducts are evident as the dissection proceeds. This procedure, however, is essentially a partially blind operation because the smaller ducts are not readily visible. Theoretical (although unproved) problems with this approach include the fact that the duct may branch into two different quadrants of the breast. It is likely that the entire duct system is not excised in many procedures. Cases have been reported where the cause of a discharge has not been excised (66). Some observers have argued that cancer deep in the breast may be overlooked, although this occurrence has never been documented. There have been cases where an intraductal papilloma causing a discharge was not excised with this type of dissection because the lesion was so close to the nipple that it was not included, but this is also unusual. The major disadvantage of this procedure is that a large amount of tissue is removed to treat a usually benign process.

Galactography

Galactography or ductography is used by some radiologists (67) to evaluate a discharging duct with varying results. Three potential advantages have been suggested for injecting contrast material into the duct. One possible advantage is the evaluation of the entire segment, regardless of which direction its branches take, and the fact that the deep branches can be evaluated. A second advantage is the potential to identify a focal abnormality that can permit either needle biopsy or needle localization and excision, avoiding the need to dissect the entire segment. The third potential benefit is the introduction of a vital dye into the duct so that the surgeon can dissect a colored duct that is more visible at surgery. None of these potential benefits has been confirmed in any prospective fashion. Anecdotally we have been able to limit the surgery by targeting a solitary filling defect and guiding the limited excision needed to remove a benign papilloma.

Performing a Galactogram. It must be possible to elicit a discharge from the duct in question at the time of the procedure so that the location of its orifice can be identified. We use a 30-gauge blunt sialogram needle that is formed with a right angle so that it can be placed into the duct opening and taped in place. Another method that appears to be successful is using a monofilament line to cannulate the duct and then passing a 0.7-mm catheter over the line to permit access to the duct (65). Standard iodinated contrast material for intravenous use (60% concentration) is drawn into a small (2- to 3-cc) syringe and flushed through the connecting tubing and sialogram needle, being careful to avoid any air bubbles because they will make pseudo–filling defects in the duct.

The patient is positioned supine, and the nipple is sterilized as for any breast needle procedure. While viewing the surface under a magnifying lens, dead cellular material is carefully cleared with the tip of the sialogram needle from the crevices that crisscross the nipple surface at the location of the discharge. The duct openings are at the bottom of the crevices. The breast or trigger point is squeezed to produce a tiny amount of discharge and the needle tip is carefully placed at that point. By holding the plastic connecting tubing, a small amount of pressure can be applied downward on the needle without exerting excessive force on the metal needle that could tear the duct. A slight rotary motion with the needle tip in the location of the discharge frequently causes the needle to slip easily into the duct opening.

The needle is gently inserted up to the bend and then taped in place so that the needle in the duct is at right angles to the flat surface of the nipple. This reduces the likelihood that the needle opening will be up against the wall of the duct. The patient is then assisted to the mammography unit taking care to not dislodge the needle, and the breast is placed on the detector with only mild compression. It remains in compression on the detector during the entire procedure.

A precontrast image is obtained and then contrast is slowly introduced. If there is resistance, the needle may be up against the side of the duct and can be carefully repositioned so that contrast flows smoothly into the duct. The injection is terminated if the patient feels any pain (possible extravasation) or fullness (the network is filled) or if the contrast begins to reflux out of the duct. A mammogram is obtained. If the network is not satisfactorily filled, additional contrast can be introduced. Once the network is sufficiently filled, views in both projections can be obtained and the study analyzed. If the findings are subtle, magnification views can be obtained. By keeping the needle in the duct, contrast can be added as needed.

If the goal is to stain the duct for surgical excision, several drops of a vital dye like methylene blue can be added to the contrast material. The duct opening is then sealed using collodion to prevent the contrast and dye from leaking out. The surgeon can then dissect out a blue duct. The patient should be alerted that the blue dye may appear in her urine.

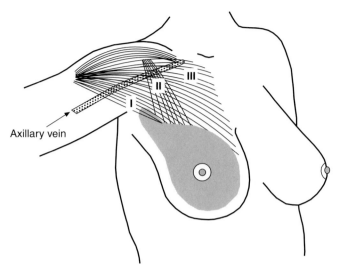

FIG. 13-136. This diagram depicts the **three regional axillary nodal groups** that are in the lymphatic drainage of the breast.

The limitation of galactography is that even if an abnormality can be defined, its etiology remains indeterminate. Breast cancer can present in several ways. It can be a single- or multiple-filling defects in the contrast. It can cause an abrupt termination of one or more ducts. Extravasation from the duct may indicate its disruption by cancer.

Axillary Lymph Nodes

Lymphatic drainage of the breast (including the medial quadrants) is primarily through the axillary lymph nodes, although there is some drainage through channels that penetrate the pectoralis muscles and some to the internal mammary chain. These latter can only be imaged by computed tomography or, as some advocate, lymphoscintigraphy.

Attempts to stage the axilla by mammography have been unsuccessful. Spread of tumor to the axillary nodes is an indication of the tumor's biological ability to metastasize and significantly worsens the prognosis and diminishes the expected long-term survival. Thus, positive axillary lymph nodes are a late, nonspecific sign of malignancy. Occasionally, palpable axillary nodes are the first indication of breast cancer. In this case a mammographic search of the breast may result in the detection of an intramammary malignant lesion that is occult to physical examination.

When malignancy that is suspicious for a breast primary is detected in axillary lymph nodes, and there is no evidence of cancer in the breast on clinical breast examination or mammography, we and others have used magnetic resonance imaging to successfully demonstrate some intramammary cancers that were otherwise occult (see Chapter 20).

Mammography with dedicated units generally provides a limited view of the axilla. The lower portion of the level

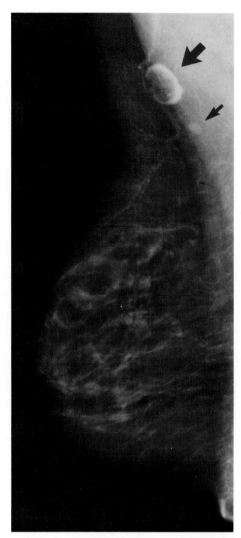

FIG. 13-137. The **fatty node in the axilla** (*large arrow*) and the smaller node below it (*small arrow*) are normal findings in the group of level I lymph nodes.

I lymph nodes (Fig. 13-136) can be seen on the MLO views (Fig. 13-137), but mammography is relatively inaccurate in determining their status (68). Normal axillary lymph nodes are <2 cm in size and have a fairly typical hilar notch or lucent center (see Fig. 13-137). When replaced by fat, axillary lymph nodes may become extremely large with only a thin rim of lymphoid tissue, but the lucent fat is obvious (Fig. 13-138). Lymph nodes without central lucency that are >1.5 to 2.0 cm in size should be considered abnormal. These are nonspecific and may be secondary to reactive hyperplasia (Fig. 13-139), but it is not possible to differentiate benign adenopathy from that due to metastatic breast cancer (Fig. 13-140) or lymphoma (Fig. 13-141). Furthermore, axillary lymph nodes may appear normal by mammography and still contain tumor. Surgical sampling is the only accurate method of assessing their true status, although positron emission tomography is fairly accurate.

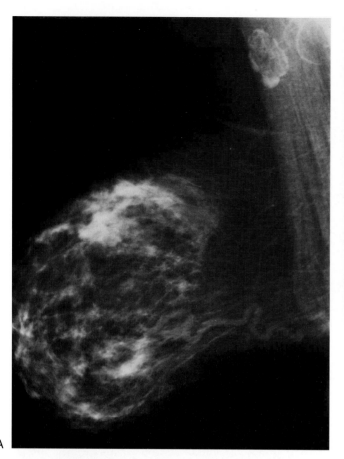

A

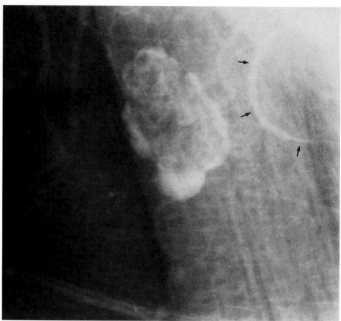

B

FIG. 13-138. Normal axillary nodes are <1.5 to 2.0 cm. Fatty replaced nodes can be extremely large, as seen in this individual. As seen on the mediolateral oblique **(A)** and photographically enlarged **(B)** images, the anterior node is still visible despite the large amount of fat that it contains. The posterior node has become a sliver (*arrows*) of tissue due to the marked infiltration with fat.

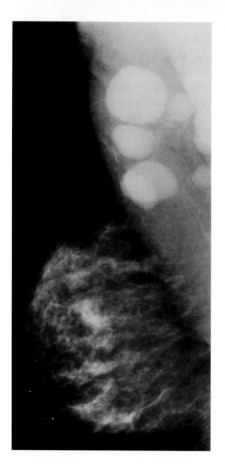

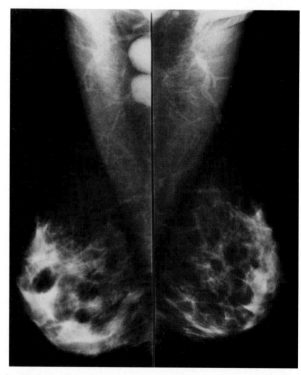

FIG. 13-139. Axillary nodal hyperplasia. Although indeterminate by mammography, these left axillary lymph nodes are very large due to benign hyperplasia in a patient with systemic lupus.

FIG. 13-140. Metastatic breast cancer to axillary nodes may cause enlargement that is visible but indeterminate by mammography. The large solid nodes on the left were due to an invasive cancer in the lower inner portion of the breast in this 34-year-old woman. The primary is seen only as subtle asymmetry.

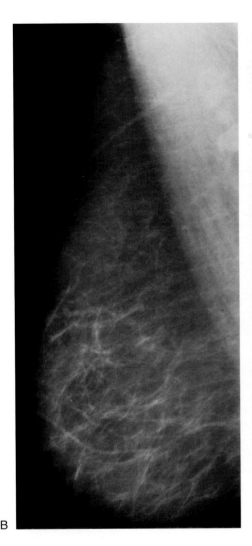
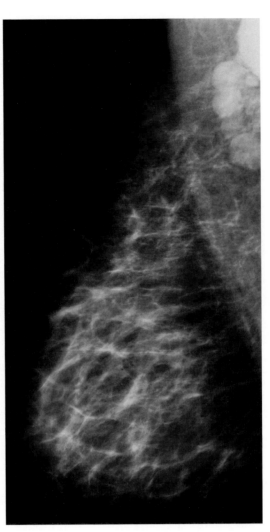

A,B

FIG. 13-141. Lymphoma is a cause of large axillary lymph nodes. In 1991 **(A)** this 60-year-old woman had a negative axilla. The lymph node enlargement that developed in 1994 **(B)** was due to lymphoma.

In a retrospective review of adenopathy detected on mammograms Walsh and associates (69) found 108 cases of mammographically abnormal axillary lymph nodes in 33,031 mammographic examinations (0.3%). Among 94 individuals pathologic (52) and clinical (42) correlations were available. Of the abnormal lymph nodes, 55% were due to malignant conditions and 45% to benign. More than half of the latter were nonspecific benign causes. Of these 94 individuals, 22 were nonspecific benign, 20 were due to metastatic breast cancer, 13 were due to chronic lymphocytic leukemia, small lymphocytic lymphoma, 6 due to collagen vascular disease, 3 to lymphoma, 3 to metastatic disease from a nonbreast site, and 3 to an unknown primary. Other cases included human immunodeficiency virus–related adenopathy, psoriasis, and infections.

Although the authors concluded that mammography could not differentiate benign from malignant adenopathy and reiterated that microscopic metastatic disease might not enlarge or deform the nodes, they reaffirmed the fact that if a node appeared spiculated or ill defined, it should then be viewed with suspicion. Although very rare, if a lymph node

contained fine, pleomorphic calcifications (not large granulomatous types) metastatic breast cancer was likely. If bilateral adenopathy was seen, then leukemia or lymphoma were likely, as would be expected.

Breast cancer can spread to the contralateral axillary nodes. It is postulated that this is either through shared lymphatics across the sternum or by a hematogenous route. Metastatic spread from other primary sites may also result in enlargement of the axillary nodes. When no tumor is found within the breast, this becomes a more significant possibility.

Calcified Axillary Nodes

On rare occasions calcifications appear in axillary nodes, but this is extremely uncommon. Large calcifications in axillary lymph nodes are of no importance (Fig. 13-142).

When fine irregular calcifications are present in axillary nodes, metastasis should be suspected, especially if tumor in the breast contains similar calcifications (70). Gold deposits in women treated with gold for rheumatoid arthritis have

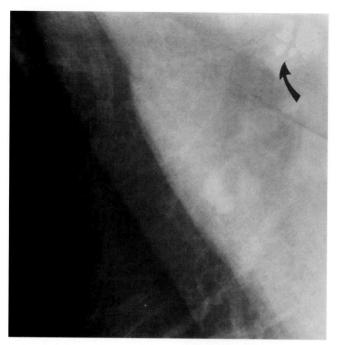

FIG. 13-142. Large calcifications in axillary nodes have no known significance, as seen in the axilla (*arrow*) of this patient.

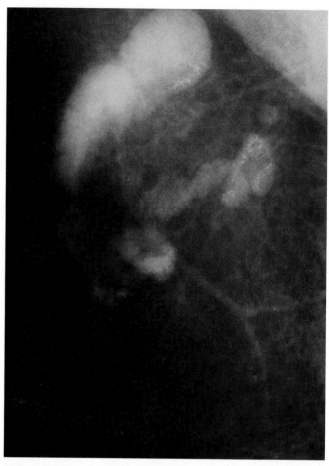

FIG. 13-143. The **tiny metallic particles** visible in this patient's axillary lymph nodes are **gold** from injections to treat rheumatoid arthritis.

been described as a rare cause of radiopaque particles in axillary nodes (71) (Fig. 13-143).

ADJUNCTIVE ASSESSMENT OF BREAST LESIONS

To arrive at a final assessment, additional techniques beyond the standard two-view mammogram may be useful. Magnification mammography results in an improvement in the sharpness of the margins of masses by reducing the contribution of noise in the image and, if the focal spot size is very small, by an increase in resolution. The morphology and number of calcifications are better appreciated using magnification. The margins of masses are seen with greater clarity, and this may aid in the assessment of these lesions. Magnification, however, should be used carefully. The focal spot must be sufficiently small to permit the amount of magnification desired without creating geometric unsharpness.

The use of the spot compression device to better spread overlapping structures can be combined with magnification, but the operator should recognize the possibility that spot compression may squeeze a true lesion out of the field of view. If a suspicious lesion seems to disappear with spot compression, this possibility should be considered.

We have also noted that, for as yet unexplained reasons, true architectural distortion may not be as evident on magnification, and we prefer to use spot compression without magnification as the first step in evaluating an area of architectural distortion. Other special views can be used to better visualize questionable lesions by rolling the breast (72) or angling the tube (see Chapter 22).

Ultrasound, described in greater detail in Chapter 16, is the most useful adjunct to mammography in analyzing mass lesions. Although many radiologists use ultrasound to assess palpable masses, this may add an unnecessary layer of expense to the workup of a mass *unless the demonstration of a cyst by ultrasound will avoid a needle aspiration.* It has been our experience that many women with a palpable mass would prefer that it be resolved. Needle aspiration simultaneously diagnoses and eliminates most cysts or confirms that the mass is solid. If the palpable mass is to be aspirated regardless of the ultrasound result, then ultrasound is superfluous. Ultrasound is efficacious when used for the palpable lesion that is thought to be a cyst but has defied clinically guided aspiration. Among this smaller number of women the ultrasound demonstration of a cyst and its confirmation by imaging-guided aspiration can avoid an open biopsy. The radiologist should be aware, however, that despite its lack of cost-effectiveness ultrasound evaluation is being promulgated as the standard of care for palpable abnormalities. As a result, we now ultrasound all palpable abnormalities out of medical/legal concerns.

Ultrasound is primarily useful in the assessment of mammographically detected nonpalpable lesions to differentiate

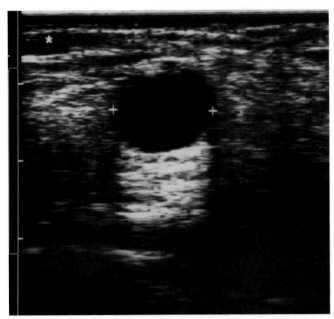

FIG. 13-144. The **ultrasound appearance of a cyst** with sharp anterior and posterior margins, no internal echoes, and enhanced through-transmission of sound, as in this 48-year-old woman with a nonpalpable mass found by mammography.

cystic from solid masses. If ultrasound is to be relied on, strict criteria must be observed to safely diagnose a cyst. The margins should be well defined with sharply defined anterior and posterior walls. There should be *no* internal echoes that suggest solid tissue (debris or proteinaceous material may cause low-level echoes, but these should be carefully analyzed before they are dismissed), and posterior acoustic enhancement should be present (Fig. 13-144). If any of these criteria is questionable, aspiration to confirm a cyst is prudent.

SUMMARY

The analysis of the mammogram should be done in a systematic fashion. If an anomaly that has benign characteristics is detected, further evaluation is not needed. Additional imaging or short interval follow-up may permit probably benign abnormalities to be classified as benign processes. Until the time that noninvasive techniques are proved reliable, lesions that remain indeterminate or suspicious should have a tissue (cytologic or histologic) diagnosis.

REFERENCES

1. Tuddenham WJ. Problems of perception in chest roentgenology: facts and fallacies. Radiol Clin North Am 1963;31:277–289.
2. Bird RE. Professional quality assurance for mammographic screening programs. Radiology 1990;177:587.
3. Tabar L, Fagerberg G, Duffy S, et al. Update of the Swedish two-county program of mammographic screening for breast cancer. Radiol Clin North Am 1992;30:187–210.
4. Thurfjell EL, Lernevall KA, Taube AAS. Benefit of independent double reading in a population-based mammography screening program. Radiology 1994;191:241–244.
5. Haus AG, Gray JE, Daly TR. Evaluation of mammographic viewbox luminance, illuminance, and color. Med Phys 1993;20:819–821.
6. Eklund GW, Cardenosa G. The art of mammographic positioning. Radiol Clin North Am 1992;30:21–53.
7. Bassett LW, Hirbawi IA, DeBruhl N, Hayes MK. Mammographic positioning: evaluation from the view box. Radiology 1993;188:803–806.
8. Stacey-Clear A, McCarthy KA, Hall DA, et al. Observations on the location of breast cancer in women under fifty. Radiology 1993;186:677–680.
9. Rosen PP, Groshen S, Saigo PE, et al. A long-term follow-up study of survival in stage I (T1 N0 M0) and stage II (T1 N1 M0) breast carcinoma. J Clin Oncol 1989;7:355–366.
10. Tabar L, Fagerberg G, Day N, et al. Breast cancer treatment and natural history: new insights from results of screening. Lancet 1992;339:412–414.
11. Bassett LW, Shayestehfar B, Hirbawi I. Obtaining previous mammograms for comparison: usefulness and costs. AJR Am J Roentgenol 1994;163:1083–1086.
12. Sadowsky NL, Semine A, Harris JR. Breast imaging: a critical aspect of breast conserving treatment. Cancer 1990;65:2113–2118.
13. Gluck BS, Dershaw DD, Liberman L, Deutch BM. Microcalcifications on postoperative mammograms as an indicator of adequacy of tumor excision. Radiology 1993;188:469–472.
14. Harris JR, Lippman ME, Veronesi U, Willett W. Breast cancer. N Engl J Med 1992;327:319–328, 390–398, 473–480.
15. Martin JE, Moskowitz M, Milbrath J. Breast cancer missed by mammography. AJR Am J Roentgenol 1979;132:737.
16. Wolfe JN. Mammography: ducts as a sole indicator of breast carcinoma. Radiology 1967;89:206.
17. Kopans DB, Swann CA, White G, et al. Asymmetric breast tissue. Radiology 1989;171:639–643.
18. Swann CA, Kopans DB, McCarthy KA, et al. Mammographic density and physical assessment of the breast. AJR Am J Roentgenol 1987;148:525–526.
19. Boren WL, Hunter TB, Bjelland JC, Hunt KR. Comparison of breast consistency at palpation with breast density at mammography. Invest Radiol 1990;25:1010–1011.
20. Le Gal M, Olliver L, Asselain B, et al. Mammographic features of 455 invasive lobular carcinomas. Radiology 1992;185:705–708.
21. Cho D, Buscema J, Rosenshein NB, Woodruff JD. Primary breast cancer of the vulva. Obstet Gynecol 1985;3(Suppl):79–81.
22. Osteen RT, Hyunds Karnell L. The national cancer data base report on breast cancer. Cancer 1994;73:1994–2000.
23. Sickles EA. Breast masses: mammographic evaluation. Radiology 1989;173:297-303.
24. Kopans DB. Re: organochlorines and breast cancer [letter]. J Natl Cancer Inst 1993;86:66.
25. Meyer JE, Ferraro FA, Frenna TH, et al. Mammographic appearance of normal intramammary lymph nodes in an atypical location. AJR Am J Roentgenol 1993;161:779–780.
26. Carter CL, Allen C, Henson DE. Relation of tumor size, lymph node status, and survival in 24,740 breast cancer cases. Cancer 1989;63:181–187.
27. Gallager HS, Martin JE. Early phases in the development of breast cancer. CA Cancer J Clin 1969;24:1170–1178.
28. Fisher B, Slack NH, Bross IDJ, et al. Cancer of the breast: size of neoplasm and prognosis. Cancer 1969;24:1071–1080.
29. Tabar L, Duffy SW, Krusemo UB. Detection method, tumour size and node metastases in breast cancers diagnosed during a trial of breast cancer screening. Eur J Cancer Clin Oncol 1987;23,7:959–962.
30. Rosner D, Lane WW. Node-negative minimal invasive breast cancer patients are not candidates for routine systemic adjuvant therapy. Cancer 1990;66:199–205.
31. Sickles EA, Herzog KA. Mammography of the postsurgical breast. AJR Am J Roentgenol 1981;136:585–588.
32. Bassett LW, Gold RH, Cove HC. Mammographic spectrum of traumatic fat necrosis: the fallibility of "pathognomonic" signs of carcinoma. AJR Am J Roentgenol 1978;130:119–122.
33. Mitnick JS, Vazquez MF, Harris MN, Roses DF. Differentiation of radial scar from scirrhous carcinoma of the breast: mammographic-pathologic correlation. Radiology 1989;173:697–700.
34. Swann CA, Kopans DB, Koerner FC, et al. The halo sign and malignant breast lesions. AJR Am J Roentgenol 1987;149:1145–1147.

35. Moskowitz M. The predictive value of certain mammographic signs in screening for breast cancer. Cancer 1983;51:1007–1011.

36. Sickles EA. Periodic mammographic follow-up of probably benign lesions: results of 3184 consecutive cases. Radiology 1991;179:463–468.

37. Varas X, Leborgne F, Leborgne JH. Non-palpable, probably benign lesions: role of follow-up mammography. Radiology 1992;184:409–414.

38. Sickles EA. Nonpalpable, circumscribed, noncalcified solid breast masses: likelihood of malignancy based on lesion size and age of patient. Radiology 1994;192:439–442.

39. Brenner RJ, Sickles EA. Acceptability of periodic follow-up as an alternative to biopsy for mammographically detected lesions interpreted as probably benign. Radiology 1989;171:645–646.

40. Bassett LW, Kimme-Smith C. Breast sonography. AJR Am J Roentgenol 156;1991:449–455.

41. McNicholas MMJ, Heneghan JP, Milner MH, et al. Pain and increased mammographic density in women receiving hormone replacement therapy: a prospective study. AJR Am J Roentgenol 1994;163:311–315.

42. Hermann G, Schwartz IS. Focal fibrous disease of the breast: mammographic detection of an unappreciated condition. AJR Am J Roentgenol 1983;140:1245.

43. Polger MR, Denison CM, Lester S, Meyer JE. Pseudoangiomatous stromal hyperplasia: mammographic and sonographic appearance. AJR Am J Roentgenol 1996;166:349–352.

44. Cohen MA, Morris EA, Rosen PP, et al. Pseudoangiomatous stromal hyperplasia: mammographic and sonographic and clinical patterns. Radiology 1996;198:117–120.

45. Rubens JR, Kopans DB. Medullary carcinoma of the breast: is it overdiagnosed? Arch Surg 1990;125:601–604.

46. Meyer JE, Kopans DB. Analysis of mammographically obvious breast carcinomas with benign results on initial biopsy. Surg Gynecol Obstet 1981;153:570–572.

47. Ganong WF. Review of Medical Physiology. Los Altos, CA: Lange Medical Publications, 1969;463–464.

48. Meyer JE, Kopans DB. Stability of a mammographic mass: a false sense of security. AJR Am J Roentgenol 1981;137:595–598.

49. Evans A, Pinder S, Wilson R, et al. Ductal carcinoma in situ of the breast: correlation between mammographic and pathologic findings. AJR Am J Roentgenol 1994;162:1307–1311.

50. Stomper PC, D'Souza DJ, DiNitto PA, Arredondo MA. Analysis of parenchymal density on mammograms in 1353 women 25–79 years old. AJR Am J Roentgenol 1996;167:1261–1265.

51. Galkin BM, Frasca P, Feig SA, Holderness BA. Non-calcified breast particles: a possible new marker of breast cancer. Invest Radiol 1982;17:119.

52. Meyer JE, Kopans DB, Stomper PC, Lindfors KK. Occult breast abnormalities: percutaneous preoperative needle localization. Radiology 1984;150:335.

53. Kopans DB, Meyer JE, Homer MJ, Grabbe J. Dermal deposits mistaken for breast calcifications. Radiology 1983;149:592–594.

54. Egan RL, McSweeney MB, Sewell CW. Intramammary calcifications without an associated mass in benign and malignant diseases. Radiology 1980;137:1–7.

55. Kopans DB. Breast Imaging. Philadelphia: Lippincott, 1989.

56. Mayr NA, Staples JJ, Robinson RA, et al. Morphometric studies in intraductal breast carcinoma using computerized image analysis. Cancer 1991;67:2805–2812.

57. Sickles EA. Mammographic features of 300 consecutive nonpalpable breast cancers. AJR Am J Roentgenol 1986;146:661.

58. Sickles EA, Abell JS. Milk of calcium within tiny benign breast cysts. Radiology 1981;141:655–658.

59. Stacey-Clear A, McCarthy KA, Hall DA, et al. Calcified suture material in the breast after radiation therapy. Radiology 1992;183:207–208.

60. Holland R, Hendriks JHCL, Verbeck ALM, et al. Extent, distribution, and mammographic/histological correlations of breast ductal carcinoma in situ. Lancet 1990;335:519–522.

61. Lev-Toaff AS, Feig SA, Saitas VL, et al. Stability of malignant breast microcalcifications. Radiology 1994;192:153–156.

62. Kopans DB, Meyer JE, Proppe K. The double line of skin thickening on sonograms of the breast. Radiology 1981;141:485–487.

63. Leis HP, Cammarata A, LaRaja RD. Nipple discharge: significance and treatment. Breast 1985;11:6–12.

64. Devitt JE. Management of nipple discharge by clinical findings. Am J Surg 1985;149:789–792.

65. Hou MF, Huang TJ, Huang YS, Hsieh JS. A simple method of duct cannulation and localization for galactography before excision in patients with nipple discharge. Radiology 1995;195:568–569.

66. Baker KS, Davey DD, Stelling CB. Ductal abnormalities detected with galactography: frequency of adequate excisional biopsy. AJR Am J Roentgenol 1994;162:821–824.

67. Cardenosa G, Doudna C, Eklund GW. Ductography of the breast: technique and findings. AJR Am J Roentgenol 1994;162:1081–1087.

68. Kalisher L, Peyster RG. Clinicopathological correlation of xerography in determining involvement of metastatic axillary nodes in female breast cancer. Radiology 1976;121:333.

69. Walsh R, Kornguth PJ, Soo MS, et al. Axillary lymph nodes: mammographic, pathologic, and clinical correlation. AJR Am J Roentgenol 1997;168:33–38.

70. Helvie MA, Rebner M, Sickles EA, Oberman HA. Calcifications in metastatic breast carcinoma in axillary lymph nodes. AJR Am J Roentgenol 1988;151:921–922.

71. Bruwer A, Nelson GW, Spark RP. Punctate intranodal gold deposits simulating microcalcifications on mammograms. Radiology 1987;163:87–88.

72. Swann CA, Kopans DB, McCarthy KA, et al. Practical solutions to problems of triangulation and preoperative localization of breast lesions. Radiology 1987;163:577–579.

Breast Imaging, 2nd ed., by Daniel B. Kopans.
Lippincott–Raven Publishers, Philadelphia © 1998.

CHAPTER 14

Benign and Probably Benign Lesions

Mammography is a screening test whose major application is the earlier detection of breast cancer; however, mammography also reveals many benign breast processes. Many of these are easily recognized, whereas others are not as easily distinguished from cancer. When a possible abnormality is detected, the first decision after determining that it is real and ascertaining its location is to try to determine what it is and whether it should raise concern. There are many findings that appear on mammograms that are clearly benign and should not elicit any further evaluation. Recognizing them and realizing that they are insignificant is an important aspect of mammographic evaluation.

The primary evaluation of a finding on the mammogram is to determine whether it is significant or can be ignored. There are a number of masses that are benign and have a typical appearance on the mammogram and rarely require any additional evaluation (Table 14-1).

Most calcifications that appear in the breast are due to benign processes. Many of these have typical morphologic characteristics and do not require any further evaluation (Table 14-2).

MASSES THAT REQUIRE NO INTERVENTION

Raised Skin Lesions

Because very little of the skin of the breast is imaged in tangent to the x-ray beam, almost anything that is on or in the skin projects over the breast tissue. The majority of skin lesions are not visible on a mammogram. However, lesions that are raised and do not flatten against the skin with compression may appear and project as masses in the breast. The most common such lesion is the seborrheic keratosis, which is a benign skin lesion associated with aging (Fig. 14-1). These appear wartlike with a verrucoid appearance that is frequently visible on the mammogram with air trapped in the irregular surface of the lesion. Air trapped around their periphery at the time of compression, which highlights their margin, is frequently what makes these lesions visible on the mammogram.

Epidermal inclusion cysts, commonly called wens, and sebaceous cysts may also appear on the mammogram (Fig.

14-2). These are circumscribed masses that are palpable immediately beneath the epidermis. An inclusion cyst is frequently accompanied by a small visible blackhead, and patients invariably attest that the blackhead has been present for many years and that periodically a foul smelling whitish material exudes from a small opening that is frequently visible on the skin. These lesions can be found on any skin surface, but it has been our experience that they are often found near the inframammary fold or near the axilla. On ultrasound they are found at the junction of the dermis and the subcutaneous fat (Fig. 14-2C).

Although the diagnosis of a skin lesion is usually obvious on the mammogram and no further analysis is required, if there is any question a radiopaque marker can be taped to the lesion. The marker remains with the projected density on the mammogram regardless of the projection. An image obtained with the beam in tangent to the lesion will confirm its cutaneous location.

The materials used to mark the skin have been termed *mole markers*. This is a misnomer as moles or nevi (pigmented lesions) are not visible by mammography unless they are raised and have an air–soft tissue interface when compressed.

Intramammary Lymph Nodes

Benign intramammary lymph nodes are evident on approximately 5% of all mammograms. They are usually well circumscribed and <1 cm in size. They have been described on histologic sectioning in all areas of the breast, but on mammography they are almost always found at the periphery of the parenchymal cone in the upper outer quadrant, usually not below the equator of the breast (1). They are seen mammographically as far as three-fourths of the way toward the nipple, but not in the subareolar area.

Intramammary lymph nodes have been reported in other parts of the breast. Meyer and associates reported two cases in which benign intramammary nodes were biopsied in the medial part of the breast (2). Since the histology of these was not provided, it is not clear whether these were true lymph nodes or rather the lymphoid tissue that we have seen in other parts of the breast.

TABLE 14-1. Masses that can be ignored

Raised skin lesions
    Seborrheic keratosis
Intramammary lymph nodes
Fat-containing lesions
    Encapsulated lucent lesions
        Lipomas
        Fat necrosis forming oil cysts
        Galactoceles
    Mixed-density lesions
        Hamartomas
        Hematomas
Multiple rounded densities
Benign calcified masses
    Calcifying involuting fibroadenomas
Benign masses with peripheral calcifications
    Calcifying involuting fibroadenomas
    Cysts with calcified walls
    Fat necrosis
Calcifying large duct papillomas
Cysts with precipitated calcium

TABLE 14-2. Calcifications that can be ignored

Lucent-centered calcifications
    Skin calcifications
    Fat necrosis
    Secretory calcifications
Milk of calcium
Vascular calcifications
Large rod-shaped calcifications
Skin calcifications
Dystrophic calcifications
Diffusely scattered calcifications (? bilateral)

Regardless, these are the only two cases of lymph nodes found in atypical locations in the breast in which histologic confirmation has been reported. The rarity of this is clear in that the two cases came from a series of more than 4,000 breast biopsies.

Intramammary lymph nodes have a fairly classic appearance, with an invaginated hilum or notch. When fatty infiltrated they have a typical lucent center (Fig. 14-3) and when in an appropriate location should not be confused with a significant abnormality. When a node becomes almost completely fatty replaced, it may appear as three or more round densities in a horseshoe arrangement (Fig. 14-4).

The diagnosis of an intramammary lymph node should not be considered when a mass is seen in any section of the breast other than the lateral portion, unless the lesion has a clearly defined lucent hilum. If an upper outer quadrant lesion does not have the characteristics of a benign intramammary node, including a lucent hilar notch and smooth, sharply defined margins, suspicion should be aroused because not all upper outer quadrant masses are benign lymph nodes and 30% to 50% of cancers are found in the upper outer quadrant.

If an intramammary lymph node is enlarged, loses its hilar notch, and becomes rounded, biopsy should be considered. Although intramammary lymph nodes can be hyperplastic or enlarged because of dermatologic problems, such as psoriasis (Fig. 14-5) or other benign inflammatory

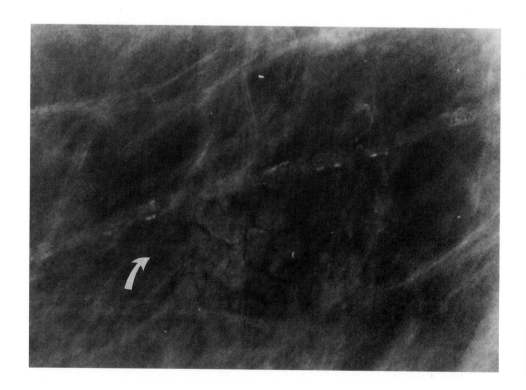

FIG. 14-1. The verrucoid appearance of this mass is typical of the benign, cutaneous **seborrheic keratosis** that is projecting over the breast.

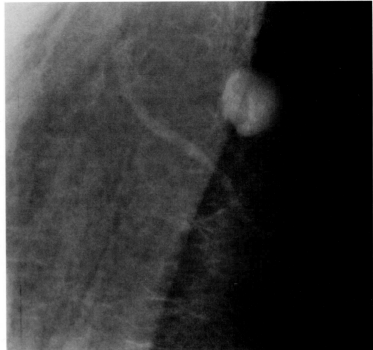

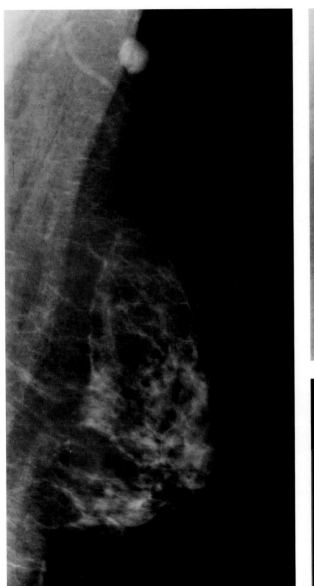

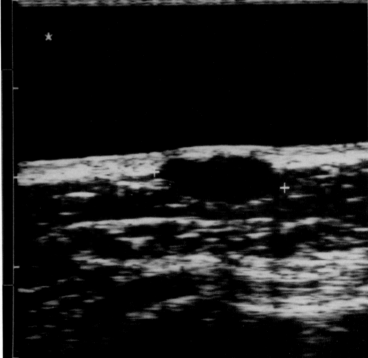

FIG. 14-2. Skin cyst. Epidermal inclusion cysts as well as sebaceous cysts are usually smooth and round unless infected. This rounded mass on the mediolateral oblique **(A)** and enlarged **(B)** corresponded to a benign sebaceous cyst evident beneath the skin. Another skin cyst on ultrasound **(C)** is sonolucent and at the interface of the dermis and the subcutaneous fat, as seen on this scan using an "off-set."

processes in the breast (3), enlargement can also be due to lymphoma or metastatic spread from an intramammary malignancy to an intramammary lymph node. Such a lesion may remain well circumscribed (Fig. 14-6) but nevertheless contain tumor cells. The breast should be carefully searched for an occult malignancy. Metastatic spread of breast can-

cer to an intramammary node carries the same worsened prognostic significance as axillary nodal involvement.

Lymph nodes can also be seen close to the chest wall. They occur in the lateral axillary chain and may extend down the chest wall in the prepectoral chain posterior to the breast.

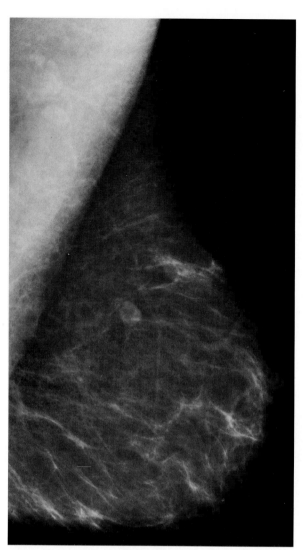

FIG. 14-3. Typical appearance of a benign, **intramammary lymph node.** It is a reniform mass with a fatty (lucent) hilum. No further evaluation is required.

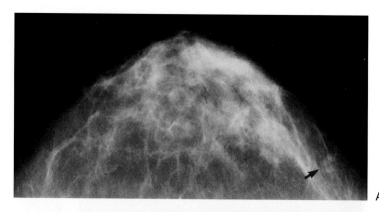

A

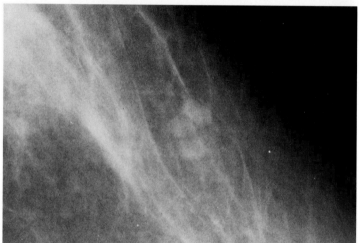

B

FIG. 14-4. Fatty replaced intramammary node. This single intra-mammary lymph node contains so much fat that it appears to be multiple masses on the craniocaudal projection **(A)** (*arrow*) and photographically enlarged **(B)**.

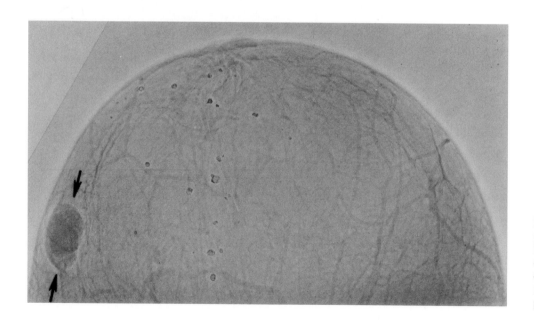

FIG. 14-5. Psoriatic dermato-pathic lymph node. This lobu-lated mass on a xerogram was excised and proved to be a dermatopathic lymph node related to the patient's known psoriasis.

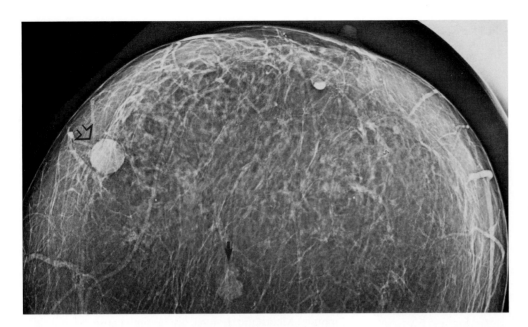

FIG. 14-6. Metastatic breast cancer to an intramammary lymph node. The circumscribed, round mass (*open arrow*) on this negative mode xerogram is an enlarged intramammary node that contained breast cancer metastatic from the irregular invasive ductal carcinoma deep in the right breast (*small arrow*).

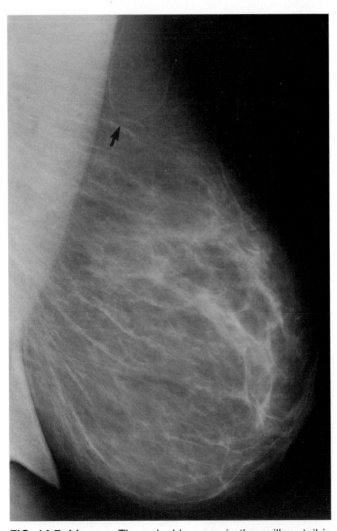

FIG. 14-7. Lipoma. The palpable mass in the axillary tail is radiolucent with a thin capsule (*arrow*). It was excised, despite the fact that it is clearly a lipoma by mammography and need not have been removed.

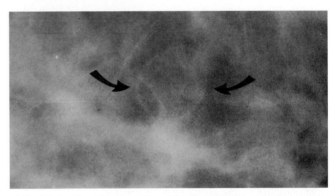

FIG. 14-8. Post-traumatic oil cyst. This palpable mass developed in an area of previous surgery. It represents encapsulated, radiolucent fat and is a form of benign fat necrosis that requires no further investigation.

Fat-Containing Lucent Lesions

Because of the low x-ray attenuation of fat, lesions that contain fat are radiolucent. Completely radiolucent lesions, including lipomas (Fig. 14-7), traumatic oil cysts (Fig. 14-8), and galactoceles (Fig. 14-9), are never malignant. Because the normal breast contains numerous locules of fat, a lipoma may not always be evident. Galactoceles are extremely rare. All of these masses may be evident on clinical breast examination (CBE), and the oil cyst in particular may present as a very hard mass. None requires surgical excision.

Mixed-Density Lesions

Encapsulated lesions that contain fat are never malignant. The mammary hamartoma (fibroadenolipoma) contains various mixtures of fat and dense tissue within a fibrous capsule (Fig. 14-10). This typical appearance defines a lesion that is

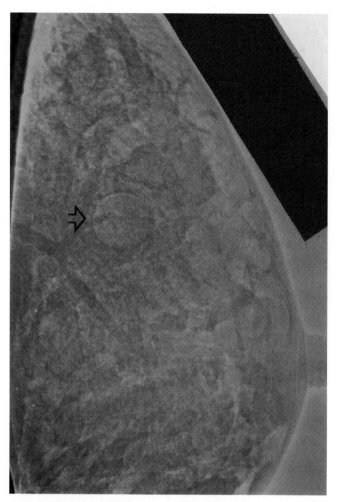

FIG. 14-9. Galactocele (*arrow*). This rare lucent lesion is a cyst containing milk with a high fat content.

never malignant. There is one case report of a lesion with similar characteristics that was reportedly a cystosarcoma (4). The term *phylloides tumor* has replaced *cystosarcoma phylloides*. Sarcomas of the breast are invariably dense lesions. Phylloides tumors are also dense. Given this single isolated occurrence, it is reasonable to state that an encapsulated lesion containing fat is always benign.

Multiple Rounded Densities

In our screening program, multiple rounded densities are found either in one breast or bilaterally in 0.5% of women. Similar findings found in multiples usually indicate a benign process.

Although the mammogram may suggest multiple rounded densities, these sometimes prove to be merely fibroglandular tissue. The rounded contours are likely due to the segmentation of the breast tissue by Cooper's ligaments (Fig. 14-11).

When true lesions are present, cysts are the most common reason for multiple rounded densities (Fig. 14-12). Multiple fibroadenomas are usually widely separated (Fig. 14-13), while cysts are usually closer together and frequently overlapping. Metastatic lesions are a rare cause of multiple rounded densities (Fig. 14-14), and the presence of a primary cancer elsewhere is almost always already known.

Our approach to multiple rounded densities in a woman being screened for the first time has been to follow her at short intervals (every 6 months for 2 years) after carefully searching to determine that a suspicious lesion (ill-defined or spiculated) is not hidden among the rounded contours.

Some advocate the use of ultrasound to evaluate multiple rounded findings, but this has never been documented in a prospective fashion as leading to earlier cancer detection; the reports are only anecdotal. Gordon and colleagues have advocated ultrasound screening of the rest of a breast that is being evaluated by ultrasound (5). They reported the detection of 15 unsuspected cancers out of 15,000 studies. However, their actual patient selection process, method of scanning, and selection of lesions to be biopsied was not documented. Furthermore, the benefit of finding these lesions was not clear since sizes and stage were not provided. The use of ultrasound to screen breast tissue is not the

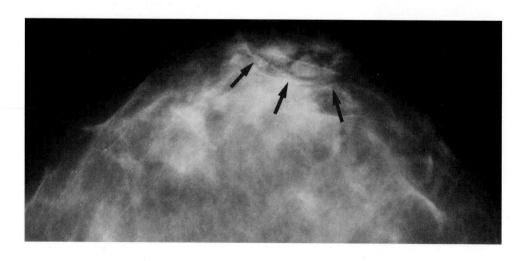

FIG. 14-10. Hamartoma (*arrows*). This mixed lesion contains fat and fibroglandular tissue. It is benign and, though palpable, requires no further evaluation.

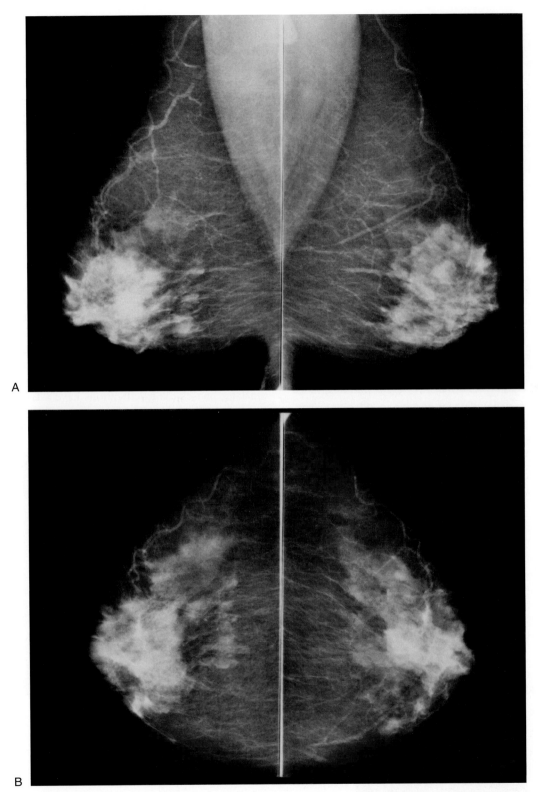

FIG. 14-11. Normal breast tissue may project as multiple rounded densities. These mediolateral oblique **(A)** and craniocaudal **(B)** mammograms of a 62-year-old woman demonstrate what appear to be rounded contours suggestive of cysts, but there were no cysts or masses by ultrasound and the tissues were unchanged 4 years later.

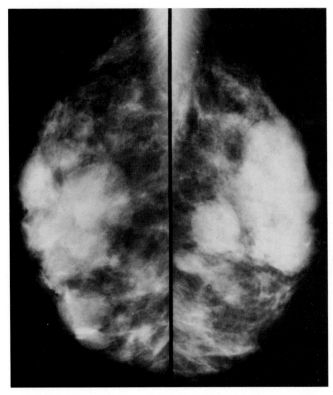

FIG. 14-12. Cysts accounting for multiple rounded densities.

standard of care (6). We use ultrasound to evaluate women with multiple rounded densities only if there is a focal area that appears to differ from the others and cyst/solid differentiation will be valuable.

If the rounded contours appear to increase or decrease in size over time but maintain their smooth shapes, they are termed *fluctuating densities* and are left alone (cancer never gets smaller).

The observer should be aware that there is always the possibility that a cancer can arise among these benign lesions. By obscuring the lesion, they can make it difficult to make an early diagnosis.

Benign Calcified Masses

Calcifying Involuting Fibroadenomas

The characteristically dense large calcifications of a benign involuting fibroadenoma, when seen within a lobulated mass, are diagnostic (Fig. 14-15). When these calcifications begin they may be very small, irregular, worrisome in appearance, and indistinguishable from malignant deposits. In such cases, biopsy may be indicated. However, in later phases the calcifications have a typical appearance that has been described as a popcorn shape. Generally

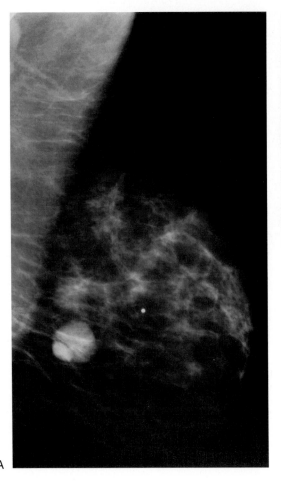

A

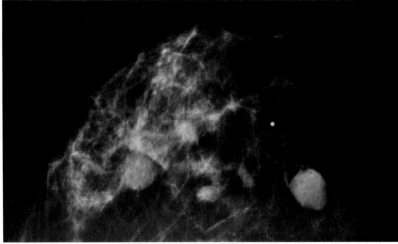

B

FIG. 14-13. Multiple fibroadenomas can account for multiple rounded densities, as seen on the mediolateral oblique **(A)** and craniocaudal **(B)** projections in this 35-year-old woman. She insisted on removal of the one that was palpable but not the two that were only visible by mammography.

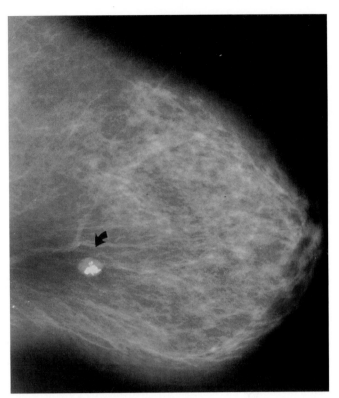

FIG. 14-15. Calcifying fibroadenoma. This calcifying mass is consistent with a benign, involuting fibroadenoma and requires no further investigation.

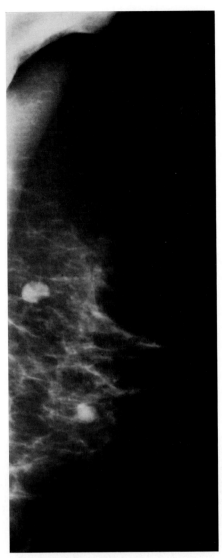

FIG. 14-14. Metastatic disease can produce multiple rounded densities. These rounded masses are metastases from ovarian cancer.

fibroadenomas calcify from the center or around their periphery and are so characteristic that they do not need to be biopsied. Some fibroadenomas, however, calcify irregularly and are indistinguishable from cancer.

It has been suggested that women who have fibroadenomas with atypical features are at increased risk for breast cancer (7). This study did not suggest that the lesion itself was at risk for malignant change, rather that it was an indicator of future overall risk. There are no data that calcifying fibroadenomas have any risk of malignant transformation. Fibroadenomas do contain epithelial elements, and consequently cancer can coincidentally develop in a fibroadenoma.

Occasionally cancer can also develop, coincidentally, immediately alongside a fibroadenoma. When other signs of malignancy such as spiculation, architectural distortion, or fine, irregular microcalcifications accompany an obvious fibroadenoma, they may signal the presence of such a coin-

cidental cancer. The calcified involuting fibroadenoma itself does not require a biopsy.

Benign Masses with Peripheral Calcifications

Masses with peripherally distributed calcifications in a rim-like pattern are virtually always benign. Fibroadenomas, cysts with calcified walls, and calcified fat necrosis commonly become calcified on their rims. Fibroadenomas usually form more irregular clumps of calcification but rarely have smooth rim-like deposits. Calcifications that define the periphery of a sphere, producing an eggshell appearance or a thicker rim, are usually seen in cysts and fat necrosis. The oil cyst can be distinguished from a fluid-filled cyst of the lobule when the mass within the calcified rim is relatively radiolucent (Fig. 14-16). Similar deposits can occur within cyst walls, but in this setting the calcified lesion is relatively radiodense because a cyst is water in its attenuation characteristics. Calcified cyst walls are usually fairly fine deposits (Fig. 14-17). Neither lesion requires biopsy.

Cysts appear to calcify in patches with a very thin layer of deposit, while fat necrosis tends to form a thicker rim. If a question persists, confirmation by aspiration is probably needed because the calcifications in the wall of a cyst can reduce the effectiveness of ultrasound in differentiating cyst from solid.

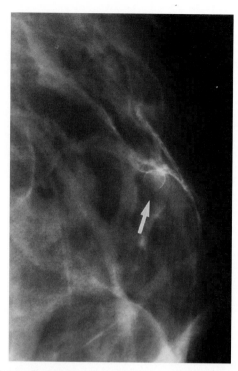

FIG. 14-16. Calcified oil cyst. This calcified mass represents an area of fat necrosis. The noncalcified portion is relatively radiolucent.

Calcified Intraductal Papillomas

It is relatively uncommon for an intraductal papilloma to be visible by mammography. In our experience, they more often present with a nipple discharge (serous or sanguineous) and are not visible on the mammogram because they conform to the duct lumen. On occasion a papilloma calcifies. It has been suggested that this is a result of infarction, but this has not been determined. In our limited experience with calcified papillomas they appear to produce shell-like deposits. They are not as round as the calcifications that are associated with cysts and appear more irregular but with lucent central areas (Fig. 14-18). A clue to the diagnosis is that they appear to be oriented in a linear fashion along a ductal course and delineate a sausage-like structure. Some papillomas present as a circumscribed mass with very fine punctate calcifications.

Benign Calcifications Without Associated Masses

Lucent-Centered Calcifications

The majority of calcifications that appear in the breast are due to benign processes and have morphologies that are

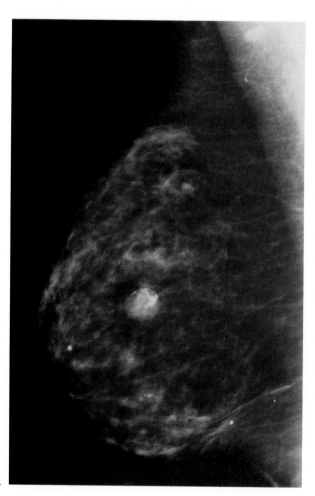

A

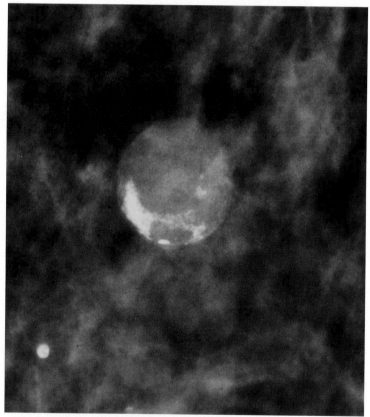

B

FIG. 14-17. These **calcifications are in the wall of a cyst** seen on contact mediolateral oblique mammography **(A)** and optically enlarged craniocaudal projection **(B)**. With this appearance, this lesion requires no further evaluation.

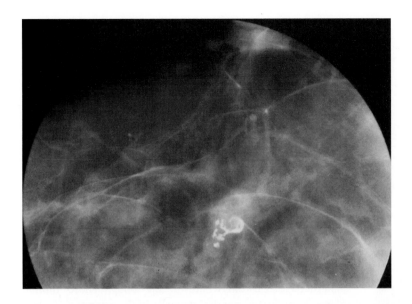

FIG. 14-18. A calcified, large-duct papilloma can appear with rimlike deposits, as seen in this magnification view. This is likely due to infarction causing necrosis at the periphery of the lesion.

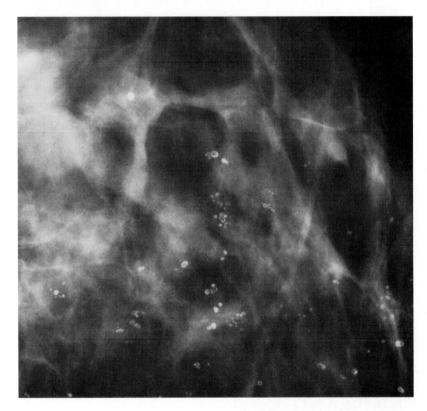

FIG. 14-19. Skin calcifications. These lucent-centered calcifications are in the skin of the medial breast.

characteristic. These do not require biopsy and usually do not require any additional evaluation. Round, hollow spheres of calcium with lucent centers are always benign. These occur in the skin (Fig. 14-19), in areas of fat necrosis (Fig. 14-20), or in association with benign calcified debris in the ducts (8). Those that occur in association with benign calcified debris in the ducts are forms of benign secretory calcification. They are almost always >0.5 mm in diameter and, although they form in the ducts, should rarely be confused with malignant calcifications. Inflammation caused by the extrusion of ductal debris into the surround-

ing stroma can produce lucent-centered tubes in the periductal tissues.

Milk of Calcium

Calcifications can form benign concretions in the lobular acini. These deposits likely account for the very small (<1 mm), smooth, round deposits that are sometimes found tightly packed together (Fig. 14-21). These acinar calcifications can on occasion be heterogeneous and difficult to differentiate from cancer. Cancer can grow back into the acini, but when

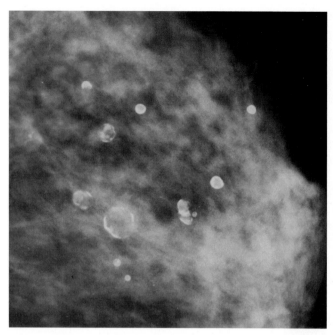

FIG. 14-20. These large, **lucent-centered calcifications** are likely due to fat necrosis.

calcifications form in these tumors they are usually in the necrotic portions of the tumor and form irregular particles.

Some forms of calcium that occur in cystically dilated lobules are characteristically due to benign processes. *Milk of calcium* is the term associated with the process in which calcium precipitates in benign cysts (9).

The calcified sediment that sometimes collects in the dependent portions of cysts may produce what initially seem to be worrisome punctate-appearing calcifications. On closer inspection, however, the diagnosis is usually easily made. Milk of calcium is diagnosed by its characteristic appearance. On the craniocaudal view, with the x-ray beam perpendicular to the floor directed down through the mobile calcium particles pooled in the bottom of the cyst, the precipitated calcium appears as small, hard-to-see, smudged dots (Fig. 14-22A). When a lateral view is obtained with the beam parallel to the floor, the calcium projects as small crescents as the beam passes from the side through the concave meniscus of the material (Fig. 14-22B). The appearance of crescent-shaped calcifications that are concave up on the horizontal beam lateral (Fig. 14-22C, D) can secure a benign diagnosis on the mammogram.

Vascular Calcifications

Vascular calcifications have the distinctive appearance of calcified arteries anywhere in the body. These intimal deposits project as parallel deposits in the arterial wall (Fig. 14-23) and are rarely confused with significant calcifications. The associated smooth, tubular, serpentine vessel is almost always distinguishable, especially on magnification views. On occasion early vascular deposits can result in calcification visible in only one side of the wall. These noncoalescent deposits may be difficult to distinguish from intraductal calcifications. Direct magnification mammography usually reveals the characteristic parallel deposits. Very small vessels may be more difficult, but these usually form very smooth, tight curves (see Fig. 14-23), which are not formed by cancer.

Arterial calcifications are virtually always related to advanced age. They are rarely seen in women in their 20s or 30s. In our experience young women who have arterial calcifications frequently have diabetes, although Sickles and Galvin found otherwise (10).

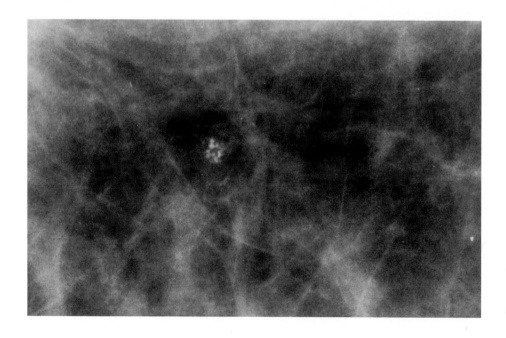

FIG. 14-21. Acinar calcifications. These calcifications have been stable for more than 3 years and are likely concretions in microcysts of the lobular acini.

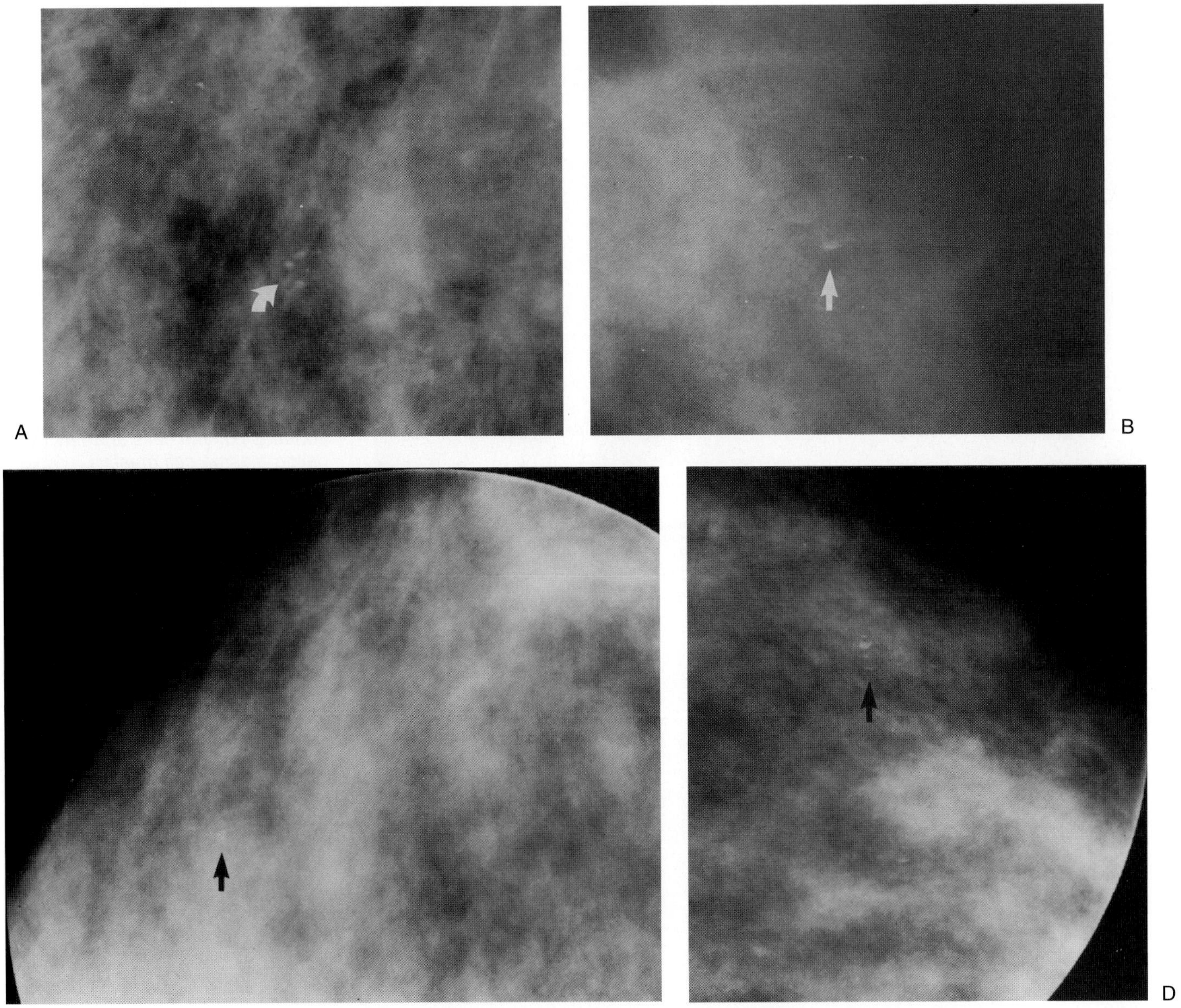

FIG. 14-22. Milk of calcium. On this craniocuadal (CC) image **(A)** the calcium that has precipitated in the bottom of small cysts appears amorphous. In the horizontal lateral image **(B)** the layering of the calcifications is evident as crescent-shaped deposits that are concave up. This second case reveals barely visible calcifications on the CC projection **(C)** and crescentic calcifications on the lateral projection **(D)**, providing a certain diagnosis of benign cysts containing milk of calcium.

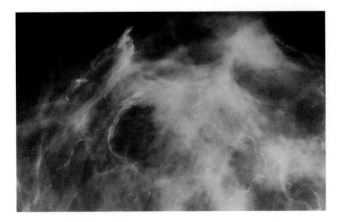

FIG. 14-23. Vascular calcifications. The serpentine deposits that can occur in the walls of large and small vessels are clearly vascular, as seen in this close-up of the front of the breast. No further evaluation is indicated.

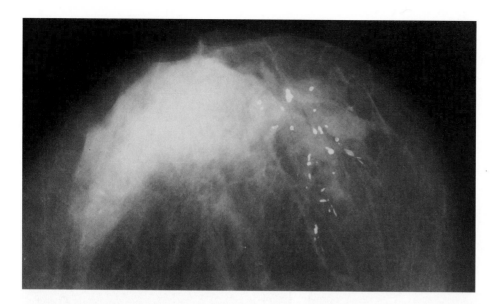

FIG. 14-24. Secretory calcifications. These large, rod-shaped calcifications of benign ductal debris are sometimes associated with a palpable inflammatory process that contains plasma cells and has been called *plasma cell mastitis.*

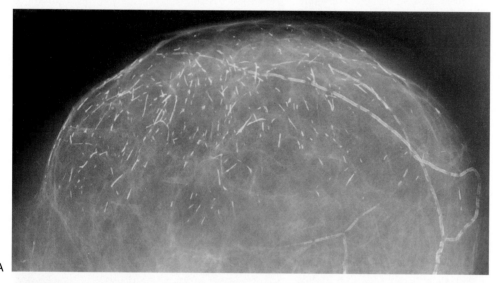

A

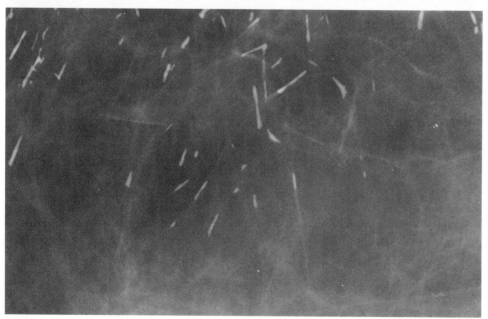

B

FIG. 14-25. Benign secretory calcifications. These linear deposits are formed in the benign cellular debris within the ducts on this craniocaudal projection **(A)** and optically enlarged **(B)**. Branching is uncommon.

Vascular calcifications, with their distinctive parallel "train track" appearance, have such typical morphologic characteristics that they can be ignored.

Large Rod-Shaped Calcifications

Rod-shaped calcifications that are >0.5 mm in diameter are due to benign processes. Sometimes they are associated with a palpable thickening of the breast (Fig. 14-24) that has been called *plasma cell mastitis* because it is accompanied by an infiltrate containing plasma cells.

Usually these benign calcifications of secretory disease are not associated with any symptoms but are found on routine mammography (Fig. 14-25). Solid rod-shaped calcifications form within the duct, but because the benign process does not narrow the lumen and may in fact distend it, these calcifications are generally larger than the deposits in the irregularly narrowed lumen of intraductal malignancy.

Tubular (lucent-centered) rods that are oriented along duct lines rarely branch and that are >0.5 mm thick are virtually always a form of benign secretory deposit within the normal or dilated ducts or the periductal stroma. They are often, although not always, bilateral. If no submillimeter fine, branching, punctate, and pointed calcifications are found to suggest coincidental cancer, then no further evaluation is necessary. When the rods have lucent centers a benign process is guaranteed.

The radiologist should exercise some caution when calcifications are extensive. The presence of an extensive benign process does not preclude a simultaneous malignancy. Regardless of the presence of benign findings, a careful search should always be made for the very fine, linear, branching (frequently associated with tiny submillimeter calcifications in single file forming a cast of the duct narrowed by tumor), or heterogeneously clustered calcifications that may herald the coincidental presence of malignant process (Fig. 14-26).

Skin Calcifications

Lucent-centered calcifications that are round or polygonal and project near the periphery of the breast are usually benign dermal deposits. Calcium deposits in the skin are usually easily recognized and should not elicit any concern. Frequently small calcified spheres with central lucencies, they may also have planar quadrilateral shapes with a central lucency (Figs. 14-19 and 14-27) when viewed *en face*. When seen in tangent, they may appear as thin disc shapes.

The exact etiology of skin calcifications is not certain, as they are not intentionally biopsied. Chronic folliculitis or inspissated material in sebaceous glands may produce these calcifications. On occasion they may be mistaken for intramammary deposits. The compression of the spherical geometry of the breast during mammography means that only a

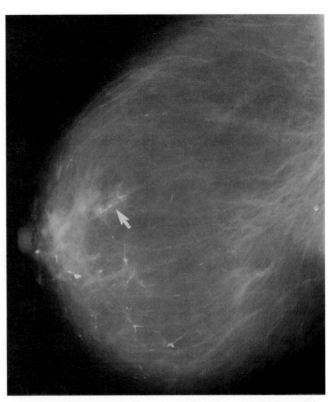

FIG. 14-26. Benign secretory calcifications and simultaneous, coincidental cancer. The anterior calcifications are due to benign secretory deposits. The deeper calcifications (*white arrow*) are in the intraductal component of an invasive cancer.

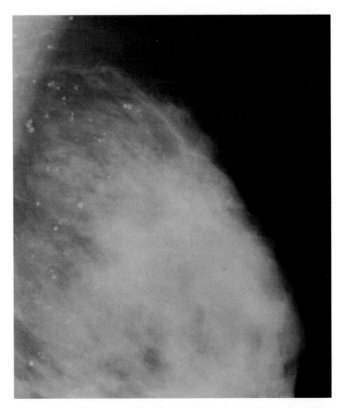

FIG. 14-27. Skin calcifications. Typical skin deposits have lucent centers with a somewhat geometric shape.

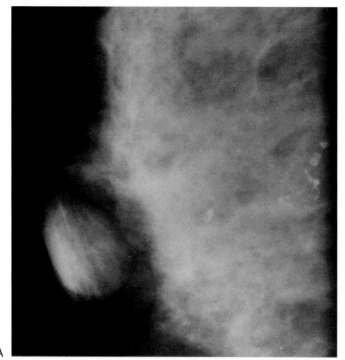

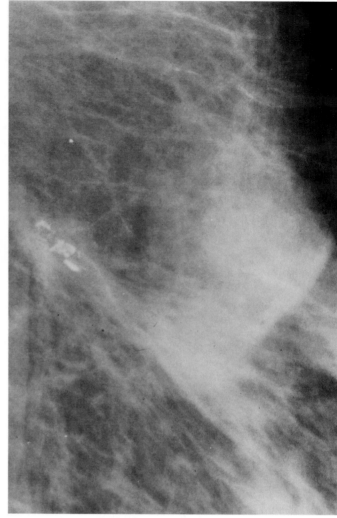

FIG. 14-28. Benign, dystrophic calcifications. These large calcifications formed following radiation therapy **(A)** in these two individuals. They frequently have lucent centers **(B)**.

small section of skin is seen tangentially in any mammographic projection and, as a consequence, structures on the skin or in the cutaneous layers can easily project as intramammary lesions.

Skin calcifications should be suspected particularly when calcifications are only visible in a single projection. If there is any doubt that peripherally located microcalcifications are in the skin, confirmation may be important. Ducts may reach through the subcutaneous fat to the skin, and cancer can (rarely) develop in these ducts in the subcutaneous fat.

A fenestrated grid can be used to place a marker on potential skin calcifications to permit tangential imaging (see Chapter 22) to confirm their dermal location. Skin deposits are always due to benign processes.

Dystrophic Calcifications

Large, solitary, solid calcifications usually represent involuted, completely calcified fibroadenomas. They are

not a cause for concern. Other large calcifications may develop, particularly in a breast that has been irradiated. These benign, dystrophic calcifications need not cause concern. They may occur up to 4 years after the surgery in as many as 30% of women who have undergone surgery and irradiation (11). These calcifications are generally at least 1 mm in size and often are larger (Fig. 14-28). They are usually not difficult to distinguish from the very small heterogeneous calcifications that signal recurrence or new cancer. Many of these postirradiation calcifications are probably related to calcified suture material and fat necrosis (see Foreign Body Reaction and Calcified Suture Material and Chapter 17).

Diffusely Scattered Calcifications

When calcifications are scattered diffusely throughout the breast and especially when they are bilateral, they almost invariably represent a benign process (Fig. 14-29). The individual radiographically visible particles are amorphous with

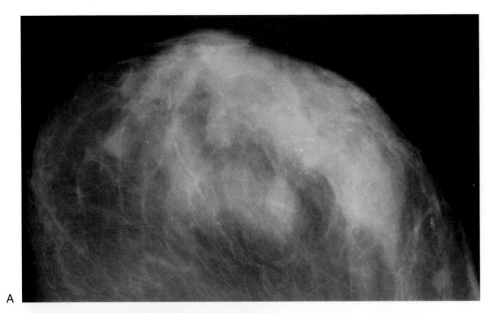

A

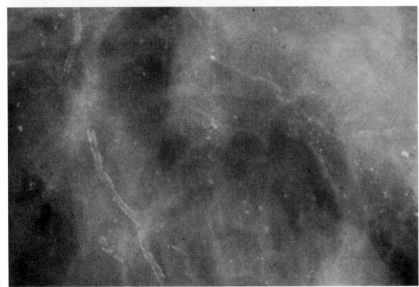

B

FIG. 14-29. Diffusely scattered calcifications are almost invariably due to a benign process. Calcifications are present throughout the breast **(A)**. On close inspection **(B)** they are amorphous, and although they vary in size their shapes are similar.

ill-defined margins. Their general shape is round. The etiology of these calcifications is not clear. Some are due to adenosis, while others are merely deposits in cysts. They are difficult to distinguish mammographically, but both are benign processes.

Foreign Body Reaction and Calcified Suture Material

Foreign bodies in the breast can elicit calcium deposition. Some forms of suture material seem to produce parallel tubular-appearing calcifications (Fig. 14-30). The etiology of these may be evident when they form a radiating pattern from a central area in the immediate vicinity of previous surgery or when they form in a relatively straight line along a suture plane (Fig. 14-31).

Calcified suture material is most common following radiation therapy but can be seen in women who have had extensive breast surgery, such as reduction mammoplasty. It is likely due to slow healing in which there is time for calcium to form on organic suture material before it is resorbed (12).

Artifacts and Skin Contaminants

Artifacts and skin contaminants can be misinterpreted as intramammary processes. Skin powders and ointments (Fig. 14-32), as well as antiperspirants, can be radiographically opaque and simulate microcalcifications (plain deodorant is not radiopaque). If their etiology is not clear, the skin should be cleansed and the image repeated.

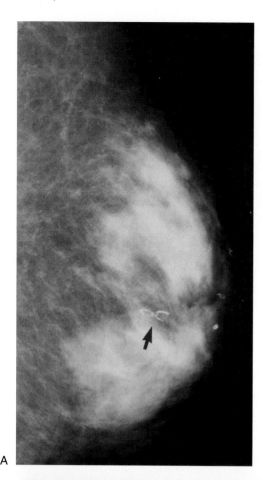

A

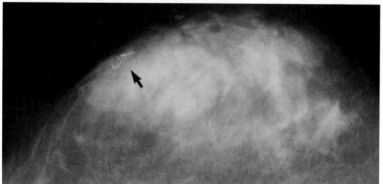

B

FIG. 14-30. Calcified suture material. The knots in the calcified suture material are evident on the medio-lateral **(A)** and cranio-caudal **(B)** projections in this individual who had been irradiated for breast cancer.

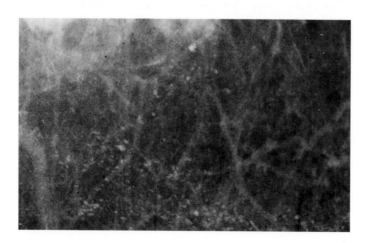

FIG. 14-31. Calcified sutures. The calcified knots are evident along the suture line following irradiation for breast cancer.

FIG. 14-32. Skin contamination. Ointment on the skin (probably zinc oxide) simulated microcalcifications.

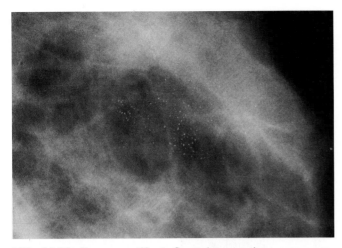

FIG. 14-33. Screen artifact. Scratches on the screen produced an artifact that simulated microcalcifications.

If what appear to be microcalcifications are visible on only a single projection, an artifact should be considered. Scratches on a screen (Fig. 14-33), dust between the screen and the film, or scratches on the film may simulate calcifications. Because light from the screen is blocked at the level of the film or the emulsion is directly damaged, these artifacts are usually sharply defined. Very tiny "calcifications" that are too sharply defined should suggest the possibility.

Foreign Bodies

As with any body structure, foreign bodies can find their way into the breast. Some are placed intentionally (Fig. 14-34). Tattoos have been reported to be visible at times (13). Nipple rings have become fashionable for some women (Fig. 14-35). As is known from needle localization procedures, the internal structures of the breast are relatively insensitive to a puncture-type injury. In several instances we have seen sewing needles that had pierced

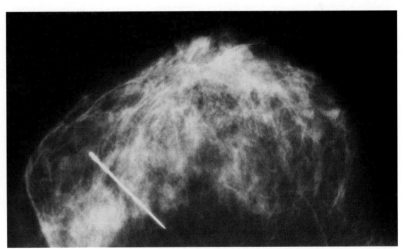

B

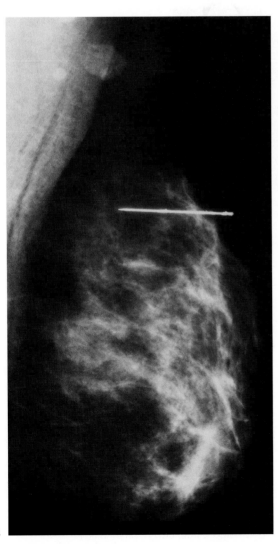

A

FIG. 14-34. Due to severe depression this patient placed **a sewing needle in her breast.** It remains unchanged 10 years later although calcifications have been deposited around it, as seen on the mediolateral oblique **(A)** and craniocaudal **(B)** projections.

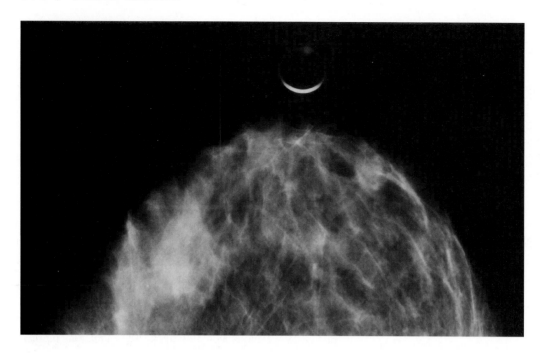

FIG. 14-35. The metallic structure at the nipple is a **nipple ring.**

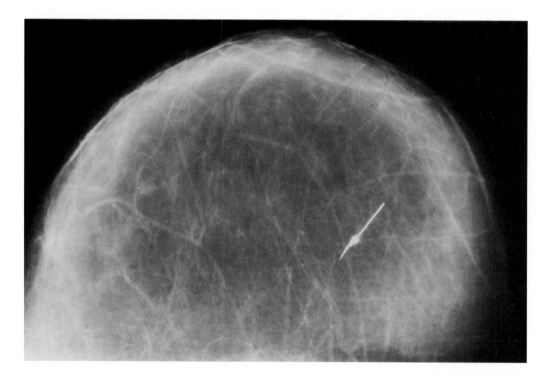

FIG. 14-36. Sewing needle in the breast. This patient was unaware that she had a broken sewing needle in her breast. Some calcium deposition near the break suggests that it had been present for some time.

the breast without the patient's noticing (Fig. 14-36). The needle was subsequently discovered by accident or presented as a thickened, sometimes painful area. Glass, pencil points (Fig. 14-37), and other foreign bodies have also been seen. These types of foreign bodies seem to be fairly well tolerated. The need for their excision, however, should be determined on an individual basis.

PROBABLY BENIGN FINDINGS APPROPRIATELY MANAGED WITH SHORT-INTERVAL FOLLOW-UP

One of the most controversial topics in mammography is the classification and management of a finding that is probably benign. These are lesions that are almost always benign, but on occasion cancer can present with a similar

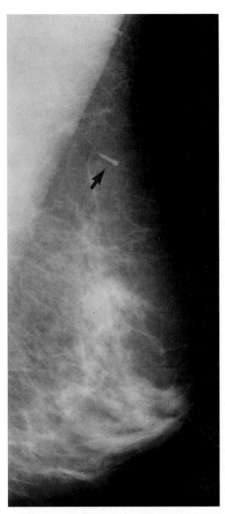

FIG. 14-37. Pencil point in the breast. This individual had fallen on a pencil 20 years earlier. The arrow points to the graphite tip of the pencil.

appearance. The probability of cancer is <5% but not zero. Many physicians believe that, based on cost and benefit, these lesions do not require biopsy but can be followed and, if they change with time, intervention can be instituted with little documented detriment to the patient.

The principle of short-interval follow-up lies in the fact that probabilities are multiplicative. Although there are cancers that can be stable for many months to even years, they are extremely uncommon. If a lesion begins with a low probability of being cancer and is then stable for several years (cancers are rarely stable), it has an extremely low probability of being malignant.

Most observers now accept the definition of "probably benign" lesions set by Sickles in a landmark paper (14). Included in his categories were round or oval circumscribed masses (Fig. 14-38), smooth, round, clustered microcalcifications (Fig. 14-39), and focal asymmetric densities that did not represent masses. Magnification mammography was used to evaluate the margins of these lesions and the morphology of the calcifications. If the circumscribed lesions

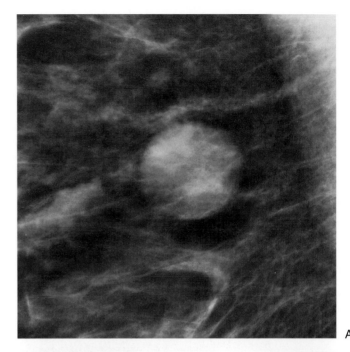

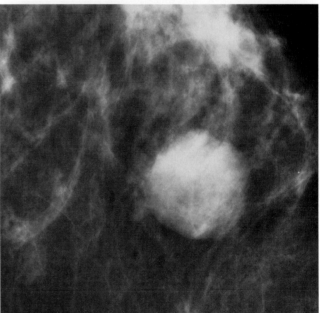

FIG. 14-38. This **round circumscribed mass with sharply defined margins** on magnification straight lateral **(A)** and craniocaudal **(B)** projections can be followed at short interval according to Sickles' data.

retained their sharp margins, the calcifications were round and regular, and the asymmetries did not form centrally dense masses fading toward their edges, Sickles found that these lesions together had only a 0.5% chance of malignancy over a 3-year follow-up period. For solitary circumscribed masses there was a 2% chance. Focal asymmetries proved to be cancers only 0.4% of the time, while rounded calcifications were associated with malignancy in only 0.1% of the cases.

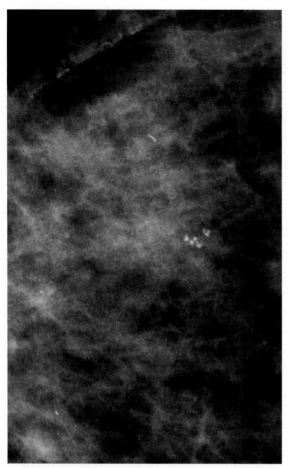

FIG. 14-39. Smooth round, clustered calcifications. These calcifications have been stable for many years and are likely deposits in benign cysts.

Varas and associates had similar results. They followed up 558 women with findings that were "probably benign" at short interval of 21,855 who had been screened (15). Among those followed for an average of 26 months, nine were found to have breast cancer (1.6%).

Sickles has argued that management by mammographic surveillance is justified by demonstrating (a) that probably benign lesions indeed have a very low likelihood of malignancy; (b) that mammographic surveillance will identify those few lesions that change in the interval that actually are malignant; and (c) that these cancers will be diagnosed early in their course, while they still have a favorable prognosis (16). It has become fairly well accepted that it is reasonable to follow a lesion that has a 2% or lower probability of cancer.

Short-Interval Follow-Up

The appropriate period of follow-up for lesions that are probably benign (<2% probability of malignancy) is uncertain. One possible approach can be arrived at by the following reasoning: (1) Given that the recommended screening interval for all women is 1 year, *and* (2) it is desirable to detect a change in a probably benign lesion as soon as possible, *but* (3) given that the average doubling time of breast cancer is 100 to 180 days *and* (4) follow-up at too short an interval may result in overlooking an increase in size because, assuming that a tumor is spherical, one doubling time (a doubling of the number of cells) only increases the diameter of the tumor by the cube root of 2 (only 1.26 times) *and* (5) given that it is reasonable to try to limit the number of radiation exposures because most of these lesions will be benign, a reasonable follow-up interval is half way to the next routine screen, or 6 months (1 to a little >1 doubling time). Since the majority of even slow-growing cancers increase in size over 2 years, it is reasonable to follow these lesions at 6-month intervals for a total of 2 years. If they remain stable over that period, then the likelihood of cancer is extremely low because the multiplied probabilities of malignancy are extremely low. Return to routine annual screening is reasonable.

Our short-interval sequence is a unilateral 6-month follow-up, bilateral follow-up and annual screen at 12 months, unilateral 18-month follow-up, and a bilateral 24-month follow-up and routine screen. This follow-up every 6 months for 2 years is not based on direct empirical data. It may one day be possible to provide a more direct measure of the appropriate interval and follow-up period. Sickles' follow-up routine was a 6-month short-interval study and then (strongly emphasized) annual mammography for 3 years. Unfortunately, 40% of the women in his study did not return for the third year of follow-up. The reader is further cautioned that short-interval follow-up only applies to a lesion that has morphology that suggests that it is almost certainly benign. Stability of a spiculated or ill-defined lesion or comedo-type calcifications *should not be reassuring*.

We have modified the approach. Although Sickles' data suggest that the likelihood of malignancy does not increase very much with the increasing size of a circumscribed solid mass (17), survival decreases with increasing size if the mass proves to be cancer (18). It appears that cancers found when they are 1 cm or smaller have the best prognosis. Thus, if one is going to intervene for a circumscribed lesion seen on the first mammogram, the intervention should be before the lesion has reached a centimeter, if possible. We have set 8 mm as an arbitrary point of intervention for these masses. If the patient's first mammogram reveals a circumscribed mass that is ≥8 mm and it is not a cyst, then we perform a needle biopsy or excisional biopsy to determine its histology.

Our data suggest that these lesions have approximately 5% probability of malignancy. Although Sickles' data did not show a strong association with cancer, our results suggest that the probability of malignancy for these lesions is significantly influenced by the age of the patient (it is possible that some of the women in his series who developed cancer were lost to follow-up). The likelihood of a solitary circumscribed lesion on a first mammogram being cancer increases with age (along with the prior probability of cancer). Ultimately, guidelines should take this into account.

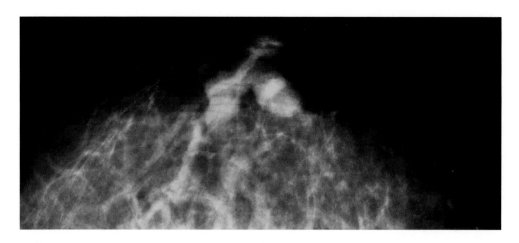

FIG. 14-40. A solitary dilated duct. Although cancer can produce a solitary dilated duct, it is extremely rare for this to occur without other signs or symptoms of cancer. The vast majority are due to duct ectasia, which is the likely diagnosis for this branching structure in the subareolar region.

Other findings that we place in the probably benign category are multiple rounded densities seen for the first time (see Multiple Rounded Densities) and a solitary dilated duct (Fig. 14-40).

In our experience, using our thresholds for intervention, it is extremely rare for a lesion that is placed in short-interval follow-up to ultimately prove to be cancer. Although short interval follow-up for probably benign lesions is an accepted approach, it is likely that if women are being screened annually and the lesions are truly probably benign, short-interval follow-up may have no advantage over annual screening (as long as the patient is diligent and returns at the appropriate times).

As has occurred in Europe, the threshold for intervention will be increasingly determined by cost. This is unfortunate. The decision to intervene or not should be made by the individual woman and her physician. It may one day be possible to provide them with probabilities based on the individual's age, other risk factors, and imaging analysis so that the patient can make an informed decision. It is conceivable that one woman may wish to follow a lesion with a 10% likelihood of malignancy, while for another even a 1% chance may be too high. The ultimate decision to intervene should be made by the individual. Efforts should continue to provide safe and accurate diagnosis so that uncertainties can be reduced at an acceptable cost.

REFERENCES

1. Meyer JE, Kopans DB, Lawrence WD. Normal intramammary lymph nodes presenting as occult breast masses. Breast Dis Breast 1982;8:30–32.
2. Meyer JE, Ferraro FA, Frenna TH, et al. Mammographic appearance of normal intramammary lymph nodes in an atypical location. AJR Am J Roentgenol 1993;161:779–780.
3. Kopans DB, Meyer JE. Benign lymph nodes associated with dermatitis presenting as breast masses. Radiology 1980;137:15–20.
4. Taupman RE, Shargo S, Boatman KK, Boggs JT. Malignant cystosarcoma with lipomatous component: a case report. Breast Dis Breast 1982;7:31–33.
5. Gordon PB, Goldenberg SL. Malignant breast masses detected only by ultrasound: a retrospective review. Cancer 1995;76:626–630.
6. Kopans DB, Sickles EA, Feig SA. Letter to the editor. Cancer 1996; 77:208–209.
7. Dupont WD, Page DL, Pari FF, et al. Long-term risk of breast cancer in women with fibroadenoma. N Engl J Med 1994;331:10–15.
8. Levitan LH, Witten DM, Harrison EG. Calcification in breast disease—mammographic-pathologic correlation. Radiology 1964;92:29–39.
9. Sickles EA, Abele JS. Milk of calcium within tiny benign breast cysts. Radiology 1981;141:655–658.
10. Sickles EA, Galvin HB. Breast arterial calcification in association with diabetes mellitus: too weak a correlation to have clinical utility. Radiology 1985;155:577–579.
11. Libshitz HI, Montague ED, Paulus DO. Calcifications and the therapeutically irradiated breast. AJR Am J Roentgenol 1977;128:1021–1025.
12. Stacey-Clear A, McCarthy KA, Hall DA, et al. Calcified suture material in the breast after radiation therapy. Radiology 1992;183:207–208.
13. Brown RC, Zuehike RL, Ehrhardt JC, Jochimsen PR. Tattoo simulating calcifications on xeroradiographs of the breast. Radiology 1981; 138:583–584.
14. Sickles EA. Periodic mammographic follow-up of probably benign lesions: results of 3184 consecutive cases. Radiology 1991;179:463–468.
15. Varas X, Leborgne F, Leborgne JH. Non-palpable, probably benign lesions: role of follow-up mammography. Radiology 1992;184:409–414.
16. Sickles EA. Management of Probably Benign Lesions. In Kopans DB, Mendelson EB (eds), Syllabus: A Categorical Course in Breast Imaging. Chicago: Radiological Society of North America, 1995; 133–138.
17. Sickles EA. Nonpalpable, circumscribed, noncalcified solid breast masses: likelihood of malignancy based on lesion size and age of patient. Radiology 1994;192:439–442.
18. Rosen PP, Groshen S, Saigo PE, et al. A long-term follow-up study of survival in stage I (T1 N0 M0) and stage II (T1 N1 M0) breast carcinoma. J Clin Oncol 1989;7:355–366.

Breast Imaging, 2nd ed., by Daniel B. Kopans.
Lippincott–Raven Publishers, Philadelphia © 1998.

CHAPTER 15

The Mammographic Appearance of Breast Cancer

Diagnosis would be greatly simplified if all cancers of the breast exhibited unique features, but unfortunately they do not. Although many cancers have specific recognizable morphologic characteristics, there is an unavoidable similarity among the shapes, margins, and densities of many benign and malignant lesions. Some cancers produce an appearance that is virtually pathognomonic of the disease, but many do not exhibit such specific morphology, and it must be accepted that benign lesions will necessarily be biopsied to find the greatest number of early cancers.

As with all of medicine, the likelihood that disease is present is a probability estimate. Some features carry a high probability of cancer, other features carry a very low or even coincidental risk of cancer, and a great number of findings are intermediate and can be present in both benign and malignant processes. The analysis of findings can be divided into three general categories: (1) findings that carry a high probability of malignancy, (2) those that have an intermediate likelihood and should be considered suspicious, and (3) others that are significant when they support or are supported by other indications of cancer.

DETECTION VERSUS DIAGNOSIS

Mammography is unchallenged as a screening test for detecting early-stage breast cancer. No other imaging technique approaches its ability to find small cancers. Because of the frequent morphologic similarity between benign and malignant lesions, however, mammography is less useful as a diagnostic test where such differentiation is paramount. The safety and low morbidity of a breast biopsy makes it difficult to postpone the biopsy of a lesion when a significant doubt exists. The increasing use of needle biopsy techniques, with their reduced morbidity and expense, increases the pressure toward more aggressive analysis of lower probability lesions.

Mammography is not sufficiently accurate to rely on for diagnostic differentiation, although a superficial analysis might suggest the contrary. Mammography appears to be highly "specific" in that a negative mammogram in an asymptomatic population of women appears to be extremely accurate. Statistical specificity, however, can be deceiving. If an asymptomatic (no signs or symptoms of breast cancer) woman has a negative mammogram, there is a >99% likelihood that she does not have cancer. This is misleading, however, since, on a purely statistical basis, it is highly unlikely that she would have cancer in the first place. For example, since only one to five women among 1,000 develop breast cancer in a given year (depending on their age), reporting a set of 1,000 mammograms as negative without even reviewing them would produce an extremely high specificity. Assuming five women would develop cancer among the 1,000, the specificity obtained by interpreting them all as negative would be 99.95% (mammograms interpreted as negative minus those that actually had cancer, divided by all the women screened = [1,000 – 5]/1,000). In this hypothetical example, the test would have extremely high specificity, but of course, all of the cancers would have been missed. Statistical measures can be misleading if they are not evaluated in the context in which they were obtained.

Suspicion Prompting a Biopsy

The quest continues to find a noninvasive test that can reliably differentiate benign from malignant. Because biopsy of the breast is so safe and, if performed properly, so accurate, if a test is to be relied on to avoid a biopsy, it would need to approach near-perfect accuracy for differentiating a benign lesion from one that is malignant.

The accuracy of a test is determined by its false-positive and false-negative rates. The thresholds used for intervention (making a tissue diagnosis) are determined by the false-negative rate; false-positive rate; size, stage, and grade of cancers at detection; and cost of making the diagnosis (physical and economic). The ideal screening test would not miss any cancers (no false-negatives). The only way to maximize the detection of cancer, however, would be to biopsy anything found by mammography that was not completely normal. This method, however, would result in an unacceptably high false-positive rate. What is evolving is that the acceptability of a test is a function of how reasonable it is for cancer to be missed. Sickles' (1) analysis of lesions that had been classified as "probably benign" and followed at short intervals has been widely accepted. This review suggested that it is reasonable to follow lesions with a 2% or lower probability of cancer. A test that can provide a 98% likelihood that a lesion is not cancer would be reasonable provided that when the missed cancers are finally diagnosed, their stage is consistent with little or no likelihood of a detrimental effect from the delay in diagnosis (early stage). There may be some detriment to this approach. What is often overlooked, however, is that when two of the 17 cancers (12%) followed by Sickles were finally diagnosed, they were characterized as stage II.

Mammography and Benign Lesions

Mammography can be diagnostic for several types of benign lesions (see Chapter 14). For example, those that appear encapsulated, contain fat, and are radiolucent by mammography are virtually always benign. A densely calcified fibroadenoma is only associated with cancer coincidentally. Intramammary lymph nodes have a characteristic shape and location and need not cause concern unless they increase in size and lose their characteristic shape. Mammography, however, is unable to differentiate, for example, a cyst from a solid lesion, and although statistically most lesions are benign, mammography can rarely be relied on to make a conclusive diagnosis of a benign process.

Mammographic criteria are also frequently insufficient to make the diagnosis of malignancy. For example, most breast cancers are radiographically very dense for their volume, but, as with all signs, this is not a uniform characteristic, and some cancers are relatively low in x-ray attenuation. Round or oval lesions with smooth, sharply defined margins are usually benign, but some cancers appear smoothly marginated.

Despite a lack of specificity for particular lesions, criteria have evolved that should alert the radiologist to the possibility of malignancy. Most of these signs are not definitive because they overlap significantly and are often exhibited by benign processes. Although mammography frequently cannot be relied on to differentiate benign from malignant lesions, when certain morphologic criteria are present it is extremely accurate.

Age and Probability of Cancer

We reviewed the biopsy results for lesions detected at screening that were clinically occult and biopsied only on mammographic suspicion. The percentage of women biopsied at each year of age from 40 years to 79 years was 1 to 2% of the women screened at that age. The yield of cancer, however, increased steadily with increasing age beginning with a positive predictive value (cancers diagnosed divided by biopsies performed) of approximately 15% at 40 years to almost 50% by 79 years. This increase is not surprising given that the prior probability of cancer (cancers available to be detected) increases steadily with increasing age. These results suggest that there are similar findings at each age that might indicate malignancy, but the likelihood that they represent cancer increases with increasing age.

TABLE 15-1. *Mammographic findings that raise the possibility of malignancy*

Neodensity or new calcifications
New masses or architectural distortion
New clustered calcifications
Findings that suggest a high probability of malignancy
Spiculated lesions
Fine, linear, branching calcifications
Findings that should arouse suspicion
A lesion with ill-defined margins
A lesion with a microlobulated margin
Architectural distortion
A distorted parenchymal edge
Density increasing over time
Clustered microcalcifications
Changing calcifications
Findings that are probably benign
Solitary circumscribed mass
Solitary asymmetric duct
Round, regular clustered calcifications
Findings that support the possibility of malignancy
Asymmetric breast tissue
Asymmetric ducts
Asymmetric veins
Skin and trabecular thickening
Nipple retraction, deviation, or inversion
Enlarged axillary lymph nodes

FINDINGS THAT RAISE THE POSSIBILITY OF MALIGNANCY

Cancer usually appears on a mammogram as a mass, architectural distortion, or cluster of calcifications. The majority of these are benign, and the radiologist must separate these from lesions that have the possibility of being cancer. Table 15-1 is a list of findings that should raise varying degrees of concern.

Neodensity or New Calcifications

The breast is a fairly stable organ that does not change dramatically from year to year except as a repository of fat with weight fluctuations. Cysts may come and go, but these are found in a minority of women. Fibroadenomas likely originate when the breast is developing, and it is unusual for a fibroadenoma to suddenly appear. Since the breast tissues of women from age 30 years and older are likely to be undergoing involutional changes, it is very uncommon for normal fibroglandular breast tissue to suddenly appear. A small percentage of women who are on hormone replacement therapy (HRT) may develop new breast tissue densities, but even this is uncommon. For this reason, a new density on a mammogram should be viewed with suspicion (Fig. 15-1), and unless the new density can be directly linked to the use of hormones, diagnostic evaluation is usually indicated.

Calcifications, on the other hand, commonly develop in the breast. The vast majority of calcifications are due to benign

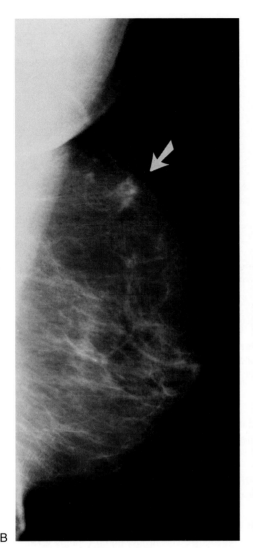
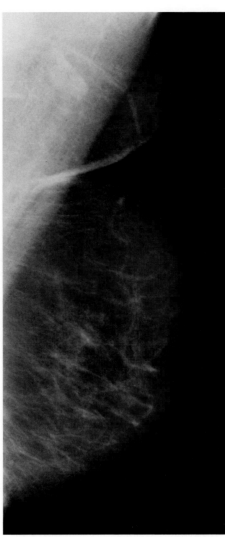

A,B

FIG. 15-1. Neodensity. (A) The density in the upper left breast (*arrow*) developed since the previous mammogram **(B)**. It proved malignant at biopsy.

processes. When new calcifications develop in clusters, however, they should be carefully evaluated to determine whether they should arouse concern.

FINDINGS THAT SUGGEST A HIGH PROBABILITY OF MALIGNANCY

Spiculated Lesion

A dense, irregular mass with a spiculated margin that is not related to prior surgery is the only combination of features that is virtually diagnostic of malignancy (Fig. 15-2). Strands of fibro-malignant tissues radiating out from an ill-defined mass producing a spiculated appearance can be considered virtually pathognomonic of breast cancer, because very few benign lesions produce a similar appearance. The spicules may extend more than several centimeters from the main tumor mass or appear as a fine "brush border" (Fig. 15-3).

They may be easily visible when the cancer is surrounded by fat or barely perceptible when the tumor grows in dense fibroglandular tissue (Fig. 15-4). The spiculations represent fibrosis that is probably related to the generalized desmoplastic response that many cancers elicit in the surrounding tissue. On occasion, only fibrosis is seen on microscopic examination of these extensions, but careful evaluation usually reveals tumor cells intimately bound and probably stimulating the fibrotic process.

A lesion with spiculated margins should be considered malignant even if it remains unchanged over time. Although rare, invasive cancers may remain unchanged on mammography for as long as 5 years (2). It is likely that cancer growth is a discontinuous process, fluctuating over time. Some lesions may exhibit slow or no growth and then suddenly accelerate their growth. A spiculated lesion that remains stable over time (up to 5 years) but cannot be explained by postsurgical change should still be considered suspicious and should be biopsied.

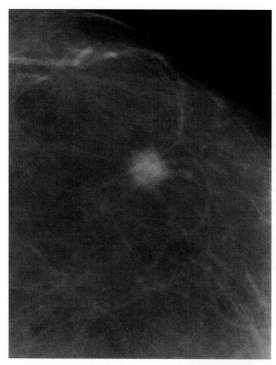

FIG. 15-2. A spiculated mass that is unrelated to surgery is almost certain to be malignant. The appearance of this 1-cm invasive breast cancer is virtually pathognomonic.

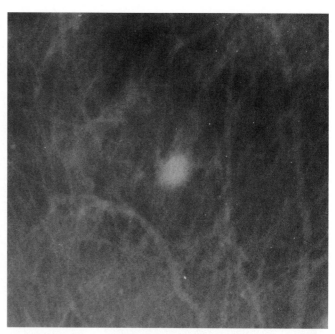

FIG. 15-3. The **very fine spiculations associated with cancer may produce a "brush border,"** which causes the ill-defined border of this invasive breast cancer.

Chapter 19) and a spiculated mass that is not clearly a scar should be biopsied.

Major Mimics of Breast Cancer

Postsurgical scarring, fat necrosis, radial scars (e.g., from elastosis or indurative mastopathy), and extremely unusual tumors such as extra-abdominal desmoid lesions and granular cell tumors may have spiculated margins that mimic those of malignancy, but with the exception of radial and postsurgical scars, these are extremely rare (see

Differentiation of a Postsurgical Scar from Breast Cancer

A postsurgical scar rarely raises significant concern. After a biopsy with benign results, the breast usually heals within 12 to 18 months, with little or no visible evidence of the previous surgery on the mammogram. On occasion, particularly if the mammogram is obtained within 1 year of the

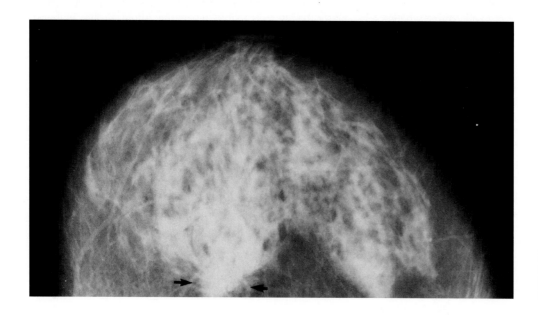

FIG. 15-4. Cancer (*arrows*) may be hidden in dense fibroglandular tissue as in this craniocaudal mammogram.

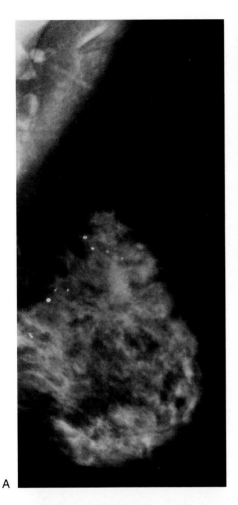

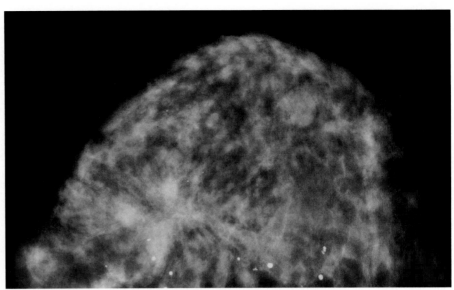

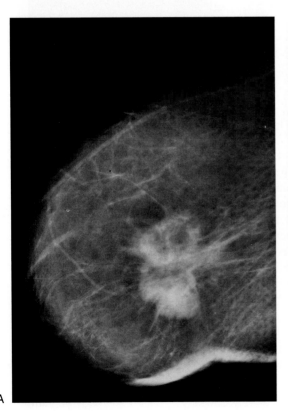

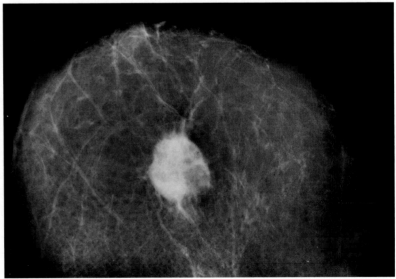

FIG. 15-5. Postsurgical change frequently almost disappears in one of the two projections. On the mediolateral oblique projection **(A)** there is little or no visible distortion, whereas on the craniocaudal projection **(B)** architectural distortion is prominent laterally from previous surgery for a benign lesion.

FIG. 15-6. Fat necrosis can be spiculated. This case is unusual. The patient had a biopsy with benign results 4 years earlier. This spiculated mass with skin retraction seen on this lateral mammogram **(A)** and the craniocaudal projection **(B)** proved to be fat necrosis. Note that the mass contains fat. Had it been completely lucent with a clear capsule, biopsy would not have been indicated.

surgery, the architecture may be distorted and spiculation may be present. Postsurgical change will almost always resolve or greatly diminish over the subsequent 6 to 12 months when the surgery has occurred for a benign process.

If the postsurgical nature of the distortion is not immediately clear, several observations can increase the confidence in the diagnosis. Postsurgical change frequently looks very different between the lateral and craniocaudal projections (Fig. 15-5). Cancer almost always looks worrisome regardless of the projection and, as a three-dimensional mass, similar in appearance on both projections, although there are occasional exceptions.

On rare occasions, fat necrosis can look like a malignancy (Fig. 15-6). If there is a clear, encapsulated, lucent structure at the center of the spiculation, benign fat necrosis is the reliable diagnosis.

Markers can be placed on the cutaneous scar to relate the incision to the underlying distortion in postsurgical change, but this may be misleading because the tissue that is removed at biopsy and the subsequent postsurgical change may be deeper in the breast and at a distance from the skin incision. Review of the preoperative mammograms, if available, provides a better comparison of the location of the distorted architecture with the location of the benign lesion as it appeared before its excision.

A review of the pathology of the removed tissues can increase the confidence that the spiculated change is merely postsurgical. It is highly improbable that a sizable cancer would develop over a 1-year period in the exact same area as a benign biopsy with no clue to its presence in the excised tissue. If there is any remaining question, the pathology should be reviewed to be certain there is no suggestion that the tissue removed might have been at the edge of a cancer that was missed at surgery. We have seen three cases in which the biopsy revealed atypical hyperplasia, and a progressive increase in calcifications in the region of the biopsy led to a re-excision that revealed intraductal cancer. This is unusual and probably related to the uncertainty that may exist in differentiating atypical hyperplasia from ductal carcinoma in situ (DCIS), but a high index of suspicion is reasonable when the biopsy reveals atypia and it is not clear that the lesion has been completely excised.

It is also important to remember that surgery may miss a visible or palpable cancer. If the mammogram preceding the biopsy revealed a very suspicious lesion, and the biopsy result was benign, it is possible that the cancer was missed at the clinically guided biopsy (3). An early (2 to 3 weeks after operation) follow-up mammogram can determine whether the lesion seen by mammography was excised.

Radial Scars

The radial scar is a fairly common benign lesion characterized by often dramatic spiculation that is very similar to that produced by cancer. Because of its name it is still confused by some with postsurgical change. They are, in fact, different lesions. The radial scar is idiopathic and unrelated

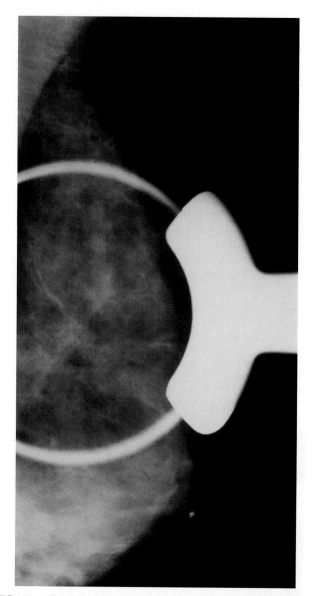

FIG. 15-7. Radial scars can appear as spiculated architectural distortion. This lesion, with long spicules seen on the spot compression lateral projection, proved to be a benign radial scar.

to known trauma. It represents a scarring process, but its etiology remains unknown. This lesion is commonly found by the pathologist reviewing breast tissue at the microscopic level. As an increasing number of women are screened, more of the larger radial scars are being found by mammography. Their appearance is indistinguishable from malignancy. They frequently have long spicules that are conspicuous because they trap fat, yet they often lack a significant central mass (Fig. 15-7). Although the diagnosis can be suggested by these characteristics, their mammographic morphology is not sufficiently distinctive to permit them to be reliably differentiated from cancer, and they should be biopsied to make a secure diagnosis. Needle biopsy has been found to be an unreliable method of diagnosing these lesions, and excisional biopsy is usually needed to safely make the diagnosis.

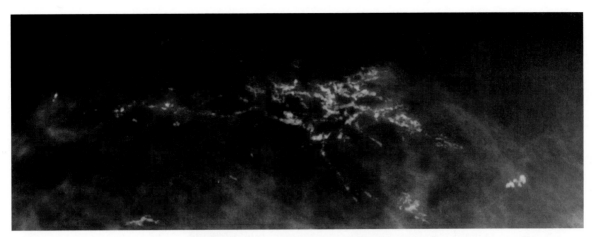

FIG. 15-8. Irregular, linear calcifications in a segmental distribution virtually guarantee malignancy. These proved to be in **high-grade ductal carcinoma in situ with comedonecrosis.**

Calcifications Associated with a High Probability of Malignancy

A wide variety of calcifications are demonstrated by mammography (see Chapter 13). Although the vast majority of calcifications are associated with benign processes, there are some patterns that are almost always due to cancer. The pattern usually associated with comedonecrosis (central necrosis of cancer filling a duct) in intraductal cancer is virtually diagnostic. Fine, linear, irregular branching calcifications are practically always due to malignancy (Fig. 15-8).

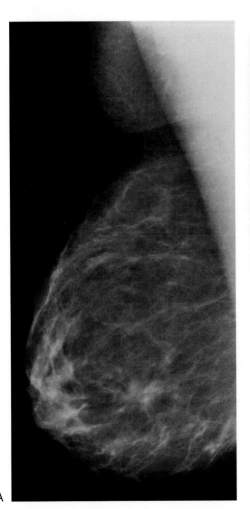

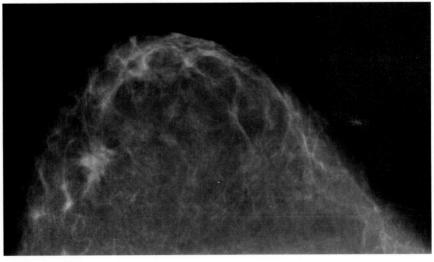

FIG. 15-9. Spiculated masses are virtually always breast cancer. This was an invasive ductal carcinoma seen in the lower left breast on the mediolateral oblique projection **(A)** and medially on the craniocaudal projection **(B).**

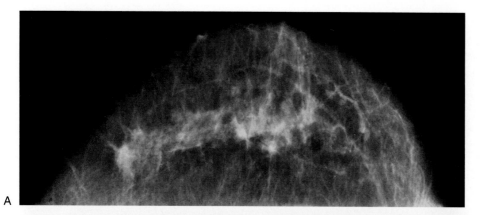

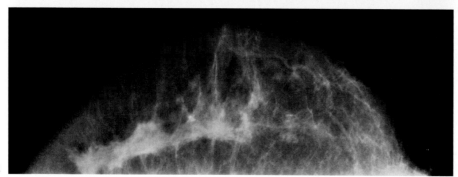

FIG. 15-10. **Asymmetric tissue density increasing over time** may indicate the insidious development of a breast cancer. Asymmetric tissue density on this craniocaudal projection **(A)** increased over 15 months **(B)** and invasive lobular carcinoma was diagnosed at biopsy. Note that the architecture remained fairly stable despite the growth of the cancer.

FINDINGS THAT SHOULD AROUSE SUSPICION

Other findings on mammography have a significant probability of being due to cancer, although many will prove to be benign. Spiculation of a mass or fine, linear, branching calcifications are the only signs that virtually always indicate cancer. All other signs can be found in association with benign lesions as well and thus are considered suspicious. Nevertheless, suspicious findings carry a significant enough risk to warrant intervention.

Lesions with Ill-Defined Margins

Ill definition of the margins of a lesion is a common, though nonspecific, characteristic that suggests a malignant process. Cancer should be considered when a three-dimensionally real volume of tissue with increased density is found whose borders are poorly demarcated from the surrounding tissue (Fig. 15-9). Many cancers do not elicit the desmoplasia that produces spiculations, but even in these cases, tumor infiltration generally is reflected in the lack of a mammographically well-defined border of the tumor as it invades the surrounding tissue.

A lesion with ill-defined margins may rarely present as a diffuse process over a large area and should be distinguished from asymmetric tissue density that is merely the accentuation of normal breast tissue. When any tumor (benign or malignant) is surrounded by dense normal fibroglandular tissue, the distinction between an invasive margin and one that is merely obscured by normal tissue becomes difficult.

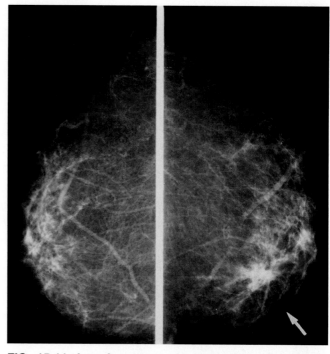

FIG. 15-11. **Invasive cancer is frequently more dense than an equal volume of fibroglandular tissue.** The invasive cancer in the right breast (*arrow*), as seen on this craniocaudal projection, is more dense than the surrounding fibroglandular breast tissue.

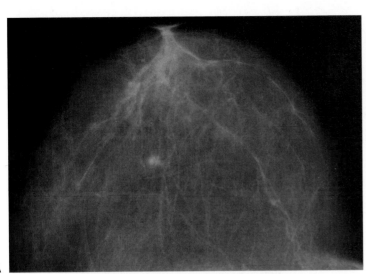

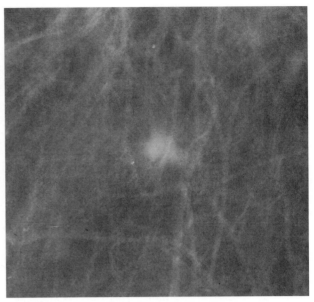

A

B

FIG. 15-12. Breast cancer is usually dense for its size. This invasive ductal cancer on the cranio-caudal projection **(A)** and photographically enlarged **(B)** is extremely small but quite dense for its size and is easily seen when surrounded by fat.

If normal breast architecture is preserved and there are no significant, associated calcifications or architectural distortion, an area of asymmetry is consistent with asymmetric breast tissue. If, however, the asymmetry is concordant with a palpable asymmetry, the area should be viewed with suspicion. If a focal area is palpable and contains no fluid on aspiration or is solid by sonography (especially with posterior acoustic shadowing), biopsy should be considered. Increasing x-ray attenuation of an area of asymmetry over time should also raise concern (Fig. 15-10).

Cancer is generally not intermingled with fat, and the attenuation of the tumor increases toward its center. When this pattern is associated with distortion of the breast architecture, the probability of malignancy is increased (Fig. 15-11). Cancer generally has higher x-ray attenuation than the same volume of fibroglandular tissue (Fig. 15-12), which is a clue to the diagnosis. However, it is not unusual for a malignant lesion to be subtle and not cause increased attenuation (Fig. 15-13). Some cancers, particularly the colloid subtypes, have even lower attenuation than an equal volume of fibroglandular tissue.

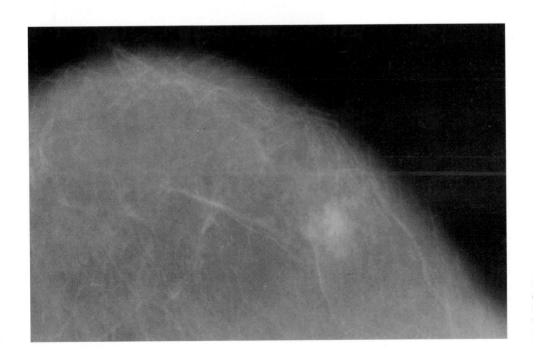

FIG. 15-13. Cancer is not always highly attenuating. This invasive cancer is not very dense for its size, as seen on this craniocaudal projection.

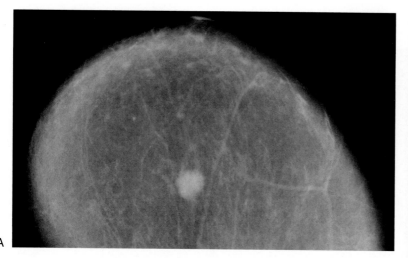

FIG. 15-14. A lesion with microlobulated margins has a high probability of malignancy. This is an example of a microlobulated mass on the craniocaudal projection **(A)** and photographically enlarged **(B)** that proved to be an invasive breast cancer.

Lesions with a Microlobulated Margin

Many well-circumscribed lesions within the breast have a degree of lobulation. Fibroadenomas, for example, are frequently not perfectly round and smooth but have undulating, lobulated margins. The more lobulated the lesion, however, the more likely it is to be malignant (Fig. 15-14). When the lobulations are multiple and measure only several millimeters or smaller, the degree of suspicion should increase. In the past, some have used the term *knobby* to describe these very small lobulations, but the American College of Radiology Breast Imaging Reporting and Data System suggests the term *microlobulation*. It is a strong indication of cancer but, once again, not pathognomonic, because benign masses can have similar margins.

Architectural Distortion

Breast cancer does not always produce a mammographically visible mass, but it frequently disrupts the normal tissues in which it develops. This distortion of the architecture may be the only visible evidence of the malignant process. This is an important but often very subtle manifestation of breast cancer. In general, the flow of structures within the breast is uniform and directed toward the nipple along duct lines. On occasion, a malignant process will produce a cicatrization of tissue pulling in the surrounding elements toward a point that is eccentric from the nipple (Fig. 15-15).

Although architectural distortion should be regarded with a high degree of suspicion and biopsy is indicated, there are also benign causes of architectural distortion. Postsurgical scarring (Fig. 15-16) and fat necrosis are the most common

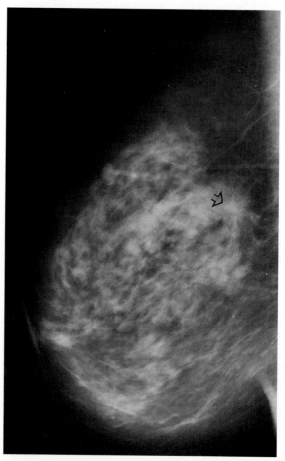

FIG. 15-15. Distortion of the tissue, particularly at the parenchymal-fat interface, can indicate cancer. This invasive ductal cancer (*arrow*) was revealed by the cicatrization of the surrounding tissue pulling the structures toward the cancer.

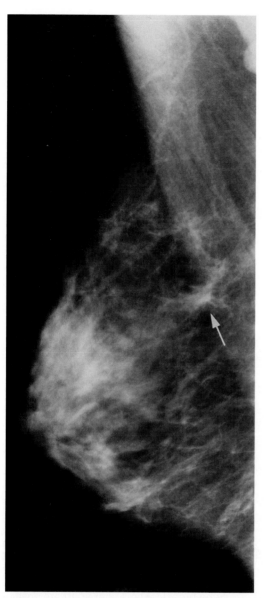

FIG. 15-16. In the **early months after surgery, architectural distortion is fairly common.** Architectural distortion (*arrow*) 1 month after the removal of a benign lesion is postsurgical and eventually disappears in most women.

nonmalignant causes, although it is surprisingly uncommon for the breast to form a permanent, radiographically noticeable, scar (in spite of palpable scarring). Unless architectural distortion clearly coincides with a region of previous surgery it should be investigated.

As noted above (see Radial Scars), similar distortion of the surrounding tissue can be seen with a radial scar (Fig. 15-17). Radial scars often present as subtle radiating lines interspersed with trapped fat and converging on a sometimes lucent zone at the center of the area. This characteristic may suggest the diagnosis, but as noted previously, the lesion still should be biopsied, because a radial scar and cancer cannot be reliably differentiated by mammography. Its gross appearance can occasionally even fool the pathologist.

Distorted Parenchymal Edge

Architectural distortion is frequently most evident at the edge of the parenchymal cone at the subcutaneous fat interface. In the normal breast the interface is scalloped by Cooper's ligaments attaching, by the retinacula cutis, to the skin. It is not unusual for cancer, which frequently develops

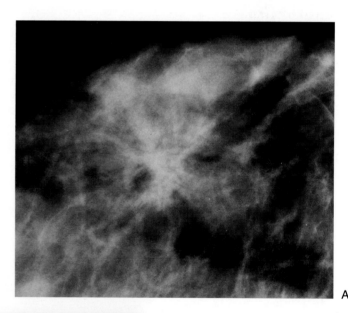

A

FIG. 15-17. **Radial scars are indistinguishable from cancer by mammography** and should be biopsied to establish an accurate diagnosis. This very suspicious spiculated mass **(A)** proved to be a benign radial scar. It is radiographically indistinguishable from this invasive ductal carcinoma **(B),** which even appears to be trapping fat, an illusion caused by overlapping breast structures.

B

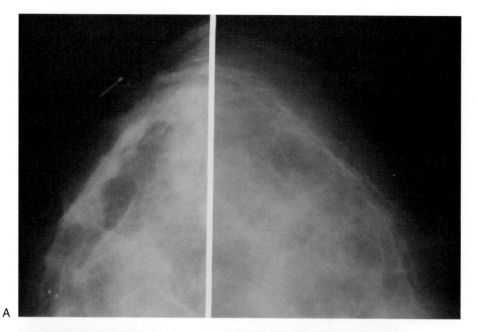

A

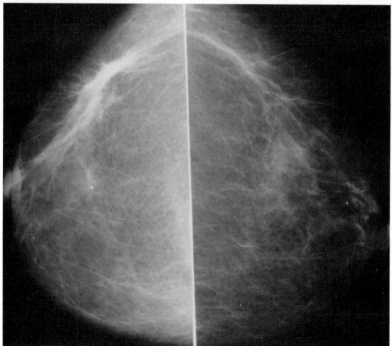

B

FIG. 15-18. The edge of the parenchyma can be distorted by cancer. In this patient **(A)**, the tissue at the edge of the parenchyma increased in density over time. Craniocaudal views of the same breast taken 1 year apart are positioned as mirror images demonstrating the increased density that has occurred in the breast tissue beneath the subcutaneous fat. This was due to invasive breast cancer. In the second patient **(B)**, there is asymmetry of the architecture in this region caused by breast cancer.

at the edge of the breast (4), to distort this relationship and cause a flattening or retraction of the parenchyma in this region. This form of architectural distortion may manifest itself as an actual pulling in or thickening or merely as a flattening or straightening of the edge (Fig. 15-18).

The opposite distortion of the parenchymal edge may also be significant. A bulge or convexity of the tissue into the subcutaneous fat, seen along the edge of the parenchyma, may also indicate a possible cancer (Fig. 15-19). Such a convex bulge, however, is more likely due to a cyst or fibroadenoma. Nevertheless, it still usually requires investigation if present in two projections.

Density Increasing Over Time

Martin and associates (5), in their review of false-negative mammograms, pointed out that the breast is an "involuting organ." Breast development likely occurs over several years, beginning in adolescence as the ducts grow and branch, ultimately forming the terminal duct lobular units and the glandular structures of the breast. A full-term pregnancy completes the development. The process reverses itself at different ages in different women. This occurs in some women early in life whereas it occurs later in other women. It is likely that for many women in their 30s, the glandular

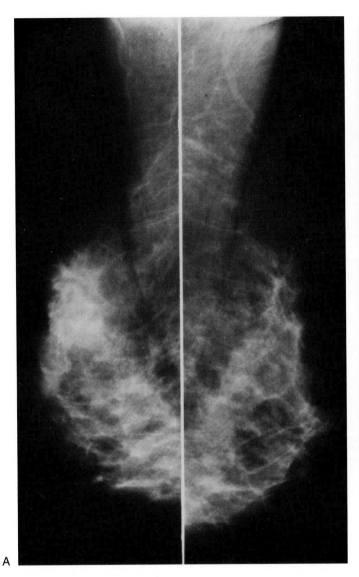

A

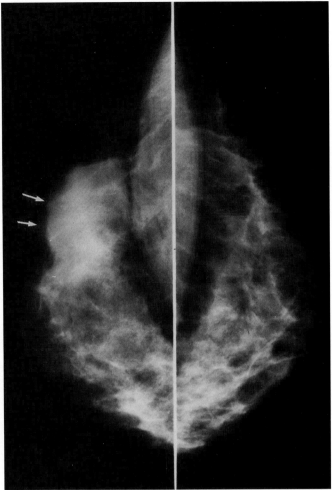

B

FIG. 15-19. Cancer can cause a bulge at the edge of the parenchyma. The invasive cancer in the left breast appears as asymmetric density on the mediolateral oblique projection **(A)**. Note on the craniocaudal projection **(B)** there is a large bulge to the contour of the parenchyma into the subcutaneous fat (*arrows*).

and fibrous structures of the breast begin to be resorbed by the process of involution. Because involution generally results in a higher proportion of fat, the breast—if it changes at all—becomes more radiolucent over time. The relative densities of the breast tissues can appear to increase over time if the patient loses a significant amount of weight. HRT can, in a small number of women, result in focal or diffuse increases in density. Focal areas in which density increases over time, however, should be viewed with suspicion and warrant careful evaluation (Fig. 15-20). If the patient is using HRT, some suggest stopping the therapy for 3 months and monitoring the density at that time. Many women prefer to continue the therapy, and in that situation, a biopsy of a focally increasing density may be warranted.

To appreciate the phenomenon of an increasing density, it is important to compare the current study with studies performed 2 or more years earlier, if they are available,

because an increasing density may not be apparent over a shorter follow-up period.

Focal Asymmetric Density

The term *asymmetric density* is a preliminary assessment. There are many asymmetric densities by mammography since the breasts are not perfectly symmetric and may not be symmetrically positioned. Most asymmetric densities prove to be benign islands of breast tissue.

A significant focal asymmetric density is distinguished from normal asymmetric dense breast tissue, which is almost always benign. When it proves to be due to cancer, asymmetric density is part of the spectrum of lesions with ill-defined margins. An asymmetric density may ultimately prove to be a mass, which is defined as a three-dimensional volume in which the density is greatest at the center and

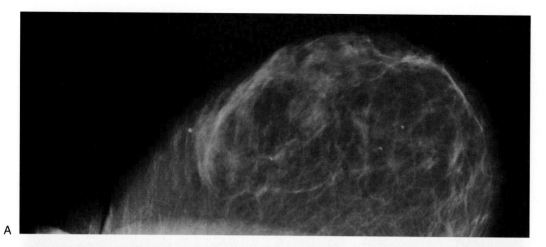

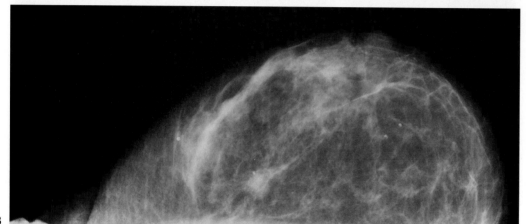

FIG. 15-20. A focal area of increased density should raise concern. The mammogram in 1988 is normal on the craniocaudal projection **(A)** in this 72-year-old woman. A new density is apparent in the lateral portion of the breast on the craniocaudal projection in 1989 **(B)**. This demonstrates the need for annual screening, even in older women.

fades toward the periphery. At times the density may be evident only because the underlying architecture is obscured and the density appears to be "trying to form a mass" (Fig. 15-21A).

A three-dimensional focal asymmetry should draw the observer's attention (Fig. 15-21B, C). Magnification views may be used to evaluate the finding and further characterize it to determine whether it merely represents an island of breast tissue or something more significant (Fig. 15-21 D–F). An asymmetric density that has the characteristics of a mass should be viewed with suspicion, and if not a cyst, biopsy should be considered.

Clustered Microcalcifications

Mammography is the only technique capable of detecting the clustered microcalcifications that, when found in isolation, frequently herald the presence of an early-stage breast cancer. The definition of clustered microcalcifications varies. The data suggest that five or more calcifications, each ≤0.5 mm in diameter isolated in a small volume of the breast, and projected within a 1-cc volume on the mammogram, warrant careful assessment.

Significance of the Number of Calcifications

There has been inordinate controversy over the significance of the number of calcifications. The number defines a cluster, but the location, morphology, and distribution of the calcifications define their significance. In trying to arrive at a reasonable threshold, the term *clustered calcifications* was developed. Loosely defined, these are calcifications that are close together in an isolated group. The question arises as to when a group of calcifications is a significant cluster.

Calcifications without an associated mass should be considered separately from calcifications within a tumor mass. It is very common to see one or more calcifications in a tumor mass, and up to 80% of breast cancers are found to contain calcium deposits on pathologic examination. It is unusual, however, for fewer than five isolated calcifications without a tumor mass to be due to cancer.

Five microcalcifications as a threshold for biopsy is not absolute. Clearly, calcium begins to be deposited at some point in time, and more than likely, a single deposit may form within a cancer. The reality, however, is that virtually all groups of calcifications containing fewer than five particles are benign. In a series by Egan et al. (11), 84% of can-

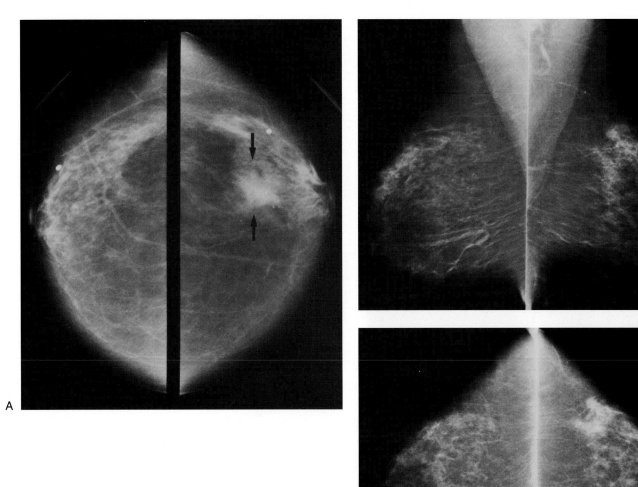

FIG. 15-21. A focal asymmetric density may need to be evaluated to determine whether it might be a mass. **(A)** In this patient, the asymmetry (*arrows*) is dense at the center and fading toward the periphery. It was three-dimensionally real, making it consistent with a mass. Biopsy revealed an invasive breast cancer. In this second patient, a focal asymmetry in the upper outer right breast is seen on the mediolateral oblique (MLO) **(B)** and craniocaudal (CC) **(C)** projections. *Continued.*

cers found only due to their associated calcifications contained >10 calcifications; they found no cancer when fewer than five calcifications were present. There are no data that indicate that cancers have been detected only by the presence of one, two, three, or four calcifications, and only anecdotal cases exist. These are likely serendipitous occurrences. Certainly the number of cases in which this happens is too small to justify routine biopsy. Unless groups of one to four calcifications are found in conjunction with other signs of malignancy or the calcifications are very suspicious morphologically (extremely fine and angular or branching), the threshold of five is appropriate.

Because the calcifications associated with breast cancer are generally very small (150- to 200-μm calcifications can be seen by contact mammography), they have been called microcalcifications even though they can be seen by the unaided eye. The possibility of malignancy increases as the size of the individual calcifications decreases (although adenosis may produce extremely small particles) and their total number per unit volume increases (3,6). The risk of malignancy increases when they are heterogeneous in size and shape. Certain patterns and types of calcifications have a strong association with breast cancer. It is their clustering at the tumor site that is significant. Most microcalcifications

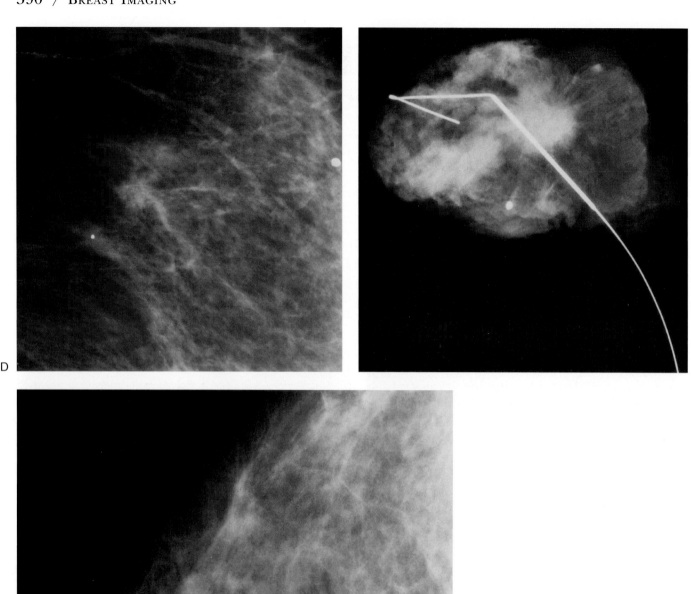

FIG. 15-21. *Continued.* Magnification of the MLO **(D)** and CC **(E)** projections suggests a spiculated lesion, and an invasive breast cancer was excised as seen on specimen radiography **(F)**.

represent benign conditions, but approximately 20% to 30% of groups that are biopsied when no palpable mass is present prove to be malignant.

Calcium deposits are extremely common in the breast. They range from several centimeters to particles smaller than 100 µm that are visible only under the microscope. The pathologist commonly sees calcifications that are not apparent by mammography. Most of the radiopaque deposits that are called calcifications contain calcium in the form of cal-

cium hydroxyapatite and tricalcium phosphate, but work done by Galkins and associates (7) has suggested that microcalcifications may also contain an array of heavy metals and may not be exclusively composed of calcium derivatives. This may be significant one day if in vivo spectral analysis can be achieved. In the near future, these heavy metals may make it possible to produce dual-energy subtraction studies using digital mammography to more easily reveal clustered calcifications.

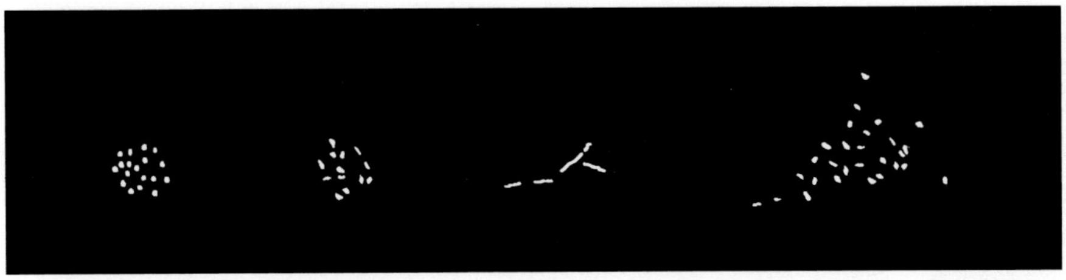

FIG. 15-22. Schematic of types of **calcifications associated with cancer.**

The cause of calcium deposition in breast cancer is still not well understood. In very large tumors the calcifications may be merely forming in necrotic tissue. However, large tumors are becoming less common. The majority of cancer-associated calcifications develop in intraductal malignancy. Many tumor-related calcifications are formed in necrotic cellular debris (6,8). This is most apparent when there is comedonecrosis in DCIS. The cells are usually poorly differentiated with high nuclear grade and a great deal of central necrosis. Other calcifications may be secondary to cellular secretions of crystalline material (9). The latter are likely the etiology of calcifications found in the cribriform spaces of the better differentiated types of DCIS. Even when a cancer is invasive, associated calcifications are usually found in the intraductal portion of the lesion.

In general, cancer-related calcifications are found in the lesion itself. On occasion the calcifications will be in benign adjacent tissue, and a cancer will be found by apparent serendipity. Since it is rare to biopsy the breast and serendipitously find cancer, the moderate frequency of this association suggests that the processes may be related and not serendipitous. Lobular carcinoma in situ (LCIS) is another example (although LCIS should not be classified as cancer). It is almost always found "coincidentally" in a biopsy, frequently for a a cluster of calcifications. The frequency of this association (10) makes it likely that the calcifications are indirectly related.

Size, Shape, and Distribution of Calcifications

Certain shapes and patterns of distribution of calcium particles are strongly associated with breast cancer (Fig. 15-22). The particles are usually ≤0.5 mm in diameter. Egan and coworkers (11) evaluated 468 lesions composed of calcifications without an associated mass. Among these, 353 were benign and 115 were malignant. They found no cancers when *all* the calcifications were >2 mm.

A second important feature of the calcifications associated with cancer is their usual clustering at the tumor site. The data indicate that the majority of cancers develop from a single cell and represent a clone of cancer cells. Cancers that have not spread extensively up and down a duct network almost always have an epicenter, and the calcifications develop about this point. Because the calcifications associated with breast cancer almost always form in the intraduc-

tal portion of the tumor, some have suggested that there is a polarity to their distribution that is somewhat triangular and aimed in the general direction of the nipple (12).

Because breast cancer is almost always a problem involving a single duct segment, calcifications that are diffusely scattered throughout the breast are almost always benign deposits. Occasionally a duct segment can be very extensive, and a comedocarcinoma involving many duct branches may produce extensive deposits. Diffusely arrayed DCIS with comedonecrosis, however, produces fairly characteristic ductal deposits that are spread in many branches of the ducts of a lobe with a characteristic, segmental distribution (Fig. 15-23). Unlike benign calcifications, they tend to be extremely heterogeneous in shape and very small. A benign process is almost assured when diffusely scattered calcifications are bilateral.

Predicting Histology

Many believe that DCIS can be subclassified and that this classification can be used to predict the future potential of these lesions. Based on the observations of Lagios et al. (13) and reaffirmed by Holland et al. (14), DCIS can be divided into lesions that have poorly differentiated features, those with intermediate or moderate differentiation, and others that can be classified as well differentiated. These classifications are based on cellular features as well as patterns of growth. These features include the nuclear grade, the architectural relationship of the cells, and the presence or absence of necrosis. The nuclear morphology in the cells is a primary prognostic indicator. Some of the features that should be evaluated are included in the system proposed by Holland et al. and listed below.

Cytologic Differentiation

1. *Well-differentiated.* Cells that are uniform in size and shape (monomorphic) with evenly distributed chromatin and absent or inconspicuous nucleoli and rare mitoses evident.

2. *Intermediately differentiated.* Some pleomorphism. The chromatin may be slightly clumped and there are nucleoli and occasional mitoses.

3. *Poorly differentiated.* Pleomorphic cells with pleomorphic nuclei, clumped chromatin, prominent nucleoli, and frequent mitoses.

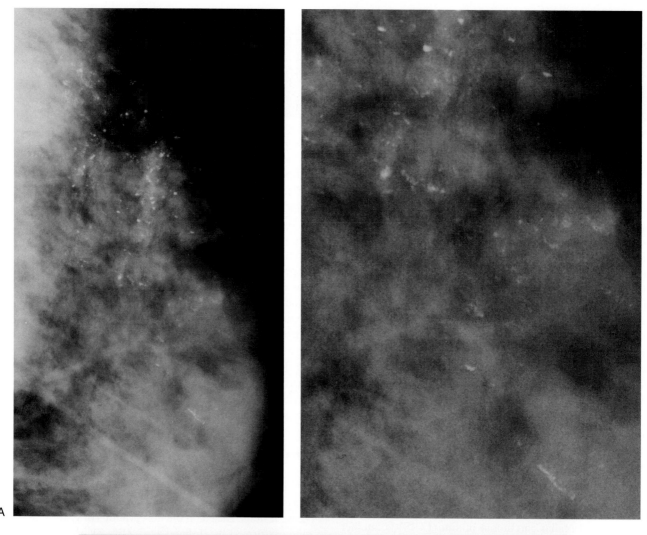

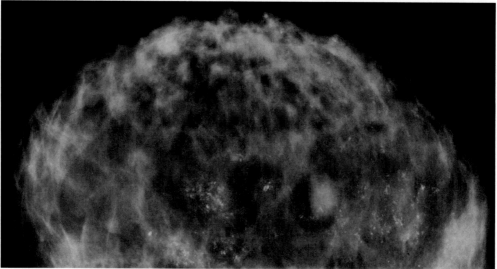

FIG. 15-23. Diffusely scattered calcifications (most likely due to a benign process) must be distinguished from segmentally distributed calcifications (more likely due to malignancy). These calcifications may initially appear to be diffusely scattered on this mediolateral oblique projection **(A)**, but more careful analysis shows that they are not found throughout the breast but rather segmentally distributed. Their morphology is pleomorphic, as seen on this photographic enlargement **(B)**, consistent with the diffuse ductal carcinoma in situ (DCIS) that was found at biopsy. **(C)** In this patient, the numerous calcifications are also not diffusely scattered but are collected in two zones and not randomly distributed. Their morphology also causes concern, and DCIS was found at biopsy.

Necrosis

Necrosis is usually present in poorly differentiated DCIS, occasionally in intermediately differentiated DCIS, and usually absent in well-differentiated DCIS. Architectural features of DCIS are as follows:

1. The polarization of the cells (orienting their long access toward a lumen) is a primary feature.

2. Highly polarized cells forming cribriform spaces or micropapillary protrusions into the lumen of the duct are associated with well-differentiated DCIS.

3. Highly polarized cells may be present without an associated lumen and can form a solid pattern of growth. This occurs occasionally with moderately differentiated DCIS.

4. Less polarization (the cells are haphazardly oriented) is associated with poorly differentiated DCIS. This may form a solid pattern with or without necrosis, or pseudomicropapillary or cribriform patterns.

Poorly differentiated DCIS is more likely to recur if incompletely treated and become invasive early (within several years of diagnosis), whereas better differentiated DCIS appears to be less likely to recur early. Protocols are being used to determine if well-differentiated DCIS can be treated less intensively. It appears to take well-differentiated DCIS longer to recur. However, Page et al. (15) reviewed 28 patients who had been biopsied in the past and incorrectly diagnosed as having a benign finding. They were, retrospectively, diagnosed as having low-grade cribriform DCIS. Among these women there were nine (36%) recurrences over a 25-year period. Seven of the women (25%) developed invasive cancers within 10 years in the same quadrant of the same breast. Two more women developed recurrences in the subsequent years. There were five deaths (18%) among this group. It must be remembered that even though these were not recognized as DCIS at the time of biopsy, these were lesions that had been excised. Many of them may have been completely excised. The fact that such a high proportion still recurred and a large percentage recurred as invasive breast cancer is strong evidence that DCIS of all grades represents a significant lesion.

As a consequence of their apparently differing natural history, there has been great interest in trying to differentiate these lesions by their mammographic appearance. This problem is compounded by the fact that many of these lesions have mixed histologies and defy simple classification. Nevertheless, when calcifications are predominantly fine, linear, and branching, they almost always represent poorly differentiated DCIS with comedonecrosis producing the calcifications. A small cluster of small heterogeneous calcifications that are not linear in their distribution may indicate well-differentiated cribriform DCIS. The reliability of predicting the histopathology of DCIS has not been established in prospective analysis, and, in our experience, it is generally unreliable with respect to low- and moderate-grade lesions.

Histologic review remains the only accurate method of establishing the histologic characteristics of DCIS.

SUSPICIOUS CALCIFICATIONS

In a population that is being screened repetitively, cancers will be found at an early size and stage. The calcifications in malignant lesions will tend to be confined to a small (1 to 2 cc) volume of tissue in relative isolation. The probability of cancer increases with the number and pleomorphism of the calcifications in the cluster.

Calcifications and the Extent of a Cancer

It should be understood that calcifications due to cancer may merely represent a small portion of the overall lesion. In fact, tumor may extend through the breast, and the only indication may be a small group of calcifications in one portion. The calcifications of the poorly differentiated comedocarcinomas come the closest to defining the extent of the lesion, but even these cancers do not always calcify, and removing only the tissue containing the calcifications does not guarantee that the entire lesion has been excised. There are no tests that can replace direct histologic analysis to define the full extent of a cancer. It is for this reason that the whole breast must be treated to reduce the likelihood that occult, residual disease will lead to recurrence.

Morphologic Characteristics of Calcifications Associated with Malignancy

The number of calcifications defines the cluster, but the shapes (morphology) and distribution of the deposits determine their importance. Despite clustering—or the equally suspicious linear or segmental distributions—if the calcifications have benign morphology, no further evaluation is needed. Malignant calcifications are irregular and heterogeneous. They have been variously described as comma-shaped, pointed, fine, linear, and branching (Fig. 15-24).

Occasionally it may be difficult to distinguish between the rod shapes of benign secretory calcifications and the fine, linear, branching calcifications of intraductal carcinoma. This difficulty is understandable because both form in debris within the ducts. Benign secretory calcifications form continuous, thick rods that usually do not branch (Fig. 15-25) and are frequently bilateral. Intraductal carcinoma generally produces irregular, fine, linear calcifications that are interrupted in a "dot-and-dash" pattern and may branch (Fig. 15-26). Careful evaluation of calcifications associated with malignancy will often show that what appear to be individual particles are made up of even smaller particles. The finer a linear calcification is, and the more irregular, angulated, and pointed individual calcifications are, the more significant they become. Furthermore, although large calcifications are

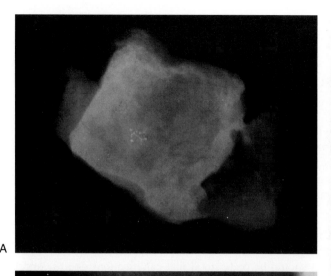

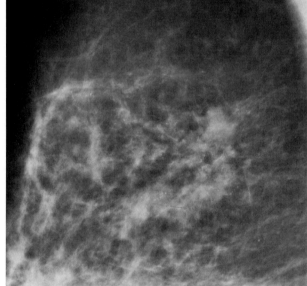

FIG. 15-24. **Fine, linear, branching calcifications** are almost always due to intraductal cancer. This tiny collection, seen on specimen radiography **(A)**, was due to a small focus of comedocarcinoma. **(B)** In this patient, these pleomorphic calcifications arrayed in a linear distribution were also caused by a comedo type of ductal carcinoma in situ (DCIS). **(C)** In this patient, the barely visible heterogeneous calcifications are all the result of DCIS of the comedo type.

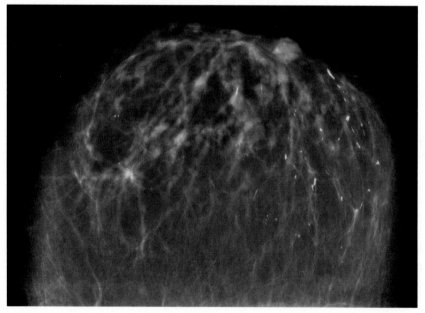

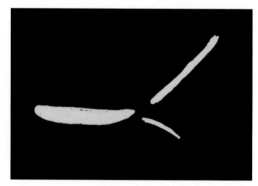

FIG. 15-25. **Segmentally distributed ductal calcifications** may be due to benign or malignant processes. **(A)** In this patient, the calcifications are benign secretory deposits. They follow a segmental distribution but are composed of solid or lucent centered rods, as represented schematically **(B)**. These are benign characteristics.

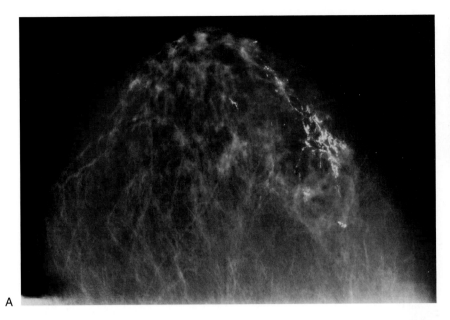

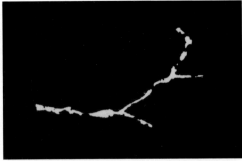

FIG. 15-26. Segmentally distributed ductal calcifications may be due to benign or malignant processes. In this patient (A), they are due to ductal carcinoma in situ. The cancer calcifications are far more abundant and are made up of multiple very small particles, as represented schematically (B). These are unlike the secretory calcifications that form solid rods.

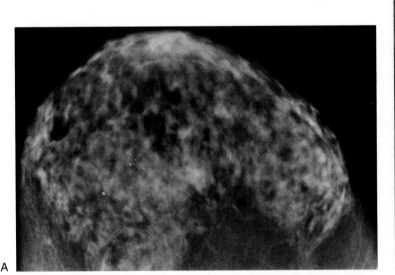

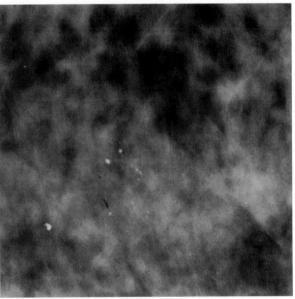

FIG. 15-27. A lesion should be judged by its most suspicious calcifications. (A) The calcifications that are easily seen in the medial right breast on this craniocaudal projection are large, round, and benign. (B) On closer inspection, there are smaller, pleomorphic calcifications adjacent to them. The latter were in ductal carcinoma in situ.

benign, if they are accompanied by small, irregularly shaped calcifications, the lesion should be biopsied (Fig. 15-27). A lesion should be judged by the smallest calcifications, not the largest.

Although a careful search for the morphologic criteria just discussed is important, the microcalcifications associated with malignancy are varied. Sickles (16) showed that, in fact, the classic, fine, linear, and branching calcifications are not the norm and are present in only 22% of the calcifications that prove to be malignant. Most microcalcifications actually represent benign processes. However, when calcifications are small, heterogeneous in size and morphology, and clustered, it cannot be determined by imaging whether they are associated with a benign (Fig. 15-28A) or a malignant process (Fig. 15-28B). Approximately 20% to 30% of grouped microcalcifications that are indeterminate by morphology and distribution that are biopsied when no palpable mass is present, prove to represent malignant lesions.

If, on the other hand, the calcifications have central lucent zones, they are always benign (Fig. 15-29). Benign skin deposits frequently have such characteristic central lucency. On rare occasions they can be misinterpreted as intramam-

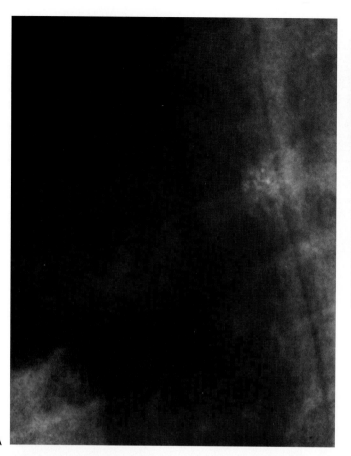

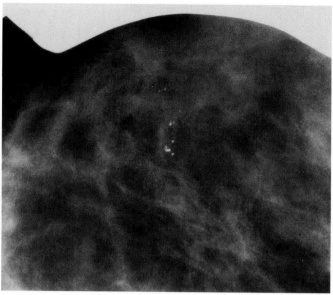

A

B

FIG. 15-28. Calcifications due to benign processes may overlap morphologically with malignant calcifications. (A) These calcifications are clustered and pleomorphic but were due to sclerosing adenosis. These rather round, benign-appearing calcifications **(B)** were due to ductal carcinoma in situ.

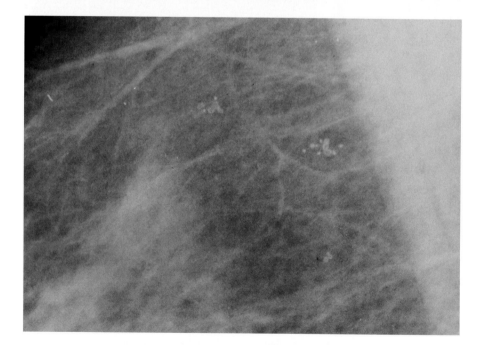

FIG. 15-29. Round calcifications with lucent centers are always due to benign processes. These are benign skin calcifications.

mary particles, but their spherical shape and peripheral location can suggest their etiology, and their location can then be verified with tangential views (17). Sickles (1) has shown that tightly clustered calcifications that are perfectly round or ovoid and smooth-surfaced on magnification views repre-

sent benign processes and do not require biopsy. Most now agree that following women with such calcifications without biopsy is reasonable since fewer than 1% will ultimately prove to be associated with cancer. Egan (11) had less success with these criteria, and only long-term follow-up of

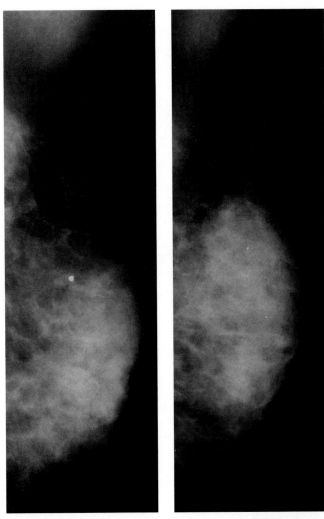

A,B

FIG. 15-30. Benign calcifications can be resorbed. The large, benign calcification in the right breast **(A)** had nearly disappeared on the mammogram 1 year later **(B)**.

these patients will determine the accuracy of this assessment. In our assessment, smooth, round calcifications are almost always benign.

Changing Calcifications

As with masses, new microcalcifications not present on previous mammograms are of particular concern. Calcifications or groups that increase in number and do not have benign morphologic characteristics usually should be biopsied. Unlike cancer masses, which may be stable over many years, it is rare for microcalcifications associated with malignancy to remain unchanged over time. Calcifications that have been stable for two years are almost always benign. As with masses that are classified as probably benign, calcifications in this category have a low probability to begin with, and stability over time markedly increases the probability that they are benign. Just as with masses, however, there are exceptions. Feig (18) has demonstrated, how-

ever, that if the morphology of calcifications is particularly worrisome, stability is not reassuring.

Disappearing Calcifications

No scientific study has been performed to evaluate the resorption of calcifications, but it has been our experience that benign calcifications may be resorbed spontaneously (Fig. 15-30). We have never seen microcalcifications in untreated breast cancer undergo resorption. Since the calcifications associated with breast cancer usually develop in the intraductal portion of the tumor, if the lesion becomes invasive, it is likely that, just as the invasive cells crowd out and kill normal cells, they likely can destroy the intraductal cells as well. We have seen at least one case in which the invasive tumor mass obliterated the calcifications of a clearly intraductal cancer that was missed on several studies but visible in retrospect (Fig. 15-31). It would be valuable if the European screening trials, which have multiple studies over many years on the same women, and also have a high threshold for intervention, would review the cases in which invasive cancer developed to determine how many had detectable calcifications on earlier studies.

After radiation therapy, cancer calcifications may increase, remain the same, or be resorbed, although at the present time most advise that all suspicious calcifications be excised before irradiation in an effort to reduce the tumor burden and the likelihood of recurrence.

FINDINGS THAT ARE PROBABLY BENIGN BUT COULD REPRESENT CANCER

There are a number of findings that are usually due to benign processes, but are, on occasion, related to a malignancy. These include the solitary circumscribed mass, solitary dilated duct, focal asymmetries, and round or oval clustered calcifications.

Solitary Circumscribed Mass

One of the major areas of disagreement in breast imaging is the management of the solitary circumscribed mass. It is extremely rare for a breast cancer to be round or oval with a sharply defined (circumscribed) margin. Unfortunately, breast cancer can be round, or oval, and well defined (Fig. 15-32). Even when the margin of a mass is so well defined that there is a lucent halo around it, due to the Mach effect, cancer cannot be entirely excluded (19).

Sickles (1) studied these lesions by following them for three years. He found that only 12 (2%) of the 589 masses that were followed at this interval proved to be cancer (1). Most now accept this (2%) as an acceptable false-negative rate and indicate short-interval follow-up for women with circumscribed round or oval masses seen on a prevalence (first) screening. If, on subsequent mammograms, the mass enlarges or its margins lose their definition, additional evaluation is indicated. If the

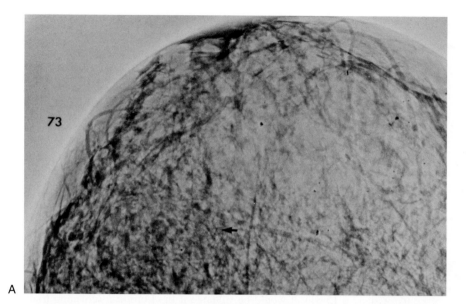

A

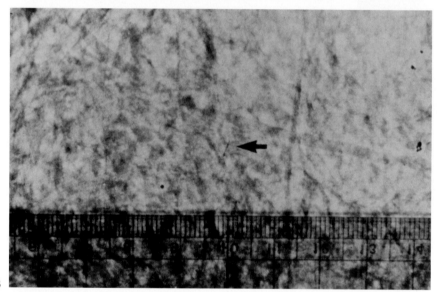

B

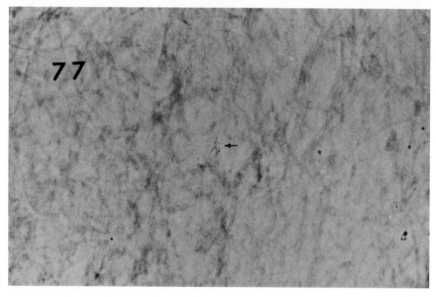

C

FIG. 15-31. The natural history of breast cancer. An invasive cancer can obliterate ductal carcinoma in situ (DCIS), replacing calcifications with a mass. On a xeromammogram in 1973 (**A** and photographically enlarged in **B**), the fine linear calcifications (*arrow*) were not seen. They were missed (appearing black) again in 1977, when they began to branch in the typical pattern of a poorly differentiated comedo DCIS (**C**). In 1981 a 2.5-cm, palpable, invasive cancer had developed and "blown apart" the calcifications (representing the in situ cancer), and a spiculated mass became visible on the xerogram (**D**). The patient died 4 years later. *Continued.*

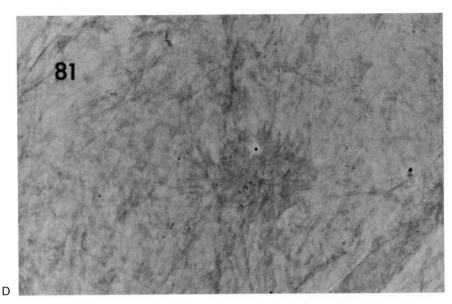

D

FIG. 15-31. *Continued.*

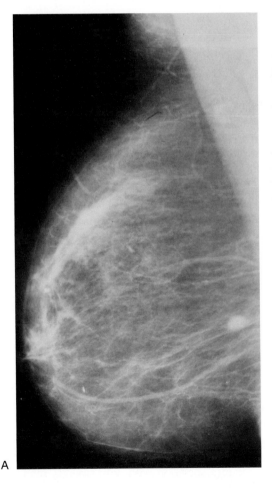

A

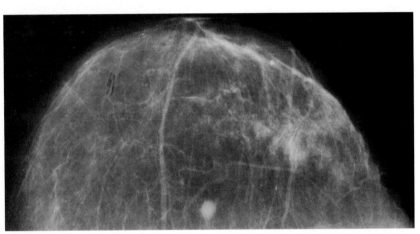

B

FIG. 15-32. Solitary round or oval masses with circumscribed margins are breast cancer <5% of the time. The mass deep in the left breast, as seen on the mediolateral oblique **(A)** and craniocaudal **(B)** projections, was well defined but proved to be invasive ductal carcinoma. The high density of the mass and the slight suggestion of ill definition along the posterior border had prompted the biopsy.

mass proves to be a cyst there is no need for additional information. If it is a solid mass, biopsy should be considered.

If such a lesion develops (neodensity), there is no logic to placing it into further short-interval follow-up and immediate evaluation should be considered. By appearing over time, a lesion that has developed has changed a priori, and investigation is warranted. Frequently ultrasound is useful for demonstrating that such a mass is a cyst and requires no further intervention. If the developing circumscribed density is solid, then biopsy should be considered.

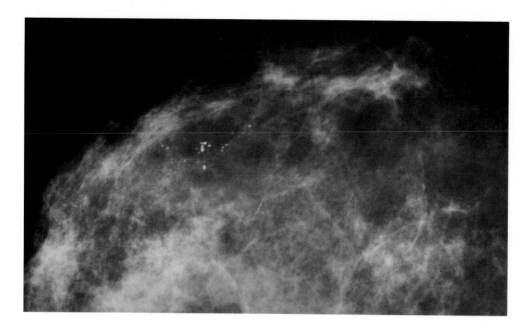

FIG. 15-33. Smooth, round, regular calcifications in a cluster are only rarely associated with breast cancer. Many of these calcifications are not only round appearing but also fairly large. Note, however, that there are several irregular calcifications as well. The cluster proved to be due to ductal carcinoma in situ.

It used to be taught that circumscribed breast cancers were of the medullary subtype and likely to be indolent. It is now known that this is not the case (20). When a breast cancer is round or oval and well defined, it is likely to be invasive carcinoma not otherwise specified, and there are no studies proving that circumscription on the mammogram predicts indolence.

Solitary Dilated Duct

As the result of a few unusual cases in which the only apparent indication of cancer was the presence of a single dilated duct, this finding became known as a secondary sign of malignancy. In fact, a solitary asymmetrically large duct is an extremely unusual finding and is rarely the only indication of cancer. Almost invariably, when cancer is present, there are other associated signs of malignancy (e.g., discharge, a mass, architectural distortion, or calcifications). Similar to other secondary signs, a solitary dilated duct usually has a benign cause.

Intuitively, one would expect that a cancer causing a dilatation of the lactiferous duct would be distal to the flow of secretions, close to the nipple, and causing duct enlargement by obstruction. This need not be the case. Cancers as well as benign lesions associated with solitary dilated ducts are in fact usually more toward the lobule. If biopsy is undertaken, the entire involved duct network (segment) should be excised.

Focal Asymmetries

It is not unusual to review the preceding mammograms in a patient diagnosed with breast cancer and discover that there was a focal asymmetric density in the region where the cancer ultimately developed. It is usually impossible to determine if this was breast tissue in which the cancer grew or a very early manifestation of the cancer. Frequently the asymmetry is one of many in a background of heterogeneous breast tissue. In his study of probably benign lesions Sickles (1) categorized 448 findings as focal asymmetric densities. In his three-year follow-up, only two (0.4%) proved to be cancers.

One of the most difficult tasks in breast imaging is to try to accurately distinguish a significant focal asymmetry from the normal heterogeneities and asymmetries that are visible on virtually every set of mammograms. Generally, if a focal asymmetry is not actually a mass and there is no associated architectural distortion or significant associated calcifications, then it is likely an island of breast tissue and does not warrant intervention.

Round Regular Calcifications

The calcifications associated with breast cancer are almost always pleomorphic, with very irregular sizes and shapes. It is extremely unusual for breast cancer to form smooth, round, regular calcifications. Once again Sickles (1) included round or oval, regular clustered calcifications (as seen on magnification mammography) in his study of short-interval follow-up. At follow-up, he found only one cancer (0.1%) among 1,234 such clusters in his study. We have only rarely seen cancer in association with only smooth, round calcifications (Fig. 15-33), and it is uncertain whether these were deposits in adjacent benign tissue and the cancer was serendipitous or whether the calcifications were due to the cancer. Regardless, the association is so uncommon that if clustered calcifications are very smooth, round (or oval), and regular, short-interval follow-up, at most, is a reasonable approach.

SIGNS WARRANTING BIOPSY ONLY WHEN PHYSICAL EXAMINATION SUPPLIES SUPPORTING EVIDENCE

Asymmetric Breast Tissue

Asymmetric breast tissue is a normal variation that is manifested by a greater volume of breast tissue in one part of one breast when compared to the same volume in the other breast; asymmetry of the pattern of tissue; or asymmetry of the density of the tissues in one part of one breast relative to its mir-

ror image on the other side. Asymmetric breast tissue should not be confused with a focal asymmetric density (Fig. 15-34).

Asymmetric tissue density can be due to breast cancer, but it is rare. Review of false-negative mammograms in women with palpable cancers will occasionally reveal an asymmetric increase in the density of the breast tissue in the region of the cancer. As a result, although nonspecific and very common in normal women, this finding is occasionally a secondary sign of malignancy.

Although an insidiously invasive cancer, such as one of lobular origin, can occasionally cause asymmetric tissue

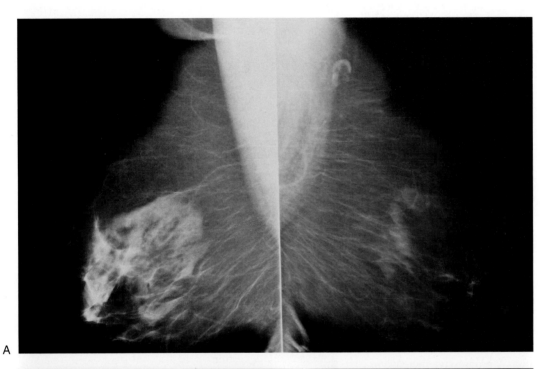

A

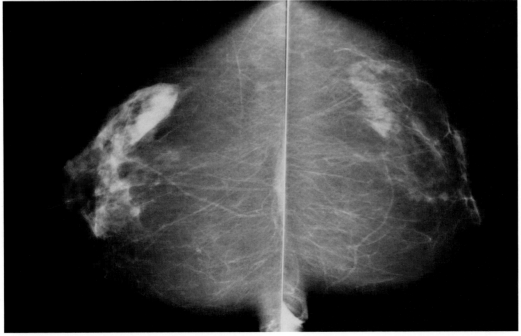

B

FIG. 15-34. Asymmetric breast tissue differs from a focal asymmetric density. This 48-year-old woman had benign asymmetric breast tissue that had remained unchanged on the mediolateral oblique **(A)** and craniocaudal **(B)** projections for at least 8 years. *Continued.*

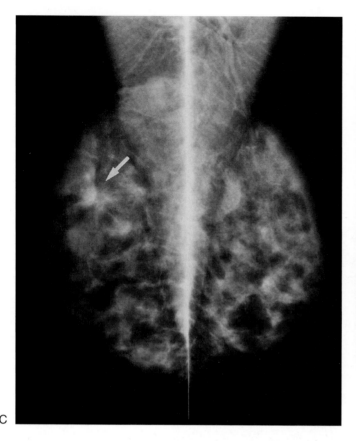

C

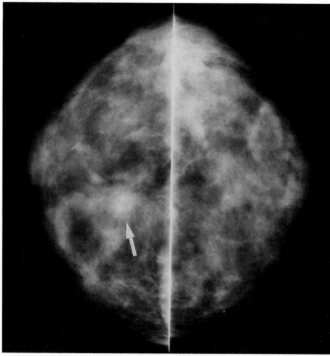

D

FIG. 15-34. *Continued.* The **focal asymmetric density** (*arrows*) in another 48-year-old woman seen on the mediolateral oblique **(C)** and craniocaudal **(D)** projections proved to be intraductal and invasive breast cancer.

density, the converse is unusual. Asymmetric breast tissue, by itself, is unlikely to be due to breast cancer. If the asymmetry is not forming a mass, the architecture is preserved, there are no significant associated microcalcifications, and there is no palpable abnormality, then asymmetric tissue is almost always a normal variation. A progressive increase in tissue density, however, particularly when focal, is of some concern. The use of HRT can also produce a focal or diffuse increase in tissue density.

In a prospective study of asymmetries, we found that at least 3% of women have prominent, three-dimensionally real, asymmetric breast tissue that appears as increased volume or density relative to the same projection and volume of the contralateral breast. This usually merely reflects normal asymmetric development. In some women, it no doubt represents the variable end-organ response of breast tissue to hormonal factors, with one part of the breast being more sensitive to hormone stimulation.

The vast majority of visibly asymmetric breast tissue is not evident on clinical breast examination. Our study showed that asymmetric breast tissue was only significant when there was a corresponding palpable abnormality on physical examination. When the mammogram and clinical examination are concordant for this type of asymmetry, it should increase the level of concern and probably prompt a biopsy (Fig. 15-35).

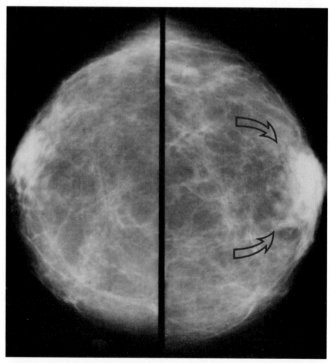

FIG. 15-35. **Mammographically visible asymmetry that is palpable should be viewed with some suspicion.** The asymmetry in the subareolar region on the right was also palpable and proved to be ductal carcinoma.

The fact that prominent asymmetric breast tissue, visible by mammography, is rarely palpable is counterintuitive unless one realizes that mammography measures different basic tissue characteristics than clinical breast examination. Mammography measures the x-ray attenuation of the atoms in the molecules that make up the tissues of the breast; the clinical breast examination measures the way the molecules are arranged and their elastic properties.

Some palpable cancers do not produce a lesion with mammographically demonstrable margins, nor do they produce calcium deposits. The only visible finding may merely be an increase in radiographic density in a volume of breast tissue. Thus, when palpable, asymmetric tissue density is a secondary sign of malignancy, but if it is not palpable and is merely asymmetric tissue density without the margins of a mass or other signs of malignancy, it is not by itself an indication for biopsy.

When assessing asymmetric density, the observer should remember that the asymmetry may be due to increased density on the ipsilateral side or to decreased tissue on the contralateral side. For example, in a woman who has had a previous biopsy, asymmetry may be due to the removal of tissue on the contralateral side rather than increased density ipsilaterally.

Asymmetric Ducts

A variant of asymmetric breast tissue is tissue that contains serpentine or nodular structures. Wolfe (21) called these *prominent ducts*, although their exact etiology likely varies. Wolfe suggested that the presence of these as asymmetric structures was an indication of possible malignancy. What Wolfe failed to evaluate was the denominator of the equation. He failed to determine how often asymmetric ducts were present without cancer. Our own analysis of asymmetric breast tissue revealed that the appearance of what has been termed asymmetric ducts was fairly common, and part of the spectrum of benign asymmetric breast tissue (22). Wolfe's observations were probably biased by the selection of cases. He never provided a reason why the areas were biopsied, but it is likely that the lesions were palpable. Our data indicate that unless associated with a palpable abnormality or other signs of cancer, asymmetric ducts are a normal variation.

A true group of ducts converging on the nipple and seen in isolation that are asymmetric from the contralateral breast can be striking. This finding usually represents benign ectasia. When associated with a malignant lesion, asymmetric ducts usually produce a palpable change. This is an extremely uncommon manifestation of cancer.

Diffuse changes that are predominantly benign but contain cancer foci are uncommon, and unless a focal lesion is visible within a large area of asymmetric ducts, the finding is probably normal and a biopsy is not necessary unless corroborative asymmetry is present on physical examination.

FINDINGS THAT MAY BE ASSOCIATED WITH BREAST CANCER

Asymmetric Veins

There are many causes for the asymmetric dilatation of vascular structures within the breast. Most of these are benign and, in fact, probably related to temporary alterations in venous flow caused by differences in mammographic compression. Vascular asymmetry, as the only sign of cancer, is not a very useful sign of malignancy. Nevertheless, if an asymmetric vein is present, the observer should be alerted. In our single experience with this very unusual finding, mammography failed to demonstrate an intramammary malignancy, but physical examination revealed a high axillary tail lesion. We have seen some advanced cancers with associated vascular engorgement, but this, too, is unusual (Fig. 15-36).

Skin Changes and Trabecular Thickening

Evaluation of the skin was considered an important component of mammographic analysis in the past when large

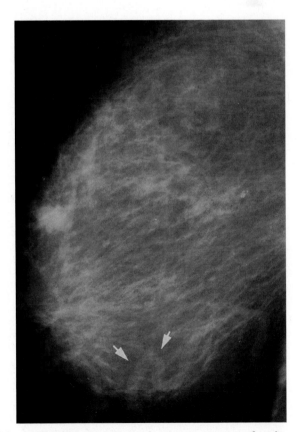

FIG. 15-36. Breast cancer is a rare cause of enlarged blood vessels. The ill-defined mass in the anterior left breast, seen on this mediolateral oblique image, was an invasive breast cancer. The serpentine structure at the bottom of the breast (*arrows*) is an enlarged blood vessel that may have been due to the increased blood flow to the tumor.

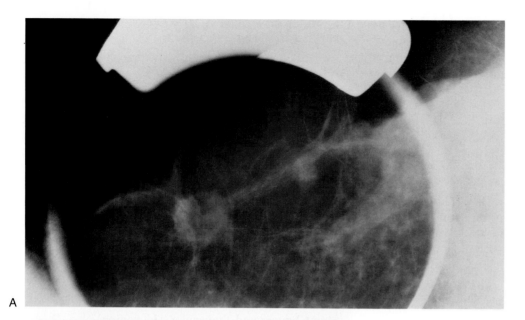

A

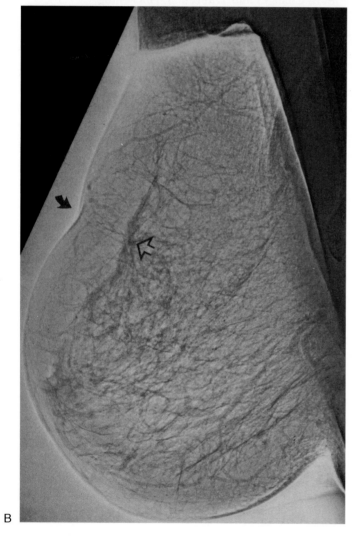

B

FIG. 15-37. Skin retraction is usually best seen by looking directly at the skin. On occasion, skin retraction can be seen by mammography, as in this case **(A)** in which the cicatrization associated with an invasive cancer beneath the skin is pulling the skin toward it. **(B)** Skin dimpling is more clearly illustrated on this old lateral xerogram, in which the cancer (*open arrow*) is pulling in the skin (*closed arrow*).

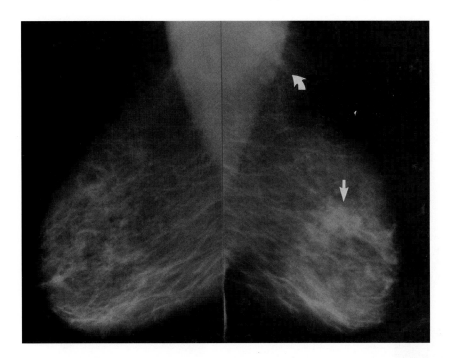

FIG. 15-38. Edema from advanced cancer can cause the trabecular structures of the breast to thicken and the overall breast density to increase. In this patient, the primary cancer is visible (*straight arrow*) in the enlarged lymph nodes in the right axilla (*curved arrow*), later found to contain tumor. The overall density of the breast (skin and trabecular thickening) is increased due to tumor in the lymphatics and edema.

cancers were more common. As the ability to detect earlier cancers has improved, evaluation of the skin has become less critical. Although the interpretation of mammograms may include an evaluation of the skin if it is visible, skin changes associated with malignancy generally occur late in the disease process with either direct invasion by the tumor or obstruction of the lymphatic or venous return. These are usually better evaluated clinically. The mammogram should be obtained to evaluate the tissues of the breast and not the skin. The best way to evaluate the skin is to view it directly.

On occasion, a cicatrizing tumor deep within the breast can cause skin retraction through the tethering of Cooper's ligaments, but in general, cancers will be found lying close beneath the pulled-in skin (Fig. 15-37). When retraction is visible on the mammogram it is usually apparent on clinical examination as a puckering or dimpling of the skin. When retraction caused by a cancer is evident clinically, the tumor mass is generally visible mammographically. If no underlying lesion is evident, the retraction is likely to be due to post-traumatic scarring.

Diffuse skin thickening associated with cancer is a late change indicating advanced disease. It is often accompanied by generalized thickening of the trabecular structures coursing through the breast (Fig. 15-38). The radiographic appearance is nonspecific and may merely reflect edema. When the thickening is due to direct tumor invasion of the dermal lymphatics, it is a poor prognostic sign. The edema may also be caused by interference with lymphatic drainage in the axilla, or even centrally in the mediastinum from obstructed vascular flow, such as that in the superior vena caval obstruction, or as a result of cardiac failure. Radiation therapy, as well as dermatologic problems, often cause skin thickening that may be self-limited or persistent.

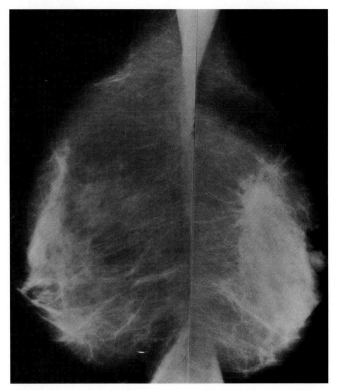

FIG. 15-39. If the nipple inverts over a short period of time, breast cancer should be considered. Nipple inversion due to cancer has become rare due to the earlier detection of most malignancies. The large cancer on the right is responsible for pulling the nipple up and back into the subareolar tissues.

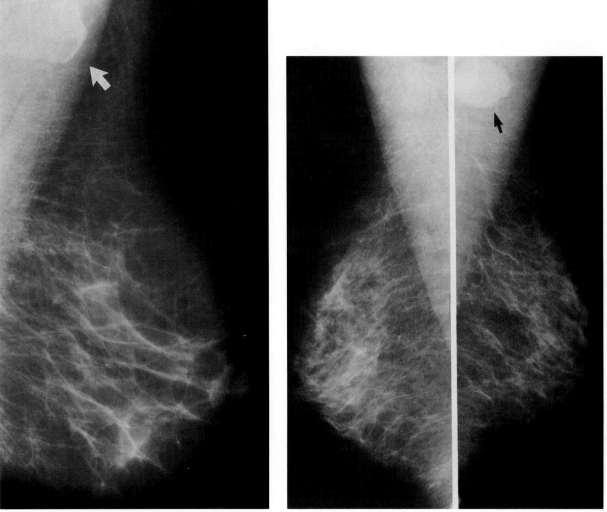

A   B

FIG. 15-40. Enlarged axillary lymph nodes seen on mammography are rarely due to breast cancer. They are usually due to fatty enlargement **(A)**, hyperplasia **(B)**, lymphoma **(C)**, and, on occasion, breast cancer **(D)**. *Continued.*

Thickened skin is part of the triad that defines inflammatory carcinoma, a highly aggressive manifestation of breast cancer in which tumor is often found permeating the dermal lymphatics. By itself, however, thickened skin is a nonspecific finding, and the diagnosis of inflammatory carcinoma is based on the clinical findings of heat, erythema, and peau d'orange (the clinical correlate of skin thickening where the thickened skin causes the pores to be prominent and resembles the skin of an orange) over ≥30% of the breast. Infection can produce similar findings and it is usually not possible to distinguish the two by mammography.

Nipple Retraction, Deviation, or Inversion

Malignant processes can cause a retraction of the nipple from the cicatrization process. If the pull is eccentric, the nipple may deviate in the direction of the cancer. In some situations the nipple may actually invert. When nipple inversion is caused by an underlying cancer, it generally occurs over a relatively short period of time. Most nipple retraction or inversion, however, is the result of benign processes and will have been present for many years. The exact cause in these cases is rarely known, but the process generally takes place over a long period.

As a secondary sign of malignancy, nipple retraction is generally associated with large cancers that are evident on the mammogram, and it is rarely the most significant indication of malignancy on a mammogram (Fig. 15-39).

Enlarged Axillary Lymph Nodes

Spread of tumor to the axillary nodes is a finding that indicates a significant worsening of the prognosis and diminishes the expected long-term survival. Although

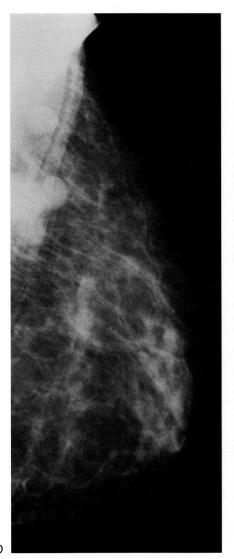

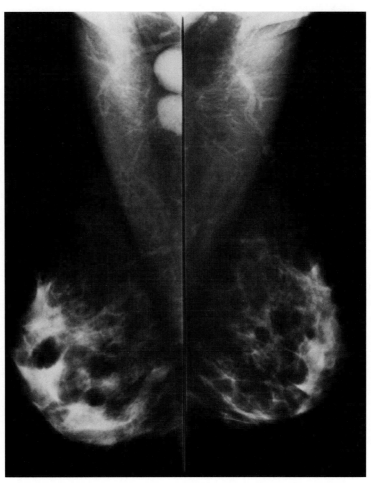

FIG. 15-40. *Continued.*

involved (positive) axillary lymph nodes may occur when tumor in the breast is microscopic, the likelihood increases with the size of the cancer (23). Mammography is not a very useful method for evaluating axillary nodes, and surgical removal of the level I and II nodes remains the most accurate way of determining whether or not they contain tumor. The need to evaluate axillary nodes as they influence treatment decisions is evolving. The demonstration and sampling of a sentinel node (see Chapter 26) may obviate the need for axillary dissection, but this still remains the best method for prognostication.

The demonstration of large nodes by mammography is nonspecific and can be due to nonmalignant causes or other malignancies, such as lymphoma. When nodes involved with breast cancer are visible by mammography, it is a late nonspecific sign of malignancy. In our experience, it is rare to see enlarged axillary nodes on mammography due to a primary breast lesion (Fig. 15-40).

In general, when metastatic disease is present in the axilla or elsewhere, the primary breast lesion is evident on mammography or to palpation. Occasionally, palpable axillary nodes are the first indication of breast cancer. In this case, a mammographic search of the breast may result in the detection of an intramammary malignant lesion that is occult to physical examination. Gadolinium-enhanced magnetic resonance imaging may be useful in finding an occult primary breast lesion.

Normal axillary lymph nodes usually are no larger than 1.5 to 2.0 cm unless they are expanded by fat (24). In the latter case, the fat will be apparent as a lucent area that in some cases almost obliterates the node, leaving a thin rim of radiodense tissue. When fat infiltration occurs, normal axillary nodes may reach 3 to 4 cm or more in size. When "solid" (non–fat-containing) enlarged nodes are found in the axilla, other causes of axillary nodal enlargement should be considered. Benign hyperplasia is indistinguishable from neoplastic infiltration. Isolated, mammographically apparent lymph nodes may indicate the presence of lymphoma.

Breast cancer occasionally may spread to the contralateral axillary nodes. It is postulated that this is either through shared lymphatics across the sternum or by a hematogenous route. Metastatic spread from other primary sites may also result in enlargement of the axillary nodes. When no tumor is found within the breast, this becomes a more significant possibility.

REFERENCES

1. Sickles EA. Periodic mammographic follow-up of probably benign lesions: results of 3,184 consecutive cases. Radiology 1991;179:463–468.
2. Meyer JE, Kopans DB. Stability of a mammographic mass: a false sense of security. AJR Am J Roentgenol 1981;137:595.
3. Meyer JE, Kopans DB. Analysis of mammographically obvious breast carcinomas with benign results on initial biopsy. Surg Gynecol Obstet 1981;153:570–572.
4. Stacey-Clear A, McCarthy KA, Hall DA, et al. Observations on the location of breast cancer in women under fifty. Radiology 1993;186:677–680.
5. Martin JE, Moskowitz M, Milbrath J. Breast cancer missed by mammography. AJR Am J Roentgenol 1979;132:737.
6. Murphy WA, DeSchryver-Kecskemeti K. Isolated clustered microcalcifications in the breast: radiologic-pathologic correlation. Radiology 1978;127:335.
7. Galkin BM, Frasca P, Feig SA, Holderness BA. Non-calcified breast particles: a possible new marker of breast cancer. Invest Radiol 1982;17:119.
8. Stomper PC, Connolly JL, Meyer JE, Harris JR. Clinically occult ductal carcinoma in situ detected with mammography: analysis of 100 cases with radiologic-pathologic correlation. Radiology 1989;172:235–241.
9. Ahmed A. Calcification in human breast carcinomas: ultrastructural observations. J Pathol 1975;117:247.
10. Sonnenfeld MR, Frenna TH, Weidner N, Meyer JE. Lobular carcinoma in situ: mammographic-pathologic correlation of results of needle-directed biopsy. Radiology 1991;181:363–367.
11. Egan RL, McSweeney MB, Sewell CW. Intramammary calcifications without an associated mass in benign and malignant disease. Radiology 1980;137:1–7.
12. Lanyi M. Diagnosis and Differential Diagnosis of Breast Calcifications. Berlin: Springer-Verlag, 1986.
13. Lagios MD, Margolin FR, Westdahl PR, Rose MR. Mammographically detected duct carcinoma in situ: frequency of local recurrence following tylectomy and prognostic effect of nuclear grade on local recurrence. Cancer 1989;63:618–624.
14. Holland R, Peterse JL, Millis RR, et al. Ductal carcinoma in situ: a proposal for a new classification. Semin Diagn Pathol 1994;11:167–180.
15. Page DL, Dupont WD, Rogers LW, et al. Continued local recurrence of carcinoma 15–25 years after a diagnosis of low grade ductal carcinoma in situ of the breast treated only by biopsy. Cancer 1995;76:1197–1200.
16. Sickles EA. Mammographic features of 300 consecutive nonpalpable breast cancers. AJR Am J Roentgenol 1986;146:661.
17. Kopans DB, Meyer JE, Homer MJ, Grabbe J. Dermal deposits mistaken for breast calcifications. Radiology 1983;149:592.
18. Lev-Toaff AS, Feig SA, Saitas VL, et al. Stability of malignant breast microcalcifications. Radiology 1994;192:153–156.
19. Swann CA, Kopans DB, McCarthy KA, et al. The halo sign and malignant breast lesions. AJR Am J Roentgenol 1987;149:1145–1147.
20. Rubens JR, Kopans DB. Medullary carcinoma of the breast: is it overdiagnosed? Arch Surg 1990;125:601–604.
21. Wolfe JN. Mammography: ducts as a sole indicator of breast carcinoma. Radiology 1967;89:206.
22. Kopans DB, Swann CA, White G, et al. Asymmetric breast tissue, Radiology 1989;171:639–643.
23. Carter CL, Allen C, Henson DE. Relation of tumor size, lymph node status, and survival in 24,740 breast cancer cases. Cancer 1989;63:181–187.
24. Kalisher L, Chu AM, Peyster RG. Clinicopathological correlation of xeroradiography in determining involvement of metastatic axillary nodes in female breast cancer. Radiology 1976;121:333–335.

Breast Imaging, 2nd ed., by Daniel B. Kopans.
Lippincott–Raven Publishers, Philadelphia © 1998.

CHAPTER 16

Ultrasound and Breast Evaluation

Breast ultrasound has undergone intensive investigation for decades. As with any modality, initial overly enthusiastic expectations have been replaced by limited, practical application derived from scientific evaluation and experience. Technical advances have steadily led to improved imaging and higher spatial resolution, but, with the exception of greater use for guiding interventional techniques, the overall efficacious use of ultrasound has remained the same. Ultrasound is primarily a method for differentiating cystic lesions from solid masses. Some believe they can use ultrasound to distinguish some benign solid masses from malignant masses. Although older studies were unable to demonstrate any efficacy for ultrasound as a screening technique, recent preliminary results suggest that improvements in technology may permit ultrasound to detect some cancers that are occult to clinical and mammographic evaluation.

METHODS

With the exception of some experimental devices, ultrasound is primarily performed using hand-held, real-time systems. With rare exception, high-frequency transducers should be used. Generally 7.5-MHz systems or higher are needed to provide the needed resolution. Little advantage can be gained by using frequencies higher than 12 to 13 MHz, and the energy deposition of higher-frequency systems may preclude their use. The transducers should be focused to permit high resolution from the skin to a depth of 4 to 5 cm. The bandwidth of the systems varies. Some systems produce multiple-frequency output that is used to obtain information from varying depths. It is unclear whether these ultimately provide any special advantage.

Ultrasound is generally performed with the patient lying supine. In most women the breast tissues can be evaluated from the skin to the chest wall by having the patient extend her arm behind her head and assume various supine oblique positions that thin the breast over the chest wall. If the breast is particularly large, the deep tissues may be difficult to evaluate. Ultrasound can demonstrate the skin, subcutaneous fat, breast parenchyma, retromammary fat, pectoralis muscle, ribs, and anterior chest wall (Fig. 16-1).

One unusual characteristic of the breast is that relative to the parenchyma, fat in the breast is hypoechoic. This poses some problems for ultrasound because, with rare exceptions, breast cancers are hypoechoic. A significant number of breast cancers are difficult if not impossible to see using ultrasound because they are isoechoic with fat or breast tissue.

Ultrasound for Screening

Ultrasound has evolved, not as a replacement for x-ray mammography, but as a study best limited to the differentiation of cystic lesions from solid and as a guide for aspiration and biopsy in specific situations. Although some investigators have described the detection of cancer by ultrasound alone, these reports have been anecdotal. The selection criteria have not been clearly defined, and the scan techniques as well as criteria for intervention have not been clearly documented. The only way to prevent bias would be blinded interpretation of the ultrasound without access to the mammogram and clinical examination (which are, presumably, negative). Gordon et al. (1) described a group of cases in which they reported evaluating the role of ultrasound-guided aspiration biopsy. Among their study group, they reported 123 women who had nonpalpable masses that were not visible mammographically. These masses, which were apparently visible only by ultrasound, were evaluated using fine-needle aspiration (FNA) cytology under ultrasound guidance. There were 10 cancers among these 123 women that were not clearly evident by clinical examination or mammography. Unfortunately, these cases were not reported in detail. It is uncertain whether they included lobular carcinoma in situ, nor is it clear how the cancers were related to the primary reason for performing the ultrasound (the women were not asymptomatic). Furthermore, it was not stated whether these were primary lesions or additional foci of cancer in women with malignancies detected by mammography or clinical breast examination. The fact that the authors did not stress the importance of these lesions by describing them in a separate report suggests that there were likely other details that reduce their significance.

In 1995 Gordon and Goldenberg (2) updated their experience and reported the retrospective results from the ultrasound evaluation of 12,706 women. The criteria by which these patients were chosen for ultrasound survey were not detailed by the authors. The breasts scanned were not asymp-

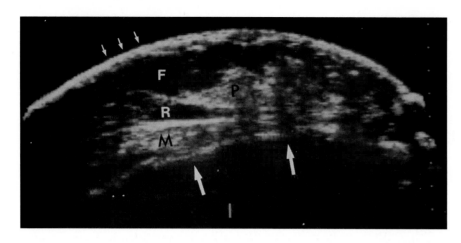

FIG. 16-1. This **whole-breast ultrasound** cross section demonstrates anatomy of the breast with the skin (*small arrows*), subcutaneous fat (F), parenchyma (P), retromammary fat (R), pectoralis muscle (M), and the chest wall (*large arrows*).

tomatic. Gordon and Goldenberg indicated that they were breasts in which concern had been raised by mammography or clinical examination. Rather than confining their evaluation to the area in question, the authors scanned the entire breast. They used hand-held equipment but did not detail their scanning technique. Ultrasound-guided FNA cytology was used to sample any solid mass that they deemed suspicious. Once again, the selection criteria were not carefully specified. Among 1,575 such solid masses that were described as nonpalpable and nonvisible by mammography, 279 had FNA. The other 1,296 masses were not aspirated because the authors thought they were not of sufficient concern. Among the criteria they provided for prompting FNA included "a mass not previously documented; an enlarging mass; a mass with worrisome sonographic features, such as taller than wide (see The L/AP Ratio in Benign and Malignant Lesions); or a stable mass causing anxiety in the patient." They used the presence of "smooth, circumscribed margins, neutral or increased through-transmission, homogeneous internal echogenicity, and wider-than-tall shape" as favorable features "but not infallible signs of benignity." Unless the patient preferred FNA, the lesions that fell into these latter categories were not biopsied but followed.

The actual follow-up of the lesions that were not biopsied was not documented, so the false-negative rate for this classification approach cannot be determined. The cytology obtained for the 279 lesions deemed suspicious by ultrasound was interpreted as definitely malignant in 22 and suspicious in 18 (six of these were found to be malignant at surgery), whereas 183 had benign cytology. The results were presented in a confusing manner. Among the 1,575, there were 44 confirmed malignancies, of which 16 were multifocal. This presumably means that there were 28 women with cancer (22 + 6) and 16 of these had multifocal lesions for a total of 44 lesions. Of the 1,575 lesions evaluated, 15 of those that proved to be cancer were in women with no other suggestion of malignancy, and the reason the ultrasound was performed proved to be a benign lesion. Fifteen other women had a malignant-appearing lesion by mammography or by clinical examination. Ultrasound found an additional focus of cancer in these women.

Summarizing these results, Kopans et al. (3) pointed out that it apparently required 12,706 ultrasound examinations to find 15 primary cancers that were not detectable—as best can be determined from the report—by clinical breast examination or mammography. Although this is the most encouraging example of ultrasound's potential as a screening technique, the data were from a retrospective review, the selection criteria were not clearly defined, the scan technique was not described in detail, and the size and stage of all the lesions were not provided (they ranged from 0.4 to 2.5 cm). Thus, it is difficult to evaluate the significance of finding these lesions, and although the authors suggested that the entire breast should be scanned if there is any indication for ultrasound, Kopans et al. pointed out that these were the most preliminary of data and needed to be confirmed by prospective study and by others before the use of ultrasound to "screen" for unsuspected cancer should be considered a standard of care.

The only modern, prospective study was first reported by Kolb et al. (4) at the Radiological Society of North America Meeting in 1996. These authors reported on 2,300 women who had radiographically dense breasts in whom they found 10 cancers by ultrasound alone, after a negative mammogram and clinical examination. This amounts to four cancers per 1,000 women, a good rate for a screened population. They reported that the cancers that were detected were similar in size (mean, 11.3 mm) to those detected by mammography (mean, 10.9 mm) as well as similar in stage (83.3% stage I for ultrasound versus 90.2% stage I for mammography). This is a significant detection rate (four per 1,000) and, coupled with the Gordon's experience (2), suggests the need to re-evaluate ultrasound as a second-level screening technique. It is possible that screening women with radiographically dense breasts using ultrasound may detect early cancers that would otherwise by missed.

Testing the efficacy of ultrasound screening needs to be performed prospectively in a triple-blind evaluation of clinical breast examination, mammography, and ultrasound with each investigator initially blinded to the findings of the other, and then with knowledge of all the available information (this is the only way to avoid significant potential for

TABLE 16-1. *Characteristics by ultrasound*

Malignant	Indeterminate	Benign
Spiculation	Maximum diameter	Absent malignant findings
Angular margins	Isoechogenicity	Intense hyperechogenicity
Marked hypoechogenicity	Mild hypoechogenicity	Ellipsoid shape
Shadowing	Enhanced sound transmission	Gentle (2–3) lobulations
Calcification	Heterogeneous internal echotexture	Thin echogenic pseudocapsule
Duct extension	Homogeneous internal echotexture	
Branch pattern		
Microlobulation		

Source: Adapted from Stavros AT, Thickman D, Rapp CL, et al. Solid breast nodules: use of sonography to distinguish between benign and malignant lesions. Radiology 1995;196:123–134.

bias). The technique of scanning needs to be defined and be reproducible. The criteria for intervention must be carefully defined because there are many ultrasound findings in any normal breast that could be mistaken for cancer and the false-positive rate could be extremely high.

Given the improvements in the technology that have taken place over the past 10 years, ultrasound should be re-evaluated as a screening technique, but until efficacy has been demonstrated, ultrasound should not be considered as a screening test.

Reliability of Differentiation of Benign and Malignant Masses Using Ultrasound

It has been said that "If your tool is a hammer, then everything is a nail." There are enthusiasts in every field, and ultrasound is no exception. Many radiologists are highly proficient in the use of ultrasound in the evaluation of the breast. Numerous papers have been written about the various ultrasound criteria that can be used to increase the likelihood that a lesion is benign. There is little doubt that oval, or slightly lobulated, sharply marginated, well-circumscribed masses with homogeneous echotexture enhanced through-transmission of sound that are longer than they are wide (measured perpendicular to the skin) have a very high probability of being benign. The problem lies in the fact that cancer can, on occasion, have all of these characteristics.

What has not been determined is how reliable a noninvasive test must be to avoid the need for tissue sampling (needle or excisional biopsy). As a consequence of the costs associated with breast biopsy (i.e., economic, psychological, and physical), there has been great emphasis placed on using imaging to avoid a biopsy. This is perfectly reasonable as long as the woman is informed of the options and has the opportunity to decide how much certainty she requires. Because the stakes may be as high as life and death, it should not be sufficient that a test such as ultrasound be able to predict the nature of a lesion, for example, 70% of the time. This leaves too much room for error. Fortunately, a breast biopsy, even surgical excision, has an extremely low morbidity and virtually no mortality. The only biopsy that is safer is a skin biopsy. The cost of a breast biopsy can be reduced, and if performed skillfully, there should be little trauma; there need be

little or no residual evidence of the surgery. If ultrasound, or any other noninvasive test, is promoted as a method to differentiate benign from malignant lesions, the false-negative rate becomes critical, and women should be properly informed of the probabilities that the test result will be incorrect, and they should be provided with their options.

How Accurate Is Accurate?

The uses of imaging in breast evaluation are fairly unique. The only proved efficacy is from using mammography to screen asymptomatic women to reduce the mortality from breast cancer through earlier detection. Given the statistical probabilities and the fact that breast cancer is fairly rare relative to the number of women at risk, the vast majority of abnormalities found by mammography or clinical breast examination prove to be benign. Investigators should constantly be reminded that in a population of women being screened repetitively, there will only be two to four new cancers each year. When the accuracy of a test is considered, it should be remembered that if 1,000 screening mammograms were reported as negative, without the radiologist even reviewing them, the accuracy would be 99.96% to 99.98%. This is a greater accuracy than virtually any other medical test. The problem, of course, is that this approach would have failed to detect the two to four cancers, and the test, although highly "accurate," would actually have been totally without value and might have even had a negative impact if the reports were used to falsely reassure the women being screened.

When a new test is promulgated it is critical to ask how its use actually alters the care of the patient, and is this alteration of benefit to the patient. Many papers and books describe how features seen on ultrasound can be used to predict whether a lesion is likely to be benign or malignant, but these are irrelevant if the lesion must still be biopsied or removed to provide certainty. If a test cannot safely alter the care of an individual, then its efficacy must be questioned.

Stavros et al. (5) have claimed that ultrasound can accurately classify "some" solid lesions as being benign such that biopsy can be avoided. They presented criteria that they claimed permitted them to accurately differentiate benign lesions from malignant lesions (Table 16-1). This publication was an unstructured report of a conglomerate of retrospective findings. The selection criteria for women who were evaluated were poorly specified and produced an aggregate of lesions that were inappropriately analyzed as a whole. They included masses that were spiculated by mammography and for which ultrasound was not indicated. They included lesions that were typically benign, and there was no blinding as to the clinical and mammographic features of the lesions. Without structure, the results are impossible to interpret, and the conclusions unsupported.

The Stavros et al. report was essentially a compilation of anecdotal observations. The authors speculated on the origin of ultrasound findings as if they were fact when they have never been substantiated. For example, they stated that an echogenic border was indicative of infiltration. This is mere speculation. They suggested that "punctate calcifications, that are sonographically visible within solid nodules, are more likely to be associated with malignant than benign lesions." This relationship has never been substantiated. They stated as fact that "markedly hyperechoic tissue that is well circumscribed and of uniform echogenicity represents fibrous tissue." This has never been documented and echogenic cancers, although rare, have been reported.

The report also mixed palpable and nonpalpable lesions indiscriminately, which reflects the failure to appreciate the efficacious use of an imaging technique. The authors stated: "Sonography helped to correctly classify 100 nodules as malignant in comparison to 38 classified as malignant with mammography." This is irrelevant because all of these lesions required a tissue diagnosis, regardless of the ultrasound classification. Once it is clear that a tissue diagnosis is needed, there is no value to additional imaging unless the additional study can safely eliminate some of that intervention. Finally, the authors relied in many instances on ultrasound-guided needle biopsies for diagnosis, and because the false-negative rate for needle biopsy remains undetermined, the accuracy of their classifications technique remains unproved.

In 1996 the Food and Drug Administration (FDA) gave premarket approval (PMA) to the Advanced Technology Laboratories (ATL) ultrasound unit. This approval incorrectly suggested that the unit had demonstrated efficacy in differentiating benign and malignant masses. Although the FDA was careful to point out that it was approving the use of the unit to "help" establish the nature of a mass, the media was led to believe that this was a method of avoiding a tissue diagnosis. The data submitted to the FDA had never been subjected to peer review. Two outside experts in breast evaluation expressed significant reservations about the approval, and the review committee contained a single retired radiologist and no one with expertise in breast imaging. The data that were reviewed constituted a series of selected cases in which the investigators were not blinded to the clinical and mammographic findings. According to the FDA, the PMA only acknowledges that this ultrasound unit has demonstrated specific capability for the evaluation of breast lesions and that it can be used specifically for this application. Other ultrasound units may have the same capabilities, but these are applications that have never been reviewed by the FDA (specifically for breast studies) and so the companies cannot claim specific applications for breast evaluation even though their equipment is used every day in breast evaluation. This raises serious questions about the value of the PMA. At the time of this writing, there is no evidence that the ATL system has any greater efficacy for breast lesion evaluation than any other ultrasound system, and there is no proof that any ultrasound device can be relied on for differentiating benign lesions from those that are malignant.

Diagnostic Ultrasound

With the exception of a simple cyst, ultrasound is not diagnostic because there is a significant overlap in the characteristics of benign solid tissues and malignant lesions. Given the safety and ease with which a cytologic or histologic diagnosis can be achieved in the breast and the greater certainty afforded by having tissue confirmation, the value of tests that rely on probabilities to avoid more definitive diagnosis is questionable. Ultimately, it is the patient and her physician who must decide how much certainty is required.

Ultrasound as a Survey Technique

In the 1970s and early 1980s, whole-breast ultrasound units were devised to permit scanning of the entire breast with the goal of screening asymptomatic women to detect early-stage breast cancer. Several large studies showed that ultrasound might be incapable of detecting cancers that were not also evident by either physical examination or mammography (6,7). As noted above, however, some investigators, using more modern equipment, have reported cancers detected only by ultrasound. Although encouraging, the studies have not been properly performed (blinded interpretation), and the scan techniques and criteria for intervention are not clearly defined.

The mounting evidence, however, suggests that ultrasound may be able to detect some early cancers that are occult on mammography and clinical breast examination. If this is the case, systems for whole-breast ultrasound evaluation will need to be developed to remove the current operator dependence of the procedure. High-quality mammography remains the only proven imaging technique that has efficacy for the detection of clinically occult early-stage cancer, but as technology improves, other tests may begin to show efficacy.

In our experience with hand-held, real-time contact breast ultrasound, as well as our original experience with whole-breast scanning with a dedicated water-path system (4,8), we frequently have had difficulty separating the hypoechoic, ill-defined appearance of breast cancer from normal, irregularly marginated, hypoechoic mammary parenchyma (Fig. 16-2). The normal structures of the breast produce findings on ultrasound that are similar to those seen with some breast cancers. Fat and some fibrous tissue can be hypoechoic and mimic the

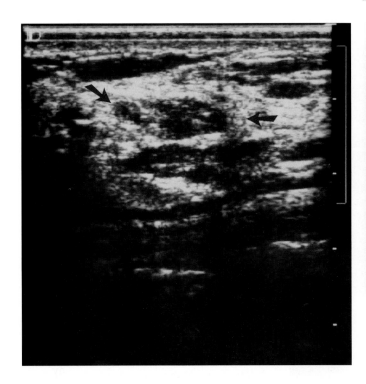

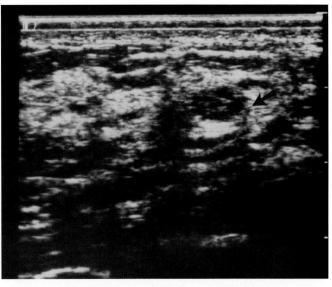

FIG. 16-2. Cancer is virtually always hypoechoic on ultrasound. Normal breast tissue can be hypoechoic and indistinguishable from cancer by ultrasound. Scanning the breast will find numerous areas that raise concern but are not cancers. The arrows point to two areas of hypoechoic tissue in a woman with normal mammography and clinical breast examination. Either one could be cancer, but both are normal breast tissue.

hypoechogenicity of breast cancer. Cooper's ligaments and other fibrous structures in the breast can produce acoustic shadowing that can also be indistinguishable from breast cancer. An additional limitation for detecting cancers with ultrasound is that microcalcifications, detectable by mammography and often associated with breast cancer, are not routinely visible with most current ultrasound technology. If ultrasound can be shown to have screening efficacy in properly performed trials, however, it could be a second-level screen, in addition to mammography, for women with dense breast tissue.

The fact that ultrasound finds lesions that mimic breast cancers but prove to be benign (false-positives) was originally demonstrated in our study of more than 1,000 women. We undertook long-term follow-up of 94 women who had suspicious lesions found *only* by ultrasound (they all had normal clinical breast examinations and mammograms). Over a 3- to 4-year period none of these women developed a clinically evident cancer (4). This study demonstrated that scanning women with normal mammograms and negative physical examinations raises concern for lesions that are invariably benign. There is, as yet, no support for surveying the entire breast by ultrasound, and with a high false-positive rate, scanning the breast is undesirable unless it is part of a research protocol. Our study used old, whole-breast ultrasound imaging, but it was prospective and the readers were blinded. The radiologist who interpreted the mammograms did not know the results of the ultrasound or the clinical examination. The radiologist who interpreted the ultrasound study (performed in a standardized fashion) was blinded to the findings on the clinical examination and the mammo-

gram. This is the only way to determine whether there is a separate, efficacious role for a test. Despite anecdotal claims, there has not yet been a prospective, blinded study of lesions detected only by ultrasound that validates its use for detecting clinically and mammographically occult breast cancer in asymptomatic women.

These observations do not negate the usefulness of ultrasound in diagnosis for evaluating lesions whose presence has been established by physical examination or mammography. Bassett et al. (9) found ultrasound as a useful adjunct to mammography, particularly in the diagnosis of cysts, to determine the need for further intervention.

Doppler Ultrasound

Numerous attempts have been made to apply Doppler ultrasound to breast evaluation. Because many breast cancers appear to have a substantial neovasculature (at the microscopic level), and most benign lesions do not have increased blood flow, the rationale for Doppler would appear to be justified. The clinical results, however, have not been particularly convincing. Many cancers can be shown to have increased blood flow, particularly at their periphery. High-velocity flow seems to be found almost only in breast cancers (10). Although preliminary reports suggested a high sensitivity and specificity for Doppler (11), other studies were not as successful, suggesting poor discrimination between normal and cancerous tissues (12). The most optimistic report by Cosgrove et al. (13) concluded that a "color Doppler signal in a lesion otherwise thought to be benign should prompt a biopsy, while the

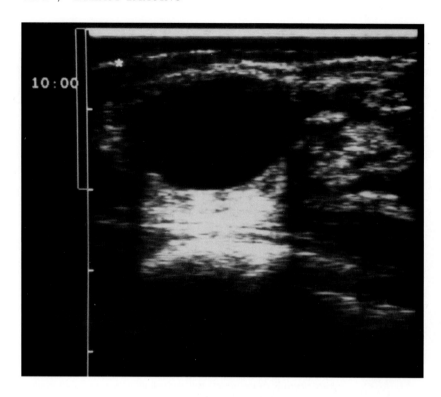

FIG. 16-3. If a lesion is round, oval, or lobulated with well-defined margins; has a clear anterior and posterior back wall; and enhances the through-transmission of sound, it is a **benign cyst,** and no further evaluation is required.

absence of signals in an indeterminate lesion is reassuring." The clinical application of this is not particularly useful. It might provide additional reassurance for women with lesions that are thought to be benign, but depending on the lesions placed in this category, the use of Doppler would only add to the cost of care because these lesions would otherwise be left alone. Indeterminate lesions would still require cytologic or histologic confirmation. Another problem with the Cosgrove et al. report was that the lesions were palpable, and evaluation of smaller lesions has not proved to be as successful.

Because benign lesions may exhibit increased flow and, more important, a significant number of cancers do not exhibit evidence of abnormal flow (14)—particularly lesions <1 cm (15)—Doppler is not yet reliable for distinguishing benign lesions from malignant lesions. There is the perplexing overlap of benign and malignant characteristics on Doppler analysis that make it difficult to avoid obtaining cytologic or histologic material (a biopsy). At this time, Doppler is not a clinically useful test for evaluating breast lesions.

Intravenous Enhancement of Breast Lesions for Ultrasound Evaluation

There is some hope that, just as with computed tomography, digital angiography, and magnetic resonance imaging (MRI), the neovascularity that develops with many cancers can be demonstrated by using intravenous (IV) contrast agents that enhance the visibility of vessels on ultrasound. A preliminary report using the IV infusion of microbubbles is encouraging (16), but this type of evaluation is still in development, with no proved efficacy for clinical care.

Ultrasound and Women with Radiographically Dense Breast Tissues

As noted in the section on Ultrasound as a Screening Technique, there is increasing evidence that ultrasound may be useful as a second-level screen for women who have radiographically dense tissues that could obscure a lesion on mammography; some palpable lesions, obscured by surrounding tissues and not visible by mammography, are visible by ultrasound. The vast majority of these lesions are palpable (that is the reason they were imaged by ultrasound), but studies by Gordon et al. (2) as well as Kolb et al. (3) suggest that some nonpalpable and mammographically undetectable cancers may be detectable by ultrasound. There is, however, no conclusive proof of any efficacy for the use of ultrasound to screen any population of women, including those with radiographically dense breasts, if they have negative mammograms and clinical breast examinations. As noted in the section on Ultrasound for Screening, the use of ultrasound to screen women with radiographically dense breast tissues needs to be properly studied prospectively. Ultrasound will likely prove useful as a second-level screen.

APPROPRIATE USE OF BREAST ULTRASOUND

Ultrasound should be considered a technique to help resolve specific management questions. If a lesion is not palpable but is detected by mammography, ultrasound can be used to analyze its composition. In particular, the ultrasound demonstration that a mammographically detected lesion is a simple cyst can obviate the need for surgery or

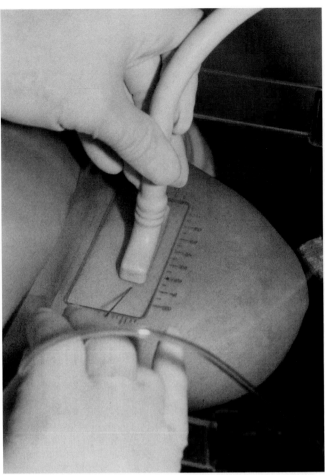

FIG. 16-4. Correlating mammography with ultrasound. By holding the breast in the mammography system and using the window compression plate, ultrasound can be performed through the window, and the abnormality can be compared using the two modalities. This can also be used to guide needle aspiration or biopsy.

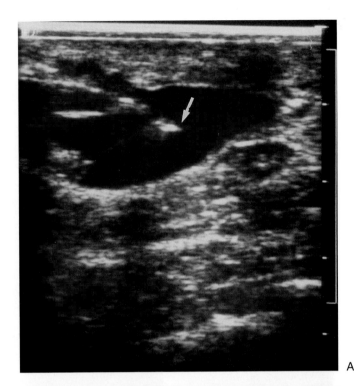

A

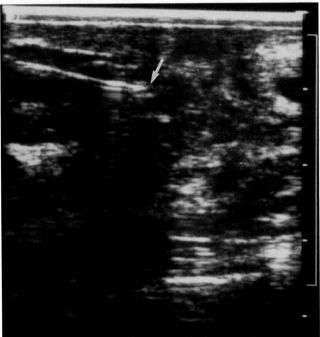

B

FIG. 16-5. Ultrasound-guided cyst aspiration. A cyst can be observed under ultrasound and a needle guided into it for aspiration under direct, real-time observation. **(A)** The tip of the needle (*arrow*) is visible in the cyst. **(B)** The fluid has been withdrawn and the cyst has collapsed.

even further intervention (Fig. 16-3). If a lesion meets the strict ultrasound criteria for a cyst, the study is diagnostic. If there is any question about the concordance of the lesion seen by ultrasound with the density on mammography, a guided aspiration followed by repeat mammography can resolve the question (see Chapter 21). Introducing a small volume of air (less than the volume of fluid removed to avoid pain) can confirm that the lesion seen using mammography was the lesion aspirated using ultrasound. We have found it helpful on occasion to evaluate the lesion with ultrasound with the breast held in the mammography unit and the lesion under the compression plate window used for needle localization (Fig. 16-4). Direct correlation can be made in this way, using the mammography coordinates from the window grid and the position of the ultrasound transducer in the window.

Ultrasound can occasionally help in the triangulation of lesions that are found in only one mammographic view. Ultrasound is very useful for guiding the aspiration of cysts (Fig. 16-5) and for obtaining cytologic material using FNA

(17,18) or histologic material using large core needle biopsy (19) (see Chapter 21). The reliability of ultrasound-guided biopsies has never been scientifically validated, and reliance on benign aspirates or cores is potentially risky due to the unknown false-negative rate, but the practice is so ubiqui-

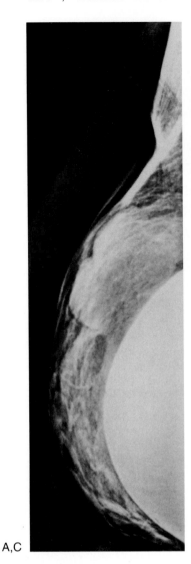

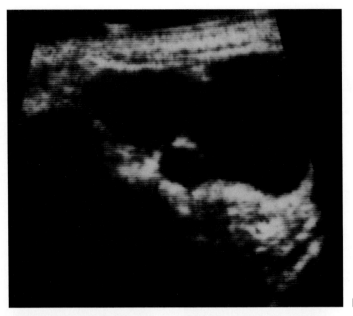

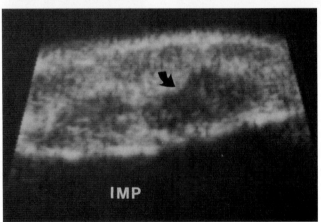

A,C

B

FIG. 16-6. Ultrasound, masses, and implants. (A) A palpable lobulated mass adjacent to the silicone implant in the upper outer quadrant. **(B)** Ultrasound confirms that the mass is a cyst, avoiding attempts at aspiration that could possibly rupture the implant. **(C)** In a second individual the mass adjacent to the implant (IMP) is solid and proved to be recurrent invasive ductal carcinoma.

tous that studies to provide scientific validation are unlikely to be undertaken. As with any imaging-guided needle biopsy, there is the potential for sampling error, and the results of the biopsy should be concordant with what was suggested by the imaging. If they are discordant, a repeat biopsy or excisional biopsy is recommended.

Ultrasound can also be used to position needles and wire guides for preoperative localization before surgical excision of sonographically visible lesions (20) (see Chapter 21).

Ultrasound and Implants

There are no data supporting the use of ultrasound to screen women with implants to detect breast cancer. Ultrasound may be helpful in evaluating women with implants if they have palpable lesions discovered by physical examination. It may be preferable to use ultrasound to determine if such lesions are cystic or solid to avoid inserting a needle that might damage the implant. Ultrasound may also be helpful for the evaluation of mammographically detected

abnormalities in women with implants to help to determine whether the such lesions are cystic or solid (Fig. 16-6).

Some have found ultrasound helpful in trying to determine whether an implant is ruptured (21). The demonstration of a "snowstorm" of echogenicity with posterior loss of information is fairly specific (see Chapter 17) and results from silicone that has extruded from the ruptured implant into the surrounding tissue (22). Rosculet et al. believe that this echogenic noise occurs when the silicone globules are so small that they are the size of a wavelength of the sound (23). Due to differences between the speed of sound in the silicone and breast tissue (sound travels slower in silicone), they hypothesize that focal areas of the beam are advanced and others are delayed as the beam passes through the tissues interspersed with silicone, and the beam becomes out of phase with the surrounding tissue. With loss of coherence, the result is a snowstorm of noise. Large globules of silicone, on the other hand, may produce hypoechoic masses. The silicone and the fibrous reaction to it from the tissues outside of the implant can cause areas of shadowing as well.

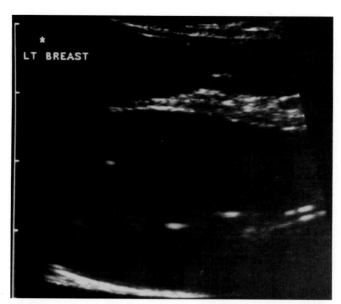

FIG. 16-7. The silicone envelope of the implant is collapsing into the gel, producing multiple levels of irregular specular reflections in the anechoic gel. This has been described as a "stepladder" pattern.

Many implants become surrounded by a fibrous capsule. When these rupture, silicone may extrude through this capsule if the capsule is incomplete or torn. This has been termed an *extracapsular rupture.* If the silicone envelope tears and collapses into the gel, which remains held in place within the fibrous capsule, it is termed *intracapsular rupture.* Intracapsular ruptures may appear normal on mammography because the contour of the silicone gel remains smooth and contained by the fibrous capsule. One of the more useful signs of an intracapsular rupture has been described on both MRI and ultrasound. As the envelope collapses into the gel, it folds on itself, and these folds can appear as a "stepladder" on ultrasound (Fig. 16-7). DeBruhl et al. (24) found that this was the most reliable sign of rupture in a series of 74 women with implants who were evaluated by ultrasound. The stepladder appearance was noted in 14 of the 20 known ruptured implants. Whether it is practical to use ultrasound to survey the entire surface of the implant for extracapsular rupture remains uncertain. We prefer to use MRI to evaluate implants for possible rupture (see Chapters 17 and 20).

Ultrasound and Asymmetric Breast Tissue

Some have advocated the use of ultrasound to evaluate women with asymmetric breast tissue. We defined normal asymmetric breast tissue as distinct from a focal asymmetric density: Asymmetric breast tissue does not form a mass, has no architectural distortion, and contains no significant calcifications or palpable abnormality (25). I would also add that the density of asymmetric breast density does not change from a previous study. If the tissues conform to this definition, scanning them with ultrasound would have no more validity than scanning a breast that was normal on mammography and clinical examination. There are no data to support the use of ultrasound to evaluate asymmetric breast tissue. If a focal asymmetric density could represent a mass, ultrasound may help, as with any mass.

EQUIPMENT

In the late 1970s and early 1980s there was an effort to use ultrasound as a screening technique to scan the entire breast. In some whole-breast ultrasound units the patient was supine with a water-path offset. In others, the patient was prone with the transducer(s) beneath in a water tank. The latter were the least desirable because they required additional, hand-held contact transducers to permit evaluation of the supine patient to guide aspiration or localization of questionable lesions. The subareolar region of the breast was particularly difficult to evaluate in prone whole-breast systems due to the unfavorable angle of incident sound unless the breast was compressed back against the chest wall (Fig. 16-8). This problem is significantly diminished in supine scanning, when the breast is naturally flattened against the chest wall. Whole-breast systems for supine scanning are bulky and unwieldy, however.

Studies finally demonstrated that whole-breast scanning was unnecessary and probably undesirable; it incurred additional expense and provided little additional information. Surveying the breast only revealed areas that raised concern but were virtually never cancerous.

Significant advances in ultrasound technology have occurred, however, and as noted in Ultrasound as a Survey Technique, studies suggest that clinically and mammographically occult cancers may be detectable by ultrasound. This will likely result in the development of ultrasound systems to permit rapid and efficient surveys of the breast.

Research has demonstrated that ultrasound is well suited for the evaluation of specific lesions, and hand-held, high-resolution systems to examine the supine patient are preferred. High-frequency (7.5-, 10-MHz, or higher frequency) transducers are necessary. These must be able to be focused from the skin to a minimum depth of 3 to 4 cm. Ultrasound of the breast is challenging because the normal breast tissues are highly attenuating and scattering while the structures to be imaged are extremely small. The ultrasound study is highly operator dependent. Skilled technologists who are closely supervised by a physician skilled in mammography and breast evaluation can perform breast ultrasound, but the intermittent application of breast ultrasound by those who are not aware of its special requirements can be problematic. We have found that it is best for the physician to be in the room closely monitoring the scanning, or (preferably) directly performing the scan. By holding the transducer in one hand and placing the fingers of the other hand against the side of the transducer, the pads of the fingers can palpate the tissues over which the transducer is moved, and the examiner can scan and determine if the area under evaluation is palpable or not.

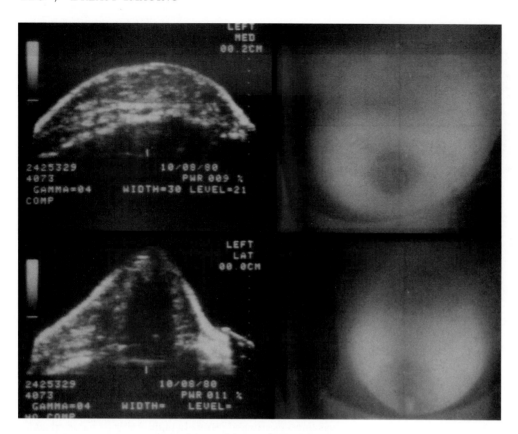

FIG. 16-8. The **nipple areolar complex.** On this whole-breast ultrasound the patient was lying prone with her breast immersed in a water bath and the transducer at the bottom of the tank. In the bottom images the breast is freely pendent and there is marked shadowing from the nipple areolar complex due to the adverse angle of incident sound relative to the fibroductal structures converging on the nipple. By flattening the breast against the chest wall as shown in the upper images the angles are flattened and sound can penetrate.

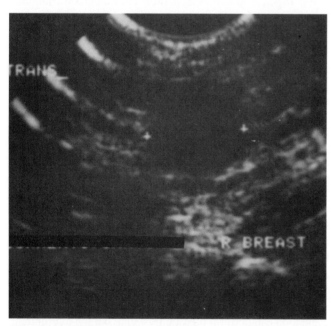

FIG. 16-9. **Improper gain settings** can eliminate important internal echoes. Because the equipment was not appropriate for breast ultrasound and the imaging parameters were not properly set, this mass was interpreted as a cyst on this outside ultrasound study. The mass proved to be a solid invasive ductal carcinoma.

Many technologists are familiar with and trained to see the cysts that are common in other organs of the body. They have the tendency to adjust the ultrasound system power and gain to artificially make lesions appear to be cystic. Some cancers produce very low-level echoes (Fig. 16-9), and the operator must be sure not to eliminate these by incorrectly setting the power or gain compensations. We believe that breast ultrasound should be performed by radiologists who are skilled in breast evaluation and technologists with similar skills.

The major prerequisite of a breast ultrasound system is that it can accurately differentiate a cyst from a solid mass and can delineate needles in the breast. The former can be a challenge in the breast because cysts may contain internal echoes, and solid masses may be extremely hypoechoic and similar to cysts except for some low-amplitude internal echoes. The most common problem with ultrasound systems used for breast evaluation is the difficulty in differentiating noise from true internal echoes. This problem may result in the operator adjusting gain settings to compensate and inadvertently eliminating significant echoes in a solid lesion so that the lesion is incorrectly diagnosed as a cyst. Because cysts are much more common than cancer this mistake is rare, but if the operator is relying on statistics instead of true imaging, ultrasound is of little added value.

Most ultrasound units provide various built-in algorithms for adjusting the gray scale mapping of the information (26). We have found that a linear map is less misleading. Other nonlinear algorithms tend to place echoes in cysts. The overall power used must be properly adjusted to maintain a good gray scale. Too much power applied to the transducer will produce spuri-

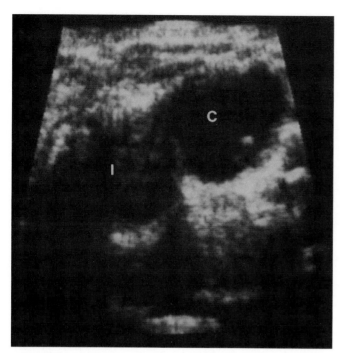

FIG. 16-10. On rare occasions **cancer can abut a cyst.** In this case an infiltrating ductal carcinoma (I) was adjacent to a benign cyst (C).

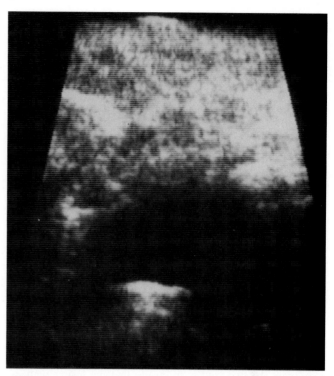

FIG. 16-11. Equipment should be appropriate for imaging the breast tissue, and tissues deep to a lesion should be visible before accurate evaluation is possible. In this case the lesion was at the bottom of the field, and the apparent deep bright reflection was an artifact. The mass was a solid cancer that was shadowing.

ous echoes. The lowest power needed to penetrate the tissues is generally desirable and the compensation algorithms should be set so that similar structures, regardless of depth, are displayed with the same signal levels. The operator must be aware that too little power risks making solid lesions appear cystic.

Because most of the tissues that must be imaged are in a zone from, and including, the skin to a few centimeters deep the transducer must be focused to this zone. If the focal zone cannot be adjusted, an offset should be used. Many transducers have a built-in fluid offset, or special pads are available that can be placed between the transducer and the breast. A soft interface with the breast will help to avoid displacement of the lesion from beneath the sound beam by the pressure of the transducer. It has been our experience that there is no preferred system for breast evaluation. The operator must become comfortable with the unit that is used and be able to use it to accurately distinguish a cyst from a solid mass.

PERFORMING BREAST ULTRASOUND

With hand-held units, patients should be supine when scanned, and efforts should be made to flatten the breast tissues overlying the lesion against the chest wall as much as possible. This reduces the amount of tissue through which the sound must travel to and from the lesion and reduces the distortion caused by passage through too much tissue. This is accomplished by rolling the patient to one side or the other, depending on the part of the breast to be studied, so that gravity thins the part to be examined. Usually the extension of the ipsilateral arm behind the head will aid in further thinning the breast. A wedge-shaped support behind the patient can facilitate oblique positioning.

Scans are then performed in standard sagittal and transverse planes of the area in question although we, ultimately, scan in whatever orientation provides the best visualization of the area in question. Breast tissues are tethered to one another, but the relative elasticity of these relationships permits easy movement when pressure is applied to the breast, and the pressure of the transducer may displace the lesion from under the sound beam. Soft stand-off pads help to avoid such displacement. It is frequently helpful to stabilize the lesion between two fingers of the nonscanning hand. This also permits a physical assessment of the tissues as they are scanned, as noted in Equipment.

Once visualized, the lesion should be completely evaluated in both planes. Some advocate imaging in a radial fashion with the long axis of the transducer aligned with the nipple. The tissues immediately abutting the lesion should be carefully assessed. In our experience, intracystic cancer is quite rare, but cancers adjacent to cysts do occasionally occur (Fig. 16-10). One should avoid interpreting a lesion if it is at the back edge of the scanned field. Valuable information is lost and mistakes can be made (Fig. 16-11) unless all the contiguous tissues are seen. A physician skilled in mammography should supervise (if not directly perform) the ultrasound examination. This is especially true if a nonpalpable, mammographically detected lesion is being assessed. Care must be exercised to carefully

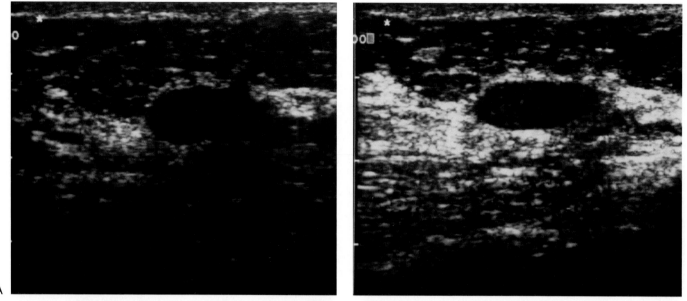

FIG. 16-12. The gain settings must be properly adjusted. This mass in a 42-year-old woman appears to be anechoic **(A)**. At higher gain, internal echoes are visible **(B)**. The mass proved to be a fibroadenoma.

coordinate the two studies to ensure that the lesion seen by ultrasound corresponds to that found by mammography as noted in the section on Appropriate Use of Ultrasound.

The presence of low-amplitude internal echoes is important in breast lesion analysis. Such echoes frequently indicate the difference between a cyst and a solid lesion, including some cancers. Solid lesions of the breast, includ-

ing malignancies, can have all the characteristics of a cyst, including posterior acoustic enhancement. Internal echoes may be the only differentiating factor. Direct involvement by the radiologist is important to avoid the possibility that a technologist may inadvertently "clean up" these internal echoes by altering scan factors and make a solid lesion appear to be a cyst (Fig. 16-12). If there is any question as

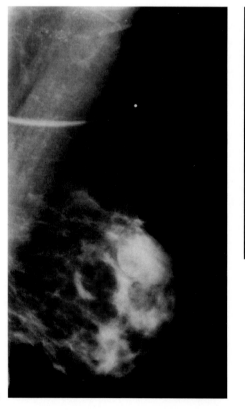

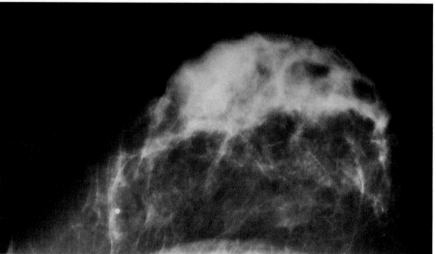

FIG. 16-13. Pneumocystography can be used to confirm on mammography what has been aspirated by ultrasound. Indeterminate densities were noted in the superolateral right breast on the mediolateral oblique (MLO) **(A)** and craniocaudal (CC) **(B)** projections. *Continued.*

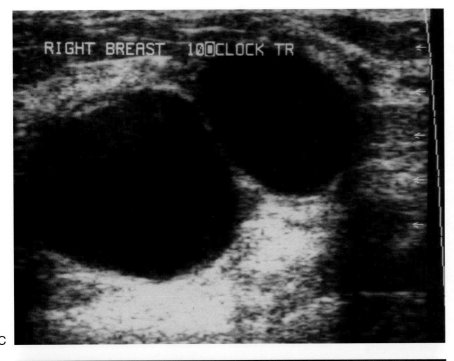

C

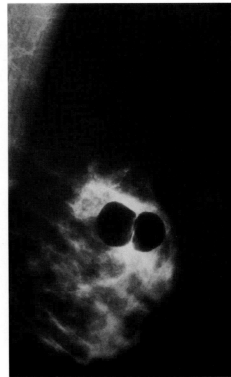

D

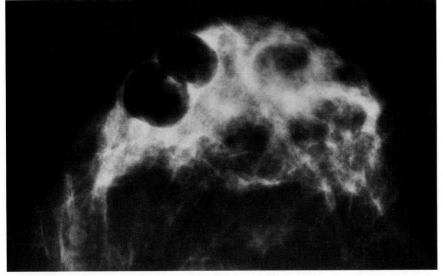

E

FIG. 16-13. *Continued.* Because of patient discomfort, these were aspirated under ultrasound guidance **(C)**, and air was introduced, not quite replacing the aspirated fluid. Postaspiration mammography in the MLO **(D)** and CC **(E)** projections clearly demonstrates the air-filled cysts and that these cysts were the cause of the pre-aspiration densities.

to whether a lesion is a cyst, the lesion should be aspirated and mammography repeated to demonstrate resolution of the lesion. If possible, we introduce into the aspirated cyst slightly less air than the amount of fluid that was removed through the aspirating needle to define on the postprocedure mammogram precisely what had been aspirated (Fig. 16-13). An alternative is to leave the needle through the aspirated lesion to identify the area on the postaspiration mammogram. Cyst aspiration is easily accomplished using ultrasound or mammographic guidance (see Chapter 21).

One must exercise great care in ultrasound evaluation of the breast. The particular characteristics of the ultrasound equipment being used should be fully understood in order to differentiate true echoes from reverberation or noise. It is a

good idea to study the ultrasound features of specific lesions that will be aspirated or biopsied to learn how cysts and solid lesions appear on a particular ultrasound system.

Acoustic Properties of Breast Tissues

The ultrasound characteristics of normal breast structures and pathologic lesions represent relative phenomena. An echogenic structure in one tissue background may appear relatively hypoechoic in different surroundings. Because normal breast tissue is extremely scattering and attenuating, a solid mass that is relatively homogeneous in its acoustic properties may facilitate the movement of sound more readily than the surrounding normal tissues, which are them-

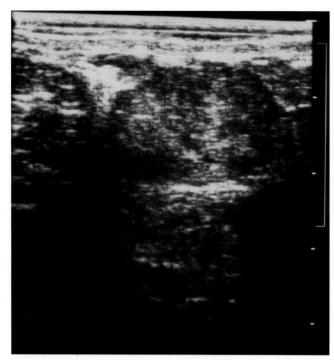

FIG. 16-14. Solid masses can produce posterior acoustic enhancement. This **fibroadenoma** not only exhibits refractive shadowing at its margins, but there is also better transmission of sound through its homogeneous structure than through the surrounding tissues, producing relative posterior enhancement.

selves more scattering and attenuating. Therefore, tissues behind some solid lesions will produce brighter echoes than the adjacent parenchyma. This phenomenon is most pronounced when the lesion is round and, acting as an acoustic lens, focuses transmitted sound and the sound reflected from the deeper tissues. As a consequence of this phenomenon, many benign as well as some malignant solid breast masses, when round or oval and sharply marginated, produce sonic effects similar to those of cysts with enhanced through-transmission of sound. Many demonstrate refractive shadowing at the edges (Fig. 16-14). Frequently the only ultrasound characteristic that distinguishes a solid lesion from a cyst is the presence of low-amplitude internal echoes.

The Normal Breast

The normal breast (Fig. 16-15) has an inhomogeneous echo texture that varies with the proportion and distribution of fibrous, adenomatous, ductal, and adipose tissues. The nipple is hypoechoic and may attenuate sound. Because of the perpendicular orientation of ducts and fibrous supporting structures beneath the nipple, sound penetration of the subareolar region may be reduced. Positioning the transducer obliquely to the nipple areolar complex often produces a more favorable angle of incident sound, enabling assessment of the subareolar tissues.

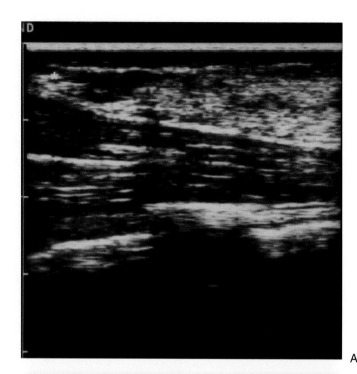

A

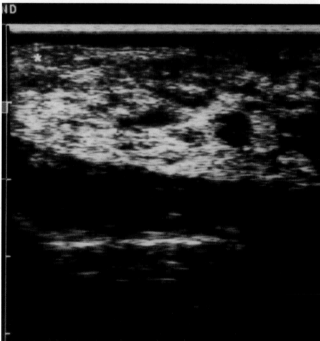

B

FIG. 16-15. Breast tissue is heterogeneously echogenic on ultrasound. These are scans in two separate areas. **(A)** A scan obtained near the axillary tail of the breast. The pectoralis muscles are quite prominent. The tightly packed echoes represent an area of dense tissue by mammography and presumably represent fibroglandular structures. Moving closer to the nipple **(B)** the heterogeneity of the tissues increases, presumably due to large duct diameters. It is impossible to tell whether the hypoechoic structures are breast tissue or masses. This is why scanning for breast cancer is not very sensitive or specific.

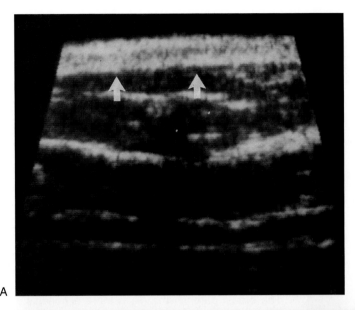

A

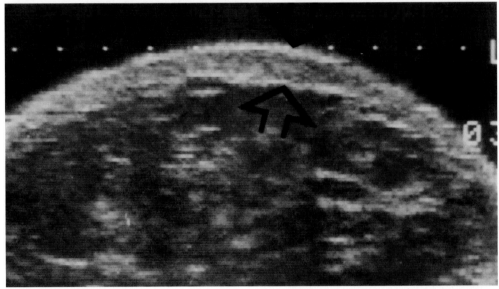

B

FIG. 16-16. The **normal skin (A)** is visible on ultrasound as a hypoechoic structure with a prominent anterior reflection at the skin-transducer interface. There is a second strong reflection at the dermal/subcutaneous fat interface (*arrows*) with dermal echoes between the two. **Skin thickening (B)** is visible by ultrasound with the separation of the two specular reflections (*arrows*).

A bright specular reflection is seen at the transducer-skin interface. The thickness of the normal skin (Fig. 16-16A) ranges from 0.5 to 2.0 mm, and abnormal thickening is visible by ultrasound (Fig. 16-16B) (27). The skin produces low-level echoes with a uniform texture. A second specular reflection occurs at the dermal–subcutaneous fat interface. When thickened, there is increased separation between the two specular reflections that is visible by ultrasound. The causes of skin thickening (edema or tumor in the lymphatics) cannot be distinguished by ultrasound (28).

Beneath the second prominent echo layer is the subcutaneous fat that surrounds the parenchymal cone of the breast (Fig. 16-17). It is a relatively hypoechoic zone whose thickness varies depending on the breast composition. Unlike fat elsewhere in the body, fat in the breast is less echogenic than the mammary parenchyma. Because echogenicity is a relative phenomenon, fat appears hypoechoic relative to the fibroglandular elements that present numerous acoustical mismatches and reflecting surfaces. In the subcutaneous tissues this presents little problem, but fat within the breast parenchyma itself can mimic hypoechoic masses, and care must be taken to avoid mistaking normal fat for a lesion. Unlike masses that have margins, collections of fat generally taper gradually as one scans through them, and they meld into the surrounding tissues. The margins of masses usually have abrupt transitions with the surrounding tissues.

The normal parenchyma varies greatly. Attempts have been made to link ultrasound tissue patterns to mammographic patterns, and to some extent this is possible (29). Fat breasts have large ovoid areas of hypoechoic tissues interspersed with more echogenic planes of Cooper's fibrous ligaments. More closely packed echoes are found in women with the American College of Radiology Breast Imaging Reporting and Data System pattern 3 (Wolfe's P2 pattern seen as fibronodular

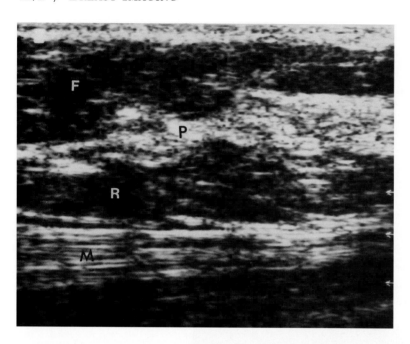

FIG. 16-17. Fat in the breast is hypoechoic. The subcutaneous fat (F) and the retromammary fat (R) in front of the pectoralis muscle (M) are hypoechoic. The breast parenchyma (P) is more echogenic in this section in a 46-year-old woman.

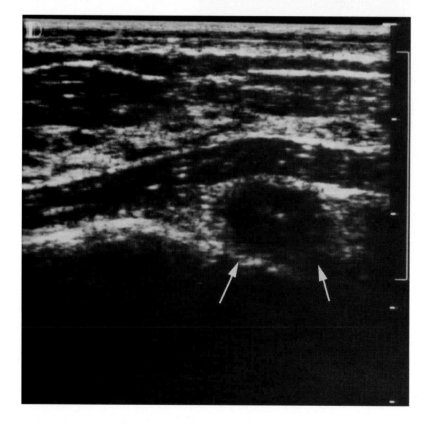

FIG. 16-18. A rib in cross section (*arrows*) is hypoechoic or can cause posterior shadowing. It can look like a mass. Note that it lies beneath the pectoralis muscle, indenting it from behind.

densities on mammograms), and breasts that are radiodense with large volumes of fibrous connective tissue may be difficult to penetrate, with many areas of blocked sound transmission. Tissue parenchymal pattern identification by ultrasound is academic, because virtually all women who have ultrasound should have had a preceding mammogram, and the pattern will already be known. Furthermore, mammographic parenchymal patterns currently have little practical signifi-

cance, although there has been some renewed interest in using the patterns as risk factors (see Chapter 12).

It is important for the practitioner to be aware that fat significantly attenuates and scatters sound and that this may make evaluation of the breast that is primarily composed of fat more difficult (30). Often such breasts are large, and their size and the sound-attenuating property of intervening tissue make it difficult to accurately assess lesions that are less than

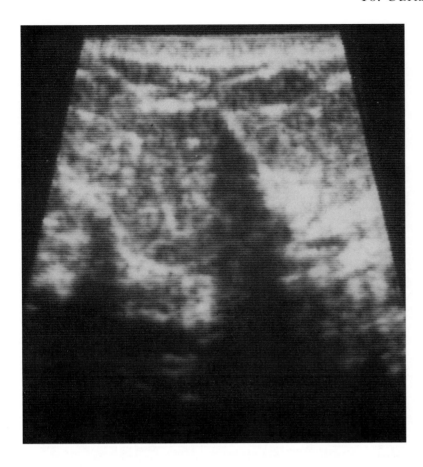

FIG. 16-19. Cooper's ligaments can cause shadowing. The incident sound can glance off the steep slopes of these connective tissue planes, resulting in shadowing behind. Changing the angle of the sound beam will eliminate this shadowing from normal ligaments.

1 cm in size if they are more than 3 to 4 cm deep. Every effort should be made to reduce the thickness of the breast in the region being evaluated by ultrasound.

Behind the mammary parenchyma is a second zone of hypoechogenicity that is of variable thickness. This is the retromammary fat. It is immediately anterior to multiple, horizontal fan-like linear reflections that define the pectoralis musculature, which is slightly more echogenic than fat and usually defined by specular reflections from fascial planes. The ribs are visible as hypoechoic structures that indent the pectoralis muscle from behind (Fig. 16-18). Along the sternum the cartilage and echogenic marrow cavity may produce a target appearance. Ribs seen in cross section should not be mistaken for intramammary lesions. They are distinguished as ribs, because muscle can be seen overlying them and separating them from the mammary parenchyma. By rotating the transducer, their linear structure can be more readily appreciated.

Cooper's ligaments coursing through the breast can create problems in ultrasound evaluation. These sloping planes of fibrous tissue cause scattering and refraction of sound and can produce shadowing (Fig. 16-19) that is difficult to distinguish from the shadowing caused by scirrhous carcinoma. By angling the transducer, a more perpendicular angle of sound is achieved, and the tissues behind the tents of Cooper's ligaments can be evaluated.

It bears reiteration that the ultrasound appearance and morphologic characteristics of a particular lesion are related

not only to the lesion's own composition but also to the properties of the normal tissue surrounding it. This probably accounts for the relative sonolucency of fat and the fact that solid masses may produce significant posterior acoustic enhancement. One must also pay close attention to the internal echo pattern of breast lesions. Cellular tumors may display only low-amplitude internal echoes, and recognition of these will avoid false identification of such a lesion as a cyst.

Calcifications, unless several millimeters in size or extremely numerous and packed closely together, usually cannot be seen in the breast with ultrasound. This is one of the major reasons ultrasound is not useful as a stand-alone screening technique. Even when calcifications are visible on ultrasound, the utility of their evaluation has never been demonstrated. There are anecdotal reports of calcifications, visible on ultrasound, being biopsied successfully under ultrasound guidance.

Ultrasound Analysis of Breast Lesions

In the early development of breast ultrasound it was believed that sonographic criteria could differentiate benign from malignant masses. Kobayashi (31) described a system of analyzing breast masses and defined ultrasound criteria to help diagnose specific lesions (Fig. 16-20). As experience increased, however, the distinctions between benign and malignant became less clear.

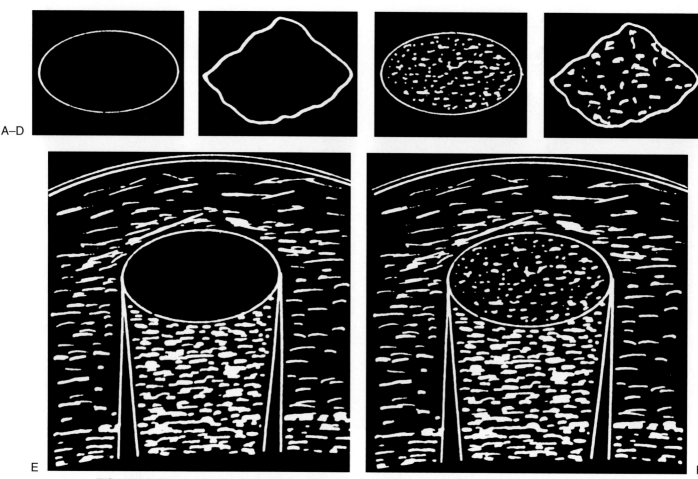

A–D

E   F

FIG. 16-20. The basic elements of the ultrasound analysis of breast lesions. It was originally hoped that ultrasound could be used to distinguish benign masses from malignant. Although there are characteristics that make a lesion much more likely to be benign or more likely to be malignant, if certainty is needed, then biopsy is necessary. Ultrasound is primarily useful for differentiating cysts from solid masses. Masses can be characterized by their shapes, margins, internal echo features, and their effect on the sound passing through and returning to the transducer. The following are general characteristics. The operator must be aware that there is an overlap between features and that benign characteristics can be found in cancers and malignant features can occur with benign lesions.

Benign masses are usually well defined and sharply circumscribed with round or oval shapes **(A)**. Malignant lesions are usually irregular in shape **(B)**. Cysts should have no internal echoes, even at high gain. Debris in cysts may cause reflections, but these reduce the certainty of the diagnosis, and aspiration may be indicated. The likelihood that a lesion is benign is increased if it is sharply defined, ovoid in shape, and has a uniform internal echo texture **(C)**. Most (not all) breast cancers have a heterogeneous internal echo texture **(D)**. Cysts must be anechoic and enhance the through-transmission of sound **(E)**. Pericystic fibrosis may attenuate and scatter the sound, and aspiration may be needed to ensure the diagnosis. Solid lesions that have a fairly uniform composition can also produce posterior acoustic enhancement **(F)** if sound traverses them with less attenuation and scattering than the surrounding breast tissue. If they are round or oval, both cysts and solid masses can cause refractive shadowing at the edges **(E, F)**. Well-defined ovoid masses with uniform internal echoes and enhanced through-transmission are usually benign. Some cancers, however, also have these characteristics. *Continued.*

Although the general morphology of breast lesions can be described by ultrasound, it should be clearly understood that cancer and benign masses can have similar characteristics. Ultrasound can accurately differentiate cysts from solid lesions, but it cannot reliably differentiate benign from malignant solid lesions.

Stavros et al. (5) have attempted to develop additional criteria and organize the characteristics for differentiating benign lesions from malignant. In their classification they developed malignant, benign, and intermediate. Any lesion that had "even a single malignant feature" was excluded from a benign classification. They required all of the criteria to be present to classify a lesion as benign (see Table 16-1).

Although their paper suggested that their study was prospective, it was described as a clinical practice situation in which the reports were retrospectively compiled. The sys-

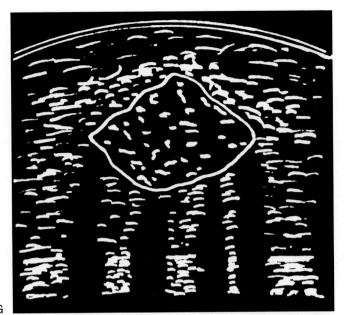

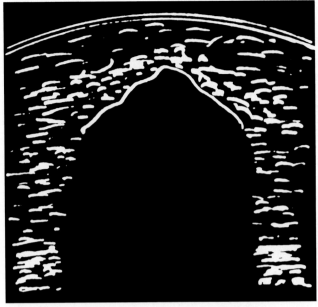

G

H

FIG. 16-20. *Continued.* **Retrotumoral attenuation of sound** is often found with cancers, although benign processes including fibroadenomas and fibrosis can block sound transmission. The shadowing can be heterogeneous **(G)** or complete **(H)**. Both should raise concern.

tem has never been applied in a prospective, blinded study that would be needed to establish the validity of the criteria.

Sonolucent Lesions

The most common sonolucent mass in the breast is the simple cyst. To make an accurate diagnosis of a benign cyst, strict criteria should be observed. Cysts should have sharply defined walls. They may be round, ovoid, or lobulated, and appear solitary or in groups. Cysts should have no internal echoes (Fig. 16-21A). It is possible to image debris suspended in cyst fluid. We have seen several cysts in which material was admixed in the fluid, causing bright echoes that moved in a churning pattern under ultrasound observation (Fig. 16-21B). We can only speculate that this movement was due to convection currents in the fluid heated by insonification. Aspiration of these lesions produced grossly unremarkable fluid. We currently suggest that lesions that are

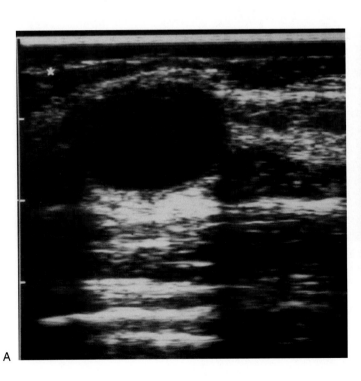

A

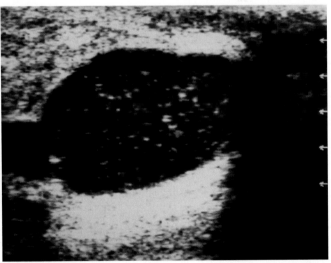

B

FIG. 16-21. (A) A **typical cyst** by ultrasound. **(B) A cyst with very bright internal echoes.** Under real-time observation, the echoes moved in a churning motion. *Continued.*

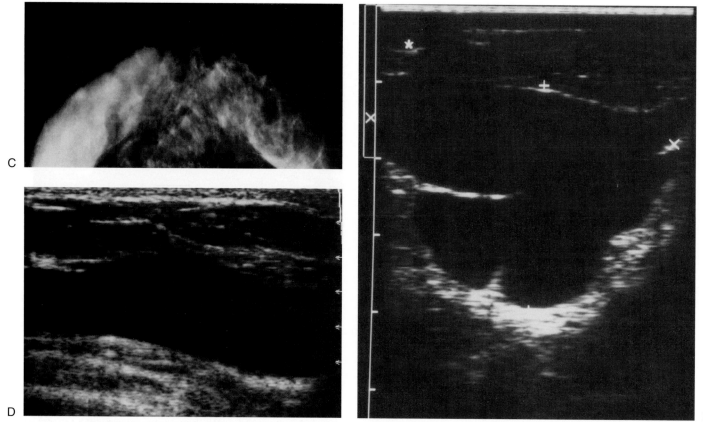

FIG. 16-21. *Continued.* The fluid appeared grossly unremarkable at aspiration. **(C)** The uniformly dense, elongated mass, seen along the medial side on this craniocaudal view is a large, patulous, anechoic cyst that is larger than the field of view, as seen by ultrasound **(D)**. **(E) Septated cysts** have no known clinical significance. They are likely due to distention of a lobule with preservation of some of the acinar architecture.

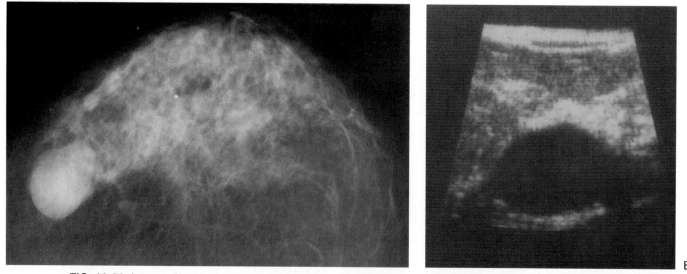

FIG. 16-22. Intracystic cancer is rare, and it is even less likely that it would not be evident by mammography or ultrasound. The sharply marginated, lobulated mass on the craniocaudal projection **(A)** has benign features. By ultrasound it was a simple cyst **(B)** but was aspirated because it was solitary and prominent (not scientific criteria). *Continued.*

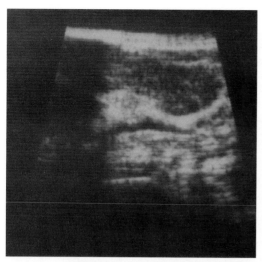

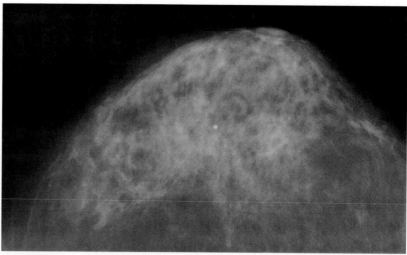

C

D

FIG. 16-22. *Continued.* The postaspiration ultrasound revealed minimal residual fluid **(C)**, and there was no mass on the postaspiration mammogram **(D)**. Nevertheless, the cytology of the fluid was suspicious, and when the cyst fluid reaccumulated, surgical excision revealed an invasive cancer that was invading the wall of a benign cyst. This is the only instance that we know of in which this has happened and it should not be considered a standard of care.

thought to be cysts but contain internal echoes be aspirated to confirm their benign origin, although there are no data that support this approach, and their management should be individually determined.

Many cysts are not round or oval but are lobulated. They may be tensely distended or patulous (Fig. 16-21C, D). Septations in cysts do not appear to have any significance (Fig. 16-21E). These are likely due to the cyst's origin. Most cysts are merely dilated lobules. The lobule is like a surgical glove blown up like a balloon. Just as the central portion of the glove enlarges and becomes spherical, some lobules dilate with fluid and become spherical cysts. The acini become incorporated in the cyst, and the entire structure becomes round. If the individual acinar structures are retained and dilate with the enlarging cysts, the separations between the acini will appear as septations.

Cysts should have a sharply defined back wall and bright posterior acoustic enhancement. Some cysts do not exhibit posterior enhancement, probably because of the scattering and attenuation from tissues lying between them and the transducer, such as pericystic fibrosis, that attenuate the beam so that the combination of attenuation from the fibrosis and the enhanced transmission from the cyst results in isoechogenicity behind the cyst. If there is any question, aspiration can eliminate the concern.

The primary importance of ultrasound is its ability to determine that a lesion represents a cyst. Ultrasound is reported to be 95% to 100% accurate in this regard if all criteria are met (32,33). Although possible, it is rare to have a simple cyst involved with cancer and not have the cancer be detected by mammography or ultrasound (Fig. 16-22). Statistically, if a lesion meets the strict criteria for a cyst, this finding can be considered diagnostic.

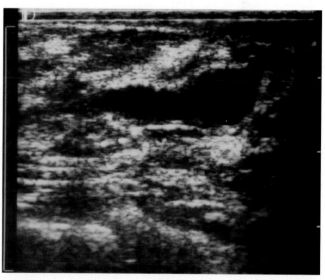

FIG. 16-23. As expected, **ectatic ducts** are tubular, as seen using ultrasound. This 51-year-old woman had tubular structures in the subareolar region. Ultrasound demonstrated fluid-filled ectatic ducts converging on the nipple.

Duct Ectasia

Duct ectasia has a variable appearance. If the duct is filled with fluid, it will be sonolucent and is indistinguishable from an elongated cyst (some cysts are actually cystically dilated ducts) (Fig. 16-23). Old cellular debris may accumulate in the duct forming a paste-like material that is hypoechoic on ultrasound. The diagnosis is readily reached because of the characteristic tubular appearance of the structure.

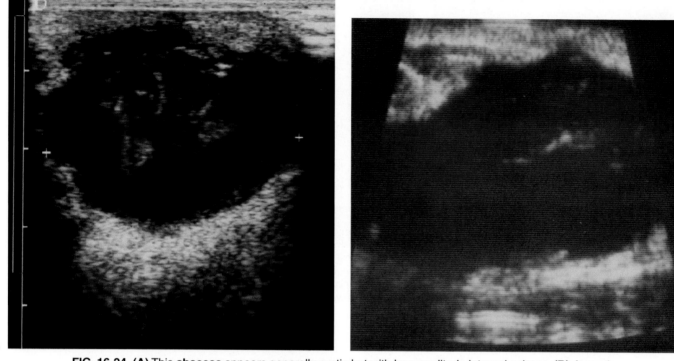

FIG. 16-24. (A) This **abscess** appears generally cystic but with low-amplitude internal echoes. **(B)** A nearly identical appearance is found in this **postsurgical hematoma.** The internal echoes are likely fibrin strands.

Fat Necrosis

Fat necrosis, in the form of post-traumatic oil cysts, can be sonolucent, although the appearance of these fat-containing cysts is variable. Their appearance is so characteristic by mammography that there is no reason to evaluate them with ultrasound (see Chapter 13).

Abscesses and Hematomas

Breast abscesses and hematomas can have similar appearances although the history usually differentiates the two. Both may also be sonolucent (Fig. 16-24), although they usually demonstrate some low-amplitude internal echoes. Some cysts appear to hemorrhage spontaneously. The diag-

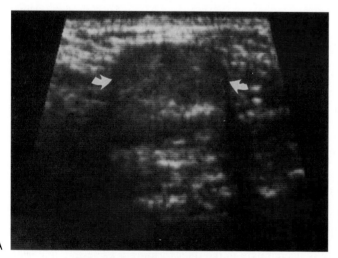

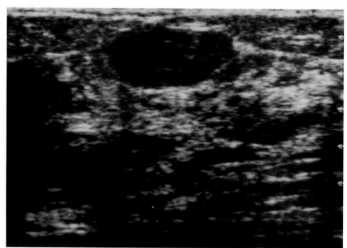

FIG. 16-25. Fibroadenomas can have multiple different characteristics. **(A)** An ovoid, well-defined fibroadenoma with a uniform echo texture and enhanced through-transmission of sound. **(B)** An ovoid, well-defined fibroadenoma that is quite hypoechoic, with low-amplitude internal echoes. The retrotumoral signal is isoechoic. *Continued.*

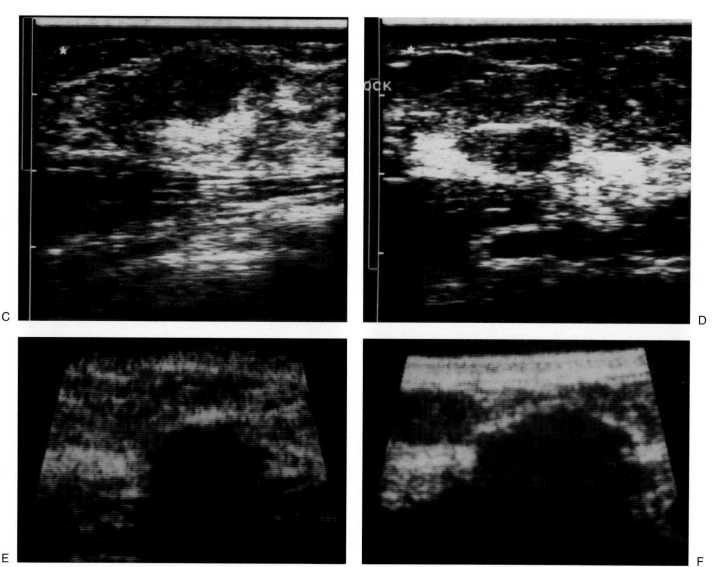

FIG. 16-25. *Continued.* **(C)** An irregularly lobulated fibroadenoma that is isoechoic with the subcutaneous fat but results in enhanced through-transmission of sound. **(D)** An irregularly shaped fibroadenoma with heterogeneous internal echoes. The retrotumoral signal is isoechoic with the surrounding tissue. **(E)** A round fibroadenoma with no internal echoes. It causes posterior shadowing. **(F)** A triangular fibroadenoma with dense posterior shadowing.

nosis can be suggested when there is irregular echogenic material adherent to the wall of the cyst with a sonolucent center. Because an intracystic neoplasm cannot be excluded in this situation, these lesions should probably be aspirated.

Circumscribed Hypoechoic Masses

Fibroadenomas are virtually always hypoechoic and usually sharply marginated (Fig. 16-25). On occasion, fibroadenomas may be isoechoic, and on very rare occasion they may be echogenic (34). In our experience and based on the few reports of circumscribed echogenic masses, these masses have all been fibroadenomas (Fig. 16-26). There have been, however, a number of cases presented at confer-

ences in which echogenic circumscribed masses proved to be cancer. Anecdotally these have been colloid cancers. In our experience, virtually all cancers are hypoechoic or isoechoic. The amplitude of the internal echoes in benign masses is variable (35).

The L/AP Ratio in Benign and Malignant Lesions

Fornage (34) attempted to differentiate fibroadenomas from malignant lesions of the breast using the ratio between the length L of the lesion (the longest diameter parallel to the skin [L]) relative to the length of the axis perpendicular to L (the diameter of the lesion perpendicular to the skin [AP]). The investigators reviewed a series of 100 fibroadenomas

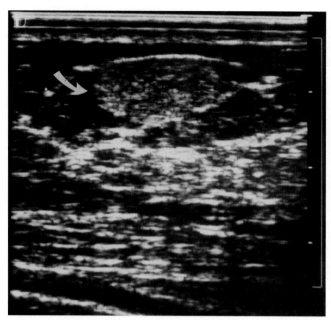

FIG. 16-26. Echogenic, circumscribed masses are extremely rare. This ovoid echogenic mass is a fibroadenoma. There have been a few cases presented at conferences that apparently proved to be colloid cancers.

(including two phylloides tumors). They found that if the long axis of a solid lesion is divided by its shortest diameter (L/AP) (Fig. 16-27), the mean for the fibroadenomas was 1.84 with a range of 0.9 to 4.14. This confirmed the well-known fact that most fibroadenomas are elongated (34). The authors noted that cancers of a similar overall size tended to be more round with an L/AP dimension ranging from 0.66 to 1.33 with a mean of 0.98. In the companion series that compared 28 cancers that were <1 cm to the fibroadenomas, 86% of the fibroadenomas had an L/AP that was above 1.4, whereas all the cancers were below this figure.

As with most tests that attempt to use gross criteria to distinguish benign from malignant lesions, there is overlap. This makes the practical use of the L/AP ratio questionable. Not only were the number of cases in the study small, but, as Fornage acknowledged, benign and malignant solids are likely to always have overlapping characteristics. Although

unusual, cancers can be elongated (Fig. 16-28A) (several of the other cancers depicted by ultrasound in this text have ratios above 1.4) and fibroadenomas can be rounded (Fig. 16-28B). This reduces the clinical usefulness of this observation. We have not seen a fibroadenoma that was vertically oriented (L/AP ratio <1.0), although they likely exist. In our experience, vertical orientation suggests a high probability of cancer (Fig. 16-28C).

Because tissue sampling in the breast is so safe and relatively simple, it is difficult to rely on a test that is less than perfect in separating benign lesions from malignant lesions. As long as women and their physicians are aware of the uncertainties in both the morphologic assessment of a solid lesion by ultrasound and the measurements derived from the ultrasound, the L/AP ratio may be used to provide probabilities, but the L/AP should not be considered diagnostic.

Shapes of Echo Texture

Although fibroadenomas are statistically by far the most common circumscribed hypoechoic masses, the histology of a given lesion cannot be determined by ultrasound. A fibroadenoma (Fig. 16-29A) cannot be distinguished from a phylloides tumor (Fig. 16-29B), infiltrating ductal carcinoma (Fig. 16-29C), or even a metastatic lesion (Fig. 16-29D). Even when the lesion is irregularly shaped it is not possible to distinguish, using ultrasound, certain fibroadenomas (Fig. 16-30A), breast carcinoma (Fig. 16-30B), lymphoma (Fig. 16-30C), an abscess (Fig. 16-30D), or even fat necrosis (Fig. 16-30E).

Even if they display posterior acoustic enhancement, virtually all lesions with true internal echoes are solid. It is not possible to accurately differentiate benign and malignant solid masses from each other except on the statistical basis that benign lesions are much more common than malignant lesions. In a study published by Egan and Egan (36), a lesion that was well-circumscribed by ultrasound was three times more likely to be benign than malignant. Nevertheless, in our own experience, 25% of cancers were sharply marginated by ultrasound (5), and this was true in the Egan series, as well as in an earlier study published by Cole-Beuglet and associates (37).

Cancers that are metastatic to the breast from other sites, such as melanoma, lung, or kidney, are frequently round and

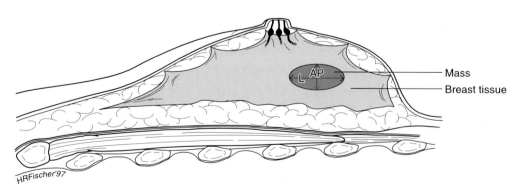

FIG. 16-27. Length-to-height ratio. This schematic demonstrates the measurements used by Fornage (36) to try to distinguish a benign solid lesion from cancer. L is the longest diameter of the lesion measured parallel to the skin and AP is the length of the axis perpendicular to L. Fornage found that most cancers have an L/AP ratio that is less than 1.4.

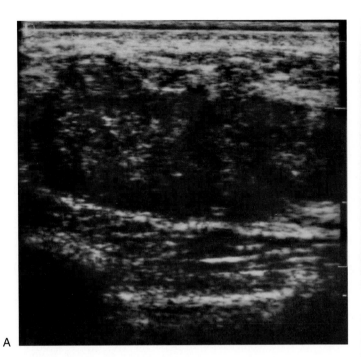

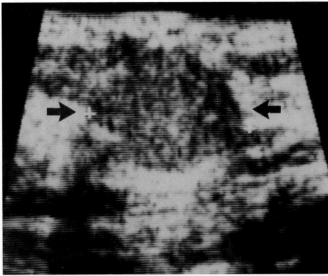

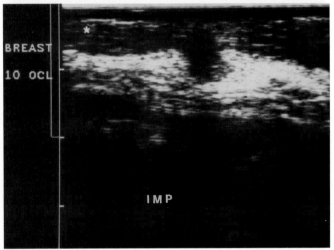

FIG. 16-28. (A) An elongated, lobulated mass that proved to be **invasive ductal carcinoma. (B)** A rounded mass that is a benign **fibroadenoma. (C)** A vertically oriented mass that was **invasive breast cancer** in a 55-year-old woman with a silicone gel implant.

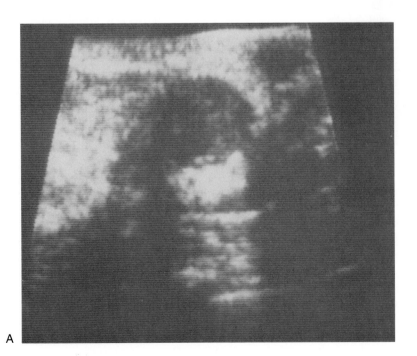

FIG. 16-29. (A) A round, hypoechoic, enhancing mass that is a **fibroadenoma.** *Continued.*

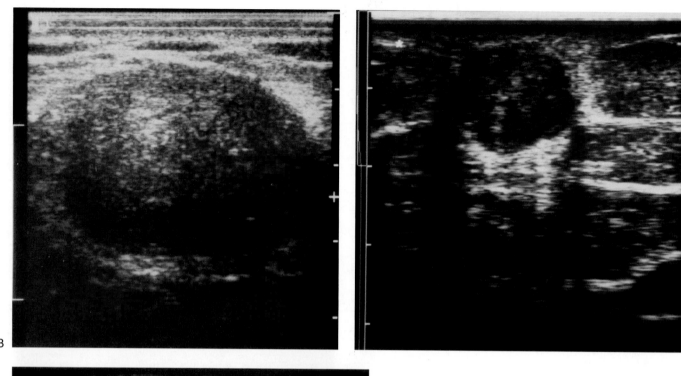

B

C

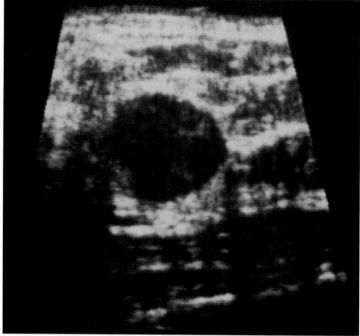

D

FIG. 16-29. *Continued.* **(B)** A round, hypoechoic mass that is a **phylloides tumor.** **(C)** A round, hypoechoic, enhancing mass that is an **invasive ductal carcinoma.** **(D)** A round, hypoechoic, enhancing mass that is **lung cancer, metastatic to the breast.**

often well circumscribed. Lymphomas may have a similar, fairly well-defined appearance. They are also always hypoechoic relative to the surrounding tissues with varying levels and heterogeneity of internal echoes. As with all solid breast lesions, metastatic lesions and lymphomas, when composed of homogeneous cells organized in a round structure, can produce posterior acoustic enhancement. Solitary metastatic lesions occur, but metastases should be considered along with multiple fibroadenomas when multiple solid lesions are found in the breast.

Other well-circumscribed lesions include lipomas, galactoceles, post-traumatic oil cysts from fat necrosis, hamartomas, and phylloides tumors. We have even seen a case of cysticercosis of the breast that formed a round, circumscribed mass.

Lipomas (Fig. 16-31) are difficult to distinguish from the surrounding normal lobules of fat in the breast. The specular reflection of their capsule is the most prominent feature. Their echo texture is similar to that of subcutaneous fat, and they are hypoechoic. Sound is attenuated and scattered sim-

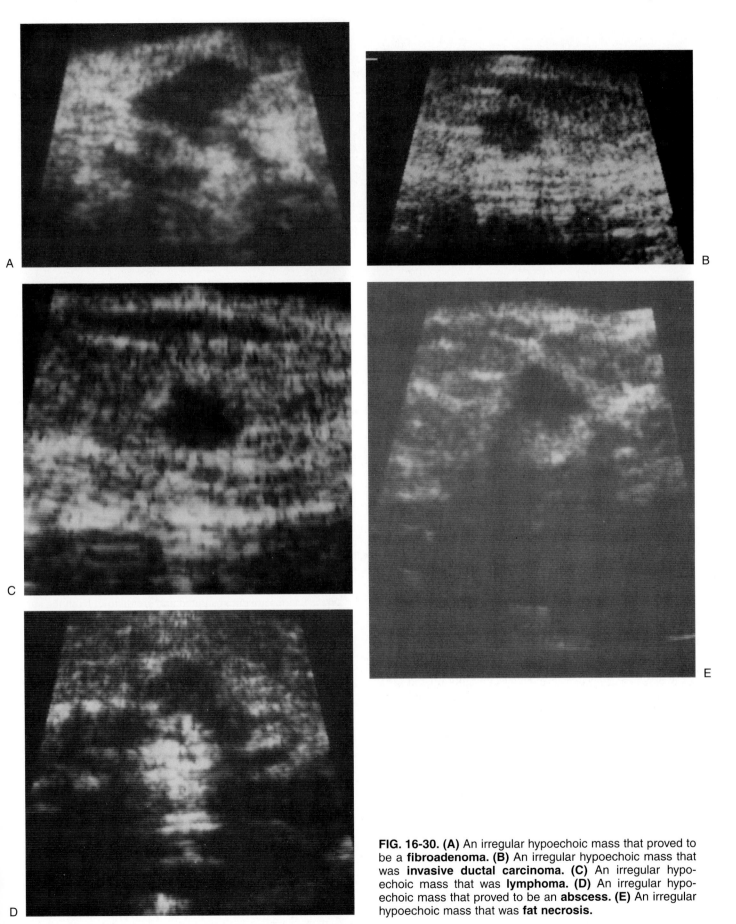

FIG. 16-30. (A) An irregular hypoechoic mass that proved to be a **fibroadenoma. (B)** An irregular hypoechoic mass that was **invasive ductal carcinoma. (C)** An irregular hypoechoic mass that was **lymphoma. (D)** An irregular hypoechoic mass that proved to be an **abscess. (E)** An irregular hypoechoic mass that was **fat necrosis.**

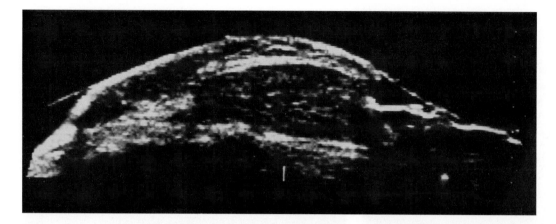

FIG. 16-31. The hypo-echogenicity of this large **lipoma** is indistinguishable from the subcutaneous fat. The features of a lipoma on mammography are so characteristic that there is no reason to evaluate these masses using ultrasound.

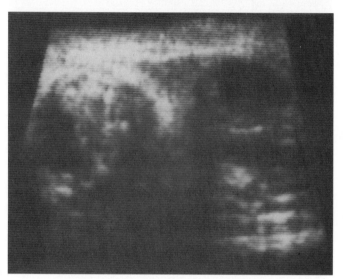

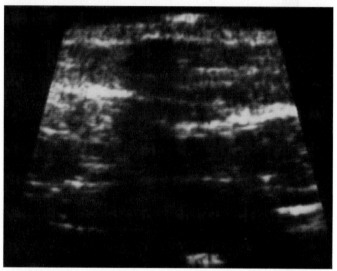

A   B

FIG. 16-32. **Oil cysts** from fat necrosis have variable appearances on ultrasound. **(A)** These are heterogeneous in their echotexture. The one on the left causes shadowing, and the one on the right causes enhancement. **(B)** This **oil cyst** was hypoechoic with a fairly dense posterior acoustic shadow.

ilar to normal subcutaneous and intramammary fat. The lipoma, however, like the oil cyst, is so characteristic by mammography that there is no reason to even evaluate it by ultrasound.

Galactoceles have been variously described as sonolucent or hypoechoic with low-level echoes possibly related to fat globule content. As fluid-filled structures, galactoceles demonstrate posterior acoustic enhancement.

Post-traumatic oil cysts, a fairly common form of fat necrosis, have a variable appearance on ultrasound but may be hypoechoic (Fig. 16-32A). They are invariably well circumscribed and may be sonolucent or hypoechoic with variable through-transmission of sound (Fig. 16-32B). As with all fat-containing lesions, the diagnosis of an oil cyst is usually evident by mammography, and ultrasound is not indicated.

The benign hamartoma (fibroadenolipoma) of the breast contains fibrous elements that may be specular in their reflections, whereas the adenomatous elements produce hypoechoic inhomogeneous structures. The fat in a hamartoma, as elsewhere in the breast, is relatively hypoechoic.

These lesions are encapsulated and are distinct from the surrounding tissues, which may be compressed around them.

The phylloides tumor is fairly uncommon and occasionally malignant. Its ultrasound appearance is similar to that of the fibroadenoma (see Fig. 16-21B). Always hypoechoic, its internal echoes may be fine or coarse, and it has a variable effect on posterior echoes. Usually well circumscribed, on occasion it is difficult to separate from surrounding fat because of its cellularity. There is one report of fluid that was visible by ultrasound in a cleft that is associated with these tumors (38). For all practical purposes, this tumor is indistinguishable by ultrasound from other solid masses.

Variable Compression

Although there has never been proof that it is diagnostically accurate, by exerting variable pressure with the transducer over a lesion, softer masses (cysts and fibroadenomas) that are more likely to be benign and change shape (Fig. 16-33), but harder masses do not deform.

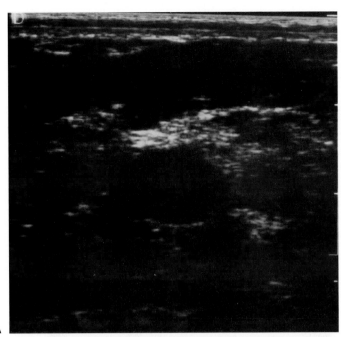

A

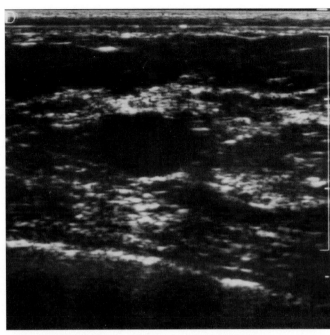

B

FIG. 16-33. Lesions that deform under compression are more likely to be benign. Note how this cyst changes with pressure from pushing on the transducer. With little pressure the cyst is rounder and has a wider cross section **(A)**. With pressure from the transducer, the cyst becomes more elongated with a smaller diameter **(B)**.

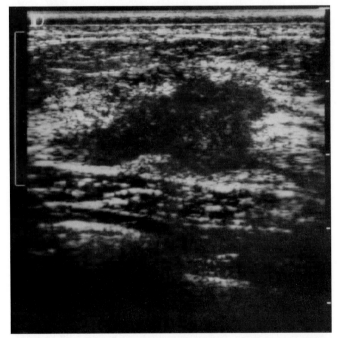

FIG. 16-34. Breast cancers are usually irregular in shape with irregular margins. This **invasive ductal carcinoma** was palpable in a 42-year-old woman with positive axillary lymph nodes.

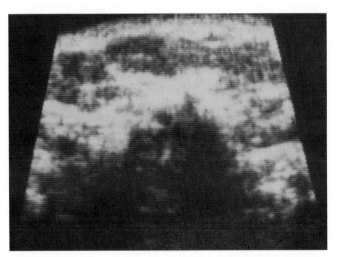

FIG. 16-35. The classic presentation of **breast cancer** on ultrasound is a mass with a triangular anterior margin and dense posterior shadowing, as with this invasive breast cancer. These generally are so characteristic by mammography that ultrasound is rarely indicated except to guide a needle biopsy or localization.

Ill-Defined Hypoechoic Masses

Lesions with ill-defined margins are more likely to be malignant. In our evaluation of 130 breast cancers, greater than 50 percent had irregular margins (Fig. 16-34) (5), and this has been true in most other series. Malignancy should be suspected, especially when the anterior margin of the lesion is somewhat triangular (Fig. 16-35). A solid mass with a tri-

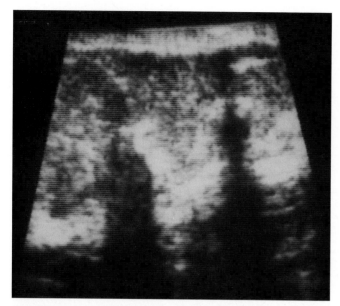

FIG. 16-36. Shadows from **Cooper's ligaments.**

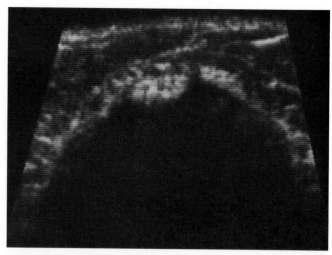

FIG. 16-37. Benign fibrosis can cause dense posterior shadowing, as in this example.

angular anterior margin is almost always malignant. Benign lesions can also have irregular, ill-defined margins.

Lesions That Produce Posterior Acoustic Shadowing

Posterior acoustic shadowing was once believed to be the sine qua non of malignancy. Although this is not the case, careful attention should be paid to lesions that cause partial or complete posterior acoustic shadowing. If a clear-cut benign etiology for such a lesion is not evident, biopsy is warranted. On occasion, ultrasound can be used to tip the balance toward earlier intervention in malignant processes.

Benign lesions, including normal structures, will scatter and attenuate sound, producing a shadow. The tent-like structures of Cooper's ligaments can cause distinct acoustic shadowing because of refraction from the steep angle of incident sound (Fig. 16-36). This shadowing may be indistinguishable from cancer and is one reason among others that screening with ultrasound may be impractical and inaccurate.

Fibrosis, as either a normal pattern (Fig. 16-37) or a postsurgical scar, can produce shadowing that is indistinguishable from cancer. Normal areas of fibrosis are found throughout the breasts but particularly in the upper outer quadrants. These tissues are attenuating and scattering and cause shadowing that can mimic that caused by the desmoplastic response to cancer. If this shadowing is asymmetric and isolated, a biopsy is warranted. If similar shadowing is present in the mirror image area of the contralateral breast, it is more than likely normal fibrosis. Such fibrosis is frequently seen in younger women (teenagers to age 35 years) and when extensive may prevent ultrasound evaluation of the deeper tissues of the breast. Even fibrocystic breast tissue with pericystic fibrosis can cause shadowing (Fig. 16-38).

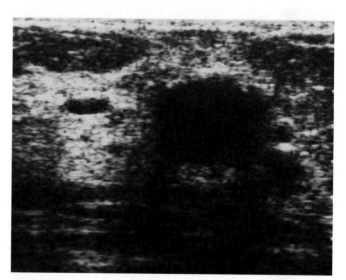

FIG. 16-38. Even a **cyst with pericystic fibrosis** can have a suspicious appearance on ultrasound. This was fibrocystic tissue in a 51-year-old woman.

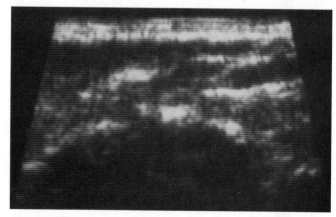

FIG. 16-39. Dense shadowing caused by a **fibroadenoma.**

Fibroadenomas can have a wide-ranging effect on posterior echoes and can cause shadowing themselves (Fig. 16-39). Oil cysts and abscesses can also produce posterior acoustic shadowing.

ULTRASOUND APPEARANCE OF BREAST CANCER

The ultrasound appearance of breast cancer can be similar to that of virtually any benign lesion found in the breast. If attention is not paid to scan factors, subtle internal echoes can be missed and a well-circumscribed cancer can even be mistaken for a cyst.

Breast cancer is always hypoechoic. It is generally irregularly marginated with heterogeneous internal echoes, and there are frequently areas that produce posterior acoustic shadowing

(Fig. 16-40). Thirty-five percent of the time the classic appearance of an irregularly shaped anterior margin with dense posterior shadowing is seen. Even this is not sufficient to establish a diagnosis of breast cancer, however, because any lesion that contains irregular fibrotic tissue can have a similar appearance. Nevertheless, an isolated lesion with this ultrasound appearance should be considered suspicious.

Twenty-five percent of cancers of the breast may exhibit well-defined margins with a lobulated contour. These may mimic the appearance of a fibroadenoma. Frequently the diagnosis of cancer is strongly suggested when the margins of the lesion appear to merge with or "invade" the surrounding tissue. Areas of shadowing increase the degree of concern.

On occasion, a cancer can be extremely well defined with subtle low-amplitude internal echoes. The ultrasound may appear similar to that of a fibroadenoma and rarely has the anechoic appearance of a cyst. Evaluation of a lesion in the

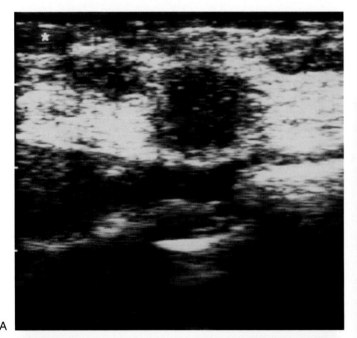

A

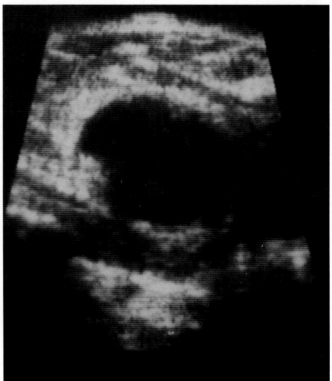

B

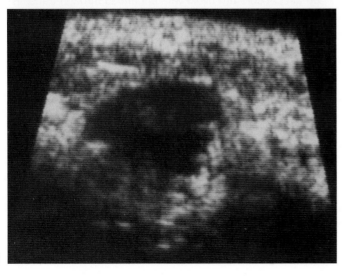

C

FIG. 16-40. Breast cancer can have many appearances on ultrasound. These are all invasive ductal cancers. **(A)** Typical invasive breast cancer by ultrasound. It is irregular in shape with ill-defined margins. **(B, C)** Breast cancer can be lobulated. *Continued.*

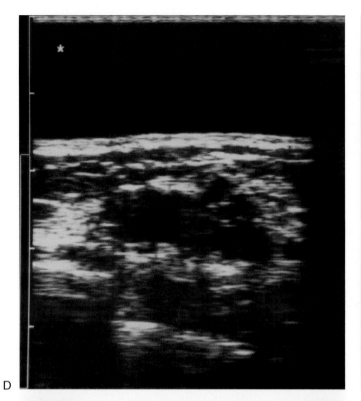

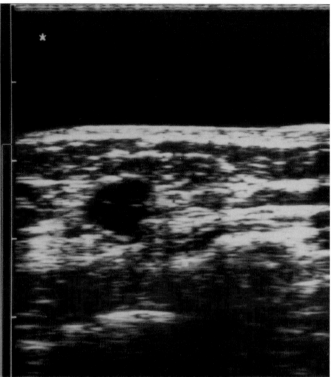

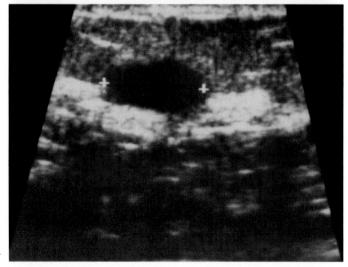

FIG. 16-40. *Continued.* **(D)** Breast cancer can be elongated. **(E)** Breast cancer with angular margins. **(F)** Some breast cancers are ovoid with enhanced through-transmission of sound.

subareolar region should be done with some trepidation, because the vertically oriented fibrous structures in this area can distort the information. Although many believe that well-circumscribed cancers are indolent medullary lesions, this is in fact not the case. Round, "garden-variety," lethal infiltrating ductal carcinoma is the usual cause of circumscribed cancer and can be indistinguishable from other lesions.

Algorithm for Breast Ultrasound

The use of ultrasound should ultimately be based on its efficacy for the individual patient and the particular situation. Our approach has evolved through studies and experi-

ence as well as the data available in the literature. Ultrasound is without demonstrable risk and is easy to perform. It does increase the cost to the patient and the health care system in general; therefore, it should be used only when the information obtained will directly and uniquely influence the care of the patient.

Nonpalpable Mammographically Detected Mass

The primary use of ultrasound is to determine whether a solitary mass, detected by mammography, is cystic or solid. Because the risk of axillary nodal metastasis and the associated diminished survival doubles for tumors >1 cm, we believe that solitary masses approaching this size should be investigated by ultrasound, aspiration, or biopsy. If the lesion is sharply marginated, contains no internal echoes, and has enhanced sound transmission, the diagnosis of a cyst can be made confidently, and the literature and our experience would suggest that no further intervention is required. If a solid lesion is demonstrated by ultrasound, then the decision to pursue further evaluation should be made in conjunction with the clinical situation, because ultrasound cannot reliably differentiate benign from malignant solid lesions.

Palpable Mass

The primary role for breast ultrasound is the evaluation of lesions that are not clinically evident, as a complement to mammography, and as a guide for needle procedures (38). The use of ultrasound in the management of palpable lesions is somewhat more controversial. The use of ultrasound for palpable lesions is cost-effective if it is coordinated with clinical decisions. As with any test, the decision to use ultrasound should be determined by the likelihood that its results will influence clinical management. If a palpable lesion is of sufficient concern to the patient or her physician that it will be aspirated or removed, regardless of the imaging analysis, then the use of ultrasound will produce an unjustified expense since the majority of these lesions will be cysts, and a cyst will be diagnosed and "treated" at the same time by clinically guided needle aspiration. If the demonstration of a cyst by ultrasound will result in no further intervention and aspiration will be avoided, its use is clinically and economically valuable as long as it does not cost more than a clinically guided aspiration.

It has been our experience that many women prefer that a palpable mass be eliminated. The majority of such masses are cysts that are easily aspirated by the referring physician after mammography. Thus, diagnosis and treatment are accomplished in a single step. The performance of ultrasound only adds a superfluous study and unnecessary expense unless aspiration is not desired. If clinically guided aspiration fails to produce fluid or resolve the mass, ultrasound can be useful. Using this approach, only a small percentage of palpable masses that defy clinically guided aspiration will require ultrasound. Aspiration may fail due to the thickness of the surrounding fibrotic tissue or the presence of fluid that is too viscid for the gauge of the needle used. The demonstration of a cyst by ultrasound makes it possible to be somewhat more aggressive in aspiration; moreover, when ultrasound guides repeat aspiration, many such lesions can be resolved without surgery.

As more and more women receive their breast evaluations from primary care physicians (PCP), who have little experience with breast problems, the use of ultrasound to evaluate palpable abnormalities has increased. Although there are no prospective, scientifically derived data, we have seen cases in which, anecdotally, the ultrasound demonstration of a suspicious solid mass may have led to earlier intervention of a palpable mass that was not thought by the PCP to be particularly suspicious. Although we do not advocate ultrasound of a palpable abnormality as a standard of care, it may be helpful in assisting clinical management.

USE OF ULTRASOUND FOR EVALUATING YOUNGER WOMEN

In the past, guidelines for breast cancer screening had suggested a baseline study at age 35 years. This was not actually based on data (since none of the screening trials included these women) but on the belief that it was desirable to have a baseline exam for future comparison obtained at a time when breast cancer is unlikely. In fact, obtaining a baseline study before 40 years is no longer supported by the American Cancer Society. Liberman et al. (40) have shown, however, that the detection rate of breast cancers by mammography for women aged 35 to 39 years is the same as for asymptomatic women aged 40 to 45 years (see Chapter 4). Although women at these ages have not been included in the randomized, controlled trials of screening, it is likely that they can benefit from earlier detection.

The role of mammography among younger women (<35 years) is less clear. Some have advocated the use of mammography in these women (41), but its efficacy has never been documented. A few studies have suggested little benefit (42). In our own review we were able to image most breast cancers using mammography in a group of 31 women under 35 years (43). Because we believe mammography may contribute to the clinical management of these women, we will perform mammograms on the few women with signs or symptoms suggesting breast cancer who are 28 years old or older. This protocol is based on our own anecdotal experience, however, and should certainly not be considered a standard of care.

Since the risk of radiation induction of breast cancer is related to the age at which the radiation is sustained (44), however, and it is preferable to avoid breast irradiation among teenage women and women in their 20s, we try to avoid mammography in younger women. The younger the woman, the higher the potential risk from radiation. For women older than 40 years, the risk from radiation is extremely low and may no longer exist at any level of exposure (45), but in younger women, there is likely a finite (although small) risk. Among younger women one must balance the exposure to the radiation against the benefit to be derived from the study. Since mammography is not sufficiently accurate to safely distinguish between benign and malignant palpable masses, its role in analyzing palpable lesions is limited. Since mammography is primarily useful for screening, its use at any age should be guided by the probability of detecting clinically occult breast cancer.

Among teenage women and women in their early 20s, breast cancer is extremely rare. Fewer than 0.3% of the annual total of 182,000 breast cancers occur in women under age 30 (500 to 600 cases). In these very young women, even the very low radiation risk may outweigh any benefit. This does not mean that mammography is not useful in caring for younger women with breast problems; it only means that there are no prospective data that support the use of mammography for screening younger women (<40 years of age). Because mammography cannot exclude breast cancer, a palpable mass must be dealt with clinically, and because there are no data to support screening women under 40 years of age, the value of mammography in these women is only anecdotal. Anecdotal experience may be reasonable to follow for an individual practice if there are no objective, prospective studies to rely on. Nevertheless, anecdotes are not sufficient to determine a national standard of care, and until such objective data are available, mammography in younger women should not be considered a standard, but dictated by individual experience. For the same reasons, any decision to biopsy a palpable mass in the breast of a woman in this age group, as in older women, remains a clinical decision.

It can be argued that imaging of any type is not useful for women <35 years of age with a palpable abnormality. Because most true masses in women under this age are likely to be fibroadenomas, even the use of ultrasound is questionable. If, however, the demonstration of a cyst will result in deferred further intervention, ultrasound is useful. If imaging is requested, we perform ultrasound for cyst/solid differentiation and do not proceed to mammography if ultrasound successfully confirms and defines the mass. If the mass is not delineated, we obtain single-view oblique mammograms to look for associated calcifications, architectural distortion, or a mass to assist in the ultimate clinical decision to intervene.

ULTRASOUND AND THE FUTURE

Ultrasound had undergone preliminary development and investigation in the 1950s through the early 1970s and evolved rapidly after Bailar's article on radiation risk (46). Kobayashi and colleagues (47), Jellins and associates (48), and others provided idealistic descriptions of the various appearances of different types of lesions seen by ultrasound that seemed specific and could categorize benign and malignant lesions. Whole-breast systems were developed to permit evaluation of the entire breast by sonography, and the criteria that had been derived were applied to these systems (49). As larger numbers of women were scanned, however, the hoped-for sharp demarcation between benign and malignant characteristics began to blur. Kopans and coworkers (8) demonstrated that only 35% of malignant lesions produced the shadowing that had been thought to be diagnostic of cancer. Furthermore, 25% of cancers were sharply marginated on ultrasound evaluation, and 12% even demonstrated retrotumoral acoustic enhancement. These latter characteristics were previously thought to indicate benign processes. The overlap between benign and malignant characteristics has been confirmed by other investigators (38,50). In a series reported by Jackson and colleagues (35),

144 masses were interpreted on sonography as fibroadenomas. Among the 59 that underwent excisional biopsy, four proved to be cancer (7%). An additional 26 masses were diagnosed as normal or suspicious, and these proved to be fibroadenomas.

Not only is ultrasound unable to differentiate benign from malignant solid masses with sufficient accuracy to avoid biopsy, but other studies have also demonstrated sonography's inability to detect breast cancer in women who have negative mammography and physical examination. Sickles and associates (7) studied 1,000 women using whole-breast ultrasound and were able to detect only 58% of the 64 biopsy-proven cancers. In this study, ultrasound detected only 48% of cancers that had not yet spread to the axillary nodes. Of the 12 cancers <1 cm, sonography failed to detect 92%. Review of other large series reveals similar data despite differing interpretations. In a similar study by Cole-Beuglet and coworkers (51), ultrasound failed to detect 31% of cancers. Data reported by Egan and Egan (52) reveal a failure to detect cancer in 32% of 31 biopsy-proven cancers.

No well-documented, blinded series has been reported in which lesions have been biopsied only on ultrasound suspicion. In 1,140 women studied in a blind comparison between physical examination, mammography, and ultrasound reported by Kopans and coworkers (6), 36% of cancers were not detected by ultrasound. In this series 94 women had normal physical examination and negative mammography but had abnormalities detected by ultrasound alone. A 3- to 4-year follow-up of these women failed to reveal any cancer.

The preceding studies are fairly old, however, more recent data, noted in Ultrasound for Screening, suggest that newer technology may increase ultrasound's ability to detect cancer. Ultrasound screening needs to be reassessed in large, prospective, blinded studies. The data at this time fail to support the use of ultrasound for screening asymptomatic women to detect cancer. Furthermore, ultrasound should not presently be used to routinely scan women who have negative physical examinations and mammography because it will only raise suspicions and will not detect cancers. This is likely to change as more studies are properly performed to reevaluate ultrasound for screening. Ultrasound should also not be relied on to differentiate benign from malignant solid lesions in a diagnostic setting.

REFERENCES

1. Gordon PB, Goldenberg SL, Chan NHL. Solid breast lesions: diagnosis with US-guided fine-needle aspiration biopsy. Radiology 1993;189:573–580.
2. Gordon PB, Goldenberg SL. Malignant breast masses detected only by ultrasound: a retrospective review. Cancer 1995;76:626–630.
3. Kopans DB, Sickles EA, Feig SA. Malignant breast masses detected only by ultrasound: a retrospective review. Cancer 1996;77:208–209.
4. Kolb TM, Lichy J, Newhouse JH. Detection of Otherwise Occult Cancer with Ultrasound in Dense Breasts: Diagnostic Yield and Tumor Characteristics. Reported at the 82nd Scientific Assembly of the Radiological Society of North America. Chicago, December 4, 1996.

5. Stavros AT, Thickman D, Rapp CL, et al. Solid breast nodules: use of sonography to distinguish between benign and malignant lesions. Radiology 1995;196:123–134.
6. Kopans DB, Meyer JE, Lindfors KK. Whole-breast US imaging: four-year follow-up. Radiology 1985;157:505.
7. Sickles EA, Filly RA, Callen PW. Breast cancer detection with sonography and mammography: comparison using state-of-the-art equipment. AJR Am J Roentgenol 1983;140:843–845.
8. Kopans DB, Meyer JE, Steinbock RT. Breast cancer: the appearance as delineated by whole breast water-path ultrasound scanning. J Clin Ultrasound 1982;10:313.
9. Bassett LW, Kimme-Smith C, Sutherland LK, et al. Automated and hand-held breast US: effect on patient management. Radiology 1987;165:103–108.
10. Cosgrove DO, Bamber JC, Davey JB, et al. Color Doppler signals from breast tumors. Radiology 1990;176:175–180.
11. Schoenberger SG, Sutherland CM, Robinson AE. Breast neoplasms: duplex sonographic imaging as an adjunct in diagnosis. Radiology 1988;168:665–668.
12. Adler DD, Carson PL, Rubin JM, Quinn-Reid D. Doppler ultrasound color flow imaging in the study of breast cancer: preliminary findings. Ultrasound Med Biol 1990;16:553–559.
13. Cosgrove DO, Kedar RP, Bamber JC, et al. Breast diseases: color Doppler US in differential diagnosis. Radiology 1993;189:99–104.
14. Dock W. Duplex sonography of mammary tumors: a prospective study of 75 patients. J Ultrasound Med 1993;2:79–82.
15. Dixon JM, Walsh J, Paterson D, Chetty U. Colour Doppler ultrasonography studies of benign and malignant breast lesions. Br J Surg 1992;79:259–260.
16. Kedar RP, Cosgrove D, McCready VR, et al. Microbubble contrast agent for color Doppler US: effect on breast masses. Work in progress. Radiology 1996;198:679–686.
17. Kehler M, Albrechtsson U. Mammographic fine needle biopsy of non-palpable breast lesions. Acta Rad Diag 1984;25:273.
18. Rizzatto G, Solbiati L, Croce F, Derchi LE. Aspiration biopsy of superficial lesions: ultrasonic guidance with a linear-array probe. AJR Am J Roentgenol 1987;148:623.
19. Parker SH, Jobe WE, Dennis MA, et al. US-guided automated large-core breast biopsy. Radiology 1993;187:507–511.
20. Kopans DB, Meyer JE, Lindfors KK, Bucchianeri SS. Breast sonography to guide aspiration of cysts and preoperative localization of occult breast lesions. AJR Am J Roentgenol 1984;143:489–492.
21. Ganott MA, Harris KM, Ilkhanipour ZS, Costa-Greco MA. Augmentation mammoplasty: normal and abnormal findings with mammography and US. Radiographics 1992;12:281–295.
22. Harris KM, Ganott MA, Shestak K, et al. Detection of silicone leaks: a new sonographic sign. Radiology 1991;181:134.
23. Rosculet KA, Ikeda Dm, Forrest ME, et al. Ruptured gel-filled silicone breast implants: sonographic findings in 19 cases. AJR Am J Roentgenol 1992;159:711–716.
24. DeBruhl ND, Gorczyca, Ahn CY, et al. Silicone breast implants: US evaluation. Radiology 1993;189:95–98.
25. Kopans DB, Swann CA, White G, et al. Asymmetric breast tissue. Radiology 1989;171:639–643.
26. Bassett LW, Kimme-Smith C. Breast sonography. AJR Am J Roentgenol 156;1991:449–455.
27. Kopans DB, Meyer JE, Proppe K. The double line of skin thickening on sonograms of the breast. Radiology 1981;141:485.
28. Meyer JE, Kopans DB. The appearance of the therapeutically irradiated breast on whole breast water-path ultrasound. J Ultrasound Med 1983;2:211.
29. Rubin CS, Kurtz AB, Goldberg BB, et al. Ultrasonic mammographic parenchymal patterns: a preliminary report. Radiology 1979;130:515.
30. Davros WJ, Madsen EL, Zagzebski JA. Breast mass detection by US: a phantom study. Radiology 1985;156:773.
31. Kobayashi T. Ultrasonic detection of breast cancer. Clin Obstet Gynecol 1982;25:409.
32. Sickles EA, Filly RA, Callen PW. Benign breast lesions: ultrasound detection and diagnosis. Radiology 1984;151:467.
33. Hilton SW, Leopold GR, Olson LK, Willson SA. Real-time breast sonography: application in 300 consecutive patients. AJR Am J Roentgenol 1986;147:479.
34. Fornage BD, Lorigan JG, Andry E. Fibroadenoma of the breast: sonographic appearance. Radiology 1989;172:671–675.
35. Jackson VP, Rothschild PA, Kreipke DL, et al. The spectrum of sonographic findings of fibroadenoma of the breast. Invest Radiol 1986;21:34.
36. Egan R, Egan KL. Automated water-path full-breast sonography: correlation with histology of 176 solid lesions. AJR Am J Roentgenol 1984;143:499.
37. Cole-Beuglet C, Soriano RZ, Kurtz AB, Goldberg BB. Ultrasound analysis of 104 primary breast carcinomas classified according to histopathologic type. Radiology 1983;147:191.
38. Cole-Beuglet C, Soriano R, Kurtz A, et al. Ultrasound, x-ray mammography, and histopathology of cystosarcoma phylloides. Radiology 1983;146:481.
39. Jackson VP. The role of US in breast imaging. Radiology 1990;177:305–311.
40. Liberman L, Dershaw DD, Deutch BM, et al. Screening mammography: value in women 35–39 years old. AJR Am J Roentgenol 1993;161:53–56.
41. Donegan WL. Evaluation of a palpable breast mass. N Engl J Med 1992;327:937–942.
42. Williams SM, Kaplan PA, Peterson JC, Lieberman RP. Mammography in women under age 30: is there clinical benefit? Radiology 1986;161:49–51.
43. Meyer JE, Kopans DB, Oot R. Mammographic visualization of breast cancer in patients under 35 years of age. Radiology 1983;147:93–94.
44. Feig SA, Ehrlich SM. Estimation of radiation risk from screening mammography: recent trends and comparison of expected benefits. Radiology 1990;174:638–647.
45. Boice JD, Harvey EB, Blettner M, et al. Cancer in the contralateral breast after radiotherapy for breast cancer. N Engl J Med 1992;326:781–785.
46. Bailar JC. Mammography: a contrary view. Ann Intern Med 1976;84:77–84.
47. Kobayshi T, Takatani O, Hattori N. Differential diagnosis of breast tumors: the sensitivity graded method of ultrasonotomography and clinical evaluation of its diagnostic accuracy. CA Cancer J Clin 1974;33:940.
48. Jellins J, Kossoff G, Reeve TS. Detection and classification of liquid-filled masses in the breast by gray scale echography. Radiology 1977;125:205.
49. Cole-Beuglet C, Goldberg BB, Kurtz AB, et al. Clinical experience with a prototype real-time dedicated breast scanner. AJR Am J Roentgenol 1982;139:905.
50. Egan R, Egan KL. Automated water-path full-breast sonography: correlation with histology of 176 solid lesions. AJR Am J Roentgenol 1984;143:499.
51. Cole-Beuglet C, Goldberg BB, Kurtz BB, et al. Ultrasound mammography: a comparison with radiographic mammography. Radiology 1984;139:693.
52. Egan RL, Egan KL. Detection of breast carcinoma: comparison of automated water-path whole-breast sonography, mammography, and physical examination. AJR Am J Roentgenol 1984;143:493.

Breast Imaging, 2nd ed., by Daniel B. Kopans.
Lippincott–Raven Publishers, Philadelphia © 1998.

CHAPTER 17

The Altered Breast: Pregnancy, Lactation, Biopsy, Mastectomy, Radiation, and Implants

MAMMOGRAPHY DURING PREGNANCY AND LACTATION

The breast undergoes significant changes during pregnancy and lactation. In the first few weeks of a pregnancy, there is a proliferation of ducts and lobules and an increase in secretions, as well as vascular engorgement and breast enlargement. As the pregnancy progresses, the lobular acini enlarge and become filled with colostrum. Several days after delivery and the cessation of placental and luteal hormone production, the pituitary gland begins to secrete prolactin, which causes the lobular acinar cells of the breast to begin to produce true milk. Under the stimulation of nursing, a neurologic loop causes the secretion of prolactin to continue. The neurologic pathway also causes the release of oxytocin from the pituitary, which, in turn, stimulates the hypertrophied myoepithelial cells whose contraction helps to propel the milk down the ducts.

There are few data on the manifestations of pregnancy and lactation on the mammogram. Swinford and associates found very few changes on the mammogram during pregnancy relative to mammograms prior to pregnancy. Three of six women showed no changes, whereas the others had some increase in radiographic density. Among six lactating women, four had no change from their prepregnancy mammograms while two showed increased density (1).

Safety

Although there are no strong data contraindicating the use of mammography during pregnancy or lactation, concerns have been raised over the possible carcinogenic effects of radiation on the epithelium, which is proliferating more actively than usual during this time. We generally avoid routine screening during pregnancy and lactation. If a mammogram is indicated during this period, however, the theoretical risk, which is not quantifiable if it exists at all, should be balanced against the potential benefit. It can be argued that mammography is not of great benefit at this time, because it is primarily a screening technique, and, if a patient has a significant clinical abnor-

mality, it would have to be resolved regardless of the results of the mammogram.

Fetal Radiation Exposure

Concerns have been raised over possible scatter radiation to the fetus. Fortunately, calculations of radiation exposure to the uterus, using dedicated mammography equipment, suggest that there would be virtually no radiation that would reach the fetus. This was determined in the following manner: The primary beam that passes through the film and screen is attenuated by the cassette holder and plate on the other side of the breast. These permit approximately $\frac{1}{5,000}$ (0.002%) of the incident radiation to pass through (approximately 0.2 mR). Assuming the fetus is 10 cm deep within the body under the film holder and plate and because the tissues attenuate the radiation by a factor of 2 (or more) per centimeter, the dose to the uterus would be about $\frac{1}{1,000}$ of the entry dose, in the craniocaudal (CC) projection. Thus, a mammogram performed in the CC projection would result in 0.0002 mR to the uterus.

Scatter radiation would add to this dose. Scatter has been measured at a distance of 12 inches from the breast surface and amounts to 1 mR per film. Assuming that there is no tissue attenuation and that the distance to the uterus is 8 inches, the dose from scatter would be approximately 2.25 mR. The attenuation of 20 cm of tissue is 1 million (i.e., 20 half-value layers). Therefore, the scatter reaching the uterus amounts to about 0.000002 mR.

Because the primary beam is directed away from the uterus in the lateral projection, scatter would be the primary source of exposure to the uterus. Thus, the dose to the uterus for each breast, from a two-view study, amounts to approximately 0.0002 mR (0.0004 mR for both breasts). Natural background radiation exposes the fetus to approximately 2 mR each week. Thus, the potential radiation exposure of a fetus from a mammogram is 5,000 times less than the weekly exposure from normal background radiation (essentially zero) (Webster E, personal communication, 1995).

Efficacy

Mammography can demonstrate abnormalities in pregnant women. What has never been shown is how the results of the mammogram influence the management of the patient. Liberman and colleagues reported on 21 women (ages 24 to 41) who had mammograms during pregnancy (2). All of the women had clinically evident abnormalities. In 21 (91%) there was a lump. One patient had a discharge, and one had diffuse enlargement of one breast with skin thickening. One woman proved to have bilateral cancers, and one had two synchronous lesions in the same breast. The mammogram showed an abnormality in 18 (78%) of the women. The unanswered question remains as to whether the mammogram influences the care of the patient.

ROLE OF ULTRASOUND IN THE MANAGEMENT OF THE SYMPTOMATIC PREGNANT OR LACTATING PATIENT

Because there is no evidence of any detrimental effect from ultrasound, its use during pregnancy and lactation is attractive. As with any breast problem, ultrasound may be of value in differentiating cystic from solid masses. There are no prospective data demonstrating that it can differentiate benign solid masses from malignant solid masses, and it should not be relied on for this purpose. As in the nonpregnant individual, ultrasound can be used to guide needle procedures.

EFFECT OF PREGNANCY ON BREAST CANCER

The data suggest that an early first full-term pregnancy reduces a woman's risk for the subsequent development of breast cancer (see Chapter 3). A woman who has her first child by the age of 18 has one-third to one-half the risk of developing a breast cancer as a woman who had her first full-term pregnancy after the age of 30. Nulliparous women are also at increased risk. Although an early full-term pregnancy does not eliminate the risk of breast cancer, the rapid completion of lobular development likely narrows the window of opportunity during which the proliferating cells of the terminal duct are more likely to be susceptible to damage from a carcinogen.

There appears to be less agreement on the effect of a pregnancy on a growing cancer. Some data suggest that the prognosis is not influenced by pregnancy (3,4). Other studies suggest that a concurrent pregnancy does worsen the prognosis. Women who are diagnosed with breast cancer during pregnancy appear to present with more advanced disease. In the review by Swinford and colleagues of Sloan-Kettering Memorial in New York, 65% of the women who were diagnosed with breast cancer during or within 1 year of a pregnancy had positive nodes at the time of diagnosis (1). This is a higher percentage than the average population.

Guinee and associates, using data from the International Cancer Patient Data Exchange System, evaluated 407 women from the ages of 20 to 29 and found that, for women whose cancer was diagnosed during pregnancy, the risk of dying from breast cancer was 3.26 times greater than for a woman who never had children (5). They also found that the risk decreased by 15% for each year between a pregnancy and the development of the cancer.

Delay in diagnosis has been suggested as an explanation for the poorer prognosis associated with pregnancy. Because the breast may become "lumpier" during pregnancy, lesions may be overlooked or dismissed and intervention delayed so that the patients are ultimately diagnosed with more advanced disease. The significance of this delay, however, is unclear. Mann and colleagues found that 58% of women who had palpable cancer (not associated with pregnancy), whose diagnosis was delayed for 2 months or more after the onset of symptoms, had positive nodes, whereas only 18% had positive nodes when diagnosis was made within 2 months of the onset of symptoms (6). The group at Sloan-Kettering, however, did not find this association in their series of pregnancy-associated cancers, and Guinee found that the poorer prognosis was only slightly affected by the size and stage of the tumor, suggesting that this was not the only explanation. There is no clear information concerning the true effects, if any, of pregnancy on breast cancer survival.

LACTATION

During pregnancy the lobules multiply and enlarge in preparation for lactation. Fat droplets begin to accumulate in the epithelial cytoplasm. The intralobular stromal elements diminish and are crowded out and replaced by the enlarging lobules, which expand to touch one another. Secretions into the acini become profuse with lactation. The multiplication and enlargement of the lobules increase the x-ray attenuation of the breast tissues.

Mammography During Lactation

Mammographically the density of the breast can increase dramatically with lactation. This is most apparent in the breast that was predominantly fat before lactation (Fig. 17-1). Lobular enlargement produces numerous lobulated and coalescent densities on the mammogram (Fig. 17-2). Although never specifically studied, this increase in heterogeneous densities likely reduces the sensitivity of mammography for detecting breast cancer.

The lactating breast produces special problems for breast imaging due to the hypertrophic changes that are present. Screening should probably be avoided while a woman is lactating. The sensitivity of the mammogram for detecting cancer earlier is almost certainly reduced, and some observers have suggested that the breast may be more sensitive to radiation. If imaging is needed to evaluate a palpable abnormality, ultrasound is used to determine if the abnormality is cystic or solid. If a mammogram is indicated, it is preferable

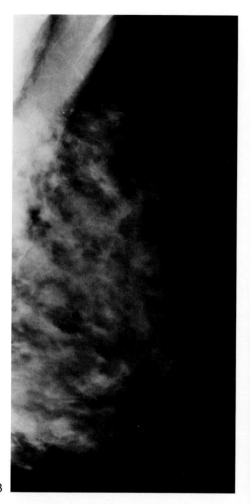
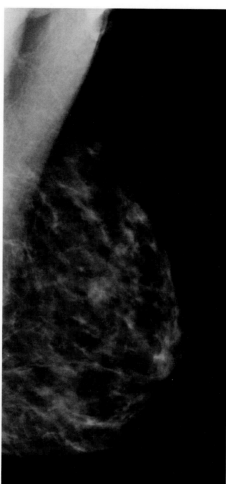

A,B

FIG. 17-1. The effect of lactation on the mammogram may be dramatic. Lactation can cause a marked increase in breast density. In this individual the breast density is markedly increased during lactation **(A)** and returned to being predominantly fat 1 year after cessation of lactation **(B)**.

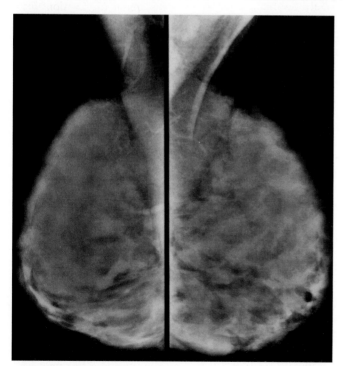

FIG. 17-2. The lactating breast frequently contains numerous lobulated densities.

for the patient to nurse immediately before the mammogram to decompress the breast and permit better compression. It probably takes at least 3 months for the breast to return to its baseline after the cessation of lactation.

BREAST BIOPSY AND ITS EFFECT ON THE BREAST

Any interventional procedure in the breast offers the opportunity of affecting the mammogram. Breast lesions can be biopsied in multiple ways.

Needle Biopsy

Needle biopsy is the least invasive of the interventional methods used to determine the nature of an abnormality. Needles can be positioned using clinical guidance (when the lesion is palpable) or imaging guidance. Needle biopsies of the breast can be performed using mammography (7), stereotactic mammography (8), ultrasound (9), computed tomography (CT) (10), magnetic resonance imaging (MRI) (11), and radionuclide imaging to guide the positioning of the needle (see Chapter 21).

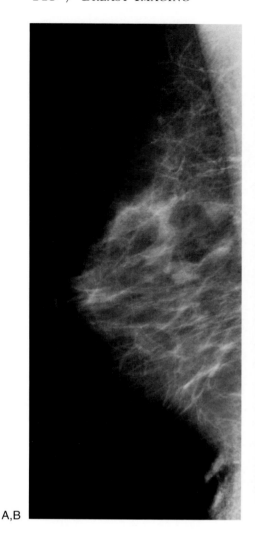
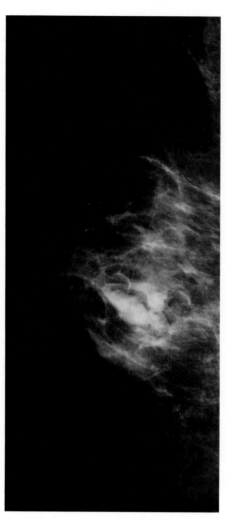

A,B

FIG. 17-3. Core needle biopsy often produces a hematoma. A mass in the medial left breast was biopsied using a 14-gauge needle. **(A)** Prebiopsy lateral mammogram. **(B)** After biopsy; the **hematoma** is obvious.

Fine-Needle Aspiration Cytology

The least traumatic method of needle biopsy involves the aspiration of cells for cytologic analysis through needles that range from 25 to 20 gauge (termed *fine needles*). The material that is removed consists of cells that have been separated from their surroundings; they are analyzed for their cytologic features. In well-trained hands, fine-needle aspiration (FNA) is extremely accurate in the diagnosis of malignancy. Because cytopathologists tend to be extremely conservative, the reported false-positive rates for FNA are extremely low. As a consequence, however, the false-negative rates (if *indeterminate* is included) are fairly high, necessitating open biopsy. Furthermore, many series have a significant number of tests in which the gathered material was insufficient for analysis. In most hands it is not possible to differentiate in situ from invasive cancers using FNA.

Core Needle Biopsy

Core needles are larger (14 to 18 gauge) and permit the removal of intact slivers of tissue that are analyzed using

standard histologic methods. Because the tissue architecture is preserved, invasive cancer can be distinguished from in situ (assuming the appropriate areas of the tumor have been sampled) using core biopsy technique.

Surgical Breast Biopsy

The most common form of diagnostic biopsy, and probably the most accurate if performed properly, is an open biopsy performed by the surgeon. This involves an incision through the skin and dissection to remove a volume of tissue. If the entire area of suspicion is removed, the procedure is termed an *excisional biopsy*. If only a portion of the tissue volume is removed, the procedure is an *incisional biopsy*. The term *lumpectomy* is usually reserved for the excision of a malignant process. The goal of lumpectomy is the removal of the tumor with an amount of normal surrounding tissue to provide margins that are free of tumor. Free margins are sought to increase the likelihood that there is little residual tumor in the breast so that radiation therapy will have a greater chance of eradicating any residual cells in the breast. Breast cancers recur after lumpectomy because the tumor

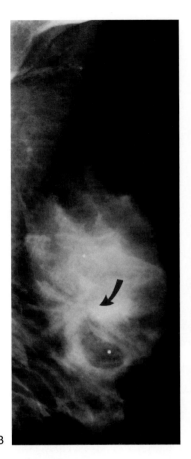
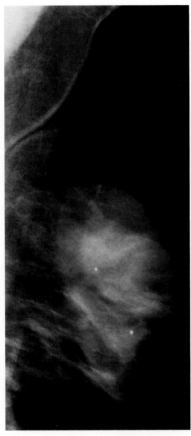

A,B

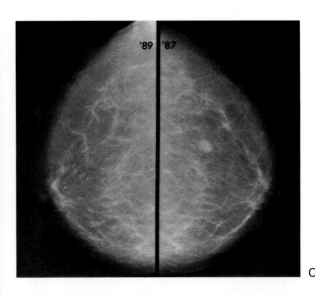

C

FIG. 17-4. The breast usually heals with no evident scar after a biopsy with benign results. This architectural distortion (*arrow*) was evident 3 months after surgery **(A)** with a benign result. Exactly 1 year later **(B)** the breast has healed completely with no radiographic evidence of the surgery. In this second case **(C)**, a mass is evident on the right in 1987. It was surgically removed and proved to be benign. There is no mammographic evidence of the surgery on the 1989 view (reversed for mirror-image comparison).

extended beyond the margins of excision and was not appreciated by the surgeon or the pathologist due to the sampling error inherent in the evaluation of excised tissue.

Changes Seen on Mammography After a Needle Biopsy

Sickles has shown that the insertion of a needle into the breast, even for a simple aspiration, can produce changes, either due to edema or hematoma, that are evident if a mammogram is performed soon after the procedure (12). It is often better to obtain a mammogram (if one is indicated) before any intervention. If, however, a needle procedure has been performed, it is prudent to wait 2 or more weeks to perform the mammogram so that any spurious tissue changes can resolve. Core needle biopsies frequently result in hematomas (Fig. 17-3), although these appear to resolve fairly rapidly with little effect noted at 6 months (13).

Postsurgical Biopsy Changes

It is a commonly repeated but fallacious belief that a surgical breast biopsy for what proves to a benign abnormality results in permanent scarring of the breast that is confusing on future mammograms (14). This is, in fact, unsubstantiated. Architectural distortion, or a spiculated mass, seen on a mammogram after a breast biopsy with benign results is

rare and is even more rarely a problem. Although the breast, as evaluated mammographically, can be a fairly slow organ to heal, there is usually little or no evidence of a biopsy at the time of the next annual screening mammogram after a biopsy with benign results.

Postsurgical changes may be visible up to a year or more after a biopsy, but for most women the breast will ultimately heal with little or no visual residual seen on the mammogram (Fig. 17-4). Healing, however, may be significantly delayed if the patient undergoes radiation therapy for cancer. Because postsurgical changes can resolve over many months, we prefer to avoid the term *scar* until it is clear that the changes have become fixed.

Among >450 women who had had breast biopsies for benign conditions, on subsequent mammograms only 11 (2%) had a visible scar that warranted any comment on the interpretation of their study (Massachusetts General Hospital, Breast Imaging Division, unpublished data). Sickles and Herzog reported a similar figure, showing that a persistent, spiculated abnormality after a biopsy with benign results is extremely rare. In their review of women who had had benign breast biopsies, only 3% of women had persistent distortion 2 to 3 years after surgery (15). These results occurred despite the fact that their data were accumulated at a time when larger volumes of tissue were routinely removed. Mitnick and associates found a similar percentage (16). There is likely a variation in the amount of persistent

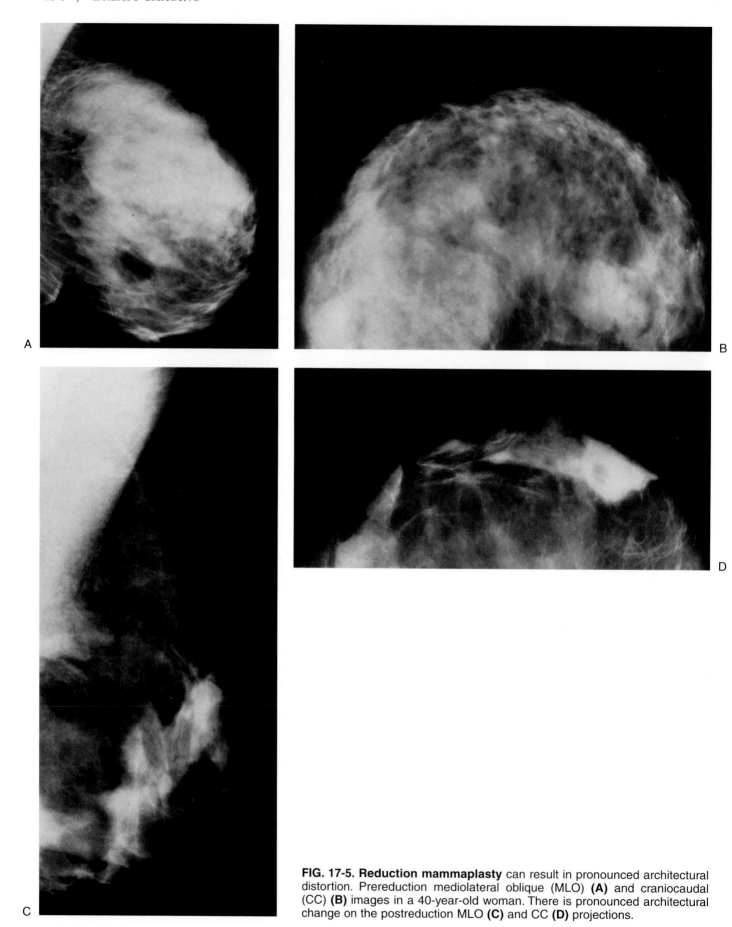

FIG. 17-5. Reduction mammaplasty can result in pronounced architectural distortion. Prereduction mediolateral oblique (MLO) **(A)** and craniocaudal (CC) **(B)** images in a 40-year-old woman. There is pronounced architectural change on the postreduction MLO **(C)** and CC **(D)** projections.

change that depends on the extent of the surgery and the postoperative course (hematoma formation or infection), but it is extremely rare for postoperative change to be apparent or confusing when the biopsy was benign.

New Baseline Mammogram After a Biopsy with Benign Results

An early postbiopsy mammogram can be obtained within days of the surgery as long as compression is carefully tailored to avoid hurting the patient and to avoid causing a wound dehiscence. The only time this type of study is warranted is if there is suspicion that the targeted lesion had not been removed. This may be obvious after needle localization when the specimen does not contain the abnormality, but it can also happen when a palpable abnormality is biopsied (17). If a lesion has not clearly been excised, then an early follow-up study is indicated.

There are some, however, who advocate an early postsurgical follow-up mammogram even when the results of the biopsy are benign. This is done to assess the extent of tissue disruption or hematoma formation from the surgery, so that on subsequent mammograms its progression to healing will be reassuring (rather than seeing change for the first time a year after the surgery). We do not advocate this approach, because postoperative change is rarely visible a year after the surgery when the patient resumes her screening program and is even less often a problem. The practice could be criticized for resulting in a significant number of unnecessary extra mammograms. For the few women who have a confusing mammogram at the first screening after a benign biopsy, short-interval follow-up (at 6 months) to monitor the area for resolution or stability will limit the overall number of women having additional studies and radiation exposure.

On rare occasion, the breast heals with a persistent area of architectural distortion. This is especially true if surgery has been extensive, such as with reduction mammaplasty (Fig. 17-5). Fat necrosis occasionally occurs, but the lucent-centered post-traumatic oil cyst that may form is easily diagnosed as a benign phenomenon (Fig. 17-6). The large, lucent-centered calcifications of fat necrosis (Fig. 17-7) are rarely confused morphologically with those produced by breast cancer.

Marking the Skin Incision

If there is any question as to whether architectural distortion is the result of postoperative change, the relationship

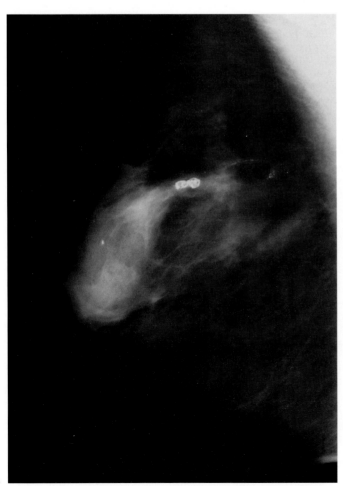

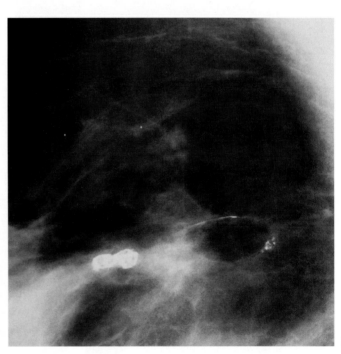

FIG. 17-6. Fat necrosis after surgery may form a typical oil cyst. The encapsulated radiolucent area on the mediolateral oblique (MLO) **(A)** and enlarged MLO **(B)** projections is a benign post-traumatic oil cyst due to fat necrosis after a reduction mammaplasty. *Continued.*

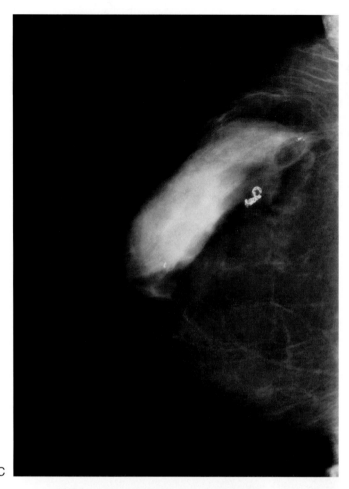

C

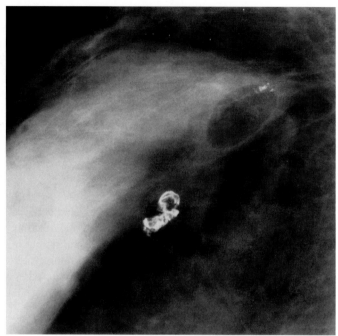

D

FIG. 17-6. *Continued.* This oil cyst was also visible on the craniocaudal (CC) **(C)** and enlarged CC **(D)** projections.

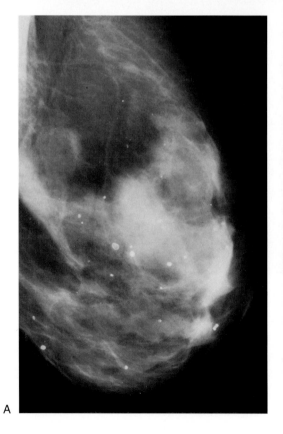

A

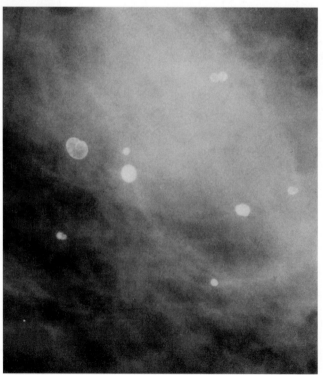

B

FIG. 17-7. Lucent-centered calcifications **(A)** are always benign. They are likely to be due to fat necrosis. **(B)** Photographically enlarged.

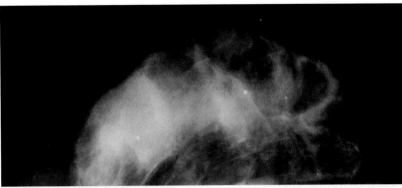

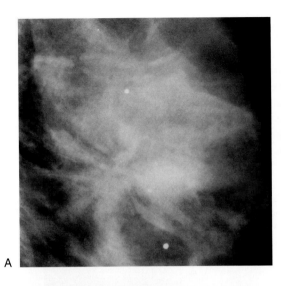

FIG. 17-8. Postsurgical change is usually more prominent on one projection than on the other. Three months after surgery, in the same patient as in Fig. 17-4, there is postsurgical architectural distortion that is more evident on the mediolateral oblique (A) projection (photographically enlarged) than medially on the craniocaudal (B).

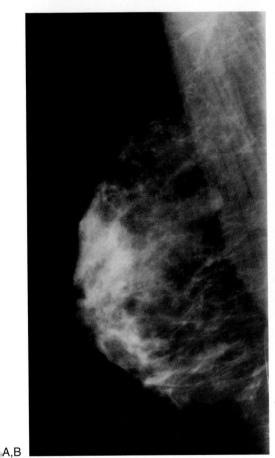

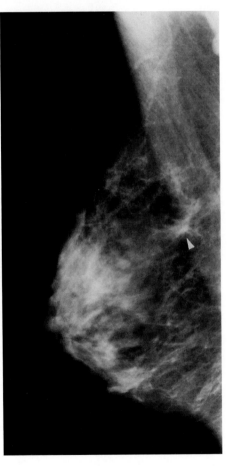

FIG. 17-9. There is usually minimal early postoperative architectural distortion after an excisional biopsy. The ill-defined density (A) in the upper left breast proved to be benign at surgery. One month (B) later there is minimal distortion (*arrowhead*) that will resolve.

of the distortion to the skin incision can be assessed by placing markers (BBs or wires) on the skin scar. Many technologists do this routinely. Because confusion is rare in our practice, we place markers only if there is a question to be resolved. Because the skin incision may be at a distance from the site of tissue removal, it is often more useful to compare the preoperative mammograms that showed the lesion and its location before its removal. This better

defines the area where architectural distortion would be expected from the surgical tissue removal.

Postsurgical Change: A Different Appearance on the Two Projections

Another helpful differential observation lies in comparing a suspicious abnormality on the two projections.

Breast cancer usually looks similarly worrisome on the two views. If it presents as a mass with spicules or as spiculated architectural distortion, it has a similar appearance in both projections. A scar or postsurgical change often has an ominous appearance on one projection but is almost imperceptible in the other projection (Fig. 17-8). Although this is not a definitive observation, in association with the other factors it is useful for differentiating postsurgical change from neoplasia.

Early Postbiopsy Changes

The only reason to perform a mammogram within days or weeks of surgery is if there is uncertainty that a lesion has been removed. If specimen radiography confirmed that the abnormality was excised and the histology was benign, there is no reason to obtain a mammogram soon after surgery. The only time that an early postoperative mammogram is needed is if there is any question as to whether the targeted lesion

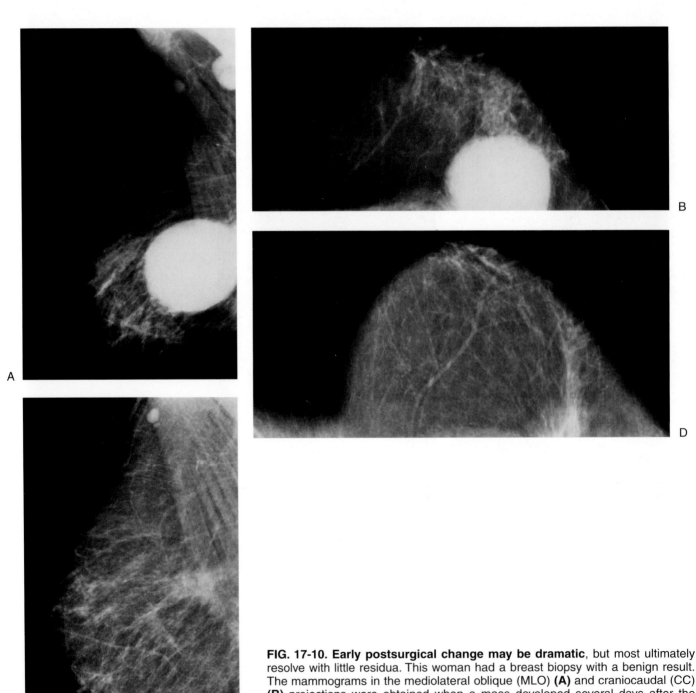

FIG. 17-10. Early postsurgical change may be dramatic, but most ultimately resolve with little residua. This woman had a breast biopsy with a benign result. The mammograms in the mediolateral oblique (MLO) **(A)** and craniocaudal (CC) **(B)** projections were obtained when a mass developed several days after the biopsy. The high density is consistent with a hematoma (the large axillary nodes are reactive) and 9 months later repeat MLO **(C)** and CC **(D)** projections show almost complete resolution.

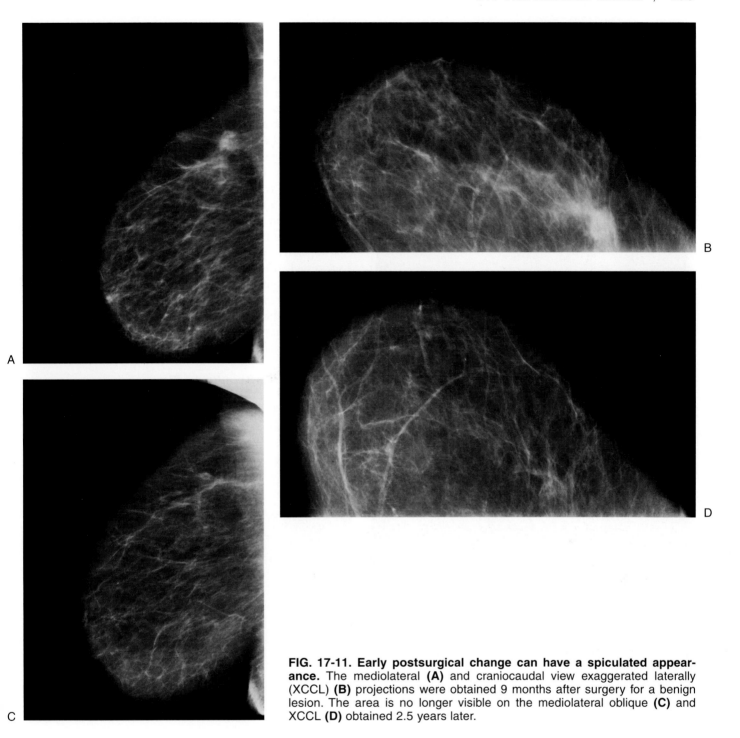

FIG. 17-11. Early postsurgical change can have a spiculated appearance. The mediolateral **(A)** and craniocaudal view exaggerated laterally (XCCL) **(B)** projections were obtained 9 months after surgery for a benign lesion. The area is no longer visible on the mediolateral oblique **(C)** and XCCL **(D)** obtained 2.5 years later.

was actually excised. There have been cases in which women have had very suspicious lesions on clinical examination and mammography. The clinically guided excision revealed a benign process. An early repeat mammogram (within days to 1 or 2 weeks after the surgery) revealed that the lesion had not been excised, and re-excision revealed malignancy (15). If the biopsy result is concordant with the preoperative diagnosis, then there is no reason to obtain an early postoperative mammogram. Unless there is a change on clinical examination to prompt earlier evaluation, there is

no reason to do any more than return to annual screening after a benign breast biopsy. It is very unusual for postsurgical change to present a problem of diagnosis a year later.

If, however, a mammogram is obtained in the early postoperative period (6 months or less) there may be prominent changes. The breast may show minimal (Fig. 17-9) or even no changes, but some women may develop a hematoma or seroma forming a mass and architectural distortion. This is not that unusual and may be dramatic (Fig. 17-10). Seromas and hematomas are usually indistinguishable. They are both

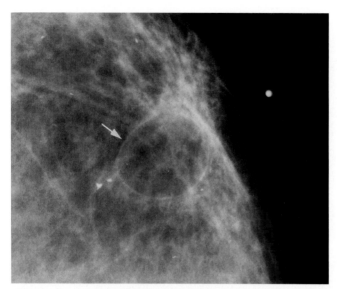

FIG. 17-12. This **post-traumatic oil cyst** (*arrow*), a form of fat necrosis, formed after a benign breast biopsy.

radiodense, although it is likely that a fresh hematoma is more attenuating than a seroma due to its iron (heme) content. The margins may be well circumscribed or ill defined. The reaction and fibrosis associated with healing may even cause the margin to be spiculated (Fig. 17-11).

Fat necrosis may result from surgery. This is easily diagnosed when an encapsulated, fat-containing lesion (Fig. 17-12) or large calcifications develop in the bed of the surgery (Fig. 17-13). The time of development of fat necrosis is variable, ranging from months to years.

If there is any question on the mammogram obtained within a year after surgery for a benign lesion, the pathology of the excised tissue should be reviewed to be certain that it was truly a bland benign lesion. If the preceding biopsy in fact removed the lesion and the tissue that was excised was clearly benign, it is extremely unlikely that a cancer was present in the bed and missed by the pathologist and developed over a few months into a large, visible breast cancer. Thus, when a mammogram is obtained in the early postoperative period after a biopsy with benign results and a spiculated lesion is present, it is virtually certain that it is only postoperative change and only short-interval follow-up is suggested to monitor its resolution (Fig. 17-14 A–F). We have found ultrasound of little value in assessing these women. The interpretation of ultrasound in the postoperative setting is difficult (Fig. 17-14G, H).

Any postoperative change should remain stable, or resolve. If it does not, intervention may be indicated.

Late Changes After a Breast Biopsy

As noted in the previous section, persistent postsurgical changes and noticeable architectural distortion that may be spiculated is unusual after a benign breast biopsy. In a few women, however, these changes persist for many years and

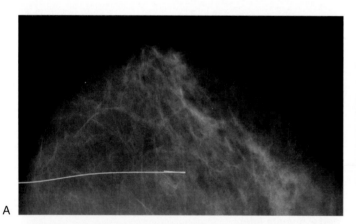

A

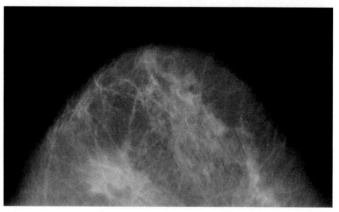

B

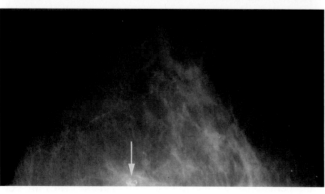

C

FIG. 17-13. Postsurgical fat necrosis can produce large calcifications. The ill-defined density **(A)** was excised and proved to be benign. Six months later there is spiculated postsurgical change **(B)** that develops a large benign calcification consistent with fat necrosis 12 months after the surgery **(C)** (*arrow*).

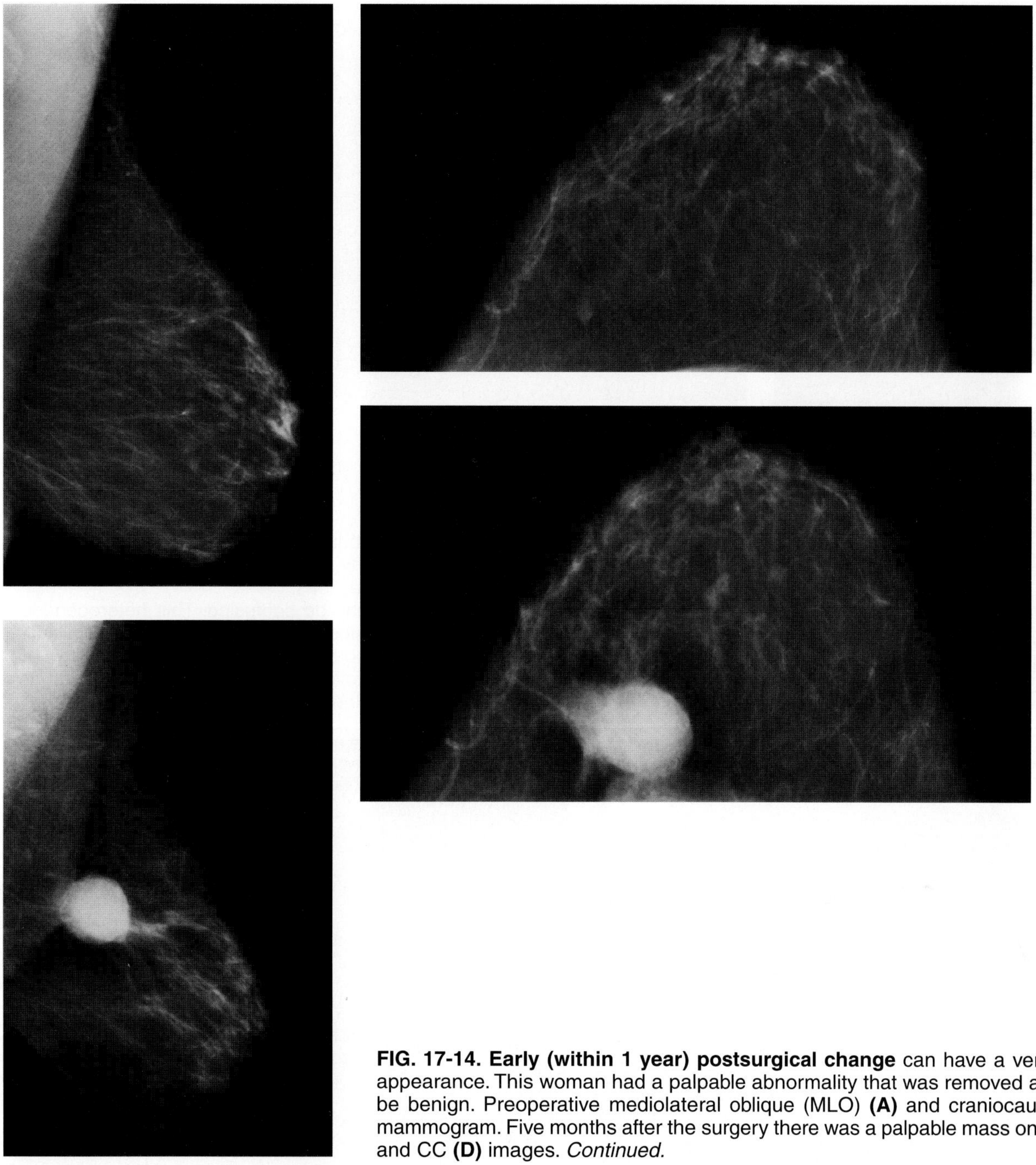

FIG. 17-14. Early (within 1 year) postsurgical change can have a very worrisome appearance. This woman had a palpable abnormality that was removed and proved to be benign. Preoperative mediolateral oblique (MLO) **(A)** and craniocaudal (CC) **(B)** mammogram. Five months after the surgery there was a palpable mass on the MLO **(C)** and CC **(D)** images. *Continued.*

presumably become a fixed scar. Some observers have suggested that this is more common if a hematoma formed postoperatively, but this has never been scientifically demonstrated. If this type of distortion causes concern, it is helpful to review the mammograms from before the surgery to determine the location of the biopsy within the volume of the breast tissue. It is also a good idea to review the pathology of the biopsy to be sure that there was no mistake and to be sure that there were no atypical changes that might indicate the possibility that the present architectural distortion is due to malignancy.

When postsurgical changes do persist after a biopsy with benign results they can be dramatic (Fig. 17-15). High-contrast mammograms overpenetrate the skin, but a careful evaluation of the incision site may reveal some skin thickening or retraction months to years after surgery. Usually subtle (Fig. 17-16) but occasionally striking architectural distortion may be present in the area of excision. There is rarely an associated mass.

After architectural distortion, fat necrosis is probably the most common long-term change caused by surgery. This may result in the development of an oil cyst with a thin wall

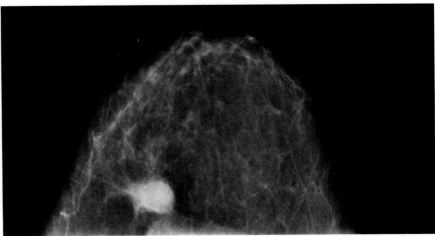

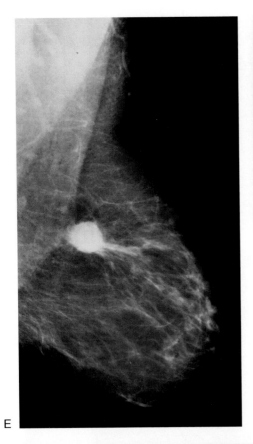

FIG. 17-14. *Continued.* Because of the benign pathology and the course over which the mass was followed, it had nearly resolved 7 months after the surgery, as seen on the MLO **(E)** and CC **(F)** projections.

Ultrasound after a breast biopsy may be confusing. This heterogeneous, hypoechoic palpable mass seen 3 months after the excision of a phylloides tumor in an 18-year-old woman was thought to represent a recurrence **(G)**. Based on the clinical evaluation, it was followed and was almost resolved at 4 months **(H)** and was no longer visible at the 7-month study.

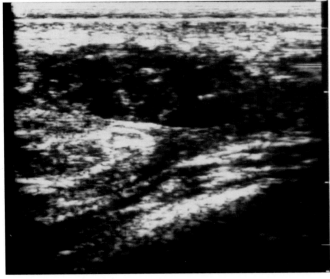

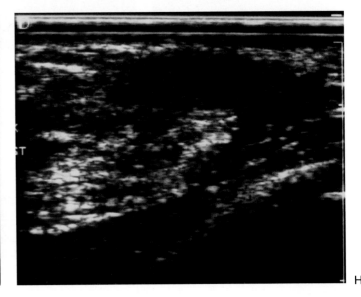

that encapsulates gelatinized, radiolucent fat within, or the process may produce large, lucent-centered calcifications. The architecture in the region of the biopsy may be distorted, and on occasion, when a large amount of tissue has been excised, the loss may be apparent on subsequent mammograms. Asymmetric breast tissue may be suggested on the contralateral side when the appearance is merely due to the excision of tissue on the ipsilateral side producing the asymmetric appearance (Fig. 17-17) (18).

With the exception of the immediate postoperative period, any changes should stabilize or improve. If the changes appear to be increasing, then intervention (biopsy) may be indicated.

Reducing the Likelihood of Postsurgical Changes

Increasing attention has been paid by surgeons to biopsy technique and has resulted in an improvement in

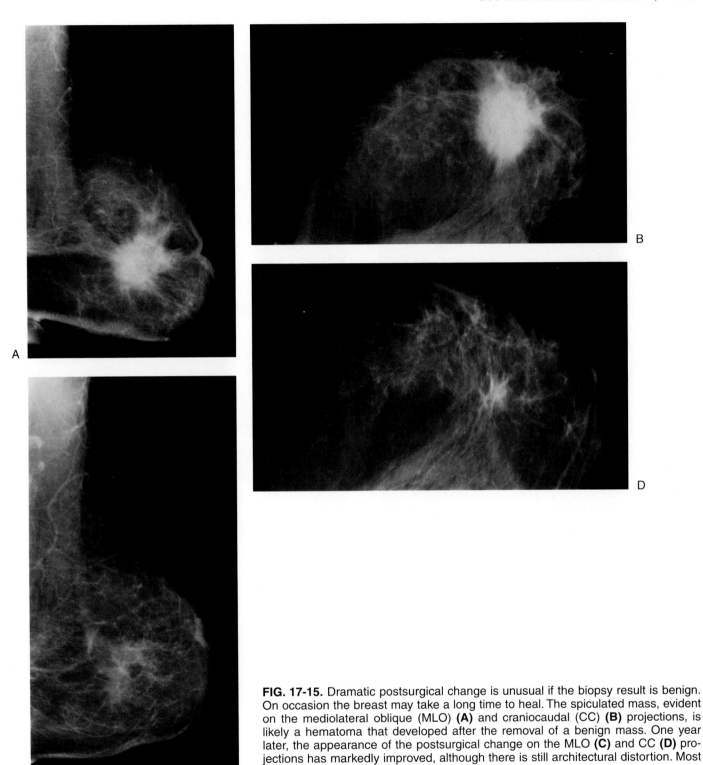

FIG. 17-15. Dramatic postsurgical change is unusual if the biopsy result is benign. On occasion the breast may take a long time to heal. The spiculated mass, evident on the mediolateral oblique (MLO) **(A)** and craniocaudal (CC) **(B)** projections, is likely a hematoma that developed after the removal of a benign mass. One year later, the appearance of the postsurgical change on the MLO **(C)** and CC **(D)** projections has markedly improved, although there is still architectural distortion. Most of this will eventually resolve.

the cosmetic results after biopsy and less permanent change on the mammogram than may have occurred in the past.

When a biopsy is performed for a nonpalpable lesion detected by mammography, accurate preoperative localization should be performed. Guides can routinely be placed within 5 mm of the lesion (19). Any farther away is unacceptable. Surgeons should be encouraged to excise the minimum amount of tissue necessary when performing a diagnostic biopsy when cancer is not anticipated.

Postsurgical tissue distortion can be reduced by not approximating the walls of the biopsy cavity with sutures, so

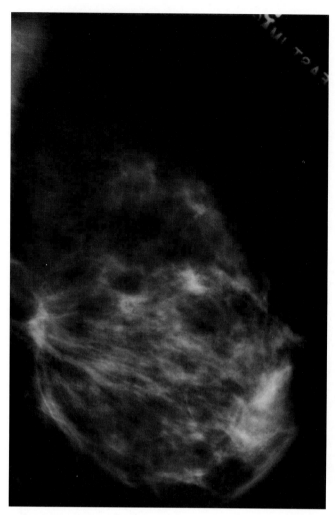

FIG. 17-16. Subtle architectural distortion several years after surgery with a benign result.

that the tissues fill in with less defect than if the walls are sutured together. Suturing the walls of the excision bed may lead to tissue distortion from the contraction of the scarring process and may result in a pronounced defect that forms a depression in the parenchyma, evident on clinical examination. Many breast surgeons use only subcuticular sutures, allowing the tissues to fall together naturally. If meticulous hemostasis has been achieved during the biopsy, there is little postoperative abnormality evident.

Calcifications After Breast Biopsy

It is fairly unusual for calcifications to form after a breast biopsy with benign results. Although large, lucent-centered calcifications can develop if fat necrosis occurs, this is fairly uncommon. Suture material can calcify, but this too is rare when a biopsy reveals a benign process. As noted in the following section, suture calcifications appear to be related to more extensive surgery, such as reduction mammaplasty, or delayed healing after radiation therapy.

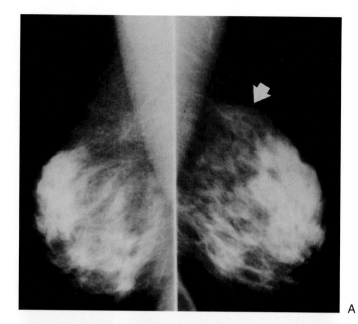

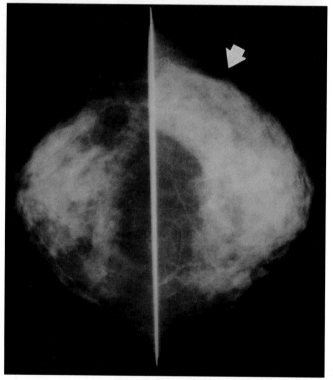

FIG. 17-17. Asymmetric tissue may be due to the surgical removal of tissue from the contralateral breast. The asymmetric tissue (*arrow*) visible in the upper **(A)** and outer **(B)** right breast was due to the earlier excision of tissue from the left breast.

MAMMOGRAPHY AFTER REDUCTION MAMMAPLASTY

The most extensive breast surgery (short of a mastectomy) undertaken for benign conditions is the removal of large amounts of tissue to reduce the size of the breast.

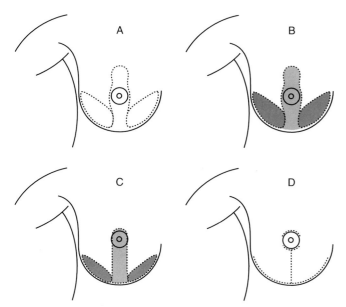

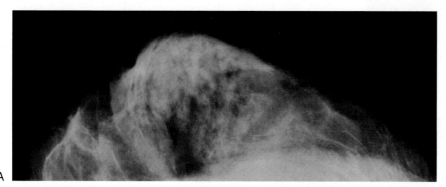

FIG. 17-18. Reduction mammaplasty surgery. This schematic demonstrates the vertical and inframammary fold incisions that are used for reduction mammaplasty. Skin and tissue are removed from the inferior and lateral incisions, and skin is removed from the midline incision. The remaining skin is elevated and pulled down to close the lower incisions and pulled together at the midline. The nipple and areola can be kept in continuity with the subareolar ducts, or they can be moved superiorly.

Reduction mammaplasty is usually performed for cosmetic and self-image purposes or because large breasts can be physically debilitating. Their weight can result in chest wall pain as well as back pain. Grooves can be worn in the individual's shoulders from the excessive weight of the breasts pulling on bra straps. Reduction mammaplasty may also be performed on the contralateral side after a mastectomy and breast reconstruction to produce more symmetric breasts.

There are several ways to reduce the volume of breast tissue while preserving cosmesis. The most common procedure involves a long incision along the inframammary fold and incisions extending from it to the 6 o'clock edge of the areola and then around the areola. Tissue is removed from the bottom of the breast and between the vertical incisions. The nipple areolar complex is moved up into a keyhole extension of the vertical incisions, which are then brought together in the midline to reform the smaller breast (Fig. 17-18).

The removal of hundreds of cubic centimeters of breast tissue can produce dramatic changes on the mammogram or be fairly unremarkable and not even noticeable. As might be expected, the fibroglandular tissues can appear redistributed from the usual upper breast location to the newly formed lower breast (20). Nonanatomic parenchymal bands and scars have been described. In our experience, there is often a swirling configuration to the remolded tissues (Fig. 17-19A),

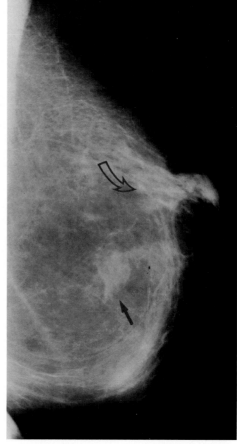

FIG. 17-19. After a reduction mammaplasty the tissues may have a swirled appearance, as in this craniocaudal **(A)** view, due to the removal of tissue and pulling together of the remaining tissues. **(B)** Isolated islands of breast tissue may result after reduction mammaplasty. In this second patient, on a mediolateral projection, there is an island of breast tissue (*solid arrow*) that is separate from the parenchyma. Note also that the nipple appears elevated (*open arrow*).

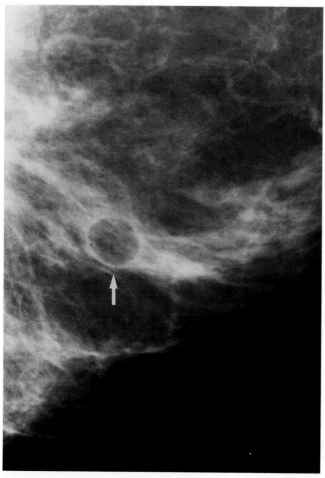

FIG. 17-20. This **post-traumatic oil cyst,** a form of fat necrosis, formed after reduction mammaplasty.

and isolated islands of breast tissue can be seen (Fig. 17-19B). Fat necrosis is relatively common with the extensive surgery involved, and oil cysts (Fig. 17-20) as well as benign calcifications can be seen after the surgery. On occasion, presumably as a result of delayed healing, suture calcifications are seen after reduction mammaplasty (Fig. 17-21). Despite the frequently dramatic changes that may be seen, in some individuals it may be difficult without previous films to tell that a reduction procedure has been performed (Fig. 17-22).

SUBCUTANEOUS MASTECTOMY

A subcutaneous mastectomy is usually performed before an individual develops breast cancer to try to reduce her risk by removing most of her breast tissue. This is a fairly drastic procedure that is usually used only when the risk of cancer is high or when the individual is extremely concerned. The surgeon attempts to remove as much tissue as possible while preserving the nipple and areolar complex and without devascularizing the skin. An implant is usually placed after tissue removal to reconstruct the breast. Because epithelial elements may extend to the skin, the complete removal of all epithelial elements would result in a compromise of the blood supply and the skin would likely slough. Thus, subcutaneous mastectomy does not usually eliminate the risk of breast cancer. Because there is residual breast tissue, we believe that mammography is still indicated for women who have had subcutaneous mastectomies.

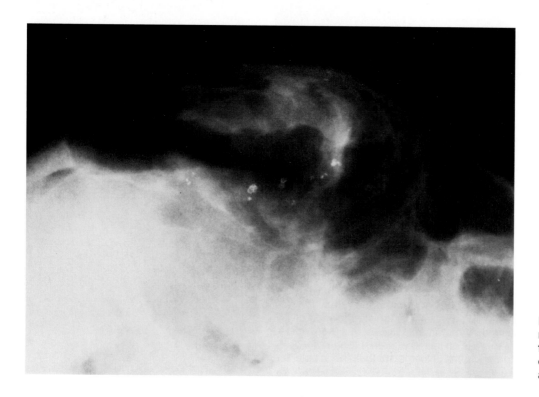

FIG. 17-21. Post–reduction-mammaplasty suture calcifications. The calcifications on this craniocaudal projection are calcified suture material.

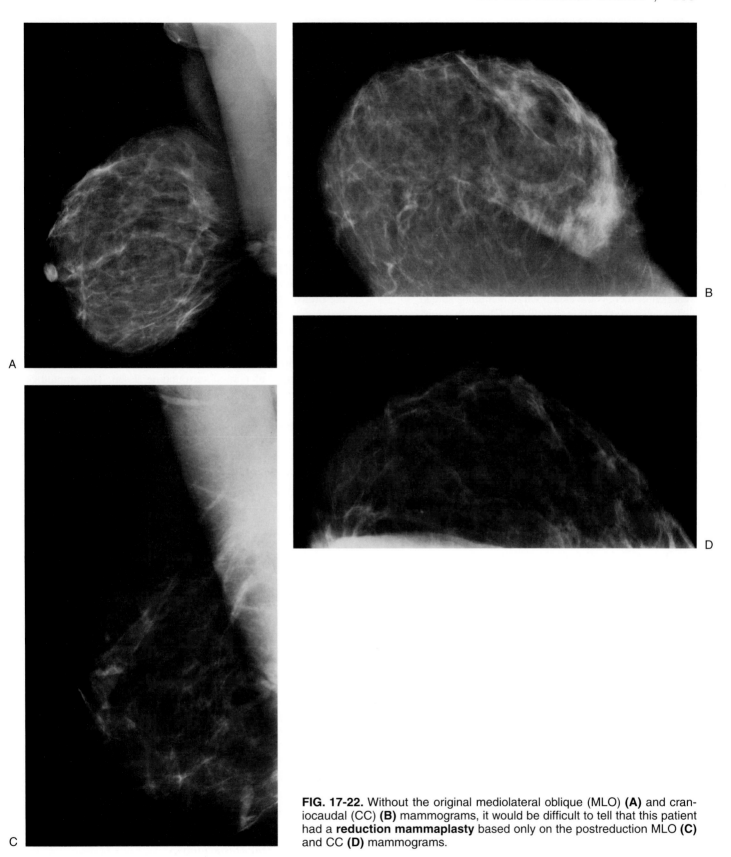

FIG. 17-22. Without the original mediolateral oblique (MLO) **(A)** and craniocaudal (CC) **(B)** mammograms, it would be difficult to tell that this patient had a **reduction mammaplasty** based only on the postreduction MLO **(C)** and CC **(D)** mammograms.

THE BREAST AFTER THERAPY FOR BREAST CANCER

Treatment for Breast Cancer

Lumpectomy and Quadrant Resection

Successful treatment of breast cancer must recognize that there are two primary treatment concerns. Local control involves treating the cancer in the breast itself, but it is metastatic disease (systemic involvement) that is the lethal component. Cancer confined to the breast cannot kill the individual. Nevertheless, its unrestricted growth can be devastating in its deformation of the breast and erosion through the skin, which can produce a weeping, ulcerated, and malodorous lesion that can be so unpleasant as to prevent social interactions. Modern treatment focuses on both local tumor control as well as systemic treatment if there is the likelihood of metastatic spread.

The use of systemic treatment (chemotherapy or hormonal manipulation using tamoxifen) is evolving. In the past, systemic treatment was used only when there was evidence of metastatic spread, such as tumor in axillary nodes. More recent analysis of the therapy trial data demonstrated evidence of a survival advantage from systemic treatment for invasive cancers >1 cm in diameter even when there was no axillary lymph node involvement (21).

Although an oversimplification of the approach to treatment, the striking fact is that treatment of the cancer locally in the breast may have little influence on overall, long-term survival. Survival from breast cancer appears to be determined by the degree of systemic involvement at the time of diagnosis and the effectiveness of systemic treatment (19).

It is generally accepted that local control involves the excision or destruction of the cancer in the breast as completely as possible. With surgical treatment the tumor as well some normal surrounding tissue is removed in an effort to reduce or eliminate any residual tumor within the breast. Radiation is used to try to eliminate any microscopic disease that may inadvertently be left behind. If too much tumor is left, the risk of local (i.e., in the breast) recurrence is increased and radiation may fail to eliminate the residual cells, leading to a high rate of cancer recurrence. Breast conservation is more likely to fail if too much gross malignancy is not eliminated before radiation therapy (22).

Margin Analysis

The surgeon frequently cannot determine where cancer ends and normal tissue begins. A crude measure of the success of tumor excision is the evaluation by the pathologist of the margins of the excised tissue. The surgeon tries to remove the tumor (and normal tissue) in a block. By staining the surface of the excised tissue with India ink or other stains, the pathologist, seeing the stain on histologic sections, can determine how close the tumor is to the margin.

Some pathologists use multiple, different colored stains to determine which margin is involved. If tumor is found in close proximity to the edge of the excised tissue or is at its margin, then the likelihood is increased that significant amounts of cancer remain in the breast.

Margin analysis is far from perfect. Because of the nature of the analysis, the pathologist is able to review only a very small sample of the margin of the excised tissue. Histologic slides provide a 4- to 5-μm–thick slice of the excised tissue. If only 1 cc of tissue was removed (usually 25–50 cc or more of tissue are removed to excise a cancer), the pathologist would have to review 2,000 slides to evaluate the entire specimen. It is not surprising that, even when the margin is believed to be free of tumor, as many as 40% of women have residual cancer in the breast. This is especially true for ductal carcinoma in situ (DCIS), where the cancer may extend down a duct from the primary tumor into another portion of the breast and the duct falls between reviewed slices so that it is not seen by the pathologist (23–25) (see Fig. 7-5).

The amount of tissue removed correlates directly with the amount of residual tumor after primary excision (26). As noted above, lumpectomy generally means the removal of the tumor with a margin of normal surrounding tissue. The amount of normal tissue varies with the surgeon. The likelihood of residual tumor can be diminished by performing a quadrant resection. The definition varies, but Italian physicians, who have had much success with extensive resections, remove a quarter of the breast (27). Shulman and colleagues found that the amount of residual tumor dropped from 40% to 14% with quadrant or segmental resection when compared to lumpectomy.

Even quadrant resection may leave tumor behind. Cancer cells grow up and down the branches of the involved breast segment (28). There is, as yet, no way of knowing whether or not the segment crosses into another quadrant of the breast such that branches of the segment (and the cancer cells contained within them) are not removed even by resecting an entire quadrant. Furthermore, the removal of such large amounts of tissue may be cosmetically unacceptable. Reconstruction is frequently used when a quadrant has been removed. Lumpectomy with clear margins, followed by radiation, has become the accepted standard in the United States.

The indications for conservation therapy (conserving the breast) have expanded over the years. It is essentially the acceptability by the individual woman of the amount of breast that will remain that determines whether the approach is undertaken. If the tumor can be excised with a margin of uninvolved tissue, then conservation therapy is an option. Although subareolar cancers usually involve the removal of the nipple/areolar complex, if the patient wishes, the remainder of the breast can be conserved.

Modified Radical Mastectomy

If the cancer is too large or the breast is too small or the cancer is extensive (multifocal), conservation therapy (exci-

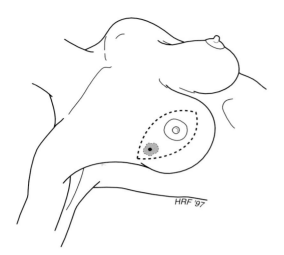

FIG. 17-23. The modified radical mastectomy. This diagram depicts the standard mastectomy incision. The breast is dissected from under the remaining skin and an axillary dissection is performed to include level I and level II lymph nodes.

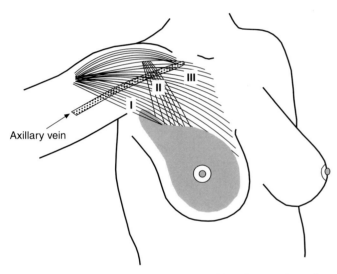

Axillary vein

FIG. 17-24. Axillary node levels. Level I nodes are lateral to and alongside the pectoralis major. Level II nodes are under the pectoralis minor muscle, and level III nodes are medial to the medial border of the pectoralis minor muscle.

sion and radiation) may not be feasible or acceptable to the patient. The modified radical mastectomy has become the most common form of mastectomy. This involves removal of the breast along with an elliptical section of skin (Fig. 17-23) as well as tissue that extends into the axilla to include level I and II lymph nodes (Fig. 17-24). Some surgeons remove the pectoralis minor muscle but preserve the pectoralis major muscle. The radical mastectomy, which removes the pectoralis major muscle, is no longer advocated as a general treatment and has no advantage over the modified radical mastectomy or lumpectomy and irradiation (29). In an effort to preserve skin to permit simplified breast reconstruction, some surgeons perform a skin-sparing pro-

cedure that removes an even smaller amount of skin along with the nipple/areolar complex.

Use of Mammography to Evaluate the Chest Wall After a Mastectomy

One study has suggested that mammography of the chest wall after a mastectomy can find clinically occult recurrences. No other review has shown a similar ability. Two reports show that there is no benefit from obtaining mammograms of the chest wall or the axilla of the side that has had a mastectomy, or both (30,31). Fajardo and associates reviewed images in 827 patients who had prior mastectomies (30). Among these, 39 (4.5%) had developed recurrent breast cancer. The mammograms showed only two of 20 recurrences at the mastectomy site, and these were evident clinically. A study by Propeck and colleagues reviewed 185 women who had prior mastectomies (31). Ten women had abnormal mammograms of the mastectomy site; only one was a true recurrence. The physical examination was also abnormal, making the mammogram superfluous. Both groups concluded that mammography of the mastectomy site and ipsilateral axilla is of no benefit.

Based on the images provided in the paper that advocated mammography after mastectomy, the difference appears to be that the mastectomies in the series that showed a benefit were not complete and left a large amount of breast tissue behind. If a mastectomy has been performed appropriately and there is no gross residual breast tissue, mammography of the chest wall has no benefit and is not a standard of care. Similarly, there are no data supporting the routine mammographic evaluation of the axilla on the side of the mastectomy.

The Breast After Radiation Therapy

The purpose of breast irradiation is not as a primary effort to destroy a breast cancer but as an adjuvant treatment to eradicate cells that have been left behind after the surgical removal of the bulk of the tumor (32). Because radiation works by "log kill," it eliminates a percentage of tumor (and normal) cells with each treatment (i.e., 90% of 90% of 90% and so on). If there are too many cancer cells, the balance between the destruction of normal cells and cancer cells by the radiation favors the malignant cells (there are too many cancer cells to kill without destroying too many normal cells), and radiation fails. Even successful radiation probably never eliminates all of the tumor cells. If the residual tumor burden after surgery (or some future primary therapy) is too great, radiation cannot eliminate the remaining cells and the tumor will recur. If the total tumor burden can be sufficiently diminished by surgery and radiation, it appears that the body's defenses can eliminate or keep in check any remaining tumor.

Overall survival and local recurrence rates appear to be equivalent for patients with early-stage lesions treated by mastectomy and those treated by breast conservation with tumor removal to clear margins followed by radiation therapy (33). There may, in fact, be some advantage to radiation as recurrence of cancer in the preserved breast does not appear to be as poor a prognostic indication as recurrence on the chest wall after a mastectomy.

Radiation Therapy Protocols

Radiation therapy generally involves the application of approximately 4,500 to 5,000 rad (45 to 50 Gy) to the whole breast in fractionated doses over a 5-week treatment period (34). Most treatment also includes a "boost" to the tumor bed and immediately adjacent tissues using an electron beam (the depth of energy deposit can be accurately determined) or temporary placement of iridium implants through catheters inserted through the tumor bed. These raise the total dose to the region where the tumor had been removed to as high as 7,500 rad (75 Gy).

There are some experimental protocols that propose to use only iridium implants so that the total dose can be delivered in a more concentrated form over a few days instead of weeks.

Imaging After Breast Irradiation

The general response of the breast to these levels of radiation is variable and often unpredictable. In some women few or, occasionally, no demonstrable changes are evident radiographically after therapeutic doses of radiation. In most women, changes are apparent. Skin and trabecular thickening occur almost universally beginning several weeks after the start of radiation therapy (Fig. 17-25). Initially these changes represent edema with engorgement of the dermal as well as intramammary lymphatics (trabecular thickening). This edema usually resolves over a period of weeks, months, or sometimes years. In some women the edema may progress to become permanent fibrosis.

Radiographically the breast appears denser. Some of this is the direct x-ray attenuation by the edematous tissues and fibrosis, whereas some is due to the fact that the swelling and soreness that are common prevent compression of the irradiated breast with an attendant increase in scatter and overlapping structures.

The radiographic appearance of the breast does not necessarily correlate with the clinical examination, and radiographically dense breast tissue may be soft on clinical examination. Conversely, the breast may be firm to palpation but exhibit only fat with thick trabeculae on mammography. Care must be taken by the technologist to avoid damaging the skin, which is more susceptible to trauma during the post-treatment period.

Depending on the extent of the surgical resection, post-treatment architectural distortion may be significant or not appreciable. Persistent scarring in the tumor bed occurs in some individuals. Because radiation slows the healing process, it is not unusual to see an area of ill-defined density or even spiculated postsurgical distortion 1 or more years after the surgery and radiation.

At times, persistent postsurgical change may be difficult to distinguish from recurrent cancer. Normally, any postsurgical change either remains stable or regresses. If a review of the pathology suggests that the tumor was excised with clear margins (there is less likelihood that gross tumor was

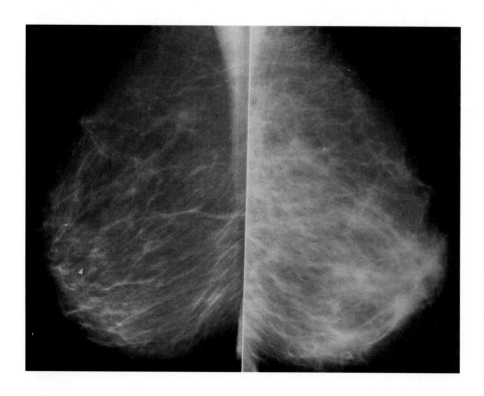

FIG. 17-25. Postradiation skin and trabecular thickening. The right breast had been irradiated 6 months earlier. The increased density is due to skin and trabecular thickening from edema. The swelling makes compression more difficult and uncomfortable, which further reduces the quality of the image.

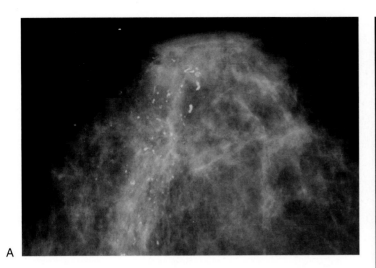

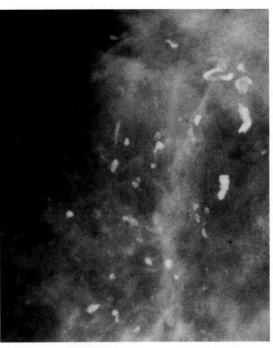

FIG. 17-26. These calcifications on the craniocaudal projection **(A)** developed after surgery and irradiation for breast cancer. They are large and coarse, and some have lucent centers on this photographic enlargement **(B)** and are typical of benign dystrophic deposits.

left in the breast), then the post-treatment change is followed at short intervals (6 months) to assess its stability, regression, or progression. If the distortion is progressive more than a year after the initial diagnosis, a biopsy may be necessary to exclude recurrent disease.

We believe that it is prudent to try to detect recurrences as early as possible, but in fact there are no data that suggest that the earlier detection of a recurrence within the breast has any effect on overall survival.

Calcifications in the Breast After Radiation Therapy

Analyzing calcifications that arise in the postirradiated breast can be difficult. Although most surgeons now try to excise all mammographically evident calcifications that may indicate residual breast cancer, no direct data support this approach. The policy has developed by inference from the apparent importance of clear margins on pathologic review. If tumor calcifications remain after surgery, they may be unaffected by radiation or undergo resorption. In some women calcifications appear after irradiation where none was previously present. There is no way of telling whether these are due to recurrent cancer or to necrosis of the original tumor from the radiation.

Benign calcifications occur in approximately one-third of irradiated breasts beginning 2 to 3 years after the therapy has been completed. They can develop as late as 4 years after the completion of treatment (35). These benign dystrophic deposits are probably due to the combination of surgical trauma and radiation. They are generally large and irregular in outline with central lucencies (Fig. 17-26) and always occur at the site of surgery.

Suture Calcifications After Irradiation

It is fairly common for sutures to calcify after radiation therapy. They are usually characteristic in that they are equally spaced along the suture line and the calcified knots are frequently evident (Fig. 17-27). In our review of these cases, we found that, among 355 women treated for breast cancer with adjuvant radiation therapy, 42 (12%) developed post-treatment calcifications and 21 of these (50%) were clearly calcified sutures (6% of all the women treated). Although the exact reason for suture calcifications has not been elucidated, we postulated that these were likely organic sutures (gut) that provided a substrate for calcium deposition and that deposits had time to form before the sutures were resorbed because radiation delays the healing process and the resorption of the sutures (36). Suture calcifications after a biopsy with benign results are extremely unusual in the breast that has not been irradiated or had extensive surgery (such as reduction mammaplasty).

Recurrent Breast Cancer After Conservation Therapy

In the United States, *conservation therapy* has come to mean excision of the tumor with a margin of grossly normal tissue surrounding it (lumpectomy) with margins that are free of tumor on histologic analysis. If the lesion is totally in situ, most surgeons do not perform an axillary dissection because truly intraductal cancer cannot spread to the axillary nodes. If the lesion is invasive, most surgeons perform a lumpectomy and axillary dissection (Fig. 17-28) to remove lymph nodes for analysis to determine the likelihood of systemic disease and the need for systemic treatment.

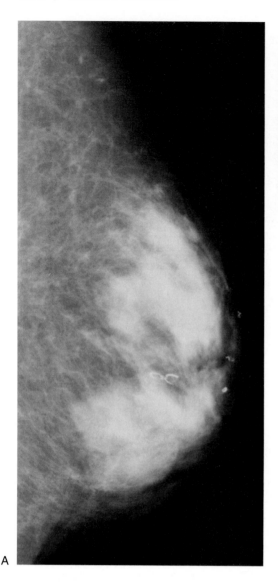

A

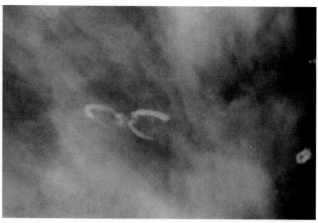

B

FIG. 17-27. Suture material may calcify after irradiation. In this patient the knots and even the trailing ends of the sutures are clearly visible on the straight lateral **(A)** and enlarged views **(B)**.

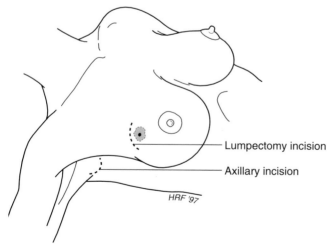

Lumpectomy incision

Axillary incision

HRF '97

FIG. 17-28. Surgery to conserve the breast involves excising the primary lesion through an excision overlying the malignancy and a separate incision to remove level I and II axillary lymph nodes.

The completeness of the primary excision of a breast cancer has an impact on the risk of recurrence. As might be expected, in one study that evaluated 503 patients the larger the tissue resection the lower the risk of residual tumor and the lower the risk of recurrence in the breast (26) (Table 17-1).

The reason for these failures is that microscopic tumor often spreads beyond the apparent edge of the lesion and the surgeon is often unaware that tumor has been cut across with residual foci remaining in the breast. The surgeon should strive for excision margins that are free of malignancy before radiation therapy to reduce the risk of recurrent breast cancer. The preoperative mammogram should be evaluated to try to determine the extent of the cancer. Calcifications frequently delineate much of the intraductal extent of the tumor, but it is fairly common for noncalcified tumor to extend beyond the visible calcifications.

Many believe that all cancer-associated calcifications should be excised to reduce the likelihood of recurrence,

TABLE 17-1. *Primary excision*

	Tumorectomy (%)	Wide excision (%)	Quadrant resection (%)
Patients	62	27	11
Residual tumor	41	14	7
Recur in	15	7	5

Source: Adapted from Harris JR, Schnitt SJ, Connolly JL. Conservative surgery and radiation therapy for early breast cancer. Arch Surg 1987;122:754–755.

although, as noted above, this has not been proved scientifically. If the specimen radiograph of the excised tissue (obtained when the lesion is not palpable) does not appear to contain all of the calcifications evident on the preoperative mammogram, a postoperative mammogram (magnification technique may be helpful) may reveal residual deposits. In one study using postoperative mammography (37), 20 of 29 women with residual calcifications visible on the postoperative mammogram had residual tumor (69%). That the mammogram cannot completely predict residual tumor is highlighted by the fact that in the same study four women of 13 who had no evident calcifications were found to have residual tumor (31%). Although the mammogram

may help to predict the presence of residual tumor after an excisional biopsy, the research on proper management and appropriate therapeutic decisions has been predicated on the pathologic analysis of the margins of the excised tissue and not the mammogram.

In addition to evaluating the mammogram to try to determine the extent of tumor, the tissue that is removed should have its surface covered with India ink or a similar stain so that when it is cut into smaller sections for histologic evaluation, the pathologist can determine how close the tumor comes to the tissue margins. If tumor is close to the margin or involves the margin, the likelihood of significant residual tumor still within the breast is high.

When there is extensive intraductal cancer with or without invasive tumor, it is frequently not possible to estimate the extent of the tumor that spreads along the segmental ducts. Because the pathologist can examine only a very small portion of the margin of the tumor, it is not surprising that cancer, spreading through microscopic ducts, may be overlooked in the sample (see Fig. 7-5). Even when margins appear clear, there is frequently residual cancer that is not appreciated at surgery or by the pathologist (38,39).

Fortunately recurrent cancer after conservation therapy is unusual. With appropriate treatment approximately 1%

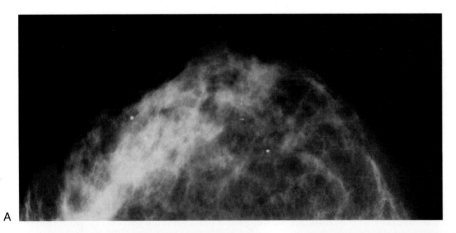

A

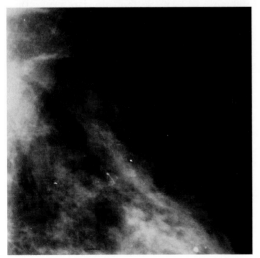
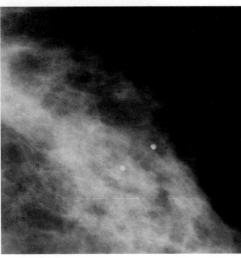

,C

FIG. 17-29. Recurrent breast cancer after irradiation is often difficult to appreciate by mammography if it only produces increased density. This patient had been treated 5 years earlier for ductal carcinoma in situ. Despite irradiation, she had a recurrence of an invasive cancer. The palpable recurrent cancer extended from the nipple to the upper outer quadrant but only caused a diffuse increase in density on the craniocaudal (CC) **(A)** projection that is imperceptible without previous examinations (the other breast had been removed for a previous cancer). The recurrence is suspected by mammography due to the calcifications that are present on the mediolateral oblique **(B)** and CC **(C)** projections. Calcifications in recurrent breast cancer are similar in appearance to those produced by a primary malignancy.

to 2% of women have a recurrence each year over a 10-year follow-up (10% to 15% over 10 years). Mendelson reported that recurrent breast cancers in the irradiated breast did not begin to appear until 30 months after the original diagnosis (39) (Fig. 17-29). This has been our experience. We have only seen a few earlier recurrences, and those have proved to be very aggressive tumors that rapidly involved the entire breast.

Follow-Up After Conservation Therapy

Women who have diffuse intraductal disease may be at an increased risk for recurrence after radiation therapy. Some investigators have determined that if 25% or more of the tumor is intraductal cancer, the woman should be classified as having extensive intraductal component (EIC) and that EIC by itself is a risk for recurrence. In women who have extensive intraductal tumor, it is more likely that cancer cells have grown down ducts that are not removed by some lumpectomies and represent too much residual tumor in the breast for the adjuvant radiation to control. As a result of this concern, it is suggested that all calcifications that are potentially associated with a cancer (the calcifications are usually in the intraductal component) be removed. Some radiologists advocate postlumpectomy magnification mammograms to evaluate the tumor bed for residual calcifications that may indicate residual tumor (40,41). This has never been shown to have any effect on overall survival.

Approximately 10% to 15% of women treated by lumpectomy and radiation can be expected to have a recurrence of cancer in the breast (local recurrence) within 10 years of treatment. As noted above, recurrences begin to appear approximately 2 to 3 years after treatment (42) and continue to appear at the rate of 1% to 2% per year. Very early recurrences (<2 years) are uncommon. In our anecdotal experience, the few that have recurred early proved to be rapidly growing and would be devastating regardless of how soon the recurrence was detected. Consequently, we obtain a new baseline 6 months after the completion of radiation therapy and then annually thereafter. There are no data to support more frequent follow-up, and routine imaging at 6-month intervals is only recommended if a question is raised on the first post-treatment study.

Six months after the completion of radiation is the time when the post-treatment changes evident by mammography are likely to be at their maximum, the breast has healed sufficiently to permit some compression, and recurrence is extremely unlikely. Subsequent to this study, the breast would be expected to improve or remain the same. There does not seem to be any scientific rationale for obtaining a mammogram sooner unless there is a clinical concern.

For the majority of patients, the expected post-treatment changes at the 6-month study do not cause any concern, and this new baseline study is the first in a return to annual screening. Because recurrences are not expected to begin to appear for at least another year, there is no reason to obtain an earlier study than the next annual screen unless a question arises sooner. If there is a questionable finding on the initial post-treatment mammogram (it is not likely to be recurrent cancer), we follow up at 6-month intervals. If the change resolves or remains stable for 2 years, we return to annual screening. Although the American College of Radiology (ACR) Standard for Diagnostic Mammography states that women who have been treated for breast cancer should not be considered candidates for screening programs (they should be evaluated in a diagnostic setting) there is no scientific rationale for this, and we have no higher recall rates for these women than the average woman evaluated in our screening program (43).

There is no rationale or any good data that support a more frequent screening interval. If there is a question as to whether a finding is due to recurrence or post-treatment change, MRI with gadolinium appears to be helpful in the analysis of the post-treatment breast changes (44). Although biopsied breast tissue can enhance in the initial few months after a biopsy, Heywang and associates found that there was rarely any enhancement 6 to 9 months after surgery (45). If the patient was treated for breast cancer and was more than a year from the treatment, Dao and colleagues found that cancer recurrences all enhanced using gadolinium (46). If it is more than a year after treatment and the abnormal area enhances, recurrent cancer should be strongly suspected.

Ultrasound

Although some observers advocate the use of ultrasound to evaluate the post-treatment breast, no data support its routine use. The only time it might be valuable is to help differentiate a fluid-filled structure from a solid structure in the region of the prior surgery. The former is almost always a seroma or hematoma that develops early in the postsurgical period, and most can be followed clinically without the need for ultrasound.

Long-Term Post-Treatment Follow-Up and Screening

Screening of the treated breast is probably a good idea. Although we believe in principle that the earlier detection of recurrences is valuable (47,48), in fact, no data prove that overall survival is influenced by the earlier detection of recurrent disease.

Because there is still the potential to develop a new breast cancer and because the ultimate survival of an individual who develops more than one breast cancer over time is determined by the stage of the worst lesion, screening the remainder of the conserved breast as well as the contralateral side for new primary cancers seems prudent.

Roubidoux and associates reviewed 69 cases in which a second primary cancer developed in the opposite breast. The second lesion occurred synchronously in 49% of the women and metachronously in 51%. They found that the second lesion had different morphologic characteristics than the first lesion 67% of the time. If the first tumor was a mass, the second might present as microcalcifications. If the first tumor was revealed due to microcalcifications, the second tumor might well present as a spiculated mass (49). Thus, screening a woman who has already been treated for a breast cancer is no different from screening any other woman.

Detection of Recurrent Breast Cancer

Recurrent breast cancer may be difficult to appreciate by mammography (Fig. 17-29A) (50). Because of the increased density from edema and fibrosis caused by the radiation, the architectural distortion caused by the surgery, and the inability to optimally compress the breast, mammography can detect approximately 60% of recurrent disease. Stomper and associates found that 35% of 45 recurrent cancers were detected only by mammography (50). Greenstein and colleagues had similar results (51). In their series, among 1,145 women treated for cancer, 102 underwent a biopsy for possible recurrence. Approximately one-third of the suspected lesions proved to be recurrent cancer (38/102). Among the 58 women who recurred who also had had a mammogram, 13 (34%) were detected only by the mammogram. Eight (21%) were evident on both mammography and physical examination, but 17 (45%) were suspected clinically and not evident by mammography. Thus, post-treatment follow-up should include clinical examination as well as mammography.

Some recurrences are evident by the development of new microcalcifications (52,53). These are usually not difficult to distinguish from the benign, dystrophic calcifications that are relatively common in the postirradiated breast (see Figs. 17-26 and 17-29). If fine (<0.5 mm), linear, or heterogeneous calcifications develop, they should be considered as a probable recurrence (Fig. 17-29B, C). The microcalcifications of new or recurrent disease frequently have the same morphology as those found in primary cancer.

The development of a mass as a sign of recurrence is unusual, but ill-defined, increasing density should raise concern. As noted above, the maximum changes from radiation therapy (distortion, density, skin and trabecular thickening) are expected approximately 6 months after the completion of treatment. These should stabilize or improve on subsequent studies. If they progress, recurrence should be suspected.

Infection may be difficult to appreciate in the treated breast, and the clinical presentation will probably dictate therapy. Skin thickening beyond 3 to 4 mm is unusual from radiation alone and causes other than the effect of irradiation should be suspected.

Radiation does not protect the breast from future cancer but merely affects the tumor that is already present. New primary cancers can occur in the irradiated breast as well as the contralateral breast, which, as noted previously, should be carefully screened with yearly mammography.

Radiation and Risk of New Breast Cancer

A concern in women who undergo radiation therapy is the possible future development of leukemia or tumors, such as sarcomas, in or near the irradiated field. Because the contralateral breast receives scatter from the breast undergoing radiation therapy, there has been some concern that the incidence of contralateral cancer might increase after radiation therapy. This does not appear to be the case for most women. At least one study has shown that, for women ages 45 and over, there does not appear to be any increased incidence of contralateral breast carcinoma from the 100 to 300 rad (3 Gy) that their contralateral breasts received from scatter during radiation therapy (54). There was a slight increase in risk for younger women.

The Breast After Primary Chemotherapy

Some large breast cancers (T3) may be too large to excise, and some may even be too large to permit a mastectomy without the risk of leaving an excessive tumor burden. Primary chemotherapy has been used to reduce the size of the local disease to permit successful mastectomy (usually followed by irradiation to the chest wall) and among some women to permit lumpectomy and radiation. In a study by Bonadonna and colleagues (55), primary "neo-adjuvant" chemotherapy was able to reduce the size of the cancers among 127 of 165 women to <3 cm, making breast conservation therapy possible. The degree of response of the tumor is inversely related to its size. They found that cancers that were hormone-receptor negative were more likely to respond better.

Frequently the response of the tumor can be seen by mammography. We have seen significant reductions in the tumor volume on mammography (Fig. 17-30). If the tumor is moderately small to begin with, it might disappear completely on the mammogram.

Segel and colleagues found that 78% of cancers treated with chemotherapy before excision or mastectomy had a moderate or excellent response (56). Of the 60 cancers monitored, 17 showed an excellent response; 88% of these cancers disappeared completely on pathologic review.

BREAST AUGMENTATION IMPLANTS

The use of silicone gel implants for breast augmentation was first reported in 1962 (57). It is estimated that over the past 30 to 40 years approximately 1 to 2 million women in the United States have undergone cosmetic breast enlargement or reconstructive procedures after mastectomy and have silicone breast implants (58). Augmentation and reconstructive procedures have evolved over the years. The injection of paraffin or free silicone was used in the past but is presently illegal in the United States. The material was free to migrate throughout the body, and many women developed granulomas and calcifications as a result of these injections (Fig. 17-31). These severely compromise clinical breast examination and mammography.

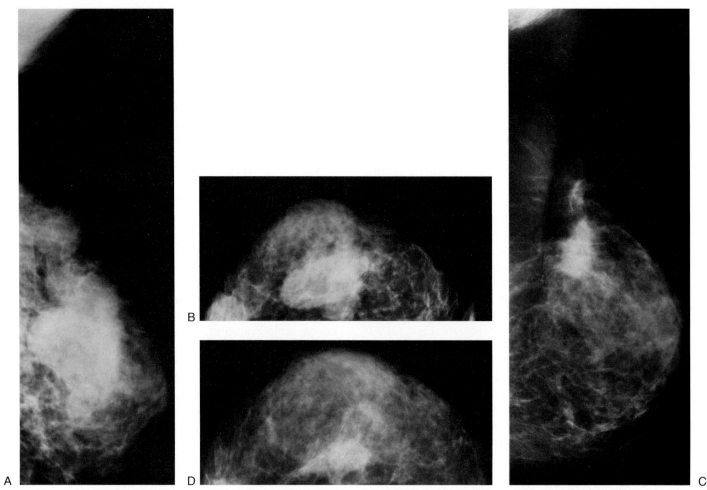

FIG. 17-30. Neo-adjuvant chemotherapy before surgery may reduce or eliminate any visible tumor in the breast. This patient had a T3 cancer that occupied much of her breast, as is apparent on these mediolateral oblique (MLO) **(A)** and craniocaudal (CC) **(B)** projections. The study was limited due to the rigidity of the breast. She was treated with four cycles of chemotherapy, and 5 months later the repeat mammogram revealed a marked reduction in the volume of tumor and a softening of the breast, as is evident on the MLO **(C)** and CC **(D)** projections.

Augmentation mammaplasty became common with the development of the silicone implant. The most commonly used implants consisted of silicone rubber bags (envelopes) that contained either saline or silicone gel. Until the Food and Drug Administration (FDA) banned their use, the placement of a silicone gel implant was the primary method of breast augmentation as well as reconstruction after mastectomy.

Despite the fact that these prosthetic devices had been in use since the 1960s the FDA determined, in 1992, that the manufacturers had not satisfactorily demonstrated their safety. The agency was concerned that, despite the lack of conclusive evidence of significant harm, there were a sufficient number of problems, potentially associated with implants, to justify the limitation of their use. The implantation of silicone gel prosthetics for augmentation or reconstructive surgery came under strict regulation. Any use of implants had to fall within the umbrella of a clinical trial, and complete documentation had to be provided for each implant.

Are Silicone Implants Harmful?

There have been anecdotal reports of connective-tissue disorders developing in women who have implants. In one report, five women with scleroderma also had implants (59). Other reports have suggested arthropathies after implantation (60). The difficulty lies in determining whether these are cause-and-effect relationships or merely coincidental associations. Studies suggest that silicone is not completely inert but may have antigenic properties. Silica may also occur in association with silicone and potentially result in silicosis.

The greatest concern has been raised over the possibility that implants may stimulate autoimmune reactions and rheumatoid syndromes, although there is an absence of any scientific proof of this. At least two reviews have failed to demonstrate any greater prevalence of these diseases among women with implants than among women without implants. In one study 749 women with implants were followed up for

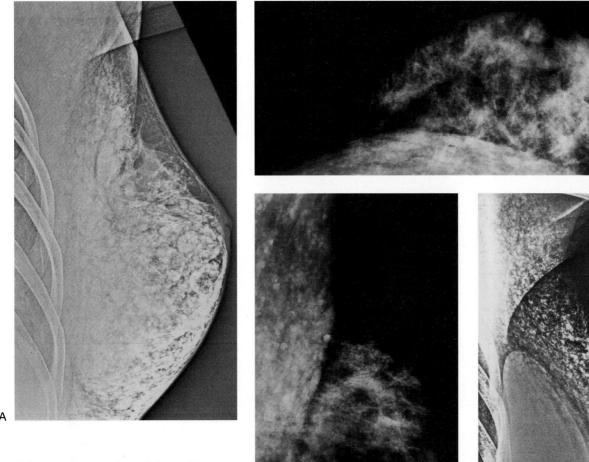

FIG. 17-31. Injection of free silicone. **(A)** These calcific densities on this negative mode xerogram are silicone granulomas that formed secondary to the injection of free silicone. Multiple calcified silicone granulomas can be seen on the craniocaudal view **(B)** and extending up into the axilla on the mediolateral oblique view **(C)** in this 49-year-old woman who had injections of free silicone 28 years prior to these mammograms. **(D)** This patient had silicone injections that have formed calcified granulomas. She subsequently had an implant added for additional augmentation.

a mean of 7.8 years after implantation. These were compared to 1,498 controls. Five women in the group with implants and 10 in control group developed connective-tissue problems (RR = 1.06). Among the women with implants, 25 had arthritis; 34 of the controls also had arthritis (RR = 1.35) (61).

In a second study involving 87,501 women, 876 had silicone gel implants. Another 170 had saline implants, and 67 had a combination of the two. With a mean follow-up of 9 years after implantation, only three of the 516 women with connective-tissue disease had implants. One individual had a gel-filled implant, one had a saline implant, and one had a combination implant. No association was found between implants and connective-tissue disease (62).

The most common problems directly attributable to implants involve the same complications expected with a surgical procedure in which a prosthetic device is implanted. Postsurgical complications such as bleeding and infection can occur, and, as with any foreign body, some individuals tolerate implants and others do not. It also appears that the silicone envelope degrades with time. A new implant can withstand up to 200 lb of pressure, but with time the strength decreases and in some women the envelope appears to disintegrate, increasing the likelihood of rupture.

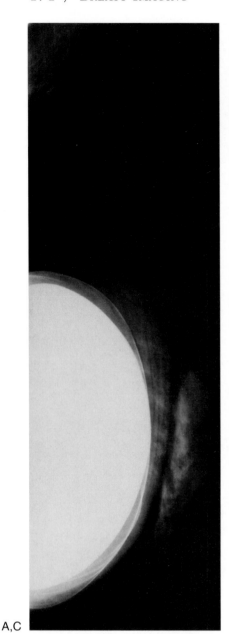

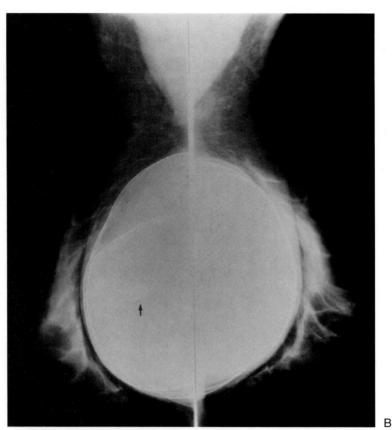

B

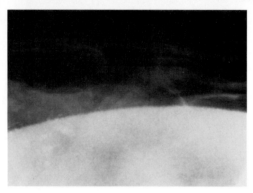

FIG. 17-32. Double-lumen implant on mammography. **(A)** Some implants such as this have an inner envelope that contains silicone gel (radiodense) with an outer envelope that is filled with saline (less dense). Implant valves may be palpable and visible on the mammogram. **(B)** The valve on this saline-filled implant is visible on the mediolateral oblique projection (*arrow*). **(C)** This implant has a textured surface that is visible on the mammogram as fine irregularity. The texturing is an attempt to reduce the development of capsular contracture.

A,C

In a follow-up study of 749 women, Gabriel and colleagues found that 208 (27.8%) underwent implant-related surgery over a mean follow-up period of 7.8 years (range, 0 to 28) (63). The most common problem was capsular contracture, which occurred in 15% of the women. Ruptured implants occurred in 3.9%. A number of problems, including hematomas and abscess formation, occur early after implantation. In capsular contraction, myofibroblasts may be responsible for pain and capsule formation, which may produce a hard implant. However, capsular contraction remains a clinical diagnosis.

There is little doubt that women who have implants are systemically exposed to silicone. Our preliminary studies have shown that silicone can be found in the blood of women with implants, and using magnetic resonance spectroscopy we have detected silicone in the livers of these women. Nuclear magnetic resonance of blood samples shows that the chemical composition of the silicone in the blood is modified from the gel polymer (64). It is not clear whether the implant must be ruptured for silicone to be detectable in the blood or liver. In addition to possibly representing a way to determine whether or not an implant is ruptured, this work has also demonstrated that the gel polymer can be chemically altered by the body. The significance of this, if any, remains to be determined. If the anecdotal problems related to exposure to silicone are shown to be real, spectroscopy may provide the most objective way to evaluate that exposure.

Despite the absence of scientific data to confirm harm, concern has remained. Because some believe that problems arise when the body is exposed to the silicone gel when an implant ruptures, there has been a great deal of emphasis placed on determining whether or not a rupture has occurred.

Types of Implants

There are numerous types of implants. The majority consist of a silicone envelope filled with silicone gel or saline. The envelope is a silicone rubber made of either polydimethylsiloxane or polydiphenylsiloxane. The gel consists of cross-linked silicone polymers. The other major type of implant is the envelope filled with saline. Combinations of the two (envelope within envelope) can be found. By placing a silicone implant within a saline implant (Fig. 17-32), the saline can be introduced in the operating room to permit adjustment of the implant size. Various valves may be present that allow for adjustment of the size of the implant that contains saline. These may be palpable and be mistaken for a mass. They may also be evident by mammography (Fig. 17-32A).

Capsular Contracture and Polyurethane Coating

It has been obvious for years that implants are not totally biologically inert. In 20% or more of women, a fibrous capsule forms around the implant (65). This can contract (capsular contracture), causing the implant to become very hard and irregular in shape. In the early and mid-1980s efforts were made to reduce the likelihood of capsular contracture by texturing or covering the surface of the implant with materials chosen to disrupt the contracture process. One approach involved texturing the surface of the usually smooth silicone rubber envelope (Fig. 17-32B). Another approach involved the application of a polyurethane foam to the implant surface. The principle was to provide the breast tissues with an irregular matrix into which they could grow in an effort to reduce the linear scarring that produced a hard capsule and contracture.

The use of polyurethane compounded the concerns raised over exposure to silicone. This coating appears to produce a prolonged foreign body reaction as the polyurethane undergoes biological degradation (57). What appears not to have been anticipated is that one of the hydrolytic degradation products of polyurethane foam is the chemical 2,4-diamino-toluene (TDA). TDA has been shown to produce liver cancer in laboratory animals (66). Another potential degradation product of polyurethane, toluene diisocyanate (TDI), as well as polyurethane itself, have also been implicated in malignancies in laboratory animals. Further complicating the problems created by the use of polyurethane is that the ingrowth of tissue into the coating makes them extremely difficult to completely remove.

Positioning of Implants in and Behind the Breast

The surgical approach to placing implants varies (67). Implants have been positioned through inframammary incisions, periareolar incisions, or from the axilla. There are two major locations relative to the breast tissue in which implants have been placed.

Retroglandular (Subglandular) Placement

Most implants have been positioned in the retroglandular location. The implant is placed behind the breast tissue but in front of the pectoralis major muscle (Fig. 17-33).

Retropectoral Placement

In another effort to reduce the development of capsule formation and contracture that commonly occurs around retroglandular implants, many implants have been placed behind the pectoralis major muscle in a subpectoral location (Fig. 17-34). The theory for this position was that the motion of the muscle over the surface of the implant would reduce the likelihood of capsular contracture. The retropectoral implant is preferable for mammography because it facilitates implant displacement imaging (see Chapter 10) and permits better compression of the breast for cancer detection.

Gel Bleed Fibrous Encapsulation and Capsular Contracture

It has been estimated that 20% to 50% of silicone implants become surrounded by a layer of fibrous connective tissue. Contracture of this encapsulation can distort the implant, cause it to feel hard, and probably cause pain. Contracture can occur weeks to years after implantation. This has been treated in the past by closed capsulotomy, in which the physician manually compresses the implant in an attempt to rupture the capsule without disrupting the silicone envelope.

The exact cause of encapsulation is uncertain. Silicone droplets have been demonstrated in the fibrous connective tissue that forms around many implants (68). It is well established that silicone can pass through the intact silicone envelope, which acts as a semipermeable membrane, of the implant into the surrounding tissue. Silicone gel is a copolymer composed predominantly of polydimethylsiloxane (PDMS) and vinylmethylsiloxane. The vinyl groups are partially cross-linked to form a three-dimensional gel structure (69). Because the groups are only partially cross-linked, the implant also contains some free PDMS. This has been shown to be able to pass through the intact implant envelope into adjacent breast tissue (70,71). Although this has been termed *gel bleed*, it is not actually the gel that passes through but rather free, unpolymerized silicone. It may be this bleeding of silicone that stimulates the production of collagen around the implant, leading to fibrous capsule formation and capsular contracture. Alternatively, capsular contracture may merely be a foreign body reaction to the implant itself. Gel bleed and free silicone have been associated with granuloma formation as well as adenopathy.

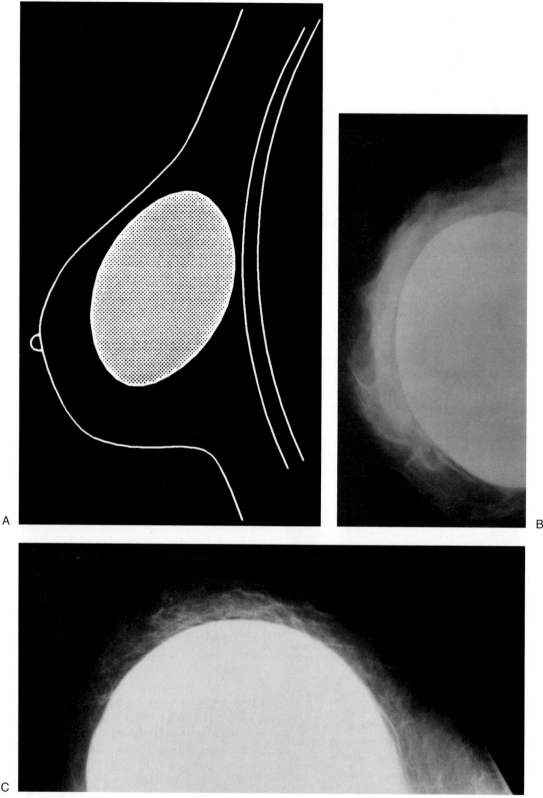

FIG. 17-33. Retroglandular (prepectoral) implant. The implant is positioned behind the glandular tissue of the breast but in front of the pectoralis major muscle **(A)** schematically and on this mediolateral oblique **(B)** projection. The implant is immediately behind the glandular tissue and anterior to the pectoralis muscle so that the muscle is not visible on the craniocaudal **(C)** projection.

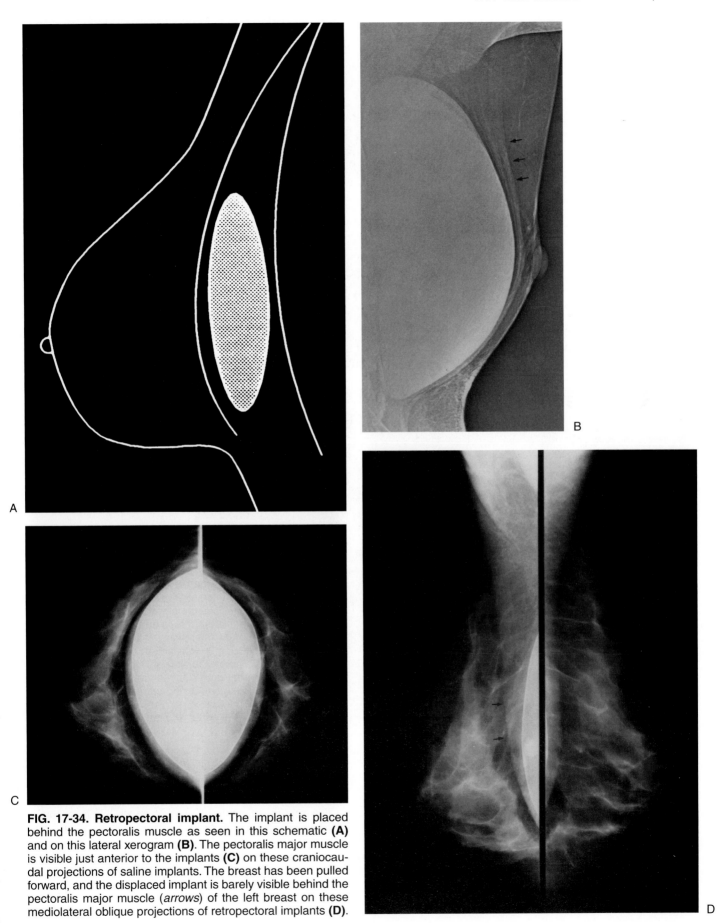

FIG. 17-34. Retropectoral implant. The implant is placed behind the pectoralis muscle as seen in this schematic **(A)** and on this lateral xerogram **(B)**. The pectoralis major muscle is visible just anterior to the implants **(C)** on these craniocaudal projections of saline implants. The breast has been pulled forward, and the displaced implant is barely visible behind the pectoralis major muscle (*arrows*) of the left breast on these mediolateral oblique projections of retropectoral implants **(D)**.

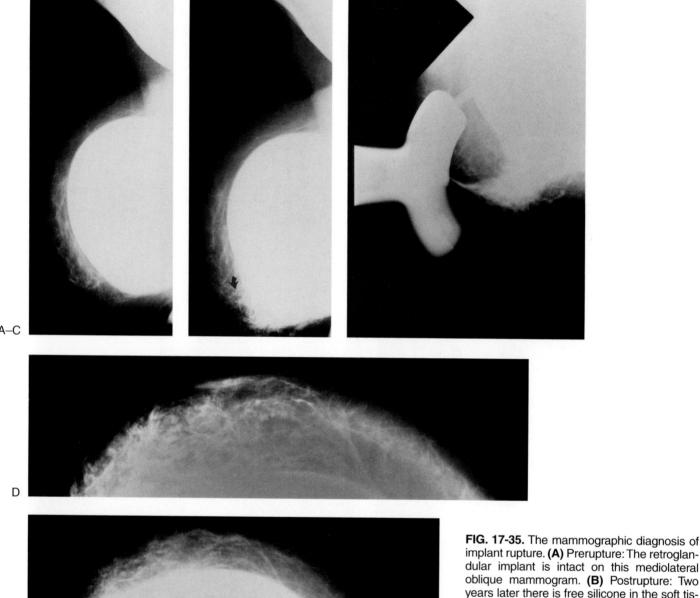

A–C

D

E

FIG. 17-35. The mammographic diagnosis of implant rupture. **(A)** Prerupture: The retroglandular implant is intact on this mediolateral oblique mammogram. **(B)** Postrupture: Two years later there is free silicone in the soft tissues of the lower left breast. The silicone is diffusely extravasated, as seen on this spot compression view **(C)** of a palpable abnormality. Extravasated free silicone is even more evident when the standard implant view **(D)** is compared to the implant displacement view **(E)** after implant rupture. *Continued.*

Fibrous contracture can turn a once pliable implant into a hard spherical object that can distort the breast and be uncomfortable for the patient. It also makes it more difficult, and often impossible, to displace the implant to permit breast compression for cancer detection by mammography.

Implant Rupture and Deformities

A great deal of concern has been raised concerning the rupture of an implant. Rupture potentially exposes the breast and

body to large amounts of the silicone gel. Although it remains to be shown that this is in fact dangerous, many physicians recommend that ruptured implants be removed (explanted).

The rupture of an implant may be dramatic or totally unsuspected. Ruptured saline implants deflate rapidly. The silicone rubber envelope of a silicone gel implant may tear, and the gel, which is extremely viscid, may be literally splattered into the surrounding tissues (Fig. 17-35 A–E). The extruded silicone in some ruptures appears to maintain some coherence and is visible as globules, some of which form

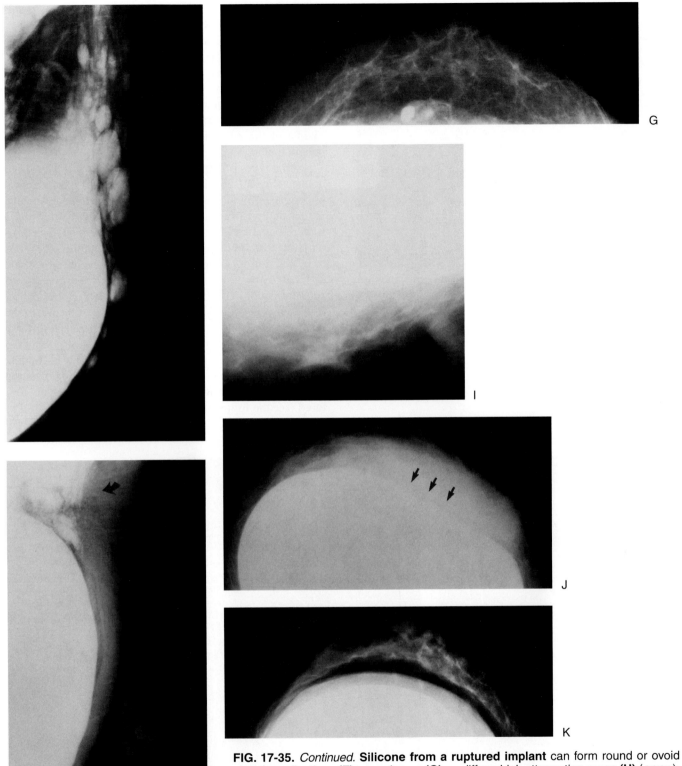

FIG. 17-35. *Continued.* **Silicone from a ruptured implant** can form round or ovoid globular collections **(F)**, granulomas **(G)**, or diffuse high attenuation areas **(H)** (*arrow*).

Clinically occult cancer can be detected among women with implants. In this individual, clustered calcifications at the bottom of the breast adjacent to the implant are barely visible on this enlargement of the lateral mammogram **(I)** (image courtesy of the New England Medical Center). They were confirmed with spot compression that displaced the implant out of the field of view and at biopsy proved to be due to ductal carcinoma in situ. Other cancers may cause a deformity in the implant, as in this patient whose palpable cancer was depressing the implant **(J)** (*arrows*), while still others may not be visible by mammography but can be imaged by ultrasound. In this patient the palpable invasive cancer was not evident on the mammogram **(K)**. *Continued.*

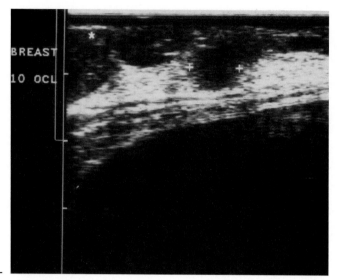

FIG. 17-35. *Continued.* However, the cancer was evident on the ultrasound **(L)** as an irregularly shaped, hypoechoic mass.

granulomas (Fig. 17-35F, G), while in some cases the silicone forms irregular masses (Fig. 17-35H).

There are other less obvious forms of implant rupture. Their manifestation is influenced by whether or not there is fibrous encapsulation of the implant and how the implant rupture relates to the capsule. Often, however, the time of rupture is indeterminate. A tear may develop and the envelope may merely retract due to its own elasticity into the middle of the gel, while the gel remains fairly contained behind the breast.

Several types of implant deformity and rupture have been defined (Fig. 17-36). Because many implants have a partial or complete fibrous capsule that forms around them, silicone may actually extravasate into the surrounding tissue from a ruptured implant (extracapsular rupture) or be contained within the fibrous capsule (intracapsular rupture).

In addition to a rupture, implants can be deformed and distorted by tissue pressures and the fibrotic reaction of capsular formation. This can produce undulations in the contour of the implant and folds in the envelope that project into the gel, forming radial folds. The latter can at times be difficult to distinguish from a rupture with the torn envelope sinking into the gel (72). Given the perceived importance of implant rupture, the challenge for imaging is differentiating distorted implants with intact envelopes from those that are truly ruptured (see the following section).

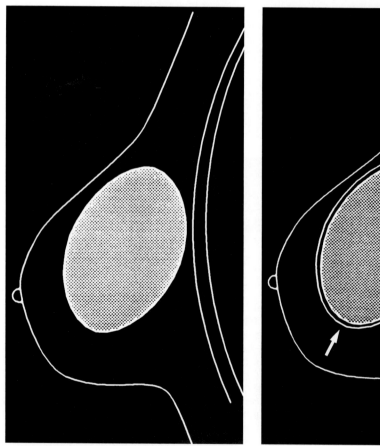
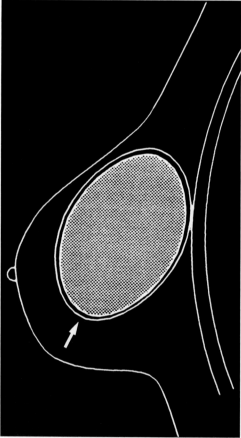

FIG. 17-36. These schematics summarize the **various changes that can occur with implants. (A)** The normal implant is round or ovoid. **(B)** A fibrous capsule can form around the implant (*arrow*). *Continued.*

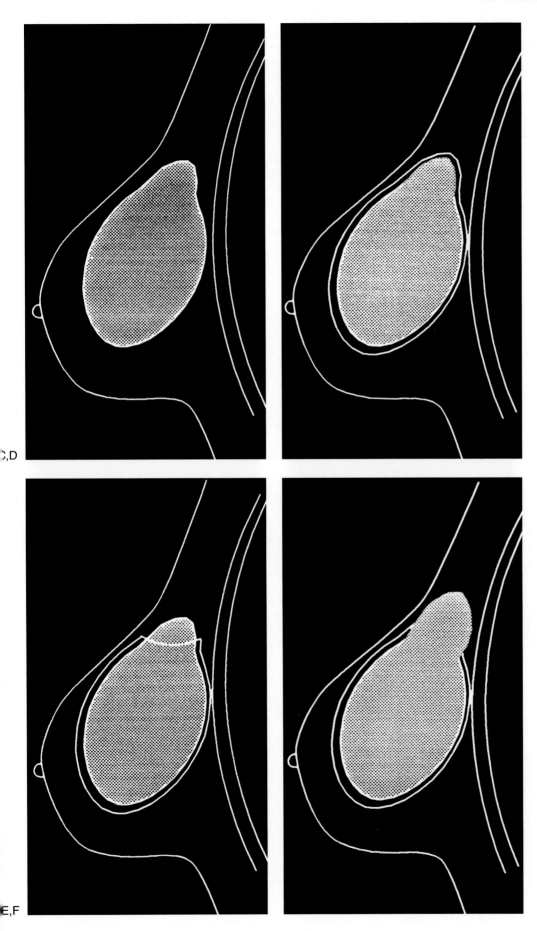

C,D

E,F

FIG. 17-36. *Continued.* **(C)** Un-encapsulated implants can bulge and deform under normal tissue pressures and still not be ruptured. **(D)** Any deformity of an intact envelope can be encapsulated. **(E)** Deformity cannot be distinguished from a herniation of the intact implant through a portion of the capsule. **(F)** Deformity and herniation cannot be distinguished from a truly ruptured implant as long as the gel maintains a smooth contour. *Continued.*

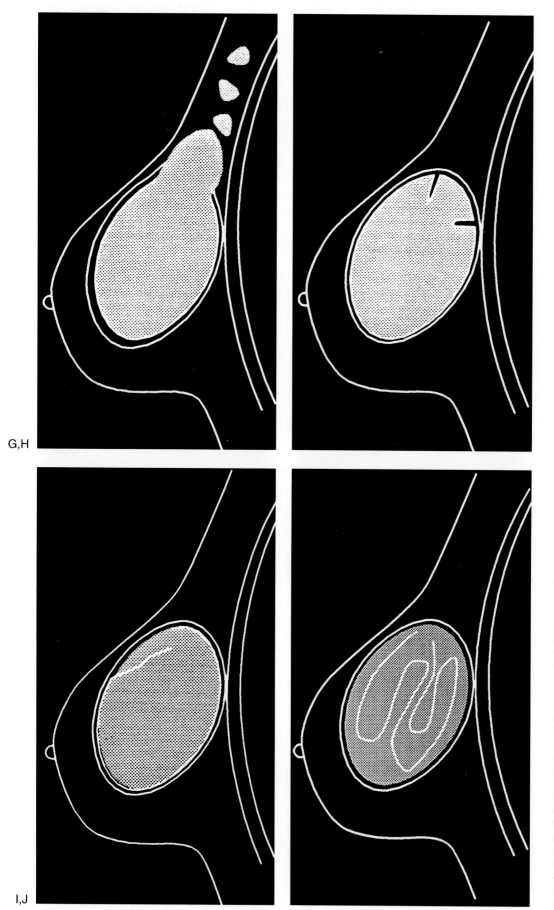

G,H

I,J

FIG. 17-36. *Continued.*
(G) Separate collections of silicone outside the implant are clear proof of implant rupture. **(H)** Normal radial folds caused by an infolding of the redundant envelope under tissue molding can be seen on ultrasound or MRI and do not represent evidence of rupture. **(I)** Intracapsular rupture. If the implant has ruptured, early retraction of the envelope may be visible on ultrasound or MRI. If the capsule is intact, it is termed an *intracapsular rupture.* **(J)** An even stronger indication of intracapsular rupture is seen by the linguine sign, in which the envelope's elastic recoil causes it to contract into the center of the gel. The smooth contour of the gel may remain intact due to its retention by the surrounding capsule, making it difficult to make the diagnosis from a mammogram.

Implants and Cancer: Risk and Detection

Implants and Risk of Developing Breast Cancer

Fears that implants might induce a malignancy in the breast have been raised, although these fears have not been substantiated in humans. In certain strains of rats, the positioning of a hard foreign body under the skin results in the development of soft-tissue sarcomas, and some investigators suggest the silicone gel causes plasmacytomas in laboratory animals. These problems have never been documented other than anecdotally in humans. As noted earlier, implants covered by polyurethane may release TDA, which has been shown to cause hepatic cancer in mice and rats (66). Although this problem has not as yet been shown in humans, concern remains, particularly in light of the fact that the coating does appear to break down over time and it is very difficult to remove these implants entirely because they were designed to encourage the tissues to grow into the coating.

Fortunately, implants do not appear to increase the risk of breast cancers. In a Canadian study, the presence of implants appears to have reduced the risk of cancer by 50% (73). Biases in that study prevent drawing absolute conclusions, but at least there is no evidence of excess breast cancer. Some very preliminary data suggest that the serum from some women with implants can kill breast cancer cells in vitro (Garrido L, personal communication, 1997). The implications, if this is true, are enormous, but it remains to be shown that this is in fact the case.

Implants and Breast Cancer Detection

It has been shown that implants may interfere with breast cancer detection by mammography. The implant can reduce the ability of mammography to image the tissues of the breast by blocking x-ray transmission. This is exacerbated by the rigidity of the breast if there is capsular contracture (74). One study suggests that as a result of implants cancers may be detected at a later stage than in women who do not have implants (75). In this study, 65% of the women who had implants and invasive cancer had positive nodes at the time of diagnosis (none were discovered by mammography alone), whereas only 28% of a parallel group of women without implants had positive nodes. This study was contradicted by another review in which 33 women with implants who developed breast cancer were compared to 1,735 women with cancer who had not had breast augmentation (76). In this second study, although 24% of the women with breast augmentation had their cancers detected by mammography as compared to 44% among those without implants, the incidence of DCIS was the same in both groups (18% vs. 15%). The sizes of the cancers were the same in both groups. Perhaps as a result of the implant pushing the tissue against the skin and aiding clinical detection, the author found that the size of the palpable cancers was smaller among women with implants. There was no good explanation for the fact that

only 19% of the women with implants had positive axillary lymph nodes as compared to 41% among those with no implants, although it was likely directly related to the detection of palpable invasive cancers at a smaller size because the node positivity rates were the same if the cancer was detected by mammography (13% vs. 15%).

Implants present a dilemma for mammography in that they obscure the breast tissue due to their high attenuation. Furthermore, the implant serves to compress the breast tissue against the skin, causing the reverse of the desired compression achieved using mammography. Pulling the breast away from the implant and displacing the implant back against the chest wall does permit improved compression of the breast tissue (see Chapter 10). However, there is still a large amount of breast tissue near the chest wall that cannot be optimally visualized even with this technique. In general, it would appear prudent to obtain tangential views to the implant using conventional mammographic positioning (mediolateral oblique [MLO] and CC) and then repeat with the implant displacement technique. Cancers may be seen in the tissues at the periphery of the implant (Fig. 17-35I). The lesion may not be visible, but it may indent the implant (Fig. 17-35J). If the mammogram is not diagnostic for a palpable mass (Fig. 17-35K), ultrasound is useful to determine if the mass is cystic or solid (Fig. 17-35L) and to guide a needle biopsy to avoid rupturing the implant.

BREAST RECONSTRUCTION AFTER MASTECTOMY

Tissue Expanders and Implants

Several methods are available to reconstruct a breast after mastectomy. The least complicated involves positioning a tissue expander under the skin covering the chest wall on the mastectomy side. This expander is essentially an implant that can have saline injected percutaneously through a valve periodically over several weeks. The skin gradually stretches to accommodate the expander and ultimately permits placement of a permanent implant.

Myocutaneous Flaps

More complicated reconstructions involve tissue transfers from other parts of the body. Although free tissue transfers can be done, it is generally better to move tissue with its blood supply intact. The use of abdominal soft tissues overlying and containing half of the rectus abdominis muscle is termed the TRAM flap (transverse rectus abdominis myocutaneous flap). A crescent of tissue is removed from the suprapubic region along with part of the rectus muscle. The blood supply to the graft is maintained by not severing the epigastric vessels. The graft on this muscle-vascular-fat-skin pedicle is then moved up to the chest through a tunnel dissected under the skin of the upper abdomen. The tissue is used to fill the space previously

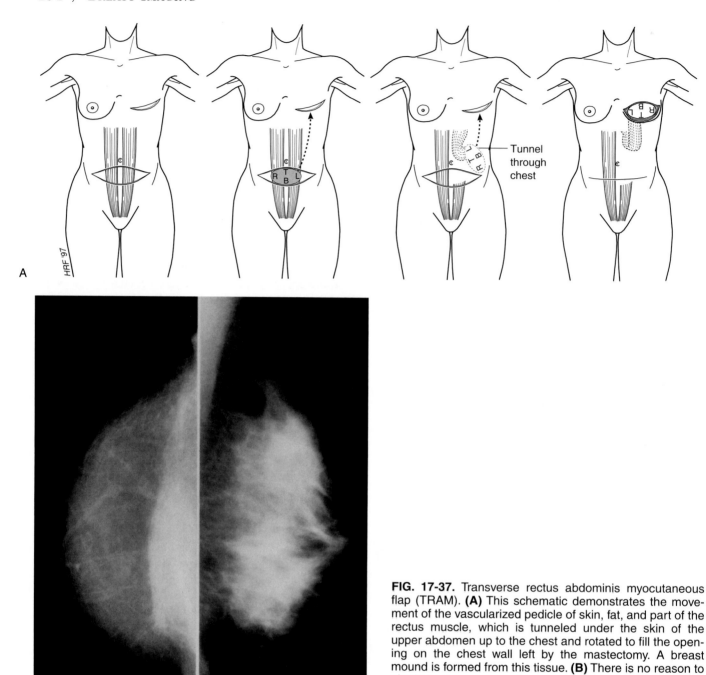

FIG. 17-37. Transverse rectus abdominis myocutaneous flap (TRAM). **(A)** This schematic demonstrates the movement of the vascularized pedicle of skin, fat, and part of the rectus muscle, which is tunneled under the skin of the upper abdomen up to the chest and rotated to fill the opening on the chest wall left by the mastectomy. A breast mound is formed from this tissue. **(B)** There is no reason to obtain a mammogram of a reconstructed breast after a total mastectomy. The breast on the right is normal. The tissue on the left is a TRAM flap imaged by mistake.

occupied by the breast (Fig. 17-37A). A mound is fashioned on the chest wall, and then various methods are used to reconstruct a nipple on this mound of tissue. The latissimus dorsi has also been used for this type of reconstruction.

Imaging After Mastectomy

Because there is no residual breast tissue after a mastectomy, breast imaging is rarely helpful in assessing the reconstructed breast (Fig. 17-37B). There are no prospective studies suggest-

ing any benefit from imaging the reconstructed breast after a mastectomy, although Loyer and associates have described various appearances of these grafts (77), and Mund and associates described a case in which recurrence in a TRAM flap was detected by a mammogram (78). Despite this single case report, because there is no breast tissue to image, mammography is of little benefit if a recurrence is suspected or for screening. If there is a concern about the graft or the surrounding tissues, CT or MRI is likely of greater value for imaging the tissues around the implant in the reconstructed breast.

IMAGING ANALYSIS OF IMPLANTS

The numerous changes that can occur after implant placement are summarized in Figure 17-36. Only a few are evident by mammography. In general MRI seems to be the best single method for evaluating implants.

Mammography

The primary reason for mammography remains the earlier detection of breast cancer. Implants make mammography more difficult. In addition to being radiopaque and obscuring visualization of portions of the breast tissue, the implant compresses the tissues toward the skin. This is exactly opposite to the compression needed to spread the tissues apart for optimal tissue evaluation.

Mammographic Positioning

The positioning of women with implants is described in detail in Chapter 10. The goal is to image as much of the tissue as possible. Mammography can aid in analyzing the status of the implants, but it is primarily used for the earlier detection of cancer in the breast. The standard views include the MLO and CC with the implant in the field of view using just sufficient compression to hold the breast as far into the field of view as possible to permit evaluation of the tissues deep and around the implant. Excess compression only pushes the implant toward the skin and compresses the tissues in the wrong direction.

The two projections are then repeated trying to displace the implants back toward the chest wall in an effort to better visualize the breast tissues (Fig. 17-38). Implant displacement views improve the ability to image the breast tissues (see Chapter 10). By displacing the implant back against the chest wall, the breast tissues can be pulled forward as with a normal mammogram. Direct compression of the breast tissues, separating overlapping structures, can then be applied with improved results. Unfortunately even these special projections do not permit imaging the entire volume of breast tissue, and usually the deep tissues are not optimally imaged.

The type of implant and its location may determine the feasibility of implant displacement imaging. Implants that are placed behind the pectoralis major muscle make it much easier to obtain mammograms with the implants out of the field of view than do implants in the retromammary position.

If an implant cannot be displaced, then views obtained tangential to it can image as much tissue as possible. This can usually be accomplished by obtaining the MLO, CC, and straight lateral (ML) projections (Fig. 17-39).

Detection of a Ruptured Implant

The FDA decision to prohibit the use of silicone gel implants for augmentation except within controlled clinical trials and the attendant concerns raised among women who already have implants has generated a great deal of interest in developing methods to detect implant rupture. At present there is no method that can prove that an implant is not ruptured. Mammography

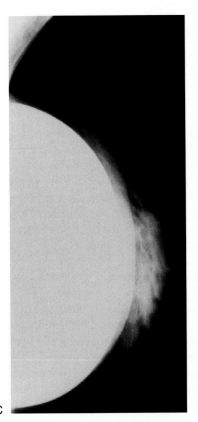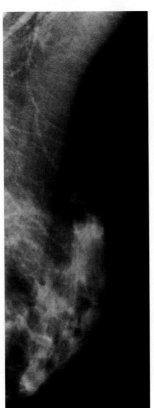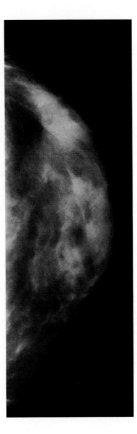

A–C

FIG. 17-38. (A) Mediolateral oblique (MLO) including the implant in the field of view. Note that the tissue is compressed toward the skin in this individual with a retropectoral implant. The implant is then displaced out of the field of view on the same MLO projection (B), as well as the craniocaudal (C) projection, so that the tissues can be better compressed and evaluated.

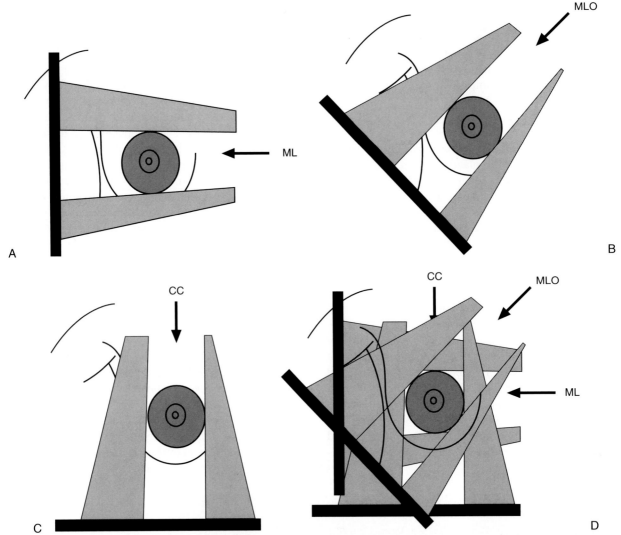

FIG. 17-39. If the implant cannot be displaced, adding the mediolateral **(A)** straight lateral projection to the mediolateral oblique **(B)** and the craniocaudal **(C)** provides tangents to the implant to permit some evaluation of most of the breast **(D)**.

remains the easiest method for detecting a rupture if the rupture produces changes that are visible on the mammogram.

Some radiologists have found CT (79) or ultrasound (80) useful in the evaluation of implants. MRI is perhaps the most useful system for evaluating implants (81). A comparison of mammography, MRI, ultrasound, and CT was performed by Gorczyca and associates, and using rabbits in which one intact and one ruptured implant was placed, they found that MRI and CT were the most accurate in detecting rupture (MR was slightly better than CT) with ultrasound and mammography considerably less accurate (82). There is no test that can determine that the envelope is intact, but each can demonstrate findings that strongly suggest rupture (see Chapters 16 and 20).

Mammography and Rupture of Implants

There has been some concern that the compression from mammography may rupture an implant. This is a theoretic

concern, but there have only been rare, anecdotal descriptions of cases where this was thought to have occurred. Implants are designed to withstand several hundred pounds of pressure. The average mammogram generates <4 lb psi. This is even less than the pressure of an examining finger, which generates 6 lb psi (83). It is no more likely that a mammogram will rupture an implant than many of the pressures on the chest encountered in daily living.

Mammographic Evaluation of Implants

The normal implant (see Fig. 17-38A) is hemi-ovoid on the lateral projection. Fibrous encapsulation tends to cause the implant to become hard and round and may make it difficult to displace the implant for imaging. The use of polyurethane-coated implants that encourage the growth of breast tissue into the surface of the implant may further complicate imaging. If a capsule has formed and

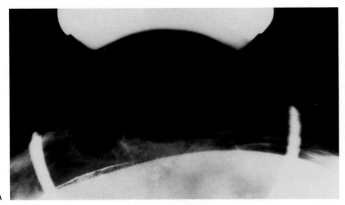

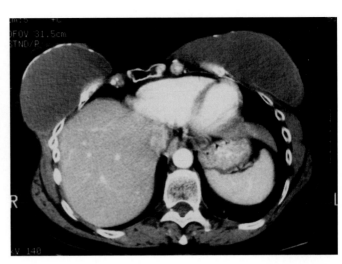

FIG. 17-40. (A) Calcifications are visible in the fibrous capsule that has formed around the implant envelope on this spot compression view. **(B)** Calcification is evident in the fibrous capsule of the left implant and, to a lesser extent, of the right implant on this CT scan of another patient.

contracted, the implant may assume a rounder, hemispherical shape. Sometimes calcifications are evident in the fibrous capsule surrounding the implant (Fig. 17-40). The surface of the implant may demonstrate bulges and depressions that are likely due to pressure deformity from the surrounding tissues or incomplete fibrous encapsulation. The intact envelope itself can fold into the gel and form a radial fold (see Fig. 17-36H). This is distinguished from a rupture forming a teardrop deformity of the envelope. The latter is not only surrounded by silicone, but it contains silicone within the fold. This can only occur if there has been a rupture.

It has been suggested that the implant, with envelope intact, can bulge through a surrounding capsule as a herniation (Fig. 17-41). A herniation cannot be differentiated from a rupture in which the gel stays together and maintains a smooth surface. In fact, the envelope of an implant may be totally disrupted and collapsed into the gel (intracapsular rupture), yet the fibrous capsule smoothly contains the gel so that the implant appears normal on the mammogram (84).

Although there is no test that can prove that an implant is not ruptured, some ruptures are apparent on the mammogram. Irregular collections of silicone may be seen outside

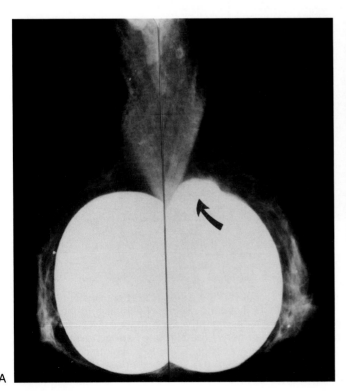

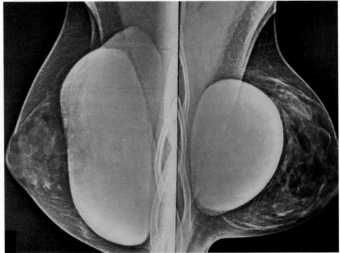

FIG. 17-41. Herniation is indistinguishable from a focal rupture if the silicone gel remains smoothly contoured. The superior bulge in this implant (*arrow*) may represent a rupture or merely a herniation of an intact implant through a discontinuous capsule **(A)**. In this second patient **(B)** the implant on the left, evaluated using xerography, is elongated and ruptured while retaining smooth contours. Rounding of the implant on the right suggests fibrous encapsulation. *Continued.*

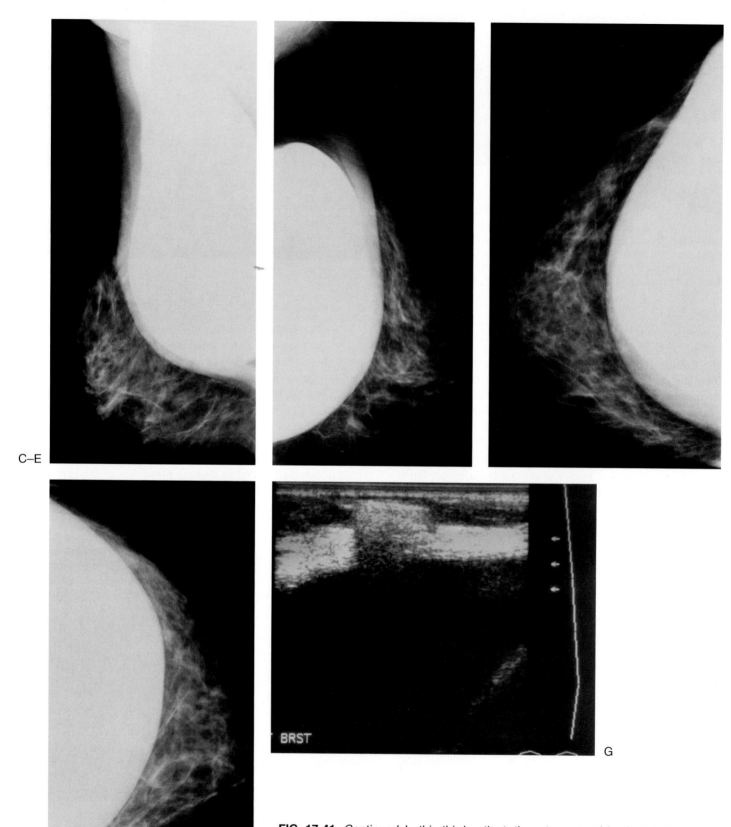

C–E

F

G

FIG. 17-41. *Continued.* In this third patient, the retropectoral implant on the left is elongated toward the axilla on the mediolateral oblique **(C)** relative to the right **(D)** and on the craniocaudal **(E)** relative to the right **(F)**. Both implants were found to be **ruptured** on MRI and confirmed by surgery. **Free silicone "snowstorm" on ultrasound.** Free silicone can produce a very echogenic appearance on ultrasound with some posterior shadowing, as in this patient **(G)** (image courtesy of Norman Sadowsky, MD, Faulkner Sagoff Breast Center, Brookline, MA).

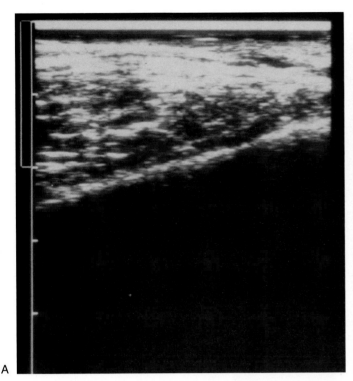

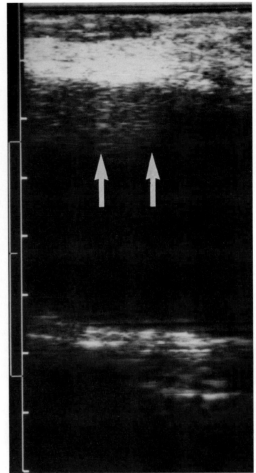

A

B

FIG. 17-42. Normal silicone gel is anechoic. The echo-free area on this ultrasound is the implant with breast tissue anterior to it **(A)**. The gel of a ruptured implant may have increased echogenicity. This must be differentiated from the reverberation artifact that can occur along the anterior undersurface of the normal implant **(B)** (*arrows*).

the implant (see Fig. 17-35). Silicone in axillary lymph nodes is a clear indication that an implant has ruptured.

Ultrasound Evaluation of Implants

Free silicone can appear as hypoechoic globules adjacent to the implant or can cause innumerable echoes adjacent to the surface of the implant. The latter has been likened to a snow storm of echoes (85) and termed *echogenic noise* (86) (see Fig. 17-41). The cause of the echogenicity is debated. It may be due to the particles themselves, reverberation, or phase shifts in the acoustic patterns as a result of the silicone in the soft tissues.

Normally silicone gel is anechoic (Fig. 17-42A). Some believe that a diffuse increase in the echogenicity of the usually sonolucent gel suggests that the implant is ruptured (Fig. 17-42B) (87). The explanation for this is uncertain. It is possible that the admixture of body fluids with the gel changes its acoustic properties. This echogenicity must be distinguished from the not uncommon reverberation artifact that can be seen beneath the anterior envelope echoes (Fig. 17-42C). This echogenicity can be distinguished from reverberation artifacts by its nonparallel configuration and the

fact that it moves independently of an up-and-down displacement of the edge of the gel by variable pressure back toward the chest wall using the transducer.

The "linguine sign" described on MRI (see the following section) that represents the ruptured silicone envelope folding back and forth on itself as it collapses into the gel (see Fig. 17-37I, J) can also be seen on ultrasound as a stepladder of specular reflections in the implant gel (Fig. 17-43).

Magnetic Resonance and Implant Evaluation

We have found that using surface coils to improve the signal-to-noise ratio and both breasts simultaneously to permit comparison is the best approach to implant imaging. A common approach is to use an axial T1-weighted gradient echo localizer with a flip angle of 30 degrees, then a sagittal fast spin echo (FSE) T2-weighted sequence, then an axial FSE with water suppression. Using an FSE inversion recovery technique, fat can be suppressed. Some find the evaluation of coronal as well as axial and sagittal planes is helpful (88). Because silicone, fat, and water have different resonant frequencies (Fig. 17-44), suppression techniques can be used to determine what is silicone on the images. On T2 imaging,

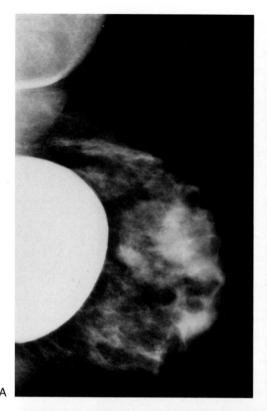

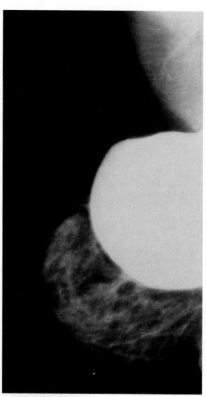

A

B

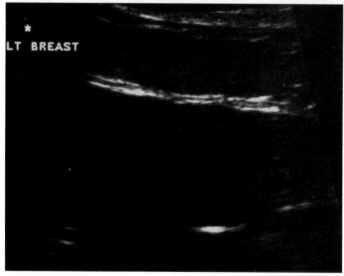

C

FIG. 17-43. The linguine sign on ultrasound. The implant in the right breast **(A)** is normal in contour. The implant in the left breast **(B)** has an abnormal bulge and undulating surface that suggests rupture. On the ultrasound **(C)** the first specular reflections are from the edge of the silicone gel. The brighter curvilinear specular reflections from within the gel are from the ruptured silicone envelope that has collapsed and is sinking into the gel.

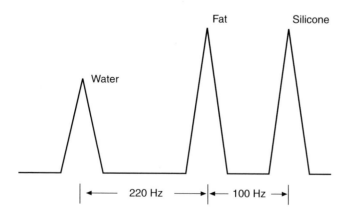

FIG. 17-44. The resonance frequencies of silicone, water, and fat are sufficiently separate to permit the use of fat- and water-suppression techniques to enhance the differentiation of silicone from the others on MRI.

TABLE 17-2. *Magnetic resonance imaging T1 and T2*

Fat: Short T1 and short T2
Parenchyma: Variable T1 and variable T2
Muscle: Variable T1 comparable to parenchyma and T2
   shorter than parenchyma
Water: Long T1 and long T2
Silicone: Long T1 and long T2

silicone and water have high signal intensity, whereas fat is lower. Water suppression improves the differentiation of silicone from fluid on the T2 images.

By using water-suppression techniques and T2 imaging, fat remains of medium signal intensity whereas the silicone gel appears as the brightest signal and cysts or peri-implant fluid collections are suppressed and have low signal. This permits the differentiation of fluid from free silicone. Double-lumen implants have a saline compartment, and water

TABLE 17-3. *Magnetic resonance imaging signal intensities*

	Fat	Parenchyma	Muscle	Saline	Silicone
	Short T1	Intermediate T1	Intermediate T1	Long T1	Long T1
T1 signal intensity	High	Intermediate	Intermediate	Low	Low
T2 signal intensity	High	Intermediate	Low	High	High

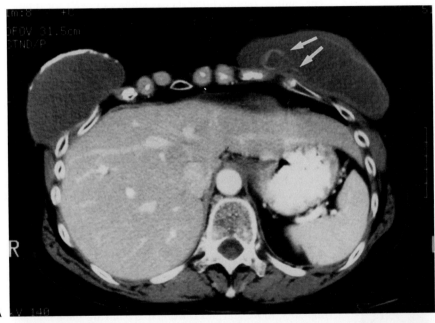

A

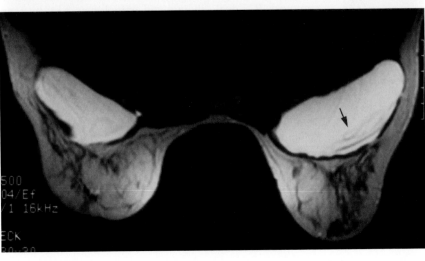

B

FIG. 17-45. The linguine sign on CT and MRI. The silicone rubber envelope can be seen folding on itself as a higher attenuation structure in the silicone gel on CT (*arrows*) **(A)**. The same phenomenon is visible in a different patient on MRI. In this patient **(B)** the silicone gel produces a high signal on these T2-weighted images. The envelope is a rope-like structure (*arrow*) folding back and forth and low in signal intensity. This is the cross-section of the **envelope that is collapsing into the gel**, forming an accordion-like structure. In both patients the envelope has ruptured and collapsed into the gel. The gel keeps its shape because it is still held in place by the fibrous capsule that had formed previously. On cross-section the envelope looks like a string of pasta. Rupture should not be confused with radial folds that are merely the crenated, intact envelope folding in on itself.

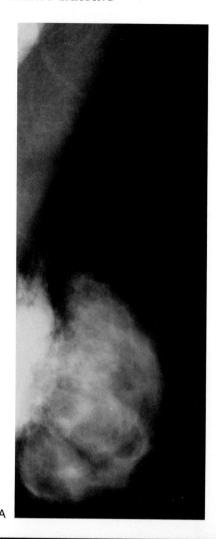

A

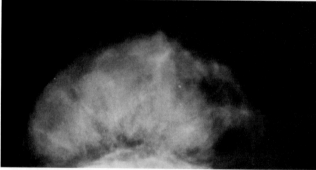

B

FIG. 17-46. Scarring after explantation. In this patient prominent scarring deep in the breast after the removal of an implant is visible on the mediolateral oblique **(A)** and the craniocaudal **(B)** projections. It is not possible to tell if there is also free silicone in the tissues, although the high attenuation is suggestive. MRI could be used to make this determination if it was needed.

suppression is useful in distinguishing this as well. The silicone envelope is low in signal intensity on T2-weighted images and is seen as a dark band.

On the T1-weighted images silicone has the lowest signal due to its long T1, whereas it is bright on T2 images because of its long T2. Fat has high signal intensity on T1 (short T1),

whereas its longer T2 contributes to its intermediate signal. Breast parenchyma has intermediate signal on both types of imaging, whereas muscle is intermediate on T1 and lower signal on T2 (Tables 17-2 and 17-3).

The Collapsing Implant Envelope

Perhaps the most accurate sign of implant rupture comes from the visualization on ultrasound (89) or MRI (81) of the envelope collapsing into the gel (90). MRI demonstrated intracapsular rupture by revealing portions of the envelope floating within the silicone gel. Gorczyca and colleagues have described this as the linguine sign because on cross-sectional imaging the rubber envelope appears to fold back and forth in the gel, having the appearance of pasta folding back and forth (Fig. 17-45). They confirmed this in an animal model (91).

The collapsing envelope is the strongest indicator of an intracapsular rupture. In Gorczyca's series of 143 women, intracapsular tears were found in 14% of the explanted prostheses. Extracapsular rupture occurred in two cases (1.4%). The authors reported that the sensitivity of MRI for rupture of either kind was 76%, with a specificity of 97%.

The collapsing envelope has also been seen on ultrasound (see Ultrasound Evaluation of Implants) in the form of a linear or series of linear specular reflections from the torn envelope as it slowly sinks into the gel, which itself remains contained within the fibrous capsule.

Everson and colleagues concluded that MRI was the best method for detecting implant rupture when they compared mammography, CT, and ultrasound (92). In their series of 32 women with 63 implants (22 found to be ruptured at surgery) mammography detected only 23% of the ruptures (with a specificity of 98%), whereas ultrasound detected 59% (specificity of 79%) with CT 82% sensitive and 88% specific. MRI was able to detect 95% of the ruptures with a specificity of 93%.

Imaging After Explantation

As a consequence of the attention paid to concerns over implants, more and more women are having their implants removed. Residual silicone and granulomas may be seen. Residual fibrous capsule has been described, as have calcifications associated with the fibrous capsule (93). We have seen what appears to be rather pronounced scarring after explantation (Fig. 17-46). If it has not also been removed, the fibrous capsule may be visible at the back of the breast (Fig. 17-47A, B). Residual silicone may be present if the explanted implant had ruptured, and the fibrous capsule may remain (Fig. 17-47 A–D).

Breast Cancer Detection in Women with Implants

The primary reason for doing mammography in women with augmented breasts is the same as for other women—the earlier detection of breast cancer. As noted earlier, some data suggest

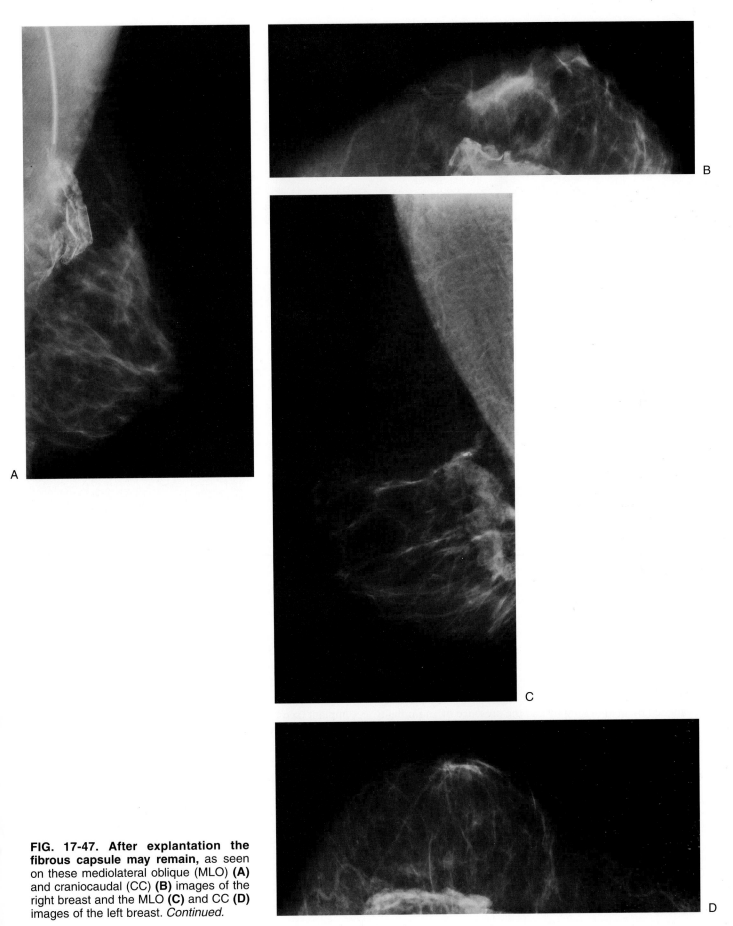

FIG. 17-47. After explantation the fibrous capsule may remain, as seen on these mediolateral oblique (MLO) **(A)** and craniocaudal (CC) **(B)** images of the right breast and the MLO **(C)** and CC **(D)** images of the left breast. *Continued.*

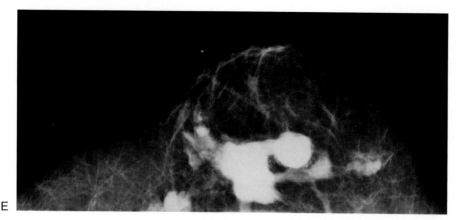

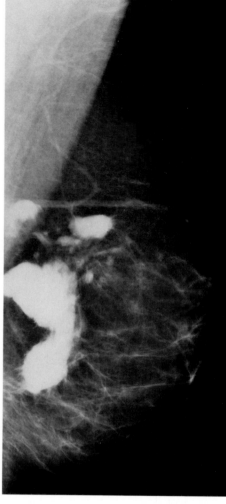

FIG. 17-47. *Continued.* In another patient **residual silicone and silicone granulomas** are visible in the right breast on the MLO **(E)** and CC **(F)** images. They were due to the rupture that led to the explantation. They were left behind when the ruptured implant was removed.

that the sensitivity of mammography is reduced in women with implants, as would be expected, but early cancers can be detected. Mammography is likely to be valuable even if a subcutaneous mastectomy has been performed, because residual breast tissue is present in which cancer can develop. The same primary and secondary signs of malignancy should be sought in a woman who has had an augmentation mammaplasty.

Although the implant may obscure some of the mammary parenchyma, a significant amount of tissue can be evaluated by mammography and the presence of an implant does not preclude the detection of cancer by mammography. In addition to the MLO and CC views that provide analysis of the tissues using x-rays tangential to the implant, implant displacement views can permit evaluation of much of the breast tissue with near standard compression. If there is no fibrous encapsulation, the implant can be pushed back against the chest wall out of the field of view and the breast can be pulled forward away from the implant. This permits compression of the breast without the implant's obstructing the image. The deep tissues may not be included, however, and the tangential views should still be obtained to try to evaluate these areas. If the implant

cannot be displaced, a straight lateral view is added to try to include all tangents to the implant.

Calcifications on occasion occur in association with the capsule that forms around the implant. When benign they generally appear as plaque-like deposits near the surface of the implant (see Fig. 17-45).

Breast cancer presents in the same fashion as in the nonaugmented breast. Clustered microcalcifications may be present. We have seen a tumor mass indent the silicone implant (see Fig. 17-44). When a mass is apparent either by mammography alone or by palpation, ultrasonography may be advisable for cyst/solid differentiation (see Chapter 16). Probing an indeterminate lesion with a needle is probably undesirable when an implant is present. Ultrasound-guided needle biopsy can be performed, because the course of the needle can be monitored in real time.

Preoperative Localization in Women with Implants

If a lesion is detected in the implanted breast, needle localization techniques can be used to insert wires tangential to the surface of the implant to avoid puncturing the implant while permitting accurate localization. This is accomplished by using fenestrated compression plates and pushing the implant back out of the field of view while pulling the area of tissue in question into the localization window. The localization is then performed in the standard fashion (94). Ultrasound can also be used to monitor the positioning of the needle and deployment of a wire (see Chapter 21).

REFERENCES

1. Swinford AK, Adler SS, Garver KA. Mammographic appearance of the breasts during pregnancy and lactation: false assumptions. Presented at the 97th Meeting of the American Roentgen Ray Society; May 4–9, 1997; Boston, MA.
2. Liberman L, Giess CS, Dershaw DD, et al. Imaging pregnancy-associated breast cancer. Radiology 1994;191:245–248.
3. Zemlickis D, Lishner M, Degendorfer P, et al. Maternal and fetal outcome after breast cancer in pregnancy. Am J Obstet Gynecol 1992; 166:781–787.
4. Petrek JA, Dukoff R, Rogatko A. Prognosis of pregnancy-associated breast cancer. Cancer 1991;67:869–872.
5. Guinee VF, Olsson H, Moller T, et al. Effect of pregnancy on prognosis for young women with breast cancer. Lancet 1994;343:1587–1589.
6. Mann BD, Giulian AK, Bassett LW, et al. Delayed diagnosis of breast cancer as a result of normal mammograms. Arch Surg 1983;118:23–24.
7. Layfield LJ, Parkinson B, Wong J, et al. Mammographically guided fine-needle aspiration biopsy of nonpalpable breast lesions. Cancer 1991;68:2007–2011.
8. Parker SH, Lovin JD, Jobe WE, et al. Nonpalpable breast lesions: stereotactic automated large-core biopsies. Radiology 1991;180:403–407.
9. Fornage BD, Fariux MJ, Simatos A. Breast masses: US guided fine-needle aspiration biopsy. Radiology 1987;162:409–414.
10. Kopans DB, Meyer JE. Computed tomography guided localization of clinically occult breast carcinoma—the "N" skin guide. Radiology 1982;145:211–212.
11. Fischer U, Vosshenrich R, Doler W, et al. MR imaging–guided breast intervention: experience with two systems. Radiology 1995;195: 533–538.
12. Klein DL, Sickles EA. Effects of needle aspiration on the mammographic appearance of the breast: a guide to the proper timing of the mammography examination. Radiology 1982;145:44.
13. Kaye MD, Vicinanza-Adami CA, Sullivan ML. Mammographic findings after stereotaxic biopsy of the breast performed with large-core needles. Radiology 1994;192:149–151.
14. The National Women's Health Network. White Paper on Breast Cancer Screening.
15. Sickles EA, Herzog KA. Mammography of the postsurgical breast. AJR Am J Roentgenol 1981;136:585–588.
16. Mitnick J, Roses DF, Harris MN. Differentiation of postsurgical changes from carcinoma of the breast. Surg Gynecol Obstet 1988;166:549–550.
17. Meyer JE, Kopans DB. Analysis of mammographically obvious breast carcinomas with benign results on initial biopsy. Surg Gynecol Obstet 1981;153:570–572.
18. Kopans DB, Swann CA, White G, et al. Asymmetric breast tissue. Radiology 1989;171:639–643.
19. Gallagher WJ, Cardenosa G, Rubens JR, et al. Minimal-volume excision of nonpalpable breast lesions. AJR Am J Roentgenol 1989;153:957–961.
20. Miller CL, Feig SA, Fox JW. Mammographic changes after reduction mammoplasty. AJR Am J Roentgenol 1987;149:35–38.
21. Early Breast Cancer Trialists' Collaborative Group. Systemic treatment of early breast cancer by hormonal, cytotoxic, or immune therapy. Lancet 1992;339:1–15, 71–85.
22. Ghossein NA, Alpert S, Barba J, et al. Breast cancer. Arch Surg 1992; 127:411–415.
23. Holland R, Solke HJ, Mravunac M, Hendriks JH. Histologic multifocality of Tis, T1-2 breast carcinomas—implications for clinical trials of breast-conserving surgery. Cancer 1985;56:979–990.
24. Holland R, Hendriks JH, Vebeek AL, et al. Extent, distribution, and mammographic/histological correlations of breast ductal carcinoma in situ. Lancet 1990;335:519–522.
25. Rosner D, Lane WW, Penetrante R. Ductal carcinoma in situ with microinvasion. Cancer 1991;67:1498–1503.
26. Shulman M, Sadfarangani GJ. Breast cancer—importance of adequate surgical excision prior to radiotherapy in the local control of breast cancer in patients treated conservatively. Arch Surg 1992;127:411–415.
27. Veronisi V, Salvadori B, Luini A, et al. Conservative treatment of early breast cancer: long-term results of 1232 cases treated with quandrectomy, axillary dissection, and radiotherapy. Ann Surg 1990;211: 250–259.
28. Ohtake T, Abe R, Izoh K, et al. Intraductal extension of primary invasive breast carcinoma treated by breast conservative surgery. Cancer 1995;76:32–45.
29. Fisher B, Redmond C, Fisher E, et al. Ten-year results of a randomized clinical trial comparing radical mastectomy and total mastectomy with or without radiation. N Engl J Med 1985;312:674.
30. Fajardo LL, Roberts CC, Hunt KR. Mammographic surveillance of breast cancer patients: should the mastectomy site be imaged? AJR Am J Roentgenol 1993;161:953–955.
31. Propeck PA, Scanlan KA. Utility of axillary views in postmastectomy patients. Radiology 1993;187:769–771.
32. Hellman S, Harris HR. Breast cancer: considerations in local and regional treatment. Radiology 1986;164:593–598.
33. Fisher B, Anderson S, Redmond C, et al. Reanalysis and results after 12 years of follow-up in a randomized clinical trial comparing total mastectomy with lumpectomy with or without irradiation in the treatment of breast cancer. N Engl J Med 1995;333:1456–1461.
34. Harris JR, Schnitt SJ, Connolly JL. Conservative surgery and radiation therapy for early breast cancer. Arch Surg 1987;122:754–755.
35. Libshitz HI, Montague ED, Paulus DO. Calcifications and the therapeutically irradiated breast. AJR Am J Roentgenol 1977;128: 1021–1025.
36. Stacey-Clear A, McCarthy KA, Hall DA, et al. Calcified suture material in the breast after radiation therapy. Radiology 1992;183:207–208.
37. Gluck BS, Dershaw DD, Liberman L, Deutch BM. Microcalcifications on postoperative mammograms as an indicator of adequacy of tumor excision. Radiology 1993;188:469–472.
38. Ohuchi N, Furuta A, Mori S. Management of ductal carcinoma in situ with nipple discharge. Intraductal spreading of carcinoma is an unfavorable pathologic factor for breast-conserving surgery. Cancer 1994; 74:1294–1302.
39. Mendelson EB. Imaging the post-surgical breast. Semin Ultrasound CT MR 1989;10:154–170.
40. Sadowsky NL, Semine A, Harris JR. Breast imaging: a critical aspect of breast conserving treatment. Cancer 1990;65:2113–2118.
41. Dershaw DD, Shank B, Reisinger S. Mammographic findings after breast cancer treatment with local excision and definitive irradiation. Radiology 1987;164:455–456.
42. Mendelson EB. Evaluation of the postoperative breast. Radiol Clin North Am 1992;30:107–138.
43. Kopans DB. Problems with the American College of Radiology Standard for Diagnostic Mammography. AJR Am J Roentgenol 1995; 165:1367–1369.
44. Gilles R, Guinebretiere JM, Shapeero LG, et al. Assessment of breast cancer recurrence with contrast-enhanced subtraction MR imaging: preliminary results in 26 patients. Radiology 1993;188:473–478.
45. Heywang SH, Hilbertz T, Beck R, et al. Gd-DTPA enhanced MR imaging of the breast in patients with postoperative scarring and silicone implants. J Comput Assist Tomogr 1990;14:348–356.
46. Dao TH, Rahmount A, Campana F, et al. Tumor recurrence versus fibrosis in the irradiated breast: differentiation with dynamic gadolinium-enhanced MR imaging. Radiology 1993;187:751–755.
47. Orel SG, Fowble BL, Solin LJ, et al. Breast cancer recurrence after lumpectomy and radiation therapy for early-stage disease: prognostic significance of detection method [see comments]. Radiology 1993;188:189–194.
48. Hassell PR, Olivotto IA, Mueller HA, et al. Early breast cancer: detection of recurrence after conservative surgery and radiation therapy. Radiology 1990;176:731–735.
49. Roubidoux MA, Lai NE, Paramagui C, et al. Mammographic appearance of cancer in the opposite breast: comparison with the first cancer. AJR Am J Roentgenol 1996;166:29–31.
50. Stomper PC, Recht A, Berenberg AL, et al. Mammographic detection of recurrent cancer in the irradiated breast. AJR Am J Roentgenol 1987;148:39–43.

51. Greenstein S, Troupin R, Patterson EA, Fowble BL. Breast cancer recurrence after lumpectomy and irradiation: role of mammography in detection. Radiology 1992;183:201–206.

52. Solin LJ, Fowble BL, Troupin RH, Goodman RL. Biopsy results of new calcifications in the postirradiated breast. Cancer 1989;63:1956–1961.

53. Rebner M, Pennes DR, Adler DD, et al. Breast microcalcifications after lumpectomy and radiation therapy. Radiology 1989;170:691–693.

54. Boice JD, Harvey EB, Blettner M, et al. Cancer in the contralateral breast after radiotherapy for breast cancer. N Engl J Med 1992;326:781–785.

55. Bonadonna G, Veronesi U, Brambilla C, et al. Primary chemotherapy to avoid mastectomy in tumors with diameters of three centimeters or more. J Natl Cancer Inst 1990;82:1539–1545.

56. Segel MC, Paulus DD, Hortobagyi GN. Advanced primary breast cancer: assessment at mammography of response to induction chemotherapy. Radiology 1988;169:49–54.

57. Cronin TD, Gerow FJ. Augmentation Mammoplasty: A New "Natural Feel" Prosthesis. In Transactions of the Third International Congress of Plastic Surgery, Amsterdam. Excerpta Medica 1964;41–49.

58. Department of Health and Human Services. Background Information on the Possible Health Risks of Silicone Breast Implants. Food and Drug Administration bulletin. Rockville, MD: Department of Health and Human Services, 1991.

59. Spiera H. Scleroderma after silicone augmentation mammoplasty. JAMA 1988;260:235.

60. Weiner SR, Paulus HE. Chronic arthropathy occurring after augmentation mammaplasty. Plast Reconstr Surg 1986;77:185–187.

61. Gabriel SE, O'Fallon M, Kurland LT, et al. Risk of connective tissue disease and other disorders after breast implantation. N Engl J Med 1994;330:1697–1702.

62. Sanchez-Guerrero J, Colditz GA, Karlson EW, et al. Silicone breast implants and the risk of connective-tissue diseases and symptoms. N Engl J Med 1995;332:1666–1670.

63. Gabriel SE, Woods JE, O'Fallon M, et al. Complications leading to surgery after breast implantation. N Engl J Med 1997;336:677–682.

64. Garrido L, Pfleiderer B, Jenkins BG, et al. Migration and chemical modification of silicone in women with breast prostheses. Magn Reson Med 1994;31:328–330.

65. Hester TR, Nahai F, Bostwick J, Cukic J. A 5-year experience with polyurethane-covered mammary prostheses for treatment of capsular contracture, primary augmentation mammoplasty, and breast reconstruction. Clin Plast Surg 1988;15:569–585.

66. Autian J. et al. Carcinogenesis from polyurethanes. Cancer Res 1975;35:1591–1596.

67. Steinbach BG, Hardt NS, Abbitt PL, et al. Breast implants: common complications and concurrent breast disease. Radiographics 1993;13:95–118.

68. Baker JL, LeVier RR, Spielvogel DE. Positive identification of silicone in human mammary capsular tissue. Plast Reconstr Surg 1992;69:56–60.

69. Picha GJ, Goldstein JA. Analysis of the soft tissue response to components used in the manufacture of breast implants: rat animal model. Plast Reconstr Surg 1991;87:490–500.

70. Winding O, Christensen L, Thomsen JL, et al. Silicone in human breast tissue surrounding silicone gel prostheses. Scand J Plast Reconstr Surg Hand Surg Suppl 1988;22:127–130.

71. Thomsen JL, Christensen L, Nielsen M, et al. Histologic changes and silicone concentrations in human breast tissue surrounding silicone breast prostheses. Plast Reconstr Surg 1990;85:38–41.

72. Soo MS, Kornguth PJ, Walsh R, et al. Complex radial folds versus subtle signs of intracapsular rupture of breast implants: MR findings with surgical correlation. AJR Am J Roentgenol 1996;166:1421–1427.

73. Berkel H, Birdsell DC, Jenkins H. Breast augmentation: a risk factor for breast cancer? N Engl J Med 1992;326:1649–1653.

74. Handel N, Silverstein MJ, Gamagami P, et al. Factors affecting mammographic visualization of the breast after augmentation mammaplasty. JAMA 1992;268:1913–1917.

75. Silverstein MJ, Handel N, Gamagami P, et al. Breast cancer in women after augmentation mammoplasty. Arch Surg 1988;123:681–685.

76. Clark CP, Peters GN, O'Brien KM. Cancer in the augmented breast. Cancer 1993;72:2170–2174.

77. Loyer EM, Kroll SS, David C, et al. Mammographic and CT findings after breast reconstruction with a rectus abdominis musculocutaneous flap. AJR Am J Roentgenol 1991;156:1159–1162.

78. Mund DF, Wolfson P, Gorczyca DP, et al. Mammographically detected recurrent nonpalpable carcinoma developing in a transverse rectus abdominus myocutaneous flap: a case report. Cancer 1994;74:2804–2807.

79. Scott IA, Muller NL, Fitzpatrick DG, Warren Burhenne LJ. Ruptured breast implant: computed tomographic and mammographic findings. Can Assoc Radiol J 1988;39:152–154.

80. Ganott MA, Harris KM, Ilkhanipour ZS, Costa-Greco MA. Augmentation mammoplasty: normal and abnormal findings with mammography and US. Radiographics 1992;12:281–295.

81. Gorczyca DP, Sinha S, Ahn CY, et al. Silicone breast implants in vivo: MR imaging. Radiology 1992;185:407–410.

82. Gorczyca DP, DeBruhl ND, Ahn CY, et al. Silicone breast implant ruptures in an animal model: comparison of mammography, MR imaging, US, and CT. Radiology 1994;190:227–232.

83. Russell DG, Ziewacz JT. Pressure in a simulated breast subjected to compression forces comparable to those of mammography. Radiology 1995;194:383–387.

84. Destouet JM, Monsees BS, Oser RF, et al. Screening mammography in 350 women with breast implants: prevalence and findings of implant complications. AJR Am J Roentgenol 1992;159:973–978.

85. Harris KM, Ganott MA, Shestak K, et al. Detection of silicone leaks: a new sonographic sign. Radiology 1991;181:134.

86. Rosculet KA, Ikeda DM, Forrest ME, et al. Ruptured gel-filled silicone breast implants: sonographic findings in 19 cases. AJR Am J Roentgenol 1992;159:711–716.

87. Levine RA, Collins TL. Definitive diagnosis of breast implant rupture by ultrasonography. Plast Reconstr Surg 1991;87:1126–1128.

88. DeAngelis GA, de Lange EE, Miller LR, Morgan RF. MR imaging of breast implants. Radiographics 1994;14:783–794.

89. DeBruhl ND, Gorczyca DP, Ahn CY, et al. Silicone breast implants: US evaluation. Radiology 1993;189:95–98.

90. Monticciolo DL, Nelson RC, Dixon WT, et al. MR detection of leakage from silicone breast implants: value of a silicone-selective pulse sequence. AJR Am J Roentgenol 1994;163:51–56.

91. Gorczyca DP, BeBruhl ND, Mund DF, Bassett LW. Linguine sign at MR imaging: does it represent the collapsed silicone implant shell? Radiology 1994;191:576–577.

92. Everson LI, Parantainen H, Detlie T, et al. Diagnosis of breast implant rupture: imaging findings and relative efficacies of imaging techniques. AJR Am J Roentgenol 1994;163:57–60.

93. Stewart NR, Monsees BS, Destouet JM, Rudloff MA. Mammographic appearance following implant removal. Radiology 1992;185:83–85.

94. Robertson CL, Kopans DB, McCarthy KA, Hart NE. Nonpalpable lesions in the augmented breast: preoperative localization. Radiology 1989;173:873–874.

Breast Imaging, 2nd ed., by Daniel B. Kopans.
Lippincott–Raven Publishers, Philadelphia © 1998.

CHAPTER 18

The Male Breast

Breast cancer in men is extremely uncommon. It accounts for <1,500 of the more than 180,000 breast cancers diagnosed in the United States each year (1). Just as with women, the prognosis for men is related to the size of the cancer and its stage (axillary lymph node status) at the time of diagnosis.

The most frequent reason for imaging the male breast, in our experience, is the clinical detection of an asymmetric thickening or a mass. The breast may be enlarged, and there may be associated pain or tenderness. This is almost always caused by asymmetric gynecomastia (Fig. 18-1). Even when gynecomastia is asymmetric, it is usually evident by mammography, to a lesser degree, in the contralateral breast. Using mammography, Chantra and colleagues, in a review of 118 cases at a referral center, observed bilateral gynecomastia in 66 male patients (55%), unilateral gynecomastia in 30 (25%), bilateral fatty enlargement (pseudogynecomastia) in nine (8%), unilateral fatty enlargement (pseudogynecomastia) in two (2%), lipomas in five (4%), normal male breast tissue in three (3%), and breast cancer in three (3%) (2).

Histologically, the normal male breast contains subareolar ducts similar to those found in prepubertal girls. When stimulated, the ducts may elongate and branch, but lobule formation is extremely rare. This accounts for the fact that lesions of the lobule (e.g., fibroadenomas) found in women do not occur in men. Cysts may develop, but they, too, are rare in men. It is unclear whether cysts in men are lobular dilatation or cystically dilated ducts. Because the male breast contains ductal epithelium, ductal carcinoma can develop.

GYNECOMASTIA

Gynecomastia is simply defined as nonneoplastic enlargement of the male breast. This condition has a range of manifestations. The breast may enlarge predominantly due to fat deposition. If the enlargement is due to firm tissue, this suggests the presence of breast tissue. This may be a diffuse thickening or a disk-like formation under the nipple. With true gynecomastia the ducts increase in number and may become dilated. Proliferation of the epithelial and myoepithelial elements occurs with the frequent development of epithelial hyperplasia. The surrounding stroma demonstrates increased vascularity and cellularity and may contain inflammatory cells. Edema is a common component of gynecomastia.

When the process becomes inactive, a hyalinized stroma may persist. Although uncommon, lobule formation can occur and secretions may be produced. This apparently is most common when exogenous estrogens are administered for prostate cancer therapy, although we have seen spontaneous cyst formation in an adolescent male as well as in a 67-year-old man (Fig. 18-2). Although atypical hyperplasia and carcinoma in situ have been found in association with gynecomastia, there is no strong evidence that this predisposes the male to the development of breast cancer.

Clinically, breast enlargement may be unilateral or bilateral. There may be skin thickening, and soreness is a common complaint. Axillary nodal enlargement may be present, despite the benign etiology of the breast changes.

Gynecomastia has a bimodal prevalence first seen around the time of puberty, with a second peak beginning around the age of 50. This is likely due to the fact that these are periods of hormonal instability. Gynecomastia has been associated with endogenous hormonal imbalance, the use of exogenous hormones, hormone-producing tumors, hepatic disease (including hepatoma), renal disease, and hyperthyroidism. Numerous drugs have been associated with the development of gynecomastia.

Transient changes are fairly common in the adolescent male (Fig. 18-3), but these are usually self-limiting and regress as hormone activity stabilizes. Drugs such as reserpine, cardiac glycosides, spironolactone, cimetidine, and thiazides, as well as marijuana, are among the many that have been associated with gynecomastia.

Testicular tumors, such as embryonal cell carcinoma, seminoma, and choriocarcinoma, may result in gynecomastia (3), and the testes should be checked when breast enlargement occurs. Other conditions that affect the testes, including Klinefelter's syndrome, have been associated with gynecomastia. Klinefelter's syndrome also has an increased association with the development of breast cancer (4). Chronic hepatic disease may result in gynecomastia, owing to the reduced ability of the liver to eliminate estro-

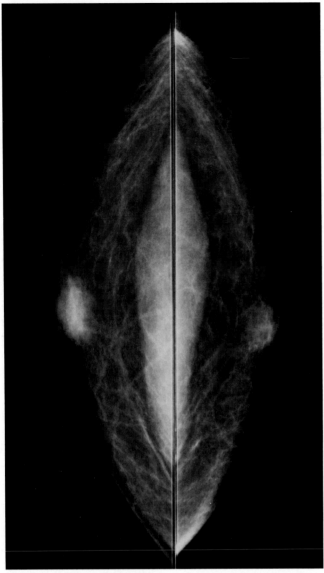

FIG. 18-1. Asymmetric gynecomastia. Most mammography in men is performed for asymmetric thickening or a mass. This 52-year-old man had asymmetric gynecomastia greater on the left than the right.

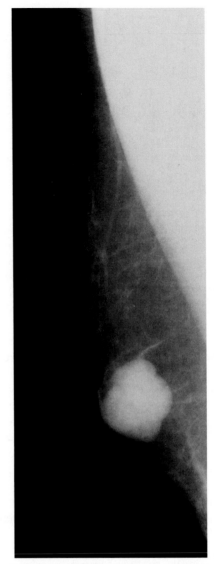

A

FIG. 18-2. Cyst in an elderly male. The palpable, lobulated mass on the mediolateral oblique **(A)** of this 67-year-old man was a cyst. *Continued.*

gen compounds that are normally produced by men. There are reports that link gynecomastia with lung diseases, including lung cancer. Finally, as might be expected, the use of exogenous estrogens produces breast development in the male.

BREAST CANCER

Breast cancer in men is extremely uncommon. Fewer than 1% of breast cancer cases diagnosed each year occur in men. As in women, its cause remains to be elucidated. Gynecomastia does not appear to increase the risk, although significant exposure to ionizing radiation does

(Fig. 18-4), and there is an increased incidence in those with Klinefelter's syndrome.

The mean age at which men develop breast cancer is approximately 5 to 10 years later than for women. In one series of 45 male cancers occurring over a 15-year period in a health maintenance organization, the age ranged from 36 to 82, with a mean of 60 and a median of 61 (5). In another series, one man of the 16 subjects with breast cancer was age 27. The others were 60 years of age or older (6).

A review of 1,429 cases of male breast cancer in the Nordic countries revealed that younger men tended to have better survivals than older men (7). Although some series have suggested a poorer prognosis for men with breast can-

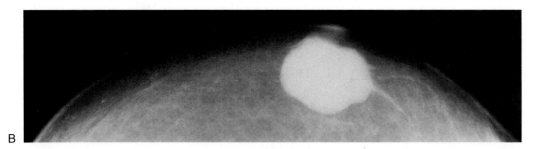

B

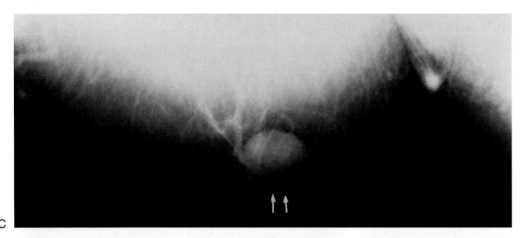

C

FIG. 18-2. *Continued.* **(B)** The mass is also seen in the craniocaudal projection. **(C)** Calcifications were collected in the dependent portion of the cyst and moved anteriorly when the patient leaned forward into the mammographic system *(arrows).*

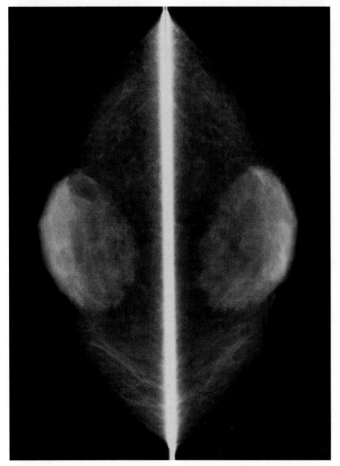

FIG. 18-3. Prominent, **symmetric gynecomastia** seen on the craniocaudal projections in a 13-year-old boy.

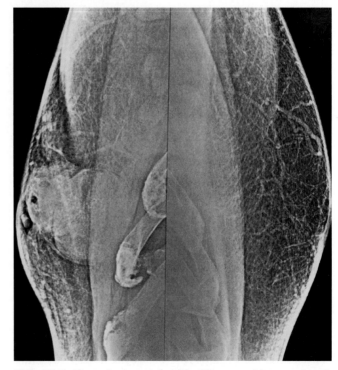

FIG. 18-4. Breast cancer in this 36-year-old man developed after irradiation as an infant for an unspecified renal tumor. He developed a large, infiltrating ductal carcinoma, visible in the subareolar region of the left breast on these lateral, negative-mode xerograms. The mass was palpable and caused nipple retraction.

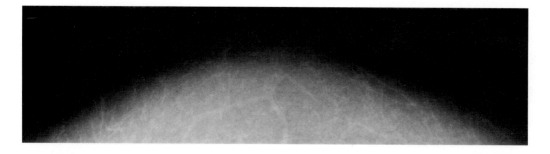

FIG. 18-5. The normal male breast, as seen on this craniocaudal mammogram, has a small nipple with only subcutaneous fat evident beneath it.

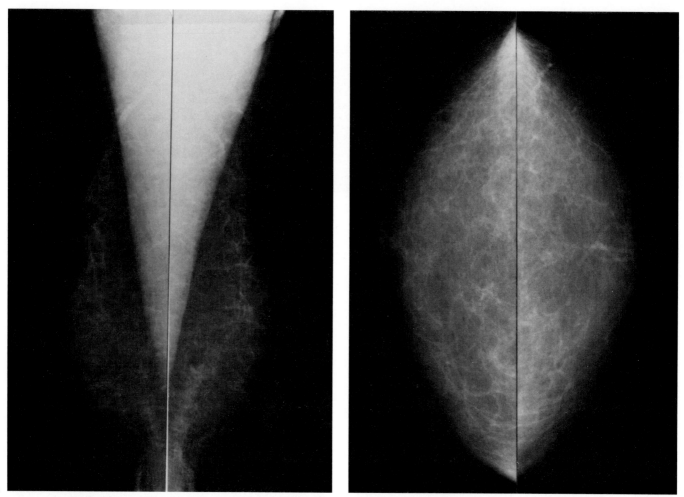

A

B

FIG. 18-6. The **normal male breast** demonstrates only subcutaneous fat, as seen in these mediolateral oblique **(A)** and craniocaudal **(B)** views of a 66-year-old man with fatty enlargement of the breasts.

cer than for women, this is probably due to case-selection bias, with more advanced disease being treated in the teaching institutions that report the data. It appears that for comparable stages, the prognosis for men is similar to that for women (8,9). In a review of 355 cases, the 5-year survival was 90% if lymph nodes were negative, 73% if one to three nodes were positive, and 55% if four or more nodes were positive, with corresponding 10-year survivals of 84%, 44%, and 14% (9).

Most male breast cancers are detected as a result of palpable masses (80% to 90%). Nipple changes are not uncommon, and in 5% to 10% nipple retraction or discharge, or both, occurs. As with women, the discharge may be serous or sanguineous. Skin ulceration does not occur with gynecomastia and is a grave sign in male breast cancer (6).

Most male breast cancers are infiltrating ductal tumors, with approximately 10% detected while still intraductal.

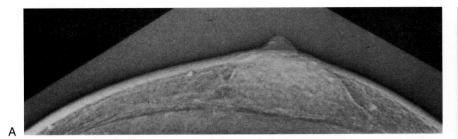

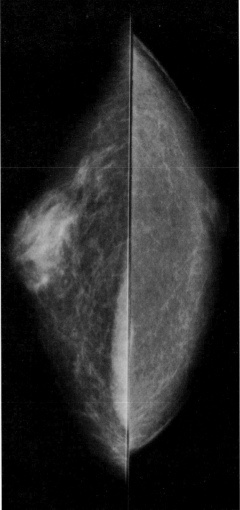

FIG. 18-7. Gynecomastia can form a fairly well-defined discoid density, as seen on this negative-mode xerogram in the craniocaudal projection **(A)**. A similar appearance is seen in the left breast of this 41-year-old man with asymmetric gynecomastia **(B)**. The right breast is almost normal.

Paget's disease of the nipple has been reported (10). Because lobule formation is rare in men, infiltrating lobular cancers are uncommon. Histologically, male breast cancer is indistinguishable from cancers of the female breast, and all ductal subtypes have been described.

IMAGING THE MALE BREAST

Development of a unilateral lump is the usual reason for referral for imaging the male breast. This is almost invariably caused by asymmetric gynecomastia. Standard mammographic projections can be obtained in males. The normal male breast reveals a small nipple, and there is only subcutaneous fat visible in the subareolar region (Fig. 18-5).

Gynecomastia

A spectrum of mammographic appearances may be found with benign male breast enlargement (11,12). There may merely be diffuse fat deposition with no radiographically visible parenchyma. Chantra and colleagues termed this *pseudogynecomastia*, because it merely represents fat deposition (Fig. 18-6). A small discoid density may be present beneath the nipple (Fig. 18-7). Often there is a very small triangular density immediately beneath the nipple (Fig. 18-8).

In our experience, the most common appearance is a fan- or flamed-shaped density that extends and expands back from the nipple toward the upper outer quadrant of the breast, reflecting the subareolar origin of the hypertrophic duct network (Fig. 18-9). In some instances the parenchymal density may appear more spherical, but in most instances the tissues fade gradually into the surrounding fat, frequently more prominent toward the upper outer quadrant and similar to the distribution of tissue seen in women. In extreme cases of gynecomastia, as may occur with exogenous estrogen administration, the male breast may be indistinguishable radiographically from the female breast (Fig. 18-10).

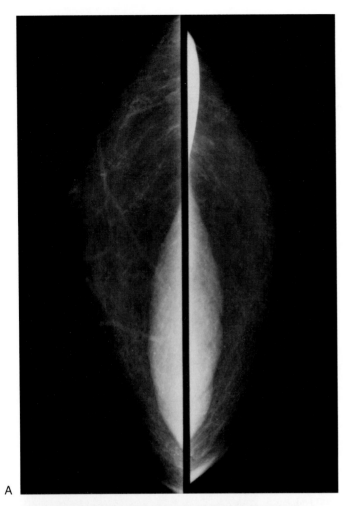

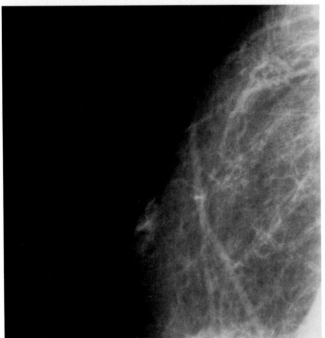

A

B

FIG. 18-8. Minimal asymmetric gynecomastia in the left subareolar region in a 54-year-old man is seen as a small triangle of density on these craniocaudal projections **(A)** and enlarged **(B)**. The right breast appears normal.

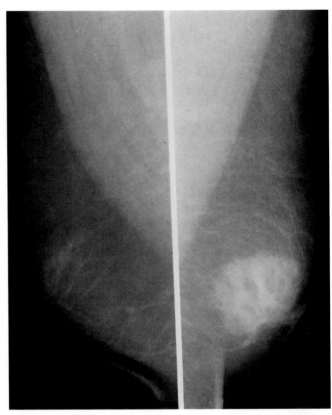

FIG. 18-9. Asymmetric gynecomastia. The right breast on these mediolateral oblique views demonstrates a typical fan-shaped density.

Despite an apparent unilaterality on clinical examination, gynecomastia is almost invariably bilateral. In most cases of gynecomastia, where clinically a mass or thickening is found on one side, the mammogram reveals a similar but smaller density on the contralateral side (Fig. 18-11). Some skin and nipple changes may be indistinguishable from those associated with breast cancer (Fig. 18-12), and biopsy may be necessary to exclude the latter.

Other Benign Lesions

Abscesses, lipomas, and sebaceous and inclusion cysts (Fig. 18-13) occur in the male breast, but they are usually diagnosed clinically and do not need imaging.

Cysts are extremely rare in the male breast, although they do occur. Ultrasound is of limited value in male breast evaluation, but if performed, gynecomastia reveals an appearance similar to that seen in the developing preadolescent female breast bud, producing round or triangular hypoechoic tissue in the subareolar region (Fig. 18-14). The shape generally conforms to the shape of the parenchymal cone seen by mammography. When male breast development is extensive, ultrasound reveals a parenchymal cone with mixed areas of echogenicity and hypoechogenicity that reflect the distribution of fibrofatty

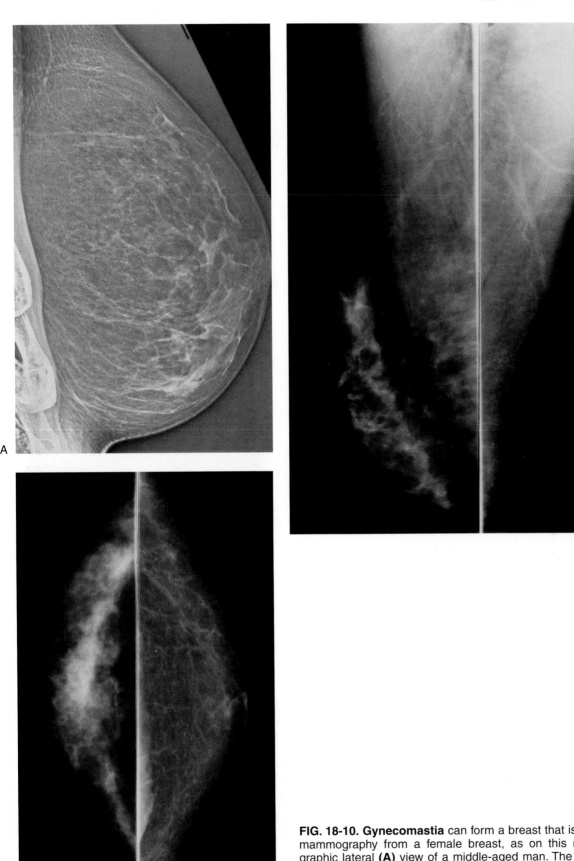

A

B

C

FIG. 18-10. Gynecomastia can form a breast that is indistinguishable by mammography from a female breast, as on this negative-mode xerographic lateral **(A)** view of a middle-aged man. The asymmetric gynecomastia in the left breast of this 35-year-old man, compared to the complete absence of tissue in his normal right breast, cannot be distinguished by mammography from breast tissue in a female on these mediolateral oblique **(B)** and craniocaudal **(C)** projections.

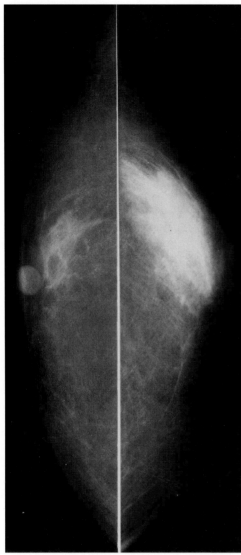

FIG. 18-11. When gynecomastia forms a palpable thickening or mass clinically on one side, as was the case in the right breast in this man, with nothing evident by clinical examination on the contralateral side, almost invariably less prominent gynecomastia is seen mammographically on the contralateral side, as is evident on these craniocaudal projections.

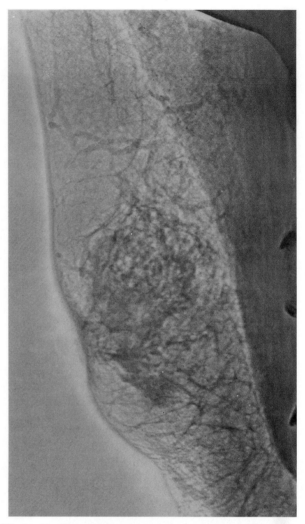

FIG. 18-12. Skin thickening and nipple retraction associated with benign gynecomastia may be difficult to appreciate on high-contrast film/screen mammography but are evident on this positive-mode, xerographic lateral image.

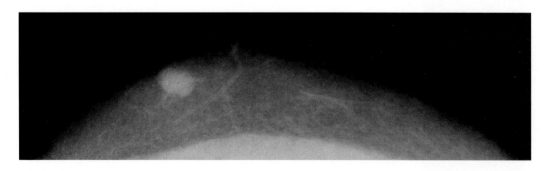

FIG. 18-13. Epidermal inclusion cyst. Intramammary cysts are very rare in men, but inclusion cysts can be seen, as on the craniocaudal view of this male breast.

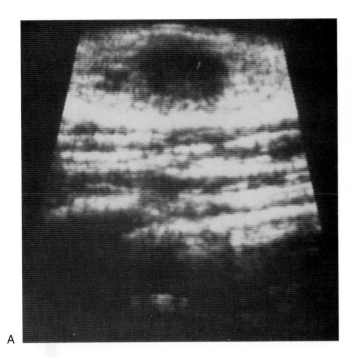

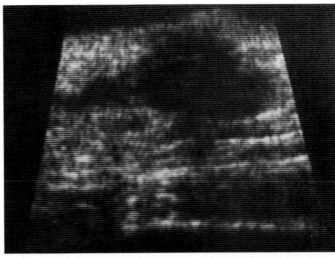

FIG. 18-14. **Gynecomastia** is hypoechoic by ultrasound. It may appear round, as in **(A)**, or triangular, as in **(B)**.

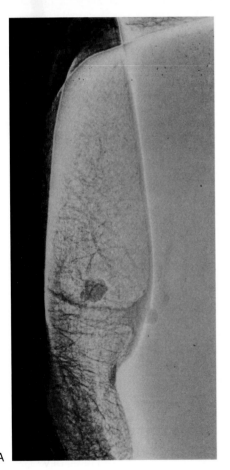

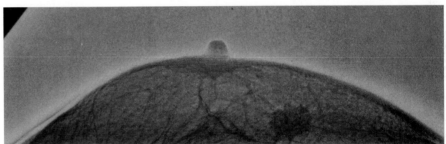

FIG. 18-15. **Male breast cancer,** seen on lateral **(A)** and craniocaudal **(B)** xerograms, is often eccentric from the nipple and can form a lobulated mass, as in this invasive ductal carcinoma.

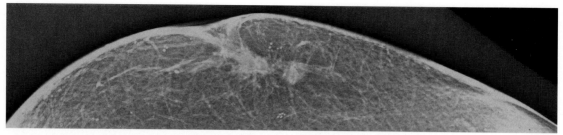

FIG. 18-16. The **male breast cancer** seen on this craniocaudal negative-mode xerogram had a spiculated margin, as seen in many female breast cancers and is causing nipple retraction.

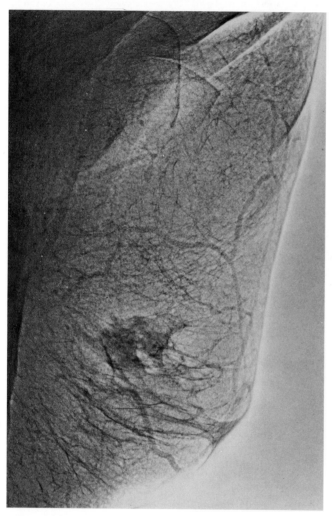

FIG. 18-17. This **infiltrating ductal carcinoma** in a man formed an ill-defined mass, as is evident on this positive mode lateral projection xerogram that was away from the nipple.

tissues and produce an appearance similar to that of the female breast (13,14).

As in women, there have been granular cell tumors described in men (15). In 1995 Rogall and Propeck described a granular cell tumor in a 35-year-old black man who presented with a palpable mass that was irregular in shape on the mammograms with a spiculated margin (16).

BREAST CANCER IN MEN

Mammography

Unlike gynecomastia, most male cancers are eccentrically located and occur away from the subareolar region, although occasionally they may develop immediately under the nipple. Of the 20 cancers in men reported by Ouimet-Oliva and colleagues (17), 60% were located eccentrically in the breast, while virtually all cases of gynecomastia produce density fanning back and are centered on the nipple. Recognition of the characteristic distribution of gynecomastia and the usual eccentric growth of breast cancer will reduce the possibility of mistaking one for the other.

The appearance of breast cancer in men is similar to that seen in women. Although male cancers more frequently tend to have lobulated margins (Fig. 18-15), they may be spiculated (Fig. 18-16) or ill defined (Fig. 18-17). Even intracystic cancer can be seen in men (Fig. 18-18). Ductal carcinoma in situ (DCIS) can be found in males, and microcalcifications can occur (Fig. 18-19). Skin calcifications are common in men and should not be mistaken for intraductal deposits. As with women, mammography does not exclude cancer, and false-negative mammograms can occur when concurrent dense gynecomastia is present (Fig. 18-20).

Dershaw and colleagues reviewed the mammograms of 23 men with breast cancer who ranged in ages from 44 to 86 (18). All were symptomatic. One had an inverted nipple, eight had a bloody nipple discharge, and 13 presented with a mass. The last patient had an occult breast cancer detected in his contralateral breast that was being screened due to his history of previous breast cancer. Only one had a first-degree relative with breast cancer. Five (20%) of the men had associated gynecomastia. One of the men (4%) had had a previous contralateral breast cancer, and two had been exposed to significant levels of radiation in the past. In 17 (74%) of the cases, there was a noncalcified mass and two (8%) patients had a mass with associated calcifications. Three (12%) of the cancers were not visible by mammography. Most of their cancers were found in the subareolar region. There were 17 (72%) invasive ductal carcinomas and six (18%) cases of DCIS.

As in women, lymphoma can occur in men. In the single case that we have seen, the ill-defined mass was indistinguishable from breast cancer.

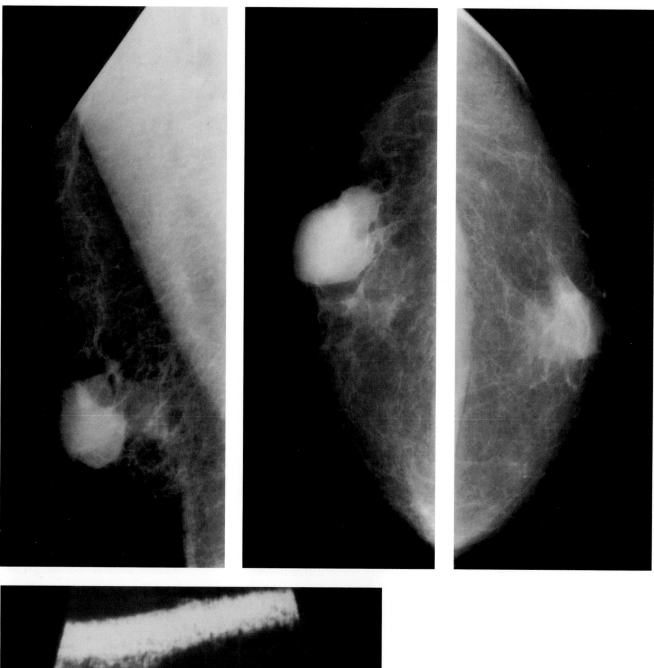

FIG. 18-18. This 66-year-old male had a palpable subareolar mass on the left that was lobulated on the mediolateral oblique **(A)** and craniocaudal (CC) **(B)** views. The appearance is different from the gynecomastia on the right, as seen in the CC projection **(C)**. Ultrasound **(D)** demonstrated a solid mass within the wall of a cyst. The diagnosis proved to be **intracystic papillary carcinoma.**

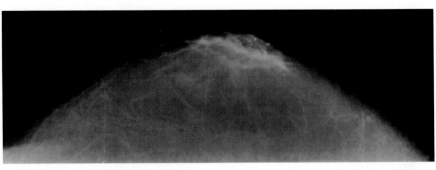

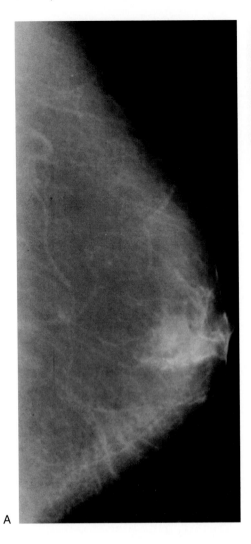

FIG. 18-19. Ductal carcinoma in situ (DCIS) in a man. Just as in women, a nipple discharge can be due to breast cancer, as in this man who, on the straight lateral **(A)** and craniocaudal **(B)** projections, has calcifications that were forming in DCIS.

Ultrasound

There is rarely a need to use ultrasound to image a mass in the male breast, but male breast cancers produce hypoechoic lesions that, as in women, reflect the shape and composition of the tumor. Spiculated lesions tend to produce irregular structures that shadow, whereas lobulated lesions may have isoechoic or enhanced posterior echoes with variable shadowing. Rare cysts have the same appearance in men's breasts as in women's.

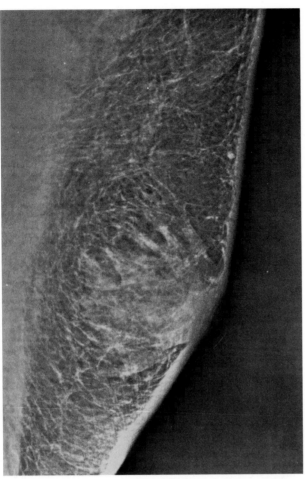

FIG. 18-20. Invasive ductal carcinoma was present at biopsy, but it was hidden on this negative-mode, xerographic lateral view in the dense tissues due to gynecomastia.

REFERENCES

1. Breast Cancer. Cancer Facts and Figures. New York: American Cancer Society, 1996.
2. Chantra PK, So GJ, Wollman JS, Bassett LW. Mammography of the male breast. AJR Am J Roentgenol 1995;164:853–858.
3. Ouimet-Oliva D, Hebert G, Ladouceur J. Radiology of breast tumors in the male. Can Assoc Radiol J 1977;28:249.
4. Jackson AW, Muldal S, Ockey CH, O'Connor PJ. Carcinoma of male breast in association with the Klinefelter syndrome. BMJ 1965;1:223.
5. Robison R, Montague ED. Treatment results in males with breast cancer. Cancer 1982;49:403.
6. Siddiqui T, Weiner R, Moreb J, Marsh RD. Cancer of the male breast with prolonged survival. Cancer 1988;62:1632–1636.
7. Adami HO, Hakulinen T, Ewertz M, et al. The survival pattern in male breast cancer. An analysis of 1429 patients from the Nordic countries. Cancer 1989;64:1177–1182.
8. Vercoutere AL, O'Connell TX. Carcinoma of the male breast: an update. Arch Surg 1984;119:1301.
9. Guinee VF, Olsson H, Moller T, et al. The prognosis of breast cancer in males: a report of 335 cases. Cancer 1993;71:154–161.
10. Serour F, Birkenfeld S, Amsterdam E, et al. Paget's disease of the male breast. Cancer 1988;62:601–605.
11. Kalisher L, Peyster RG. Xerographic manifestations of male breast disease. AJR Am J Roentgenol 1975;125:656.
12. Dershaw DD. Male mammography. AJR Am J Roentgenol 1986; 146:127.
13. Cole-Beuglet C, Schwartz GF, Kurtz AB, et al. Ultrasound mammography for male breast enlargement. J Ultrasound Med 1982;1:301.
14. Jackson VP, Gilmore RL. Male breast carcinoma and gynecomastia: comparison of mammography with sonography. Radiology 1983; 149:533.
15. DeMay RM, Lay S. Granular cell tumor of the breast. Pathol Annu 1984;19:121–148.
16. Rogall B, Propeck P. Granular cell tumor of the male breast. AJR Am J Roentgenol 1995;164:230.
17. Ouimet-Oliva D, Hebert G, Ladouceur J. Radiographic characteristics of male breast cancer. Radiology 129:37,1978.
18. Dershaw DD, Borgen PI, Deutch BM, Liberman L. Mammographic findings in men with breast cancer. AJR Am J Roentgenol 1993; 160:267–270.

Breast Imaging, 2nd ed., by Daniel B. Kopans.
Lippincott–Raven Publishers, Philadelphia © 1998.

CHAPTER 19

Pathologic, Mammographic, and Sonographic Correlation

Cancer is, without question, the most important pathologic process that affects the breast. Its early diagnosis is the paramount reason for performing a breast biopsy. Other abnormalities that occur in the breast are important primarily because they concern the patient or physician and must be differentiated from malignancy. Of less clinical importance, but of potentially great value, has been an effort by investigators to predict which women are more likely to develop breast cancer by identifying histologic changes that may indicate a higher risk for subsequent malignancy. These efforts have been complicated by difficulty in distinguishing pathologic processes from the wide range of physiologic processes that occur. Even the distinction between benign atypical hyperplasia and ductal carcinoma in situ (DCIS) is frequently disputed.

Certainly one of the major goals of imaging would be the ability to noninvasively differentiate benign lesions from malignant lesions. This is likely to be an unattainable goal until molecular probes become available that can be used with imaging. After all, breast cancer cells are merely modifications of normal cells that perform abnormally. Even the pathologist cannot always predict how cells will behave even though they can examine them individually. Unless the phenotype of the cell reflects its genotype (which determines its capability), even directly viewing the cell may not be informative. It should be no surprise that the radiologist is frequently unable to make these distinctions at a grossly lower level of resolution.

The purpose of this chapter is to provide an overview of the current state of understanding of the pathologic processes that occur in the breast and their appearance on imaging. Even though the ability to image tissues changes, the processes themselves do not change, and many observations of the past continue to hold true.

THE NORMAL BREAST

There is a lack of clear-cut understanding of what constitutes the normal breast, and this has been reflected in the frequently unsatisfactory terminologies that have been coined to describe various, probably physiologic, changes that occur as part of a spectrum of normal variation. Such terms as *mastopa-thy, cystic mastitis, dysplasia,* and the all-encompassing *fibrocystic disease* are indicative of a lack of true understanding of where normal physiology ends and true pathology begins.

Imaging and the Menstrual Cycle

At a cellular level, the breast is a dynamic organ that is continually changing with the cyclic fluctuation of hormones, causing cell proliferation (particularly in the terminal duct lobular unit [TDLU]) followed by apoptosis (programmed cell death), with the process repeated cycle after cycle. These primarily microscopic alterations have never been demonstrated by mammography. Some magnetic resonance imaging data using gadolinium to enhance the visibility of the vasculature suggest that normal tissues may have increased enhancement in the later phases of the menstrual cycle, presumably reflecting hyperemia (1). The physiologic changes are reflected clinically in many women by cyclic pain and swelling.

The breast is also a heterogeneous organ. Further complicating breast analysis is the variable end-organ response of its cellular constituents. Some tissues are extremely sensitive to hormonal fluctuations while others appear to be affected very little. This is true even within the same breast. This heterogeneous response can result in clinically apparent lumps that may merely reflect disproportionate stimulation of a volume of breast tissue, resulting in a prominence that distinguishes the particular tissue volume from the surrounding, less affected, tissues. These physiologic lumps usually change with the menstrual cycle.

Involutional Changes

Histologically, the breast involutes with age, and the periodic variations described above appear to be superimposed on the long-term involutional changes. There has been a great deal of misinformation concerning the involution of the fibroglandular tissues and their replacement by fat. This is not a uniform sequence. It occurs in different women to differing degrees at different ages. The actual process of involution is rarely obvious mammographically, although at times, replacement of the fibroglandular elements by fat can be fairly dramatic. The available data suggest that some of the dense patterns are associated with active glandular tissues although most of the attenuation of breast tissue is due to fibrous connective tissue.

Histologically, involution results in replacement of the fibroglandular structures by fat, but it is not clear that there are any fewer lobules in women with fatty breast patterns on mammography when compared to those with dense patterns. Dense pattens are associated with younger women, while a higher percentage of older women have fatty patterns, but it is rare to see a pattern change by mammography from one year to the next; many young women (even younger than 40 years) have predominantly fat breast tissues while many older women, even into their 70s and 80s, have extremely dense patterns. When a pattern change is evident mammographically, it is usually a gradual process occurring slowly over several years. Rapid change is usually due to weight gain or loss because the breast is a repository for fat.

Prechtel (2) has shown the same phenomenon histologically. The collagen-supporting structures of the breast and the glandular tissues are gradually replaced by fat beginning in the second decade of life and progressing steadily throughout life. For many women, no changes occur in the breast's tissue pattern with age (see Chapter 12).

"Fibrocystic Disease" and "Mammary Dysplasia"

The lack of uniform definitions of pathology has only added to the confusion. By circular reasoning, any lump that develops and is excised, for whatever reason, becomes, by definition, abnormal tissue. Faced with these biopsies, pathologists needed to find the pathology, and thus developed "wastebasket" categories. The terms *fibrocystic disease* and *mammary dysplasia* have been used to categorize histologic variations that range from normal physiologic responses to true premalignant proliferative growth.

Clinicians and radiologists, optimistically trying to assure themselves that they could predict histopathology from their clinical breast examination (CBE) and from the mammograms, adopted these terms with little justification. The examining fingers feel tissue inhomogeneities and elasticity that are more often than not the normal variations of a heterogeneous organ. The mammogram reflects the x-ray attenuation of the tissues producing shadows that relate more to the water content of the structures than to their cellular composition. With the exception of the ultrasound diagnosis of a cyst, the calcification of an involuting fibroadenoma, or the spiculated margins of some cancers, imaging techniques are rarely able to accurately define true histology, owing to the overlapping appearance of many processes. The normal and the neoplastic may produce identical morphologic change, and inferring specific histology from physical examination or imaging is a statistical guess in most instances.

Terms such as *fibrocystic disease* and *dysplasia* should not be used because they have been compromised by lack of specificity. More than 50% of women will have breast tissue that meets the loose criteria of these terms (3). Dupont and Page (4) have shown that it is only the small subcategory of proliferative histologies and, specifically, the atypical proliferative changes within the category of fibrocystic disease that carry a higher risk for future malignant change. The College of American Surgeons, in their 1985 review and consensus statement (5), discouraged the use of the term *fibrocystic disease*, but added: "If used, the terms 'fibrocystic changes' or 'condition' should be used." They outlined subcategories and defined the relative risks of the various histopathologies.

Relative Risk for Invasive Breast Cancer Based on Pathologic Examination of Benign Breast Tissue (5)

1. *No increased risk:* Women with any lesion specified below in a biopsy specimen are at no greater risk for invasive breast carcinoma than comparable women who have had no breast biopsy.

> Adenosis, sclerosing or florid
> Apocrine metaplasia
> Cyst
> Duct ectasia
> Fibroadenoma
> Fibrosis
> Hyperplasia, mild (more than two but not more than four epithelial cells in depth)
> Mastitis (inflammation)
> Periductal mastitis
> Squamous metaplasia

2. *Slightly increased risk (one and one-half to two times):* Women with any lesion specified below in a biopsy specimen are at slightly increased risk for invasive breast carcinoma relative to comparable women who have had no breast biopsy.

> Hyperplasia, moderate or florid, solid or papillary
> Papilloma with fibrovascular core

3. *Moderately increased risk (five times):* Women with any lesion specified below in a biopsy specimen are at moderately increased risk for invasive breast carcinoma relative to comparable women who have had no breast biopsy.

> Atypical hyperplasia (borderline lesion)
> Ductal
> Lobular

Cysts are of no consequence unless they occur in women with a family history of breast cancer. Dupont and Page (4) found that this combination increases a woman's risk two- to threefold.

The most important histologic risk factor, beside ductal and lobular carcinomas in situ, appears to be atypical epithelial hyperplasia. According to Dupont and Page, and corroborated by Kriger and Hiatt (6) and Connelly (7), women with this proliferative disorder are approximately five times more likely to develop breast cancer than are women with no proliferative changes, and when found in women with a family history of breast cancer, the relative risk increases 11-fold.

With these important exceptions, no useful correlations exist between the broad category of fibrocystic change and breast cancer risk. Furthermore, atypical hyperplasia can only be diagnosed by breast biopsy and as yet cannot be predicted by mammography, although Stomper et al. (8) have shown that biopsies performed for mammographically detected calcifications reveal a higher percentage of women with atypical hyperplasia than any other test.

The terms *fibrocystic disease* and *mammary dysplasia* cause unnecessary fear and carry an unsubstantiated prejudicial connotation. They certainly do not belong in an imaging lexicon. They should probably be eliminated altogether and replaced by specific histologic categories.

MAMMOGRAPHIC AND SONOGRAPHIC FEATURES OF PATHOLOGIC PROCESSES

Those involved in breast imaging will be confronted with the various benign and malignant lesions found in the breast. A working understanding of these will aid in image interpretation and patient management.

Collagen and Imaging

Although no quantitative comparisons are available, collagen is the most common factor in x-ray attenuation and the major component of radiographic density. Collagen production appears to be a common response to many processes in the breast, including part of normal development. Not only do malignant lesions frequently elicit a fibrous reaction, but most benign lesions also have fibrosis as an integral element. Collagen overgrowth occurs on an idiopathic basis in many lesions, whereas in others it may be a postinflammatory response to cellular debris extruded from cysts or ducts. Because fibrous tissue is a major constituent of the breast, it is at times difficult to determine whether the quantity of collagen is normal or related to the lesion being investigated. Nevertheless, it is likely that the tactile and radiographic differences that are created between collagen and the adipose elements of the surrounding tissue are the major reason benign and malignant lesions are detectable.

Overview of the Duct Network and Pathologic Processes

Benign and malignant lesions of the breast may be categorized by the level within the duct network in which they occur. Some processes arise from the cells of the ducts, whereas others develop from the components of the lobules. Few important lesions arise in the extra(inter)lobular stroma.

Proximal and Distal

By convention, the location within the duct should be described from the point of secretion. *Proximal* is the portion of the duct in close proximity to the lobule; *distal* indicates a position near the nipple. The following list summarizes changes that occur in the distal portion of the

duct working back to the lobule. This is followed by a more detailed description of the abnormalities grouped into benign and malignant processes.

The duct network can be divided into four major sections:

1. Nipple and lactiferous sinus
2. The major ducts
3. The minor ducts (segmental branches)
4. The terminal duct

The blunt-ending ductules that form the acini of the lobule are a part of the duct network, but they can appropriately be considered separately.

The nipple is occasionally the site of breast disease. Nipple adenomas are related but considered distinct from the large duct papillomas that may occur immediately beneath the nipple or in the lactiferous sinuses.

Paget's disease of the nipple is a manifestation of breast cancer. The skin of the nipple is continuous with the lining epithelium of the duct. It is not surprising that ductal cancer occasionally spreads into the large ducts and out through the duct into the nipple. This type of ductal carcinoma is frequently detected early owing to its spread into the nipple and the eczematoid crusting that develops on the nipple. The diagnosis is made when the characteristic large cells first described by Paget are found in the dermis of the nipple. Clinically, Paget's disease often produces an eczematoid nipple lesion. This form of intraductal carcinoma has a favorable prognosis because of its early presentation. Some pathologists have speculated that Paget's disease may be a primary nipple lesion in some women because an underlying ductal cancer is not always identified.

Other lesions develop in the major ducts of the breast. Nonspecific duct ectasia is a dilatation of the lactiferous sinus and the major collecting duct beneath the nipple, although the process can extend throughout the breast. Duct ectasia can be seen by mammography and ultrasound as tubular structures in the subareolar region converging on the nipple.

Solitary, large duct papillomas are benign growths found in the major ducts. Smaller and multiple peripheral papillomas are changes of the smaller, minor ducts.

The terminal duct as it enters the lobule may be the most significant element of the breast. Using three-dimensional analysis of whole-breast sections, Wellings and Jensen (9) demonstrated the earliest malignant lesions of breast cancer developing in the TDLU. It is not clear whether cancers arise in the extralobular or intralobular portion of the duct, but they speculated that the site of origin might be at the junction of the intralobular and extralobular terminal duct or the junction between the intralobular terminal duct and the branches of the intralobular acini (ductules).

Benign hyperplasia of the epithelium in the distal duct and lobular ductules is relatively common. Its frequent association with cysts may be the cause and effect relationship of a benign obliteration of the duct blocking lobular drainage and leading to cyst formation, although, as noted below, cyst formation probably does not require ductal obstruction.

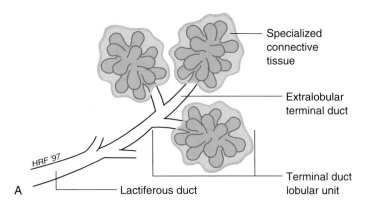

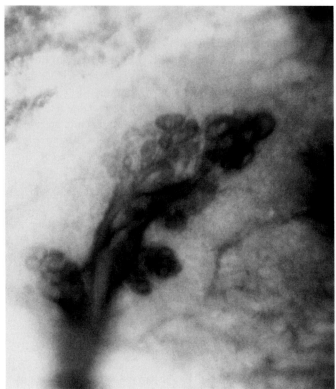

B

FIG. 19-1. The **terminal duct lobular units** (TDLUs) form the glandular elements of the primary unit in the breast. **(A)** The TDLU is shown schematically. **(B)** A 40× magnification of a thick section of tissue that has been defatted and stained to demonstrate several **terminal ducts and lobules** forming TDLUs. *Continued.*

Gallager and Martin (10) have theorized that hyperplasia represents a nonobligatory, reversible, preliminary step toward neoplasia. Even when atypical changes develop, hyperplasia still appears to represent a reversible process, but in a significant proportion of women, atypical ductal epithelial hyperplasia is more likely to progress to intraductal carcinoma (carcinoma in situ). Atypical hyperplasia likely represents a large number of cells that are genetically unstable. Their number and instability increase the chance that one will develop additional alterations that convert it into a full malignancy.

Another form of proliferation, papillomatosis, has been described in the distal ducts. Microscopic multiple papillomatous growths can be found in this region. Pathologists believe that these growths represent a different process than the solitary papillomas of the large ducts or even the multiple peripheral papillomas. They may represent part of a continuum of hyperplastic lesions, and some believe that multiple peripheral duct papillomas of this type represent a premalignant change.

Intraductal carcinoma (DCIS) elicits much controversy. Teleologically, some believe that it is the last step in a continuum that ends in frank invasion (infiltrating ductal carcinoma). Some do not believe in this progression but instead argue that intraductal cancer and infiltrating ductal cancer are two separate processes, with the latter metastasizing very early and the former having a prolonged and indolent growth within the duct (see Chapter 7).

The fact that mammography detects many preinvasive cancers (DCIS), and mammographic screening results in decreased deaths from breast cancer suggests that some of the mortality decrease is due to elimination of these lesions. Breast cancer growth is likely a continuum with an invasive phase that varies from individual to individual. It is likely that DCIS is not always directly linked to invasive cancer because the intraductal phase may be short lived before an invasive clone of cells dominates and eliminates any traces of the in situ form. It is also likely that, at times, a normal cell is transformed to a malignant genotype over a short period of time and that its clones are fully capable of invasion and metastasis without any intermediate stages.

Once a cancer has developed the ability to pass through the basement membrane it becomes invasive or infiltrating ductal carcinoma. These lesions have been subcategorized according to their phenotypes (perhaps reflecting differing amounts of dedifferentiation) in an attempt to better characterize the prognosis associated with each type of lesion.

The most common benign lesions—fibroadenomas, cysts, and adenosis—arise in the lobule. The lobule comprises the multiple terminal branches of the duct network that are blind-ending and form glandular acini that resemble the fingers of a glove (Fig. 19-1). The lining cells of the acini differ from those lining the ducts. Surrounding the acini, defining the lobule, and distinct from the interlobular con-

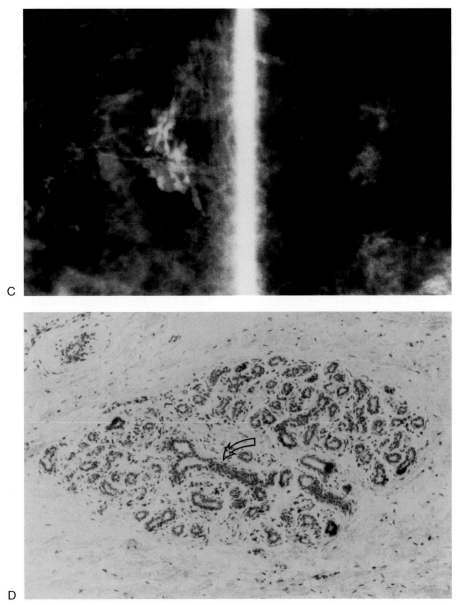

FIG. 19-1. *Continued.* **(C)** Two craniocaudal (CC) projections of the same breast have been placed back to back. The image on the right is an enlarged portion of a mammogram in the CC projection near the chest wall. Contrast material was introduced through a discharging duct and the image on the left (reversed for comparison) is the same area, but the vague density has become opacified revealing several **ductules forming the acini of a TDLU. (D)** A TDLU seen on hematoxylin and eosin histologic cross section. The terminal duct (*arrow*) is visible entering the lobule that is composed of acini and surrounded by specialized connective tissue.

nective tissue is the specialized connective tissue of the lobule. No membranous structure separates the intralobular connective tissue from the extralobular connective tissue, but their composition is clearly and visibly different on histologic staining. Fibroadenomas are believed to be predominantly abnormal overgrowth of this specialized connective tissue of the lobule.

Cysts are sometimes dilated large ducts but are usually dilated lobular acini. These range in size from microscopic to those containing many cubic centimeters of fluid. They are likely due to an imbalance of secretion and resorption, usually secondary to apocrine metaplasia of the acinar lining cells, presumably causing hypersecretion and leading to distention of the duct or of the acinar structure of the intralobular terminal ducts. The role of duct obstruction in the genesis of cysts is unclear.

Adenosis is a benign proliferation of the stromal and epithelial elements of the lobule producing an increased

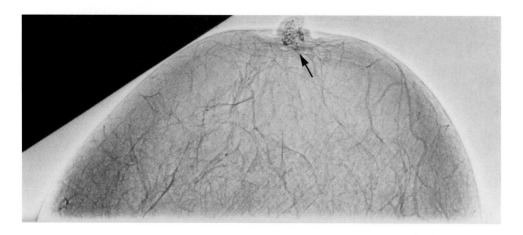

FIG. 19-2. Nipple calcifications (*arrow*) are due to a **pleomorphic adenoma.**

number of acinar structures. Adenosis is a benign process, but when associated with fibrous architectural distortion (sclerosing adenosis), it can be confused with malignant change.

Although most breast cancers appear to originate in the TDLU (in either the extra- or intralobular portion of the duct) and are designated as ductal in origin, some resemble the epithelial cells that line the acini within the lobule and are correspondingly called *lobular carcinomas*. Because the relationship of lobular carcinoma in situ (LCIS) to invasive lobular carcinoma remains unclear, some prefer to call the noninvasive lesion *lobular neoplasia*. Invasive cancer that resembles the cells lining the lobule are designated invasive lobular carcinoma.

BENIGN BREAST LESIONS

Nipple Adenomas

Nipple adenomas are fairly uncommon lesions (11). They are distinct from the large duct papillomas that may occur immediately beneath the nipple and the papillomatosis that may occur in the lactiferous sinuses. They are composed of varying epithelial proliferations mixed with fibrous tissues. Although considered distinct entities, nipple adenomas appear to have similarities to large duct papillomas. They contain mixed elements of adenosis, hyperplasia, and papillomatosis. Apocrine metaplasia can occur and cysts in the nipple with squamous lining have been described (12). Nipple adenomas are characterized by continuity with the squamous epithelium of the nipple surface. They are most common in middle-aged women but may occur in women of any age. Nipple adenomas may cause symptoms similar to Paget's disease, with nipple crusting, surface irregularity, or discharge.

Mammography will generally not demonstrate these subtle changes, but calcifications may develop in these lesions in the nipple (Fig. 19-2). Treated by excision, recurrence is rare and likely due to incomplete excision.

Benign Lesions of the Major Ducts

Large Duct Papilloma (Intraductal Papilloma)

One of the most common causes of a serous or bloody nipple discharge is the large duct papilloma, a benign proliferation of ductal epithelium that projects into the lumen of the duct and is connected to the epithelium by a fibrovascular stalk (Fig. 19-3). Usually found in the subareolar region within a major lactiferous duct, solitary papillomas can grow large enough to be visible by imaging methods when they distend the duct. They are only occasionally palpable. As noted earlier, these represent a proliferative process, and their presence signifies a slightly increased risk of breast cancer that ranges from one and one-half to two times the risk of a woman who has nonproliferative changes (5). These lesions are unlikely to be "precursor" lesions, but their development may indicate an unstable epithelium that may be slightly more prone to malignant transformation.

Intraductal papillomas, as their name implies, are contained within the duct. They commonly extend longitudinally through its lumen and are found only on microscopic section. They are either discovered coincidentally in a biopsy for some other reason or they cause a serous or bloody nipple discharge. Some pathologists believe that their vascular supply is fragile, which leads to areas of necrosis, infarction, and bleeding (and possibly the calcification that is occasionally seen by mammography). The duct around them can dilate and form a cystic structure. This is the origin of the intracystic papilloma. Histologically, they are usually not difficult to differentiate from papillary carcinomas, which lack a myoepithelial layer.

Intraductal papillomas are usually solitary, but they can be multiple. The latter should not be confused with papillomatosis, which is a form of epithelial hyperplasia. Pathologists have not agreed on the description of papillomatosis. Solitary papillomas are usually in the subareolar region, whereas multiple papillomas are usually

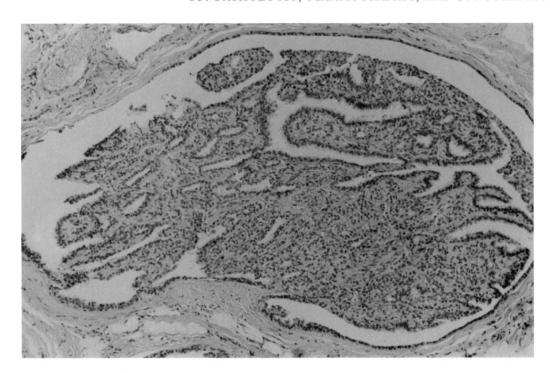

FIG. 19-3. The fronds of this **intraductal papilloma** are apparent on this photomicrograph.

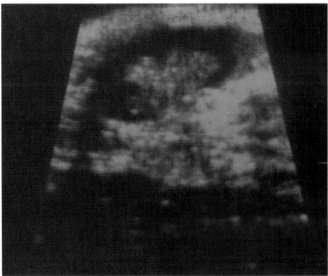

B

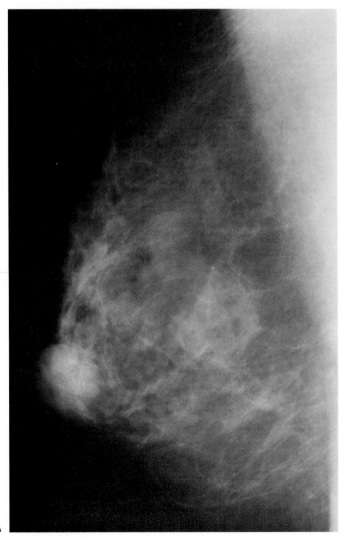

A

FIG. 19-4. **Intracystic papillomas** are probably actually in cystically dilated ducts. A rounded mass is visible under the nipple on the lateral mammogram **(A)**. The mushroom-like appearance of an intracystic papilloma is evident on ultrasound **(B)** within the cyst, although a biopsy is necessary to make the diagnosis. *Continued.*

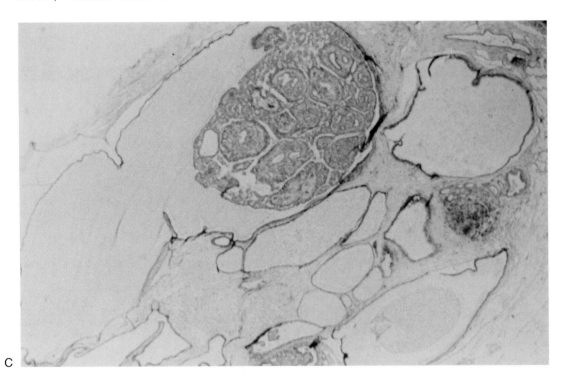

FIG. 19-4. *Continued.* Another **intracystic papilloma** is evident on this photomicrograph **(C)**.

C

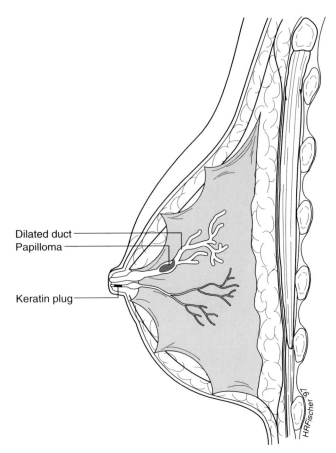

Dilated duct
Papilloma

Keratin plug

FIG 19-5. This schematic demonstrates the usual relationship of the **papilloma** relative to the nipple. **Ductal dilatation** is likely not due to obstruction but secretion that is not balanced by resorption.

more peripheral. Rosen and Oberman suggest that women with multiple papillomas are usually younger than those with solitary papillomas (13). Solitary intraductal papillomas are generally discovered in the peri- and postmenopausal years.

Multiple peripheral duct papillomas are less common and are believed to arise in the TDLU. Multiple peripheral duct papillomas are associated with an increased likelihood of atypical changes and carcinoma.

Mammographic Appearance

Because they are confined within the duct and conform to it, most papillomas are not visible by mammography. They frequently extend over a long length of the duct lumen without expanding it and may follow segmental branches. Occasionally they will present as a lobulated mass distending the duct and forming a fairly well-circumscribed mass (Fig. 19-4A), but these cannot be differentiated from other lobulated lesions. When visible, they are almost always in the anterior part of the breast because they are usually lesions of the large ducts. Sometimes they are found within a cyst, and it is the cyst that is evident on the mammogram. Although these are called *intracystic papillomas*, they are actually cystically dilated portions of the duct containing a papilloma. The origin of these cysts is likely different from the cysts that arise in the lobule.

The role of obstruction in the formation of these cysts is unclear. Although they can occasionally be found in the nipple itself, papillomas usually develop in the large duct several centimeters proximal to the nipple. The duct is

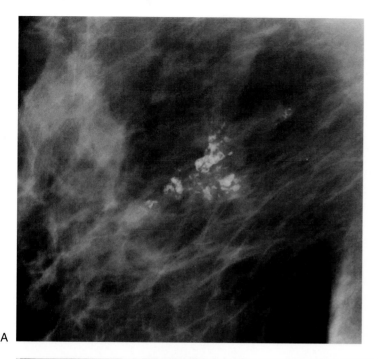

A

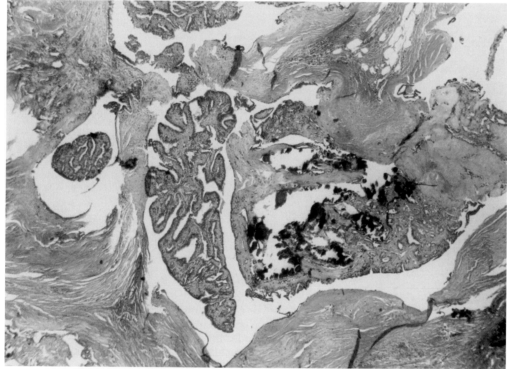

B

FIG. 19-6. These "shell-like" calcifications in a branching pattern **(A)** were due to partial **calcification of a large duct papilloma.** In another case, the calcifications in a large duct papilloma are evident on the photomicrograph (darkly stained material) **(B).** Some of the calcium has been chipped out during the tissue sectioning.

sometimes dilated in association with a papilloma, but the papilloma is usually not right in the distal portion of the dilated duct (near the nipple), making it unlikely that the duct is dilated due to obstruction. Because the ducts are almost always obstructed by keratin plugs in the nipple, cystic ductal dilatation is likely more complex than mere obstruction: It is likely due to a combination of increased secretion (perhaps from the papilloma or irrita-

tion due to it) that is not balanced by resorption, causing the duct to dilate in accordance with Laplace's law (its widest portion) (Fig. 19-5).

Solitary papillomas of the major ducts calcify infrequently. Occasionally they produce a nonspecific cluster of microcalcifications. "Shell-like," lucent-centered, calcific deposits in the subareolar region are almost certainly due to partial calcification of a large duct

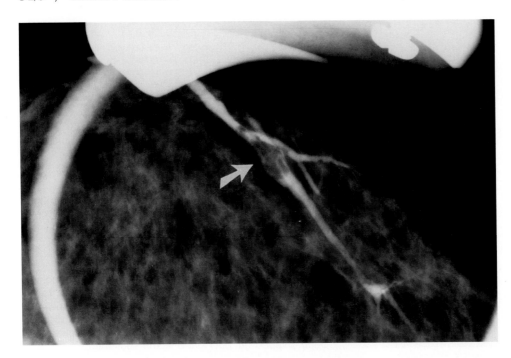

FIG. 19-7. The filling defect (*arrow*) in the duct filled with contrast proved to be an **intraductal papilloma.**

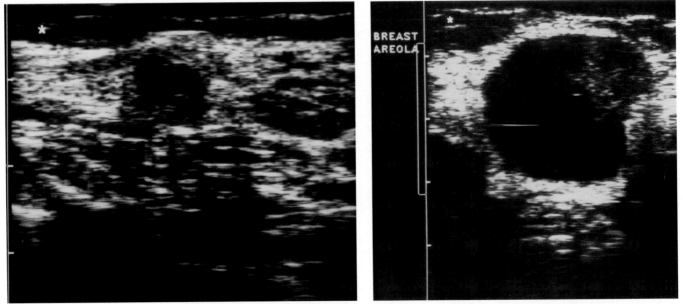

A

B

FIG. 19-8. An intraductal papilloma is rarely seen using ultrasound unless it is within a cyst. **(A)** An irregularly shaped, hypoechoic mass that proved to be an **intraductal papilloma.** The mass in this cyst **(B)** proved to be an intracystic papilloma. Although not diagnostic, intracystic papilloma is suggested by the frond-like appearance of the mass.

papilloma (Fig. 19-6). Infarction with hemorrhage is thought to be the reason that papillomas sometimes produce a bloody discharge (14). This process, which pathologists say is rare, also likely accounts for the rare, but distinctive shell-like calcifications.

Ductography, to evaluate nipple discharge, may reveal a filling defect that proves to be an intraductal papilloma (Fig. 19-7), but because intraductal papillomas cannot be distinguished from cancer on the ductogram, a biopsy is needed to establish the diagnosis. Both breast cancer and papillomas may produce a filling defect in the contrast column, extravasation, or complete obstruction to retrograde flow on ductography.

Five percent of solitary duct discharges are due to cancer, and most believe these discharges should be investigated surgically. A filling defect delineated by galactography can

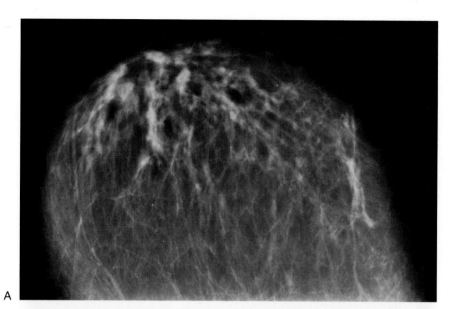

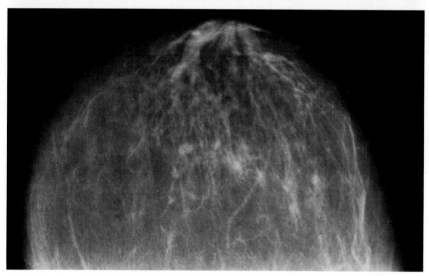

FIG. 19-9. (A) An example of **duct ectasia** with tubular structures appearing to converge toward the nipple. A similar appearance of duct ectasia is seen in **(B)**. *Continued.*

be targeted and a needle biopsy performed. These lesions (filling defects) can be needle localized, just as with any other lesion evident by mammography, and the lesion can be excised, limiting the amount of surgery needed if it proves to be a papilloma (see Chapter 21).

Ultrasound Appearance

Papillomas are solid, hypoechoic, usually lobulated masses when they are large enough to be seen by ultrasound (Fig. 19-8A). Because they are intraluminal lesions, they may be associated with excess fluid production (or decreased fluid reabsorption), which may account for their occasional location within a cystically dilated duct (intracystic papilloma).

When found within a cystic structure, the frond-like shape of the papilloma's surface may be more recognizable (see

Fig. 19-8), although any cyst that contains such a growth should be biopsied, because cancer cannot be excluded.

Duct Ectasia

Duct ectasia primarily affects the major ducts in the subareolar region, but sometimes the smaller segmental ducts are involved. There is a nonspecific dilatation of one or more ducts that may be palpable or merely visible by mammography.

The distended ducts are filled with fluid or thick, unresorbed secretions and cellular debris. Periductal fibrosis may be found in association with an inflammatory infiltrate.

The cause of this benign process remains obscure. Duct dilatation may be secondary to periductal inflammation or the cause of it. The duct may be weakened by the surrounding inflammation and become patulous, filling with unresorbed cellular debris. Conversely, the duct may be

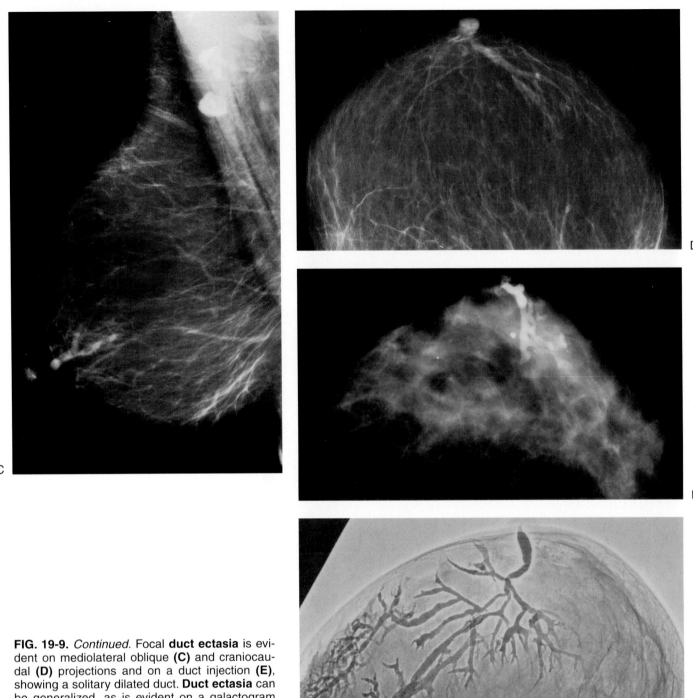

FIG. 19-9. *Continued.* Focal **duct ectasia** is evident on mediolateral oblique **(C)** and craniocaudal **(D)** projections and on a duct injection **(E)**, showing a solitary dilated duct. **Duct ectasia** can be generalized, as is evident on a galactogram imaged using xeroradiography **(F)**.

primarily distended with cellular debris, and a secondary inflammation may be triggered when this material is extruded out of the duct into the periductal tissues.

The thickened ducts and chemically induced aseptic inflammation may produce a palpable mass that may lead to biopsy. This inflammation is frequently associated with an infiltrate that contains plasma cells and has been termed *plasma cell mastitis*. Collected debris in the ducts may calcify and produce characteristic calcifications that are visible

by mammography. Duct ectasia does not predispose to future malignancy.

Ducts are present in all breasts, but they are frequently too small to be resolved by mammography or may be obscured by surrounding tissues of similar x-ray attenuation. Ducts may become thicker and more visible when ectatic or thickened because of periductal collagen deposition. Dilated, thickened ducts are relatively common, and when symmetrically distributed, are of no concern. They usually appear as tubular, serpentine structures converging on the nipple in the subareolar region (Fig. 19-9A). Ectasia involves a single duct (Fig. 19-9B, C) or multiple ducts (Fig. 19-9D).

Secretory Deposits

The mastitis that can accompany duct ectasia (or be the cause of it) may result in distinctive calcifications that have been called *secretory deposits*. These appear in one of three patterns. Intraluminal debris may calcify and produce thick, continuous, solid, rod-shaped deposits oriented along duct lines diffusely (Fig. 19-10A) or in a segmental distribution (Fig. 19-10B). Other rods may have a central lucency (Fig. 19-10C), and are probably periductal calcifications with a noncalcified luminal center. The third type of calcification commonly seen with this entity are spherical or globular deposits with lucent centers (Fig. 19-10D). The latter are common benign deposit that probably arise in small areas of

fat necrosis or in ductal debris. When these deposits are extensive, and particularly if they are associated with an inflammatory mass, they have been called *plasma cell mastitis*, owing to the plasma cell infiltrate that can be seen histologically as part of the inflammatory response.

Secretory calcifications may be confined to one duct network, but they are usually diffuse and bilateral. Even though this benign process is not associated with an increased risk of cancer, one must not overlook the possibility that a cancer can develop coincidentally. Occasionally secretory calcifications may be difficult to distinguish from malignant deposits. Cancer calcifications are not as regular. They lack lucent centers and are finer and more delicate linear forms with diameters <1 mm, rather than having the thicker, benign rod shapes (Fig. 19-11). The deposits are usually distinctively different. The benign ductal calcifications are continuous and thick and rarely branch, whereas those caused by cancer are usually discontinuous and fine (made up of very small particles) and

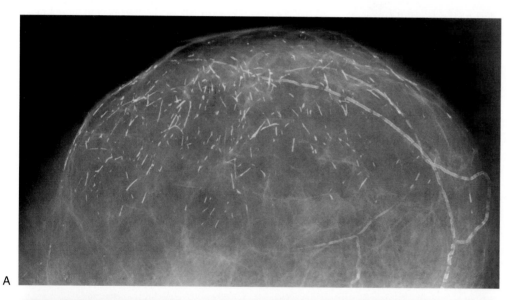

A

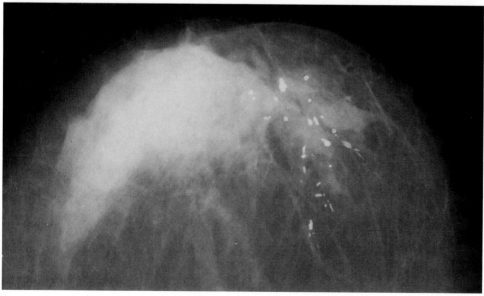

B

FIG. 19-10. Secretory deposits may form linear rods of calcified debris that are diffuse **(A)** or segmental **(B)** in their distribution. *Continued.*

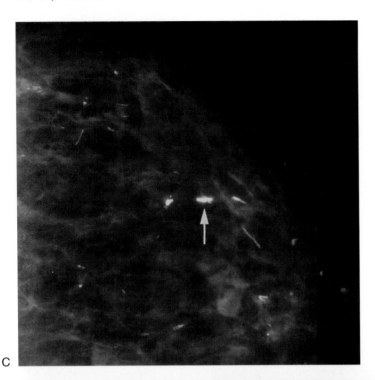

C

FIG. 19-10. *Continued.* Calcifications can form around a duct. **(C)** The duct may be responsible for the central lucency in some tubular calcifications (*arrow*). **(D) Secretory calcifications** are not always rod-shaped but may be globular, as on this craniocaudal projection. At times secretory deposits form calcified spheres with lucent centers that are indistinguishable from calcifications due to fat necrosis.

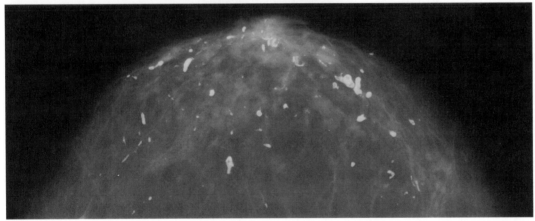

D

often branch, producing a discontinuous "dot-dash" pattern (see The Mammographic Appearance of Breast Cancer).

Ultrasound of these dilated ducts is as might be expected. If there is fluid in the distended duct, it will appear as a tubular lucency that may have visible branches (Fig. 19-12). If the duct is filled with debris, it will produce a solid-appearing tubular structure with a fairly homogeneous echotexture, although we have also seen ectatic ducts produce a target appearance with greater central echogenicity (Fig. 19-12B).

Benign Lesions of the Extralobular Terminal Ducts

Hyperplasia

Ducts are normally lined by a single layer of epithelium. Also termed *epitheliosis*, ductal hyperplasia is a benign pro-

liferation of the epithelial cells lining the ducts and producing multiple cell layers. Its cause is unknown. It usually occurs in the prelobular terminal ducts but may also develop in the lobular epithelium (lobular hyperplasia). Hyperplasia, as defined by Page and Anderson (14), is when there are at least three cell layers above the basement membrane.

Pathologists divide this process into mild, moderate, and florid. The cells may even form bridges across the duct similar to in situ cancer. The presence of myoepithelial cells helps distinguish hyperplasia from intraductal cancer in which the myoepithelial cells are absent. The overgrowth and heaping up of epithelial cells may almost completely occlude the duct lumen with a heterogeneous population of cells. Hyperplasia is fairly common and estimated to be present in 15% to 20% of the population (15). It can occur at all ages but is uncommon before 40 years of age and appears to increase in prevalence with age, although this may be

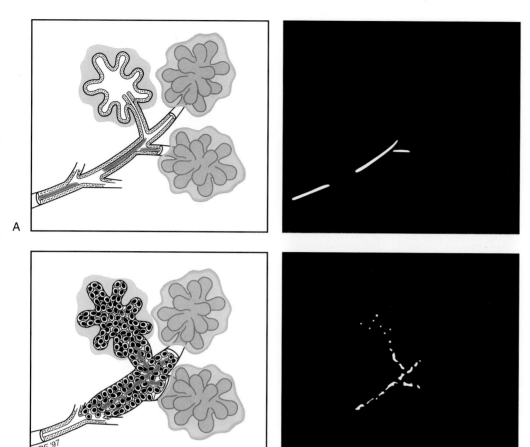

FIG. 19-11. Schematic comparing the relative size and morphology of **calcifications in necrotic cancer when compared to those in secretory disease.** Secretory calcifications are usually thicker, and the rods are uniformly calcified, whereas ductal carcinoma in situ produces finer linear deposits that are interrupted.

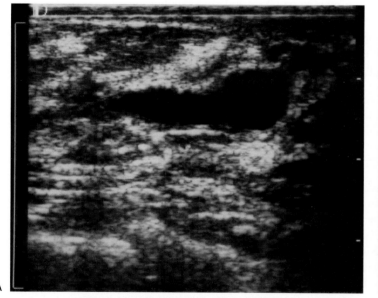

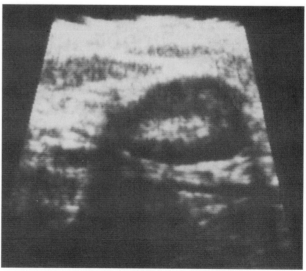

FIG. 19-12. Ultrasound of an ectatic duct may reveal an anechoic, fluid-filled tubular structure such as this duct **(A)**, which is converging on the nipple that is causing shadowing at the right edge of the image. This duct was ectatic and filled with **cellular debris that produced a target-like appearance** when imaged transversely on ultrasound examination **(B)**.

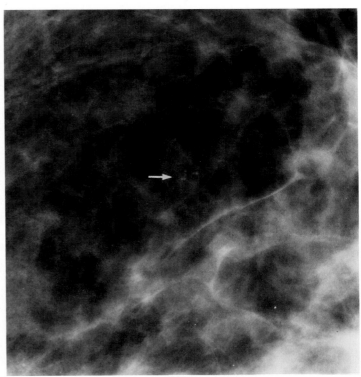

FIG. 19-13. These pleomorphic calcifications in a segmental distribution **(A)** were found to be caused by **hyperplasia** at biopsy. They cannot be differentiated from those associated with some cancers. **(B)** A small cluster (*arrow*) that proved to be due to a **peripheral papilloma**.

skewed by the selection bias of the autopsy series from which this observation was made. Page suggests that it is found in almost 50% of biopsies performed in perimenopausal women.

Hyperplasia does not usually form a palpable mass but is discovered histologically in association with other lesions such as cysts that are biopsied due to clinical or mammographic suspicion. Among the group of lesions that have, in the past, been included in the category of risk factors, hyperplasia alone only slightly increases the subsequent risk of breast cancer.

Atypical Ductal Hyperplasia

If a single layer of epithelium is normal, then hyperplasia represents an abnormal proliferation of cells. Most hyperplastic proliferations, however, probably never evolve further. The exact relationship of hyperplasia, atypical ductal hyperplasia (ADH), and DCIS remains uncertain. It has been suggested that in some women with hyperplasia, atypia develops and the risk of future breast cancer is increased. There is no question that ADH represents an increased risk for breast cancer, but its origin is unclear.

ADH probably represents a nonobligatory step in the development of carcinoma in situ. In other words, this lesion may be able to revert to normal epithelium. It is theorized, however, that, in some women, ADH progresses to irreversible intra-

ductal malignancy. Atypical changes are difficult to classify but are a group of lesions that probably constitute a spectrum leading to frank in situ carcinoma. Because the classification is based on observation that requires the removal of the lesion, the exact relationships to future cancer development are speculative. In fact, the differentiation between atypical hyperplasia and carcinoma in situ is often related to the amount of the process (10). According to the definition by Page and Anderson, DCIS requires all of the following (14):

1. A uniform population of cells
2. Smooth geometric spaces between cells or micropapillary formations with even cellular placement
3. Hyperchromatic nuclei

If only a few of the necessary elements are present, the process is termed ADH.

Atypical Lobular Hyperplasia

Pathologists make a distinction between ADH and atypical lobular hyperplasia (ALH). In the pathologist's evaluation, these are lesions that look similar to but do not fulfill all of the requirements of LCIS. Once again, according to Page, ALH is diagnosed when the cells have the cytologic features of LCIS but less than half of the acini are "filled, distorted and distended with a uniform population of characteristic cells."

Atypical Hyperplasia Increases the Risk of Breast Cancer

Atypical changes may involve the duct (ADH) or the lobule (ALH). In a large landmark study by Dupont and Page, women with atypical hyperplasia had five to six times the risk of developing breast cancer within 10 years when compared to women with nonproliferative changes (4). When atypical hyperplasia was found in women with a family history of breast cancer, the risk was increased 11-fold.

Mammographic Appearance

Bland hyperplasia rarely causes any mammographic changes. Atypical hyperplasia can produce masses, but it typically produces microcalcifications that are indistinguishable from breast cancer on a mammogram (Fig. 19-13A). Helvie et al. (16) reviewed 58 cases and found that among the 45 women who had mammographically identified lesions, 27 lesions caused calcifications, eight appeared as nodules, five were associated with spiculated masses, two were calcifications associated with architectural distortion, one was a nodule containing a calcification, one was asymmetric density and one was an area of architectural distortion.

Multiple Peripheral Papillomas

Multiple peripheral papillomas are hyperplastic lesions that project into the lumen of the distal ductal epithelium just proximal to the lobule (17). This entity differs from a solitary ductal papilloma, which is always benign and occurs singly in the major ducts.

These lesions lack the fibrovascular core that distinguishes the large duct papilloma. A multifocal epithelial proliferation in the small ducts, multiple peripheral papillomas are usually diagnosed only on histologic assessment. They are significant from an imaging point of view in that, as with hyperplasia and malignancy, they may produce mammographically detectable clustered microcalcifications. The association of this entity with increased risk for subsequent cancer development has been suggested but remains to be confirmed.

Mammographic Appearance

Usually papillomatous lesions are not seen on the mammogram because they are microscopic changes. Occasionally they produce focal clustered microcalcifications of varying morphology that are indistinguishable from cancer calcifications and require biopsy for diagnosis (Fig. 19-13B). We believe that they may occasionally form multiple small masses that are visible on mammograms, but this has never been confirmed.

Ultrasound Appearance

Occasionally found in conjunction with cysts, hyperplastic and papillomatous lesions are usually too small to be detected by ultrasound. They may be associated with irregular hypoechoic tissue, but this is probably due to surrounding fibrosis.

Benign Lesions of the Lobule

Fibroadenoma

The fibroadenoma is the most common benign solid lesion of the breast that prompts a biopsy. The fact that it is fairly common in teenage women suggests that it is likely a lesion that develops with the breast (18). It is extremely rare to have a fibroadenoma appear later on in life in breast tissue in which there was clearly no evidence of it in the past, although enlargement of a fibroadenoma is not that uncommon (19). Any solid lesion that appears de novo in an older woman, however, should be considered suspicious and not dismissed as a fibroadenoma.

Fibroadenomas are the result of an overgrowth of the specialized stromal connective tissue of the lobule. As this lesion enlarges, the acini and the epithelial lining cells of the acini are stretched and elongated (Fig. 19-14). These elongated acini have been termed *canaliculi* by pathologists, although this term is rarely used. The acini and the intralobular terminal duct are surrounded and compressed by this idiopathic proliferation of collagen within the lobule. This proliferation may produce a palpable mass that expands the lobule, resulting in a rounded, lobulated lesion whose margins are usually clearly separable from normal breast tissue.

The fibroadenoma is freely movable on physical examination, and at surgery it can frequently be extruded from the surrounding tissue. Regrowth has been reported if a small margin of surrounding tissue is not removed with the lesion,

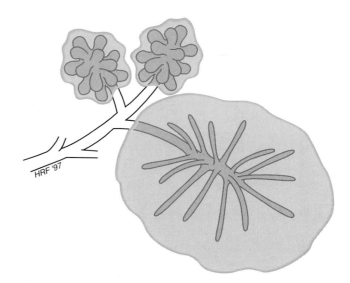

FIG. 19-14. Schematic of a fibroadenoma shows how the enlarging volume of the specialized, intralobular connective tissue stretches and thins the acinar structures.

but this is extremely uncommon. If a fibroadenoma regrows, the original diagnosis should be questioned because the tumor was likely not a fibroadenoma to begin with, but rather a phylloides tumor, which is likely a variant of the benign fibroadenoma.

The proportions of stromal elements found in a fibroadenoma may vary, producing very cellular adenomas with fibroblastic proliferation, or a fibrotic lesion with a preponderance of sclerotic, collagenous tissue. Fibroadenomas range in size from microscopic, incidental findings to extremely large masses that occupy much of the volume of the breast.

When very large, ≥10 cm, they are termed *giant fibroadenomas*. This designation is only a recognition that these benign masses can be very large and still not represent phylloides tumors. When a fibroadenoma grows rapidly and becomes very large (often occupying much of the breast) in an adolescent, it is termed a *juvenile fibroadenoma*. Histologically it has fewer stretched acini, probably reflecting the fact that the lobules are not completely developed in the adolescent. Otherwise, except for their rapid growth, these lesions are apparently not different from the standard fibroadenoma. Giant fibroadenomas are usually found in the adolescent. The lesion is not invasive but may grow to occupy most of the breast and produce asymmetric enlargement of the affected breast.

Fibroadenomas have been reported in prepubertal girls, but because these lesions appear to be hormone dependent, their prevalence increases with menarche. According to Haagenson (20), it is the most commonly excised lump in teenaged women and women in their 30s. As in any part of the breast, cancer can occur by serendipity alongside a fibroadenoma, but there is no good evidence to suggest a direct association between this lesion and the development of cancer. The fibroadenoma is itself always benign, with no increased malignant potential. Because it contains epithelium, however, cancer may arise within a fibroadenoma (21). Both ductal and lobular carcinomas have been found arising in some fibroadenomas (22). Just as malignant cells may spread from the ducts back into a lobule, cancer arising adjacent to a fibroadenoma may spread back into it.

Dupont et al. (23) have suggested that certain types of fibroadenomas, which they termed *complex*, indicate an increased risk for the future development of breast cancer. The authors reviewed 1,835 cases. If the fibroadenoma contained cysts, sclerosing adenosis, epithelial calcifications, or papillary apocrine changes, they were classified as complex. They found that having a complex fibroadenoma increased a woman's risk three times (relative risk [RR], 3.10). A family history of breast cancer raised the RR to 3.72, and if there was benign proliferative disease adjacent to the fibroadenoma the RR rose to 3.88. These elevated risks remained elevated for decades after the fibroadenoma had been removed. There was no increased risk if the fibroadenoma was not complex. It is likely that the complex fibroadenoma is similar to atypical hyperplasia in that it is a phenotypic reflection of a genetically unstable epithelium whose cells are more prone to malignant transformation. It is probably

not the fibroadenoma that is of significance but the epithelial changes contained within. There is no evidence that these fibroadenomas themselves ever transform (they were all removed to make the diagnosis), but the complex fibroadenoma appears to be an indicator of higher risk.

Although fibroadenomas have no directly established malignant potential, they may be difficult to distinguish from a phylloides tumor. The phylloides tumor is probably a related lesion and can be locally recurrent and invasive and may occasionally metastasize. The exact relation of the two lesions is not clear. Phylloides tumors were more common in the past, and their present greater rarity may be due to the fact that surgeons have been more aggressive in biopsying abnormalities found on clinical and mammographic evaluation, and small phylloides tumors are being removed and mistakenly diagnosed as fibroadenomas.

The fibroadenoma appears to be sensitive to hormones. They seem to be less common in postmenopausal women (24), although they are the cause of 22% of the needle localizations that we perform in women younger than 50 years of age and 15% of the biopsies that we perform on women aged 50 years and over (the percentage decreases steadily with increasing age).

Involution of Fibroadenomas

Many fibroadenomas undergo involution. The exact timing and causes of their involution and its relationship to menopause is not clear. Involuting, hyalinized fibroadenomas are seen in premenopausal women, and enlarging fibroadenomas are found in postmenopausal women. In a series of 26 clinically occult, mammographically detected fibroadenomas that had enlarged, Meyer et al. (25) found that half were in women aged 46 to 60 years. Loss of hormonal support likely results in atrophy and hyalinization, but this is not completely clear. It is also unclear whether infarction plays a role. Involution is the usual cause for the development of mammographically distinctive calcifications.

Mammographic Appearance

Mammographically, the fibroadenomas are usually sharply circumscribed, well-defined lesions that are round, ovoid, or smoothly lobulated. They often have one or more flattened surfaces. Fornage et al. (26) have shown that on ultrasound, fibroadenomas are usually not round, but elongated (see Chapter 16), but this may be, in part, an artifact of pressure from the transducer and tethering by breast tissue with the patient in the supine position. As with all breast lesions, the margins of a fibroadenoma may be obscured by the surrounding normal tissue. Because it does not infiltrate, the fibroadenoma only distorts the surrounding tissue by occupying space. Fairly commonly, a thin, lucent halo may surround it (Fig. 19-15A), but this is not a diagnostic sign because it can accompany other circum-

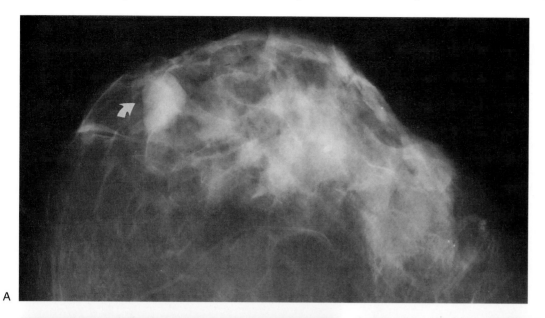

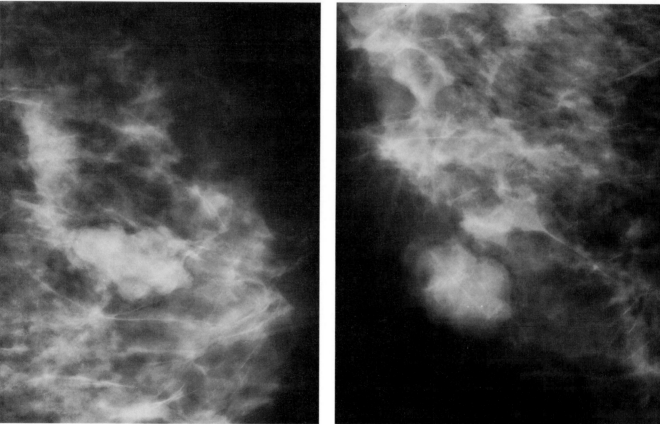

FIG. 19-15. The **classic fibroadenoma** has a smooth, sharply defined margin **(A)**. It is often lobulated with flattened edges. The thin, dark, lucent line surrounding this fibroadenoma (*arrow*) has been termed a *halo*. It is due to the optical illusion created by the Mach effect (the suppression of retinal cones adjacent to an area of abrupt transition).

Some **fibroadenomas** are lobulated and concern is increased, as for this mass seen on the mediolateral oblique **(B)** and craniocaudal **(C)** projections in a 36-year-old woman that proved, at biopsy, to be a benign fibroadenoma.

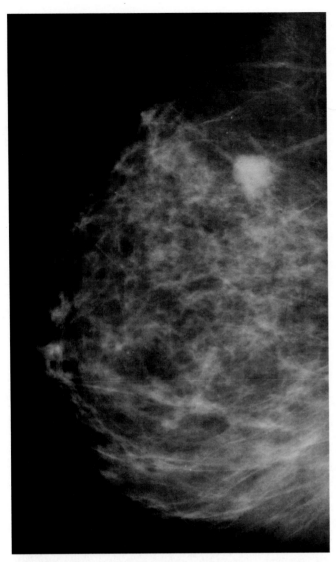

FIG. 19-16. This mass with very small lobulations proved to be a **fibroadenoma.** Nevertheless, this type of microlobulated margin should raise the concern and biopsy should be performed.

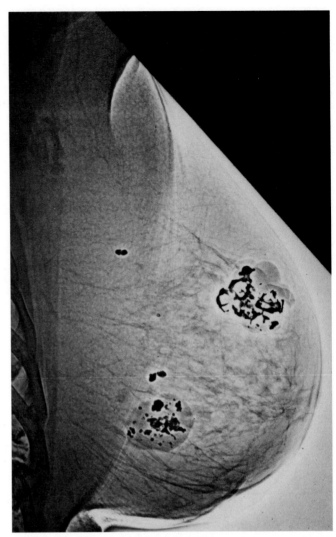

A

FIG. 19-17. Large calcified masses (dark black) shown on a xerogram **(A)** have the typical appearance of multiple benign **involuting fibroadenomas.** *Continued.*

scribed lesions, including malignancy. The halo reflects an abrupt density transition between the lesion and the surrounding tissue producing an optical illusion caused by the Mach effect (27). Fibroadenomas may have somewhat flattened contours, which, if present, help to distinguish them from cysts, although ultrasound and aspiration are the only accurate methods of distinguishing cysts from solid lesions.

Because they recapitulate the structure of the lobule, fibroadenomas are often lobulated (Fig. 19-15B, C). Occasionally they may have a microlobulated border, with frequent small undulations of their surface (Fig. 19-16). Because some cancers have similar margins, however, the level of suspicion must increase with this morphologic characteristic.

Fibroadenomas may develop anywhere in the breast where there are lobules, and occasionally they are multiple and bilateral. If they undergo involution leading to hyalin-

ization, they may calcify (Fig. 19-17). The cause of the calcifications is unclear. Although most calcified fibroadenomas are found in postmenopausal women, they are not uncommon among premenopausal women.

Calcifications in fibroadenomas usually begin inside the mass (Fig. 19-18 A–D) and increase centripetally (Fig. 19-18E, F), but they may calcify along their periphery as well (Fig. 19-18G, H). Some residual mass may be visible, or the lesion may completely calcify. When heavily calcified, fibroadenomas have a pathognomonic appearance as popcorn-shaped large calcifications (Fig. 19-19). Occasionally early calcifications may be fine and irregular and indistinguishable from cancer, and because they are indistinguishable from those forming in cancer, require biopsy to ensure the diagnosis (Fig. 19-20). Fibroadenomas may grow to an extremely large size, but they usually maintain a round or ovoid shape.

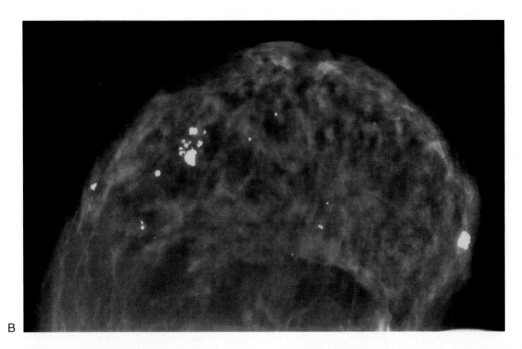

FIG. 19-17. *Continued.* In a 70-year-old patient **(B)**, the large calcifications are due to multiple, **involuting fibroadenomas.**

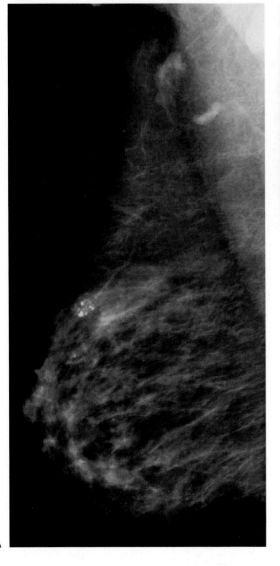

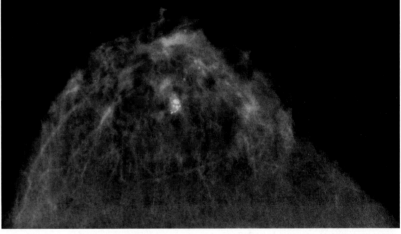

FIG. 19-18. Typical appearance of an **involuting fibroadenoma** on the mediolateral oblique (MLO) **(A)** and craniocaudal (CC) **(B)** projections in a 76-year-old woman. *Continued.*

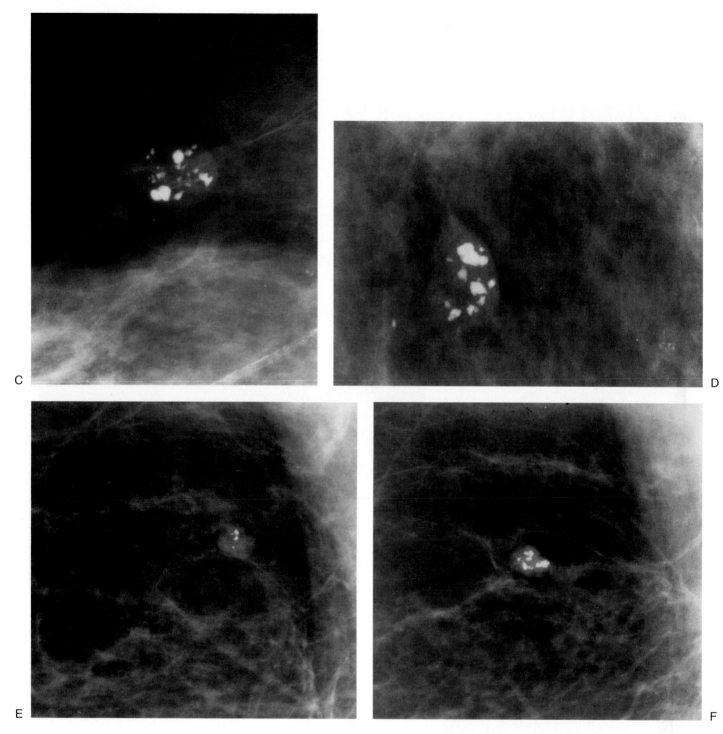

C

D

E

F

FIG. 19-18. *Continued.* The lesion is also seen on magnification MLO **(C)** and magnification CC **(D)** projections. The calcifications forming in this **involuting fibroadenoma** are seen in the lesion in a 62-year-old woman **(E)**. Several years later more large calcifications are evident **(F)**. *Continued.*

Cancer can serendipitously arise alongside a fibroadenoma, and it may envelope the lesion. Cancer arising in a fibroadenoma is also likely serendipitous (Fig. 19-21). Because there is epithelium within fibroadenomas, cancer can develop just as it can in normal ductal epithelium (28). Baker et al. found that ill-defined margins, clustered micro-

calcifications, and large size or an increase in size should raise concern (22).

Fibroadenomas can grow to very large sizes (Fig. 19-22). Pathologists define a variant of large fibroadenomas that may occur soon after puberty. These are termed *juvenile fibroadenomas* and appear to be more cellular than the adult

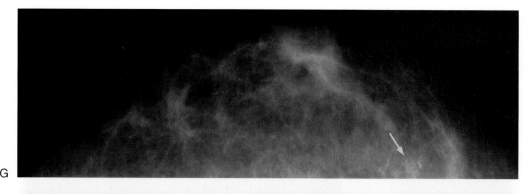

G

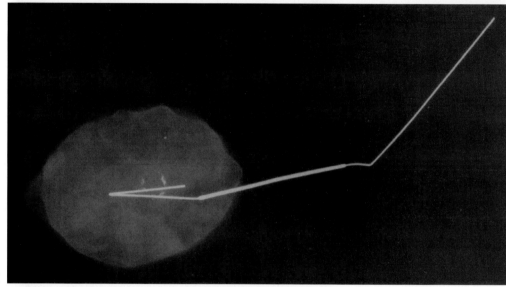

H

FIG. 19-18. *Continued.* **Pleomorphic calcifications** (*arrow*) in another case **(G)** that proved to be forming in an involuting fibroadenoma with calcifications around its periphery. This is better seen on the specimen radiograph **(H)**.

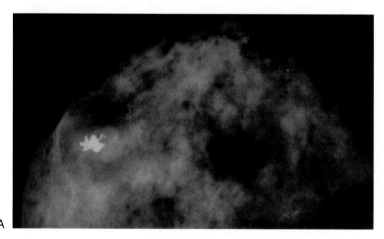

A

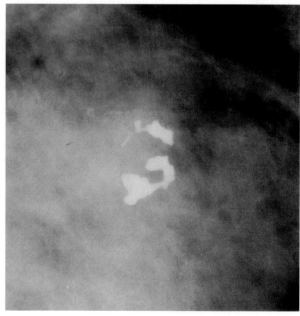

B

FIG. 19-19. Typical "popcorn" calcifications of an involuting fibroadenoma may form in a visible mass **(A)** or appear alone **(B)**.

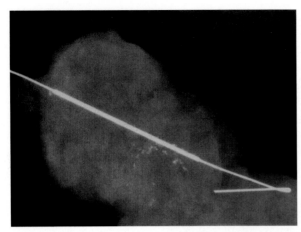

FIG. 19-20. Early calcifications in a fibroadenoma may be indistinguishable from the pleomorphic clustered calcifications of intraductal cancer. Even on this specimen radiograph calcifications that proved to be in an involuting fibroadenoma are highly suspicious.

type of fibroadenoma. Although there has been some confusion in the past, the giant fibroadenoma appears to be distinct from a phylloides tumor.

Ultrasound Appearance

Sonographically, fibroadenomas may produce every imaginable combination of echo characteristics (29). Their appearance is extremely variable, and morphologically, a given fibroadenoma is indistinguishable by ultrasound from other lesions, including cancer. Fibroadenomas are typically ovoid, well-circumscribed, hypoechoic lesions that are longer than they are high (width from the side facing the skin to the side facing the chest wall with the patient supine), with margins that are usually sharply distinguished from the surrounding tissue (Fig. 19-23A). Their borders, on occasion, merge with the surrounding tissues and may appear ill defined. They may have a notch in their surface contour.

Although some believe that fibroadenomas can be differentiated from cancers using ultrasound, this has never been proved in a prospective fashion. Fibroadenomas have a markedly variable appearance, and there is an overlap with some malignant lesions. As with other masses that are round or oval, fibroadenomas may exhibit lateral wall refractive shadowing (Fig. 19-23B).

The internal echo pattern may be homogeneous or irregular, with high-amplitude echoes (Fig. 19-23C), or if the lesion is cellular, the echoes may be sparse, making it possible to mistake a fibroadenoma for a cyst if the gain settings are not appropriate (Fig. 19-23D, E). Occasionally a fibroadenoma is isoechoic with the surrounding parenchyma and not visible, or barely visible using ultrasound (Fig. 19-23F). In a series of 100 fibroadenomas, Fornage et al. (26) described four that were hyperechoic, although this appears

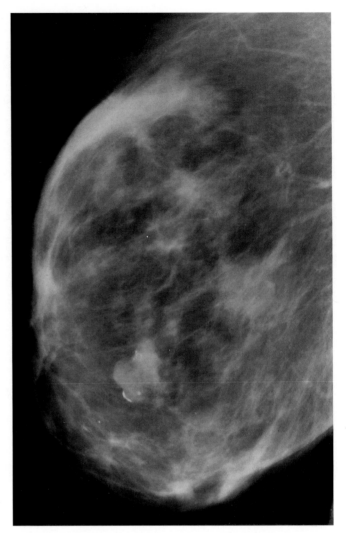

FIG. 19-21. Cancer developing within a fibroadenoma is very unusual and apparently serendipitous. This benign fibroadenoma, calcifying along its periphery, contained an intraductal cancer. It was biopsied because of its overly lobulated shape.

to be extremely rare. We have seen only one fibroadenoma that was more echogenic than breast tissue.

Echoes posterior to these lesions are frequently enhanced, particularly when the adenoma is cellular and round and acts as an acoustic lens focusing the sound. The retrotumoral echoes are often isoechoic with the surrounding breast tissue. A lesion containing abundant fibrosis may produce posterior acoustic shadowing that is indistinguishable from the classic shadowing found with some cancers (Fig. 19-24).

Some believe that fibroadenomas can be differentiated from cancer using ultrasound: This is probably a statistical phenomenon. Fornage et al. (26) found that most cancers were more round than ovoid, whereas fibroadenomas tended to be ovoid. They measured the longest axis of the mass and compared it to the axis of the mass perpendicular to the skin and found that if the ratio was ≥1.4, the likelihood of malignancy was extremely small. Clearly this is a probability argument because there are cancers that are elongated. Sim-

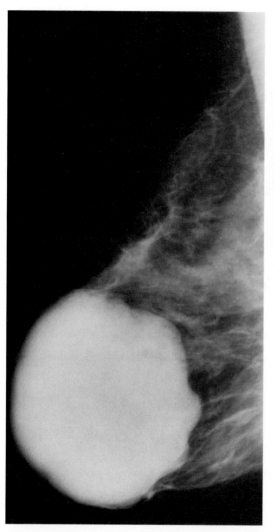

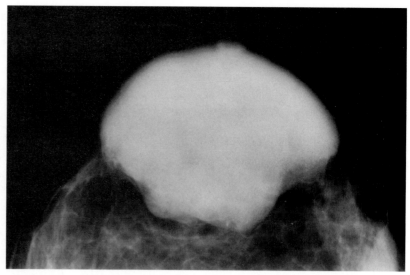

FIG. 19-22. This large, palpable mass seen on the mediolateral (A) and craniocaudal (B) projections was a **benign, giant fibroadenoma** in a 34-year-old woman.

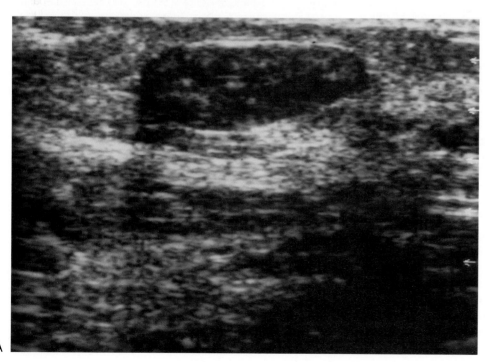

FIG. 19-23. (A) A palpable mass in a 32-year-old woman has the typical appearance of a **fibroadenoma by ultrasound.** It is a mass that is longer than it is deep, ovoid in shape with sharply defined margins, and has a fairly uniform internal echo texture. *Continued.*

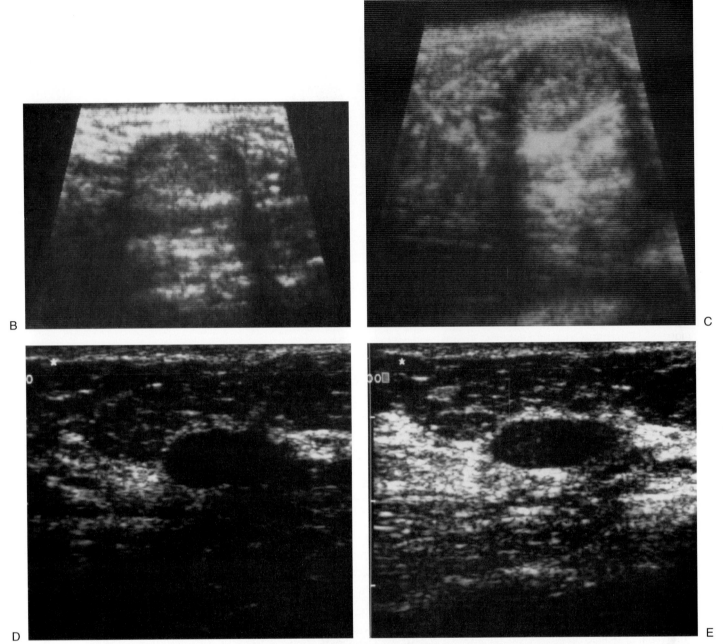

FIG. 19-23. *Continued.* The oval shape of a fibroadenoma can focus the sound and produce enhanced through-transmission of sound as well as **refractive, lateral wall shadowing (B)**, as in this **fibroadenoma.** There are **prominent internal echoes in some fibroadenomas and posterior acoustic enhancement** can be dramatic despite the fact that the lesion is solid **(C)**. The internal echoes are not visible in this fibroadenoma **(D)** until the gain is set properly **(E)**. *Continued.*

ilarly, others have claimed that the combination of high resolution ultrasound and Doppler can differentiate fibroadenomas from cancer. This, too, is a claim that is based more on probability than the ability to differentiate benign lesions from malignant lesions. If a lesion is round or oval and well circumscribed on a mammogram and is not a cyst, there is only a 2% to 5% chance that it represents cancer. If it is these lesions that are chosen for ultrasound with other obvi-

ously benign lesions such as intramammary lymph nodes included in the study, then ultrasound can be made to seem very accurate. Without even performing the ultrasound, the specificity would start at 98% if all of the lesions were called benign. The problem with this type of approach is that it is the two cancers that need to be found early, and allowing them to pass through the screen because ultrasound gave improper reassurance may reduce the benefit of screening.

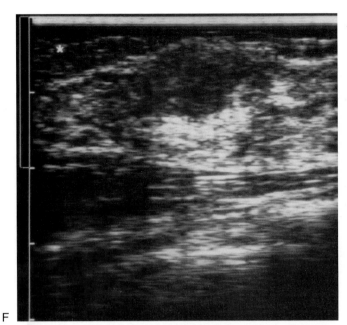

F

FIG. 19-23. *Continued.* This **fibroadenoma (F)** is barely distinguishable from the subcutaneous fat.

Cysts

Cysts can be found in women of all ages, but their peak prevalence is in women aged 30 to 50 years. Although some cysts are actually distended large ducts, most cysts form in the lobule and represent dilatation of the lobular acini. In postmenopausal women, some are thought to be part of the involutional process. As the lobular epithelium atrophies, the acini coalesce, producing fluid-filled spaces surrounded by the sclerotic specialized connective tissue of the lobule. Through progressive distention the lobule becomes obliterated and replaced by the fluid-containing cyst.

The role of duct obstruction in the formation of cysts is unclear. Because the duct orifices in the nipple, in most women, are normally blocked by keratin plugs, the ducts are "blocked" all of the time, yet this does not result in cyst formation. It is more likely that cysts form as a result of an imbalance between secretion and resorption. Active secretion occurs throughout the duct and lobular system even in the nonlactating individual. It has been shown, experimentally, that these secretions are handled by a balanced reabsorption. It is believed that many cysts form as the result of a change that takes place in the cells lining the lobule. The cells enlarge and secretions appear to increase. This is termed *apocrine metaplasia* (Fig. 19-25). If secretion increases but resorption lags behind, the resulting imbalance produces dilatation of the terminal ductules (acini) within the lobule (Fig. 19-26A). Progressive effacement of the acinar structure of the intralobular terminal ductules replaces the lobule with a group of small cysts that may, ultimately, coalesce into a large cyst (Fig. 19-26B, C).

Because hyperplasia is a frequently associated finding, it is postulated that some cysts form when the extralobular duct becomes occluded, but the association is not clear because occlusion may also be secondary to pressure on the terminal duct from the enlarging cyst. Occlusion is clearly not required

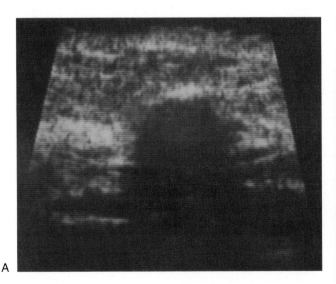

A

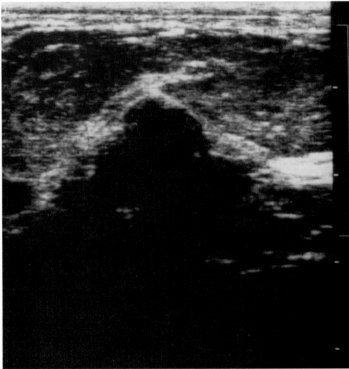

B

FIG. 19-24. **(A)** A fibroadenoma with a rounded contour and dense posterior acoustic shadowing. **(B)** An irregular, **triangular fibroadenoma** with low-amplitude internal echoes and marked posterior acoustic shadowing, making it indistinguishable from breast cancer by ultrasound.

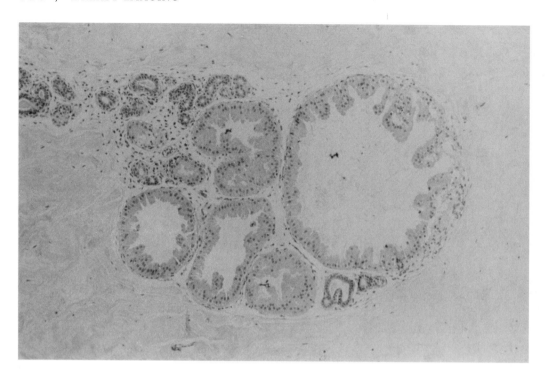

FIG. 19-25. Most **cysts likely form as a result of apocrine metaplasia,** producing secretions that are not balanced by resorption, which leads to progressive dilatation of the acini. Histologic section (hematoxylin and eosin) shows several acini of a lobule whose lining cells are large having undergone apocrine metaplasia. Secretions fill the microcystically dilated acini. It is unclear why some of the acini have not undergone metaplasia even though they appear to be part of the same lobule. Progressive accumulation of fluid may dilate the acini so that they coalesce and become a detectable cyst.

for cyst formation because there is frequently free communication between a cyst and the duct. We have seen this on ultrasound and galactography (Fig. 19-27). Fluid accumulation may increase dramatically, occasionally reaching >100 ml. It is likely that many cysts merely represent the most distensible portion of a network that is experiencing increased secretion.

Cysts may be solitary but are often multiple. A single layer of cuboidal epithelium defines their walls. As noted above, apocrine metaplastic transformation of the lining cells is felt

to play a role in the development of cysts. The metaplasia may persist, or the epithelium may revert to a cuboidal or flattened epithelium. In autopsy studies, between 20% and 50% of women are found to have visible cysts.

Carcinoma is rarely found in a cyst. When it occurs, the relationship remains obscure. Intracystic cancer is potentially just coincidental. Most (of the rare) intracystic cancers, however, are papillary. The surrounding cysts are likely formed from the larger ducts. Perhaps the duct becomes cys-

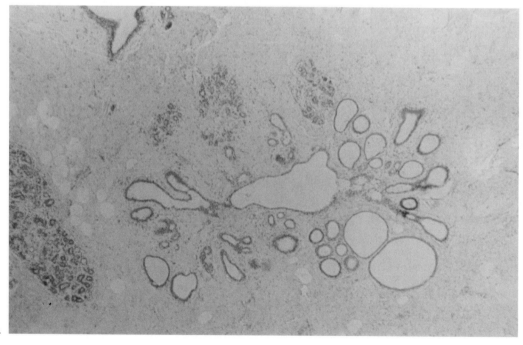

A

FIG. 19-26. In this photomicrograph, the **acini of the lobules are markedly dilated (A).** *Continued.*

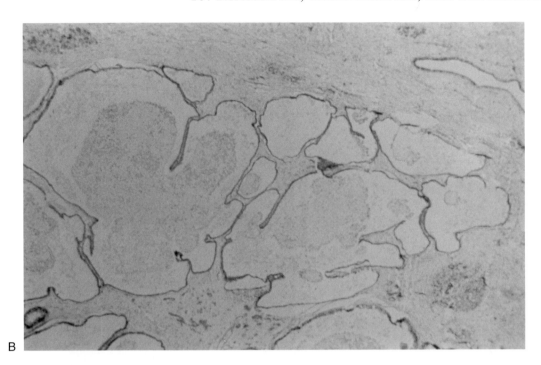

B

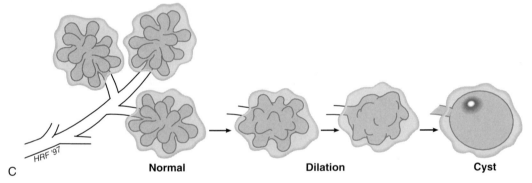

C   **Normal**   **Dilation**   **Cyst**

FIG. 19-26. *Continued.* In another case, they are coalescent **(B)**. The process may continue so that acini of the lobule may ultimately coalesce to form a cyst as represented schematically **(C)**.

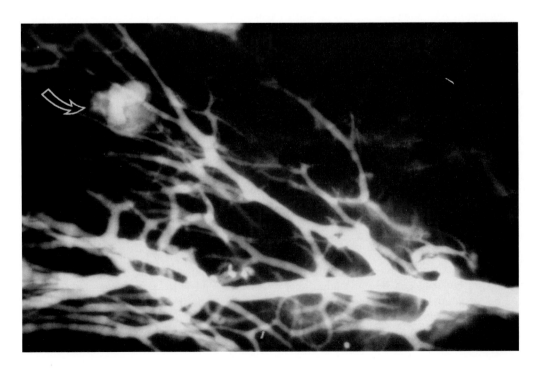

FIG. 19-27. Cysts may communicate with the ducts. Obstruction is not a prerequisite for cyst formation. **Contrast material flowed into this lobulated cyst** (*arrow*) from a retrograde injection into a discharging duct.

tically dilated due to hypersecretion by the tumor. Alternatively, cancer could be the source of duct obstruction. In our experience intracystic cancer is found in <0.2% of cysts.

Cysts may be soft, or they may be under tension from undrained secretions. If cyst fluid leaks into the surrounding stroma it can elicit inflammation that may result in pericystic fibrosis. This can produce ill-defined margins on mammography although cysts are usually sharply demarcated and freely movable.

Cyst Fluid and the Management of Cysts

Cyst fluid is rarely colorless and "sparklingly" clear; rather, it is usually turbid yellow or green. When viewed through the cyst wall, the fluid appears blue, leading to the term *blue-domed cyst.* Cyst fluid may be thin and easily aspirated, or it may have the viscosity of thick mucus or gelatin and resist removal even through large-gauge needles.

Hemorrhagic Cyst Fluid. When cyst fluid is maroon or brown, previous hemorrhage should be suspected. Hemorrhage into a cyst may be idiopathic, secondary to an intracystic papilloma, or due to a rare intracystic cancer. Although controversial, most surgeons believe that cysts containing old hemorrhagic fluid (not fresh blood caused by the introduction of the needle) should be excised because of the small possibility of intracystic carcinoma. The majority of focal intracystic lesions, when they occur, prove to be benign papillomas. Intracystic cancer is extremely uncommon. As with any other part of the breast, malignancy can arise alongside a cyst, even if it is not the direct cause of it. Some surgeons argue that a large cyst might obscure an adjacent malignancy and they aspirate some cysts for this reason (the documentation of this approach is obscure).

The appropriate handling of nonhemorrhagic cyst fluid is also a source of controversy. Many surgeons believe that there is no reason to send fluid for cytologic analysis unless it contains old blood, because the prevalence of benign cysts is so much greater than the rare intracystic cancer (30). Furthermore, a negative cytologic analysis of breast cyst fluid does not exclude the possibility of intracystic cancer. Some argue that when the fluid is unremarkable, cytology is not cost-effective. Meyer et al. found that if no old blood is present, cytologic evaluation is of no value. Many surgeons are satisfied if the lesion that is drained is completely resolved by the aspiration. If the cyst recurs, many would reaspirate, and if it recurred again, many would excise it. The scientific reason for this approach is unclear. Most agree that if the ultrasound evaluation of a mass reveals all of the characteristics of a simple cyst, no further intervention is needed. This is certainly true for nonpalpable masses that are diagnosed as cysts using ultrasound.

Cysts and Menopause. Common in the perimenopausal years, cysts may regress after menopause, but they can be found in women of all ages and are not uncommon in postmenopausal women. Hormone replacement therapy (HRT) has been linked to the development of postmenopausal cysts,

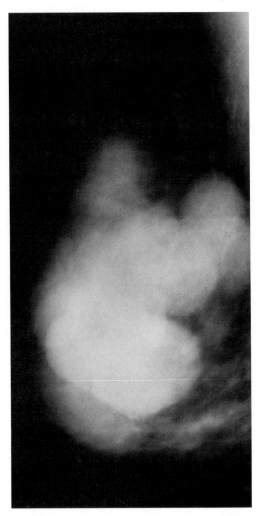

FIG. 19-28. The rounded contours are due to **multiple cysts.**

but postmenopausal women not infrequently develop cysts for no apparent reason or significance. Some past studies have linked cysts with increased breast cancer risk, probably due to selection bias and a skewed population. Dupont and Page found an increased risk of breast cancer only when cysts occurred in women with a family history of breast cancer (31).

If a circumscribed mass meets the criteria for a simple cyst as described below, there is rarely any reason for further evaluation. Cyst aspiration (imaging guided for nonpalpable or difficult to aspirate lesions) is a fairly simple and very safe procedure, and if there is any question one can quickly determine the composition of a lesion. If the aspirated lesion disappears on ultrasound (and mammography, if indicated) and the fluid is not hemorrhagic, the likelihood of an intracystic cancer is extremely low with no reported cases.

Cyst Recurrence After Aspiration. Although some surgeons believe that a cyst that recurs following aspiration should be reaspirated and if it recurs again should be excised, the data supporting this are not clear and the practice appears to be anecdotal. As already stated, intracystic cancers are extremely rare. In our (anecdotal) experience,

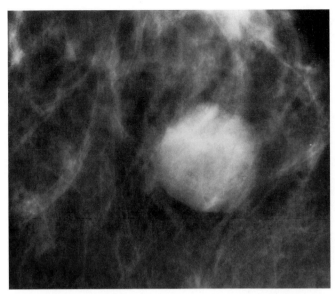

FIG. 19-29. Most cysts are round or ovoid, as seen in this 39-year-old woman.

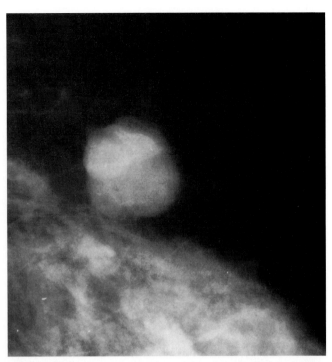

FIG. 19-30. Cysts are occasionally lobulated, as in this postmenopausal woman. The lobulation is likely a recapitulation of the lobular architecture from which the cyst arises.

they are usually associated with large (>2 cm in diameter), hemorrhagic cysts. When we aspirate a cyst, the fluid is unremarkable, and the cyst is no longer visible by the imaging modality on which it appeared (i.e., ultrasound, mammography, or both) the patient is encouraged to return to annual screening. If the cyst recurs, it is merely commented on but does not elicit any additional evaluation unless there are new, worrisome associated findings.

Mammographic Appearance

Cysts frequently appear as multiple, rounded densities (Fig. 19-28). They may occupy much of the breast volume and produce numerous overlapping rounded contours.

Solitary cysts are not uncommon. They are normally round or ovoid (Fig. 19-29) but may be lobulated (Fig. 19-30). They are usually well defined with circumscribed margins that may be obscured by the surrounding tissue. Pericystic fibrosis from inflammation may cause cyst margins to be obscured. A lucent halo may be seen around them (Fig. 19-31) but, as with other circumscribed lesions, this is not a diagnostic feature. This halo is a Mach effect in which the cones of the retina, when exposed to a bright object with a sharp margin, suppress the adjacent cones so that the signal generated by these adjacent cones at the margin is lower than it should be, and the effect is the illusion of a dark zone adjacent to the edge of the bright object.

Whether single or multiple, cysts may remain for many years or spontaneously resorb. Brenner et al. (32) reported that, among 5,000 consecutive women screened, 53 (1%) had developed cysts at one time or another. More than half of these cysts regressed or spontaneously resorbed within one year, and more than two-thirds had diminished over two

years. They found that only 12% had not shown some diminution in size over 5 years. Cysts may be resorbed over time. This resorption may occur rapidly (Fig. 19-32). Pennes and Homer (33) suggested that cysts may rupture with mammographic compression although this has not been our experience.

When multiple, cysts may overlap and look irregular, but they usually do not distort the basic breast architecture except by displacement.

Calcifications and Cysts

Cysts cannot be accurately diagnosed by mammography, because they cannot be distinguished from other well-circumscribed masses unless they display several characteristic patterns of calcification.

Occasionally the wall of a cyst may calcify, producing egg-shell–thin "rim" deposits (Fig. 19-33). Other cysts may contain precipitated calcium in the form of milk of calcium. Small radiopaque calcium particles can precipitate from cyst fluid and gravitate to the dependent portion of a cyst. This produces a concave crescent of density when viewed tangentially in the upright lateral projection (Fig. 19-34) (see Chapter 13), and concomitant amorphous dots of calcium, when seen, en face in the craniocaudal projection, owing to their dependent position pooled in the bottom of the cyst. This appearance is pathognomonic of milk of calcium, and biopsy is not indicated (34). On occasion, the precipitated

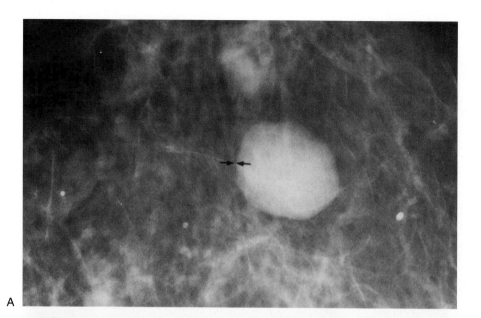

A

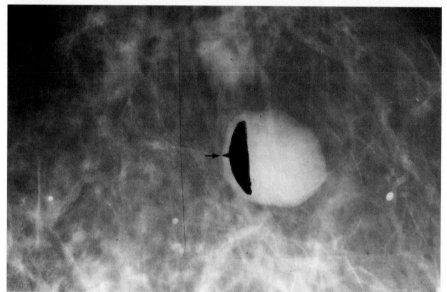

B

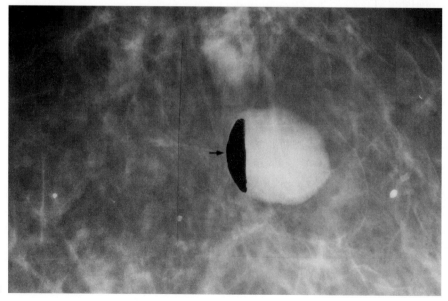

C

FIG. 19-31. (A) A cyst with a sharp line surrounding its margin, forming a "halo" (the dark band between the two arrows). The halo is an optical illusion due to the **Mach effect.** Note that the halo disappears as the lesion immediately beneath the edge is covered **(B, C)** (note that the halo itself was not covered).

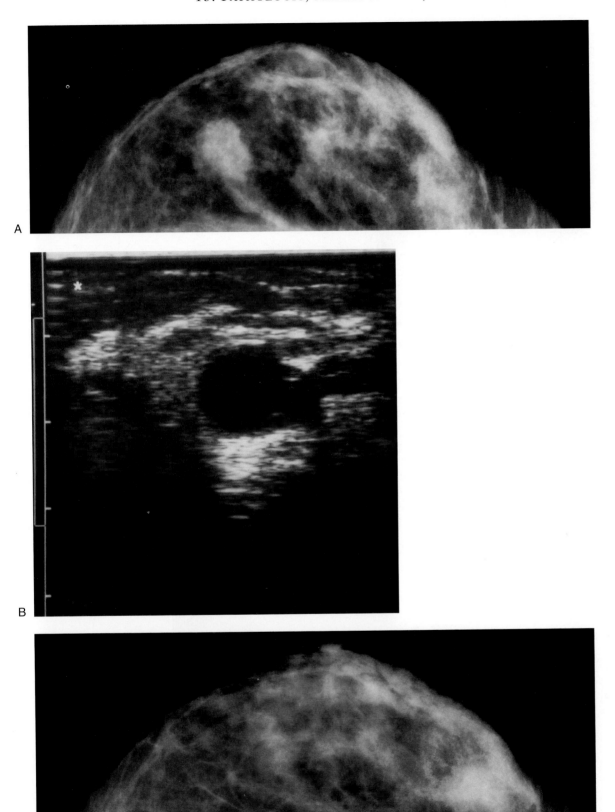

FIG. 19-32. Cysts can be resorbed spontaneously. This mass, seen on craniocaudal projection **(A)** was a cyst by ultrasound **(B)**. It resolved spontaneously over 2 months **(C)**.

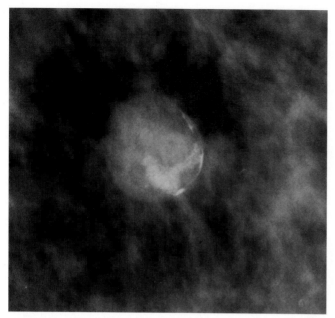

FIG. 19-33. Fine-curve, linear, **"egg-shell"** calcifications are usually in the wall of a **benign cyst.**

calcium aggregates into small balls that literally roll in the dependent portion of a cyst.

Aspiration of cyst fluid is generally therapeutic, particularly if all the fluid is removed, although we have found that approximately 40% of cysts will recur over a 2-year period after aspiration. After aspiration, cysts should no longer be visible on the mammogram. If there is a residual mass, biopsy should be considered to exclude a concomitant malignancy, although this is extremely rare.

Ultrasound Appearance

Ultrasound is the simplest way to diagnose a cyst. To do this accurately, strict criteria must be observed. Cysts should be sharply marginated and contain no internal echoes (Fig. 19-35). This is critical. Solid lesions, including cancer, may have only subtle internal echoes and be otherwise indistinguishable from cysts (Fig. 19-36). Internal echoes cannot be ignored. Cysts may be round, ovoid, flattened, or lobulated. They may occur singly. When multiple, they may overlap on ultrasound, and because their refractive shadowing may be projected onto one another, accurate assessment can be difficult.

Septated Cysts

Truly septated cysts are unusual. A large cyst may appear septated because of the lobulations that may occur with the distention of the acinar structures (Fig. 19-37). Frequently a cyst that appears septated can be completely aspirated with a single puncture because all sections communicate. Septations in cysts that are not due to recent hemorrhage or infection are of no significance.

Cysts should have bright posterior acoustic enhancement, although this relative phenomenon may be diminished by attenuation from tissues anterior or posterior to the cyst. Cysts may be lobulated or septated. Under real-time ultrasound, debris may be seen floating within.

On very rare occasions we have seen cyst fluid begin to move and develop dramatic turbulence under ultrasound observation. We believe that this is due to the generation of heat by the sound beam, causing convection currents in the cyst fluid or perhaps mechanical motion from the sound is induced.

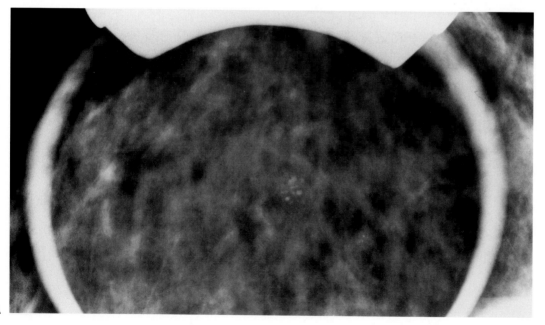

A

FIG. 19-34. Milk of calcium is precipitated calcium forming fine or round particles that can fall to the dependent portion of a cyst and outline its curved inner margin in the lateral projection. These calcifications are amorphous in the craniocaudal projection **(A).** *Continued.*

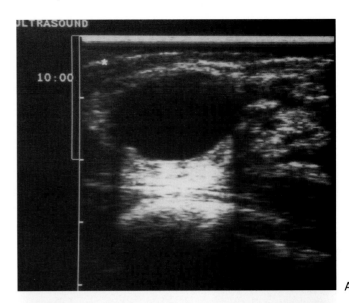

A

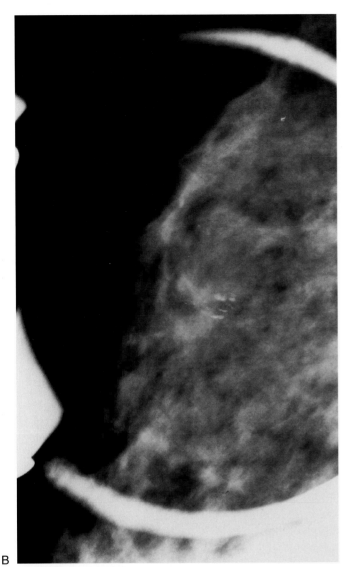

B

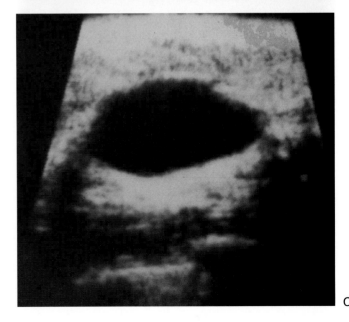

B

FIG. 19-34. *Continued.* The calcifications of milk of calcium are concave up in the lateral magnification mammogram **(B)**. These shapes are due to their location in the dependent portion of benign cysts.

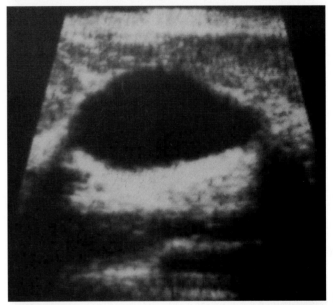

C

FIG. 19-35. To make the confident diagnosis of a cyst by ultrasound, the mass should be round, oval, or smoothly lobulated, with sharply defined margins, no internal echoes, and enhanced through-transmission of sound, as seen in this cyst **(A)**. There may be some reverberation artifact that accounts for echoes in the anterior portion of the cyst.

(B) Ideally, **a cyst,** seen here at proper gain, **should not fill in with echoes** when the gain is increased **(C)**. With modern ultrasound units, however, low-level echoes may be seen in cysts, which may indicate that the fluid is extremely viscid. When there is a question, ultrasound-guided aspiration can resolve the problem.

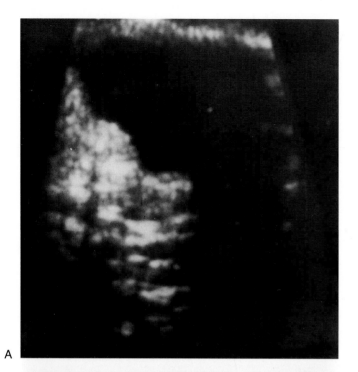

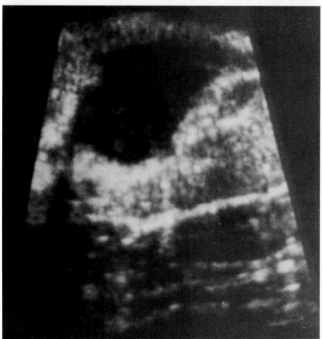

FIG. 19-36. Cancer may have only low-level echoes. The shadowing on the right of this invasive ductal carcinoma **(A)** was due to the nipple. The solid lesion appears cystic by ultrasound with no internal echoes until it is imaged from a better angle with increased gain to show that there are true echoes **(B)**.

Occasionally, a cyst may contain blood. Fresh blood from an acute bleed may resemble cyst fluid on ultrasound. As fibrin begins to organize, internal echoes develop, and what appear to be septations may arise. An older, organized clot can resemble solid tissue (Fig. 19-38A). Although a rare

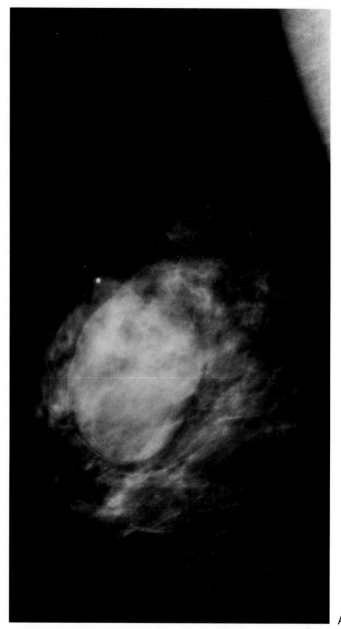

FIG. 19-37. Septations in a cyst are of no major significance unless they are due to previous hemorrhage. **(A)** An ovoid mass was seen on the mediolateral oblique projection. *Continued.*

phenomenon, an older clot may produce irregular low-amplitude echoes around the inside periphery of the cyst (Fig. 19-38B). Any suggestion of a lesion within a cyst should prompt excision, although cancer is very rare and an intracystic lesion is most likely a benign intracystic papilloma (Fig. 19-39). If a lesion is indeterminate by ultrasound, complete aspiration will determine that it is a cyst.

Adenosis

Adenosis, a relatively common benign lesion of the breast, when combined with distortion from sclerosis (sclerosing

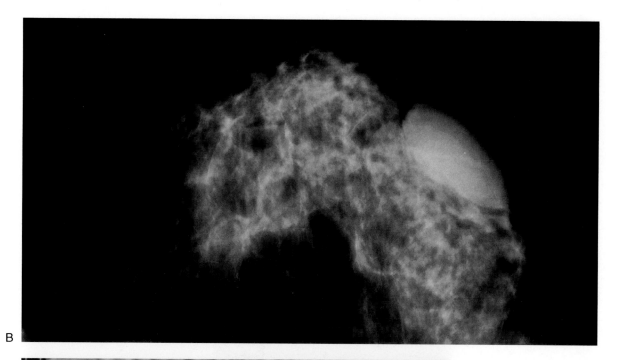

B

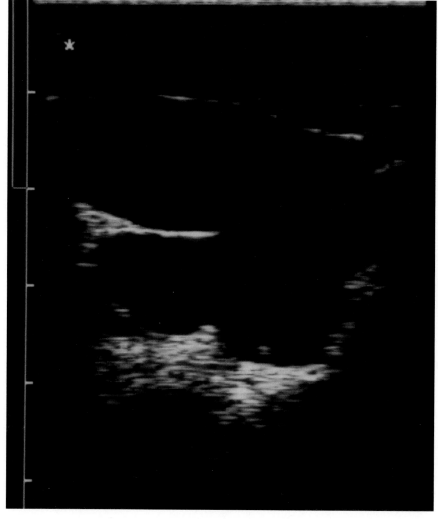

C

FIG. 19-37. *Continued.* The **cyst,** also seen in the craniocaudal projection **(B),** was a benign **cyst with septations** on ultrasound **(C).** If there is no suggestion of an internal mass, no further evaluation is needed.

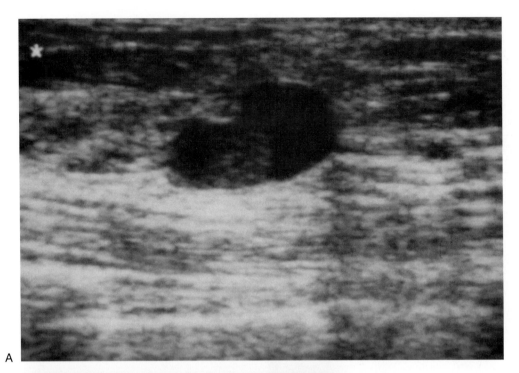

A

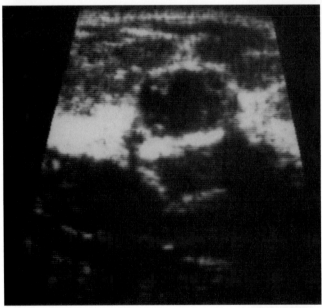

B

FIG. 19-38. A **blood clot** can form in a cyst that has spontaneously bled. The clot forms the area of low-level echoes at one end of this cyst **(A)**. In a second cyst, **echoes** within the periphery **(B)** were **due to a clot.**

adenosis) may pose problems for the pathologist in its similarity to cancer, particularly on frozen-section analysis. A range of lobular lesions constitute adenosis. Jensen et al. (35) categorize sclerosing adenosis along with the other "proliferative breast diseases without atypia." They suggest that a woman who has a biopsy that reveals sclerosing adenosis has a relative risk for the subsequent development of breast cancer that is 1.5 to 2.0 times that of a woman with a nonproliferative lesion at biopsy. They derived this relative risk by following 349 women who had benign breast biopsies between 1950 and 1968. The average period of follow-up was 17 years. They ascertained which women had subsequently developed breast cancer and arrived

at this relative risk figure. Perhaps contributing to this increased risk was the relatively common association of sclerosing adenosis with atypical hyperplasia, a lesion that also carries an increased risk for breast cancer development.

In its simplest form, adenosis merely represents an enlargement of the lobule secondary to a benign proliferation of the blunt-ending intralobular ductules (acini) (Fig. 19-40). This proliferation within the TDLU is primarily an elongation and multiplication of the acini accompanied by an overgrowth of the epithelial, myoepithelial, and connective tissue elements in the lobule. Hypertrophic changes occur in the epithelium as well, and secretory activity may increase. Cys-

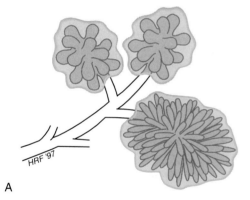

FIG. 19-39. The hypoechoic mass in this cyst proved to be a **benign intracystic papilloma.** This can only be diagnosed by a biopsy.

A

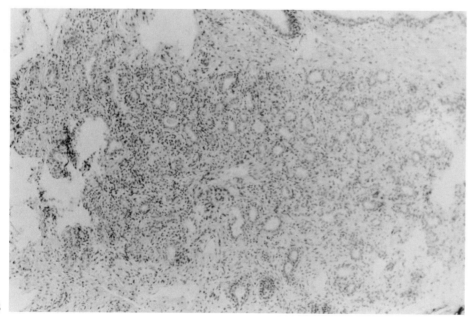

B

FIG. 19-40. This schematic **(A)** depicts **adenosis.** In its simplest form, it represents an idiopathic proliferation of the acini (terminal ductules). On three-dimensional microscopy the lobule has the appearance of a porcupine, whereas on two-dimensional micrographs **(B)** the innumerable acini are seen in cross section, as in this hematoxylin and eosin preparation. If there is excessive fibrosis accompanying the adenosis it is termed *sclerosing adenosis.*

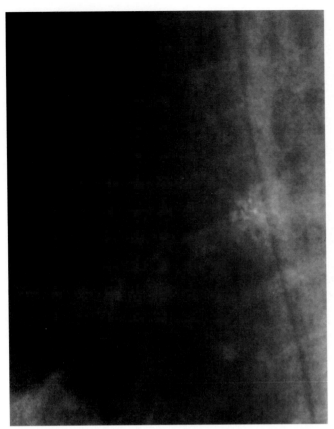

FIG. 19-41. This cluster of **calcifications** was indistinguishable from those produced by cancer, but at biopsy, they proved to be forming in **benign adenosis.**

tic dilatation of the acini is likely the location for calcium precipitation and clustered calcifications that may be found by mammography, although truly microscopic calcifications may be seen in the ductules.

Although benign, with no known predisposition toward malignancy, adenosis can have a locally infiltrative appearance. Proliferation of the epithelium and myoepithelial layer distorts the lobule, and when dense hyalinization (sclerosis) occurs, it leads to compression and distortion of the epithelium and may be mistaken for malignant change. When a large volume is involved, a palpable lump may be detected. Adenosis with or without sclerosis (sclerosing adenosis) has been termed a *weak risk factor*, but there are no data to suggest that the lesion itself carries any major predisposition for future cancer development.

Mammographic Appearance

Mammographically, adenosis rarely forms a visible mass. On occasion it may be the cause of isolated clustered microcalcifications. These are extremely small deposits that can precipitate in the thinned, increased acini of the lobule and their cystically dilated ends. The very small calcifications seen using mammography are often a projected superimposition of the even smaller particles that are beyond the resolution of mammography. Because the deposits are frequently heterogeneous, they are indistinguishable from those associated with breast cancer (Fig. 19-41).

Adenosis is usually indistinguishable from normal nonadipose breast tissue. Diffuse adenosis has been suggested as one of the causes of diffuse calcifications seen using mammography, but it is likely that this is uncommon if it ever occurs. Diffusely scattered calcifications are more likely nonspecific deposits in the lobules or even in the stroma. These latter deposits are characterized by monotonous, relatively round and regular calcifications with indistinct amorphous shapes (Fig. 19-42).

When adenosis produces an isolated cluster of calcifications, the diagnosis can be suggested because the individual particles, seen at the relatively low resolution of mammography, are frequently composed of smaller and smaller particles when viewed with magnification as would be expected from the porcupine-like development of the lobular acini and the calcifications that form within. Although the diagnosis can be suggested, we continue to recommend their biopsy because they cannot be reliably distinguished from

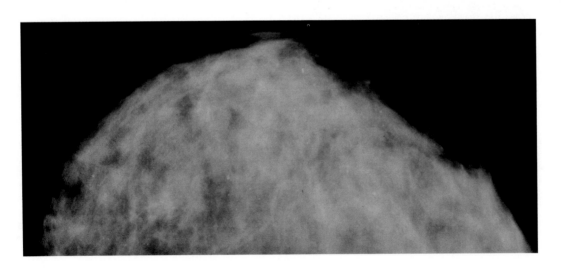

FIG. 19-42. **Diffusely scattered calcifications** may be due to adenosis. These calcifications, scattered throughout the breast, are thought to be due to adenosis, although the data supporting this are inconclusive.

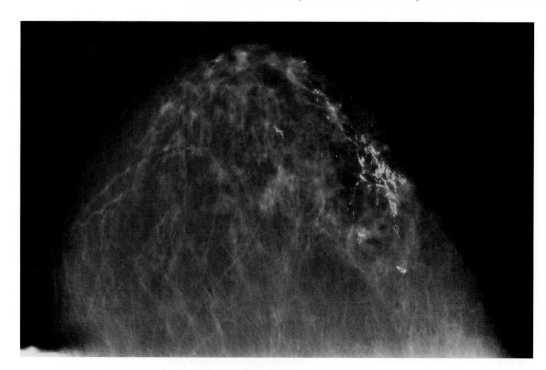

FIG. 19-43. Calcifications produced by high-grade comedocarcinoma are usually obvious in the marked heterogeneity of the size and shape of the particles and their segmental distribution.

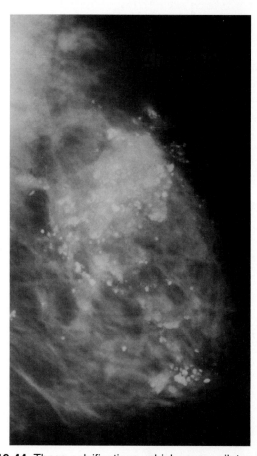

FIG. 19-44. These calcifications, which were unilateral, form a very rare manifestation of **diffuse carcinoma.** Many of the forms suggest a benign process such as milk of calcium, but the overall "wild" appearance and unilaterality should arouse suspicion. This proved to be diffuse intraductal cancer with apocrine features.

deposits due to malignancy. When calcifications are diffusely distributed throughout the breast, however, and especially when bilateral, biopsy can be avoided.

Numerous calcifications may occur with extensive comedocarcinoma, but in contradistinction to the round, intralobular calcifications of adenosis, comedo calcifications are usually irregular in shape and frequently have associated fine linear and branching forms that suggest their ductal distribution (Fig. 19-43). We have described rare cases of diffuse breast cancer that contain many varying and often benign forms of calcifications (36). These are very uncommon and are distinguished by the wild appearance that they produce and the fact that they are extensive and unilateral (Fig. 19-44). We noted that these cancers frequently had malignant cells with apocrine features (not true apocrine cancers—see Apocrine Carcinoma), and we postulated that it might be this feature that accounted for the profusion of calcifications.

Ultrasound Appearance

Adenosis is not visible by ultrasound as a distinct entity, although, as with other processes that elicit a fibrotic response, tissues containing adenosis may be hypoechoic and produce shadowing by attenuation and scattering of the beam.

Other Benign Lesions

Lipomas

Fat is frequently the preponderant tissue in the lobes of the breast, making it difficult to distinguish a true lipoma

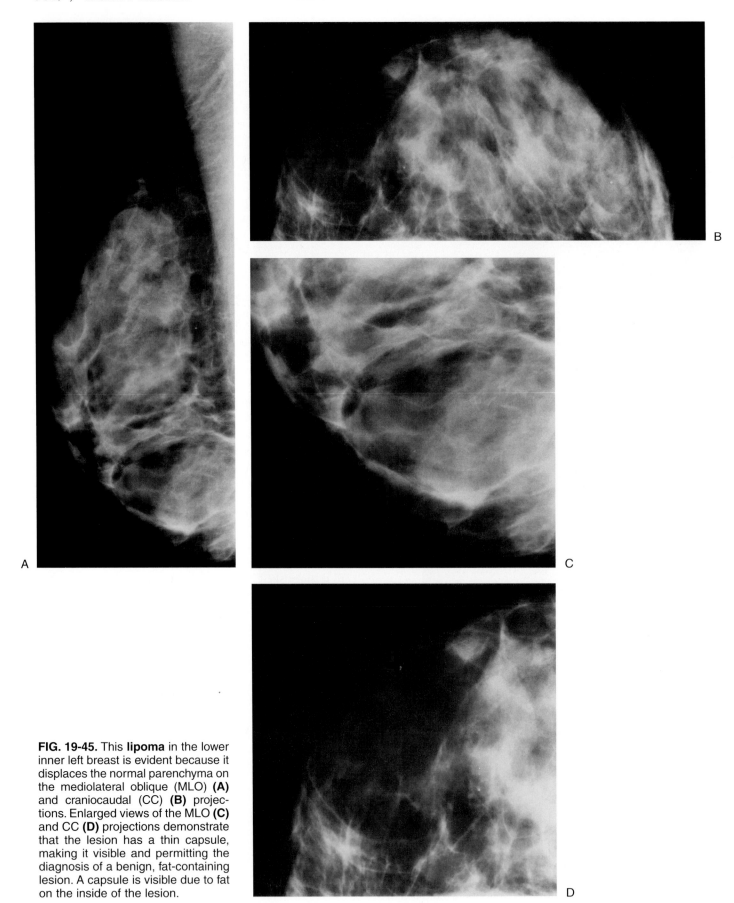

FIG. 19-45. This **lipoma** in the lower inner left breast is evident because it displaces the normal parenchyma on the mediolateral oblique (MLO) **(A)** and craniocaudal (CC) **(B)** projections. Enlarged views of the MLO **(C)** and CC **(D)** projections demonstrate that the lesion has a thin capsule, making it visible and permitting the diagnosis of a benign, fat-containing lesion. A capsule is visible due to fat on the inside of the lesion.

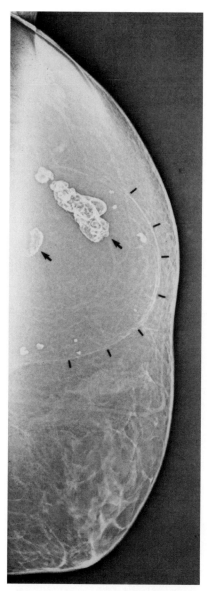

from normal fat surrounded by the fibrous septa of Cooper's ligaments. Lipomas are generally superficial, found around the periphery of the breast parenchyma, and always encapsulated. The presence of this capsule leads to the noninvasive diagnosis of this benign lesion. As elsewhere in the body, lipomas are freely movable and generally soft. They may distort the breast architecture by displacing normal structures but do not infiltrate and have not been shown to undergo malignant degeneration. Liposarcoma is much rarer than the lipoma. Clinically, it usually is firm to hard and (unless very well differentiated) radiographically dense so that there is usually no difficulty distinguishing a benign lipoma from a liposarcoma. As with any collection of fat, necrosis can occur and calcifications may result (see Scarring and Fat Necrosis).

Mammographic Appearance

Lipomas have a typical radiolucent mammographic appearance that permits the diagnosis of a benign lesion. Although they cannot always be distinguished from other fat-containing lesions, this is of no consequence because encapsulated, fat-containing lesions are all benign. The lipoma has a thin capsule (Fig. 19-45) that is visible because of fat on the inside as well as on the outside. Lipomas may cause distortion of the surrounding architecture by displacement, or they may themselves be molded by the surrounding breast. Harder, round, lucent lesions are generally either post-traumatic oil cysts secondary to fat necrosis or galactoceles. Lipomas, as with all fat, are subject to possible necrosis, and occasionally they may contain the typical spherical calcifications of fat necrosis (Fig. 19-46).

Ultrasound Appearance

Ultrasound is usually not indicated when a lipoma is suspected because the diagnosis is usually apparent and the lesion is clearly benign by mammography. Lipomas are

FIG. 19-46. Fat necrosis in this lipoma (*short lines*), seen on this negative-mode xerogram, produced typical-appearing, lucent-centered calcifications (*large arrows*).

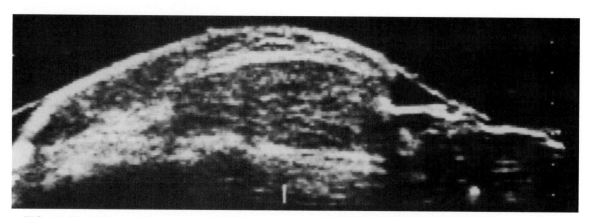

FIG. 19-47. Ultrasound is rarely needed to evaluate a lipoma. The capsule of this **lipoma** is evident on ultrasound and distinguishes the mass from the similar echotexture of the subcutaneous fat.

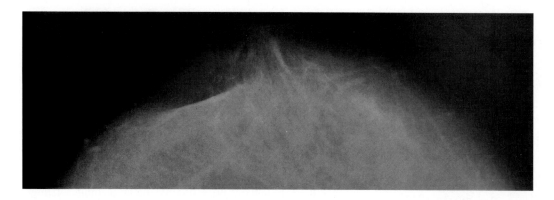

FIG. 19-48. Postsurgical fat necrosis can cause **scarring and skin retraction,** as seen medial to the nipple on this craniocaudal projection.

hypoechoic and similar in echotexture to subcutaneous fat. They may be distinguished from the subcutaneous fat by the demonstration of the specular reflection from the capsule (Fig. 19-47). If present, the calcifications in necrotic areas may cause shadowing.

Scarring and Fat Necrosis

Focal fat necrosis is quite common in the breast, probably owing in part to the large quantities of unprotected adipose tissue that constitute much of the gland. Fat necrosis may produce several differing results. Basically a nonsuppurative inflammatory response to fat cell damage, the process may produce a palpable, sometimes painful mass with skin thickening or retraction. Most commonly it develops unnoticed by the patient, revealed only by mammography as a new density, architectural distortion, calcium deposition, or oil cyst.

As in other parts of the body, fat necrosis is seen histologically as damaged fat cells that have lost their nuclei and are interspersed with histiocytes containing phagocytized fat in their cytoplasm. This inflammation may elicit a fibrotic response and occasionally, as with a scar, can produce a gross appearance that is similar to the desmoplasia of cancer as well as calcium deposition that can also mimic cancer.

Occasionally, necrosed fat may form a gelatinous mass that becomes encapsulated by a thin, smooth, fibrous wall. Because of the frequent history of antecedent trauma, particularly after surgery, this form of fat necrosis has become known as the *post-traumatic oil cyst.* Oil cysts may feel extremely hard on CBE and thus cause concern, but their appearance is pathognomonic on mammography and they are always benign.

Mammographic Spectrum

Fat necrosis can produce changes that are radiographically similar to those of cancer (37). Cicatrization and spiculation may result from the fibrotic reaction that may accompany the process. They can occur especially in a scar formed after surgery, and even skin retraction may result (Fig. 19-48).

Despite a history of trauma or even surgery, radiographically visible scar formation is relatively rare in the absence

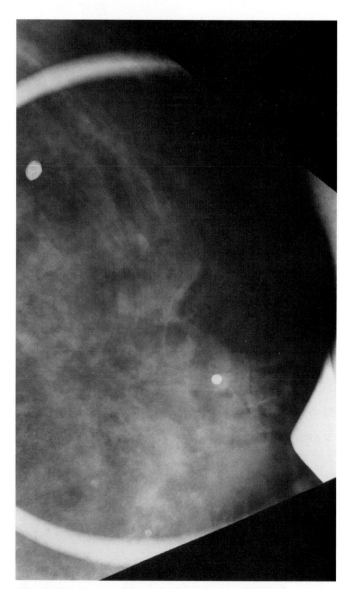

FIG. 19-49. Postsurgical change rarely has a central mass. The subtle architectural distortion in an area of previous surgery for a benign lesion converges on a lucent zone. This is consistent with **postoperative change.**

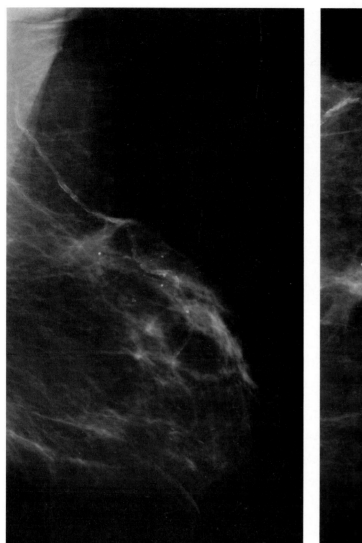
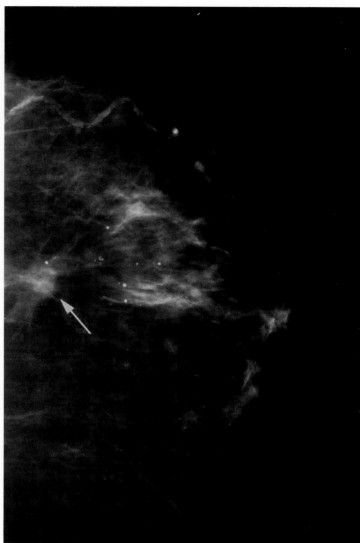

A

B

FIG. 19-50. Architectural distortion that is dramatic on one view but not on the other is **usually due to postsurgical change.** In this case, the patient was treated for breast cancer 3 years earlier with excision and irradiation. The postsurgical change is not very striking on the mediolateral oblique projection **(A)**, but it is quite obvious on the craniocaudal projection **(B)**.

of treatment for breast cancer. In the immediate postoperative period, however, architectural distortion is common, and in some instances this may persist for up to 6 to 12 months (38), but long-term fixed changes are the exception.

Differentiating Postbiopsy Change from Cancer. When scarring does occur after surgery, it may rarely produce architectural changes that are indistinguishable from those of cancer. Several clues may help avoid biopsy. If a lesion has been excised and shown to be completely benign, it is extremely unlikely that an occult cancer will coincidentally develop in the same area at a later date, particularly within 1 to 2 years of the biopsy. Thus architectural distortion in an area of previous surgery need not elicit concern unless the previous biopsy revealed a borderline lesion, such as atypical hyperplasia, papillomatosis, or carcinoma in situ. Furthermore, architectural distortion associated with scarring

can be suggested when the center of the process is lucent fat (Fig. 19-49) and not a nidus of dense tissue, as is the case with most cancers. Usually, a spiculated mass due to postsurgical change appears striking in one projection, but is almost imperceptible in the other (Fig. 19-50).

Post-Traumatic Oil Cysts. The most readily diagnosable form of fat necrosis is the traumatic oil cyst. This usually appears on the mammogram as a round, radiographically lucent lesion that is defined only by its capsule (Fig. 19-51). Containing gelatinized fat and usually surrounded by fat, the capsule is visible as a thin circle with a diagnostic appearance.

Calcium deposition occurs frequently with fat necrosis and may produce several patterns. At times a shell forms around the necrotic tissue, producing a spherical appearance that is characteristically benign. These may be only several millime-

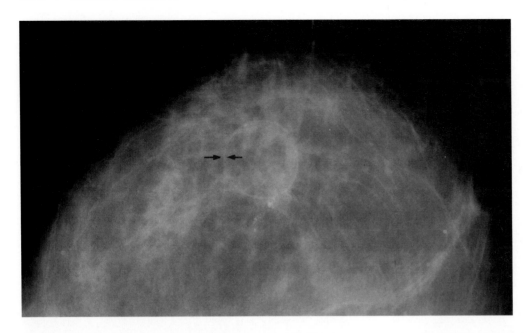

FIG. 19-51. The appearance of a **post-traumatic oil cyst** is usually pathognomonic. This patient had undergone a biopsy for what proved to be a benign lesion. The surgery resulted in fat necrosis, which formed a gelatinized mass whose margins are demarcated by its encapsulation (*arrows*). Radiolucent, encapsulated masses are always benign.

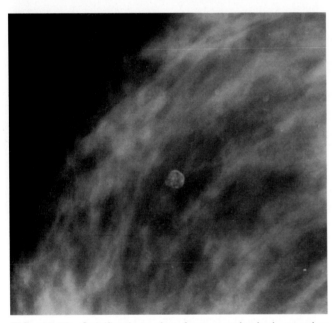

FIG. 19-52. Calcifications that form a spherical grouping around a lucent center, as in this enlarged view, are probably the result of fat necrosis. This type of calcium distribution is an indication of a benign process.

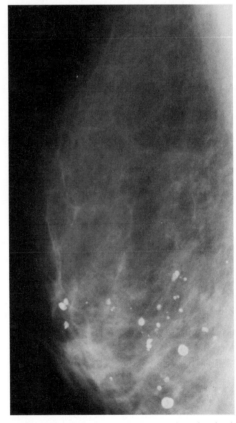

FIG. 19-53. These large, lucent-centered, spherical calcifications are almost certainly due to fat necrosis.

ters in diameter (Fig. 19-52) or calcified spheres ≥1 cm in size (Fig. 19-53). The latter can usually be distinguished from the calcified wall of a cyst because the rim calcifications of fat necrosis surround a lucent tissue volume, whereas cysts are water density. Cyst wall calcifications are generally more delicate in appearance than those of fat necrosis.

Numerous, irregular, clustered deposits have been described as forming in fat necrosis that are indistinguishable from those associated with cancer (39). This is extremely uncommon in our experience.

Ultrasound Appearance

Little has been written concerning the sonographic appearance of fat necrosis with the exception of the post-traumatic oil cyst (40). When oil cysts are formed, they are invariably well-

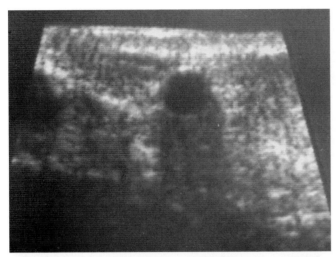

FIG. 19-54. This **post-traumatic oil cyst** on ultrasound produced posterior shadowing despite its sonolucent appearance.

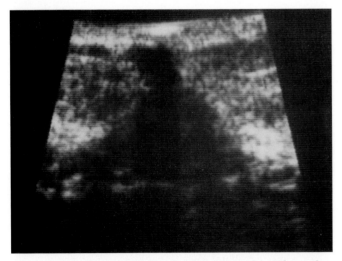

FIG. 19-55. Postsurgical scarring may be triangular, hypoechoic, and produce posterior shadowing, as seen on this ultrasound. The fact that the shadowing extends from the skin supports the benign nature of the finding, but if there is a significant question, only a biopsy can provide certainty.

circumscribed lesions. They may have the sonolucent appearance of cysts with good through-transmission of sound, or they may contain low-amplitude internal echoes and produce posterior acoustic shadowing (Fig. 19-54). When a true scar is formed, it scatters and attenuates sound and is indistinguishable from cancer (Fig. 19-55). Ultrasound is usually not indicated, because the mammographic appearance of most forms of fat necrosis is so characteristic.

Galactocele

Occasionally a milk-containing cystic structure develops during lactation or in the months after the cessation of nursing. This usually occurs in women in their late 20s or early 30s, probably as a result of an obstructed duct. The proximal (lobular) segment becomes distended with inspissated milk, the composition of which varies with differing proportions of protein and fat. Clinically, a galactocele is indistinguishable from other pathologic processes that form palpable round masses. If the milk-filled cystic mass has sufficient fat content, it may be visible by mammography as a well-circumscribed radiolucent mass against the water density of the lactating breast. As with other lucent lesions, these are always benign. They are usually resolved by aspiration.

Mammographic Appearance

The galactocele may be indistinguishable from other fat-containing lesions of the breast when it contains sufficient fat to be relatively radiolucent. All fat-containing breast masses are benign, and a precise diagnosis is not necessary. Usually surrounded by the dense tissue of the lactating breast, such a lesion will appear as a round, radiolucent zone (Fig. 19-56). Galactoceles are well circumscribed and only distort the surrounding tissues by occupying space. Fat fluid levels have been described in upright lateral mammograms. A mottled appearance similar to that of a hamartoma has been described with some galactoceles and likened to curdled milk (41). Some galactoceles are not radiolucent but are low in x-ray attenuation and indistinguishable from cysts.

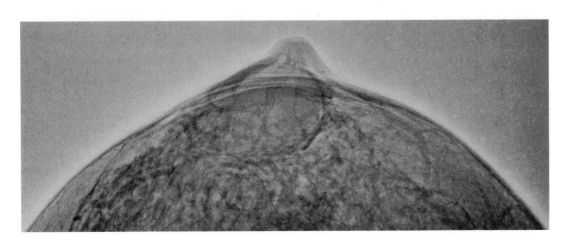

FIG. 19-56. Galactoceles may have varying density and are rare. This is the only one that we have seen, imaged here with positive-mode xeroradiography. It is evident as a radiolucent mass in the subareolar portion of the breast.

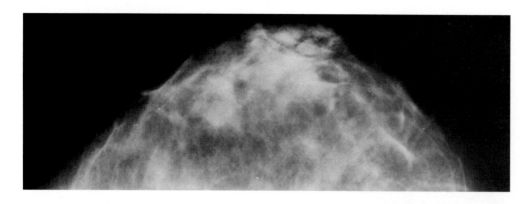

FIG. 19-57. The mass in the subareolar region of the right breast, seen on craniocaudal projection, has the typical appearance of a **mammary hamartoma.**

Ultrasound Appearance

Galactoceles appear as well-circumscribed masses. They contain low-level internal echoes, may produce refractive lateral wall shadowing, and may demonstrate posterior acoustic enhancement. This appearance makes it impossible to differentiate them from a well-circumscribed, solid breast tumor. If characteristic mammographic findings are not present to make the diagnosis, aspiration is indicated.

Unusual Benign Lesions

Numerous unusual lesions occur in the breast. The following are a sampling that may occasionally be mistaken for cancer by imaging modalities or, as in the case of the hamartoma, can be diagnosed with certainty by mammography as a benign lesion.

Mammary Hamartoma (Fibroadenolipoma)

The hamartoma is a proliferation of fibrous and adenomatous nodular elements in fat surrounded by a capsule of connective tissue. This lesion has been described under various names that are permutations of its component parts (e.g., *fibroadenolipoma, lipofibroadenoma, adenolipofibroma*). It is a relatively uncommon benign lesion. In one series (42), 16 cases were diagnosed in 10,000 mammographic studies. Because the fibroadenolipoma contains the major constituents of the breast in an encapsulated lesion, it is believed to represent a mammary hamartoma, although some believe it merely represents a lipoma with trapped breast elements. Containing ducts, lobules, and fibrous and adipose tissue, it may present as a palpable mass or as an incidental finding on mammography. Unless the capsule is appreciated, the lesion may go undiagnosed or be misdiagnosed as a fibroadenoma. The importance of this benign lesion lies in its typical diagnostic appearance by mammography, obviating the need for surgery.

Mammographic Appearance

On mammography, hamartomas are usually characteristic in appearance, and the diagnosis can be made with certainty

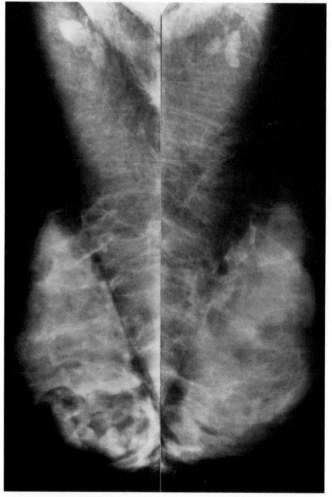

FIG. 19-58. A **hamartoma** in the lower inner left breast is seen in the mediolateral oblique (MLO) **(A)** projection. *Continued.*

by mammography. Composed of fat, these lucent lesions contain varying water density structures of fibrous and adenomatous elements (Figs. 19-57 and 19-58). With the exception of a single case report of a sarcoma with a similar appearance (43), this lesion is always benign. They are sharply marginated and surrounded by a thin capsule, which will be evident if there is fat outside the lesion. Lobulated

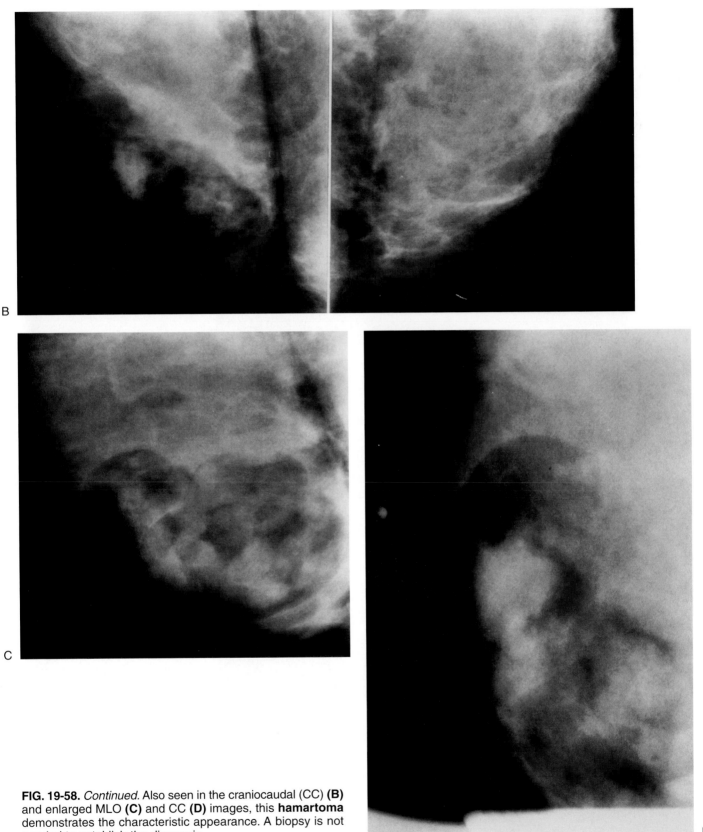

FIG. 19-58. *Continued.* Also seen in the craniocaudal (CC) **(B)** and enlarged MLO **(C)** and CC **(D)** images, this **hamartoma** demonstrates the characteristic appearance. A biopsy is not needed to establish the diagnosis.

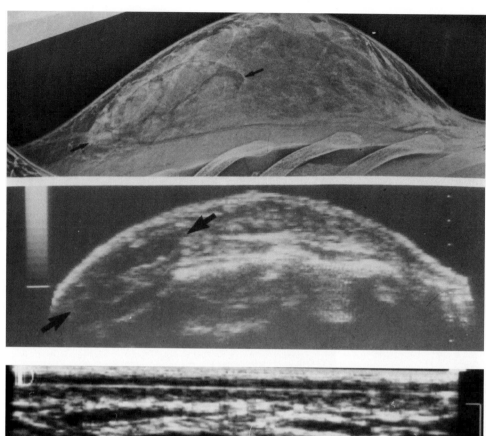

A

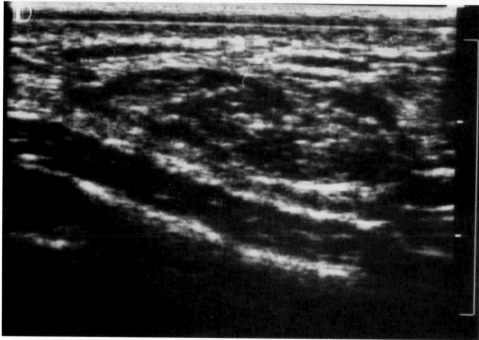

B

FIG. 19-59. (A) This hamartoma (*arrows*) is well demarcated by the capsule surrounding it as seen (top) in this lateral, negative-mode xerogram (dark represents fat). On whole-breast ultrasound (bottom), the tissues of the hamartoma are relatively sonolucent with respect to the interspersed, echogenic, fibrous, and glandular tissue. This ultrasound **(B)** is from the evaluation of the lesion in Fig. 19-58. The ultrasound appearance of a hamartoma is not diagnostic, whereas the mammogram usually is.

densities dispersed within the encapsulated fat give the hamartoma its characteristic appearance that some have likened to a slice of salami.

Ultrasound Appearance

As with a lipoma or oil cyst, the mammographic appearance of the hamartoma is so characteristic that there is usually no indication for the use of ultrasound in the analysis of this lesion. If obtained, the ultrasound appearance parallels the radiographic morphology of the lesion (Fig. 19-59). The mass is sharply defined and displaces surrounding structures. It contains sonolucent zones as well as echo-producing fibrous structures with a heterogeneous internal echo pattern.

Granular Cell Tumors

Formally called *granular cell myoblastomas* because they were thought to originate from muscle, these benign lesions are now called *granular cell tumors*. Usually occurring in

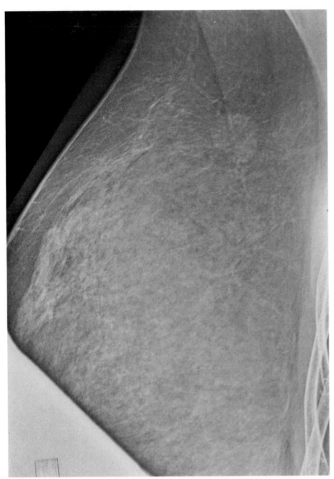

FIG. 19-60. The round density with ill-defined margins seen in the upper breast on this negative-mode xerogram is a rare, benign, **granular cell tumor.**

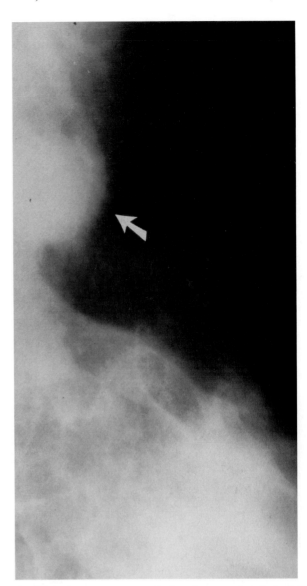

FIG. 19-61. This irregular, spiculated mass that is indistinguishable from breast cancer proved to be a **benign granular cell tumor.**

the tongue, only 5% to 6% of these extremely rare lesions are found in the breast (44). Its progenitor is unclear, although most now believe in a neurogenic origin from the Schwann cells of peripheral nerves. These tumors are benign but may be locally infiltrative and are indistinguishable from cancer clinically and using imaging. They are very fibrous, firm or hard to palpation, and fixed to the surrounding tissue. On occasion they even produce skin retraction. They rarely occur in the lower breast, but are generally found in the upper half. Histologically, they contain spindle cells and are distinguished by a characteristic granularity to the cell cytoplasm from which they derive their name. The granules are periodic acid–Schiff positive. Wide excision is usually sufficient therapy.

Mammographically and on gross inspection, this lesion may mimic cancer. It forms a mass with an irregular shape, and its margins appear infiltrative. We have seen a lesion that had very fine, short, brush border–type spiculations (Fig. 19-60), as well as a granular cell tumor with long spiculations that were indistinguishable from those usually associated with malignancy (Fig. 19-61).

Focal Fibrosis

Fibrosis is a common component of many breast lesions (Fig. 19-62A). When it occurs in isolation, it is usually unclear whether an isolated palpable or mammographically detected island of fibrous tissue represents a new proliferation or merely an involution of the normal lobules with persisting residual intralobular fibrous stroma. This entity is uncommon and benign. It is significant from an imaging perspective because it may present as a nonpalpable, irregular mass with ill-defined margins that cannot be distinguished from cancer (45). Usually palpable, these lesions are rubbery and freely movable. They do not have a capsule and are visible mammographically when in contrast with surrounding fat. Histologically, they are merely isolated areas of abundant fibrous stroma and have no association with cancer.

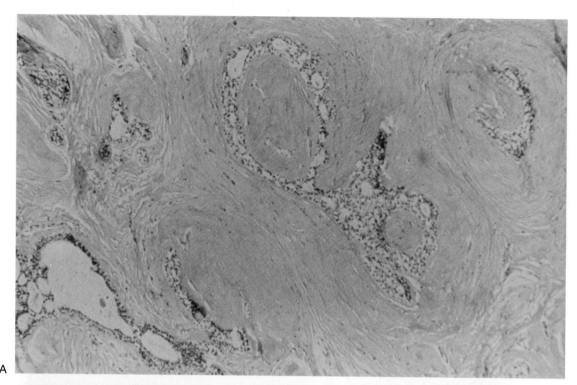

A

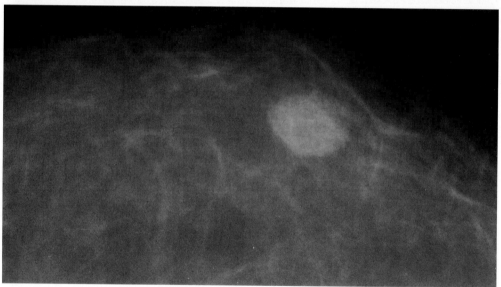

B

FIG. 19-62. (A) Photomicrograph (hematoxylin and eosin) of a **benign fibrous lesion** that is composed primarily of connective tissue. **(B)** An ovoid, fairly well-defined, focal mass on mammography that proved to be **benign focal fibrosis.**

Mammographic Appearance

This uncommon lesion may present as a well-circumscribed mass (Fig. 19-62B) or as an ill-defined lesion that is indistinguishable from breast cancer.

Ultrasound Appearance

There is little information on the ultrasound findings in these lesions, but in our experience, they parallel the shape of the lesion seen by mammography. A well-circumscribed focus will be the same on ultrasound and exhibit the internal echoes of a solid lesion (Fig. 19-63). When irregular and ill defined by mammography, shadowing is probably due to attenuation and scattering of the sound.

Diabetic Mastopathy

Diabetic mastopathy is a fibrous "tumor" that has been reported with increased frequency after first being described in 1984 (46). Originally described in association with type I insulin-dependent diabetes, it has also been diagnosed in

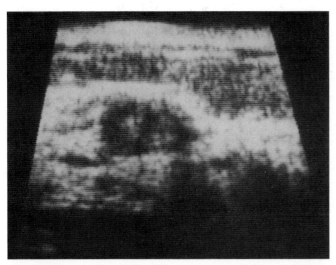

FIG. 19-63. On ultrasound, this ovoid area of **focal fibrosis** was indistinguishable from a fibroadenoma or carcinoma.

women with type II diabetes. It is a lesion that usually occurs in adolescents and young women but has been found in women as old as their early 50s. The lesion presents as a firm, nontender mass that can range from millimeters to many centimeters in diameter. Histologically, there is an increased density of fibroblasts in the stroma. Lymphocytes are characteristically found collected around and in the walls of small blood vessels. These lymphocytes are apparently predominantly B cells. These lesions may be multiple.

Mammographic Appearance

In 1989 Logan and Hoffman (47) reported on 36 women who were diagnosed with what the authors called *diabetic fibrous breast disease.* Among the patients, all had dense breast tissue patterns. The lesions were not visible on mammography but were palpable. The tissue was extremely firm making fine-needle aspiration difficult.

Ultrasound Appearance

The appearance of diabetic mastopathy is characteristic but nonspecific. It is a hypoechoic, irregular lesion with extremely dense posterior acoustic shadowing. The visible anterior margin may have a flame shape with multiple irregular peaks. Unfortunately, although the diagnosis can be suggested, histologic confirmation is needed.

Pseudoangiomatous Stromal Hyperplasia

Vuitch et al. (48) first described pseudoangiomatous stromal hyperplasia (PASH) in 1986. It is a benign lesion (49) that is probably more common but is only found when it forms a mass that it is described as a distinct entity. Because

it appears to occur only in premenopausal women, it is likely hormone related.

The lesion is usually well defined with a smooth border and can be as large as 10 cm. It appears to be a benign overgrowth of the fibrous, connective tissue stroma of the breast that separates the lobules and ducts. The proliferation of the stroma produces numerous anastomosing spaces that resemble vascular structures but do not actually represent blood vessels. Care must be taken to differentiate the lesion from a low-grade angiosarcoma. As with angiosarcoma, most women with PASH are premenopausal, further complicating differentiation. Unlike angiosarcomas, however, the spaces in PASH have myofibroblasts along one side. The PASH spaces contain a mucopolysaccharide material, whereas angiosarcomas contain red blood cells. It has been postulated that these benign tumors are tissues that are hyperresponsive to progesterone in the normal menstrual cycle, although a few of these lesions have been reported in postmenopausal women who were not using HRT. PASH is apparently more commonly seen on microscopic analysis than by mammography or CBE (49). Among the cases reported, a number have been shown to enlarge over time. If not completely excised, PASH can recur.

Mammographic Appearance

Although PASH has been reported with increased frequency since it was first described, it remains uncommon. Polger et al. (50) reported seven cases out of 1,661 breast biopsies. The patients ranged in age from 36 to 61 years. Of the seven women diagnosed with PASH, 43% of the masses were palpable while the others were detected by mammography. The masses ranged from 1.1 cm to as large as 11 cm. They tend to be round or oval with margins that range from well defined to indistinct (or obscured).

Ultrasound Appearance

PASH has been described as being round or oval and hypoechoic. As with most round or oval solid masses, posterior echoes may be attenuated (shadowing), isoechoic, or enhanced.

In one case of PASH, the patient presented with a palpable mass. It was ovoid and well defined on ultrasound with a uniform internal echotexture (Fig. 19-64). The diagnosis was made using ultrasound-guided core needle biopsy.

Extra-Abdominal Desmoid Tumor

The extra-abdominal desmoid tumor is extremely rare in the breast. It usually arises in the muscle and fascia of the abdominal wall. In the abdomen, they are locally invasive and may be difficult to distinguish from fibrosarcomas. Trauma is frequently a preceding event. There is little experience with these lesions in the breast (51). Their major significance is

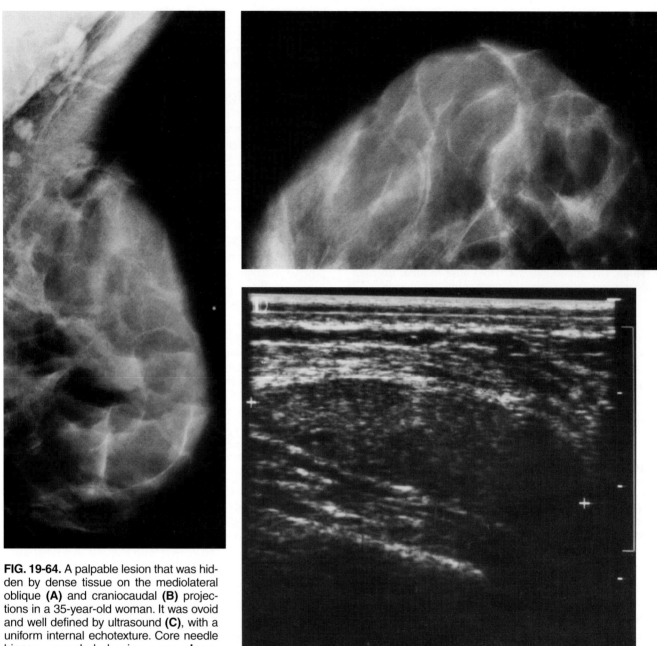

FIG. 19-64. A palpable lesion that was hidden by dense tissue on the mediolateral oblique **(A)** and craniocaudal **(B)** projections in a 35-year-old woman. It was ovoid and well defined by ultrasound **(C)**, with a uniform internal echotexture. Core needle biopsy revealed benign, **pseudoangiomatous stromal hyperplasia.**

that they are among the rare benign processes that can have spiculated margins on mammography and can be indistinguishable from breast cancer. Histologically, the lesion consists of hypocellular dense fibrous tissue that locally invades adjacent muscle. In the breast, the reported cases are all in proximity to the pectoralis muscles. Wide excision is reported to be sufficient, with no documented metastatic potential.

Mammographic Appearance

This very rare benign lesion forms a mass that can be spiculated and ill defined on mammography (Fig. 19-65A).

None has been reported to demonstrate microcalcifications. In our limited experience, the diagnosis can be suggested by the proximity of the lesion to the chest wall and by the relatively long projections radiating from it that are thicker than the spicules often associated with cancer. These are clearly visible in Fig. 19-65B, which may be the only reported case of an extra-abdominal desmoid tumor that was found by screening mammography. Although the diagnosis can be suggested, because cancer is much more common, and the morphologies overlap, biopsy of any spiculated lesion is required to make the diagnosis.

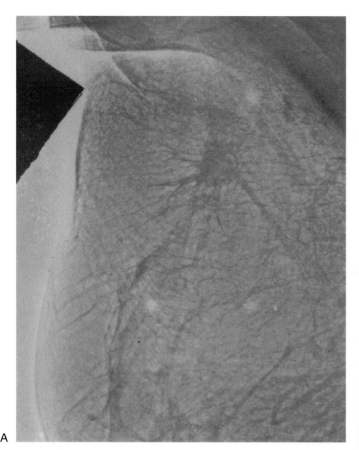

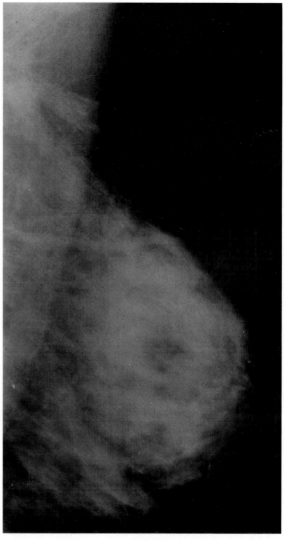

FIG. 19-65. The spiculated mass near the pectoralis major muscle seen on this lateral xeromammogram **(A)** proved to be an **extra-abdominal desmoid tumor.** Another irregular mass **(B)** with long spicules was detected by mammography and was not palpable. It proved to be an **extra-abdominal desmoid tumor.**

Ultrasound Appearance

There are no descriptions of this lesion in the literature, but it is likely to be hypoechoic, with scattering and attenuation producing posterior acoustic shadowing and an appearance that is indistinguishable from breast cancer.

Radial Scar (Elastosis, Indurative Mastopathy, Radial Sclerosing Lesion, Sclerosing Duct Hyperplasia)

The radial scar is one of the few benign lesions that can form spiculations similar to those formed by some cancers. It gained significance in the literature (52) when it was suggested that the radial scar was a post-traumatic precursor of breast cancer, but this seems to have been refuted. Its major significance lies in the difficulty of distinguishing it from cancer by mammography, CBE, and, indeed, by gross histology.

When palpable, these lesions are firm but movable. Reports of the prevalence of this entity vary. It is often coin-

cidentally found when biopsy material is evaluated histologically, and the more carefully breast tissue is evaluated the more commonly the lesion is found (13). Rosen and Oberman (13) reported that Wellings and Alpers (53) found radial scars in 14% of breasts, while Nielson et al. (54) found these lesions in 28% of women at autopsy. As mammographic studies increase, there have been more reports of radiographically detected lesions, although many more are found, coincidentally, by the pathologist.

This benign lesion is spiculated in gross as well as mammographic studies, with a chalky appearance that is similar to cancer, and connective tissue spicules radiating from a central nidus. The nidus is distinguished histologically by a predominant elastic tissue component mixed with fibrosis. The surrounding ducts are distorted, and there is frequently adenosis and epithelial proliferation that often has a papillary pattern. The radial scar results in a distortion of the surrounding tissue, mimicking cancer (55). These lesions even occasionally contain microcalcifications that likely arise in the associated adenosis.

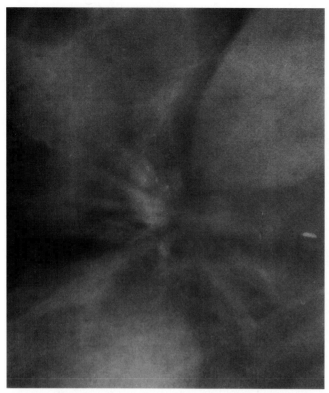

FIG. 19-66. This is an enlargement of **a radial scar** in the left breast. It has an ill-defined center with long associated spicules and some calcifications. An excisional biopsy is needed to establish the diagnosis.

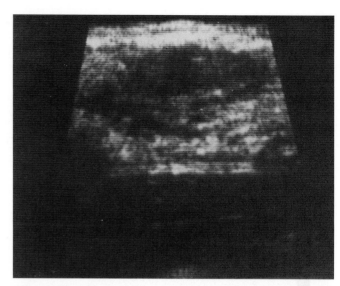

FIG. 19-67. Ultrasound is generally not indicated in the evaluation of a spiculated mass such as this **radial scar** because biopsy is needed. In this case, however, the area appeared as a hypoechoic mass with irregular margins and good sound transmission.

Mammographic Appearance

The radial scar has a worrisome appearance mammographically, as an area of architectural distortion with spiculations radiating from a central point. There may be accompanying microcalcifications (Fig. 19-66) (56). Cancer generally has a central core that has grown irregularly in all directions such that if a mass is present, it has a similar appearance in differing projections. The radial scar does not generally have a central mass, but is usually just an area of architectural distortion with elastic tissue at its center (57). It frequently looks different, depending on the projection. The center of the lesion frequently contains lucent zones of fat that may have been trapped by the cicatrizing process. Although the diagnosis may be suggested by this entrapment of fat and the long spicules with little if any central density, the radial scar cannot be distinguished from some cancers and this lesion still requires excision for confirmation. Radial scars cannot be accurately diagnosed by core needle biopsy, and stability over as many as 5 years is not reassuring. The differentiation of this lesion from cancer can only be made by excisional biopsy.

Ultrasound Appearance

The one radial scar that we have scanned presented as hypoechoic, poorly defined tissue (Fig. 19-67). Because the lesion is suspicious by mammography, has no sizable mass, and has no similarity to a cyst, ultrasound has no useful role in the evaluation of this lesion.

Superficial Thrombophlebitis (Mondor's Disease)

Thrombophlebitis of a superficial vein of the breast, first described by Henri Mondor in 1939 (58), is an uncommon phenomenon. Some cases have been associated with trauma (including surgery). Because it has been reported in association with breast cancer, the presence of thrombophlebitis should provoke a careful search for an associated malignancy, but it is usually an idiopathic event. The process may not be evident by mammography, and the diagnosis is usually made clinically by a thickened linear ridge that is associated, at times, with a linear dimpling, both of which resolve with time. Skin retraction can raise concerns of possible malignancy. The process is self-limited.

Mammographic Appearance

Occasionally the mammogram may be characteristic. The thrombosed vein can have a rope-like, or even more diagnostic, beaded appearance similar to a string of sausages (Fig. 19-68). The process may be asymptomatic or may cause pain.

Ultrasound Appearance

Conant et al. (59) have described the sonographic appearance of superficial thrombophlebitis as reflecting the mammographic findings. The vein may be seen as a hypoechoic tubular structure that has alternating constricted and dilated segments.

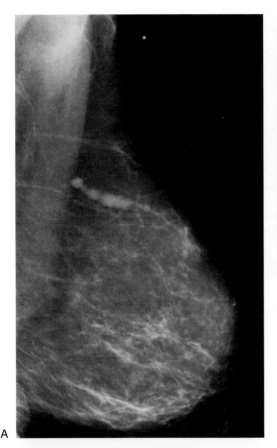

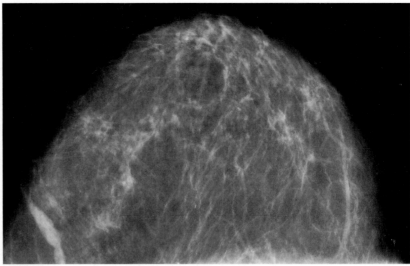

B

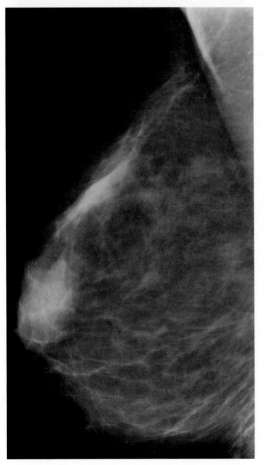

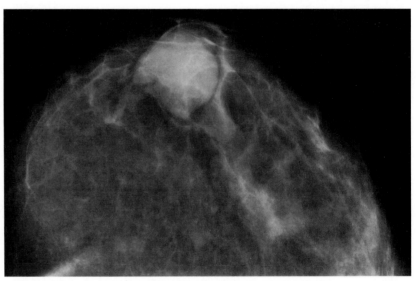

D

FIG. 19-68. Mondor's disease—thrombophlebitis of a superficial vein of the breast—may have a typical string-of-beads appearance on mammography, as seen on these mediolateral oblique **(A)** and craniocaudal (CC) **(B)** projections.

This **myoid hamartoma** is indistinguishable from any other round mass on these lateral **(C)** and CC **(D)** projections.

C

Myoid Hamartoma

The myoid hamartoma is an extremely unusual breast tumor. Rosen and Oberman group it with the general category of myoepitheliomas (13). These are benign lesions that contain smooth muscle that presumably arise from the myoepithelium of the duct (60). They are a combination of adipose tissue, fibrous tissue, and smooth muscle. Erlandson and Rosen (61) described their ultrastructure as containing (1) round or spindle-shaped cells (2) that are partially invested by basal lamina, (3) with pinocytotic vesicles along cell membranes, (4) arrays of microfilaments in the cytoplasm, (5) fusiform densities along arrays of microfilaments, and (6) cells joined by mature desmosomes.

Mammographic Appearance

We have seen only one myoid hamartoma (Fig. 19-68C). As a lobulated, fairly well-circumscribed mass, it was indistinguishable from other solid breast masses.

Ultrasound Appearance

We are unaware of any descriptions of myoid hamartomas by ultrasound.

Bacterial Infections

Breast infections are fairly common during the childbearing years and are usually associated with breast-feeding. In our experience, they are usually treated clinically and do not benefit from imaging. The usual organism is *Staphylococcus,* introduced through a crack in the skin around the nipple areolar complex. Ultrasound may be useful if an abscess is suspected. Ultrasound-guided aspiration can be accomplished to obtain material for culture. Drainage of an abscess is often therapeutic. Surgery runs the risk of transecting ducts and causing secondary abscesses in the branches of the duct system.

Tuberculosis has been reported in the breast (62). Given the increasing number of tuberculosis cases in the general population, tuberculous breast infections may become more common.

Mammographic Appearance

The mammographic appearance of a breast infection is nonspecific. There may be trabecular thickening, and skin thickening is commonly seen, but none of these is diagnostic. We have seen an ill-defined mass that proved to be an abscess, although abscesses are generally hidden in the dense breast tissue.

Ultrasound Appearance

Ultrasound is useful for delineating an abscess so that purulent material can be obtained for analysis and culture and a drain inserted to speed treatment. Infected breast tissue

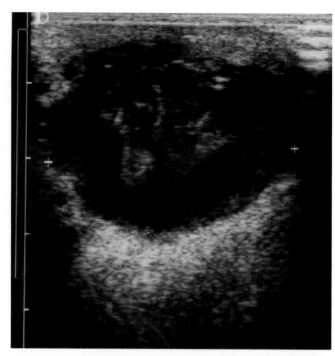

FIG. 19-69. This **breast abscess** following a breast biopsy presented as a complex mass with fluid- and solid-appearing components.

is hypoechoic and nonspecific in appearance (Fig. 19-69). The skin thickening seen clinically and by mammography is also visible by ultrasound. An abscess is a complex or hypoechoic mass that often has ill-defined margins but may have better defined margins as organization takes place. Generally, the internal structure is mixed in appearance with fluid-filled portions as well as more solid-looking tissue.

Parasitic Infections

Parasitic infections involving the breast are fairly uncommon in the United States.

Blastomycosis

A case of blastomycosis, a fungal infection endemic to the Mississippi and Ohio River basins, has been reported in a 56-year-old woman (63). The woman presented with multiple skin lesions and bone involvement and a palpable 1.4-cm circumscribed mass with an obscured border in the upper outer quadrant of the right breast that was solid on sonography. The mass disappeared after a course of amphotericin B.

Schistosomiasis

Schistosomiasis is caused by a parasitic fluke that is endemic in the tropics and subtropics. The parasite causes granulomas and fibrosis. It is extremely rare in the breast, but does occur (64).

We have seen this infection manifest as calcifications in a linear distribution. In the case reported by Gorman et al. (64), the calcifications were "fine," "innumerable," and tightly packed.

MALIGNANT LESIONS OF THE BREAST

Breast malignancy can be subdivided into four major histologic categories. These include tumors of the ductal epithelium and those of the lobular epithelium, and malignant lesions of the stromal tissues of the breast, which are extremely uncommon. Finally there are malignancies that develop in other organs that can metastasize to the breast.

The various types of primary breast cancer are summarized below. These categories are defined by pathologists who have found that certain morphologic characteristics can be used to group lesions.

I. Tumors of ductal epithelial origin
   A. DCIS (the classification of DCIS is evolving—see Chapter 7)
      1. Poorly differentiated DCIS—intraductal cancer—usually comedocarcinoma, with extensive necrosis
      2. Moderately well-differentiated DCIS—large cell—solid
      3. Well-differentiated DCIS—small cell—micropapillary and cribriform
   B. Invasive duct carcinoma—not otherwise specified (NOS)
   C. Paget's disease—tumor cells involve the nipple
   D. Tubular carcinoma—"attempts" to form ducts
   E. Papillary carcinoma—often in a cystically dilated duct
   F. Colloid carcinoma—extensive mucin production
   G. Medullary carcinoma—syncytial growth with extensive lymphocytic infiltrate
   H. Apocrine cancer
   I. Inflammatory carcinoma—aggressive invasive cancer with early dermal lymphatic invasion
   J. Adenoid cystic carcinoma
II. Tumors of lobular origin
   A. Lobular carcinoma in situ—may not be "real" cancer
   B. Infiltrating lobular carcinoma
III. Stromal malignancy
   A. Phylloides tumor
   B. Fibrosarcoma
   C. Liposarcoma
   D. Angiosarcoma
   E. Osteogenic sarcoma
   F. Malignant fibrous histiocytoma
IV. Tumors of lymphoid origin: primary lymphoma
V. Metastatic disease to the breast
   A. Melanoma
   B. Lymphoma
   C. Lung
   D. Renal
   E. Other

Stalsberg and Thomas (65) reviewed the age distribution of the various types of breast cancer. Using data from the Surveillance, Epidemiology, and End Results program (SEER) of the National Cancer Institute for the years 1973–1984, they looked at the number of cancers per 100,000 women diagnosed at each age each year (incidence), the total number at each age, and the relative frequency (what part of the total is comprised of the specific cancer). These are summarized in Table 19-1.

Cancer of the Ductal Epithelium

Cancers of the breast have many different manifestations, but the majority are believed to originate from the ductal epithelium. Lesions that remain confined within the duct and its basement membrane are termed *intraductal*. When the cells have developed the ability to leave the duct and invade the surrounding tissues they become *infiltrating* or *invasive*

TABLE 19-1. *Distribution of cancer types*

Histologic types of invasive cancer	Number of women	Percent of the total (%)	Median age at diagnosis (yrs)
Ductal and other (NOS)	98,930	83.9	61
Lobular	8,755	7.4	60
Medullary	3,677	3.1	53
Mucinous (colloid)	2,661	2.3	71
Paget's disease	1,217	1.0	62
Papillary	1,100	0.9	68
Tubular	743	0.6	61
Inflammatory	580	0.5	58
Metaplastic	150	0.1	59
Apocrine	72	0.06	59
Signet-ring	54	0.05	68
Secretory	9	0.01	67
Total	117,948	100.00	61

NOS = not otherwise specified.
Source: Adapted from Stalsberg H, Thomas DB. Age distribution of histologic types of breast cancer. Int J Cancer 1993;54:1–7.

TABLE 19-2. *Characteristics of the various forms of DCIS*

Features	Differentiation in DCIS		
	Poor	Moderate	Well
Nuclear	Highly pleomorphic; varying size and spacing	Moderately pleomorphic; less variation	Uniform
Chromatin	Coarse, clumped	Fine to coarse	Uniform/fine
Nucleoli	Prominent	Evident	Insignificant
Mitoses	Often present	Occasionally present	Rarely present
Architectural differentiation (polarization of cells)	Absent	Present	Marked
Frequently associated features			
Necrosis	Present	Variable	Absent or minimal
Growth pattern	Solid, clinging	All patterns; micropapillary/cribriform	Rarely solid
Calcifications	Amorphous	Amorphous or laminated	Laminated or psammoma-like

Source: Adapted from Holland R, Peterse JL, Mills RR, et al. Ductal carcinoma in situ: a proposal for a new classification. Semin Diagn Pathol 1994;11:167–180.

ductal carcinoma. Invasive ductal carcinoma accounts for 84% of all invasive breast cancers (65).

Ductal Carcinoma In Situ (Intraductal Carcinoma)

Before the use of mammography to screen asymptomatic women, the diagnosis of DCIS was made infrequently. Fewer than 5% of cancers diagnosed in the 1970s were DCIS. Mammography has made it possible to detect these lesions, usually by their associated deposition of calcium, so that they now comprise 20% to 30% of the cancers detected in a screening program. Although the detection of DCIS increases with the age of women being screened, it does not increase as rapidly as the increase in the detection of invasive breast cancer (66), which may indicate that the cases of DCIS that occur among younger women become the invasive cancers found among older women. The actual relationship of DCIS to invasive breast cancer, however, remains controversial.

Our understanding of the noninvasive forms of ductal carcinoma is evolving. Previously grouped according to gross histologic characteristics, Lagios found that by adding an analysis of histologic grade he could further characterize some of these lesions as being apparently more indolent, whereas others were more prone to earlier invasion if not treated properly (67). Schwartz et al. (68) had a similar experience. Holland et al. (69) have proposed a new scheme for categorizing these lesions, dividing them into poorly differentiated, intermediately differentiated, and well differentiated (Table 19-2).

Silverstein et al. (70) have proposed the Van Nuys Prognostic Index for DCIS. This scheme assigns points for the size of the lesion, the width of normal tissue removed as the margin, and the pathologic classification. One point is assigned if the lesion is ≤15 mm, the width of the margin is >10 mm, or the pathologic classification is not high grade

and there is no necrosis. A size of 16 to 40 mm is assigned two points, as is a margin 1 to 9 mm. Non–high grade with necrosis also gets two points. If the size is ≥41 mm, the lesion is assigned three points. Three points are assigned for a margin of <1 mm, and high grade with or without necrosis also receives three points. The authors found that a total score of three or four points had only a 2% recurrence rate, whereas a score of five, six, or seven points resulted in a 19% recurrence, and a score of eight or nine points resulted in a 57% recurrence. There were no deaths among the 101 women with a score of three or four points; three deaths out of the 209 women with scores of five, six, or seven points; and no deaths among the 23 women with a score of eight or nine points. As has been shown in other series, the larger the volume of DCIS the greater the recurrence rate.

There are only preliminary data that evaluate all of these classification systems. To be validated, the systems need prospective analysis. Furthermore, these studies will take many years to complete because the recurrence rate of DCIS appears to increase as patients are followed over a longer period of time. Solin et al. (71) found that the rate of recurrence among women with low-grade DCIS was 2% at 5 years, 5% at 8 years, and 15% at 10 years. Nevertheless, many therapists are treating high-grade DCIS more aggressively than low-grade DCIS.

The earliest stage DCIS is thought to originate in the terminal duct at its junction with the lobule or just inside the lobule. Histologically, the cells of ductal carcinoma may distend the duct to many times its normal size and extend into the lobules and down other branches of the duct network. Still contained by the basement membrane, these are classified as *intraductal lesions*. If the duct wall is slightly breached they may be termed *microinvasive*.

Most pathologists recognize several histologic types of DCIS. The most common form of DCIS appears to be made up of large cells that fill and distend the ducts with frequent central necrosis of the tumor. This type of comedonecrosis has provided the name *comedocarcinoma* for this form of DCIS. Comedocarcinomas produce the most distinctive calcifications on mammography (see Poorly Differentiated Comedocarcinoma).

The next most common types of DCIS are made up of small cells. When these form cribriform spaces (resembling a sieve), they have been termed *cribriform DCIS*, and when they produce papillary growths they are termed *micropapillary DCIS*. Lennington et al. (72) found that these lesions are frequently not uniform but contained cells that were more poorly differentiated at the center and better differentiated at the periphery with atypical hyperplasia at the edges. They concluded that these lesions develop from a central focus and expand peripherally.

Using his classification scheme to grade DCIS, Lagios et al. (73) studied DCIS detected by mammography alone and measuring <25 mm in diameter. These lesions were treated by local excision only. He found that comedocarcinoma was more likely to recur or become invasive in a 10-year follow-up period than were the micropapillary or cribriform types. Among the comedocarcinoma lesions with high nuclear grade (poorly differentiated), 19% (6 of 31) recurred within 26 months of surgery, whereas only one of the 10 intermediate-grade (cribriform) lesions recurred over an average of 18 months, and none of the 33 patients with micropapillary/non-necrotic cribriform types and low nuclear grade had a recurrence. Schwartz et al. (68) had a similar result among 70 patients with DCIS followed for a median of 47 months. Among the 15% of women who had recurrences, 14 of the 15 had high-grade lesions.

Morrow (74) has speculated that it is the time to recurrence that varies and not the actual rate. High-grade lesions tend to recur early (within 5 years), whereas low-grade lesions take longer to recur. She pointed to the work of Betsill (75) reported in 1978. Among 25 patients with low-grade DCIS who had been treated by biopsy only, seven of 10 women who were followed for an average of 21.6 years recurred and six of the seven recurred as invasive breast cancer. These data suggest that given enough time, a high percentage of DCIS will recur, and many will recur as invasive cancer. What is not known is the effect of using minimal treatment for these lesions and risking an invasive recurrence that has the potential to be lethal versus overtreating low-grade lesions that have a high likelihood of cure with excision alone.

The fact that there may be prognostic differences between the histologically distinctive forms of DCIS is gaining support. Until better methods are defined, it appears likely that these lesions will be categorized by the pathologist's estimation of their level of differentiation.

Because most DCIS is not clinically evident, the increased use of mammography has resulted in a marked increase in the diagnosis of this early lesion. Using results from the SEER program of the National Cancer Institute, Ernster et al. (76) compared the increase in incidence (diagnosis) of DCIS between 1973 and 1983 with the increase in incidence between 1983 and 1992. For women aged 30 to 39 years, the incidence increased by only 0.3% during the first period, although it increased by 12% during the second period. For women aged 40 to 49 years, it rose from 0.4% to 17.4% and, as these authors often have done, they grouped all women aged 50 years and older, showing that the incidence increased from 5.2% to 18.1%.

The total number of DCIS diagnosed in the United States in 1992 was 23,368. This was twice the number expected based on the rates from 1973 to 1983. There is little doubt that the increased incidence is due to the increased use of mammography and detection of more in situ lesions. The authors, however, blamed mammographic screening for the fact that many of these women with the earliest form of breast cancer are still treated by mastectomy. This is a case of shooting the messenger: It is not mammography that is at fault, but the fact that pathologists and oncologists have not been able to agree on the best treatment for these lesions.

It is fairly clear that there are some women who have DCIS that never affects them during the course of their lives, and if it was never discovered they would have never been troubled by the lesion. There are also cases of DCIS that progress to invasion and death, however. Most of the data on the long-term follow-up of DCIS are from studies in which the lesions were removed, improperly categorized as benign, and, thus, incompletely treated. Their long-term follow-up has been used to estimate the natural history of untreated DCIS. This is very inaccurate. In addition to the fact that some of the women have been lost to follow-up, it is frequently forgotten that the surgery that removed these lesions may have removed the entire focus of DCIS so that the follow-up may underestimate the significance of these early cancers.

The fact that DCIS is far from innocuous was highlighted by the long-term follow-up of low-grade DCIS in a study by Page et al. (77). Among a group of 28 women who were followed up for almost 30 years after the incorrect diagnosis of a benign lesion that was actually DCIS, nine women developed invasive breast cancer (30%) in the same location from which the previous lesion had been removed. Among these nine women, seven (25%) developed invasive breast cancer within 10 years of the biopsy. Two more women developed invasive breast cancer after more than 10 years. One developed invasive cancer 23 years after the biopsy, whereas another developed invasive cancer 31 years after the initial biopsy. This latter individual developed metastatic breast cancer and died as a result at the age of 79 years. Among the 28 women with so-called low-grade DCIS who had uncertain treatment, nine (32%) subsequently developed invasive breast cancer and five (20%) died from breast cancer. Two of the deaths came within 5 years of the biopsy, four came within 10 years, and the fifth occurred 34 years after the initial missed diagnosis. Some have used this report to suggest that DCIS is not an important lesion, but the authors estimate that, even for these "indolent forms" the risk of invasion was 25% to 50%, and the risk continued beyond 30 years after the missed diagnosis.

In a study conducted by the National Surgical Adjuvant Breast Project (NSABP), a multicenter collaborative program, lumpectomy alone was compared to lumpectomy with adjuvant radiation therapy (Trial B-17) (78). The NSABP randomly assigned 818 women to the two groups. The protocol called for lumpectomy with histologically clear margins for all the women. The irradiated group received 5,000 rads (50 Gy). The mean follow-up was <4 years (only 43 months) with a range of 11 to 83 months. Among the women who received irradiation, the event-free (i.e., no recurrent or new cancers, no regional or distant metastatic cancer, and no cancer deaths) was 84.4% at 5 years, whereas it fell to 73.8% among the women who were not irradiated. Among the 391 women treated by the surgery alone, 64 (16.4%) had recurrences and 32 of these were invasive cancers (50% of the recurrences and 8.2% of the total). Among the 399 women treated with surgery and irradiation, 28 (7%) recurred, with eight being invasive cancer (29% of the recurrences and 2% of the total). From these data it would appear that approximately 10% of women with DCIS will recur within 5 years of excision alone (no irradiation). The long-term survival of these women remains to be determined.

Even with this large study, there is still controversy. The authors only found that comedonecrosis and uncertain margins were associated with recurrence and did not feel that the newer measures of differentiation were of predictive value (79), but their review was criticized for not properly grading the lesions and analyzing combinations of factors (80).

Moriya and Silverberg (81) approached the question of the significance of the various types of DCIS from a different perspective. They compared the histologic findings of lesions that were pure DCIS with invasive cancers that had residual elements of DCIS. Solid DCIS with and without necrosis was seen more frequently in the mixed cancers than in pure DCIS. The authors also found periductal inflammation and multifocality to be more common in the mixed lesions. The DCIS in mixed lesions was poorly differentiated and had a higher mitotic rate. The authors concluded that a solid growth pattern with a high nuclear grade (poor differentiation) was a feature that would likely predict earlier progression to invasion.

The controversies associated with DCIS will likely continue for many years. The available data, however, strongly suggest that these are the earliest identifiable forms of breast cancer and that clones with invasive potential arise from these in situ lesions, and these can lead to death. The exact risk is unknown. The available data suggest that invasion is more likely to occur early in the course of poorly differentiated lesions, but even well-differentiated DCIS can lead to invasive cancer, and the risk appears to be lifelong. Although mammography has been criticized for finding DCIS at increased frequency in younger women, these women also have the longest life expectancy and will likely live long enough for invasive cancers to develop. Mammography should not be faulted for finding DCIS. Rather, oncologists need to determine how best to treat these lesions. It is hoped that one of the grading systems described above will ultimately prove accurate in differentiating the various forms of DCIS and their natural history so that therapy can be tailored appropriately.

DCIS is usually detected because of associated calcifications. Some believe that the various types of DCIS can be differentiated by their patterns of calcium deposition, but no one has provided convincing evidence that this is the case. There are some patterns that are very characteristic, however, such as the fine linear branching calcifications that frequently occur in the necrotic portions of poorly differentiated comedocarcinomas. Many in situ ductal cancers produce fewer characteristic calcifications that may be similar in appearance to those produced by benign processes. In a review of 100 consecutive cases of DCIS, Stomper et al. (82) found that 72% produced microcalcifications, 10% produced small masses, and 12% were a combination. The authors found that 35% of the lesions had the typical fine linear branching structures (usually due to comedocarcinoma), whereas 52% were less typical "granular" types of calcifications, and 13% were mixed.

Ikeda and Anderson (83) found a group of 73 cases (out of 190) of DCIS that did not manifest calcifications. Among these, 60 were clinically evident and 30 had a negative mammogram. DCIS in this group included 15 lesions that were round masses, 12 that were focal nodular densities, one indicated by asymmetric density, two as ill-defined masses, one as dilated ducts, four as architectural distortion, three as subareolar masses, and four as developing densities.

Kinkel et al. (84) found that the density that may surround comedo DCIS that presents with mammographically evident calcifications may not represent invasion but is often an inflammatory reaction.

Evans et al. (85) reviewed 54 mammographically detected in situ ductal cancers and 77 that were clinically evident. DCIS represented 5% of clinically evident cancers diagnosed over the period 1978 to 1992, whereas DCIS represented 24% of the screen mammographically detected cancers. The clinically evident lesions were more extensive. Diffuse DCIS was present in 13% of the symptomatic group but none of the screen-detected lesions. None of the screen-detected cases had Paget's disease, whereas 22% of the symptomatic cases had Paget's lesions. Eight of the clinically evident cancers (11%) were cribriform-micropapillary large cell cancers. None of the screen-detected DCIS was of this type. Comedocarcinoma was more common among the mammographically detected cancers. Among the symptomatic lesions, 20 of 77 (26%) were of the comedo type, whereas among the mammographically detected lesions, 23 of 54 (43%) were comedocarcinoma.

Poorly Differentiated Comedocarcinoma

Comedocarcinoma is merely gross descriptive terminology for a ductal carcinoma that is characterized by abundant cells that fill the ducts of the involved lobe with frequent areas of necrosis that often calcify. When cut in cross section (Fig. 19-70), this necrotic debris is extruded from the

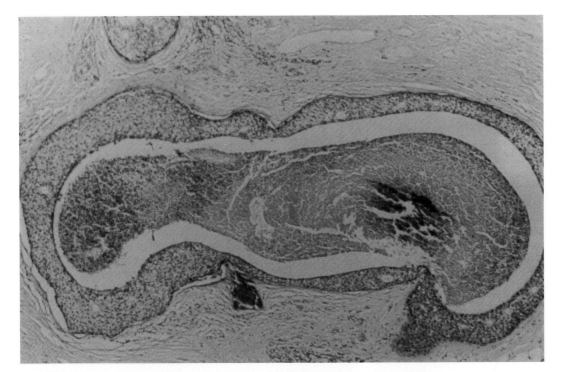

FIG. 19-70. A duct that is cut in cross section. It has been distended by **ductal carcinoma in situ of the comedo variety,** which can be seen in irregular layers lining the duct. In the center, the necrotic portion of the tumor has separated in the preparation. The dark area that appears fractured is irregular calcium deposition. It is this irregular pattern of necrosis and calcium deposition that produces calcifications that are often characteristic of this in situ cancer.

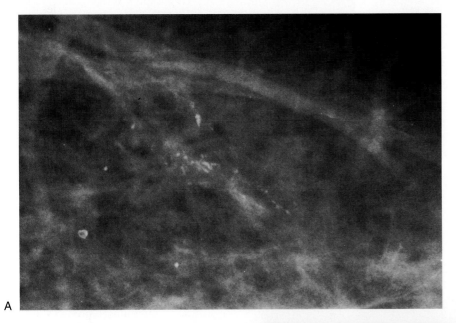

A

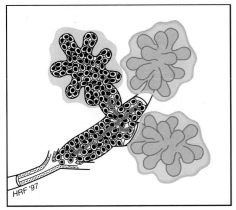

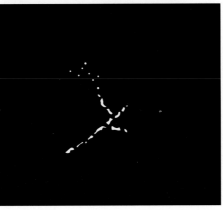

B

FIG. 19-71. (A) High-grade comedocarcinoma often produces typical linear, branching, pleomorphic calcifications in a linear distribution, as in this 67-year-old woman. **(B)** The process is rendered schematically.

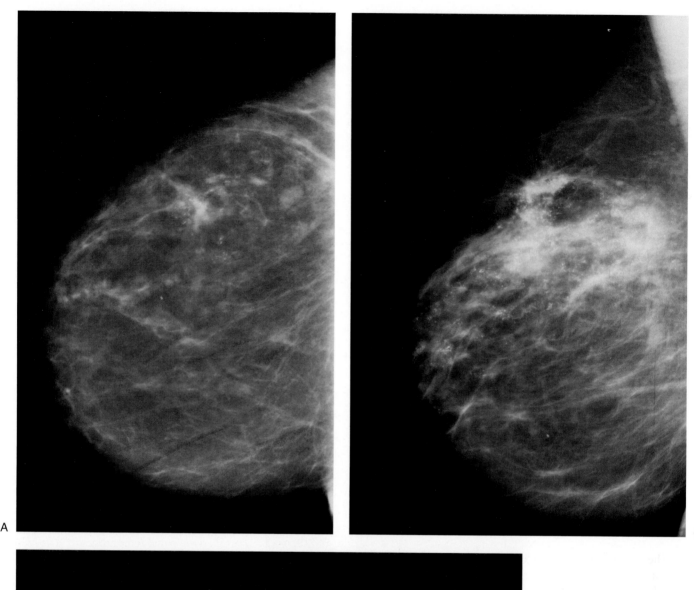

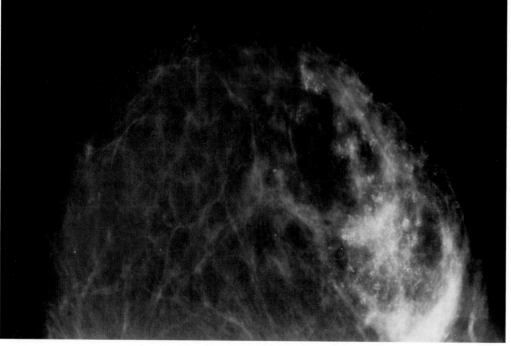

FIG. 19-72. High-grade ductal carcinoma in situ progresses rather rapidly. The patient refused investigation of the calcifications seen in the lateral aspect of the left breast in 1987 on this craniocaudal (CC) projection **(A)**. She returned 2½ years later with extensive calcifications occupying the upper outer left breast, seen here on the CC **(B)** and mediolateral oblique projections **(C)**. Biopsy revealed extensive intraductal carcinoma with areas of invasion.

duct like a comedo, hence the name. As with other ductal cancers, it may be confined to the ducts or be associated with varying degrees of invasion. The lesion may present as a palpable mass or be only detected by mammography. Although usually characterized by an extensive intraductal growth, the larger the volume of duct involvement, the greater the likelihood of an area of invasion. Although it has a favorable prognosis when confined to the ducts, as with any invasive ductal cancer, if there is associated invasion it may metastasize and be lethal. Newer classifications of DCIS are being devised that grade the lesion based on the cytologic features of the cells and the structural distribution of the cells. These lesions with necrosis are generally associated with poorly differentiated (high-grade) DCIS.

Mammographic Appearance

High-grade comedocarcinoma characteristically produces exuberant calcification in the necrotic cellular debris that accompanies the lesion (Fig. 19-71). Frequently there are innumerable calcium deposits that fill the ducts and may extend over large areas of the breast (Fig. 19-72). The calcifications are heterogeneous, displaying varying irregular shapes and sizes. Because this form of ductal carcinoma tends to arise or spread through the ducts, the general distribution of the calcifications is characteristically along the duct lines. Comedo elements may accompany any ductal cancer with or without invasion, and thus these characteristic calcifications may also be seen in association with a tumor mass (Fig. 19-73).

Ultrasound Appearance

The mammographic appearance of diffuse comedocarcinoma is usually so characteristic that ultrasound is not indicated. No particular ultrasound features have been defined to characterize this lesion. If no tumor mass is present, it is unlikely that the ductal tumor or calcifications will be seen by ultrasound, although some have been able to image the calcifications when they are profuse and close together. Some have used ultrasound to guide the needle biopsy of these lesions.

As with any cancer forming a tumor mass, one would anticipate nonspecific hypoechoic irregular tissue. If calcifications are sufficiently dense or there is a significant fibrotic component to the lesion, shadowing may result.

Well-Differentiated Ductal Carcinoma In Situ (Micropapillary and Cribriform Lesions)

As described in Ductal Carcinoma In Situ, the evaluation of DCIS is evolving. Well-differentiated DCIS appears to have a better prognosis than poorly differentiated DCIS (or is at least later to infiltrate), and moderately differentiated

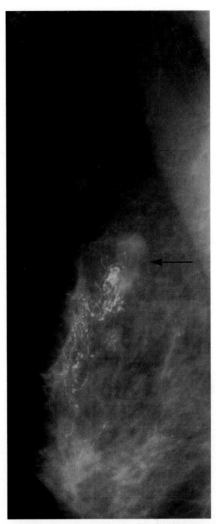

FIG. 19-73. If left long enough, **ductal carcinoma in situ (DCIS)** will likely develop **an invasive component.** The high-grade DCIS in this patient is evidenced by calcifications on the mediolateral oblique projection. There is an associated tumor mass indicative of the invasive tumor that has arisen, presumably from a clone of the DCIS.

DCIS is in between. These lesions tend to comprise smaller, more uniform cells. It would appear that they are better differentiated, and their effort to form cribriform spaces may be their disorganized effort to build ducts and lobules.

Mammographic Appearance

Some have claimed that the calcifications of poorly differentiated DCIS can be distinguished from those produced by well-differentiated cancers (86). This has not been our experience. Certainly the classic fine, linear branching calcifications described above almost always predict comedonecrosis, but predicting degrees of differentiation of DCIS by mammography has been less successful. The more granular appearance

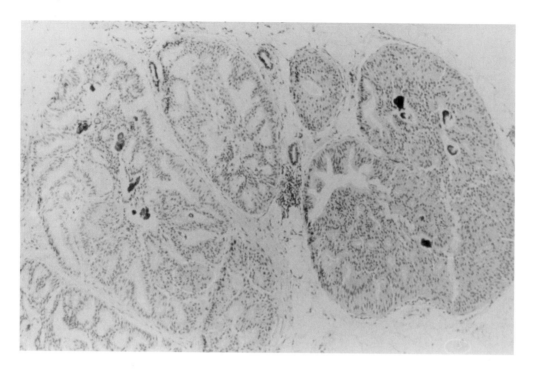

FIG. 19-74. A photomicrograph (hematoxylin and eosin) demonstrates a well-differentiated type of ductal carcinoma in situ. The lesion is forming cribriform spaces, indicating some attempt at differentiation. The calcifications are the dark-staining material and appear to form in the cribriform spaces.

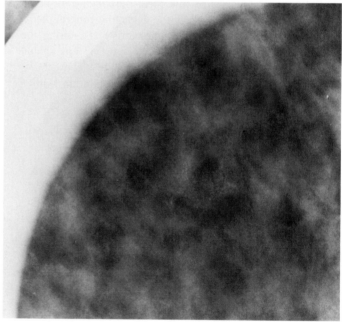

A

B

FIG. 19-75. Occasionally the calcifications seen by mammography reflect the pattern of growth **for low-grade ductal carcinoma in situ (DCIS).** The calcifications seen here on magnification lateral **(A)** and craniocaudal projections **(B)** are nondescript, pleomorphic deposits in a cluster. This proved to be due to a well-differentiated cribriform type of DCIS in a 57-year-old woman.

and clustered distribution that others have attributed to well-differentiated micropapillary and cribriform DCIS have only rarely held up in our cases (Figs. 19-74 and 19-75). Part of the problem is likely due to the fact that many DCIS lesions are not purely a single type but have multiple forms within the same lesion and their categorization is difficult.

Infiltrating Ductal Carcinoma (Invasive Ductal Carcinoma)

Infiltration may be present in tumors of any size, forming invasive, or infiltrating, ductal carcinoma. Once they invade, cancers of ductal origin develop additional characteristics that permit grouping. Some of these have prognostic significance.

Invasive Ductal Carcinoma Not Otherwise Specified

The majority of invasive breast cancers are nonspecific forms of carcinoma that originate in the ductal epithelium probably in the terminal duct at its junction with the lobule. The better differentiated forms of invasive ductal carcinoma create specific patterns that have been subclassified, but the majority of ductal malignancies fall into the general category of lesions that are undifferentiated and have no particular distinguishing features histologically. When a cancer does not fit into any of the defined subtypes it is termed *not otherwise specified* (NOS). According to data from the SEER program, invasive ductal carcinoma NOS accounts for 65% of the breast cancers diagnosed in the United States (65). The relative frequency of these lesions appears to remain fairly constant regardless of age. In general, infiltrating ductal carcinoma NOS elicits a fairly vigorous desmoplastic response with cicatrization and fibrosis. This produces a very hard mass on palpation and what has best been described as a gritty texture when the lesion is cut across. Many are associated with abundant fibrosis, leading to the nonspecific designation of scirrhous carcinoma.

Because screening mammography continues to be underused, many of these cancers are still found by the woman herself. In general, these are firm to hard lesions that may be tethered to the skin or to the deep structures of the chest wall. Vascular and lymphatic spread ulti-mately result, and if left untreated, carcinoma may eventually erode through the skin of the breast itself, producing an ulcerated mass. Dermal lymphatic involvement with tumor can occur early in the course of the disease, signaling the poor prognosis associated with inflammatory carcinoma, or it may be a late result of a neglected tumor. Sometimes skin thickening is present, but if only edema is found, it is most likely caused by obstruction of the axillary lymphatics.

Within this general category of undifferentiated invasive lesions, pathologists have devised subclassifications that help predict prognosis. The predominate cell types may be classified from low-grade (I) fairly uniform cells that show some degree of differentiation (mucin production or tubule formation) to high-grade tumors (III), in which anaplastic, pleomorphic cells predominate (see Chapter 2).

Collagen production is a prominent feature of many breast cancers, and calcium deposition is common within the tumor. These are responsible for the characteristic firm, gritty nature of these lesions. The desmoplasia associated with many ductal cancers produces the distinctive, irregular, spiculated appearance seen on gross inspection histologically (Fig. 19-76) and using mammography.

Mammographic Appearance

The mammographic appearance of breast cancer is varied (see Primary, Secondary, and Supporting Signs of Malignancy in Chapter 5). The diagnosis is virtually certain when an irregular mass with a spiculated margin is present (Fig. 19-77A).

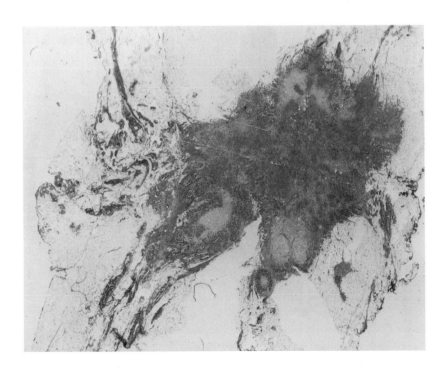

FIG. 19-76. The irregular shape of this **invasive ductal carcinoma (not otherwise specified)** is evident in this low-power photomicrograph (hematoxylin and eosin).

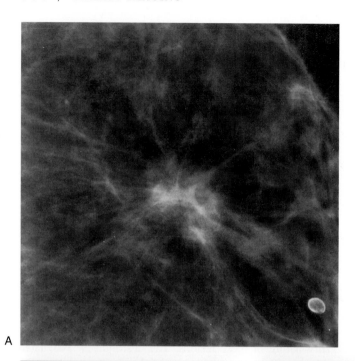

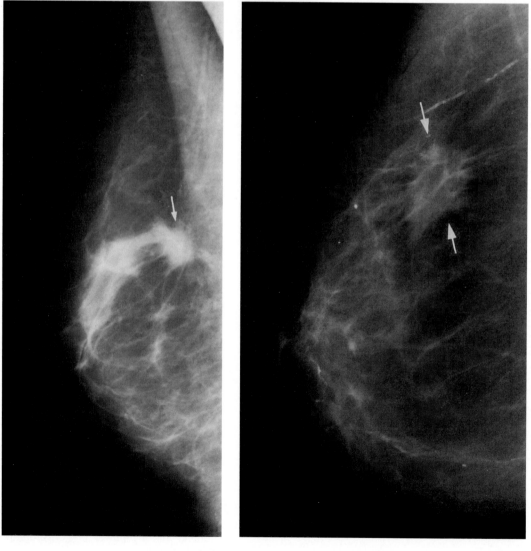

FIG. 19-77. (A) Classically, **invasive ductal carcinoma** presents as an irregular mass with spiculated margins detected only by mammography, as in this lesion in a 59-year-old woman. **(B)** Cancer is usually high in x-ray attenuation, as in this invasive ductal carcinoma. **(C)** It can occasionally be fairly low in attenuation, as in this large, palpable cancer (*arrows*). Note that attenuation can be influenced by x-ray technique.

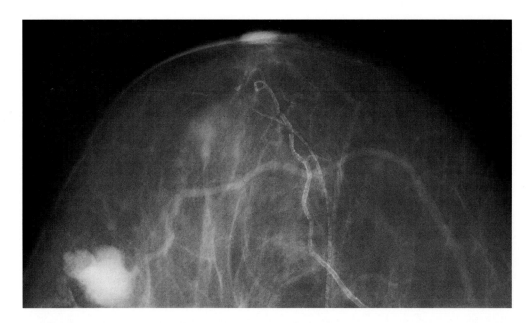

FIG. 19-78. Invasive ductal carcinoma with a lobulated margin.

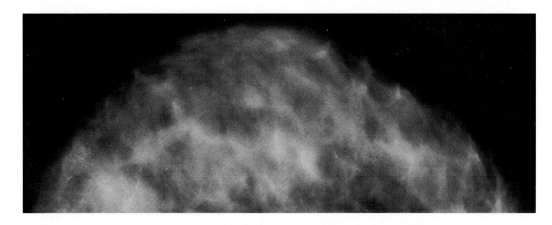

FIG. 19-79. The calcifications in the lateral half of the breast of a 33-year-old woman who had a palpable mass following delivery were the only mammographic indication of **an invasive and intraductal carcinoma.**

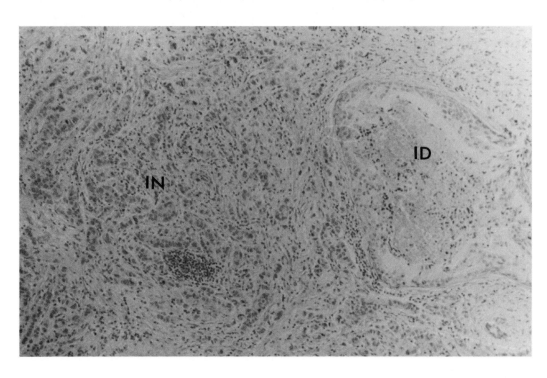

FIG. 19-80. This photomicrograph (hematoxylin and eosin) demonstrates the continued growth of **ductal carcinoma in situ** within the duct (ID) while invasive cancer grows around the duct (IN).

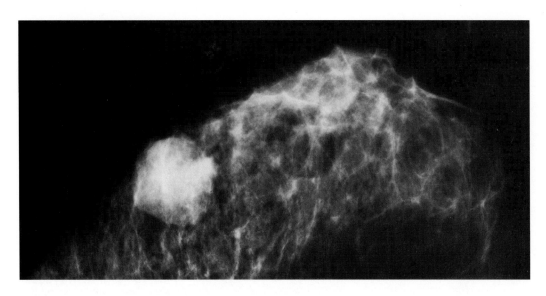

FIG. 19-81. Breast cancer can be round. This rounded mass proved to be **invasive ductal carcinoma.**

Lobulated shapes are fairly common, and the more undulating the border, the more suspicious the lesion (Fig. 19-78). The mass can be high in x-ray attenuation (Fig. 19-77B).

Some ductal cancers reveal their presence early by the deposition of calcium (Fig. 19-79), which is due to either direct cellular secretion or cell necrosis (87). When calcifications are present in association with a typical tumor mass, the diagnosis is even more certain. Although an invasive clone may have developed and produced a tumor mass, intraductal cancer clones may continue to grow confined to the ducts (Fig. 19-80). When calcifications are found in association with an invasive lesion detected only by mammography, the calcifications will invariably be found in the intraductal portions of the cancer. The fibrosis, desmoplasia, and cicatrization that accompany many ductal cancers may produce distortion of the surrounding architecture with or without an apparent tumor mass, and this process may lead to skin or nipple retraction.

Breast cancer usually produces an ill-defined shadow, but even "garden variety" infiltrating ductal carcinoma may produce a sharply circumscribed mass that is indistinguishable from a benign lesion (Fig. 19-81). The generally greater x-ray attenuation relative to its volume often distinguishes the malignant lesion.

Some cancers infiltrate without distorting the normal breast architecture and without calcium deposition. If the normal parenchyma abutting the tumor is the same radiographic density, the tumor may be undetectable by mammography. Occasionally the only indication of the presence of cancer is nonspecific asymmetric density. If this is focal, additional imaging may reveal the lesion (Fig. 19-82). Asymmetric breast tissue (i.e., no mass, significant calcifications, or architectural distortion), however, is a normal variation. It must be palpable before the diagnosis of cancer is considered (88).

Ultrasound Appearance

Just as there is a spectrum of mammographic presentations, the ultrasound appearance of breast cancer is extremely variable (89). The classic description of breast cancer is an irregularly shaped hypoechoic structure that frequently has a triangular anterior margin and attenuates and scatters sound, producing retrotumoral shadowing (Fig. 19-83). This is fairly characteristic of the spiculated scirrhous lesion, but there is rarely any reason to ultrasound such a lesion. Furthermore, it is not the only way that cancer can present. In 130 cancers studied by whole-breast ultrasound, this appearance was seen only 35% of the time. Virtually every other shape and pattern has been seen. Cancers are almost always irregular, frequently lobulated (Fig. 19-84), and hypoechoic. Their internal echo pattern may vary from sparse and heterogeneous (Fig. 19-85) to very prominent and homogeneous (Fig. 19-86). At least two colloid cancers have been described at meetings that were hyperechoic relative to the normal parenchyma, although we have only seen fibroadenomas that were hyperechoic.

There may be retrotumoral shadowing, or the posterior tissues may appear isoechoic. If the tumor is relatively homogeneous and round or ovoid, the posterior echoes may be enhanced relative to the scattering and attenuation caused by the surrounding normal breast tissue (Fig. 19-87).

Fornage (90) has demonstrated that breast cancers tend to be more vertically oriented relative to the skin layer on supine ultrasound evaluation, whereas benign lesions tend to be more horizontally oriented and elongated, but there are always exceptions. Fibroadenomas may be vertically oriented, whereas cancer can be elongated (Fig. 19-88), and because a tissue diagnosis is so safe it is dif-

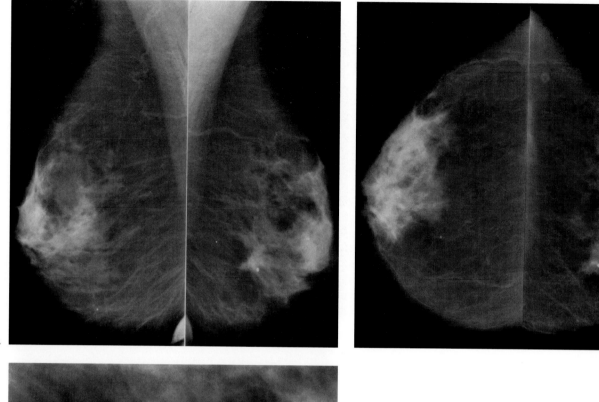

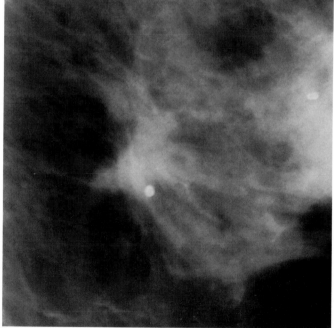

FIG. 19-82. A **focal asymmetry** may prove to be breast cancer. Note the focal asymmetry, which on the mediolateral oblique is in the lower right breast **(A)** and on the craniocaudal is in the medial right breast **(B)**. Spot compression **(C)** reveals an irregular, spiculated mas that proved to be **invasive ductal carcinoma (not otherwise specified)**.

ficult to forgo an almost certain tissue diagnosis for one that is based on statistics. In general, ultrasound cannot be used to make a firm diagnosis that a lesion is benign because of the broad range of appearances and the overlap between benign and malignant lesions. Ultrasound should only be used to differentiate cystic breast lesions from solid ones and to guide needle positioning for interventional procedures.

Distinctive Cancers of Ductal Origin

Although most cancers that arise from the epithelium of the duct are undifferentiated adenocarcinomas, a small percentage are sufficiently well differentiated or distinctive enough to be subclassified. These may be artificial distinctions in a continuum, and it is not unusual for differentiated and undifferentiated cell lines to be found in the same tumor.

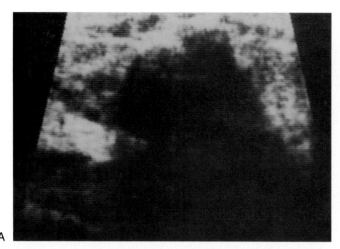

A

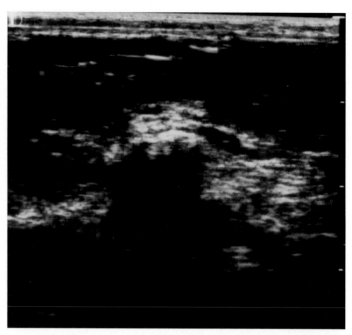

B

FIG. 19-83. (A) The "typical" appearance of breast cancer on ultrasound is an irregular mass with a triangular anterior margin, heterogeneous low-level internal echoes, and posterior acoustic shadowing. **(B)** A variation of an irregular shape with dense posterior shadowing is seen in this invasive cancer that was not palpable but was detected by mammography in a 54-year-old woman.

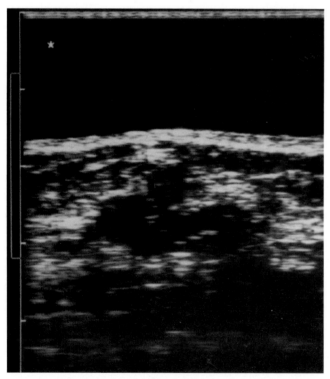

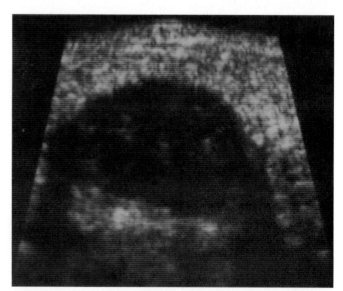

FIG. 19-85. This invasive ductal carcinoma had sparse, low-level internal echoes. Note that its shape is fairly round and regular making it impossible to differentiate this malignant lesion from a benign lesion by ultrasound.

FIG. 19-84. This invasive and intraductal carcinoma was lobulated, with a heterogeneous internal echo texture on ultrasound. There is some posterior acoustic shadowing.

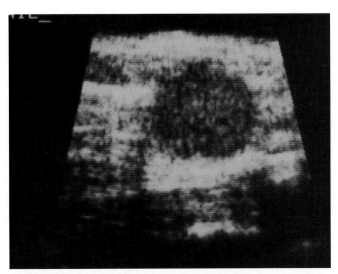

FIG. 19-86. This small, **invasive breast cancer** has a prominent, homogeneous internal echo texture. Note there is also posterior acoustic enhancement.

The common association is that all appear to arise from epithelial cells of the ducts.

Paget's Disease

Paget's disease, a form of ductal carcinoma that involves the epidermal layers of the nipple, was first described by Sir James Paget more than 100 years ago. Although some cases of pure nipple involvement without an intraductal lesion have

been described, most pathologists agree that this carcinoma is merely a ductal malignancy that spreads along the ducts out onto the nipple, because the ductal lining is continuous with the nipple. Consequently, the breast cancer that produces Paget's disease presents itself at an early stage. The resulting eczematoid reaction on the nipple causes women to seek evaluation early. Histologically, the tumor is characterized by large, pleomorphic cells in the nipple. Occasionally a palpable mass is present, but frequently no tumor mass is evident. The prognosis is generally favorable because of the early presentation. Overall survival depends on whether the underlying lesion is in situ or infiltrating at the time of diagnosis, and, as with all cancers, relates to the stage of the lesion.

Mammographic Appearance

It is not unusual for Paget's disease to be clinically apparent with no mammographic abnormality. Because this is a carcinoma that spreads along the ducts and out onto the nipple, occasionally a mass will be visible deeper in the breast with typical malignant characteristics (Fig. 19-89). Microcalcifications may be seen within the ducts in the subareolar region directed toward the nipple (Fig. 19-90). The diffuse pattern of ductal calcifications associated with the comedo form of ductal carcinoma may also be seen.

Ultrasound Appearance

Paget's disease is not visible by ultrasound per se. The underlying cancer may be visible by ultrasound and appear

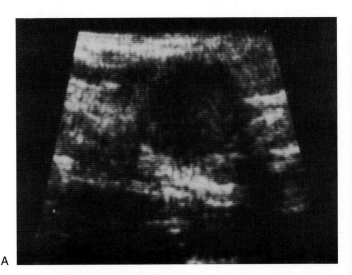

A

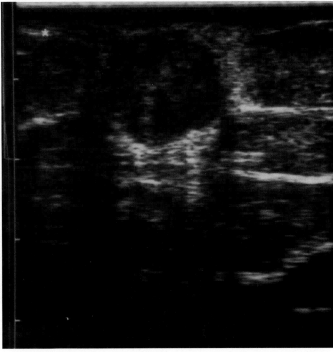

B

FIG. 19-87. (A) This round **invasive ductal carcinoma** has posterior acoustic enhancement, as does this **invasive cancer (B)** in another woman.

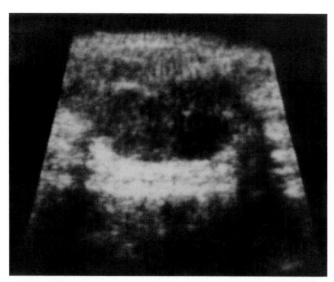

FIG. 19-88. This lobulated, circumscribed lesion was elongated and had enhanced through-transmission of sound with a uniform echo texture. Although these are benign characteristics, this proved to be an **invasive ductal carcinoma.**

as any other malignant lesion. It is likely that a tumor visible by ultrasound will also be evident on physical examination, and in general, ultrasound is not indicated when a patient presents with a nipple abnormality.

Tubular Cancer

Tubular carcinoma is a well-differentiated form of invasive ductal carcinoma. It makes up 0.6% of invasive breast cancers (68). Although it is an invasive cancer, its differentiation results in the production of what appear to be poorly formed ductal structures consisting of haphazardly arranged tubules lined by a single layer of cuboidal epithelium. The pathologist may, on occasion, have difficulty distinguishing tubular carcinoma from benign adenosis. Although sometimes palpable, the lesions are frequently detected by mammography. They are slow growing and are usually very small when detected (91). Perhaps because of its differentiation (it is attempting to form ducts), tubular cancer has a favorable prognosis with a low metastatic potential and the axillary nodes are rarely involved. In Tabar's data (92) tubular carcinoma accounted for 6% to 8% of all cancers (invasive + DCIS). Stalsberg and Thomas (65) suggest that the relative frequency of tubular cancer increases to a peak among women in their late 40s followed by a small dip and then a slow increase after the age of 64 years.

Nothing distinguishes the lesions of tubular cancer from other cancers except that on average, perhaps owing to slow growth, they are found at a very small size. Because of length bias sampling (it is more likely that screening at periodic intervals will find slower growing cancers) the slower growing tubular carcinoma is the likely diagnosis when a very small (5 mm) spiculated lesion is found by mammog-

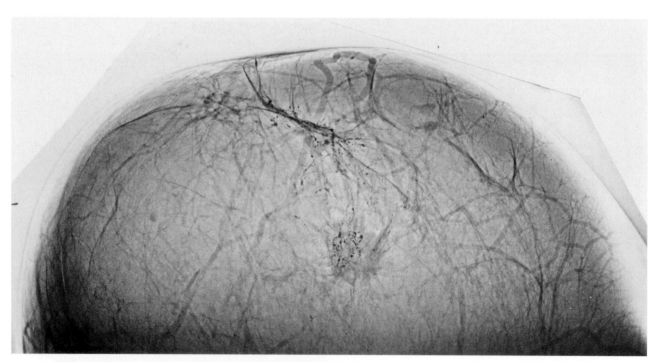

FIG. 19-89. This patient **presented with Paget's disease.** The xeromammogram (dark is dense, light is fat) reveals an **invasive cancer deep in the breast,** with calcifications indicative of intraductal carcinoma extending to the nipple.

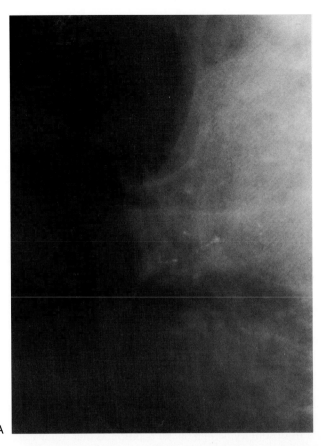

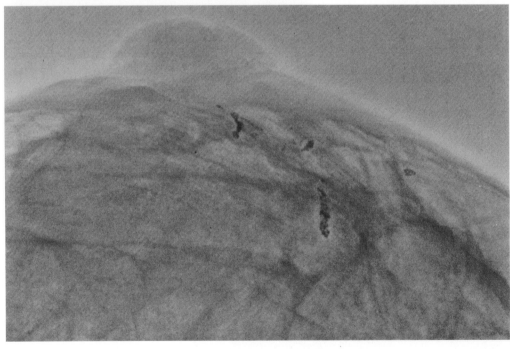

FIG. 19-90. Calcifications in ductal carcinoma in situ (A) are visible extending toward the nipple in this 70-year-old woman with Paget's disease. A similar appearance is seen on this positive-mode xerogram in another patient with **Paget's disease (B).**

A

B

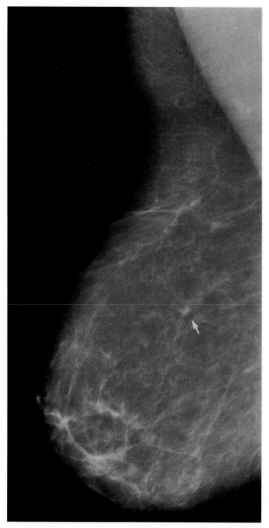

FIG. 19-91. This tiny spiculated mass (*arrow*) was a **tubular carcinoma** in a 59-year-old women that was detected by screening mammography.

raphy (Fig. 19-91). The majority of tubular carcinomas are <1 cm at the time of diagnosis and have a central mass with ill-defined or spiculated margins (Fig. 19-92). Axillary lymph node metastases are rare. Feig and colleagues (92) reported that none of 17 tubular cancers was well circumscribed or merely areas of asymmetric density. Leibman et al. (93) found that 11 of 13 tubular cancers were ≤1.7 cm with an average diameter of 0.8 cm. Although not a characteristic feature, some contain microcalcifications.

Papillary Carcinoma

Relatively rare, papillary cancer is a form of ductal malignancy in which the epithelium proliferates into villous-like projections that eventually fill the lumen. These lesions comprise approximately 0.9% of invasive cancers (68) and their relative frequency increases with patient age. Papillary carcinoma can develop as an intracystic lesion although it is likely that the "cyst" is merely a cystically dilated portion of the duct rather than a dilated lobule. Unlike comedocarcinoma, papillary carcinoma remains viable within the duct and does not necrose as readily. Pathologists can confuse this lesion with atypical papillomatosis. It is unclear whether this represents a continuum beginning with benign peripheral small-duct papillomas or whether these are de novo lesions. Papillary carcinomas are not generally thought to arise from solitary benign ductal papillomas that usually are found in the major ducts. Papillary carcinoma has a slow growth rate. It is not aggressively infiltrative and does not tend to produce the profuse fibrotic reaction associated with other cancers of the duct. Generally well circumscribed (due to the cystic structure that often surrounds it) and movable, it is usually not particularly hard on palpation.

As with any intraductal cancer, papillary carcinoma may become invasive. Some have reported a low rate of axillary nodal involvement and a favorable prognosis. Others report

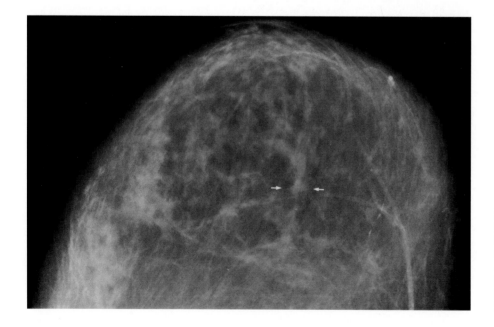

FIG. 19-92. Tubular carcinoma is slow growing and the most likely diagnosis when a very small, spiculated cancer is detected at screening. Periodic screening is more likely to detect slow-growing cancers (length-biased sampling), as in this patient with a tubular carcinoma (*arrows*).

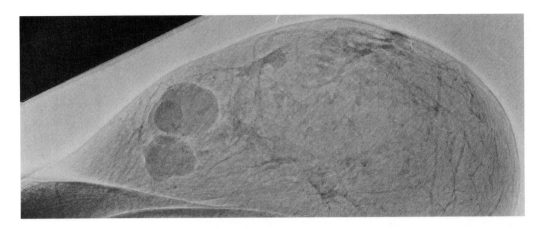

FIG. 19-93. These **papillary cancers** seen on positive mode xeroradiography (dark is dense and light is fat) appear round because they are growing in cystically dilated ducts. It is the cysts that are round.

a stage-for-stage prognosis similar to that of ductal carcinomas in general.

Mammographic Appearance

While still intraductal, papillary carcinoma is generally not evident mammographically. These tumors do not tend to produce the fibrotic proliferation associated with other forms of ductal carcinoma. As papillary carcinomas enlarge, however, they tend to produce fairly well-circumscribed masses. We have seen papillary carcinoma with a surrounding lucent halo (Fig. 19-93), again confirming the fact that this is not a diagnostic criterion for a benign process but rather the result of an abrupt transition in density associated with a smooth margin. Papillary carcinoma growing within a cyst is indistinguishable from a solitary cyst unless there is some distortion of the circumference by the tumor. The diagnosis is made only by microscopic assessment. If the cancer bleeds, the cyst may be extremely dense on the mammogram because of the iron content.

Ultrasound Appearance

Because this is a rare lesion, there is little specific information concerning the sonographic appearance of papillary carcinoma. One would predict that these well-circumscribed homogeneous masses would have a uniform internal echo-texture and probably result in isoechoic or posterior acoustic enhancement. When intracystic, the tumor will produce an appearance that is indistinguishable from that of an intra-cystic papilloma, with multiple fronds projecting into the lumen of the cyst. The few cases that we have seen have presented as hemorrhage into what appears to be a cyst, and the ultrasound appearance is that of a complex mass with cystic and solid properties.

Colloid or Mucinous Carcinoma

The presence of abundant mucin production is characteristic of the relatively uncommon colloid, or mucinous carcinoma. These account for approximately 2% to 3% of all invasive breast cancers (68) with their relative frequency

increasing with increasing age. Although many ductal cancers produce some mucin, the abundant production by this lesion is felt to indicate its greater degree of differentiation. This differentiation is thought to explain the better survival for patients with this form of duct cancer.

The cells produce mucin while still intraductal. As the tumor enlarges, it forms a firm, but not particularly hard mass to palpation that may be relatively smooth. When not part of a less well-differentiated cancer, pure colloid carcinoma tends to have a more favorable prognosis, with a lower rate of axillary nodal metastases and a 5-year survival of 70% to 80%. Stalsberg and Thomas (65) report that the relative frequency of these cancers is low until approximately age 60 years at which age a steady increase in the frequency of the diagnosis of these lesions begins.

Mammographic Appearance

There are no particular features that distinguish colloid carcinoma from other cancers of the breast. A review by Conant et al. (94) suggested that the lesions tend to be better circumscribed but may be ill-defined, and some have spiculated margins. The latter tended to be higher in nuclear grade with lower mucin production and infiltrating margins. Cardenosa et al. (95) reviewed 10 cases of colloid cancer. The ages of the individuals ranged from 31 to 88 years with a mean of 67 years. The majority of the cancers (70%) were not palpable but were detected by mammography. Their cases ranged from poorly defined lobulated masses to a cluster of lobulated masses that resembled a tight group of cysts. In some tumors the contour demonstrates very small lobulations (Fig. 19-94). When mucin production is profuse these tumors tend to be less dense radiographically than more scirrhous forms owing to the lower attenuation of the mucin.

Ultrasound Appearance

The appearance of colloid carcinoma is nonspecific. By ultrasound, these are hypoechoic lesions with posterior echoes that depend on the architecture of the tumor and the uniformity of the cellular composition.

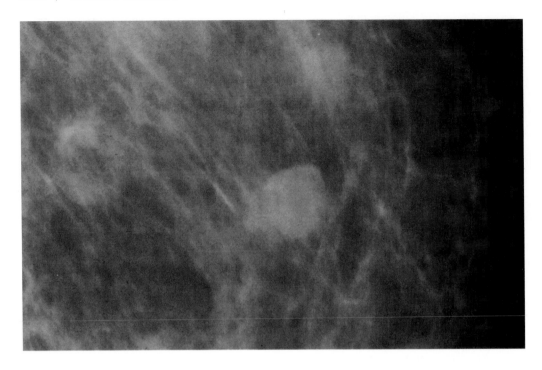

FIG. 19-94. Colloid carcinoma is frequently round or oval and may be relatively low in x-ray attenuation.

Medullary Carcinoma

Another relatively uncommon cancer, medullary carcinomas make up approximately 3% of all breast cancers. SEER data suggest that the relative frequency of medullary carcinoma rises rapidly during the third decade of life (women in their 20s) and then decreases relatively steadily after that (68). These cancers are distinctive in that they frequently grow quite large before being detected. Often round or lobulated and fairly distinct from the surrounding tissue, they are relatively soft on physical examination. Because they do not infiltrate aggressively, they tend to be freely movable in the breast.

Histologically, they comprise large cells with basophilic cytoplasm, large nuclei and frequent mitoses. True medullary carcinoma has a favorable prognosis, but only if specific histologic criteria have been met. These have been described by Ridolfi et al. (96). True medullary carcinoma must have a syncytial growth pattern with "pushing" margins (Fig. 19-95). Another characteristic feature of medullary carcinoma is the abundant infiltration of the lesion by lymphocytes and other

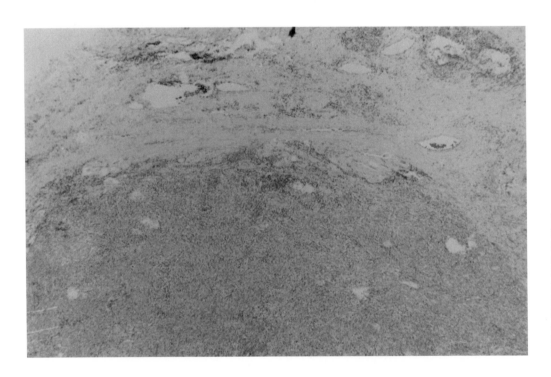

FIG. 19-95. This is a photomicrograph (hematoxylin and eosin) of the margin of a medullary carcinoma. Note that, although the margin is "pushing," it is not sharply defined, and these lesions usually are not sharply marginated by mammography contrary to earlier teaching.

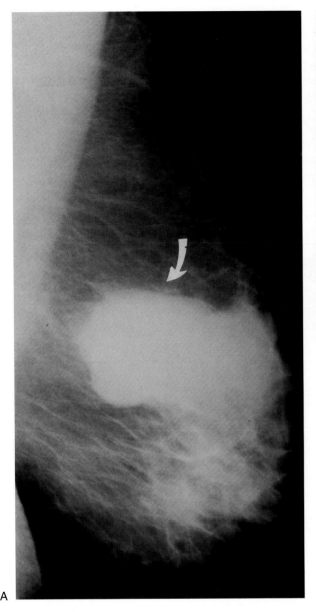

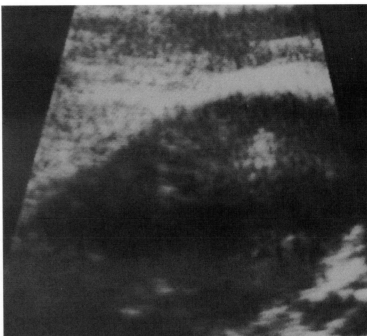

FIG. 19-96. (A) The **medullary carcinoma** in this right breast grew to a large size because it was relatively soft. The margins of medullary carcinoma are not well defined. On ultrasound **(B)** this medullary cancer is fairly well defined with a heterogeneous internal echo texture and good through-transmission of sound. Note that it is elongated.

inflammatory cells. It has been speculated that this is some form of immunologic response by the host to the tumor and may account for frequent necrotic areas within the tumor. To be a true medullary carcinoma, the tumor must have no ductal or glandular features.

Many tumors have been inappropriately classified as medullary when they are either atypical medullary cancers or merely invasive ductal carcinoma NOS (97,98). According to Ridolfi et al. (99), the atypical medullary cancers have a prognosis that is in between the true medullary and carcinoma NOS.

Mammographic Appearance

Medullary carcinoma is classically described as a fairly well-circumscribed, smooth, round, or ovoid mass (100). Although it used to be taught that sharply defined cancers were generally

medullary, this is not the case. Medullary carcinoma is frequently not sharply demarcated by mammography, but has a somewhat ill-defined margin (Fig. 19-96A). The fact is that most sharply circumscribed cancers are infiltrating ductal carcinoma (NOS) and are not medullary carcinoma. Although these lesions frequently exhibit necrosis histologically, calcifications are not a particularly significant feature of medullary cancer.

One case of enlarged lymph nodes in the axilla has been reported appearing in association with a medullary carcinoma that was clinically and mammographically suspicious for metastatic spread but proved to be benign, reactive adenopathy.

Ultrasound Appearance

Medullary carcinomas by ultrasound are generally well-circumscribed, frequently lobulated, hypoechoic lesions (Fig.

19-96B). They contain low-amplitude internal echoes, although the internal echoes may be quite heterogeneous. Probably because of their uniform cellular composition and circumscribed shape, posterior acoustic enhancement is not unusual in medullary cancer.

Apocrine Carcinoma

The various subtypes of breast cancers recognized by pathologists are due to the various ways that normal cells dedifferentiate into abnormal phenotypes that almost cer-tainly are a reflection of their abnormal genetic composition. One form of altered differentiation is seen in rare cancers that have a large percentage of cells with apocrine features. These have been termed *apocrine carcinomas*, and they make up approximately 0.06% of invasive cancers (68). Many cancers have some cells that have apocrine metapla-sia. To be termed *apocrine carcinoma*, however, the major-ity of the cells should have apocrine characteristics.

These are very rare tumors probably accounting for <1% of ductal cancers. Aside from their histologic features they appear to behave in a similar fashion to ductal carcinoma NOS.

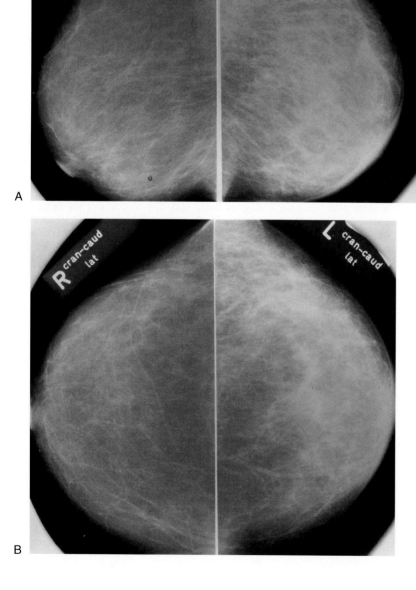

FIG. 19-97. **Inflammatory carcinoma** is indistin-guishable from other causes of inflammation of the breast. In this case, the left breast is diffusely denser due to edema and skin thickening as seen on the magnification lateral **(A)** and craniocaudal **(B)** projec-tions. Note that the right breast is on the left and the left breast is on the right in these figures.

Mammographic Appearance

Although the experience with these tumors is limited, their mammographic appearance does not appear to be distinctive (101). They most commonly present as masses with ill-defined margins. Some have fairly well-defined margins. Some have associated calcifications, but none has any distinctive characteristics that would aid in their mammographic diagnosis.

Ultrasound Appearance

There do not appear to be any characteristics of apocrine carcinoma that would be distinctive on ultrasound.

Inflammatory Carcinoma

The definition of inflammatory carcinoma is somewhat elusive. Many believe that the diagnosis should be made on the clinical manifestations of increased warmth, erythema, and the classic peau d'orange (skin of an orange) appearance of the thickened skin. The latter is named because of the accentuation of the depressions around the hair follicles caused by skin edema. This appearance can be mimicked by benign inflammatory processes. Frequently the diagnosis is difficult to make and a biopsy is required. Antibiotic therapy may improve the clinical changes in both benign and malignant disease. Histologically, inflammatory carcinoma represents diffuse early invasion of the dermal lymphatics by an aggressive form of infiltrating carcinoma. In its pure form, the underlying primary lesion is frequently not evident. Fortunately, it is fairly uncommon, making up approximately 0.5% of invasive breast cancers. Although the incidence of inflammatory cancer increases with age, its relative frequency is highest in young women, peaking around age 30 years (68).

Although recent aggressive therapy (i.e., chemotherapy, mastectomy, and radiation therapy) may have produced some improvement, patients with inflammatory carcinoma generally have a poor prognosis. Pure inflammatory carcinoma appears to carry a worse prognosis than an infiltrating ductal carcinoma that has, secondarily, locally invaded the skin.

Mammographic Appearance

The mammographic appearance of inflammatory carcinoma is indistinguishable from that of other processes that cause skin thickening (Fig. 19-97). In our experience it is unusual to find a mass or tumor-associated calcifications, although in a series of 22 women Dershaw et al. (102) found a mass or significant calcifications in every patient. Inflammatory carcinoma in association with an underlying mass is probably a separate entity representing a later-stage progression of an infiltrating tumor mass with secondary invasion of the dermal lymphatics (Fig. 19-98). There appears to be a predilection for these cancers to develop in the left breast. In the Dershaw et al. series, 67% of the inflammatory cancers first involved the left breast. As with any process that overwhelms the lymphatic drainage, diffuse trabecular thickening and an overall increase in x-ray attenuation may produce a diffuse increase in radiographic density in the affected breast.

Ultrasound Appearance

There is no major role for ultrasound in the evaluation of inflammatory carcinoma unless an abscess or a deep mass is suspected (Fig. 19-99). Inflammatory carcinoma produces nonspecific skin thickening, which is indistinguishable from thickening from any other cause when imaged by ultrasound. The separation of the specular reflections produced by the transducer-skin interface and the second specular reflection at the dermal-subcutaneous fat interface is widened. Low-amplitude echoes are seen within this space, but plain edema cannot be differentiated from actual tumor infiltration.

Ultrasound can be useful in distinguishing infection from inflammatory cancer if an abscess is evident. This can be confirmed by aspiration. The diagnosis of inflammatory cancer is based on the clinical constellation and pathologic proof of breast cancer.

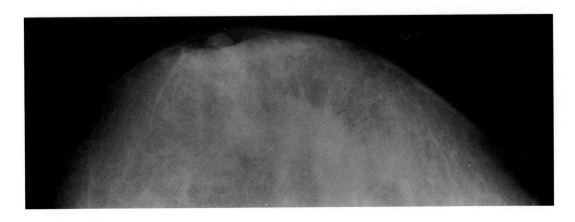

FIG. 19-98. A large **invasive cancer** deep in the breast is responsible for the nipple retraction and skin thickening in this patient.

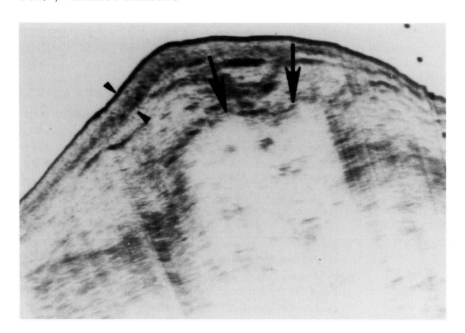

FIG. 19-99. Diffuse skin thickening from inflammatory carcinoma is evident (*small arrows*) on this ultrasound image (black on white) of a patient with a large invasive carcinoma (*large arrows*).

Malignant Lesions of the Lobule

Lobular Carcinoma In Situ

In 1941 Foote and Stewart (103) described a neoplastic process involving the lobule, which they termed LCIS. The lesion consisted of a filling up of the lobule with numerous cells of uniform appearance with round nuclei and relatively clear cytoplasm (Fig. 19-100). Rosen and coworkers (104) noted the high risk of subsequent development of invasive breast cancer (either invasive lobular or invasive ductal) among women with this lesion. The investigators followed up 99 women with LCIS over an average of 24 years. Thirty-nine invasive cancers were diagnosed in 32 women. Half were in the same breast as the LCIS and the other half were in the opposite breast. It is this latter relationship that makes

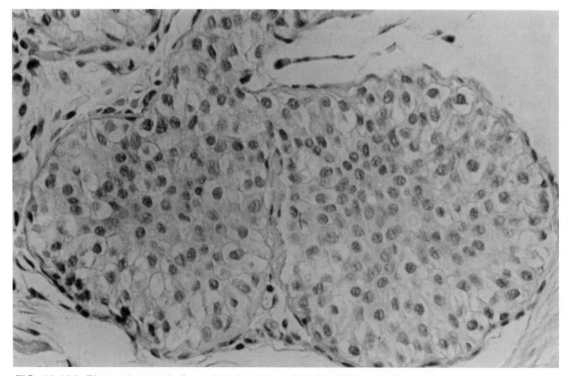

FIG. 19-100. Photomicrograph (hematoxylin and eosin) of **lobular carcinoma in situ** shows the lobular acini distended by a uniform population of round cells with round nuclei and clear cytoplasm.

LCIS such a perplexing lesion because, unlike DCIS, which is primarily a lesion that indicates an ipsilateral risk for invasive cancer (a direct precursor), LCIS represents a lesion that indicates a bilateral risk of invasive cancer. A woman with LCIS has approximately a 15% chance of developing an invasive breast cancer in the breast in which the LCIS is discovered, but she also has a similar risk (15%) in the other breast, for a total risk of developing an invasive cancer in either breast of 30% over the next 20 years and beyond (105,106). According to Rosen et al. (104), a woman with LCIS has nine times the risk of the general population of developing invasive breast cancer and 11 times the risk of dying from breast cancer

LCIS has been described as a serendipitous finding. It does not form palpable masses or lesions that are reproducible on mammography and is generally found coincidentally when a biopsy is performed for some other reason. It is of interest, however, that when LCIS is found coincidentally after a biopsy instigated by concerns raised on a mammogram, the reason for the biopsy is often nonspecific clustered calcifications. This was the experience of Pope et al. (107) and Beute et al. (108), and it has been our experience as well. It remains to be seen how the calcifications actually relate to the LCIS.

Because it has been difficult to relate LCIS directly to invasive breast cancers, some have suggested that it be considered a risk factor such as atypical hyperplasia (which is also a bilateral risk) rather than true breast cancer. Haagensen (109) suggested that LCIS should actually be termed *lobular neoplasia*. Although the terminology has not been universally accepted, most physicians now favor the latter implication. Although LCIS has remained the terminology of choice, LCIS is not counted as breast cancer in reports of breast cancer trials.

Because the exact relationship of LCIS to invasive breast cancer remains to be defined, it is generally not treated. Although the risk of subsequent cancer is high, the majority of women will still not be affected. Thus, when LCIS is found, most now recommend careful follow-up with annual mammography, and at least annual, if not more frequent, CBE. Any more aggressive treatment would legitimately have to involve both breasts because the risk of subsequent invasive breast cancer is equal for both breasts. Whether careful follow-up will prove to be the best course of action remains to be seen.

Beute et al. (108) found that LCIS was more commonly found in younger women than ductal carcinoma. Our anecdotal experience agrees with theirs. It has also been our experience that LCIS is found more commonly in women with radiographically dense breasts. Beute et al. found the same. Their review indicated that 85% of women with LCIS had breast tissues that were >50% dense. They went as far as to speculate that the persistence of dense breast tissue patterns in postmenopausal women might indicate a higher percentage with LCIS and an increased risk for breast cancer. This remains to be proved. Given the difficulty in finding early cancer in women with dense breast tissue and the propensity for LCIS to be in dense breast tissues, the success of close follow-up remains to be proved.

Mammographic Appearance

Lobular carcinoma in situ is generally a histologic diagnosis and more than likely a serendipitous association with lesions seen mammographically. Most investigators who have reviewed large numbers of cases have concluded that LCIS is a serendipitous finding. As already noted, however, calcifications are a common occurrence in benign tissue adjacent to the LCIS. On occasion, calcifications are found within the LCIS. The exact relationship of these calcifications to the underlying process remains to be elucidated, but it is likely that LCIS represents a field abnormality in which cells throughout the breast (and often bilaterally) have undergone changes that predispose them to future malignant change. The calcifications are likely a reflection of this field phenomenon. A tumor mass is rarely seen. As noted above, it is our impression that LCIS is more common in the radiographically dense breast.

Ultrasound Appearance

The ultrasound findings of LCIS are also not well characterized. Some have described hypoechoic tissue with associated posterior acoustic shadowing, but it is unclear whether this represents the lesion itself or adjacent tissues that were beside the serendipitous, histologically detected LCIS.

Infiltrating (Invasive) Lobular Carcinoma

Infiltrating lobular carcinoma (ILC) was first described in 1946 by Foote and Stewart (110). Pathologists have since recognized forms of invasive breast cancers whose cytologic features suggest that they arose from the epithelium of the lobule. ILC accounts for <10% of breast malignancies. Some studies have suggested that ILC is more often bilateral than invasive ductal carcinoma (111). This perhaps reflects the propensity for LCIS to be bilateral, although the exact relationship of LCIS to ILC is unclear.

Histologically, ILC is often insidious in its development. It frequently invades the normal tissues without invoking the vigorous desmoplastic response that usually accompanies infiltrating ductal cancer, and is characterized by similar cells forming into linear invasive columns. This may account for the fact that ILC is frequently less apparent on mammograms than invasive ductal carcinoma. Because it is not as readily detected as is invasive ductal carcinoma, ILCs are generally somewhat larger at diagnosis. In a comparison between invasive duct cancers and ILCs, Silverstein et al. (112) found that the average size at diagnosis for 1,138 invasive ductal cancers was 23 mm, whereas the average size of the 161 ILCs was 29 mm.

Although most have suggested that ILC has a similar prognosis as invasive duct carcinoma, a review by Le Gal et al. (113) and the one by Silverstein et al. suggest that ILC may have a slightly more favorable prognosis with fewer women with positive nodes at diagnosis. When ILC does metastasize, there are some data that suggest a propensity for spread to endocrine organs such as the adrenals (114).

Mammographic Appearance

ILC is notoriously difficult to detect early (115,116). It frequently develops insidiously and is diagnosed at a later stage than most invasive ductal cancers. There are no features that characteristically distinguish an ILC from an infiltrating ductal carcinoma. When visible mammographically, these lesions generally have ill-defined margins and distort the architecture in a manner similar to that of their ductal counterparts. Calcifications can occur, but once again, this is not a particularly distinguishing feature. Le Gal et al. (113) found little differences between the mammographic appearance of ILC when compared to invasive ductal carcinoma. Mendelson et al. (117) described five patterns in 50 patients, half of whom had palpable cancers:

1. Asymmetric density without definable margins was the most common pattern.
2. A high-density mass with spiculated margins was the next most common presentation.
3. Dense breast tissue with no tumor discernible by mammography was fairly uncommon in their series.
4. Microcalcifications: 25% of the lesions contained calcifications, but calcifications alone were rarely the reason for biopsy and more than half the time the calcifications were in contiguous, benign tissue.
5. Round, discrete mass was a rare presentation for ILC.

These patterns seem indistinguishable from those of invasive ductal carcinoma. The fairly common presentation of asymmetric density without a definable mass and the cases in which there is no abnormality by mammography, however, contribute to the fact that ILC is frequently more difficult to diagnose at a small size.

Although ILC can form typical spiculated masses, it frequently appears as an area of progressively increasing density in an area of radiographically dense breast tissue. Krecke and Gisvold (118) found that because it frequently does not form a demonstrable mass or distort the architecture or commonly produce calcifications, and is frequently isodense with normal tissue, it is not unusual for ILC to go undetected on sequential mammograms until it becomes clinically evident (Fig. 19-101). Retrospective review of the mammograms will sometimes show a subtle and gradual increase in density over several years with little architectural distortion in the area of the ILC, although the distortion ultimately becomes evident. Most investigators agree that ILC often does not produce a central tumor mass that is visible by mammography as is frequently the case for invasive ductal carcinoma.

Ultrasound Appearance

ILC cannot be distinguished from infiltrating ductal carcinoma by ultrasound. The morphology of the two lesions is similar both grossly and by imaging techniques, and on ultrasound, hypoechoic tissue is seen with varying degrees of posterior acoustic shadowing.

Other Unusual Malignant Lesions

Malignant lesions of other than ductal origin occur within the breast, but most are extremely rare.

Sarcomas of the Breast

The remaining malignant lesions of the breast arise from the stromal structures. Sarcomas of the breast are extremely uncommon, constituting <1% of all malignant breast tumors. Included in this category are the occasionally malignant phylloides tumor, previously called *cystosarcoma*, angiosarcomas, and non–epithelium-containing stromal sarcomas.

Phylloides Tumor

The phylloides (or phyllodes) tumor is an unusual stromal tumor, and many believe it is related to the fibroadenoma. Although listed here among the sarcomas, most now do not classify it as a sarcoma, although the malignant form metastasizes to the lung as does a sarcoma and not to the axillary lymph nodes. The term is due to its "leafy" pattern of growth. Most are indolent and benign, but approximately 25% will recur locally if treated incompletely and approximately 10% can be expected to metastasize. Some divide the malignant lesions into low and high grade. The phylloides tumor has been described in women at virtually all ages, although its peak prevalence between ages 30 and 50 years occurs earlier than breast cancer (119). Its prevalence appears to have diminished over the past years, and it has been suggested that this may be the result of more aggressive removal of solid breast lesions. Pathologists can mistake phylloides tumors for benign fibroadenomas.

In general, a phylloides tumor presents as a rapidly enlarging mass that is many centimeters in size when diagnosis is made. It normally has smooth, lobulated contours and remains relatively mobile even when very large. Although sharply defined, it does not have a true capsule. The phylloides tumor appears to arise, as does the fibroadenoma, from the specialized connective tissue of the lobule. The convoluted hypercellular overgrowth found in this lesion causes elongation and distortion of the ducts that produce slit-like, epithelium-lined clefts and cystic spaces that have contributed to the older terminology of *cystosarcoma*. The tumor is usually more cellular than a fibroadenoma. This is particularly evident in the stroma adjacent to the

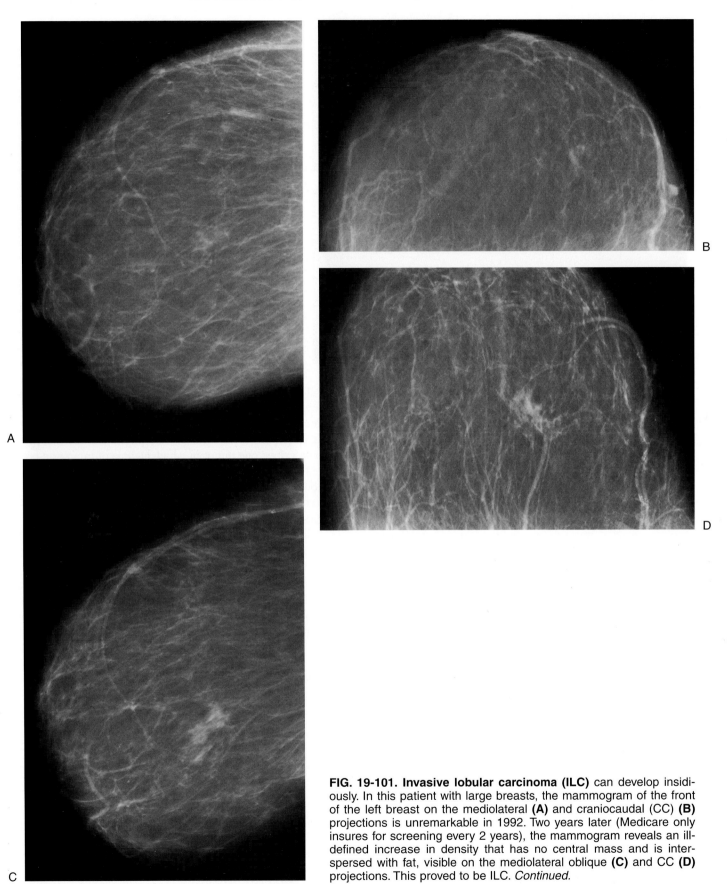

FIG. 19-101. Invasive lobular carcinoma (ILC) can develop insidiously. In this patient with large breasts, the mammogram of the front of the left breast on the mediolateral **(A)** and craniocaudal (CC) **(B)** projections is unremarkable in 1992. Two years later (Medicare only insures for screening every 2 years), the mammogram reveals an ill-defined increase in density that has no central mass and is interspersed with fat, visible on the mediolateral oblique **(C)** and CC **(D)** projections. This proved to be ILC. *Continued.*

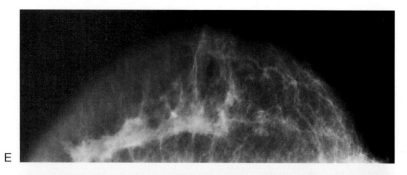

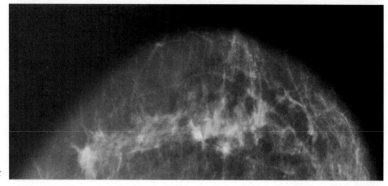

FIG. 19-101. *Continued.* When **ILC** arises in denser tissue, it can go undetected for a longer period of time as in this second case. The CC projection in 1994 **(E)** is unremarkable except when compared to the CC projection **(F)** from 15 months earlier. The entire parenchymal density has increased, due to ILC but the architecture is fairly well preserved. It is fairly common with ILC for the architecture to be preserved because the cells infiltrate in columns often with normal tissue in between, and the tumor frequently appears to elicit little desmoplastic response.

stretched ducts found within the tumor. Increased mitoses characterize the malignant forms.

Malignant phylloides tumors contain sarcomatous elements. The majority resemble fibrosarcomas. Liposarcomatous differentiation is the next most common finding, with chondrosarcomas being the least common. There are insufficient data available to make accurate comparisons, but because these sarcomatous elements arise from the cells of the specialized connective tissue of the lobule (intralobular), their prognosis is likely different from the usual (although rare) sarcomas of the breast that arise from the extralobular stroma, or interlobular connective tissue.

Most phylloides tumors are benign, but the differentiation of benign from malignant is only possible by histologic analysis of mitotic activity, cytologic atypia, and infiltrative versus pushing margins. Phylloides tumors can be locally invasive and recur if not completely excised. When metastases occur, they are usually hematogenous and not to the axilla by way of the lymphatics.

Wide excision may be sufficient to eliminate this lesion. If the tumor recurs, more radical wide excision or mastectomy appears to be the treatment of choice.

Mammographic Appearance. Phylloides tumors are indistinguishable by mammography from other well-circumscribed breast lesions. Although their margins may be obscured by the surrounding parenchyma (Fig. 19-102), they are generally well-defined lesions (Fig. 19-103). Spiculation does not occur, and microcalcifications are not a feature of this lesion. A halo may be seen surrounding the tumor, but once again, this is merely related to the macroscopically smooth margin.

Liberman et al. (120) found that there were no traits evident by mammography or ultrasound that could be used to differentiate benign from malignant phylloides tumors, although tumors >3 cm were more likely to be malignant. In their review of 46 women with 51 phylloides tumors, they also described one tumor in which an area of infarction produced calcifications that resembled the type of large calcifications found in involuting fibroadenomas. They also described a case of a phylloides tumor arising in a hamartoma. We believe that this is an extremely rare occurrence.

Ultrasound Appearance. The ultrasound appearance of phylloides tumors is usually identical to that of fibroadenomas. They are generally well-circumscribed lesions, distinguished only by their relatively large size. Variable low-amplitude internal echoes are present (Fig. 19-103A, B). Occasionally they may even be difficult to distinguish from the surrounding fat using ultrasound (Fig. 19-104). Retrotumoral echoes may be diminished, isoechoic, or increased. Fluid-filled, slit-like spaces are sometimes seen (121), but diagnosis remains speculative, and the lesion requires biopsy to establish the diagnosis.

Fibrosarcoma and Liposarcoma

Sarcomas of the breast are extremely rare. We have no experience with fibrosarcomas or liposarcomas.

Angiosarcoma

Fortunately a rare malignancy, angiosarcoma has a very poor prognosis. It is generally seen in younger age groups, although it may occur in women at any age. On CBE the tumor presents as a palpable mass or thickening. If it is close

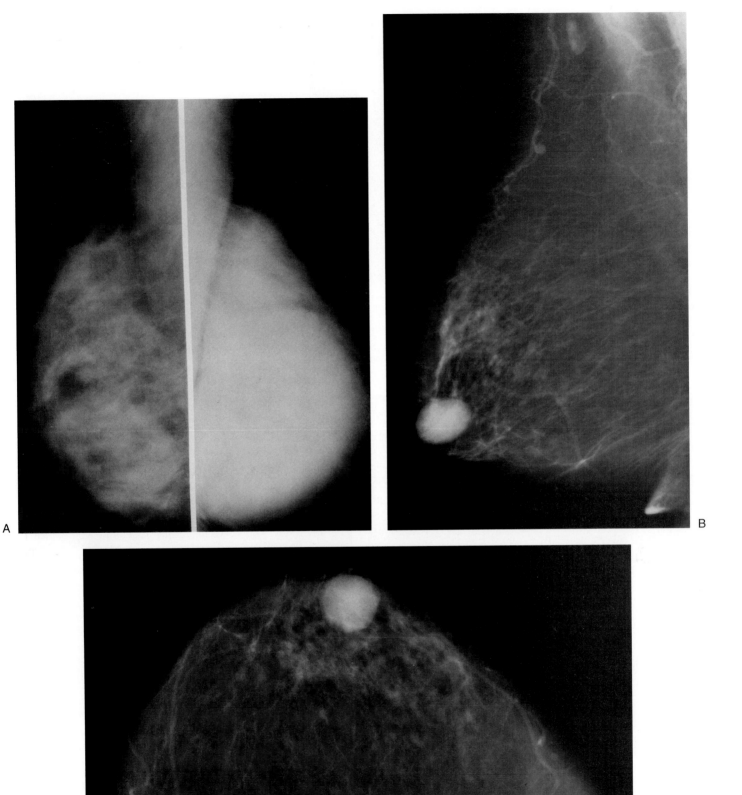

FIG. 19-102. The large mass **(A)** in the right breast in this 28-year-old woman is obscured by the surrounding dense tissue. It had grown rapidly over several months and proved to be a **phylloides tumor.**
    This phylloides tumor in a 71-year-old woman was a well-defined circumscribed mass seen on this mediolateral oblique **(B)** and craniocaudal **(C)** projection. *Continued.*

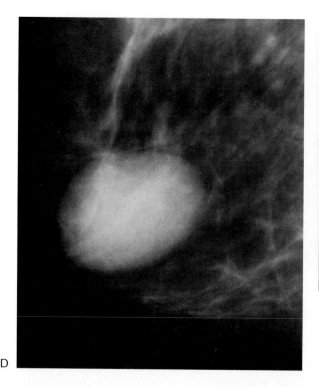

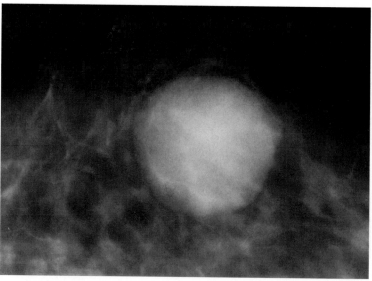

D

E

FIG. 19-102. *Continued.* The images are enlarged **(D, E)** to show the sharply defined border. This mass had grown rapidly over a 7-month period.

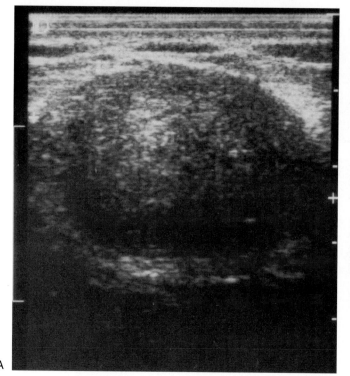

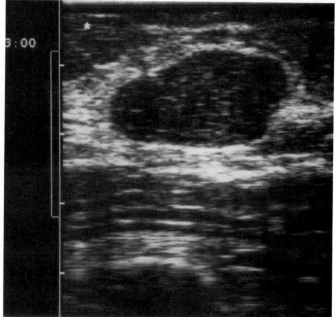

A

B

FIG. 19-103. (A) This **phylloides tumor** was found in an 18-year-old woman. On ultrasound, it is ovoid with a uniform internal echo texture. **(B)** Ultrasound of the phylloides tumor in Fig. 19-102 B–E. It is smoothly lobulated with a uniform internal echotexture and enhanced through-transmission of sound.

to the skin, there may be a blue discoloration in the skin. The lesions are firm and composed of vascular channels that may be similar in appearance to those of benign hemangiomas. As with tumors of capillary origin, the diagnosis is made by the cytologic analysis. Pathologists now divide angiosarco-mas into low, intermediate, and high grade (122). Benign hemangiomas occur in the breast, but they are invariably <2 cm, whereas angiosarcomas are usually >2 cm.

Angiosarcomas are almost uniformly fatal with rapid metastatic spread, and survival beyond 5 years is extremely

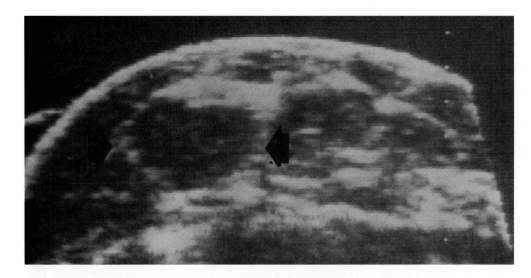

FIG. 19-104. On whole-breast ultrasound, this phylloides tumor (*arrows*) was almost indistinguishable from the normal surrounding fat.

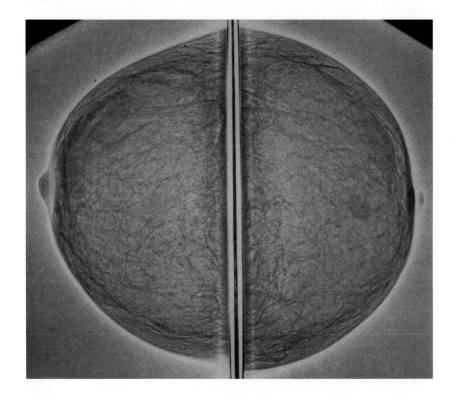

FIG. 19-105. The lobulated mass in the anterior right breast on this positive mode xerogram (dark areas are dense; light areas are fat) proved to be an angiosarcoma. (Reprinted with permission of William Ladd, M.D.)

rare, although the more recent division of the lesions by grade suggests that women with low- and intermediate-grade lesions may have better survival. Because these lesions spread as sarcomas, axillary dissection is not indicated.

When seen mammographically, angiosarcomas appear somewhat lobulated and ill defined (Fig. 19-105). Microcalcifications and spiculations are not distinguishing features.

Osteogenic Sarcoma

Primary osteogenic sarcoma can occur in extraosseous locations and has been reported in the breast (123). They are rare but can occur in an area that was previously irradiated.

It has been postulated that they arise from mesenchymal cells in fibroadenomas.

A lesion reported by Watt et al. (123) was densely ossified with thread-like spiculations of sarcoma-produced osteoid. We have seen two cases of osteogenic sarcoma in the breast. One was a well-defined mass with somewhat unusual calcifications (Fig. 19-106); the other was irregularly shaped.

Malignant Fibrous Histiocytoma

A very rare breast lesion, malignant fibrous histiocytoma (MFH) of the breast has been associated with a history of

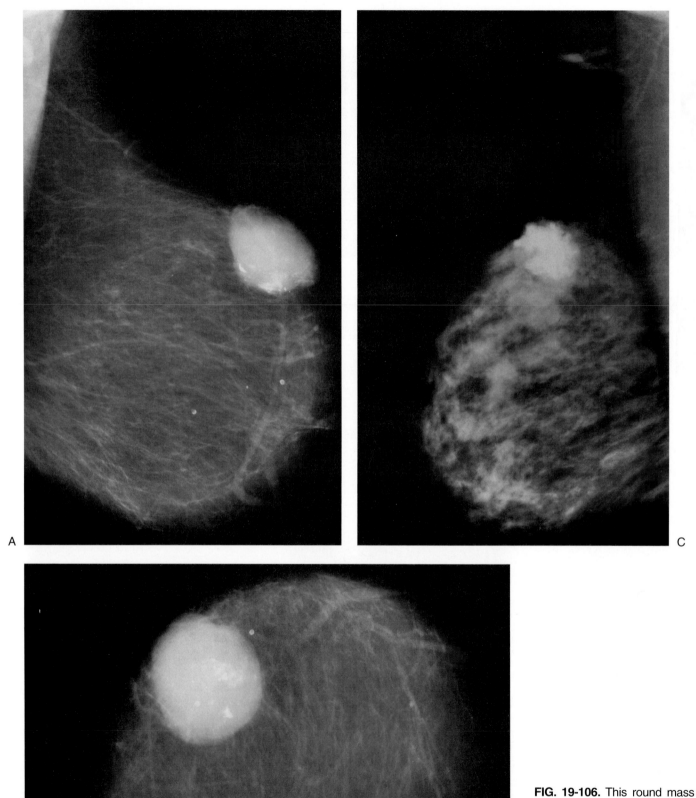

FIG. 19-106. This round mass with ossifications on the lateral **(A)** and craniocaudal **(B)** projections proved to be an **osteogenic sarcoma.** A second, irregular and irregularly calcified mass on the mediolateral **(C)** projection also proved to be an **osteogenic sarcoma.**

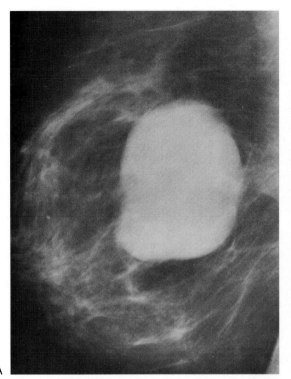
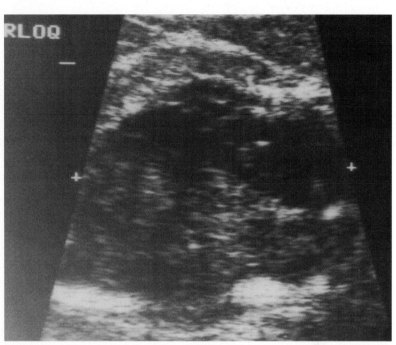

A   B

FIG. 19-107. This large smoothly lobulated mass **(A)** proved to be a malignant fibrous histiocytoma. On ultrasound **(B)**, it appeared complex, with a heterogeneous internal echo texture that was indistinguishable from a carcinoma, abscess, or hematoma.

previous radiation therapy, but a few cases have been reported without this association (124). This form of sarcoma is much more likely to arise in the connective tissue of the extremities, abdominal cavity, or retroperitoneum. Composed of spindle cells and histiocytes, MFH carries a fairly good prognosis, although it may recur locally and can metastasize and be lethal.

The reported cases presented as bulky masses. Metastatic spread appears to be hematogenous, because the axillary nodes are rarely involved. Wide excision is the minimal suggested treatment, but mastectomy is preferred. Tumors that occur in the postirradiated breast appear to have a poorer prognosis.

Mammographic Appearance. The literature on malignant fibrous histiocytoma in the breast is not extensive. When

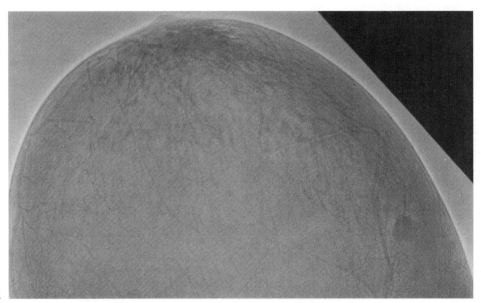

A

FIG. 19-108. **(A)** Adenoid cystic carcinoma may be fairly well circumscribed, as seen on this craniocaudal positive-mode xerogram (dark is dense; light is fat). *Continued.*

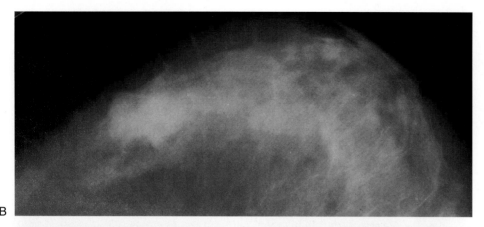

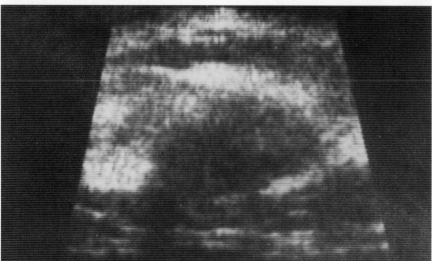

FIG. 19-108. *Continued.* In a second case of **adenoid cystic carcinoma (B)**, the lesion presented as an ill-defined obscured mass. On ultrasound **(C)**, the second case was an ovoid mass with somewhat irregular margins but a uniform internal echo texture. This is a nonspecific appearance.

mammograms have been obtained, the lesion appears to be large and fairly well circumscribed with lobulated margins (Fig. 19-107). Spiculations and microcalcifications have not been described.

Ultrasound Appearance. There is no large experience with the ultrasound appearance of MFH. Our one case of MFH had a nonspecific appearance that reflected its circumscribed lobulated shape (Fig. 19-107B). It is impossible to distinguish this appearance from a carcinoma, abscess, or hematoma.

Adenoid Cystic Carcinoma

Adenoid cystic carcinoma is generally associated with the salivary glands, but occasionally, these lesions develop in the breast. They represent extremely indolent processes, and although death from adenoid cystic carcinoma of the breast has been reported, it is extremely rare.

The diagnosis is made by histologic analysis, and special stains are used to reveal the mucin that is associated with the pseudocysts found in the tumor.

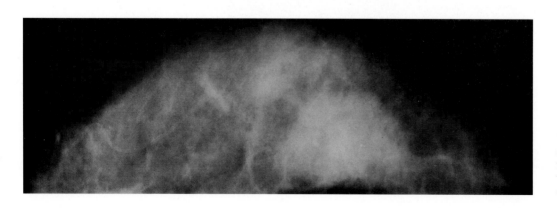

FIG. 19-109. This large spiculated mass in a 63-year-old woman proved to be an **adenoid cystic carcinoma**.

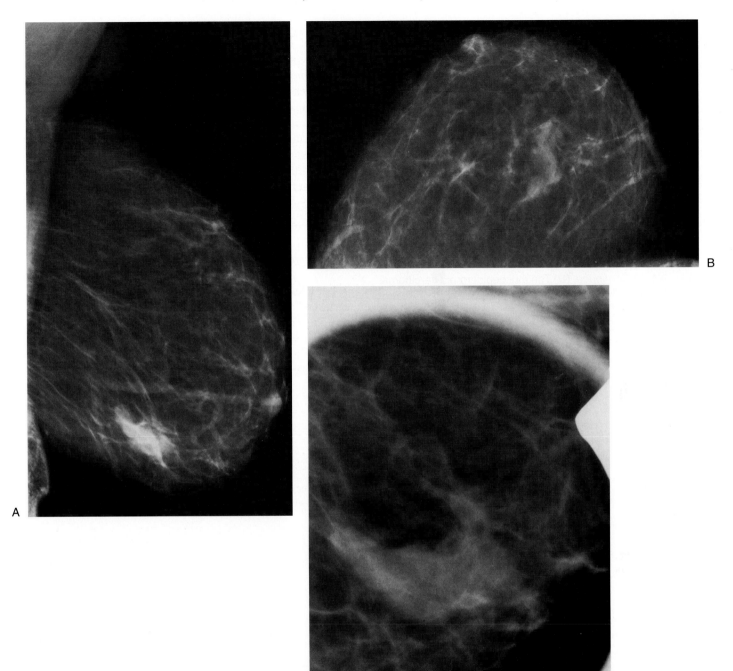

FIG. 19-110. A **mucoepidermoid carcinoma** in a 51-year-old woman seen on the mediolateral **(A)**, craniocaudal **(B)**, and spot magnification lateral **(C)** projections. *Continued.*

Mammographic Appearance. There is a limited experience with these lesions reported in the literature. Our three cases were all somewhat different. One presented as a small, fairly well-defined, slightly lobulated mass (Fig. 19-108A), whereas the second was larger with a much more ill-defined margin (Fig. 19-108B). The third was a large spiculated lesion (Fig. 19-109).

Mucoepidermoid Carcinoma

Mucoepidermoid carcinoma is another extremely rare lesion in the breast with no particular prognostic significance. It is a tumor that is generally found in the salivary gland, although it has been described in the breast (125).

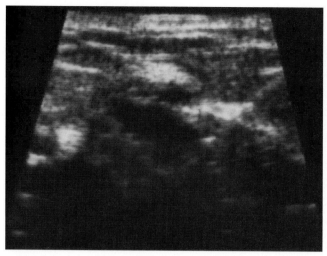

D

FIG. 19-110. *Continued.* **(D)** The mucoepidermoid carcinoma on ultrasound was nonspecific in appearance. It is hypoechoic with posterior shadowing.

Page and Anderson (14) suggest that these may be variants of mucinous carcinoma. These lesions contain mucin-secreting cells, as well as epidermoid cells and myoepithelium.

Mammographic Appearance. We have seen a single case of this lesion (Fig. 19-110 A–C). The lesion was lobulated and elongated with no distinguishing features.

Ultrasound Appearance. The ultrasound of our single case of mucoepidermoid carcinoma demonstrated that the elongated mass was not a cystically dilated duct; otherwise it was of little value. It demonstrated an irregular, hypoechoic mass that blocked the transmission of sound (Fig. 19-110D).

Tumors of Lymphoid Origin

Lymphoma of the Breast

Lymphoma of the breast can occur primarily or as a metastatic lesion from elsewhere in the body. It is extremely rare for lymphoma to appear in the breast without evidence of the disease elsewhere in the body. These lesions account for only approximately 0.1% of breast malignancy (126). Secondary involvement is more common, although it, too, is

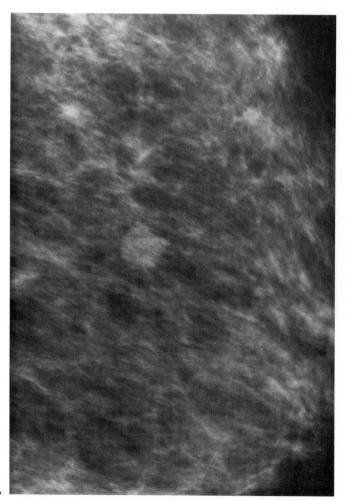

A

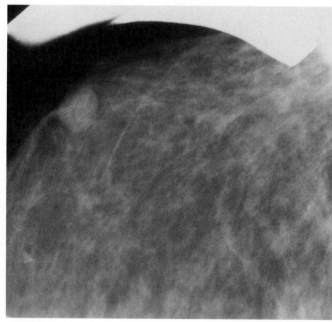

B

FIG. 19-111. This nodule, seen on the magnification lateral **(A)** and the spot magnification craniocaudal **(B)** projections proved to be **lymphoma** at biopsy in a 56-year-old woman with no other sites of involvement.

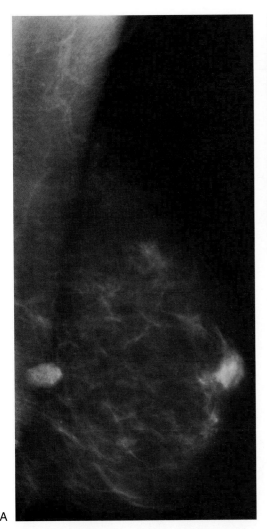

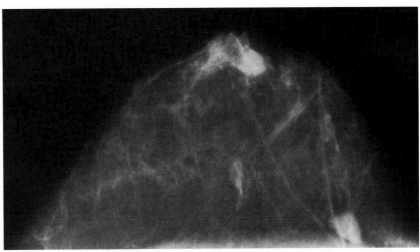

A

B

FIG. 19-112. These are multiple nodules of lymphoma seen on the mediolateral oblique **(A)** and craniocaudal **(B)** projections in the breast of a woman who has had known **lymphoma** for 5 years.

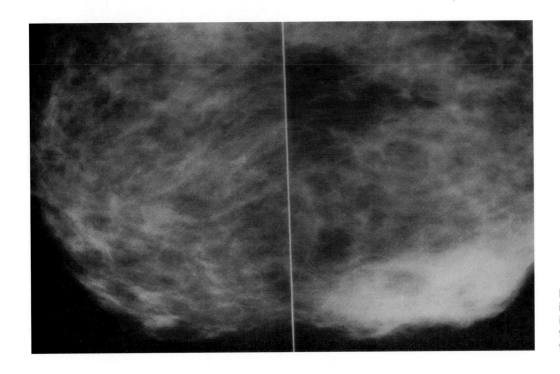

FIG. 19-113. The diffuse increase in density medially in the right breast seen on these craniocaudal projections was due to **lymphoma.**

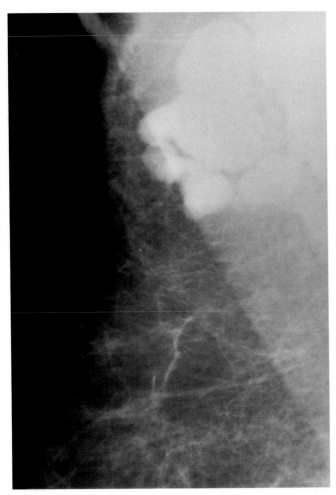

FIG. 19-114. The large axillary nodes in this patient were due to lymphoma.

unusual. Lymphoma presents as either a discrete palpable mass or diffuse thickening. When large axillary nodes are present at the same time as a palpable intramammary mass, the diagnosis should be considered.

Mammographic Appearance

Mammary lymphoma may produce a single discrete nodule (Fig. 19-111) or multiple nodules (Fig. 19-112). It may also produce a diffuse increase in radiographic density (Fig. 19-113). Nodules may be well circumscribed or have margins that fade into the surrounding tissue. The lesion's borders may be ill defined, but spiculations are not a feature of lymphoma. A diffuse increase in density can also occur, and although the presence of large axillary nodes should raise the possibility of lymphoma (Fig. 19-114), axillary nodal involvement is radiographically indistinguishable from diffuse ductal cancer with regional nodal involvement (Fig. 19-115) or even lymphoid hyperplasia (Fig. 19-116). We have seen lymphoma in the breast resolve with therapy (Fig. 19-117).

Lieberman et al. (127) reviewed 32 lesions in 29 women. Two-thirds of the lesions were primary. In 69% of the

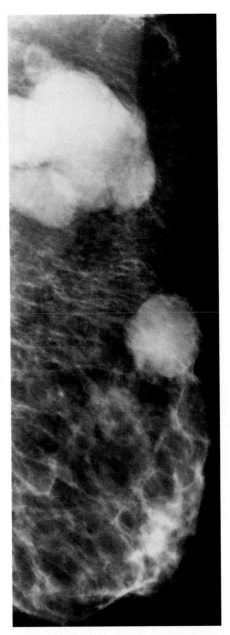

FIG. 19-115. Lymphoma is indistinguishable from breast cancer metastatic to the axillary nodes, although, in our experience, lymphoma is more commonly seen by mammography. The round mass in the breast of this 78-year-old woman on this axillary tail view was **invasive ductal carcinoma,** and the large axillary masses are lymph nodes involved with tumor in the axilla.

cases, the lesion was solitary, and three women had multiple masses.

Ultrasound Appearance

Lymphoma in the breast produces a nonspecific hypoechoic mass (Fig. 19-118) with variable through-transmission of sound. The lesion is clearly solid, containing low-amplitude echoes but cannot be diagnosed by ultrasound.

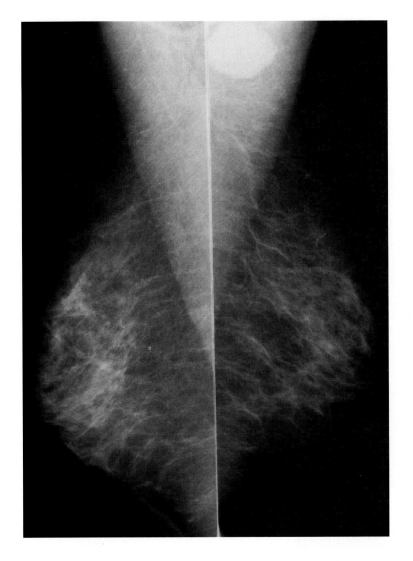

FIG. 19-116. The large axillary node on the right in this patient proved to be **benign lymphoid hyperplasia.**

Metastatic Lesions to the Breast

Cancer from other organs can metastasize to the breast (128). Melanoma is the most common tumor to produce this relatively rare event. It is of interest that breast cancer cells (of ectodermal origin) may produce pigment, and histologically, there can be confusion between melanoma and breast cancer. Excluding sarcomas and lymphomas, the next most common tumor to metastasize to the breast is lung cancer, followed by stomach, ovary, and kidney, with at least one case reported from most other common cancer sites, such as ovary, cervix, thyroid, colon, uterus, and bladder. Prostate cancer in males has been known to appear in the breast.

There is clinically little to distinguish these lesions except for the history of an antecedent primary malignancy.

Mammographic Appearance

Lesions that metastasize to the breast may produce changes similar to those of primary breast cancer, but they are more likely to be multiple; are frequently bilateral; and, perhaps, owing to their centripetal growth, form a nidus of tumor cells that are usually round with fairly well-defined margins (Fig. 19-119). Microcalcifications are not a distinguishing feature, and although their margins may be ill defined, spiculations are not commonly found.

Ultrasound Appearance

Lesions that metastasize to the breast have ultrasound findings that reflect their shape and composition (129). Usually round or ovoid with some degree of lobulation, they have variable internal echoes ranging from scattered low-amplitude signals to heterogeneous fairly prominent reflections (Fig. 19-120).

The posterior echoes are usually preserved, and as with all round solid breast masses, relative enhancement may occur.

Metaplastic Bone Formation

Actual bone formation in the breast is unusual, but it can be seen in benign processes, such as hematomas and fat necrosis.

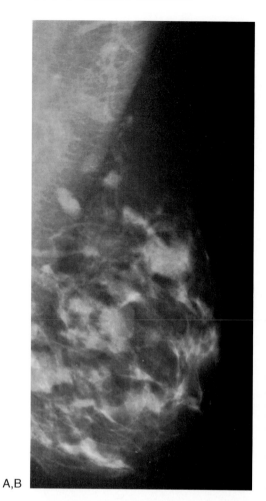 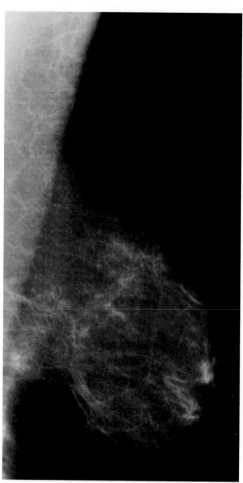

A,B

FIG. 19-117. Masses due to lymphoma may resolve with therapy. The masses seen here **(A)** disappeared after chemotherapy for lymphoma **(B)**.

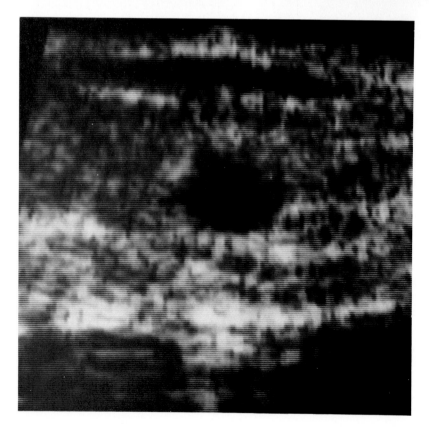

FIG. 19-118. Lymphoma by ultrasound is hypoechoic, with a shape that is consistent with its appearance on mammography. If the mass is round, it will be round by ultrasound. If it is irregular, it will be irregular by ultrasound. The internal echoes are low level and through-transmission is variable.

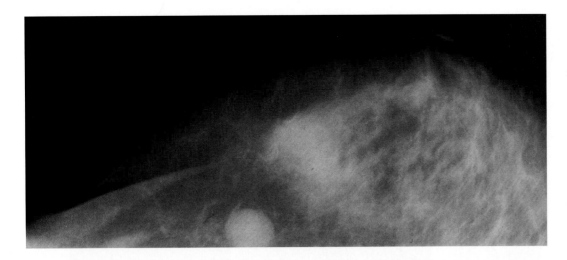

FIG. 19-119. Lesions that are metastatic to the breast from other organs are frequently fairly well defined. This round density was **metastatic melanoma.**

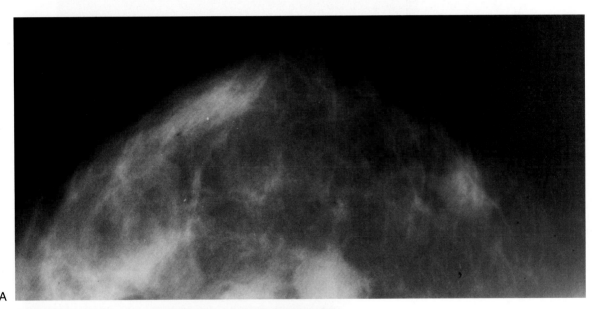

A

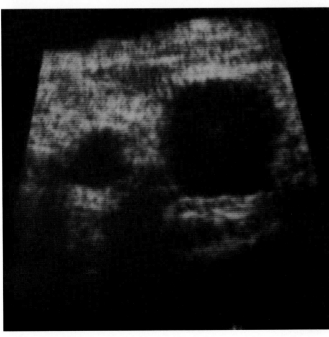

B

FIG. 19-120. (A) Metastatic renal cell carcinoma formed round masses on the mammogram. **(B)** On ultrasound the masses could almost be mistaken for cysts. They are round and regular with extremely low-level internal echoes and enhancement of the posterior echoes.

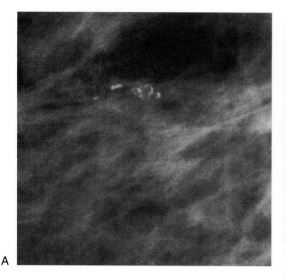

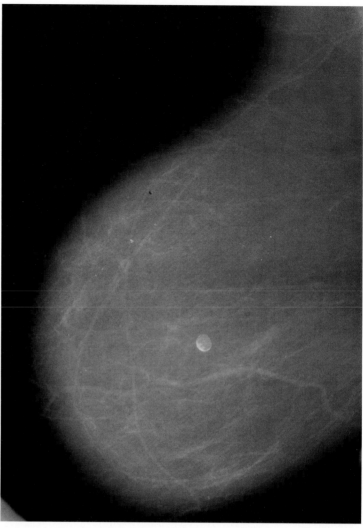

FIG. 19-121. (A) **Metaplastic bone** was found in association with intraductal carcinoma at the biopsy of this collection of irregularly shaped calcifications. **(B)** Metaplastic bone was found in the wall of this benign cyst.

A

B

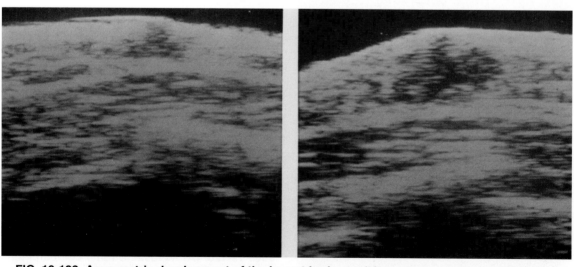

FIG. 19-122. **Asymmetric development of the breast buds** at adolescence is not unusual. The triangular, hypoechoic tissues in this adolescent girl are the breast buds developing asymmetrically. Asymmetric development should not be mistaken for a mass because its removal will preclude future breast development.

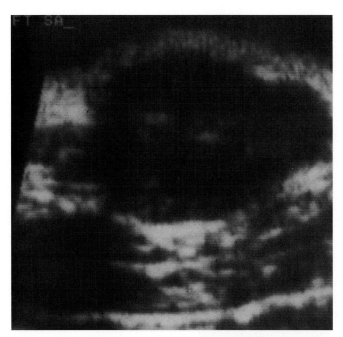

FIG. 19-123. An unusual **secretory carcinoma** was diagnosed in this 5-year-old girl who had a palpable mass that was eccentric to the nipple. It was a lobulated, hypoechoic mass, as seen on this ultrasound.

Malignant lesions, including sarcomas as well as adenocarcinomas, also have been known to develop bone. Osteogenic sarcoma is described above. The mechanism of bone formation in breast tumors is probably due to cellular metaplasia (130), although in some tumors it may be the result of alterations in the primitive cells. Bone in the breast has been known to take up radionuclide bone-scanning agents.

Mammographic Appearance

Metaplastic bone formation is an uncommon entity. It can be suspected when the matrix of the calcifications is unusual, forming coarse deposits (Fig. 19-121), but the diagnosis can only be made by biopsy.

Tumor Masses in Preadolescent Females

It should be emphasized that significant breast pathology is extremely unusual in preadolescent females. On occasion the breast bud will develop asymmetrically and present as an enlarging unilateral subareolar mass. There is no indication for mammography in such patients. Ultrasound can demonstrate hypoechoic, triangular tissue and will probably demonstrate smaller but similar tissue on the contralateral side (Fig. 19-122). This subareolar tissue should not be excised, because removal of the breast bud will prevent future breast development.

Significant breast pathology is uncommon before puberty. Fibroadenomas can occur and usually present as

well-circumscribed masses eccentric from the nipple. A rare form of breast cancer is found in this age group, but fortunately it is indolent.

Secretory Carcinoma

Secretory carcinoma is a rare form of ductal carcinoma that may occur in the adult, but it is a rare form of breast cancer that has been described in the preadolescent as well. The tumor usually presents a hard mass eccentric to the nipple.

Histologically, its abundant secretions are similar to lactation, producing eosinophilic-staining material. It rarely metastasizes, but some cases of this tumor have been lethal.

Mammographic Appearance

Mammography is not indicated in preadolescent and adolescent girls. Cancer is virtually unheard of and radiation risk for the breast is high at these young ages.

Ultrasound Appearance

Our only experience with secretory carcinoma was in a 5-year-old girl who developed a mass eccentric to the nipple. Because of the patient's age, mammography was not performed. Ultrasound demonstrated a hypoechoic lesion with heterogeneous internal echo texture and posterior acoustic enhancement, indistinguishable from a fibroadenoma (Fig. 19-123).

Other Breast Problems

Poland's Syndrome

Poland's syndrome was first described in 1841 as an absence of the pectoralis major muscle (131). According to Samuels et al. (132), it affects one in 36,000 to 50,000 people (men and women are equally affected). Absence or underdevelopment of the breast is common as are anomalies of the thoracic bones and costal cartilage (133). Vascular compromise during intrauterine growth has been postulated, but the cause remains idiopathic.

Mammographic Appearance

In the case described by Samuels et al. (132), one breast was considerably smaller than the other with no pectoralis major visible on the affected side. They performed a computed tomography scan that confirmed the absence of pectoralis major muscle on the affected side. In the single case that we have seen, there was a virtual absence of the breast (Fig. 19-124) with no visible pectoralis major.

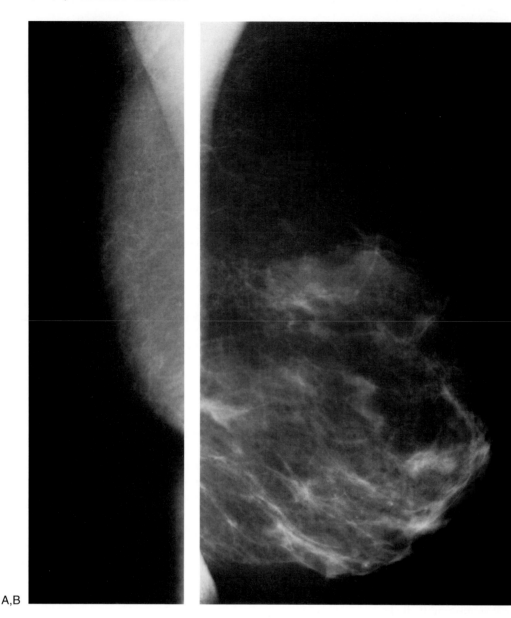

A,B

FIG. 19-124. Poland's syndrome. Note the marked difference in the size and development of the abnormal left breast **(A)** relative to the normal right breast **(B)** in this patient with congenital absence of the chest wall muscles and soft tissues.

Ultrasound Findings

There is no indication for routine ultrasound in women with Poland's syndrome, but Sferlazza and Cohen (134) reported that the absence of the pectoralis major muscle could be demonstrated by ultrasound.

REFERENCES

1. Harms SE, Flamig DP, Hesley KL, et al. Fat-suppressed three-dimensional MR imaging of the breast. Radiographics 1993;13:247–267.
2. Prechtel K. Mastopathic und Altersabhangige Brystdrusen Verandernagen. Fortschr Med 1971;89:1312–1315.
3. Love SM, Gelman RS, Silen W. Fibrocystic disease of the breast—a nondisease? N Engl J Med 1982;307:1010.
4. Dupont WD, Page DL. Risk factors for breast cancer in women with proliferative breast disease. N Engl J Med 1985;312:146.
5. Cancer Committee of the College of American Pathologists. Consensus Meeting—"Is 'fibrocystic disease' of the breast precancerous?" October 3–5, 1985. Arch Pathol Lab Med 1986;110:171–173.
6. Kriger N, Hiatt RA. Risk of breast cancer after benign breast diseases: variation by histologic type, degree of atypia, age at biopsy, and length of follow-up. Am J Epidemiol 1992;135:619–631.
7. Connolly J, Schnitt S, London S, et al. Both atypical lobular hyperplasia and atypical ductal hyperplasia predict for bilateral breast cancer risk. Lab Invest 1992;66:13A.
8. Stomper PC, Cholewinski SP, Penetrante RB, et al. Atypical hyperplasia: frequency and mammographic and pathologic relationships in excisional biopsies guided with mammography and clinical examination. Radiology 1993;189:667–671.
9. Wellings SR, Jensen HM. On the origin and progression of ductal carcinoma in the human breast. J Natl Cancer Institute 1973;50:111.
10. Gallager HS, Martin JE. Early phases in the development of breast cancer. CA Cancer J Clin 1969;24:1170.

11. Fechner RE, Mills SE. Breast Pathology: Benign Proliferations, Atypias and In Situ Carcinomas. Chicago: American Society of Clinical Pathologists Press, 1990;45–49.

12. Peerizin KH, Lattes R. Papillary adenoma of the nipple. A clinico-pathologic study. Cancer 1972;29:996–1009.

13. Rosen PP, Oberman HA. Tumors of the Mammary Gland. Atlas of Tumor Pathology. Washington, DC: Armed Forces Institute of Pathology, 1992.

14. Page DL, Anderson TJ. Diagnostic Histopathology of the Breast. New York: Churchill Livingstone, 1987.

15. Sloane JP. Biopsy Pathology of the Breast. New York: Wiley, 1985.

16. Helvie MA, Hessler C, Frank T, Ikeda DM. Atypical hyperplasia of the breast: mammographic appearance and histologic correlation. Radiology 1991;179:759–764.

17. Ohuchi N, Abe R, Takahashi T, Tezuka F. Origin and extension of intraductal papillomas of the breast: a three-dimensional reconstruction study. Breast Cancer Res Treat 1984;4:117.

18. Hughes LE, Mansel RE, Webster DJT. Abnormalities of normal development and involution: a new perspective on pathogenesis and nomenclature of benign breast disorders. Lancet 1987;2:1316–1319.

19. Meyer JE, Frenna TH, Polger M, et al. Enlarging occult fibroadenomas. Radiology 1992;183:639–641.

20. Haagenson CD. Diseases of the Breast. Philadelphia: Saunders, 1971.

21. Pick PW, Iossifides IA. Occurrence of breast carcinoma within a fibroadenoma: a review. Arch Pathol Lab Med 1984;105:590.

22. Baker KS, Monsees BS, Diaz NM, et al. Carcinoma within fibroadenomas: mammographic features. Radiology 1990;176:371–374.

23. Dupont WD, Page DL, Pari FF, et al. Long-term risk of breast cancer in women with fibroadenoma. N Engl J Med 1994;331:10–15.

24. Foster ME, Garrahan N, Williams S. Fibroadenoma of the breast: a clinical and pathological study. J R Coll Surg Edinb 1988;33:16–19.

25. Meyer JE, Frenna TH, Polger M, et al. Enlarging occult fibroadenomas. Radiology 1992;183:639–641.

26. Fornage BD, Lorigan JG, Andry E. Fibroadenoma of the breast: sonographic appearance. Radiology 1989;172:671–675.

27. Swann CA, Kopans DB, McCarthy KA, et al. The halo sign and malignant breast lesions. AJR Am J Roentgenol 1987;149:1145–1147.

28. Pick PW, Iossifides IA. Occurrence of breast carcinoma within a fibroadenoma: a review. Arch Pathol Lab Med 1984;108:590.

29. Jackson VP, Rothschild PA, Kreipke DL, et al. The spectrum of sonographic findings of fibroadenoma of the breast. Invest Radiol 1986;21:34.

30. Chalas E, Valea F. The gynecologist and surgical procedures for breast disease. Clin Obstet Gynecol 1994;37:948–953.

31. Dupont WD, Page DL. Risk factors for breast cancer in women with proliferative breast disease. N Engl J Med 1985;312(3):146–151.

32. Brenner RJ, Bein ME, Sarti DA, Vinstein AL. Spontaneous regression of interval benign cysts of the breast. Radiology 1994;193:365–368.

33. Pennes D, Homer MJ. Disappearing breast masses caused by compression during mammography. Radiology 1987;165:327–328.

34. Sickles EA, Abele JS. Milk of calcium within tiny breast cysts. Radiology 1981;141:655.

35. Jensen RA, Page DL, Dupont WD, Rogers LW. Invasive breast cancer risk in women with sclerosing adenosis. Cancer 1989;64:1977–1983.

36. Kopans DB, Nguyen PL, Koerner FC, et al. Mixed form, diffusely scattered calcifications in breast cancer with apocrine features. Radiology 1990;177:807–811.

37. Bassett LW, Gold RH, Mirra JA. Nonneoplastic breast calcifications in lipid cysts: development after excision and primary irradiation. AJR Am J Roentgenol 1982;138:335.

38. Sickles EA, Herzog KA. Mammography of the postsurgical breast. AJR Am J Roentgenol 1981;136:585.

39. Bassett LW, Gold RH, Cove HC. Mammographic spectrum of traumatic fat necrosis: the fallibility of "pathognomonic" signs of carcinoma. AJR Am J Roentgenol 1978;130:119.

40. Morgan CL, Trought WS, Peete W. Xeromammographic and ultrasonic diagnosis of a traumatic oil cyst. AJR Am J Roentgenol 1978;130:1189.

41. Gomez A, Mata JM, Donoso L, Rams A. Galactocele: three distinctive radiographic appearances. Radiology 1986;158:43.

42. Hessler C, Schnyder P, Ozzello L. Hamartoma of the breast: diagnostic observations of 16 cases. Radiology 1978;126:95.

43. Taupman RE, Shargo S, Boatman KK, Boggs JT. Malignant cystosarcoma with lipomatous component: a case report. Breast Dis Breast 1982;7:31–33.

44. Bassett LW, Cove HC. Myoblastoma of the breast. AJR Am J Roentgenol 1979;132:122.

45. Hermann G, Schwartz IS. Focal fibrous disease of the breast: mammographic detection of an unappreciated condition. AJR Am J Roentgenol 1983;140:1245.

46. Soler NG, Khardori R. Fibrous disease of the breast, thyroiditis, and cheiroarthropathy in Type I diabetes mellitus. Lancet 1984;1:193–195.

47. Logan WW, Hoffman NY. Diabetic fibrous breast disease. Radiology 1989;172:667–670.

48. Vuitch MF, Rosen PP, Erlandson RA. Pseudoangiomatous hyperplasia of the mammary stroma. Hum Pathol 1986;17:185–191.

49. Ibrahim RE, Sciotto CG, Weidner N. Pseudoangiomatous hyperplasia of the mammary stroma. Some observations regarding its clinico-pathologic spectrum. Cancer 1989;63:1154–1160.

50. Polger MR, Denison CM, Lester S, Meyer JE. Pseudoangiomatous stromal hyperplasia. Mammographic and sonographic appearances. AJR Am J Roentgenol 1996;166:349–352.

51. Kalisher L, Long JA, Peyster RG. Extra-abdominal desmoid of the axillary tail mimicking breast carcinoma. AJR Am J Roentgenol 1976;126:903.

52. Rickert RR, Kalisher L, Hutter RVP. Indurative mastopathy: a benign sclerosing lesion of breast with radial scar which may simulate carcinoma. CA Cancer J Clin 1981;47:561.

53. Wellings SR, Alpers CE. Subgross pathologic features and incidence of radial scars in the breast. Hum Pathol 1984;15:475–479.

54. Nielson M, Jensen J, Andersen JA. An autopsy study of radial scar in the female breast. Histopathology 1985;9:287–295.

55. Cohen MI, Matthies HJ, Mintzer RA, et al. Indurative mastopathy: a cause of false-positive mammograms. Radiology 1985;155:69.

56. Orel SG, Evers K, Yeh IT, Troupin RH. Radial scar with microcalcifications: radiologic-pathologic correlation. Radiology 1992;183:470–482.

57. Ciatto S, Morrone D, Catarazi S, et al. Radial scars of the breast: review of 38 consecutive mammographic diagnoses. Radiology 1993;187:757–760.

58. Mondor H. Tronculotie Sous-cutanee Subaigue de la Paroi Throacique Antero-laterale. Mem Acad Chir 1939;65:1271–1278.

59. Conant EF, Wilkes AN, Mendelson EB, Feig SA. Superficial thrombophlebitis of the breast (Mondor's disease): mammographic findings. AJR Am J Roentgenol 1993;160:1201–1203.

60. Daroca PJ, Reed RJ, Love GL, Kraus SD. Myoid hamartomas of the breast. Hum Path 1985;16:212–219.

61. Erlandson RA, Rosen PP. Infiltrating myoepithelioma of the breast. Am J Surg Pathol 1982;6:785.

62. Graeme-Cook F, O'Brian DS, Daly PA. Unusual breast masses: the sequential development of mammary tuberculosis and Hodgkin's disease in a young woman. Cancer 1988;61:1457–1459.

63. Propeck PA, Scanian KA. Blastomycosis of the breast. AJR Am J Roentgenol 1996;166:726.

64. Gorman JD, Champaign JL, Sumida FK, Canavan L. Schistosomiasis involving the breast. Radiology 1992;185:423–424.

65. Stalsberg H, Thomas DB. Age distribution of histologic types of breast cancer. Int J Cancer 1993;54:1–7.

66. Kopans DB, Moore RH, McCarthy KA, et al. The positive predictive value of mammographically initiated breast biopsy: there is no abrupt change at age 50 years. Radiology 1996;200:357–360.

67. Lagios MD, Margolin FR, Westdahl PR, Rose MR. Mammographically detected duct carcinoma in situ: frequency of local recurrence following tylectomy and prognostic effect of nuclear grade on local recurrence. Cancer 1989;63:618–624.

68. Schwartz GF, Finkel GC, Garcia JC, Patchefsky AS. Subclinical ductal carcinoma in situ of the breast: treatment by local excision and surveillance alone. Cancer 1992;70:2468–2474.

69. Holland R, Peterse JL, Millis RR, et al. Ductal carcinoma in situ: a proposal for a new classification. Semin Diagn Pathol 1994;11:167–180.

70. Silverstein MJ, Lagios MD, Craig PH, et al. A prognostic index for ductal carcinoma in situ of the breast. Cancer 1996;77:2267–2274.

71. Solin LJ, Kurtz J, Fourquet A, et al. Fifteen year results of breast conserving surgery and definitive irradiation for the treatment of ductal carcinoma in situ (intraductal carcinoma) of the breast [abstract]. Proc Am Soc Clin Oncol 1995;14:107.

72. Lennington WJ, Jensen RA, Dalton LW, Page DL. Ductal carcinoma in situ of the breast: heterogeneity of individual lesions. Cancer 1994;73:118–124.

73. Lagios MD, Margolin FR, Westdahl PR, Rose M. Mammographically detected duct carcinoma in situ: frequency of local recurrence following tylectomy and prognostic effect of nuclear grade on local recurrence. Cancer 1989;63:618–624.

74. Morrow M. The natural history of ductal carcinoma in situ. Implications for clinical decision making. Cancer 1995;76:1113–1115.

75. Betsill WL, Rosen PP, Liuberman PM, Robbins GF. Intraductal carcinoma: long-term follow-up after biopsy alone. JAMA 1978;239:1863–1867.

76. Ernster VL, Barclay J, Kerlikowske K, et al. Incidence of and treatment for ductal carcinoma in situ of the breast. JAMA 1996;275:913–918.

77. Page DL, Dupont WD, Rogers LW, et al. Continued local recurrence of carcinoma 15–25 years after a diagnosis of low grade ductal carcinoma in situ of the breast treated only by biopsy. Cancer 1995;76:1197–1200.

78. Fisher B, Costantino J, Redmond PHC, et al. Lumpectomy compared with lumpectomy and radiation therapy for the treatment of intraductal breast cancer. N Engl J Med 1993;328:1581–1586.

79. Fisher ER, Costantino J, Fisher B, et al. Pathologic findings from the National Surgical Adjuvant Breast Project (NSABP) Protocol B-17. Cancer 1995;75:1310–1319.

80. Page DL, Lagios MD. Pathologic analysis of the National Surgical Adjuvant Breast Project (NSABP) B-17 Trial. Cancer 1995;75:1219–1222.

81. Moriya T, Silverberg SG. Intraductal carcinoma (ductal carcinoma in situ) of the breast. A comparison of pure noninvasive tumors with those including different proportions of infiltrating carcinoma. Cancer 1994;74:2972–2978.

82. Stomper PC, Connolly JL, Meyer JE, Harris JR. Clinically occult ductal carcinoma in situ detected with mammography: analysis of 100 cases with radiologic-pathologic correlation. Radiology 1989;172:235–241.

83. Ikeda DM, Anderson I. Ductal carcinoma in situ: atypical mammographic appearances. Radiology 1989;172:661–666.

84. Kinkel K, Gilles R, Feger C, et al. Focal areas of increased opacity in ductal carcinoma in situ of the comedo type: mammographic-pathologic correlation. Radiology 1994;192:443–446.

85. Evans AJ, Pinder S, Ellis IO, et al. Screening-detected and symptomatic ductal carcinoma in situ: mammographic features with pathologic correlation. Radiology 1994;191:237–240.

86. Holland R, Hendricks JHCL. Microcalcifications associated with ductal carcinoma in situ: mammographic-pathologic correlation. Semin Diagn Pathol 1994;11:181–192.

87. Ahmed A. Calcification in human breast carcinomas: ultrastructure observations. J Pathol 1975;117:247.

88. Kopans DB, Swann CA, White G, et al. Asymmetric breast tissue. Radiology 1989;171:639–643.

89. Kopans DB, Meyer JE, Steinbock T. Breast cancer: appearance as delineated by whole breast water-path ultrasound scanning. J Clin Ultrasound 1982;10:303–322.

90. Fornage BD, Lorigan JG, Andry E. Fibroadenoma of the breast: sonographic appearance. Radiology 1989;172:671–675.

91. Feig SA, Shaber GS, Patchefsky AS, et al. Tubular carcinoma of the breast. Radiology 1978;129:311.

92. Tabar L. The impact of breast cancer screening with mammography in women aged 40–49 years. Presented at the Falun Conference, March 21–22, 1996, Falun, Sweden.

93. Leibman AJ, Lewis M, Kruse B. Tubular carcinoma of the breast: mammographic appearance. AJR Am J Roentgenol 1993;160:263–265.

94. Conant EF, Dillion RL, Palazzo J, et al. Imaging findings in mucin-containing carcinomas of the breast: correlation with pathologic features. AJR Am J Roentgenol 1994;163:821–824.

95. Cardenosa G, Doudna C, Eklund GW. Mucinous (colloid) breast cancer: clinical and mammographic findings in 10 patients. AJR Am J Roentgenol 1994;162:1077–1079.

96. Ridolfi RL, Rosen PP, Port A, et al. Medullary carcinoma of the breast: a clinicopathologic study with 10 year follow-up. Cancer 1977;40:1365–1385.

97. Rapin V, Contesso G. Medullary breast carcinoma: a reevaluation of 95 cases of breast cancer with inflammatory stroma. Cancer 1988;61:2503–2510.

98. Rubens JR, Kopans DB. Medullary carcinoma of the breast: is it over-diagnosed? Arch Surg 1990;125:601–604.

99. Ridolfi RL, Rosen PP, Port A, et al. Medullary carcinoma of the breast: a clinicopathological study with 10 year follow-up. Cancer 1977;40:1365–1385.

100. Meyer JM, Amin E, Lindfors KK, et al. Medullary carcinoma of the breast: mammographic and sonographic features. Radiology 1989;170:79–82.

101. Giles R, Lesnik A, Guinebretiere J, et al. Apocrine carcinoma: clinical and mammographic features. Radiology 1994;190:495–497.

102. Dershaw DD, Moore MP, Liberman L, Deutch BM. Inflammatory breast carcinoma: mammographic findings. Radiology 1994;190:831–834.

103. Foote FW, Stewart FW. Lobular carcinoma in situ. A rare form of mammary cancer. Am J Pathol 1941;17:491–496.

104. Rosen PP, Kosloff C, Lieberman PH, et al. Lobular carcinoma in situ of the breast. Am J Surg Pathol 1978;2:225–251.

105. Wheeler JE, Enterline HT, Roseman JM, et al. Lobular carcinoma in-situ of the breast: long term follow-up. Cancer 1974;34:554–563.

106. Webber BL, Heise H, Niefeld JP, Cosa J. Risk of subsequent contralateral breast carcinoma in a population of patients with in-situ breast carcinoma. Cancer 1981;47:2928–2932.

107. Pope TL, Fechner RE, Wilhelm MC, et al. Lobular carcinoma in situ of the breast: mammographic features. Radiology 1988;168:63–66.

108. Beute BJ, Kalisher L, Hutter RVP. Lobular carcinoma in situ of the breast: clinical, pathologic, and mammographic features. AJR Am J Roentgenol 191;157:257–265.

109. Haagensen CD, Lane N, Lattes R, Bodian C. Lobular neoplasia (so-called lobular carcinoma in situ) of the breast. Cancer 1978;42:737–769.

110. Foote FW, Stewart FW. A histologic classification of carcinoma of the breast. Surgery 1946;19:74–99.

111. Dixon JM, Anderson TJ, Page DL, et al. Infiltrating lobular carcinoma of the breast: incidence and consequence of bilateral disease. Br J Surg 1983;70:513–516.

112. Silverstein MJ, Lewinsky BS, Waisman JR, et al. Infiltrating lobular carcinoma: is it different from infiltrating duct carcinoma? Cancer 1994;73:1673–1677.

113. Le Gal M, Ollivier L, Asselain B, et al. Mammographic features of 455 invasive lobular carcinomas. Radiology 1992;185:705–708.

114. Bumpers HL, Hassett JM, Penetrante RB, et al. Endocrine organ metastases in subjects with lobular carcinoma of the breast. Arch Surg 1993;128:1344–1347.

115. Holland R, Hendriks JHCL, Mravunac M. Mammographically occult breast cancer: a pathologic and radiologic study. Cancer 1983;52:1810–1819.

116. Sickles EA. The subtle and atypical mammographic features of invasive lobular carcinoma. Radiology 1991;178:25–26.

117. Mendelson EB, Harris KM, Doshi N, Tobon H. Infiltrating lobular carcinoma: mammographic patterns with pathologic correlation. AJR Am J Roentgenol 1989;153:265–271.

118. Krecke KN, Gisvold JJ. Invasive lobular carcinoma of the breast: mammographic findings and extent of disease at diagnosis in 184 patients. AJR Am J Roentgenol 1993;161:957–960.

119. Hart WR, Bauer RC, Oberman HA. Cystosarcoma phyllodes: a clinicopathologic study of twenty-six hypercellular periductal stromal tumors of the breast. Am J Clin Pathol 1978;70:211.

120. Liberman L, Bonaccio E, Hamele-Bena D, et al. Benign and malignant phyllodes tumors: mammographic and sonographic findings. Radiology 1996;198:121–124.

121. Cole-Beuglet C, Soriano R, Kurtz A, et al. Ultrasound, x-ray mammography, and histopathology of cystosarcoma phylloides. Radiology 1983;146:481–486.

122. Rosen PP, Oberman HA. Tumors of the Mammary Gland. Atlas of Tumor Pathology. Washington, DC: Armed Forces Institute of Pathology, 1992.

123. Watt CA, Haggar AM, Krasicky GA. Extraosseous osteogenic sarcoma of the breast: mammographic and pathologic findings. Radiology 1984;150:34.

124. Langham MR, Mills SA, DeMay RM, et al. Malignant fibrous histiocytoma of the breast: a case report and review of the literature. Cancer 1984;54:558.

125. Kovi J, Duong HD, Leffall LD Jr. High grade mucoepidermoid carcinoma of the breast. Arch Pathol Lab Med 1918;105:612–614.

126. Meyer JE, Kopans DB. Xeromammographic appearance of lymphoma of the breast. Radiology 1980;135:623–626.

127. Liberman L, Giess CS, Dershaw DD, et al. Non-Hodgkin's lym-

phoma of the breast: imaging characteristics and correlation with histopathologic findings. Radiology 1994;192:157–160.

128. Toombs BD, Kalisher L. Metastatic disease to the breast: clinical, pathologic, and radiologic features. AJR Am J Roentgenol 1977; 129:673.

129. Derchi LE, Rizzatto G, Guiseppetti GM, et al. Metastatic tumors in the breast: sonographic findings. J Ultrasound Med 1985;4:69.

130. Cole-Beuglet C, Kirk ME, Selouan R, et al. Bone within the breast. Radiology 1976;119:643.

131. Poland A. Deficiency of the pectoral muscles. Guys Hosp Rep 1841;6:191–193.

132. Samuels TH, Haider MA, Kirkbride P. Poland's syndrome: a mammographic presentation. AJR Am J Roentgenol 1996;166:347–348.

133. Ravitch MM. Poland's syndrome: a study of an eponym. Plast Reconstr Surg 1977;59:508–512.

134. Sferlazza SJ, Cohen MA. Poland's syndrome: a sonographic sign [letter]. AJR Am J Roentgenol 1996;167:1597.

Breast Imaging, 2nd ed., by Daniel B. Kopans.
Lippincott–Raven Publishers, Philadelphia © 1998.

CHAPTER **20**

Magnetic Resonance Imaging

Carol A. Hulka and Daniel B. Kopans

Magnetic imaging (MRI) of the breast has undergone two cycles of investigation. In the initial testing it was apparent that some cancers were easily seen when surrounded by fat (Fig. 20-1) on T1-weighted images, and cysts were easily identified on T2 images (Fig. 20-2). However, despite initial optimism, it was found that the differences in the relaxation times between benign and malignant tissues overlapped and were frequently insufficient to provide any clinical benefit for MRI, used without contrast material, as a diagnostic procedure.

Many breast cancers were even indistinguishable from normal breast tissue. When gadolinium-diethylene triamine pentaacetic acid (Gd-DTPA) became available as a contrast agent, a second round of breast MRI investigation began leading toward potentially clinically useful applications. The role of MRI in the detection of breast cancer and the evaluation of breast lesions is becoming better defined. Because of improvements in MR technology and imaging techniques and with the increased interest in developing ways to detect early breast cancer as well as differentiate benign from malignant lesions, there has been a surge in research using breast MRI for breast cancer detection and diagnosis.

A second use for MRI was stimulated by the controversy that arose over the possible significance of silicone gel implants and their potential relationship to autoimmune disease. Emphasis was placed on trying to identify implants that had ruptured. It became apparent that MRI is particularly useful in the evaluation of implants and may be the best method for detecting certain types of rupture.

CLINICAL RELEVANCE OF MRI

Imaging of implants has already become an accepted method of analysis. Although many investigators still feel that MRI for lesion analysis is experimental, some now incorporate MRI into the clinical management of breast lesions using gadolinium enhancement to analyze specific lesions to try to determine the extent of breast cancer, to search for a primary lesion when metastatic disease has been found, and to detect intramammary recurrence after primary conservation therapy. Because it appears that virtually all invasive breast cancers demonstrate enhancement after the intravenous administration of gadolinium, some radiologists use the lack of enhancement to reinforce the likelihood that a specific lesion is not an invasive breast cancer. This latter approach, however, has yet to be demonstrated in sufficiently large prospective series that include, in particular, small (<1 cm) nonpalpable cancers. Potentially compounding the reliance on MRI to exclude cancer is the fact that normal tissues enhance, and ductal carcinoma in situ (DCIS) may not always enhance.

STAGING BREAST CANCER AND DETERMINING THE EXTENT OF THE LESION

A number of trials have now shown that MRI can demonstrate additional occult foci of breast cancer in a breast in which a cancer has been detected, and some physicians use MRI in the staging process, once breast cancer is diagnosed, to try to establish its extent. This becomes somewhat more difficult in that benign lesions can also enhance, and, although sensitivity is high, specificity of MRI is moderate to low and separating true positive foci of cancer from falsely positive tissue is problematic.

MRI as a Possible Second-Level Screen

Another possibility that has yet to be proved is the use of MRI to detect breast cancer in asymptomatic, healthy-appearing women with negative mammograms. The fact that some clinically and mammographically occult cancers can be detected by MRI also suggests the possibility of MRI as a second level screening technology that may be able to

Portions of this chapter were previously published in Hulka CA. MRI of the Breast. In Taveras JM, Ferrucci JT (eds), Radiology: Diagnosis, Imaging, Intervention. Philadelphia: Lippincott–Raven, 1996;1–10. Reprinted with permission.

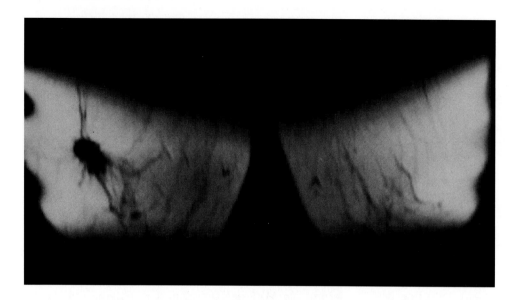

FIG. 20-1. Invasive breast cancer visible on T1-weighted image because of the surrounding fat.

detect early cancers that at present are mammographically as well as clinically occult.

CURRENT USES OF MRI

MRI of Breast Implants

Background

Until 1992, when the U.S. Food and Drug Administration (FDA) halted the routine use of silicone gel implants except within specific scientific protocols, silicone gel implants were the most commonly used prosthetic device for augmenting the breast and for reconstructing the breast after mastectomy. It has been estimated that between 1 and 2 million women in the United States have had breast augmentation or reconstruction with silicone gel implants.

Most of the implants used for these purposes were composed of a silastic elastomer envelope filled with a viscid, cohesive silicone gel. These were placed either behind the glandular tissue (Fig. 20-3A) and in front of the pectoralis major muscle or behind the muscle in front of the thoracic wall (Fig. 20-3B) (see Chapter 17).

The retropectoral location was used in an effort to prevent the implant from becoming hard due to fibrous encapsulation. As with any foreign body, implants can stimulate breast tissue to form a fibrous capsule around the implant (Fig. 20-3C). The contraction of this surrounding membrane could cause the implant to feel hard. When placed behind

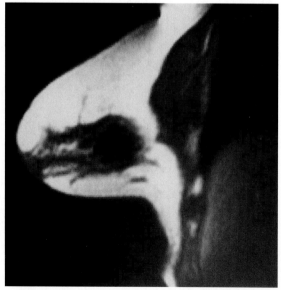

A

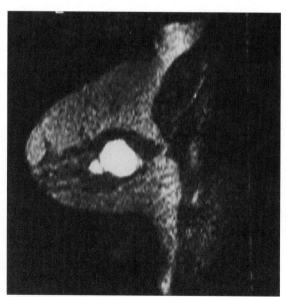

B

FIG. 20-2. On MRI this cyst had a characteristically low signal intensity (*black*) on this T1-weighted image **(A)** and a high signal intensity (*white*) on the T2-weighted image **(B)**.

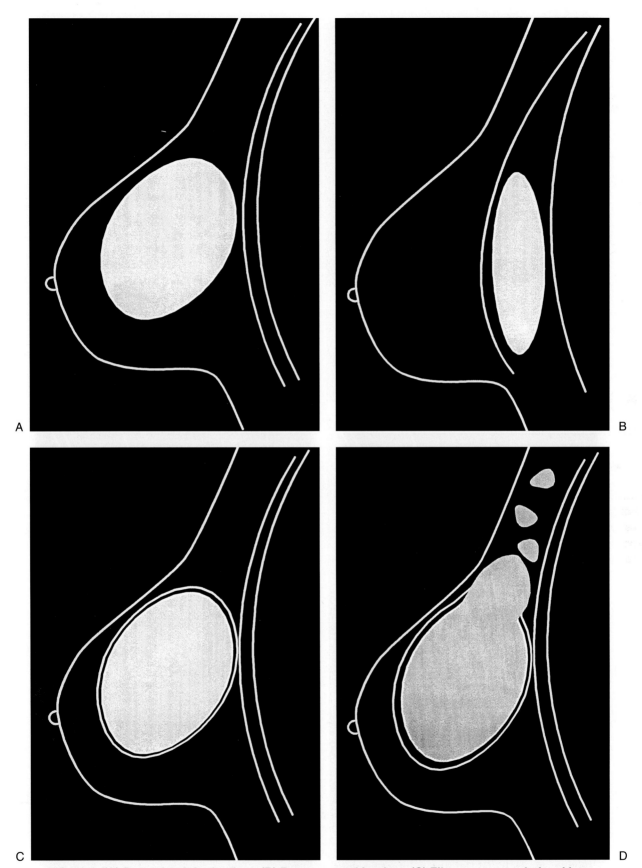

FIG. 20-3. (A) Retroglandular implant. (B) Retropectoral implant. (C) Fibrous encapsulation. Many implants develop a surrounding fibrous capsule. **(D) Ruptured implant.** An implant is clearly ruptured when there are drops of silicone gel in the surrounding tissue. *Continued.*

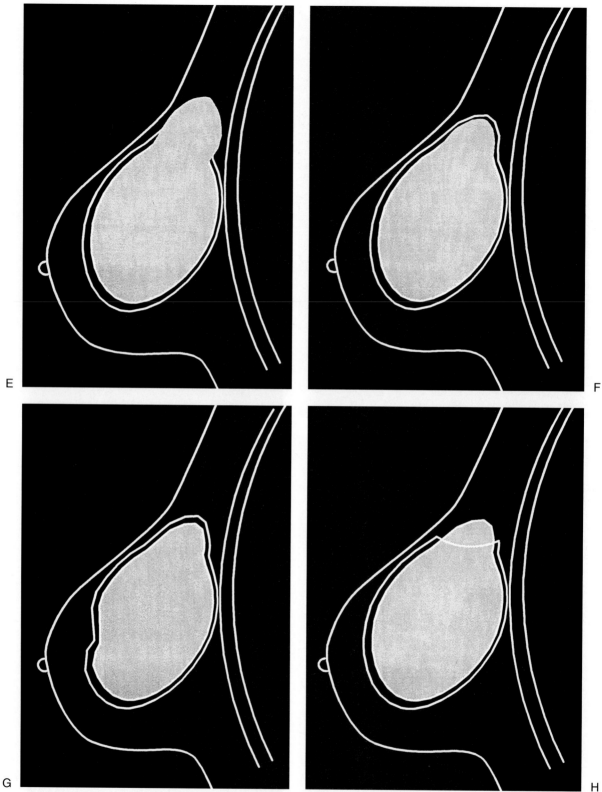

FIG. 20-3. *Continued.* **(E) Extracapsular ruptured implant.** This schematic demonstrates rupture of the implant with extrusion of silicone out of the envelope, through the surrounding capsule (extracapsular rupture) into the surrounding tissue but with its smooth surface maintained. **(F) Intracapsular rupture.** The same appearance as in **(D)** can occur if the rupture is contained by the capsule (intracapsular rupture; see **H, I**). **(G) Deformed, intact implant.** The same appearance may merely be due to deformity of the implant with an **intact envelope. (H) Herniated implant.** Extruded silicone or deformity of the implant may be indistinguishable from a herniation of an intact implant through a torn or incomplete fibrous capsule. *Continued.*

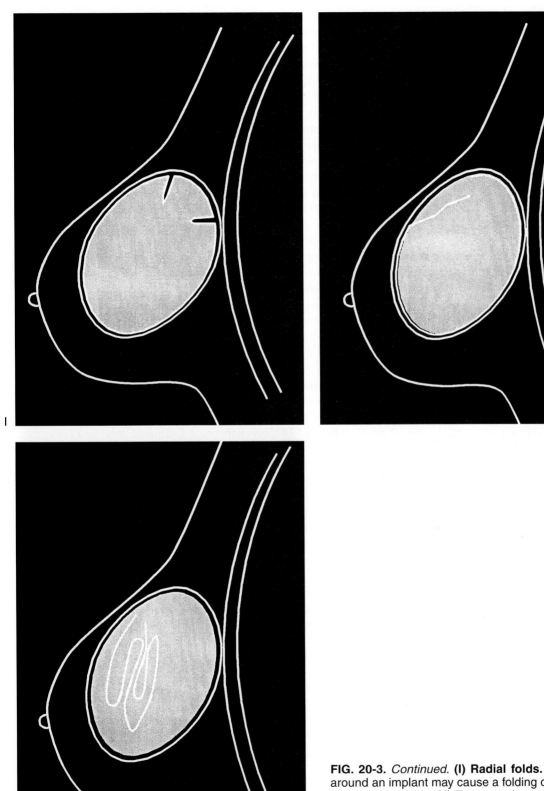

FIG. 20-3. *Continued.* **(I) Radial folds.** Pressure from the tissues around an implant may cause a folding of the pliable envelope, producing radial folds. **(J) Torn envelope.** When an implant envelope tears, the envelope may begin to fall into the gel. **(K) Ruptured implant.** The envelope may collapse completely into the gel, which may appear smoothly contained if there is a surrounding fibrous capsule.

the muscle, it was felt that motion of the muscle over the surface of the implant would reduce capsule formation.

When concerns were raised that implants might also trigger more systemic responses, such as autoimmune reactions and so-called adjuvant diseases, a great deal of emphasis was placed on detecting ruptured implants because it is believed that direct exposure of the tissues to the silicone gel was a major reason for these problems.

Until fairly recently, mammography, clinical history, and physical examination were the only methods of diagnosing breast implant rupture. The demonstration of implant rupture by mammography, however, may be difficult as silicone is highly attenuating and blocks most of the low-energy x-rays used in mammography. Consequently, only the contour of the silicone gel is visible on the mammograms. If a capsule has formed around the implant, the envelope may have completely disintegrated but the implant appears intact on the mammogram because the gel is contained by the fibrous capsule.

Even contour abnormalities can be misleading on the mammogram because normal tissue pressures, as well as the formation of a capsule, can distort the implant contour. When an implant ruptures, silicone may be obvious in the surrounding tissues by mammography (Fig. 20-3D), but this is unusual. Although bulges in the implant contour may suggest a rupture with extrusion of silicone into the tissues (Fig. 20-3E) or contained by a capsule (Fig. 20-3F), the same appearance may be caused by distortion of the intact implant by the surrounding tissues (Fig. 20-3G) or even a herniation of an intact implant through a gap in the fibrous capsule (Fig. 20-3H). Consequently, mammography is not very sensitive to implant ruptures.

Because MRI is a cross-sectional technique that can differentiate the low signal intensity of the envelope and fibrous capsule from the high signal intensity of the silicone gel, imaging of these structures is possible. As a consequence of this capability, MRI has been shown to be able to diagnose many ruptures. Ultrasound is another useful method of implant imaging (see Chapter 16) (1); however, the overall anatomic and structural detail provided by MRI appears to be superior to that of ultrasound for implant evaluation (2).

Although many types of implants have been used, silicone gel with a 200- to 300-μm outer silicone rubber envelope was the most commonly used device. Saline implants are composed of an outer silicone envelope filled with saline, which may have rings or valves in the envelope for filling or positioning. Double-lumen implants have saline surrounding an internal silicone-filled implant, and a reverse double-lumen implant contains silicone surrounding saline. Rarely, triple-lumen implants have been used, with silicone and saline mixed within a single envelope and multiple devices placed within each breast. The patient history and knowing what type or types of implants are in place are very useful for interpreting implant MR images, although many women do not know detailed information concerning their implants.

Silicone gel is a copolymer composed predominantly of polydimethylsiloxane (PDMS) and vinylmethylsiloxane. The vinyl groups are partially cross-linked to form a three-dimensional gel structure (3). Because the groups are only partially cross-linked, the implant also contains some free PDMS. This has been shown to be able to pass through the intact implant envelope into adjacent breast tissue (4,5) and is termed *gel bleed*. It is believed that it is this free PDMS material that stimulates the host fibroblasts and results in the formation of the fibrous capsule around the implants in many women (4–7).

In addition to positioning the implant behind the pectoralis muscle, in an effort to prevent fibrous encapsulation and concomitant hardening of the implant, the implant envelopes have been modified in various ways. The most common envelopes are smooth silicone rubber that often become surrounded by strong fibrous capsules. Silicone envelopes with rough textured surfaces were designed to decrease the amount of fibrous encapsulation. Polyurethane-covered shells were designed to permit the fibroblasts to grow into the coating in a more irregular pattern to form a less cohesive capsule, keeping the implant soft. This latter type of envelope is less common. The fact that there is ingrowth of tissue into the coating makes it more difficult to remove the implant. There is also concern about the long-term effects of the polyurethane coating. A degradation product of polyurethane, 2,4 diamino toluene (TDA), has been shown to cause liver malignancies in laboratory animals (see Chapter 17), although to date none has been reported in humans.

Because of the ongoing concern about the safety of silicone implants, only saline-filled implants have been available for aesthetic augmentation since April 1992 (8). However, silicone implants are available for patients with a certified medical need who are enrolled in clinical trials. Silicone implants are also allowed for patients with temporary expanders awaiting permanent placement (those patients undergoing reconstructive surgery at the time of mastectomy and those patients with ruptured implants needing replacement). Given the concerns over exposure to silicone the detection of ruptured implants has become a major effort.

Imaging Techniques for Silicone Implants

The implant controversy is beyond the scope of this review. The association of silicone with autoimmune or connective tissue diseases is primarily anecdotal due to isolated case reports (9). Large cohort studies have not reported any significant association between silicone implants and connective tissue diseases (10). Nevertheless, efforts continue to detect rupture and MRI has become integral to that effort.

A dedicated breast coil is preferred for MR breast imaging, because it provides a better signal-to-noise resolution than a body coil. Imaging both breasts simultaneously permits comparison of both sides; however, some coils are

TABLE 20-1. *Relative signal intensities of silicone, fat, and water on MRI of the breast*

Pulse sequence	Silicone	Fat	Water
Fast spin-echo T2-weighted (TR/TE, 5,000/200)	High	Medium	Very high
Fast spin-echo with water suppression	High	Medium	Low
Inversion recovery fast spin-echo (TR/TE, 5,000/90; T1, 140)	High	Low	Very high
Inversion recovery, fast spin-echo with water suppression	High	Low	Low
Three-point Dixon, silicone only	High	None	None

Source: Adapted from Mund DF, Farria DM, Gorczyca DP, et al. MR imaging of the breast in patients with silicone-gel implants: spectrum of findings. AJR Am J Roentgenol 1993;161:773–778.

TABLE 20-2. *Tissue T1 and T2 in breast imaging*

Tissue	T1	T2
Fat	Short	Short
Parenchyma	Variable	Variable
Cancer	Variable	Variable
Fibroadenoma	Variable	Variable
Muscle	Similar to parenchyma	Usually shorter than parenchyma
Blood (vascular hemorrhage)	Arterial is long, venous is long Early is long Late (days or longer) methemo-globin causes shortening at the periphery	Arterial is long, venous is short Early is long Late (days) methemoglobin causes shortening at the periphery
Fluid	Long	Long
Silicone	Long	Long

designed such that only one breast can be imaged at a time. The imaging is improved if the patient lies in the prone position with the breasts pendent in the coil. The effect of gravity helps to separate the tissues and provides a greater understanding of anatomic relationships than if the patient is lying supine with the breast flattened on the chest wall.

A variety of techniques and pulse sequences have proved useful. The simplest sequence includes a T1-weighted gradient echo localizer with a flip angle of 30 degrees, a T2-weighted fast spin-echo (FSE) sequence, and a T2-weighted FSE sequence with water suppression (11). Because silicone and water have similar signal intensity on T2-weighted imaging, water suppression allows for differentiating cysts and other fluid collections from extruded silicone. The more T1-weighted images obtained, the more information regarding the presence of any blood components (Tables 20-1 and 20-2).

This group of sequences is fast, allowing completion of an examination within 30 minutes. Because fat and silicone both have bright signal intensity, fat suppression methods such as inversion recovery or three-point Dixon techniques can be added to decrease the fat signal relative to the silicone for better silicone imaging (12).

Because the MR frequencies of silicone and fat are close (100 Hz) (Fig. 20-4), concern has arisen that fat suppression may also suppress some silicone using certain methods. This does not, however, appear to be a problem in a clinical setting. Small series using silicone-selective pulse sequences have also been described (13,14). Echoplanar imaging, an ultrafast method of imaging, is one method of imaging silicone alone by suppressing water and fat; however, the sig-

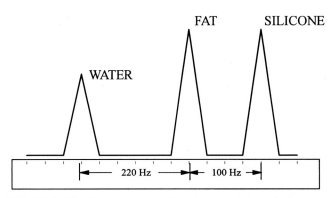

FIG. 20-4. The frequency peaks of water, fat, and silicone at 1.5 T are close but due to their separation permit suppression of water or fat to help distinguish silicone.

nal-to-noise resolution is inferior to conventional imaging techniques, and we presently rely on conventional imaging to evaluate implants.

A conventional method of silicone-selective imaging using standard inversion recovery techniques for fat suppression and a chemical-shift-selective excitation pulse for water suppression has been reported in a small group of patients and showed promising results, although some experimental software was used (10).

Some limitations of MRI include a chemical-shift artifact at the silicone/tissue interface that may be confused with encapsulation of the implant. As with most MR studies, motion of the patient can be an additional problem. Encouraging the patient to remain as still as possible during imaging is effective, but the prone position ultimately creates

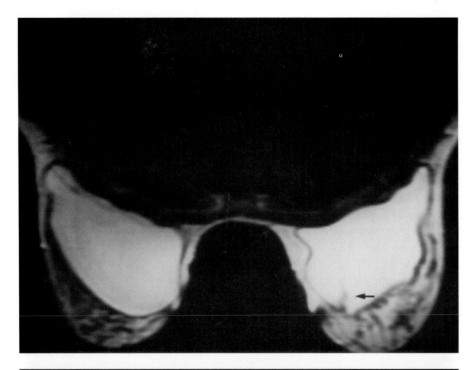

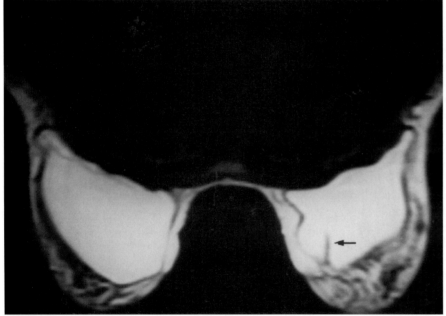

FIG. 20-5. Radial fold. Consecutive axial T2-weighted images show a linear low–signal-intensity structure within the anterior aspect of the right breast implant. This appearance is due to infolding of the intact envelope (radial fold). (With permission from Taveras JM, Ferrucci JT [eds]. Radiology: Diagnosis, Imaging, Intervention. Philadelphia: Lippincott–Raven, 1996.)

shoulder stiffness and discomfort that after a certain time period result in patient movement.

Cardiac motion during scanning produces a significant artifact. This can be effectively reduced by choosing the appropriate phase-encoding direction. By encoding in a right-to-left direction with the patient in the prone position, the cardiac motion is placed across the posterior chest wall and not out into the breasts and implants. The phase direction can be tailored to each study. If, for example, much of the implant remains in a more posterior axillary location, even in the prone position, the phase direction can be placed in the anterior-to-posterior direction.

MRI Appearance of Silicone Implants

Normal implants usually have a smooth implant-tissue interface on MRI. The silicone rubber envelope and reactive fibrous capsule around the implant envelope produce a low signal intensity band surrounding the implant. Undulations of the implant contour are common due to normal surrounding-tissue pressures. Without other MR abnormalities and without gross asymmetry between the two sides, these are not considered abnormal. Occasionally, a small amount of reactive fluid surrounds the implant, despite the fact that it is intact (15). Some implants (especially those that have a

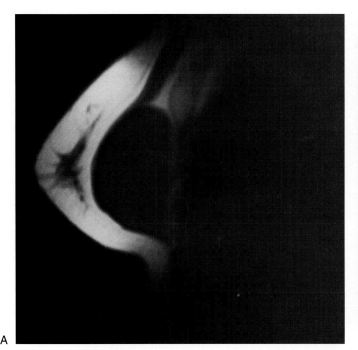 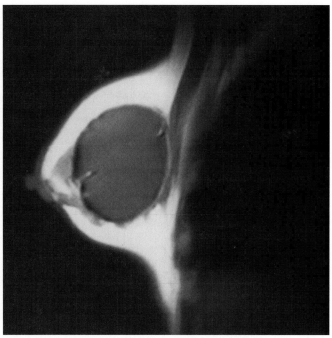

A   B

FIG. 20-6. Retropectoral and retroglandular placement of implants on MRI. Sagittal T1-weighted images of two different patients with silicone implants. **(A)** The pectoralis muscle is draped over the subpectoral implant. **(B)** The pectoralis muscle is posterior to the subglandular implant. Note the radial folds extending to the periphery of the implant **(B)**. (With permission from Taveras JM, Ferrucci JT [eds]. Radiology: Diagnosis, Imaging, Intervention. Philadelphia: Lippincott–Raven, 1996.)

polyurethane envelope and often those with saline) have linear and curvilinear, low–signal-intensity structures protruding into the gel or saline from the surface in a radial fashion. These radial folds are merely creases in the implant envelope due to tissue pressure or contraction of the fibrous capsule. They appear as low–signal-intensity linear bands extending from the periphery of the implant into the gel or saline (see Figs. 20-3I and 20-5).

Sagittal images are obtained to best determine the location of the implant as subpectoral or subglandular (Fig. 20-6). The pectoralis muscle may be so thin as it stretches over the implant that it may be difficult to appreciate using axial images alone. The sagittal plane is also excellent for evaluation of the axillae in relation to the pectoralis. If bilateral implants are present, overall symmetry can be checked.

Silicone shows the lowest signal intensity on T1-weighted images due to its long T1 value and appears bright on T2-weighted images because of its long T2 value. Fat can be distinguished due to its relatively shorter T1 value (high signal intensity on T1-weighted images) and longer T2 value. Breast parenchyma is of intermediate signal intensity on both T1- and T2-weighted images, and muscle has intermediate signal intensity on T1-weighted images and low signal intensity on T2-weighted images. Uncomplicated fluid and the various blood products appear as expected on MRI.

The complications involving breast implants are varied (see Fig. 20-3). An intracapsular rupture is defined as a disruption of the implant envelope with the implant contents contained by the surrounding fibrous capsule. The fibrous capsule may become discontinuous, allowing protrusion of the implant through the opening with an intact implant envelope, resulting in herniation. If both the fibrous capsule and implant envelope are disrupted, free silicone gel extrudes into the surrounding tissue and is termed an *extracapsular rupture*.

In some cases, rather than a true bursting of the envelope, it appears that the silicone envelopes become thinned over time and they can disappear, so that rupture may occur without a history of trauma. Free silicone may produce silicone granulomata from long-standing rupture. Granulomata can also occur with direct silicone injection, but this is illegal in the United States. Silicone can also be seen in the axillary lymph nodes.

The preceding are usually long-term problems associated with implants. Postoperative complications after implantation are fairly common. In a study of 749 women, 208 (27.8%) underwent implant-related surgery over a mean follow-up period of 7.8 years (16). The most common problem was capsular contracture in 112 (14.9%) of the women. Ruptured implants occurred in 29 (3.9%). A number of problems occur soon after implantation, including hematomas and abscess formation. In capsular contraction, myofibroblasts may be responsible for pain and capsule formation, which may produce a hard implant. However, because there are no proven correlates of capsular contracture on imaging, the diagnosis remains a clinical diagnosis.

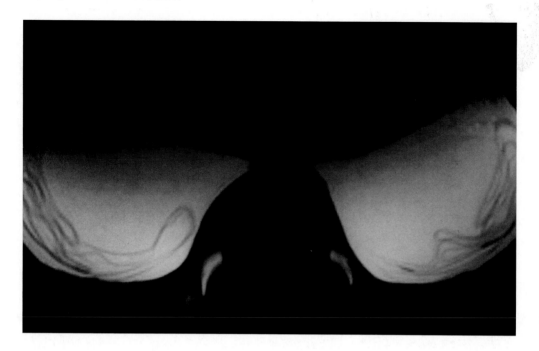

FIG. 20-7. The linguine or fallen envelope sign. Axial T2-weighted image with fat suppression using the inversion recovery technique of a patient with bilateral silicone implants. The multiple curvilinear low–signal-intensity areas within the anterior implants are the disrupted envelopes that have fallen into the gel in this patient with bilateral intracapsular ruptures. (With permission from Taveras JM, Ferrucci JT [eds]. Radiology: Diagnosis, Imaging, Intervention. Philadelphia: Lippincott–Raven, 1996.)

The MR appearance of intracapsular rupture was described by Gorczyca and associates (11). They described fine, serpentine, low–signal-intensity linear bands within the silicone implant as indicative of a disrupted envelope collapsing and falling into the gel. In cross section it was thought to look like a piece of pasta weaving back and forth on a plate and was termed the *linguine sign*. Others call it the *fallen envelope sign* (Fig. 20-7) (7,8). In an intracapsular rupture, the implant gel is held in place by the fibrous capsule, which may or may not be identified on the MR images. The MRI of extracapsular rupture includes globules of silicone outside the expected location of the implant either separate or contiguous with the implant (see Fig. 20-3D, E). Without an associated fallen envelope and where the protruding silicone surface is continuous with the implant (Fig. 20-8), herniation may remain difficult to distinguish from extracapsular rupture. The linguine sign is the best evidence of a ruptured implant. Several series show a high correlation of the linguine sign with rupture, reporting 76% to 94% sensitivities (predictive of rupture) and 97% to 100% specificities (no rupture when the sign is not present) (11,12,14).

MRI OF BREAST LESIONS

Background

Early studies demonstrated that MRI of the breast was not useful in distinguishing normal breast tissue from benign or malignant lesions due to poor spatial resolution and the overlap in lesion morphology and signal intensities using the normal tissues' T1 and T2 values (17). Noncontrast MRI could easily distinguish cysts and blood products based on

their T1 and T2 values (see Table 20-1) and MR behavior, but the ability to detect or aid in the diagnosis of breast cancer was lacking. Heywang and associates were among the first to demonstrate that intravenous contrast material could help distinguish an abnormality from normal breast parenchyma on MR images (18,19). Since that time, the experience using Gd-DTPA enhancement suggests that the vast majority of malignancies demonstrate enhancement. Unfortunately, some benign entities also enhance. The use of enhancement to separate the normal from the abnormal is somewhat complicated by the fact that normal breast parenchyma also enhances, but the amount of normal parenchymal enhancement is much less than that of malignancies or some benign lesions in the early period after an intravenous bolus injection. An additional problem that is not often accounted for is that signal intensities of normal tissue can also vary with the time in the menstrual cycle during which the scanning is performed (20). It has been suggested that maximum enhancement of the normal tissues of the breast occurs in the luteal phase, the week prior to menstruation (21), as well as in the first week of the cycle (22,23). Unfortunately, cyclic enhancement is not uniform but can be nodular, and some tissues can have rapid enhancement similar to malignant processes. If there is a choice, it would appear that MRI of the breast is best performed between days 7 and 20 of the menstrual cycle.

Despite the fact that the experience with contrast-enhanced MRI of the breast has greatly increased, much of the data are anecdotal. The lack of large prospective studies to scientifically define the efficacy of MRI in breast evaluation has kept it largely a research tool. The cost of the study and limited access to the magnets has greatly slowed the research. Specific uses, however, are emerging.

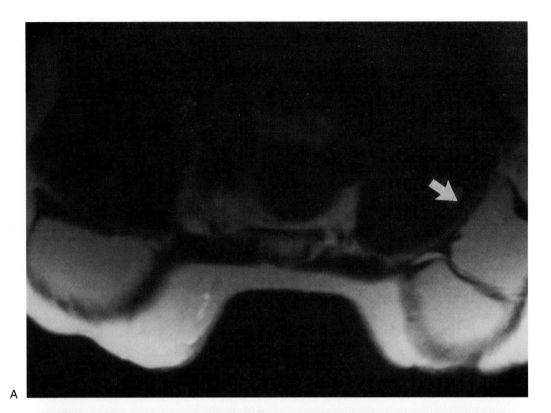

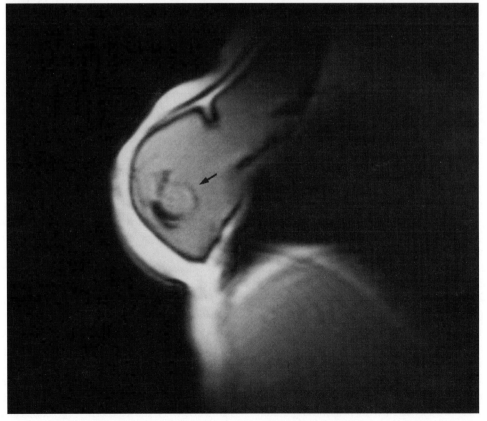

FIG. 20-8. Linguine sign. Axial T2-weighted image **(A)** shows protrusion of the right silicone implant laterally. The sagittal image shows the axillary extension and the fallen envelope inferiorly **(B)** in this patient with an extracapsular rupture. (With permission from Taveras JM, Ferrucci JT [eds]. Radiology: Diagnosis, Imaging, Intervention. Philadelphia: Lippincott–Raven, 1996.)

Although film-screen mammography remains the method of choice for detecting breast cancer, the ability of mammography to differentiate benign from malignant lesions is low. Many lesions detected mammographically and by physical examination are indeterminate, requiring biopsy to exclude cancer, and 70% to 80% of biopsies result in benign diagnoses (24,25). Even the addition of ultrasound plays a limited role in excluding cancer, providing cyst-versus-solid differentiation. The mammographically dense breast also presents limitations, as cancer may not be visible in this group of patients.

MRI may have diagnostic value in the separation of benign from malignant entities. It remains to be seen whether this application will be efficacious, given the safety and relatively inexpensive imaging-guided needle biopsy techniques that are now available. Experience with MRI in the evaluation of known malignancies and the fact that MRI can detect associated foci of cancer that are otherwise occult offers the possibility of detecting cancers de novo that are presently not detectable by mammography or clinical breast examination (CBE). Before MRI can be applied to screening, however, much work is needed to validate its efficacy. More immediate uses of breast lesion MRI include staging of local disease by determining the extent of tumor involvement and the evaluation of women who have already been treated for cancer in an effort to detect local tumor recurrence in the postsurgical scar site (11,26–29).

Imaging Techniques

As with implants, a dedicated breast coil is preferable for breast MRI. A single or double coil may be used. We prefer a double coil because it permits simultaneous comparison between the two sides. Just as with mammography, symmetry of the tissues, or more specifically, lack of symmetry, may be significant in detecting malignancy. If, however, a specific question is to be answered, a single coil is appropriate because it provides a better signal-to-noise ratio. A variety of coils are available, including receive-only and transmit-receive coils. Whether transmit-receive coils significantly improve imaging remains to be proved.

The coils are designed such that the patient is imaged in the prone position, supported by the coil and table, with the breasts pendent in the coil. This position reduces motion artifact from respiration and allows gravity to pull and separate the structures of the breast while maintaining an anatomic orientation and configuration that facilitates interpretation.

Before the patient is positioned in the coil, an intravenous line maintained with 0.5% saline with a stop-cock apparatus is connected to a power-injector filled with Gd-DTPA. If a power injector is not available, the second line can be connected to a Gd-DTPA–filled syringe. This preliminary setup reduces changes in position between the pre- and postcontrast set of images and diminishes the amount of time the patient is within the scanner.

The optimal dose of Gd-DTPA may range from 0.1 to 0.2 mmol per kg body weight, depending on the imaging sequence selected. Higher doses have been suggested. Heywang-Koebrunner and associates found that improved imaging could be achieved using 0.16 mmol/kg (30). Weinreb and Newstead, however, speculated that this may have been a function of the technique and pulse sequence used by the authors (21). If a power injector is used, the rate may vary up to 3 ml per second.

A variety of MR sequences for contrast-enhanced breast imaging can be used. The most effective technique with high sensitivity for enhancing lesions includes three-dimensional imaging such as 3D FLASH (fast low-angle shot), FISP (fast imaging with steady precession), FATSS (fast adiabatic trajectory in a steady state), and GRASS (gradient-recalled acquisition in a steady state) (31–35). The same sequence is performed before and after injection with Gd-DTPA. These sequences allow volumetric coverage of the breasts resulting in thin, contiguous slices (1 to 2 mm).

Small lesions are better detected with three-dimensional sequences than with two-dimensional techniques because the latter produce gaps between slices that may miss a small lesion. We use a T2-weighted sequence before the pre- and postenhancement sequences for distinguishing blood products from fluid or fibrosis.

Because of the high signal intensity of both fat and enhancing lesions on gradient echo images, methods of eliminating fat from MR images include chemical-shift imaging and image subtraction of the precontrast images from the postcontrast images (21,27,36–38). To optimize the chemical-shift techniques, maximizing the field homogeneity of the imaging volume is necessary. Shimming before imaging may be needed to reduce the field inhomogeneities that commonly occur in breast imaging. Some vendors now offer automated shimming for this purpose.

One effective method of fat suppression uses the RODEO (rotating delivery of excitation off-resonance) pulse sequence (21,27,39). This sequence requires a transmit-receive coil, which is usually unilateral.

Because fat does not enhance very much, subtraction of the precontrast images from those following contrast can be used to cancel out the fat signal. However, for subtraction to work, alignment of the two sets of images must be accurate. Any motion of the patient compromises the method.

One method of dynamic scanning during the injection of Gd-DTPA uses standard (two-dimensional) radiofrequency spoiled gradient echo (SPGR) or FLASH imaging at frequent time intervals (every 10 to 15 seconds) at a single level of interest. A report using partial k-space sampling with three-dimensional imaging for dynamic scanning in a small group of patients had promising results (40). However, concern over the reliability of distinguishing benign from malignant lesions with these techniques remains.

Echoplanar imaging (EPI), an ultrafast method of acquiring MR data (41), is another method of imaging that can provide rapid information on the dynamics of the tissue enhancement. It also can account for basic tissue variability

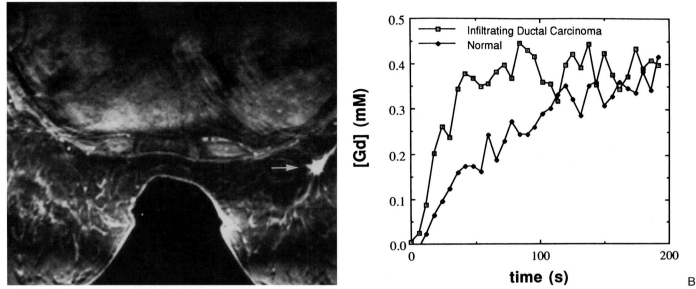

FIG. 20-9. Enhancing invasive cancer. Axial three-dimensional gradient echo image with fat suppression after **(A)** injection of Gd-DTPA shows an enhancing spiculated mass in the posterior right breast. A region-of-interest marker was placed on the lesion and normal breast parenchyma in the patient shown in **(B)**. Concentration of Gd-DTPA was calculated using dynamic echoplanar techniques. The course shows rapid initial tumor accumulation of contrast within the first 50 seconds of injection.

such as underlying T1 values (42,43). EPI uses rapidly changing gradients to sample all of k-space with a single excitation, producing images in as little as 50 msec. This permits physiologic imaging that covers multiple levels throughout the entire breast, after contrast infusion, to study the dynamics of contrast enhancement at intervals as often as 6 seconds. EPI, however, is not currently widely available and remains a research tool.

MR Enhancement Behavior of Breast Lesions

It appears that almost all invasive malignancies enhance with Gd-DTPA, and some research has shown that with dynamic MR imaging techniques malignancies may enhance at much more rapid initial rates than benign lesions (11,19,27,44–47) (Fig. 20-9). This rapid initial enhancement rate of malignancies is likely due to tumor angiogenesis. Malignant lesions are known to require the recruitment of a large concentration of tumor neovessels to permit their continued growth beyond a few millimeters (48). New vessels recruited by the tumors also have abnormal basement membranes that cause vessel leakiness and an increase in surrounding interstitial fluid pressure (49). The increased concentration of vessels at the tumor site and their leakiness likely account for the rapid accumulation of Gd-DTPA in breast cancers. Some benign breast lesions also enhance with Gd-DTPA (Fig. 20-10). This may also be due to higher vascularity, although whether the enhancement is due to increased concentrations of vessels or large feeding vessels in some benign entities is not clear (Fig. 20-11). The initial

enhancement rate (within the first minute) is usually less rapid in benign diagnoses than in malignancies, offering the opportunity to distinguish benign lesions from malignant by their enhancement pattern (see Fig. 20-10) (11,19,27,28,42,43). It is important to note that if MRI is delayed and scanning begins even only minutes after the injection of Gd-DTPA, some benign lesions will show a higher signal intensity than malignant lesions. It is not the absolute enhancement that permits separation of benign from malignant lesions, but the dynamics of the enhancement. It should be remembered that if the goal is to use MRI to differentiate benign from malignant lesions, the analysis of the enhancement soon after injection of the contrast appears to be critical.

Some investigators have disputed the consistency of early dynamic MR in distinguishing benign from malignant lesions, as several benign lesions demonstrated a more rapid rate of enhancement than expected (28,50–52). Furthermore, several invasive cancers, including several infiltrating lobular carcinomas, two malignant phylloides tumors, one tubular carcinoma, and colloid and mucinous carcinomas have been reported as having slow enhancement profiles (19,28,43,53,54). Although differences in vessel density may be the explanation for such variation, studies correlating low vessel density with slow enhancement of certain cancer cell types have not been performed. However, pathologic studies have shown a low expression of endothelial growth factor receptor messenger RNAs in infiltrating lobular carcinomas (as opposed to strong expression in invasive ductal carcinomas), which may account for decreased vascularity of this cell type (55).

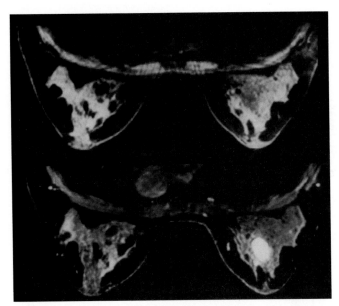

FIG. 20-10. Enhancing fibroadenoma. No mass is seen before gadolinium infusion. The brightly enhancing mass following the infusion proved to be a fibroadenoma.

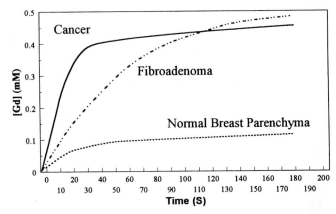

FIG. 20-11. These **idealized enhancement curves** demonstrate the difference in enhancement rates between benign and malignant lesions and the normal breast tissues. In general, cancers tend to enhance more rapidly.

Some of these variations in enhancement may also be the result of the MR technique used to calculate enhancement. If conventional techniques are used and simple changes in enhancement (or percent enhancement) from pre- and post-contrast scans are calculated, an overlap in benign and malignant values may result as this method does not account for the varying baseline of the T1 values of benign and malignant lesions before injection (the reason MR could not distinguish benign from malignant lesions without Gd-DTPA). For example, a lesion with a longer baseline T1 value would show greater relative enhancement than a lesion with a shorter baseline T1 value at 1 minute, even though the concentration of Gd-DTPA within the first lesion (longer T1) may be less than the concentration of Gd-DTPA in the second lesion (shorter T1). As some benign lesions have longer initial T1 values than cancers, this baseline T1 variation may explain the overlap described by some researchers.

Improved techniques for estimating the actual concentration of Gd-DTPA in lesions and accounting for baseline T1 values as well as correlation with vessel density are under investigation (27,42,43).

Some authors report that the morphology of the lesion and its pattern of enhancement may permit the separation of benign from malignant processes (19,26,30). As has been demonstrated by mammography and ultrasound, cancers demonstrate more irregularly shaped borders than benign tumors. However, because neither mammography nor ultrasound has been able to morphologically differentiate many lesions with sufficient accuracy to avoid a tissue diagnosis, it is unlikely that MRI will be any more successful. Nevertheless, morphologic studies using MRI bear careful evaluation because MRI provides cross-sectional morphology that, com-

bined with enhancement dynamics, may improve its accuracy. Nunes and colleagues constructed a flow chart model to try to use these enhancement and architectural characteristics to differentiate benign lesions from malignant (56). They used the results from 98 cases to produce the model and then tested it on 94 different cases. They found that a lesion was likely to be cancer primarily if it enhanced. A high degree of enhancement, an irregular pattern of enhancement, irregular borders, and the lack of any internal septations were associated with malignancy. Cancer was very unlikely if the lesion was not visible after gadolinium infusion, if its borders were smooth or lobulated, if the mass was irregular in shape, or if it had nonenhancing internal septations.

The early results from trials are frequently the most successful. More work is necessary before applying patterns of enhancement shape, rate, or combination of MR data with mammography and sonography before benign and malignant lesions can be distinguished with sufficient accuracy to avoid a safe tissue diagnosis.

MRI and Ductal Carcinoma in Situ

The MR behavior of DCIS is not clear, as enhancement varies from a rapid rate to no enhancement. This variation in enhancement behavior may be due to the variation of neovessel recruitment in DCIS. Despite the fact that these are intraductal lesions, some DCIS can stimulate neovascularity (28,57). Harms and colleagues have suggested that all DCIS can be detected. Others have not been as successful because some cases of DCIS do not appear to enhance. In a review of 13 patients with pure DCIS, Orel and associates were able to identify 10 of the lesions on the MRI scans. In six cases, curvilinear enhancement was termed *ductal*. In three of the cases there was segmental or regional enhancement, and in one case the enhancement was termed *peripheral*. Three lesions were not evident on their scans and two other lesions were not identified in six additional patients

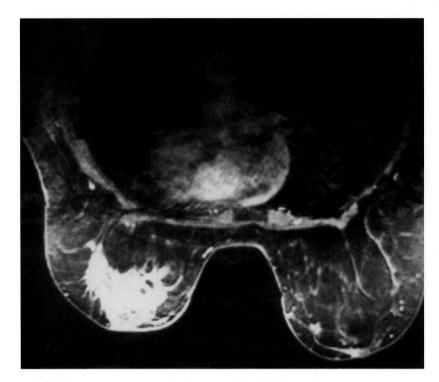

FIG. 20-12. Invasive lobular carcinoma. Axial three-dimensional gradient echo image with fat suppression before and after Gd-DTPA injection (2.5-mm slice thickness) shows extensive involvement of the left breast with an enhancing mass. Pathologic examination of the mastectomy specimen confirmed multifocal infiltrating lobular carcinoma. (With permission from Taveras JM, Ferrucci JT [eds]. Radiology: Diagnosis, Imaging, Intervention. Philadelphia: Lippincott–Raven, 1996.)

who had both invasive and intraductal cancer (58). Giles and colleagues evaluated 36 women with DCIS and contrast enhancement evaluation using the subtraction technique. They were able to identify 34 of the lesions, but failed to demonstrate two cases of comedocarcinoma (59). One problem that complicates some of the studies is the fact that there is a difference between knowing where DCIS was found histologically and finding it on an imaging study versus identifying the lesion prospectively and having it confirmed by the histology.

The ability of MRI to detect DCIS, particularly poorly differentiated DCIS, is important. Not only do these lesions tend to progress to invasion sooner (see Chapter 7), but the demonstration of DCIS is critical for assessing the extent of the cancer. If DCIS is not recognized extending away from a primary invasive tumor, then excision or even destroying the primary tumor in vivo (e.g., laser, cryotherapy, high-frequency ultrasound) is likely to fail to achieve local control because residual, undetected (and hence untreated) tumor will lead to high recurrence rates.

Specific Applications of Breast Lesion MRI

The roles for MR in evaluating breast lesions are being defined. The ability to distinguish benign from malignant lesions on the basis of their dynamic enhancement pattern and their morphologic characteristics using the variety of techniques discussed remains under investigation in the United States. MRI is already being used by some physicians for tumor staging and to differentiate scar tissue from cancer recurrence.

Tumor Staging

Tumor staging is done to determine the extent of disease within the breast, which is important to permit complete excision or tumor destruction if conservation therapy is chosen.

Determining the extent of tumor involvement (multifocality or multicentricity) within the breast with an imaging technique may be useful to the surgeon, radiation therapist, and oncologist. This added information may alter or guide surgical planning and radiation or chemotherapy (26,35). Using the conventional three-dimensional techniques with Gd-DTPA and fat suppression described in the previous section provides a detailed map of tumor involvement with high anatomic detail and signal-to-noise resolution (Fig. 20-12).

The extent of tumor involvement is not confined to staging of breast cancers, as some benign lesions may be quite large (Fig. 20-13). In such cases, mammography or ultrasound may not adequately delineate the tumor size and location, whereas MRI gives an excellent three-dimensional map for surgical planning.

Differentiation of Scar Tissue from Cancer Recurrence

Sometimes, a patient who has undergone lumpectomy or radiation therapy, or both, for cancer later presents with a suspicious mammogram or physical examination in the region of prior surgery. Some of these patients undergo re-excision of the scar due to the concern for local recurrence, although local recurrence only occurs in 1% of such patients each year (60). MRI may be useful in distinguishing scar tissue from local recurrence at the specified post-

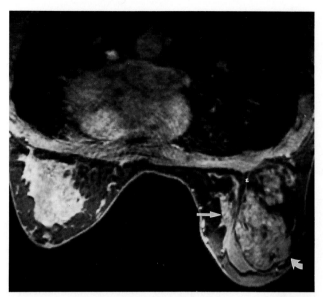

FIG. 20-13. Hamartoma. Axial three-dimensional gradient echo image with fat suppression after Gd-DTPA injection of a patient who desired removal of a right breast mass that had been present for many years. A large mass in the lateral right breast shows fat and parenchymal components and a low–signal-intensity fibrous capsule compressing the adjacent parenchyma medially. The posterior relation of this mass to the chest wall was not appreciated on mammography or sonography, and the MRI aided the surgeons in removal of this tumor. A hamartoma was confirmed at pathologic examination of the surgical specimen. (With permission from Taveras JM, Ferrucci JT [eds]. Radiology: Diagnosis, Imaging, Intervention. Philadelphia: Lippincott–Raven, 1996.)

operative time interval. Although immediately after surgery and during the course of radiation therapy a high density of new vessels from wound healing can result in enhancement on MRI, some small series have suggested that scar tissue does not enhance with Gd-DTPA on MRI. Dao and colleagues have suggested that MRI can be used to follow women treated conservatively with excision and irradiation (61). Areas of surgery frequently enhance if studied within 6 to 12 months after treatment. After that period of healing, fixed fibrosis does not enhance, but recurrent breast cancer frequently does (27). If any enhancement is visualized in a scar older than 12 months, the possibility of recurrence increases. Although the early detection of recurrence in the breast may have useful therapeutic value, it has yet to be shown that detecting recurrences earlier alters mortality. Nevertheless, in the absence of data, early detection of recurrent breast cancer would seem to be a good idea.

Other Applications

Chest wall imaging, searching for a primary malignancy, and following the response of breast cancers to chemotherapy are other areas in which some physicians find MRI of the breast to be useful. The detection of chest wall recurrence may be a problem after mastectomy and reconstruction with an implant or a TRAM (transverse rectus abdominis myocutaneous flap) procedure (Fig. 20-14). As noted earlier, we and others have found MRI to also be useful for searching for a primary breast cancer in patients with

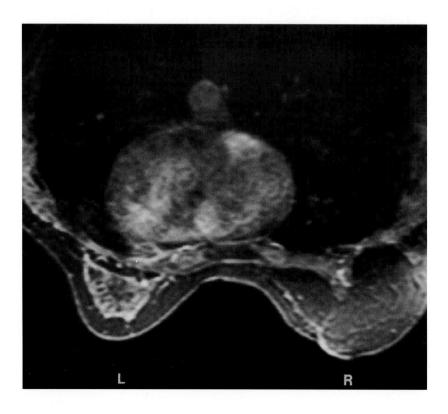

FIG. 20-14. TRAM flap. Axial three-dimensional gradient echo image with fat suppression after Gd-DTPA injection of a patient with a TRAM-flap reconstruction of the right breast after mastectomy for cancer. The posterior muscle and enhancing associated vascular pedicle are identified. (With permission from Taveras JM, Ferrucci JT [eds]. Radiology: Diagnosis, Imaging, Intervention. Philadelphia: Lippincott–Raven, 1996.)

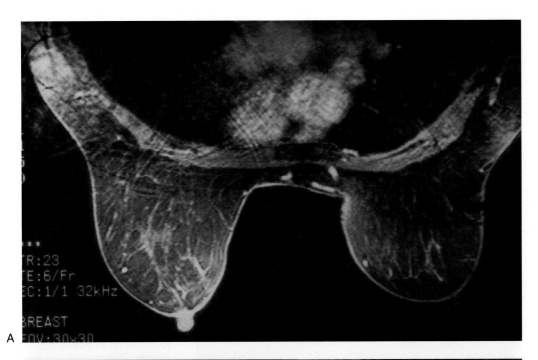

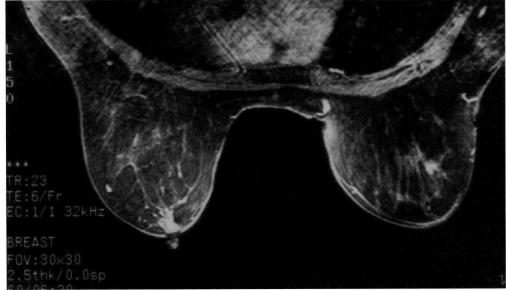

FIG. 20-15. Detection of occult malignancy. This patient had a positive axillary lymph node with a negative clinical examination and negative mammogram. T1-weighted images after the intravenous administration of gadolinium showed marked left nipple **(A)** and subareolar **(B)** enhancement that was much greater than the normal nipple enhancement. Clinically there was subtle crusting of the nipple. **Intraductal and invasive breast cancer** was found at surgery.

metastatic disease of unknown origin or in those with axillary adenopathy highly suspicious for a breast malignancy (Fig. 20-15).

The evaluation of local tumor response to chemotherapy with MR breast imaging may also provide useful information to oncologists or surgeons.

Future of Breast MRI

At present, MRI of silicone implants has a defined role in the evaluation of implant rupture. Contrast-enhanced MRI of the breast is also useful in solving specific problems, such as distinguishing scar from cancer recurrence

12 or more months after surgery and in local staging of breast cancer. MRI is also useful in searching for a primary breast cancer when the patient presents with metastatic disease.

Differentiation of benign from malignant breast disease with dynamic MRI remains an area of research. If successful, MRI could reduce the number of biopsies for benign lesions and could possibly provide a means for earlier cancer detection in a limited group of patients.

Because of its cost, the need to inject contrast material, and the complexity of the examination, MRI is not likely to be a universal screening test. Nevertheless, MRI may be useful to screen selected groups of patients with mammographically

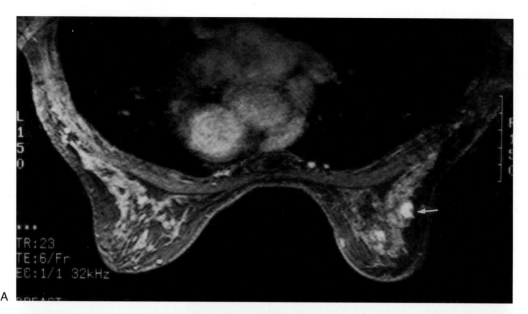

A

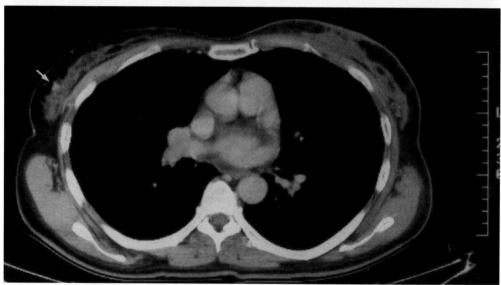

B

FIG. 20-16. Detection and localization of occult breast cancer. This patient was participating in an MRI research study. She had what proved to be invasive breast cancer detected by mammography on the left *(arrow)*. T1-weighted MRI after gadolinium revealed an unsuspected enhancing lesion in the right breast **(A)** that could not be seen, even in retrospect, on mammography and was not visible on ultrasound. The lesion was localized using its enhancement on computed tomography **(B)** after contrast enhancement *(arrow)*. It proved to be a tubular carcinoma.

dense and complex breast tissue or those at very high risk for developing breast cancer (Fig. 20-16A).

Because of its high sensitivity and ability to image small lesions, but its still rather low specificity, methods to guide tissue diagnosis and localization of MRI-detected lesions are necessary. These lesions may not be seen with mammography or sonography, and methods need to be devised to guide needle localizations, fine-needle aspiration, and core biopsies with MRI. Researchers have developed methods to guide needle procedures with MRI, but they remain fairly cumbersome (11,62–66). We have used computed tomography and contrast enhancement with iodinated contrast material to replicate enhancement seen by MRI and to guide needle procedures (Fig. 20-16B).

It remains to be seen whether digital mammography with contrast subtraction will be a low-cost alternative to enhanced MRI (see Chapter 26).

REFERENCES

1. Harris KM, Ganott MA, Shestak KC, et al. Silicone implant rupture: detection with ultrasound. Radiology 1993;187:761–768.
2. Gorczyca DP, DeBruhl ND, Ahn CY, et al. Silicone breast implant ruptures in an animal model: comparison of mammography, MR imaging, US, and CT. Radiology 1994;190:227–232.
3. Picha GJ, Goldstein JA. Analysis of the soft tissue response to components used in the manufacture of breast implants: rat animal model. Plast Reconstr Surg 1991;87:490–500.
4. Winding O, Christensen L, Thomsen JL, et al. Silicone in human breast tissue surrounding silicone gel prostheses. Scand J Plast Reconstr Surg Hand Surg Suppl 1988;22:127–130.
5. Thomsen JL, Christensen L, Nielsen M, et al. Histologic changes and silicone concentrations in human breast tissue surrounding silicone breast prostheses. Plast Reconstr Surg 1990;85:38–41.
6. Brandt B, Breiting VB, Christensen L, et al. Five years experience of breast augmentation using silicone gel prostheses with emphasis on capsule shrinkage. Scand J Plast Reconstr Surg Hand Surg Suppl 1984;18:311–316.
7. Gylbert L, Asplund O, Jurell G. Capsular contracture after breast

reconstruction with silicone and saline-filled implants: a 6-year follow-up. Plast Reconstr Surg 1990;85:373–377.

8. Kessler DA. The basis of the FDA's decision on breast implants. N Engl J Med 1992:326:1713–1715.

9. Weiner SR. Silicone Augmentation Mammaplasty and Rheumatic Disease. In Straymeyer ME (ed), Silicone in Medical Devices. Bethesda, MD: Department of Health and Human Services, 1991;81–102. FDA publication 92-4249.

10. Sanchez-Guerrero J, Colditz GA, Karlson EW, et al. Silicone breast implants and the risk of connective-tissue diseases and symptoms. N Engl J Med 1995;332:1666–1670.

11. Gorczyca DP, Sinha S, Ahn C, et al. Silicone breast implants in vivo: MR imaging. Radiology 1992;185:407–410.

12. Gorczyca DP, Schneider E, DeBruhl ND, et al. Silicone breast implant rupture: comparison between three-point Dixon and fast spin-echo MR imaging. AJR Am J Roentgenol 1994;162:305–310.

13. Garrido L, Kwong KK, Pfleiderer B, et al. Echo-planar chemical shift imaging of silicone gel prostheses. Magn Reson Imaging 1993;11:625–634.

14. Monticciolo DL, Nelson RC, Dixon WT, et al. MR detection of leakage from silicone breast implants: value of a silicone selective pulse sequence. AJR Am J Roentgenol 1994;63:51–56.

15. Berg WA, Caskey CI, Hamper UM, et al. Diagnosing breast implant rupture with MR imaging, US and mammography. Radiographics 1993;13:1323–1336.

16. Gabriel SE, Woods JE, O'Fallon M, et al. Complications leading to surgery after breast implantation. N Engl J Med 1997;336:677–682.

17. El Yousef SJ, Duchesneau RH. Magnetic resonance imaging of the human breast: a phase I trial. Radiol Clin North Am 1984;22:859–868.

18. Heywang S, Hahn D, Schmidt H, et al. Magnetic resonance imaging of the breast using gadolinium-DTPA. J Comput Assist Tomogr 1986;10:199–204.

19. Kaiser WA, Zeitler E. MR imaging of the breast: fast imaging sequences with and without Gd-DTPA. Radiology 1989;170:681–686.

20. Nelson TR, Pretorius DH, Schiffer LM. Menstrual variation of normal breast NMR relaxation parameters. J Comput Assist Tomogr 1985;9:874–879.

21. Weinreb JC, Newstead G. MR imaging of the breast. Radiology 1995;196:593–610.

22. Muller-Schimpfle M, Ohmenhauser K, Stoll P, et al. Menstrual cycle and age: influence on parenchymal contrast medium enhancement on MR imaging of the breast. Radiology 1997;203:145–149.

23. Kuhl CK, Bieling HB, Gieseke J, et al. Healthy premenopausal breast parenchyma in dynamic contrast-enhanced MR imaging of the breast: normal contrast medium enhancement and cyclical-phase dependency. Radiology 1997;203:136–144.

24. Kopans DB, Swann CA. Preoperative imaging-guided needle placement and localization of clinically occult breast lesions. AJR Am J Roentgenol 1989;152:1–9.

25. Spivey GH, Perry BW, Clark VA, et al. Predicting the risk of cancer at the time of breast biopsy. Am J Surg 1982;48:326–332.

26. Orel SG, Schnall MD, Powell CM, et al. Staging of suspected breast cancer: effect of MR imaging and MR-guided biopsy. Radiology 1995;196:115–122.

27. Dao TH, Rahmouni A, Campana F, et al. Tumor recurrence versus fibrosis in the irradiated breast: differentiation with dynamic gadolinium-enhanced MR imaging. Radiology 1993;187:751–755.

28. Gilles R, Guinebretiere JM, Shapeero LG, et al. Assessment of breast cancer recurrence with contrast enhanced subtraction MR imaging: preliminary results in 26 patients. Radiology 1993;188:473–478.

29. Heywang SH, Hilbertz T, Beck R, et al. Gd-DTPA enhanced MR imaging of the breast in patients with postoperative scarring and silicon implants. J Comput Assist Tomogr 1990;14:348–356.

30. Heywang-Koebrunner SH, Haustein J, Pohl C, et al. Contrast-enhanced MR imaging of the breast: comparison of two different doses of gadopentate dimeglumine. Radiology 1994;191:639–646.

31. Harms SE, Flamig DP, Hesley KL, et al. MR imaging of the breast with rotating delivery of excitation off resonance: clinical experience with pathologic correlation. Radiology 1993;187:493–501.

32. Heywang-Kobrunner SH. Contrast-enhanced magnetic resonance imaging of the breast. Invest Radiol 1994;29:94–104.

33. Frahm J, Haase A, Mattai D. Rapid three-dimensional NMR imaging using FLASH technique. J Comput Assist Tomogr 1986;10:363–368.

34. Oppelt A, Graumann R, et al. FISP: Eine neue schnelle pulssequenz fur die kernspintomographie. Elektromedica 1986;54:15–18.

35. Pierce WB, Harms SE, Flamig DP, et al. Three-dimensional gadolinium-enhanced MR imaging of the breast: pulse sequence with fat suppression and magnetization transfer contrast. Radiology 1991;181:757–763.

36. Rubens D, Totterman S, Chacko AK, et al. Gadopentate dimeglumine-enhanced chemical-shift MR imaging of the breast. AJR Am J Roentgenol 1991;12:19–24.

37. Oellinger H, Sander B, Quednean U, et al. Three dimensional reconstruction of subtraction images in female breast imaging. J Magn Reson Imaging 1993;3:109.

38. Harms SE, Flamig DP. MR imaging of the breast: technical approach and clinical experience. Radiographics 1993;13:905–912.

39. Harms SE, Flamig DP, Helsey KL, Evans WP. Magnetic resonance imaging of the breast. Magn Reson Q 1992;8:139–155.

40. Chenevert TL, Helvie MA, Aisen AM, et al. Dynamic three-dimensional imaging with partial k-space sampling: initial application for gadolinium-enhanced rate characterization of breast lesions. Radiology 1995;196:135–142.

41. Petersein J, Saini S. Fast MR imaging: technical strategies. AJR Am J Roentgenol 1995;165:1105–1109.

42. Cohen MS, Weisskoff RM. Ultra-fast imaging. Magn Reson Imaging 1991;9:1–37.

43. Hulka CA, Smith BL, Sgroi DC, et al. Benign and malignant breast lesions: differentiation with echo planar imaging. Radiology 1995;197:33–38.

44. Stack JP, Redmond OM, Codd MB, et al. Breast disease: tissue characterization with Gd-DTPA enhancement profiles. Radiology 1990;174:491–494.

45. Hachiya J, Seki T, Okada M, et al. MR imaging of the breast with Gd-DTPA enhancement: comparison with mammography and ultrasonography. Radiol Med (Torino) 1991;9:232–240.

46. Gilles R, Guinebretiere JM, Lucidarme O, et al. Nonpalpable breast tumors: diagnosis with contrast-enhanced subtraction dynamic MR imaging. Radiology 1994;191:625–631.

47. Fobben ES, Rubin CZ, Kalisher L, et al. Breast MRI techniques with commercially available techniques: radiologic-pathologic correlation. Radiology 1995;196:143–152.

48. Folkman J. What is the evidence that tumors are angiogenesis dependent? J Natl Cancer Inst 1990;82:4–6.

49. Negendank WG, Brown TR, Evelhoch JL, et al. Proceedings of a National Cancer Institute workshop: MR spectroscopy and tumor cell biology. Radiology 1992;185:875–883.

50. Kelcz F, Santyr G, Cron GO, Mongin S. Application of a quantitative model to differentiate benign from malignant lesions detected by dynamic gadolinium-enhanced magnetic resonance imaging. J Magn Reson Imag 1996;6:743–752.

51. Schnall M, Orel S, Muenz L. Analysis of time intensity curves for enhancing lesions [abstract]. 1993.

52. Orel SG, Schnall MD, LiVolsi VA, Troupin RH. Suspicious breast lesions: MR imaging with radiologic-pathologic correlation. Radiology 1994;190:485–493.

53. Boetes C, Barentsz JO, Mus RD, et al. MR characterization of suspicious breast lesions with a gadolinium-enhanced turbo FLASH subtraction technique. Radiology 1994;193:777–781.

54. Piccoli CW, Mitchell DG, Schwartz GF, Vinitski S. Contrast-enhanced breast MR imaging with dynamic and fat-suppression techniques. In the program of the annual meeting of the Society for Magnetic Imaging; 1993;47–48. San Francisco.

55. Brown LF, Berse B, Jackman RW, et al. Expression of vascular permeability factor (vascular endothelial growth factor) and its receptors in breast cancer. Hum Pathol 1995;26:86–91.

56. Numes LW, Schnall MD, Orel SG, et al. Breast MR imaging: interpretation model. Radiology 1997;202:833–841.

57. Guidi AJ, Fischer L, Harris JR, Schnitt SJ. Microvessel density and distribution in ductal carcinoma in situ of the breast. J Natl Cancer Inst 1994;86:614–619.

58. Orel SG, Mendonca MH, Reynolds C, et al. MR imaging of ductal carcinoma in situ. Radiology 1997;202:413–420.

59. Giles R, Zanfrani B, Guinebretiere J, et al. Ductal carcinoma in situ: MR imaging-histopathologic correlation. Radiology 1995;196:415–419.

60. Kurtz JM, Amalric R, Brandone H, et al. Local recurrence after breast-conserving surgery and radiotherapy: frequency, time-course, and prognosis. Cancer 1989;63:1912–1917.

61. Dao T, Rahmouni A, Servios V, Nguyen-Tan T. MR imaging of the breast in the follow-up evaluation of conservatively treated breast cancer. Magn Reson Imaging Clin N Am 1994;2:605–622.

62. Hussman K, Renslo R, Phillips JJ, et al. MR mammographic localization work in progress. Radiology 1993;189:915–917.

63. Fischer U, Vosshenrich R, Keating D, et al. MR-guided biopsy of suspect breast lesions with a simple stereotaxic add-on device for surface coils. Radiology 1994;192:272–273.

64. Heywang-Kobrunner SH, Huynh AT, Viehweg P, et al. Prototype breast coil for MR-guided needle localization. J Comput Assist Tomogr 1994;18:876–881.

65. Orel SG, Schnall MD, Newman RW, et al. MR imaging-guided localization and biopsy of breast lesions: initial experience. Radiology 1994; 193:97–102.

66. Fischer U, Vosshenrich R, Kopka L, et al. Preoperative MR mammography in patients with breast cancer: impact on therapy. In the scientific program of the 80th scientific assembly and annual meeting of the Radiological Society of North America; 1994;121.

Breast Imaging, 2nd ed., by Daniel B. Kopans.
Lippincott–Raven Publishers, Philadelphia © 1998.

CHAPTER 21

Imaging-Guided Needle Placement for Biopsy and the Preoperative Localization of Clinically Occult Lesions

The primary objective of mammography is the detection of clinically occult cancer of the breast at an early stage in its growth in the hope of interrupting the natural history of the malignancy before it has successfully metastasized to other organs and preventing or delaying death from the cancer. In addition to mortality reduction, earlier detection can permit less aggressive forms of therapy and allows breast-preserving cancer treatment options. Early detection requires the screening of asymptomatic, apparently healthy women who have no signs or symptoms of breast cancer.

Because the time of successful metastatic spread cannot be determined, there is no guarantee that a given individual can be cured of breast cancer, even if her cancer is discovered and treated early; but the interruption of the growth of a breast cancer at as early a time as possible in its development is generally desirable. Failure to aggressively pursue subtle signs of malignancy and a high threshold for intervention, in which the radiologist recommends intervention only when classic signs of cancer are present, will result in permitting early cancers to pass through the screen and will compromise the benefit (1,2). Similarly, if an early lesion is detected but the diagnostic test is falsely negative, the benefit of screening and earlier detection may be lost. The false-negative rate for cancer is very important for determining the value of a diagnostic test.

The screening process results in the detection of a myriad of breast changes, many of which are not due to cancer. There is as yet no test that can reliably differentiate benign from malignant lesions with the same accuracy as histologic analysis, and consequently, before appropriate treatment can be instituted histologic diagnosis is usually required. To obtain cells or tissue for diagnosis, needles, in one form or another, must be placed into the breast as either a primary method of tissue sampling or to place guides to assist a surgical procedure. These are required for cytologic analysis, core needle histologic sampling, incisional biopsy, or excisional biopsy diagnosis. The accurate positioning of needles is critical for accurate diagnosis and will likely be needed even if in vivo ablative therapies become efficacious. This chapter describes the various techniques for needle positioning for all of these procedures.

OVERLAP BETWEEN BENIGN AND MALIGNANT LESIONS

Although it is frequently described as a diagnostic test, mammography is primarily a screening test. Despite its ability to find earlier stage, clinically occult breast cancer, it is usually not able to permit the differentiation of benign findings from malignant, because the morphologic characteristics of benign and malignant lesions may be similar. Lesions that are round or ovoid and that have sharply defined margins are statistically very likely to be benign (3), but some cancers have similar shapes and margins. The abrupt transition in tissue density at these margins can result in a Mach effect that causes the observer to see a thin, dark, lucent halo around the lesion. The halo was once thought to indicate a benign process, but even this characteristic sharply defined margin indicating an abrupt transition between tissues does not always guarantee a benign process (4).

At the other end of the spectrum, even the classic lesion with a spiculated margin, which is almost invariably due to malignancy, can on occasion be a benign change such as a radial scar, an area of postsurgical change, fat necrosis (5,6), or an unusual lesion such as an extra-abdominal desmoid tumor. In addition the calcifications associated with cancer are frequently morphologically indistinguishable from those produced by benign processes (7). Because many benign lesions detected by mammography are indistinguishable from cancer by any noninvasive assessment, a cytologic or histologic diagnosis is usually sought for lesions that cannot be classified as benign or probably benign.

POSITIVE PREDICTIVE VALUE OF A BREAST BIOPSY AND THE HEALTH CARE CONTROVERSY

The cost of health care has become a major factor in the delivery of services. The goal of most health planners is to keep down the cost of health care. The goal of breast cancer screening is to save lives by finding as many cancers at as early a stage as possible. These goals often conflict. Not only does screening have an economic cost, but it leads to breast biopsies, which add to the overall expense. Biopsies also induce less quantifiable costs, such as the anxiety to the individual woman who fears that she may have breast cancer and the physical trauma from a biopsy needed to determine whether an abnormality is benign or malignant.

The difference between the health-planner perspective and the medical goal was seen at a meeting organized by the National Cancer Institute to review the data on double reading. The health planners were most interested in the use of double reading as a way to reduce the rate at which women are called back for additional evaluation and as a way to reduce the number of breast biopsies. The physicians involved in caring for women with breast cancer viewed double reading as a way to improve the detection of small cancers. It is difficult to predict how these contradictory perspectives will ever be resolved.

Because of the costs involved, the number of biopsies performed as a result of mammography has become a major issue. Many planners and radiologists are interested in the accuracy of mammography. One measure is the positive predictive value (PPV) for biopsies. The PPV for biopsies prompted by mammography is the ratio of the number of cancers diagnosed to the number of biopsies recommended. Because many of the biopsies reveal benign histology (false positives) the number of biopsies recommended can be defined as the true positives plus the false positives. Thus,

$$PPV = \frac{\text{True positives}}{\text{True positives} + \text{false positives}} = \frac{\text{Cancers diagnosed}}{\text{Biopsies performed}}$$

Because of the broad overlap in the morphologic appearance of benign and malignant lesions, it is impossible to avoid benign biopsies if the goal is to diagnosis breast cancers earlier. The ability to separate benign from malignant lesions by their morphology is limited, and historically the PPV for a suspicious, nonpalpable abnormality seen by mammography has ranged from 15% to 35% (8–10).

The PPV, however, cannot be considered in isolation (11). It must be evaluated in conjunction with other factors. One of the primary elements that influences the PPV is the prior probability of cancer in the population (the *actual* number of cancers in the population being evaluated). Because the prior probability of cancer increases with the age of the population of women being screened, PPV is influenced by age. In a review of 36,000 screening studies, we found that approximately the same percentage of women, at any age, were recommended for a biopsy, but that the PPV for mammographically generated biopsies rose steadily with the age of the women. PPV was 10% to 15% for women at age 40 but rose steadily to almost 50% by age 79. These results are a reflection of the gradual increase in incidence of cancer in the population that occurs with the increasing age of the population. If there are more cancers to be detected, mammography will detect them. Thus, the risk factors of the population being evaluated greatly influence the PPV, and,

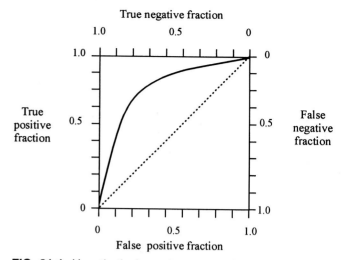

FIG. 21-1. Hypothetical **receiver operating characteristic curve.** Unless the observer has unique information, all trained interpreters operate on the same curve. The only way to reduce interventions that prove to be benign lesions (false positives) is to permit some cancers to pass through the screen (false negatives).

because age is a major risk factor, the age of the population being screened has a great influence on the PPV.

There has been concern that mammographic screening leads to too many biopsies with benign results. These have even been termed *unnecessary biopsies*. There are no agreed on methods to determine what an acceptable PPV should be. All well-trained radiologists operate on a similar receiver–operating-characteristic (ROC) curve. This means that, unless one radiologist has unique information that permits more accurate differentiation of benign from malignant lesions by mammography, the only way to increase the PPV (reduce the biopsies with benign results) is to alter the threshold for recommending an intervention by increasing the false-negative rate and permitting cancers to slip through the screen (2,12) (Fig. 21-1). If the threshold for intervention is high and the radiologist only recommends a biopsy when strong indicators of malignancy are present, the yield of cancers will be high (the PPV will be high) but cancers will be missed. By having a high threshold for intervention, small cancers pass through a screen and mortality reduction is compromised. This is one of the reasons that some screening trials, such as the program in Nijmegen in the Netherlands (for women under the age of 50), have not been successful in reducing breast cancer mortality.

It is not sufficient to compare PPVs in isolation. A key measure is the success of the screening program at detecting small cancers and not missing cancers. The sensitivity of the screening is perhaps the most critical of factors. This is defined as the percentage of the cancers that are diagnosed in the population over a defined (usually 1 year) period that are detected by the screen. Cancers that are missed by the screen but become apparent in the interval between screens (found by the patient or her doctor) are called *interval cancers*. A successful screening program should have a high sensitivity (>80%) and a low interval cancer rate (<20%). Sensitivity is directly influenced by thresholds for intervention; therefore, the size and stage of the cancers that are detected must also be considered when evaluating the success of a screening program.

One method of evaluating the sensitivity of a screening program is to determine the number of cancers detected for every 1,000 women screened for the first time (prevalence) and the number detected in each subsequent year (incidence). A successful program that screens an average population of women from the ages of 40 to 80, will detect anywhere from 6 to 10 cancers per 1,000 women screened in the prevalence screen and then 2 to 3 cancers per 1,000 in each subsequent incidence screen. These figures vary depending on the actual cancer rate in the population being studied. A high-risk population or an older population (naturally at higher risk) will have larger numbers of cancers in the prevalence screen and in each incidence screen, whereas a low-risk group will have lower numbers. A program, for example, that only detects one cancer per 1,000 women screened among a high-risk group is certainly not a successful screening program.

The difference between the prevalence rate and the incidence rate, assuming the same women return each year for screening, is a crude measure of the lead time gained by screening (how much earlier screening detects cancer). Thus, the number of cancers detected in each screening provides an indication of how much earlier screening detects breast cancer. The first screening (prevalence screening) detects cancers that had been growing and were possibly detectable for many years but were not detected because the women were not being screened. Cancers that could only have been detected for the first time during that year would also be detected. These are the new cancers that appear each year at whatever the level of detection (incidence). Thus, the cancers detected in the first screening can be considered to represent a sum of the cancers that could have been detected in the year before the first screening plus those that could have been detected 2 years before the first screening plus those detectable 3 years earlier, and so on, up to N years earlier. This N is the lead time for the screening. It represents how much earlier cancers can be detected by the screening program compared to routine care without screening.

Because the cancers detected in the first screening (prevalence) are the sum of cancers that could have been detected each year for N years earlier, lead time can be calculated by subtracting the number of cancers detected in an incidence screening from the number of cancers detected in the prevalence screening and then dividing the result by the average number of cancers detected in the incidence screenings. A measure of lead time can be summarized by the following equation:

$$\text{Lead time} = \frac{\text{Prevalent cancers} - \text{incident cancers}}{\text{Incident cancers}}$$

This formula is a crude measure because it is merely an estimate and does not account for the interval cancers. It does provide an indication of the success of a screening program.

For example, if a screening detects two cancers each year in every 1,000 women screened and in the first (prevalence) screening six cancers are detected, this implies that two cancers per year were accumulating in the population in the years before the first screening but were undetected by the patients' usual care. At the time of the first screening, the mammogram found the two that would have surfaced without screening. Two more would have surfaced in the next year, and the final two would have surfaced in 2 years. This suggests that the mammographic screening detected cancers approximately 2 years before they would have become apparent without screening. The lead time gained by screening is 2 years (see Chapter 4).

Using our data of eight to ten cancers detected per 1,000 at the first screening and two or three in subsequent incidence screenings implies that our screening is detecting breast cancers, on average, 1.7 to 4.0 years earlier [(8 – 3)/3 to (10 – 2)/2] than was the case before the women began being screened. For a screening program to be successful, it must at the least detect cancers earlier. If, for example, a program detected four cancers per 1,000 in the prevalence screening and two in the incidence screening, the lead time would be about 1 year and this would likely be less successful at reducing mortality than a program with a 2- to 3-year lead time.

One European screening program that screened every 3 years prided itself on detecting six cancers per 1,000 women each time. What they failed to realize is that this meant that they had no lead time (they weren't detecting cancers much earlier than without screening) and that screening was unlikely to have any benefit. At their prevalence screening and at each subsequent screening six cancers are found per 1,000 women. This means that the program is providing the women with little or no benefit. The lead time equals (6 – 6)/6 = 0 years. They are discovering the cancers at about the same time that the women would have discovered them if there was no screening. The goal should be to have an incidence rate at detection that is one-third or lower than the prevalence screen.

In addition to the sensitivity of the screening, lead time can be affected by the background detection rate. If women in a population usually present with very late stage disease, then even a crude screening will improve the early detection rate. At the time of the Health Insurance Plan of New York trial (HIP), there was little attention paid to early detection. Many women delayed seeking care for breast cancer. This accounts for much of the success of the HIP trial, where the control women presented with a high percentage of advanced cancers. Any form of screening that lowered the stage at diagnosis would provide a benefit. This made it easier to demonstrate a benefit from screening in the HIP.

The more recent screening programs have found it more difficult to show a benefit because the control women were being more carefully monitored routinely (by themselves or their doctors). Many of them even had mammography on their own outside the trial (contamination), making it more difficult among the screened women to have their cancers found at a smaller size and earlier stage.

Sensitivity

Sensitivity alone does not indicate the success of the screening program. The sensitivity of a program may be fairly high, because all significant cancers ultimately become evident and if women are relying on screening most cancers will eventually be found by the screen. The benefit, however, may be low. It is the detection of the small, early cancers that determines the success of a screening program. If, for example, increasing the PPV (fewer false positives) results in permitting small cancers to pass through the screen and results in the detection of mostly stage II cancers, the sensitivity may be high and the PPV may be high but the benefit of screening is lost. To be successful screening must find cancers at a smaller size and earlier stage than care without screening.

Early Intervention

The size, stage, and histologic grade of a cancer are the main predictors of outcome. Survival is improved when cancers are found at a small size and when there is no evidence of spread to the axillary nodes or to other organs (13). Even within stages, size is a further indication of prognosis. Rosen has shown improved survival for small stage I cancers in comparison to larger stage I cancers. Invasive malignancies that are 1 cm or smaller have a statistically significantly better prognosis than stage I cancers 1.1 to 1.9 cm in size (14). Although Tabar recommended that the median size of invasive cancers in a screening program should be 1.5 cm, his data also suggest that the detection of cancers 1 cm or less in diameter is an important goal (15). He found that women whose cancers were detected at 1 cm or smaller had uniformly excellent survivals of >95%. Furthermore, he found that, although histologic grade was a prognostic factor for women with cancers that were >1 cm, women with a cancer <1 cm all did well, regardless of grade.

If screening is to have benefit, a large percentage of cancers must be found at an earlier stage than the usual care without screening. Mortality can be reduced if as many invasive cancers as possible are found when they are <1 cm in size. The only true value of mammography is in the detection of cancers at a smaller size and earlier stage.

In summary, comparisons of PPVs should include an evaluation of the population being screened and how many cancers are expected in that population (prior probability); the sensitivity of the screening (what percentage of the cancers are detected earlier); the number of cancers detected per 1,000 women screened at the first screen (prevalence) and at subsequent screens (incidence); and the size, stage, and histologic grade of cancers detected.

Interval Cancers and Detection Targets

Ideally, although the figures are difficult to determine outside of a funded screening trial, the true interval cancer rate (cancers detected between screenings) is also an important measure of the value of the screening effort. In our own screening program, mammography detects 90% to 95% of the cancers present in a given year (this is an estimate, because the true false-negative rate cannot be accurately determined). In programs such as that of the University of California at San Francisco, where the program has access to regional cancer registries, the sensitivity is approximately 85%. This figure includes cancers that surface within 1 year of a negative mammogram. In Arizona, Linvers, with links to the regional tumor registry, found the same sensitivity of approximately 85% to 88% (15a).

Among our screened patients, 30% of the cancers detected by mammography are ductal carcinoma in situ (DCIS) (LCIS is not included in our cancer statistics), and >50% of the invasive cancers are 1 cm or smaller with <20% of the women having positive axillary nodes. We detect approximately eight to ten cancers per 1,000 women being screened for the first time (all ages combined) and two to three cancers per 1,000 women in subsequent screenings (all ages combined). Of course it is difficult to compare a screening program such as ours that takes only physician-referred women with population-based screening programs. There are likely biases that are introduced by the selection of our patients, but these targets can be achieved. However, they require active investigation of lesions while they are still small and often do not have the characteristics of cancer. The benefits of screening will be compromised if thresholds for additional evaluation are determined by politics and economics and not by the goal of finding as many cancers as early as possible.

Determining Appropriate Positive Predictive Value

An ideal PPV would be 100%, with all cancers being detected at a curable stage. In other words, all biopsies would reveal cancers (there would be none performed for benign lesions), and all cancers detected would be curable. At present, this cannot be achieved. There is no absolute method for determining an appropriate PPV. A frame of reference is found in the historical PPV for clinically detected abnormalities. A review of the published data (generally the best experiences) concerning the PPV for a suspicious clinical breast examination (CBE) that leads to a biopsy is revealing (16–18). For a general population of women, the PPV for biopsies instigated by CBE ranges from as low as 5% to about 25%.

In our own practice, the PPV for a biopsy instigated by a CBE of asymptomatic women is >50% lower than for lesions detected by mammography. In a group of women who were originally deemed to be asymptomatic, approximately 100 were biopsied over the course of a year for clinically suspicious abnormalities (negative mammograms) and only 7% of the biopsies revealed a cancer (PPV = 7%). Among the same women, approximately 400 biopsies were performed for mammographically detected problems, and approximately 80 of these were cancers (PPV = 20%).

Not only is the PPV similar (if not higher) for mammographically detected lesions, but, when a cancer is detected by mammography alone, it is more likely to be detected at a smaller size and earlier stage (19) with a better prognosis (20) than a lesion detected by CBE. Thus, if the goal is to reduce the number of biopsies performed that have benign results, screening using CBE should be the first test to eliminate, although I do not advocate its elimination.

As should be apparent from the earlier discussion, the PPV is meaningless without the other information described earlier and a single figure without this information should not be the target.

Alternatives to breast biopsy have been suggested. Many benign biopsies can be avoided by monitoring lesions categorized as probably benign through short-interval follow-up (mammograms at some time interval that is less than the standard time between screenings) (21). Although society may eventually decide on the basis of cost who should be offered biopsy, it would be best to provide the individual woman with the probability for a given lesion's being cancer and permit her to decide how certain she would like to be in determining its significance. For one woman, a probability of 5% may be sufficiently low that she would be comfortable following the abnormality, whereas another women might find the probability of 1% too high and prefer to have a firm tissue diagnosis from a biopsy. Efforts should be made to improve tissue diagnosis at a lower cost and with less trauma so that women have these options without reducing the accuracy of the test.

SURGICAL BIOPSY: THE GOLD STANDARD

An open surgical excisional or incisional biopsy has always been the gold standard for diagnosis in the breast. The breast is one of the safest organs to biopsy. The morbidity associated with a properly performed breast biopsy is minimal. With rare exception these can be outpatient procedures performed using local anesthesia.

Postsurgical Scarring After a Biopsy for a Benign Lesion

It has been argued that screening leads to biopsies of findings detected by mammography, many of which prove to be benign, and that these biopsies scar the breast so that future mammography is compromised. This is a myth. The breast, after a biopsy with benign results, is not left with permanent scarring that complicates the interpretation of future mammograms, although much has been made of the potential postsurgical changes that may be seen after a surgical biopsy. The fact is that, if the surgery is performed properly and the biopsy reveals a benign process, the breast heals with little or no evidence of previous surgery by mammography. It is extremely rare that persistent postsurgical changes are confusing on subsequent mammography if the lesion removed was benign. Sickles found that 2 years after a breast biopsy with benign results <5% of women had any significant residual tissue distortion (22). In an informal survey we found that, among 1,200 women who provided a history of having had a previous benign breast biopsy, it was rare that postsurgical changes were even evident prospectively, and it was even less likely that the changes that were evident caused any confusion on subsequent mammograms. Mrose and associates have had a similar experience (personal communication, 1996). None of our patients has required a biopsy because of postsurgical change after a biopsy with benign results. These were rarely confusing on a mammogram.

THE NEEDLE BIOPSY CONTROVERSY

Needle biopsies (fine-needle aspiration and core needle biopsy [CNB]) have become increasingly popular as a substitute for surgically performed excisional breast biopsy because of their potential to reduce the trauma to the patient and their potential to decrease cost. Because of sampling errors (the needle may miss the malignancy), however, the accuracy of needle biopsies will likely never equal the accuracy of excisional biopsy after needle localization.

The controversy over reliance on these techniques arose when their use was promulgated without having undergone scientific validation (23). Proponents of needle biopsy failed to realize that when a new technique is being considered as a substitute for one with established efficacy it should be compared in a properly designed, prospective fashion with the gold standard to ensure that the two approaches are equal, particularly when the gold standard is extremely safe and efficacious, and overlooking a cancer may have significant consequences.

The only studies that have compared needle biopsies directly to needle localization and excision have compared high-quality needle biopsy to inaccurately performed needle localization and excisional biopsy. In our review of 1,000 radiographically detected cancers diagnosed after needle localization and excision, five cancers were not excised by the first procedure. The localization and surgical procedures were performed by residents, fellows, and staff physicians using the standard approach (24) outlined later in this chapter. Using this approach, not only was the error rate only 0.5%, but, by performing specimen radiography, it was apparent when a lesion had been missed and rebiopsy was performed expeditiously.

Unfortunately, the true accuracy of imaging-guided CNB is not known. Because of the zeal with which this less inva-

TABLE 21-1. *Summary of the early papers on core needle biopsy*

Author	Year	Modality	Patients (no.)	Core and biopsy	Cancers	False-negative core (no.)	False-negative core (%)	No long-term follow-up	No long-term follow-up (%)
Parker	1990	Stereotaxis	103	101	15	1	7	—	—
Parker	1991	Stereotaxis	102	102	23	1	4	—	—
Dronkers	1992	Ultrasound and stereotaxis	70	53	45	4	9	17	24
Parker	1993	Ultrasound	181	49	34	0	—	132	73
Elvecrog	1993	Stereotaxis	100	100	36	1	3	—	—
Caines	1994	Stereotaxis add on	254	121	75	5	7	—	—
Gisvold	1994	Stereotaxis	166	104	47	5	11	—	—
Burbank	1994	Ultrasound and stereotaxis	105	7	13	—	—	81	77
Doyle	1994	Ultrasound and stereotaxis	225	—	39	—	—	124	55
Parker	1995	Ultrasound and stereotaxis	6,152	1,363	984	15	2	4,789	77

sive approach has been adopted, most of the reports of its use in the literature have relied on the results of the needle biopsy, and patients have not gone on to have the targeted lesion excised for confirmation. Few of the reported studies have long-term follow-up of these lesions; the miss rate, therefore, remains undetermined (Table 21-1).

The data are obscured by the comparison of benign needle biopsies with those of excised lesions. It is not the accuracy of determining the histology of a benign lesion that is important. What is important is the ability to accurately determine whether a lesion is benign or malignant and, in particular, whether it is malignant. The true false-negative rate for cancer will probably never be known because many of the women who have negative needle biopsies and are subsequently shown to have breast cancer are lost to follow-up by the centers in which they had their biopsies. Increasing litigation over these missed cancers may reveal some information, but the technology has been so accepted that the true miss rate for cancer will never be accurately determined.

Many physicians began to rely on imaging-guided needle biopsies in the early 1990s, ignoring the fact that the only way that the efficacy of the procedure could be established was through a prospective trial in which all participants (selected because they would normally be expected to have an excisional biopsy) had a needle biopsy and then an accurately performed needle localization and excisional biopsy or were followed for a minimum of 3 years with no evidence of breast cancer.

Only a few of the early investigators performed both needle biopsy and excisional biopsy on every one of a small number of patients. Dowlatshahi had a fairly high error rate for diagnosing breast cancer using a core needle (25). Parker had very encouraging results (26). He performed needle biopsies on 102 women with mammographically suspicious, nonpalpable lesions using stereotactic guidance and CNB. He compared the needle biopsy results to the results among the same women who underwent stereotactically guided localization and exci-

sional biopsy for the same lesions. The diagnosis of cancer was made in 23 of the women. In this series, Parker missed one invasive cancer by CNB (4%). He concluded that CNB, using stereotactic guidance, was as accurate as needle localization followed by excisional biopsy, because his surgeons also missed a cancer at surgery after needle localization. The fallacy in his conclusion lay in the fact that needle localization followed by excisional biopsy should have a cancer error rate of <1%. In his series a cancer was missed at excisional biopsy because his needle localizations were performed using inaccurate stereotactic localization. Thus, he had compared accurate needle biopsy with inaccurate needle localization.

If the localizations had been performed properly, needle biopsy would be approximately six times less accurate for the diagnosis of breast cancer than needle localization and excision. Because the error rate is so low for both procedures, however, needle biopsy may be justified to reduce trauma and cost, but women and their physicians should be aware that the error rate for diagnosing cancer for needle biopsy is higher than it is with excisional biopsy after a properly performed needle localization.

Although the number of cancers missed by needle biopsy in a given practice will be low, if only 30% of the 180,000 cancers (60,000) diagnosed in the United States each year were subjected to diagnosis by needle biopsy, 2,400 cancers would be misdiagnosed by needle biopsy whereas only 300 would be missed by excisional biopsy, and the majority of the latter would be immediately apparent on the specimen radiograph. If needle biopsy is substituted for excisional biopsy after localization, women should be informed of the lower accuracy of the former.

Of the series that have been reported in which *selected* patients underwent needle biopsy and also excisional biopsy (26–28), the lowest error rate for needle biopsy remains 3% (10), six times the error rate for excision. A large series performed under the guidance of the National Cancer Institute unfortunately did not require excision of all lesions and permitted localizations where the localization guide was as far as 1 cm from the lesion. This is much lower than the easily achievable accuracy. If a needle localization is performed using the appropriate technique, the guide should be no further than 5 mm from the target lesion (29).

Error Rate for Needle Biopsy

The error rate (missed cancers) for needle biopsy has never been determined. Most of the studies that have been reported did not include the excision of the lesions after a properly performed needle localization as the gold standard for comparison. A majority of the women who have been included in the studies have not been followed up for >1 year, and, as a result, the true false-negative rate for needle biopsies is unknown. In a study of 77 cancers undergoing stereotactic biopsy with an add-on device, Caines and colleagues made a benign diagnosis with core biopsy of five (6%) lesions that proved to be cancer (30); 14 lesions that were thought to be cancer on core proved to be benign. Half of their patients did not have excisional biopsies because the core suggested a benign process and at the time of the report had not even had 6 months of follow-up. A Mayo Clinic study of 160 lesions revealed 93 (58%) benign lesions and 67 (42%) malignancies. In this series, five (11%) cancers were called *benign* out of 47 in which five or more stereotactically guided core samples were obtained (28).

The largest CNB series was reported by Parker and associates (31) in 1994, in which a consortium of 20 institutions reported core needle biopsies of 6,152 lesions. The biopsies were guided by stereotactic needle positioning in 4,744 of the lesions, whereas ultrasound was used to guide the biopsy of 1,408 lesions. Unfortunately the data were retrospectively as well as prospectively acquired, and the data from the two guidance approaches were combined. Most of the women had only core biopsies, and only 1,363 (22%) had confirmatory excisional biopsies. More than 35% of the women had not returned for even a 6-month follow-up, and none had been followed for 2 or more years. Thus, there is no way of knowing the actual false-negative rate for this series.

At the time of publication of the Parker et al. series, 15 of the 910 cancers (1.6%) were known to be falsely negative on CNB. The difficulty in interpreting these results is that the truth is not known for 77% of the women because most of the lesions were not excised to provide truth. This type of review unfortunately does not provide the confirmation suggested by the authors (23). There will likely be many more cancers that will surface in this population over time that were falsely diagnosed as benign by CNB due to sampling error.

Because of surgeons' unwillingness to accept benign CNB diagnosis early in the experience at each site or because of continued suspicion, 253 surgical biopsies were performed. Ten (4%) lesions deemed benign by needle biopsy were found to be malignant, and an additional five also proved to be cancer after benign results by CNB

because they increased in size at the 6-month follow-up. Without knowing the actual false-negative rate, this study missed 15 (2%) cancers out of 910 in which histology was confirmed by surgery.

Most other series profess to analyze the accuracy of needle biopsy but fail to provide definitive diagnosis or long-term follow-up to confirm the accuracy for these techniques (30,32,33) (Table 21-1). Many determined the overall accuracy of the procedure by comparing the results for core and excision (benign and malignant). This merely dilutes the numbers. The key answer that remains unknown is the actual false-negative rate for cancers.

Although many of the women in these studies will be followed up, a large number will likely be lost to follow-up. The problem with this approach is that it is entirely possible that many of the cancers missed by needle biopsy will be diagnosed in women who go elsewhere for their cancer care, and the investigators will not be aware of the errors.

The only way to determine the true accuracy of needle biopsy as a substitute for excisional biopsy after imaging-guided needle localization is to compare needle biopsy directly to the gold standard. The best method is to perform a needle biopsy on all women who would ordinarily undergo excisional biopsy and then perform the excisional biopsy in the usual fashion after needle localization. This is difficult to accomplish because many women will refuse to participate in the study because it will not directly benefit their care.

Other biases can enter into a study of this type. The consortium cited above merely collected the results of biopsies from multiple centers. The selection of patients who participated was not clear. If, for example, many of the women had lesions that were likely to be benign to begin with, then the study would suggest that a benign result was accurate when, in fact, it was merely due to the fact that there were few cancers to be missed. Selection bias is important because a study may validate needle biopsy for a narrower category of lesions than would ultimately be targeted by the technique, and the results from the narrow application may not hold when applied to the general population.

The way to reduce selection bias that may result is to randomly chose women with suspicious lesions for participation. This reduces but does not completely eliminate the problem of bias that may occur from the women who refuse. As with all prospective studies, the needle biopsy should be interpreted by the pathologist blindly without the knowledge of the excisional biopsy results. The national study cited above, based on the preceding rationale in which all lesions are excised or the women are followed for at least 3 years, may clarify the accuracy of needle biopsy. Unfortunately, there will also be women in that study who are lost to follow-up (more than likely the false negatives), and the true false-negative rate will not be known.

Any study that compares needle biopsy to excision after needle localization should require that the localization guides be placed no more than 0.5 cm from the lesion. This accuracy is easily achievable. Any reduced accuracy will favor core biopsy in the results, and CNB will be compared to needle localization that is not as accurate as can easily be achieved.

Needle biopsy involves fairly random sampling of a targeted lesion. Usually five core samples are removed from as many portions of the targeted tissue. Sampling error, in which the needle is not positioned in the cancer but in nearby tissue, is difficult to avoid and can result in a false-negative test. Because the goal of excisional biopsy is to remove the entire lesion, sampling error is not an issue. The difficulty with needle biopsy is that, if the pathology is benign, a false-negative biopsy will go undetected until the patient returns (or presents somewhere else) with a larger cancer. With excisional biopsy, the specimen radiograph provides immediate proof that the targeted lesion has been removed.

The use of imaging-guided needle biopsy to differentiate benign from malignant breast lesions is an attractive approach. Partly in response to the effort to reduce the cost of health care, and in an effort to reduce the level of invasion and trauma needed to make a diagnosis and partly in response to the mythologic belief that open biopsy causes permanent scarring, practitioners developed imaging-guided needle biopsy procedures.

Summary of the Needle Biopsy Controversy

As a consequence of intense marketing pressures that also pitted radiologists against surgeons in a turf battle over who should do breast biopsies, imaging-guided needle biopsy has been accepted as an alternative to excisional biopsy despite the lack of scientific validation. Despite the fact that the available data demonstrate that needle biopsy is less accurate than properly performed needle localization and excisional biopsy, imaging-guided breast biopsies have been widely advocated and are in widespread use.

If a needle biopsy is to be substituted for a needle localization and excisional biopsy, the woman should be informed of the diminished accuracy so that she can give informed consent. It remains to be seen whether the false-negative rate for needle biopsies will be acceptable when women with false-negative CNBs begin to surface.

APPROACHES TO NEEDLE BIOPSY OF BREAST LESIONS

Fine-Needle Aspiration Biopsy

Fine-needle aspiration involves the placement of thin (20- to 25-gauge) needles into suspicious lesions in an effort to aspirate cells that can be used to determine the significance of the lesion in question. Breast cancer cells tend to be less cohesive and break off more easily than normal tissues. These cells can frequently be removed by agitating a very thin needle in the lesion. They can then be smeared onto a slide, allowed to air dry, or fixed in fixative for interpretation and diagnosis.

Because cytopathologists tend to be very conservative, it is extremely rare for a skilled cytopathologist to make a false-positive diagnosis. As a result of this conservatism and the sampling error inherent in the technique, false-negative cytology can be as high as 20%.

For many years European physicians have used stereotactically guided fine-needle aspiration biopsy (FNAB) to determine whether a breast lesion is benign or malignant. This approach appears to be quite accurate in highly skilled hands. In 1989, Azavedo and colleagues reported on stereotactically directed FNAB of 2,594 nonpalpable lesions (34). Benign cytology was found in 2,005 (77.3%). With 14 months of follow-up, only one (0.04%) of the lesions that were determined by FNAB to be benign turned out to be a false negative when cancer was diagnosed.

Although there have been a number of studies that have purported to compare FNAB to excisional breast biopsy, none have been properly designed to evaluate the approach scientifically (35–38). Because not all of these women actually had their lesions excised and many have been lost to follow-up, most series do not actually know the false-negative rate for imaging-guided FNAB.

Advantages

FNAB is advantageous because it is virtually atraumatic and fairly simple to perform. It is rare to even cause a hematoma with a small needle. There are no reports of tracking cancer cells and seeding another part of the breast using FNAB.

Disadvantages

There are also disadvantages to FNAB. The technique is extremely dependent on the skill of the individual performing the procedure and the individual interpreting the smears. This includes the amount of suction, if any, that is applied during the aspiration and the vigor with which the needle is oscillated in the targeted tissue. Many observers have found that unless skilled cytotechnologists or cytopathologists do the actual aspiration, prepare the slides, and evaluate the results while the patient is still available for additional aspirates, there is a high percentage (20% to 30%) of unsatisfactory aspirates.

It is generally possible for the cytopathologist to make only the diagnosis of breast cancer, and it is unusual to be able to determine whether the cells represent invasive or in situ cancer. Furthermore, analysis of cytologic preparations is extremely dependent on the skill and experience of the individual interpreting the smears. There are few cytopathologists in the United States who are skilled in the cytologic interpretation of breast lesions. Although there are practices that rely on FNAB, most have adopted CNB because it is less operator dependent and easier for the average pathologist to interpret.

Core Needle Biopsy

CNB involves the actual removal of slivers of breast tissue using needles that range from 18 gauge to as large as 11 gauge. The slivers are prepared and analyzed as histologic samples.

Advantages

There are several advantages to CNB. Even using large needles, there is considerably less trauma from a needle biopsy than a surgical incision and biopsy. Imaging-guided CNB is considerably less expensive than an open biopsy. Because it uses spring-loaded needles or suction-driven cutting systems, CNB is more mechanical than FNAB and less operator dependent. Because the material is histologic, it can be interpreted by most pathologists who interpret breast pathology. If invasive cancer is sampled, the presence of invasion can be determined from the core although invasive cancer cannot be excluded if the core reveals only in situ cancer.

Disadvantages

The major disadvantage of CNB is that, as with any needle biopsy procedure, the needle may miss the cancer and provide a false-negative result. Using the larger needles adds the greater likelihood of bleeding and a hematoma. There has been at least one reported case of seeding of tumor cells in the track of a large-bore CNB (39), although the viability of those cells was never proved. Because the needles are large, they can displace large pieces of cancer. Some inexperienced pathologists have misinterpreted intraductal cancer that got pushed into the normal stroma as invasive cancer when there was not true invasion.

IMAGING GUIDANCE FOR NEEDLE BIOPSY

Because of the marketing hype that occurred with the introduction of stereotactically guided needle biopsy, many physicians confused the needle biopsy with the imaging guidance. There are numerous ways to guide needles to a significant abnormality for FNAB, CNB, cyst aspiration, or needle localization. The biopsy systems are, for the most part, independent of the imaging-guidance systems. Thus, needles can be placed for virtually all these procedures using mammography, stereotactic mammography, ultrasound, computed tomography (CT), magnetic resonance imaging, and nuclear medicine studies.

INDICATIONS FOR NEEDLE BIOPSY

The indications for needle biopsy will likely evolve as new approaches to the diagnosis and treatment of breast cancer are developed. Although more and more palpable lesions are being biopsied under imaging guidance, in the unsub-

stantiated belief that this will be more accurate than clinically guided biopsy for these lesions, the following is a review of the use of imaging-guided needle biopsy for nonpalpable lesions.

Nonpalpable Lesions That Can Be Considered for Needle Biopsy

1. Lesions that have a finite probability of cancer that is >2% and warrant surgical biopsy
2. Lesions with a high probability of cancer
3. Lesions that are probably benign, but the patient's anxiety is too high to permit short-interval follow-up or the needle diagnosis can be shown to be more cost-effective than short-interval follow-up

Most proponents of needle biopsy agree that lesions that are of sufficient concern to warrant an excisional biopsy may benefit from imaging-guided needle biopsy. In the American College of Radiology BIRADS system, these are lesions in category 4 (i.e., Suspicious: Biopsy should be considered) and category 5 (i.e., High probability of malignancy).

If a lesion that carries some suspicion of malignancy can be shown to be benign with a high degree of accuracy, then needle biopsy can be used to avoid an open biopsy. The difficulty comes in determining when a benign result is reliable. Proponents of needle biopsy caution that if a benign result is not concordant with an expected diagnosis of malignancy, then the needle biopsy should be ignored and the needle biopsy should be repeated or the lesion should be surgically removed. What has never been elucidated is the fact that all category 4 and 5 lesions are considered suspicious for malignancy. What constitutes a concordant benign biopsy result becomes a subjective decision.

It is probably safe to rely on a needle biopsy that reveals a fibroadenoma if the lesion that is biopsied is round, oval, or lobulated. If the majority of calcifications are removed using a needle biopsy system from a small lesion and the results are adenosis or fibrocystic tissue with calcifications, these are likely sufficiently concordant. If no calcifications are removed or only a few are removed or the suspicion of malignancy is high, the operator should probably not rely on a benign needle biopsy result.

If the needle biopsy reveals atypical hyperplasia, an excisional biopsy is indicated as a high percentage of these prove to be DCIS when the lesion is removed (28). If an area of spiculated architectural distortion produces a benign needle biopsy result, excision should still be undertaken because the diagnosis of a radial scar cannot be made reliably on needle biopsy and the lesion might still represent a malignancy.

If a lesion has a high likelihood of malignancy, a benign result is not reliable and an excisional biopsy is suggested. The advantage of making the diagnosis of cancer with the needle biopsy is that it permits the surgeon to discuss the options with the patient before any major surgery. If the patient elects lumpectomy and radiation, there is the opportunity to perform only a single surgical procedure with a wide excision and axillary dissection and a single anesthesia. Similarly, if she elects a mastectomy, the surgical biopsy can be avoided and only a single surgical procedure and anesthetic are required.

The weakness of this approach is that, armed with the knowledge that the patient has cancer, the surgeon may remove a much larger piece of tissue than is necessary to try to ensure free margins at a single operation whereas he or she might have removed the lesion with only a small amount of surrounding tissue as an excisional biopsy prior to any diagnosis. This small excision might, in fact, suffice if the margins are clear.

Conversely, even knowing that the patient has a breast cancer may not avoid two surgical procedures. If the margins are positive after the therapeutic biopsy, then re-excision or mastectomy may be required as a second operative procedure and the needle biopsy would have added an unnecessary layer of expense.

If the ability to rely on the evaluation of the first draining axillary nodes (sentinel node, see Chapter 26) as an indication of nodal status is reliable, then full axillary dissection will be unnecessary. The sentinel nodes can be removed under local anesthesia. It is also possible that nodal evaluation will become unnecessary. These developments will affect the benefit of needle biopsy and its value may be diminished.

ACCURATE NEEDLE POSITIONING

Safety and accuracy are of primary importance in performing any biopsy. Even in situations where needle biopsy is used to establish a diagnosis, malignant lesions must still be excised and accurate guidance for the surgeon is important. Because the lesions detected by mammography are not palpable, methods have been devised to position needles for sampling and to place guides to direct the surgeon to the suspected tissue.

NEEDLE LOCALIZATION AND EXCISIONAL BIOPSY

As needle biopsy procedures become more common, needle localization and excisional biopsy will become less common for diagnostic purposes and more commonly used to direct the excision or ablative treatment of cancers diagnosed by needle biopsy or to guide other, potentially less invasive diagnostic procedures. Nevertheless, because accurate needle sampling cannot always be achieved, there will still be numerous instances in which excisional biopsy after a needle localization procedure is necessary for diagnosis and treatment.

The procedure of needle localization and excisional biopsy should be extremely safe and, if performed properly, extremely accurate. As new techniques are devised to differentiate benign from malignant lesions, they should be compared to the accuracy of needle localization and surgical excision to determine their accuracy and efficacy.

Preoperative Needle Localization for an Excisional Biopsy

Clinically occult, mammographically detected lesions are likely to be at an earlier stage than palpable lesions, and an aggressive approach is justified if early-stage lesions are to be diagnosed. Criteria that should prompt a biopsy are continually being refined. It is likely that refined morphologic analysis, coupled with fine-needle aspiration cytology or CNB, will reduce the need for open, excisional biopsy. Nevertheless, if performed properly, excisional biopsy after needle localization remains the most precise diagnostic method. The false-negative rate for guided excision should be very low. The failure to remove a breast cancer after a needle localization should be <1%.

Not only is properly performed localization safe and accurate, but specimen radiography can immediately confirm whether the lesion has been removed so that if a lesion is missed, the biopsy can be repeated expeditiously. Having surgically excised tissue, pathologists can provide a more complete assessment of the lesion than from needle biopsy material. Even if needle biopsies are used for primary diagnosis, once a cancer is detected, accurate needle localization is needed to guide the optimal surgical removal of the lesion for therapy.

Particularly for diagnostic biopsies, very accurate guidance for the surgical excision of breast lesions is important, not only to ensure that the lesion is removed but also to minimize morbidity and cosmetic damage. Quadrant resection for diagnostic purposes is absolutely contraindicated, because it is inaccurate and results in the removal of unnecessarily large amounts of tissue. The majority of mammographically detected lesions are benign. Consequently, when the degree of suspicion is low the goal of excisional biopsy should be to remove as little breast tissue as is necessary to make an accurate diagnosis. If the morphologic criteria strongly suggest malignancy, a wider excision is recommended to try to obtain margins that are free of tumor to reduce the need for re-excision.

As for all procedures, safety for the patient should be a prime consideration. Techniques used for needle placement for preoperative localization can also be used to accurately position needles for needle biopsy.

Estimating the Location of a Lesion

It is inaccurate to try to relate the actual position of a lesion when the patient is lying supine on the operating table based on mammograms in which the breast was vigorously compressed and pulled away from the chest wall with the patient upright. Indicating the location of the lesion with marks on the skin is reliable only if the lesion is immediately beneath the skin. There is too much elasticity of the internal structures of the breast to permit accurate localization by skin coordinates.

To minimize the volume of tissue excised, the goal of accurate preoperative localization should be positioning the needle through or alongside the lesion (Fig. 21-2). Using the

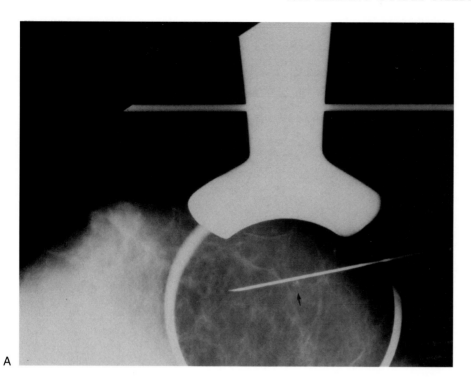

A

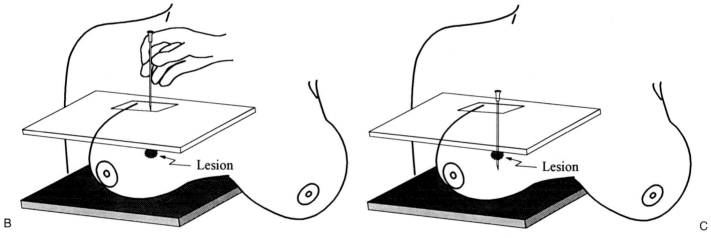

B

C

FIG. 21-2. Accurate localization should be routine. In this case a needle has been placed alongside a group of calcifications (*arrow*) in the left breast **(A)**. The basic goal is to pass a needle parallel to the chest wall **(B)** and transfix the lesion with the needle **(C)** or ultimately with a wire guide. The needle should never be >5 mm from the lesion if surgical excision is planned.

technique described in the following section, a needle can be routinely placed within 0.5 mm of a lesion (29). Any distance that is further than this should not be acceptable. If cytologic evaluation or core samples are to be obtained, then the needle must be placed in the lesion.

Locating an Occult Lesion Three Dimensionally

A recommendation for the biopsy of a nonpalpable lesion should not be made unless the location of the lesion is understood in three dimensions. The three-dimensional location of a lesion within the breast is usually apparent from the standard views. The standard screening lateral is the mediolateral oblique (MLO), and, consequently, the location of a lesion may be somewhat distorted. A straight lateral (orthogonal to the craniocaudal [CC]) image is useful before needle placement.

On occasion a lesion is visible in only one projection. Before recommending a biopsy, the radiologist should be confident of the ability to place a needle tip at the lesion. If a lesion is seen in only one projection the radiologist must be confident that the lesion is real (see Chapter 22).

It is generally best to return to the projection on which the lesion was seen and work from there. Coned-down spot compression can be used to mechanically spread overlapping structures (40). Changing the angle of the incident beam by rotating the tube relative to the breast or rolling the breast tissue to reorient the overlapping structures can assist in differentiating a true lesion from an overlap of benign structures (summation shadow) (41). Using these parallax techniques and the apparent shift of a lesion relative to the other breast structures, one can verify a lesion and also simultaneously determine its location in the breast.

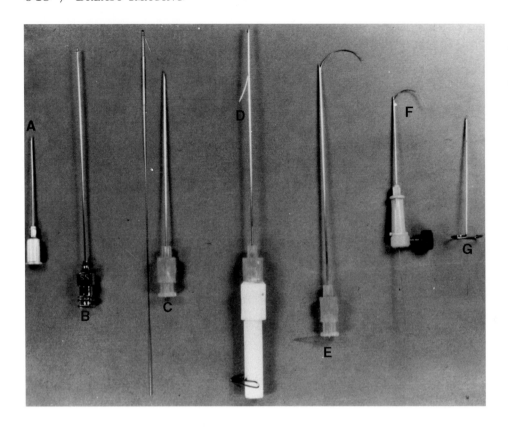

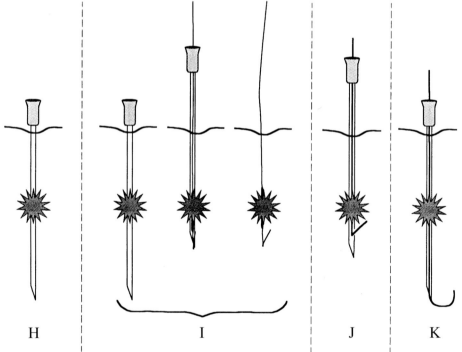

FIG. 21-3. **Localization guides** vary. A simple hypodermic needle **(A)** or a longer spinal needle **(B)** can be used. Hookwires can be placed through needles **(C)**. Needles can be held in place by a wire that comes out the side of the needle **(D)** or curved wires that come out the end of the needle **(E, F)**. Some surgeons prefer a needle with a flat head **(G)** (see Fig. 21-4). These are seen schematically as they are positioned through a lesion. A hypodermic needle is passed through and beyond the lesion **(H)**. After the needle is properly positioned, a spring hookwire can be placed **(I)**. When the hook comes out the side of the needle, there is often a long segment of needle that protrudes from the breast **(J)**. A needle with a curved wire coming out its end has little holding power and is not much better than a hypodermic **(K)**.

Once the location of a lesion is determined, it can usually be accurately demonstrated on an orthogonal view. If the general location of the lesion is known, an alternative method of needle placement using very simple stereotaxis and the plain geometric relationship of similar triangles can be used to perform an accurate localization (see Parallax Needle Localization) (42). This may be particularly useful when a lesion is difficult to project in two orthogonal planes.

If these methods fail or a more anterior approach is desired, ultrasound can be used to locate masses (43) and guide localization. If rotated views and ultrasound fail to triangulate a lesion, CT can be used to guide localization (44) (see Chapter 22). A mass that is surrounded by fat is usually identifiable by CT. This technique is generally not capable of demonstrating clustered microcalcifications unless there are a sufficient number in an isolated volume of breast tissue to avoid attenuation dilution by volume averaging. If the lesion can be located by CT scanning, guides for the surgeon can be positioned under CT observation.

General Considerations for Preoperative Needle Localization

Many approaches to guiding the surgeon to a nonpalpable lesion have been devised, but all accurate methods require the positioning of a needle in or through the tissue volume in question.

Although a great deal of attention has been focused on needle localization, surgeons have rarely discussed the advantages and disadvantages of various surgical approaches. Most published reports in the surgical literature on needle localization and surgical excision have come from series where the surgeon required that the guides be placed from the front of the breast. This is inherently inaccurate and has led to the perception that large amounts of tissue needed to be removed. Accurate localization can permit the need to remove only a small amount of tissue.

The surgeon must understand that biopsies of clinically occult lesions require some thought and attention to detail. Careful surgical dissection avoids dislodging needles or cutting wires. The radiologist, surgeon, and pathologist must work closely together. The radiologist is responsible for recognizing the features of lesions that should arouse concern and should avoid recommending biopsy of lesions that are characteristically benign or probably benign. Safe, accurate

localization techniques permit the aggressive evaluation of indeterminate lesions while they are small and result in a reduction in the stage at diagnosis and a commensurate reduction in overall mortality from breast cancer.

Choice of Localization Guide

The actual choice of the mechanical guide that is used depends on the preferences of the radiologist and surgeon. Many systems are available, ranging from off-the-shelf hypodermic needles to specially designed localization devices (Fig. 21-3).

Conventional Hypodermic Needles

A conventional hypodermic needle is the simplest guide for preoperative breast lesion localization. The needle must be of sufficient length to pass through (or immediately alongside) and beyond the lesion when the needle is imaged with compression perpendicular to its course to ensure that the suspect tissue does not slip off the tip of the needle.

Advantages

Conventional needles are extremely simple guides to place in the breast. Because they are stiff, the surgeon can torque the shaft and feel the needle to discern its course within the breast tissue. A straight needle is easily removed or repositioned if its relationship to the lesion is suboptimal.

Disadvantages

The disadvantage of a simple needle is that it can be easily and accidentally dislodged from the tissues. Furthermore,

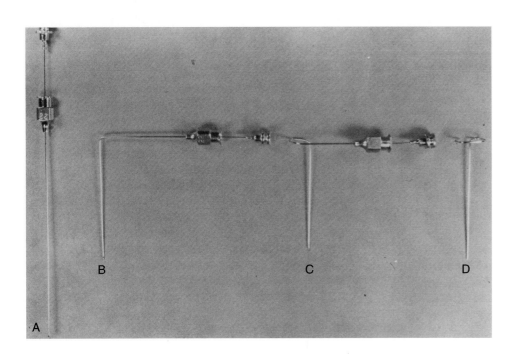

FIG. 21-4. A flat-head needle can be made from a standard 22-gauge spinal needle. **(A)** Pull the stylet back 1 cm. **(B)** Bend the needle 90 degrees at the desired length. **(C)** Make the next bend as a spiral, perpendicular to the shaft of the needle. **(D)** Cut off the excess needle and hub with wire cutters.

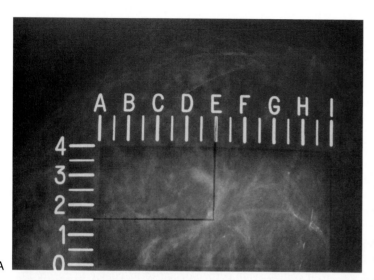

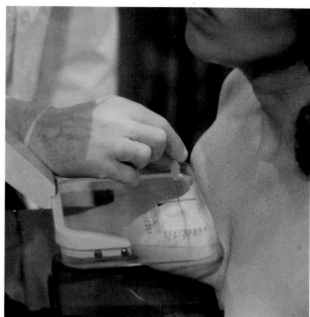

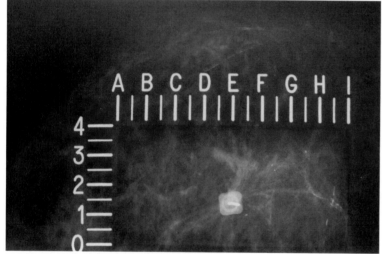

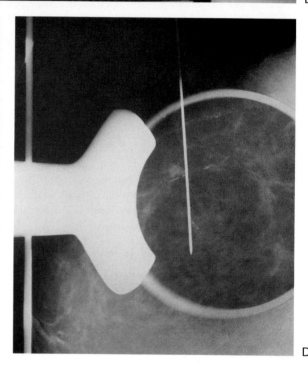

FIG. 21-5. Standard needle localization. Using spring hookwire systems, the lesion is positioned so that it is projected through the window of a fenestrated compression paddle with grid markers **(A)**. The coordinates are used to guide the passage of the needle through or alongside the lesion **(B)** in the first projection and advanced beyond the lesion and confirmed, as seen here **(C)** looking down the shaft of the needle. The patient is removed from the window compression system. Ensure that the tip of the needle stays beyond the lesion by advancing the needle and pulling the breast up around it as compression is slowly released. The gantry is rotated 90 degrees and using a spot-compression device the breast is recompressed to show the relationship of the lesion to the tip of the needle **(D)**. *Continued.*

it does not provide a three-dimensionally stable indicator of the depth of the lesion. The protrusion of the needle hub above the skin may result in its being inadvertently caught and pulled out of the breast prematurely. We have modified a hypodermic needle to avoid this problem by forming a flat pushing surface out of its proximal shaft (Fig. 21-4).

This flat-head needle is accomplished by bending a standard 22-gauge spinal needle. The stylet is pulled back from the needle tip but is left in the needle for strength when the needle is bent. The hub is removed and the proximal portion of the shaft is bent at right angles and then into a spiral. This creates a flat-head needle (that can be

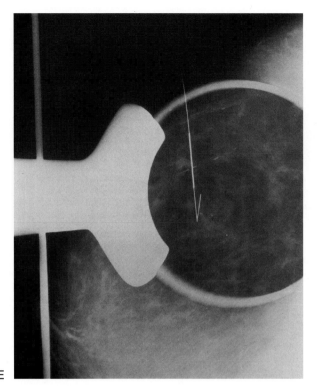

E

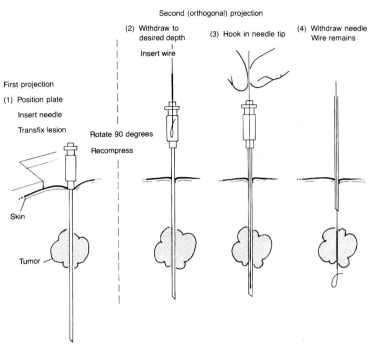

F

FIG. 21-5. *Continued.* The needle is withdrawn so that the tip is positioned where the wire is to engage the tissue, and the wire is afterloaded. The wire is held firmly, and the needle is withdrawn so that the wire engages the tissue with the lesion on the thickened segment **(E)**. The sequence is summarized schematically **(F)**.

fashioned at varying lengths) that can be inserted flush to the skin similar to a long thumbtack. Because the proximal spiral is made from the needle, the lesion can be imaged through it.

Many surgeons find a straight needle sufficient, but it only provides two-dimensional accuracy. The surgeon must estimate the distance of the lesion along its shaft. There is also the chance that movement of the breast may cause the lesion to slip off the needle.

Hookwire Systems

In 1979, Hall and Frank described the use of a wire with a hook formed at its end. This was introduced near the lesion to anchor in the tissue and to guide the surgeon to a nonpalpable abnormality. In their system, the wire was placed in a needle with the hook protruding from the pointed end and bent back along the needle shaft. The system required a skin incision and then the needle, with the hook protruding, was forced into the breast tissues. Because the hook was outside the needle tip, the needle could only be advanced forward. Once the needle was pulled back, the hook became embedded in the tissue and could be not be withdrawn (45). It provided a three-dimensionally stable anchor for the wire guide.

The hookwire concept was modified to permit more accurate positioning. By overbending the end of the wire a spring was formed. This permitted the hook to be contained entirely within the needle (46). These needles can be positioned (and repositioned) until the desired location relative to the lesion is accurately attained. Once a satisfactory position is achieved the wire can be inserted through the hub and down the shaft of the needle. By withdrawing the needle over the wire, the compressed hook is released and engaged in the appropriate tissue volume (Fig. 21-5). Because the delivery device is essentially a hypodermic needle lesions can be aspirated through the same needle, so that if the lesion proves to be a cyst and fluid is aspirated the biopsy can be terminated. If the lesion proves to be solid and not a cyst, a wire can be afterloaded to anchor in the tissue without introducing a second needle (47).

Advantages

Hooked wires afford the most three-dimensionally accurate localization guides. They have the additional advantage of flexibility so that nothing projects above the skin, making it more difficult to dislodge them. Once positioned, wires are comfortable for the patient and the surgeon can apply gentle traction to assist in the dissection.

Disadvantages

Because wires are flexible, they are difficult for the surgeon to feel. Unless followed directly from the skin insertion site into the breast, some surgeons find it difficult to locate wires within the breast. This difficulty may be overcome by passing a cannula over the wire in the operating room (29). This stiffens the wire and permits it to be more easily palpated.

Surgeons should be cautioned not to use wires as retractors because with sufficient traction they can be pulled out of the breast. Wires are stable in fibroglandular tissue but may be moved in fat if there is no firmer tissue in which to anchor, because fat is almost liquid at body temperature.

All wires can be cut with scissors, and fragments have been left in the breast. Surgeons should be urged to use scalpel dissection. We routinely advise the patient that the wire may be transected, although this has happened only 10 times in >6,000 localization procedures. There does not appear to be any harm from small fragments of wire being left in the breast. They do not appear to move within the tissues (48), but long fragments with intact hooks that have been initially positioned from the front of the breast have been reported to have migrated to other parts of the body (49).

The surgeon should be cautioned to dissect carefully. Scalpels cannot cut most wires but scissors can. Contact of a wire with the electrocautery theoretically can result in a thermal injury along the course of the wire or cause the wire to fracture and should be avoided. This is also true for all needle systems used for localization.

The length of a wire is important. Wires that are too short should not be used, and care should be exercised if a wire is shortened (cut) after it has been positioned in the breast. Wires must be of sufficient length so that when the breast is in its natural position the wire will not be enveloped completely by the breast and drawn beneath the skin. This possibility seems to be most likely if the needle is positioned from the front of the breast and the wire is engaged while the patient is supine. When the patient sits up, there is the danger that the re-expanded breast will completely envelope the wire. This is important to consider when performing guide placement under ultrasound or CT guidance from the front of the breast. To be safe, the length of the wire should exceed by several centimeters the maximum distance from the skin entry site to the lesion.

The length of the needle and wire can be estimated from the mammographic projection where the breast will be compressed orthogonal to the direction of needle insertion by measuring the distance of the lesion from the skin surface through which the needle will be passed (Fig. 21-6). This distance may in actuality be shorter than the final distance because of the curvature of the breast, but it cannot be longer. If the length of wire is chosen properly and insertion is performed parallel to the chest wall, there is no need to anchor the protruding end of the wire. Firmly anchoring the wire is

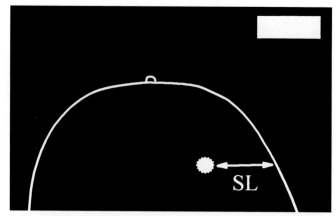

FIG. 21-6. Needle length is chosen by measuring distance from the skin to the lesion in the projection that is orthogonal to the expected course of the needle. If, for example, the needle is to be introduced from the lateral side of the breast, the needle length can be estimated in the craniocaudal projection. The actual distance to the lesion may prove to be shorter, but a needle that is longer than the distance from the skin to the lesion (SL) should be used.

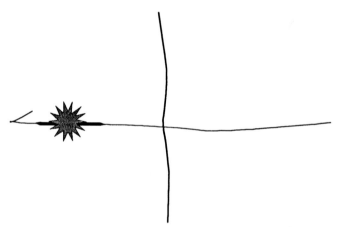

FIG. 21-7. When using spring hookwires, the lesion is optimally placed on the thickened segment of wire so that the surgeon, on reaching the thickened segment, knows that the lesion is in the next volume of tissue.

actually contraindicated because movement of the breast may cause the wire to be pulled out of the lesion. The wire should be loosely taped to the skin to permit movement in and out of the skin so that the hook is not under any tension.

The Thickened Distal Segment

To reduce the difficulty for the surgeon who might have problems estimating the distance to the lesion, a 2-cm thickened segment was added to the wire just proximal to the hook. This facilitates the procedure. The wire guide is positioned so that the lesion is along this segment with the hook on the other side of the lesion (Fig. 21-7). The surgeon can then dissect down the wire to the thickened section. The thickened segment acts as a palpable and visual mark indicating that the hook is 2 cm farther down the wire. Knowing that the lesion is along the next portion of wire, the tissue around this thickened portion can be excised along with the distal hook. The removal of the lesion with a surrounding rim of normal tissue is facilitated (24). Placing the hook beyond the lesion is important. Although the surgeon should not pull on the wire, if there is traction on the wire it will pull into the lesion rather than away from it.

Anchored Needles

Hooked wires have been combined with needles in an effort to provide a three-dimensionally stabilized stiff needle in the breast.

Curved Wires That Protrude from the Needle Tip

Some surgeons use a curved-end wire that can be retracted into the tip of the introducing needle as a guide. Because the wire can be retracted into the needle, the needle can be repositioned. A commercially available system contained wires that were initially described as uncuttable and three-dimensionally stable (50). As experience with these increased, it became apparent that the wires could be cut and that they were not stable.

Advantages

A needle with a protruding wire with a tight curve has the advantage of being repositionable even after the hook is advanced by permitting retraction of the hook back into the needle. The repositioning capability is useful for accurate positioning, and the stiffer target is helpful for the surgeon.

Disadvantages

Unfortunately, there are trade-offs with all guides. The ability to straighten out the curve and pull the wire back into the needle weakens its holding power. Our own investigations into the development of this type of configuration led us to discard the technology. A wire that can be pulled into the tip of the needle can be pulled out of the breast.

When using the commercially available system, to prevent the wire from being cut it is recommended that the needle be left protecting it. This may result in a large portion of the needle protruding from the skin (see Fig. 21-3J) because the depth of a lesion can never be accurately determined ahead of time. This increases the chance that the needle will be dislodged. Since the original description of the commercial system, the recommendation has changed so that it is advised that the introducing needle be left in to protect the wire from transection (51). By leaving the needle on the wire, it is more likely that the system will inadvertently be pulled out of the breast; it is therefore recommended that the introducing needle be pushed completely into the breast flush to the skin

before advancing the hook. Unfortunately this causes a loss of the third dimension in the localization, and using this system in this fashion may have little advantage over a straight needle because the surgeon must once again estimate the location of the lesion along the needle shaft.

Side-Port Protruding Hookwire

The combination of needles and wires has been thoroughly explored. The greatest holding power for a needle that can be repositioned after deployment of a hook comes from having the wire hook protrude from a side hole near the tip of the needle. Because the hook can be pulled back into the needle, this configuration permits the radiologist to reposition the needle and provides a stiff guide with three-dimensional stability for the surgeon. When we explored this type of system, we discarded the approach because there were varying amounts of the needle that projected from the skin, making it likely that the proximal portion could become snagged. The commercially available needle comes with a clamp that is fastened at the skin surface to prevent the advance of the needle deeper into the breast tissue. The external portion should be protected. Some radiologists tape a paper cup over it to prevent dislodging the system.

Advantages

The major advantages of this system are the stiffness of the guide for the surgeon and the ability to reposition the needle. A stable, three-dimensionally accurate localization can result. Studies have demonstrated that a wire protruding from the side of a needle has one and one-half times the holding power of a flexible springhook wire anchor and six times the holding power of a curved wire protruding from the end of the needle (52,53).

Disadvantages

The major drawback to this system is that it is not flexible. Three-dimensional positioning results in variable lengths of needle protruding from the breast. This must be protected to prevent the protruding portion from being inadvertently hit and dislodged or damaging the tissues.

POSITIONING NEEDLES AND GUIDES

Preparing the Patient

Needle localization procedures should be safe and as atraumatic as possible. Patients are often extremely anxious. Most fear that they have breast cancer, and the thought of having a needle placed in the breast is psychologically disturbing. Compassionate support throughout the procedure is mandatory. As with any procedure, the technologist and radiologist should remember that although the procedure is routine for them it is a unique and often frightening experience for the patient.

Premedication is usually not needed and is contraindicated because full cooperation is required. Local anesthesia can be used, although in our experience it is frequently more uncomfortable than the actual localization procedure. It requires a needle for injection and initially produces burning pain. Mixing sodium bicarbonate (8.4%, 1 mEq/ml) with lidocaine (1 part sodium bicarbonate to 9 parts anesthetic) can reduce the burning.

Reynolds and colleagues have shown that local anesthesia may be used, but for the majority of women it is not needed and may be more painful than the localization itself (54). These investigators also found that discomfort was higher among premenopausal women who underwent localization premenstrually rather than during the first part of the menstrual cycle. There may be a psychological benefit from using a local anesthetic. The perception that pain relief is being withheld is upsetting to some patients, and we now offer anesthetic and reinforce the goal that the procedure *should not be painful*. Although local anesthesia may not be needed, it should be readily available.

Breast compression during the procedure produces some numbness. Many women are not even aware of the placement of the needle. It has been our *anecdotal* experience that women whose breasts are predominantly fat experience less discomfort than those with dense breast tissue.

Efforts should be made to make the procedure as painless as possible. We remind the patient that if at any time she experiences discomfort, anesthetic can be injected. Many localization needles permit the injection of anesthetic without the need to insert an additional needle. The patient should be cautioned that she will still feel pressure and movement, but we ask her to inform us immediately if the procedure becomes painful so that we can administer anesthetic.

Before the start of the localization, the procedure should be explained to the patient by a physician in as nonthreatening a manner as possible but with sufficient detail so that she is fully informed. Despite the fact that most biopsies performed for diagnostic purposes provide benign results, many patients are convinced that they have breast cancer. In addition, the anticipation of having a needle positioned in their breast is extremely threatening. Calmly and supportively discussing the various steps of the procedure should include reassurance that the majority of lesions found in this way are benign (unless, of course, a prior needle biopsy suggests malignancy). Patients may also find it reassuring if the very small size of the lesion is stressed. If the placement of the guide is to be undertaken in a manner that is parallel to the chest wall, the patient can be reassured that it is an extremely safe procedure.

The patient should be supported with kindness and compassion and be attended at all times. Vasovagal reactions are uncommon, but they should be anticipated. These events can be kept to a minimum by distracting the patient with continuous pleasant conversation and by preventing her from viewing the needle. Syncopal episodes should occur in <2% of women undergoing needle localization. We have never required medication to treat these rare episodes. Placing the patient supine for several minutes is usually all that is required, and the procedure can then be completed.

Anteroposterior Approach to Guide Placement

There are basically two approaches to needle placement: anteroposterior and parallel to the chest wall.

Freehand Localization from the Front of the Breast

Because surgeons are trained to operate down toward the table, they prefer that guides be positioned from the front of the breast, back toward the chest wall to a suspected abnormality so that they can follow the wire directly down when the patient is supine in the operating room. Methods have been described that attempt to accomplish this using measurements from compressed radiographs and transposing them to the uncompressed breast. This cannot be done precisely, but with experience proponents report accurate results.

Various methods are used with the patient either seated or supine. The methods involve the transposition of measurements from the compressed mammogram to the uncompressed breast and suggest that by measuring the distance of the lesion from the nipple in the two projections the true location of the lesion can be estimated. The radiologist must then transfer these measurements to the patient. The needle is introduced at this estimated point and directed back toward the lesion. Because the needle is inserted toward the chest wall, the radiologist must exercise caution to avoid entering the pectoralis muscle or the thorax.

Due to the elasticity of the breast, its distortion from compression, and variable magnification on the mammogram, the initial placement of a guide from the front of the breast can only be an approximation. Some radiologists have tried to compensate for this by adding a magnification factor.

Once the guide has been first positioned, orthogonal mammograms are obtained. Based on estimates of the relationship and distances of the needle tip to the lesion, the needle is then repositioned to better approximate the location of the lesion. Confirmatory mammograms are again obtained (55). The needle is then readjusted to move it closer to the lesion. This sequence of orthogonal views and repositioning is repeated until the needle is in the desired relationship to the lesion.

In general, positioning needles from the front of the breast freehand under mammographic guidance cannot be accomplished with the same accuracy or safety as positioning guides using the parallel-to-the-chest-wall approach (PCW). There are some add-on devices that can be used with stereotactic devices that have improved the accuracy of localizations from the front of the breast. With the patient seated, stereo x-ray pairs are obtained, and the depth of the lesion is determined in the standard fashion. A rigid arm that is designed to fit onto the needle guide of the stereo device protrudes parallel to the film plane and then has a bend that is directed perpendicularly toward the film plane. By matching the length of this perpendicular arm to the stereo device (just as the device is calibrated for specific needle lengths), the needle guide at the end of this arm will aim the needle at the proper location of the lesion. Theoretically, a needle inserted through this guide, parallel to the film plane, can be positioned from any direction from the front of the breast to the lesion. There have, as yet, not been any prospective analyses of the accuracy of these devices, but we found that a similar system that we devised many years ago was not accurate because the breast was compressed and accordioned parallel to the plane of the needle insertion. Any deflection of the needle as it passed through the breast tissue was amplified when the breast was uncompressed and the needle ended up in a different plane than the plane of the lesion. Any needle deflection compromises the accuracy of guide placement for surgical excision.

Advantages

Most breast surgeons prefer that guides be placed in an anteroposterior direction to facilitate their surgery. They prefer to dissect directly down the needle or wire guide to the lesion. Because many surgeons believe that a circumareolar incision leaves the most cosmetic scar, some even prefer that the needle be inserted at the limbus of the areola. A circumareolar approach also facilitates the inclusion of the surgical track in a mastectomy if this is the ultimate therapeutic choice.

If the breast is sufficiently flexible so that it can be positioned with the anterior surface and the lesion in a line that can be simultaneously and directly imaged, circumareolar needle positioning can be done with a high degree of accuracy. The breast is rotated so that the anterior surface or the limbus of the areola is positioned in the window compression. If the lesion lies beneath, then an accurate needle localization can be performed. Ultrasound and CT also permit positioning the needle from the front of the breast.

Disadvantages

Positioning guides from the front of the breast directed back toward the chest wall can be dangerous. Freehand needle localization is extremely operator dependent. Although some individuals claim a high degree of accuracy, it has never been shown that this method is as generally accurate as the PCW. Most practitioners of this method accept a needle that is approximately 1 cm from the lesion. This is too far as it necessitates the removal of large volumes of tissue by the surgeon to ensure that the lesion has been removed. It is fairly common to have the surgeon remove additional tissue samples using this guidance, because the lesion is frequently missed with the first excision.

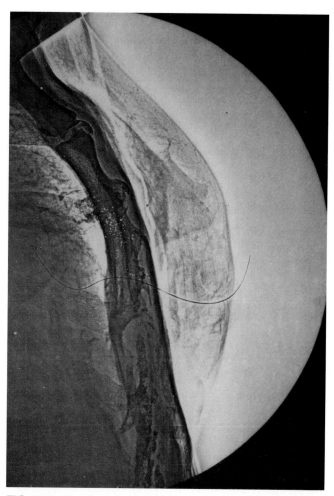

FIG. 21-8. Freehand needle localization from the front of the breast can be dangerous. In this patient a wire was placed by freehand technique with the patient lying supine. She was rolled into the lateral projection for this xerogram. The hooked end of the wire projects over the lung. Fortunately it was not in her lung, but it was hooked into the pectoralis major muscle; when she sat up, her breast re-expanded and completely enveloped the entire wire. Not only did the lesion have to be relocalized, but the surgeon had to be guided to the wire.

Freehand localization is a technique that cannot rely on geometry but only on the artistry of the operator. It relies on successive approximations and requires a degree of skill and luck if accurate localizations are to result, particularly for lesions that are deep in the breast.

Anteroposterior needle insertion can be dangerous, particularly if the target lesion is close to the chest wall. Needles introduced back toward the chest wall have been inserted into the pectoralis muscles (Fig. 21-8) or into the pleural space (56), lung, or mediastinum. Introducing needles in this fashion has caused pneumothorax, and there has purportedly been a case in which a wire was placed into the aortic valve, ultimately requiring replacement of the valve.

If positioning from the front of the breast is desired, ultrasound or CT should be used.

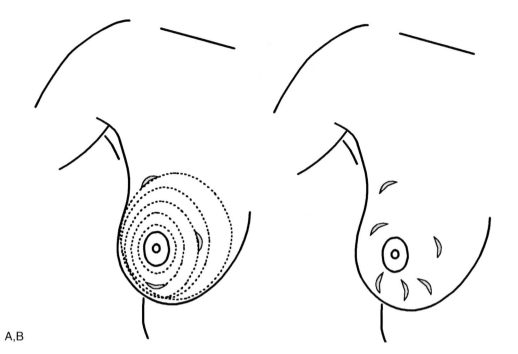

A,B

FIG. 21-9. This schematic shows **the natural lines of skin tension (A), known as Langer's lines.** Small incisions should follow these lines for the best cosmetic results. If large amounts of tissue are removed, surgeons advise following radial lines in the lower breast **(B)**.

Wire Migration

If needle localization procedures are performed properly, problems should be rare. Some have suggested that wires may migrate from their original position. This is an illusion. Wires do not migrate unless they are left in the breast and not removed. Wires can be *placed* inappropriately—and they have been positioned by radiologists into the muscle, lung, and mediastinum—but they do not migrate there. Wire guides can appear to move once they are anchored. If wires are placed with the patient supine, the thickness of the breast may be greatly underestimated as it spreads on the chest wall. If the wire is too short for the true depth of the lesion, when the patient sits up and the breast re-expands, a wire placed in this fashion may be enveloped by and completely disappear into the breast (giving the appearance of migration). There have been reports of wires that have not only been completely enveloped by the breast but were not retrieved by the surgeon. Over a period of time, some of these have been massaged by body motion into other parts of the body (49). Our review suggests that this happens only when wires have been placed directed back toward the chest wall, although in general it is best to remove all of the wire guide.

Caution

The anteroposterior approach should be used with great caution and is probably best suited for superficial lesions. There is no reason to suspect that breast cancer cells are easily seeded along thin needle tracks, but this remains a theoretic possibility. We have found no evidence that needle localization with 20-gauge or smaller needles poses any risk of needle track seeding in the breast (57), but the potential inadvertent tracking of cells into the pleural space during an anteroposterior localization has never been investigated and remains a potential problem with this approach.

Complications can be avoided by positioning guides with approaches parallel to the chest wall (24). Surgeons may initially be reluctant to accept this approach, but it should be stressed that it is a much safer and much more accurate way of positioning a guide, because the lesion can be held away from the chest wall in the mammography unit so that it can be pierced by the inserted needle. The parallel approach is precise with no estimation required.

Circumareolar Incision

Although some surgeons believe that a circumareolar incision is cosmetically preferred, this is not necessarily the case. If incisions are made in appropriate relation to the contours of the breast (Langer's lines) (Fig. 21-9), peripheral incisions fade and become virtually imperceptible. Dragging a breast cancer through a large volume of the breast to remove it through a circumareolar incision is not recommended and may preclude conservation therapy with radiation. If this maneuver contaminates an unacceptably large volume of normal breast tissue, requiring a larger volume of tissue to be boosted to the highest doses by the radiation therapist, a mastectomy may be required. The surgeon should be aware of this and use incisions that permit the most accurate removal of a lesion and provide good cosmetic results, without compromising treatment options.

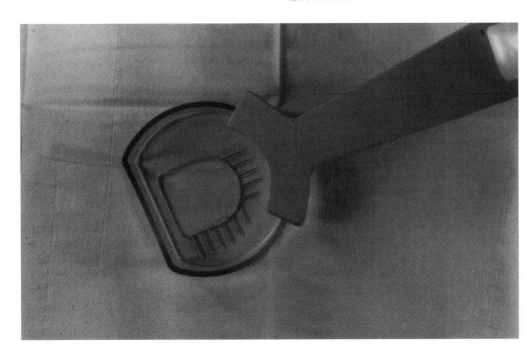

FIG. 21-10. A spot compression plate with a window can facilitate needle placement near the nipple.

Guides Introduced Parallel to the Chest Wall

Most complications associated with needle localization can be avoided if guides are placed using safe and accurate techniques. The safest and most accurate methods involve positioning needles parallel to the chest wall (24). The PCW procedure can be performed using any standard mammography system.

Fenestrated Compression Plates

Compression plates that have holes or cutouts make accurate needle positioning possible. The compression paddle holds the breast firmly to prevent motion so that needles can be introduced very accurately. Virtually all mammography units come with compression plates that have a series of holes or a fenestration with calibration marks along the side that permit access to the breast and to the lesion through the opening while the breast is held in compression. We have found that a single fenestration with calibrations along the sides is the most convenient and accurate to use. Some radiologists prefer multiple holes. It has been our experience that when multiple holes are used the targeted lesion invariably ends up under the plastic between holes and the breast must be repositioned or the localization is inaccurate.

Variations of these paddles are very useful. A spot compression device with a window is useful for the front of the breast (Fig. 21-10). We have found that a spot compression plate with a window on a sliding track that can be locked at any position is very helpful. Windows cut in the corner of a large compression paddle facilitate the positioning and localization of lesions that are high in the axillary tail of the breast (Fig. 21-11).

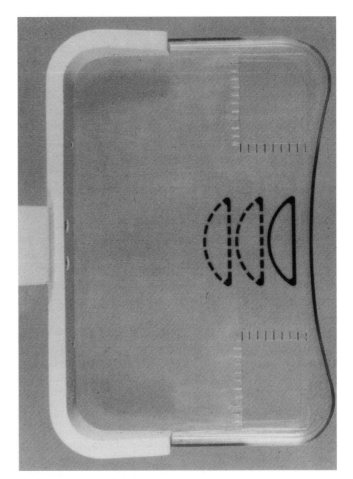

FIG. 21-11. Metallic markers along the edge of **windows in the corners of a compression paddle** can facilitate needle placement for lesions in the axillary tail.

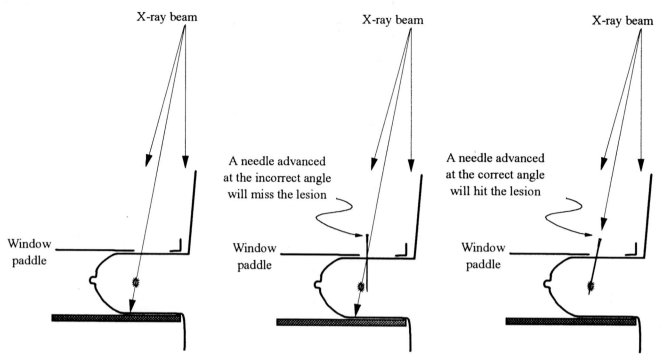

FIG. 21-12. When positioning needles it is important to remember that **the x-ray beam is divergent and is only perpendicular to the film at the center of the chest-wall side of the detector.**

Alignment of the Centering Light

Accurate needle localization requires the alignment of the centering light in the collimator of the x-ray tube with the x-ray beam. The x-ray beam in all mammography systems is divergent. In most units it is perpendicular to the film plane only at the center of the chest-wall edge of the compression plate (Fig. 21-12). Because the centering light is used to advance needles in the direction that the x-ray beam passes through the breast and the lesion, the centering light must be aligned with the x-ray beam. It is very simple to determine if the beams are aligned.

Checking the Alignment. Using a fenestrated compression plate, a piece of sponge is compressed in the mammography system as a simulated breast. With the centering light on, needles are placed at the corners of the window (Fig. 21-13) in the plate (or through the holes that are most commonly used if a multi-hole plate is used). The needles should be pushed into the rubber so that the shadow of their hubs in the centering light is centered on the shadow of the needle tips (if one could sit in the gantry at the light source, one would be looking straight down the bore of the needles). If this is done properly, the needles are tilted from the perpendicular because the light is divergent. If the light is properly aligned, the needles are also aligned with the divergent x-ray beam. An x-ray exposure is made, and, if the centering light is properly aligned with the x-ray beam, the needles are projected as if the operator is looking straight down their lumens. If this is not the case, the light should be aligned so that it coincides with the x-ray beam.

Needle Introduction from the Skin Surface Closest to the Lesion

To reduce the amount of tissue that must be traversed by the surgeon, the shortest distance to the lesion from the skin that will permit the skin surface and the lesion to be in the window while the breast is held in the compression device of the mammography system should be chosen. This is determined by evaluating the location of the lesion based on the screening mammograms. If the only mediolateral image that is available is the MLO projection, it is useful to obtain a straight lateral view. The straight lateral and the CC projections permit the most accurate estimate of the actual location of the abnormality in the breast (Fig. 21-14).

If the lesion proves to be closest to the medial surface of the breast, the initial needle positioning is accomplished in a mediolateral approach with the medial skin surface in the window of the compression device, inserting the needle from the medial skin surface (Fig. 21-15). If the lesion is closest to the lateral surface of the breast, a lateromedial approach is used with the window over the lateral surface of the breast. A lesion near the top of the breast is localized from the CC projection, whereas one at the bottom of the breast can be localized using a caudocranial projection by turning the gantry upside down.

If the gantry does not rotate into the caudocranial projection or if the patient and radiologist are more comfortable, the patient can be placed on her side on a stretcher with the gantry turned as if for a straight lateral projection. The breast can then be positioned with the fenestrated compression permitting access to the inferior breast surface.

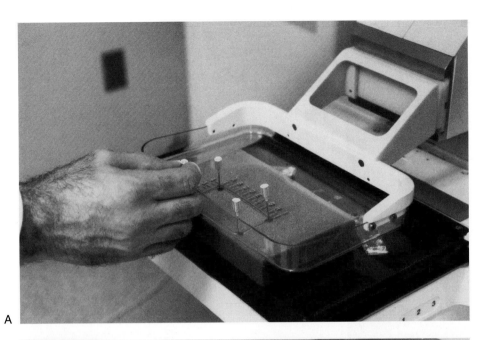

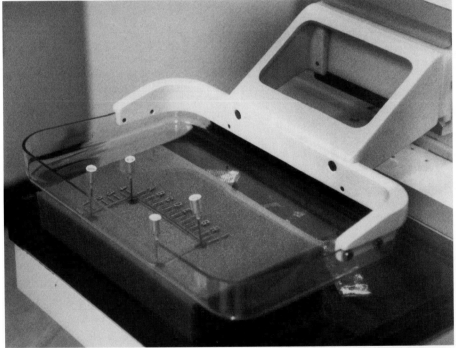

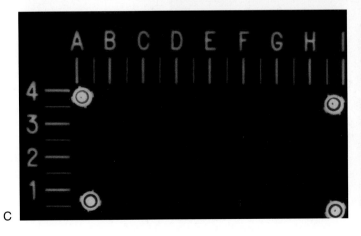

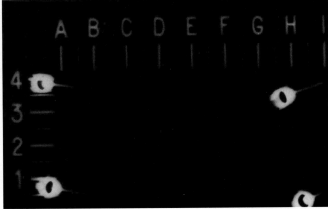

FIG. 21-13. The centering light should be aligned with the x-ray beam. A sponge is compressed under the fenestrated compression, and needles are placed using the centering light to align their hubs over the point of entry into the sponge **(A)**. Needles are advanced into the sponge **(B)**. If the light and tube are aligned, a subsequent x-ray will look down the lumen of the needles **(C)**. If the light is not aligned with the x-ray beam, then an x-ray of the needles will suggest that they are tilted **(D)**. The light should be realigned.

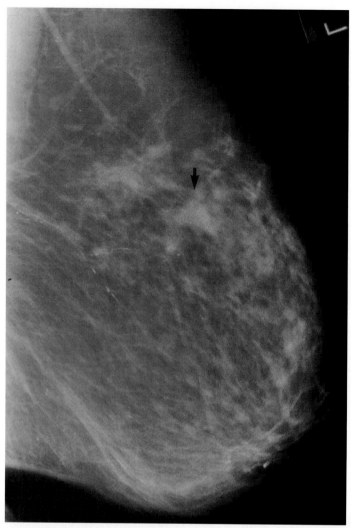

A

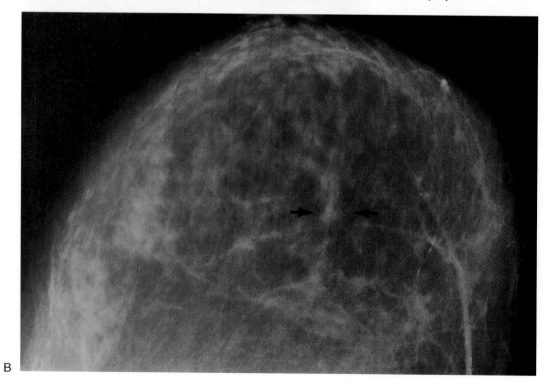

B

FIG. 21-14. The entry point for the needle is determined by evaluating the location of the lesion on a straight lateral (mediolateral [ML]) projection and a craniocaudal (CC) view. Unless there are other considerations, the shortest distance to the lesion should be chosen. In this case the lesion (*arrows*) is closest to the top of the breast, as is evident on the ML **(A)**, and fairly far from the medial or lateral surfaces, as seen on the CC **(B)** projection. The best approach is from the top with the patient in the CC projection.

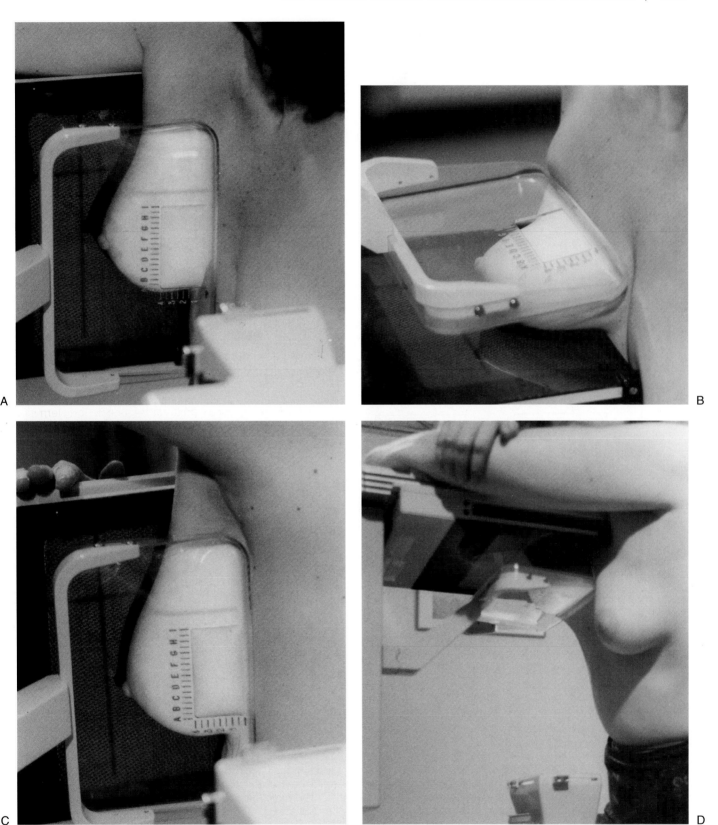

FIG. 21-15. If a lesion is medial, then the window compression is positioned over the medial skin surface **(A)**. If the lesion is at the top of the breast, then the craniocaudal approach is used **(B)**. For laterally located lesions, the lateromedial approach is used **(C)**, and if the lesion is in the lower breast the window can be placed on the under side with the gantry turned upside down **(D)**. It is not necessary to choose one of these directions. The window can be positioned anywhere in between as long as the lesion can be positioned in the field of view.

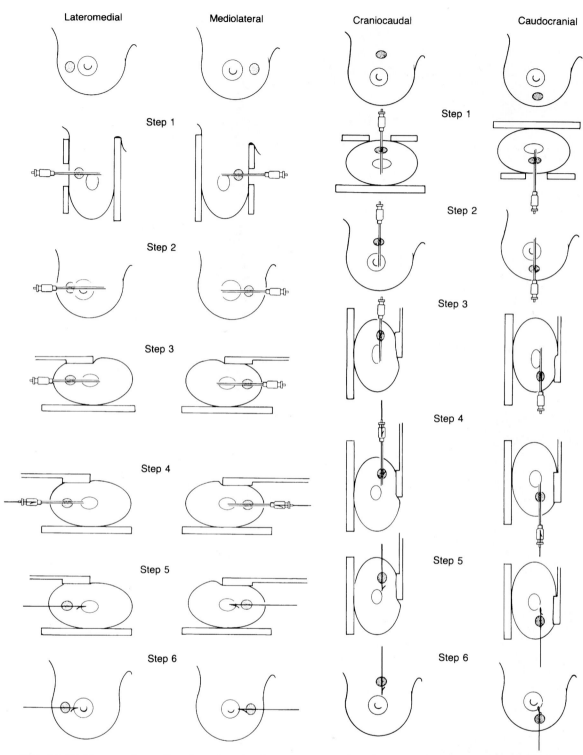

FIG. 21-16. These schematics show the step-by-step approach to lesions, depending on their position in the breast. *Step 1.* The breast is compressed using a fenestrated plate, affording the shortest approach to the lesion, and the needle is inserted. *Step 2.* The needle is passed through or alongside the lesion, and the breast is uncompressed, with the lesion transfixed by the needle. *Step 3.* The breast is recompressed with a spot compression. If a straight-needle technique is used, the localization is complete. On this second view, the distance of the lesion along the needle can be measured. *Step 4.* If the hookwire technique is used, the needle is withdrawn so that the tip is the desired distance beyond the lesion. *Step 5.* The hookwire is afterloaded and advanced to the needle tip. By holding the wire and withdrawing the needle, the hook will engage where the needle tip has been. Ideally this is just beyond the lesion. *Step 6.* The breast is removed from compression and the hook will be just beyond the lesion.

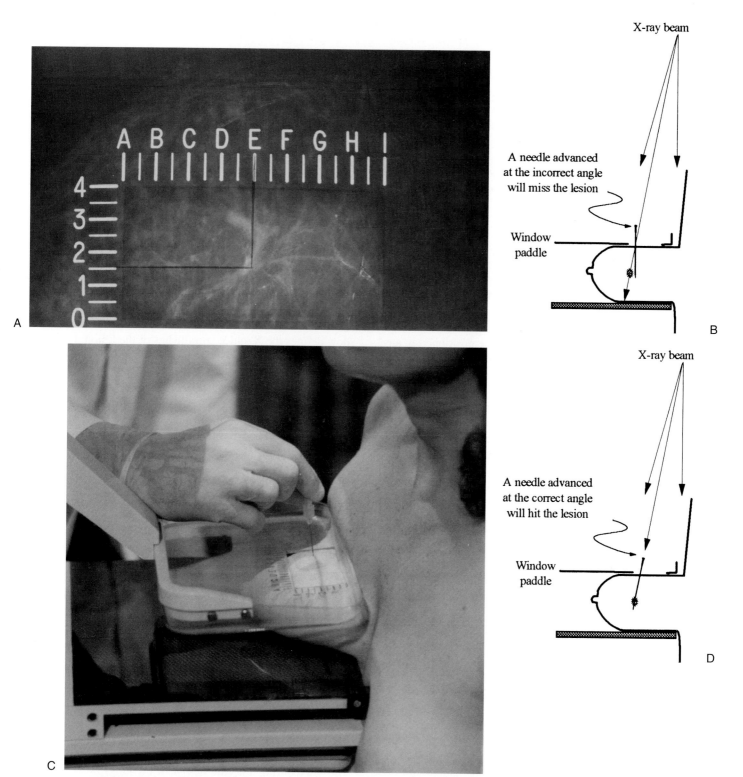

FIG. 21-17. The breast is positioned so that on the scout film **(A)** the lesion projects in the window of the compression paddle. The lines drawn on the film using a wax marker define its coordinates, using the grid markings at the edge of the window **(B)**. If the needle is advanced perpendicular to the film, it will miss the lesion because the x-ray beam is divergent. The needle tip should be placed at the intersection of the cross-hairs as they project on the skin, having been adjusted to the proper coordinates **(C)**. The needle should be advanced at the appropriate angle (using the centering light) in the direction of the x-ray beam to hit the lesion **(D)**. *Continued.*

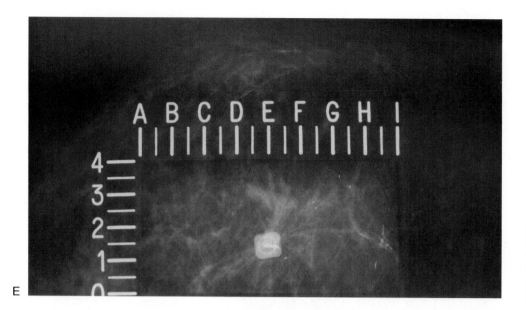

FIG. 21-17. *Continued.* The fact that the alignment was correct can be checked on the subsequent x-ray, where the needle and its hub are superimposed on the lesion **(E)**.

It should be clear that the breast can be positioned in any way that affords access to the lesion through the window while the breast is held in compression (Fig. 21-16). The gantry or the breast can be rotated to permit access from any direction (see Fig. 21-15). In some patients, the lesion can even be localized from the front of the breast if the breast is sufficiently flexible that it can be turned so that the desired anterior surface is in the window and the lesion is also visible in the window of the compression plate on the x-ray.

Once the shortest distance has been determined, the patient is seated facing the unit. With her face turned away from the side to be localized, the breast is compressed within the mammographic unit using the fenestrated compression plate so that the preliminary mammogram will project the lesion in the opening of the compression plate (Fig. 21-17).

Because viewing the needle can produce a vasovagal response, the patient should be instructed to keep her head turned away from the localization procedure. This should be done in a supportive manner. Rather than reminding the patient that she might faint seeing a needle in her breast, we find that it is best to suggest that we merely do not want her face to project in our pictures.

The patient should be advised of the importance of not moving her breast and staying in the mammography machine. She should be informed of each step of the procedure so that she is not startled. We also position an aide or the technologist so that she can talk to the patient and distract her from the procedure. It is often useful to mark the skin of the breast with an ink marker at the corners of the window to help to determine whether the patient moves during the procedure.

Using the preliminary image, lines are drawn perpendicular to the edges of the window through the center of the image of the lesion (see Fig. 21-17A). The intersection of these lines with the calibrations along the edge of the window defines the X and Y coordinates of the lesion. If a compression plate containing multiple holes rather than a single opening is used, the holes must be large enough to permit the needle hub to pass through (or special hubless needles that can pass through the holes must be used). The breast should be repositioned if the lesion is not visible in a hole.

After suitable skin preparation (we have always used three Betadine wipes and an alcohol wipe), the coordinates of the lesion as seen on the preliminary film are identified on the compression plate. Most modern mammography systems have linear cross-hairs or a laser light in the collimator of the tube housing that can be projected onto the fenestrated compression and the breast. By aligning the cross-hairs with the coordinates from the film, the skin entry for the needle can be determined. Because the x-ray beam that made the preliminary film is divergent, the only place that it is perpendicular to the film plane is at the center of the compression plate along the edge closest to the chest wall. If a needle is introduced *perpendicular* to the film plane at any other location, it will miss the targeted lesion (see Fig. 21-17B). Using a properly aligned centering light or appropriately aligned laser device, the needle tip is positioned at the intersection of the cross-hairs on the skin (see Fig. 21-17C) and then aligned in the direction of the x-ray beam (see Fig. 21-17D) by positioning the shadow of the hub on the skin directly over and centered on the point of the needle (the centering light is used in a similar fashion as a fluoroscope during a needle biopsy of the lung).

If the centering light is appropriately aligned with the x-ray beam and the shadow of the hub cast by the centering light is centered over the shadow of the needle, then the needle can be advanced in the same direction as the x-ray beam that made the image of the lesion, and the needle will pass through the targeted lesion. This can be confirmed by a repeat x-ray (see Fig. 21-17E). Using this technique, we have shown that even if the needle does not pass directly

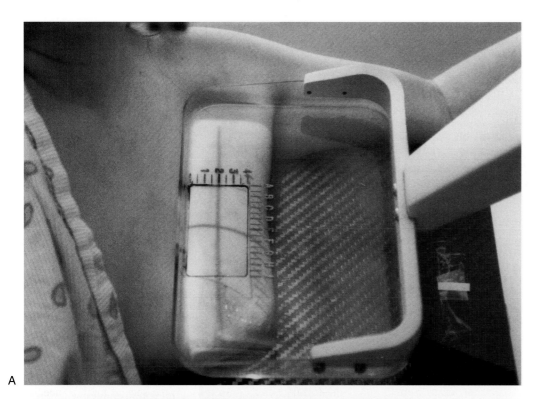

A

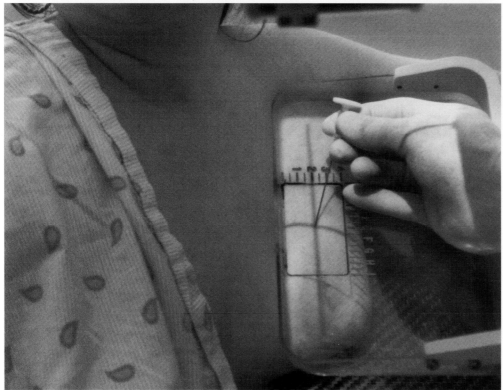

B

FIG. 21-18. (A) The cross-hairs are projected onto the skin at the appropriate grid coordinates, and the tip of the needle is placed on the intersection of the cross-hairs, as in this localization from the mediolateral oblique projection **(B)**. *Continued.*

through the lesion, the shaft of the needle will never be >5 mm from the lesion (28).

To facilitate positioning the needle, we developed a small disk that can be placed on the hub of the needle. This disk, which we call a TARGET, permits the cross-hairs to be pro-

jected onto its flat surface. Based on the scout film, the cross-hairs are projected onto the skin at the appropriate grid coordinates (Fig. 21-18A) and the needle tip is positioned at the skin entry site at the intersection of the cross-hairs on the skin surface in the routine fashion (Fig. 21-18B). While maintain-

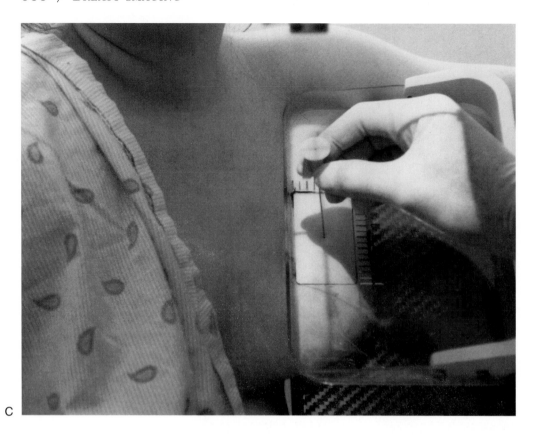

C

FIG. 21-18. *Continued.* While maintaining the needle tip on the skin entry point, the needle is angled up so that the cross-hairs project onto and are centered on the TARGET **(C)** and so that the needle can be advanced into the breast while maintaining alignment with the x-ray beam.

ing the needle tip in position on the skin, the needle is then tilted so that the cross-hairs are projected onto the center of the TARGET disk (Fig. 21-18C) on the needle hub. If the centering light is properly aligned with the x-ray beam, the needle will be positioned in direct alignment with the path that the x-ray beam followed to generate the preliminary film.

The needle can then be passed through the skin in a rapid motion (particularly if no local anesthetic has been used) to minimize any discomfort (generally the skin is the most sensitive to the passage of the needle). The needle is then advanced into the tissues in a smooth motion, keeping the cross-hairs centered on the TARGET, ensuring accurate positioning.

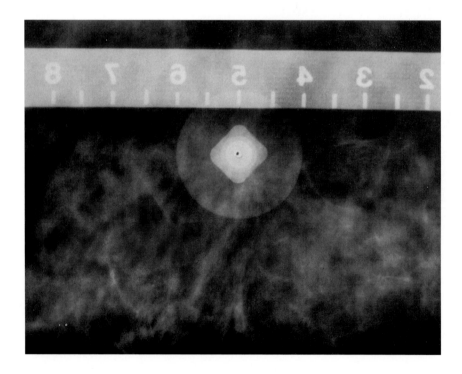

FIG. 21-19. The TARGET is radiolucent so that it can remain on the needle, because the lesion can be imaged through it, as seen in this case. The hub of the needle is the dense square in the center of the circular density, which is the target.

Regardless of the method, it is important to pass the needle through and beyond the suspected lesion so that it is either skewered by the needle or immediately adjacent to it. This method permits extremely accurate needle positioning. Unless the patient moves, it is virtually impossible for the needle to be any >0.5 mm from the lesion. The TARGET can be removed if desired, or, because it is radiolucent, the lesion can be imaged through it (Fig. 21-19) to confirm the X and Y coordinates of the needle position. The central hole in the target facilitates the introduction of a hook-wire into the needle cannula during a localization procedure (Fig. 21-20A).

Once the relationship of the needle to the lesion has been confirmed (X and Y coordinates), *there is no reason to return to this first projection.* If the needle is passed beyond the lesion and is in appropriate position on the second film, an engaged wire must be in the same relation to the lesion as the needle through which it was introduced and, therefore, *there is no reason to return to the first projection once a hookwire is engaged.* It is, in fact, not a good idea to return to this projection once a wire has been deployed, because compressing a wire in the direction of its insertion may result in moving it.

If the initial placement is suboptimal, the needle can be partially withdrawn, the insertion angle changed, and the needle reinserted without repuncturing the skin to achieve a more accurate position. If the breast had moved during the procedure, a new skin puncture may be necessary if the localization needle will be >5 mm from the lesion.

Occasionally the breast tissues are extremely firm and resist the passage of a needle. Generally a constant, firm pressure on the needle will ultimately permit it to pass through this type of tissue.

Once the X and Y coordinates are confirmed and are satisfactory with respect to the lesion, compression is slowly released. The radiologist should reach between the compression plates and hold the breast in one hand while holding the needle hub (on the other side of the plate) with the fingers of the other hand. It is *very important* that as compression is slowly released the radiologist advances the needle into the breast while simultaneously pulling the breast up around the needle (Fig. 21-20B), so as to ensure that the tip of the needle remains beyond the target and that the lesion remains on the shaft of the needle. If the lesion comes off the shaft of the needle (Fig. 21-20C), accurate localization is lost and the procedure should be started again. It is generally possible and desirable for needle stability to push the hub flush with the skin. The needle should have been chosen such that, when this is accomplished and the breast is compressed perpendicular to its course, the needle tip is at least 1 cm beyond the lesion.

After complete release of the breast from the compression system, the patient is moved from the mammography unit.

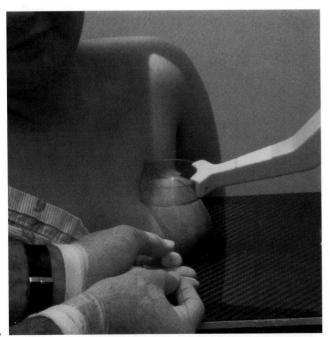

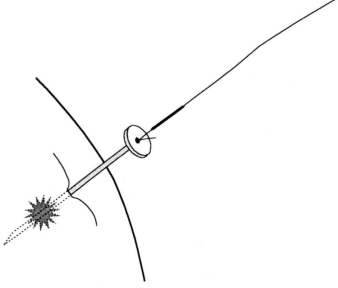

A

B

FIG. 21-20. The central hole in the TARGET can facilitate the introduction of a hookwire into the needle cannula during a localization procedure. Here **(A)** the radiologist is afterloading the wire through the hole in the center of the TARGET. Having advanced the needle as the breast is uncompressed, the tip will have stayed deep to the lesion, and the lesion will maintain its relationship to the needle **(B)**. *Continued.*

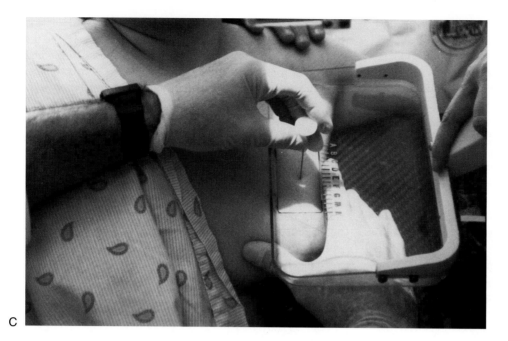

C

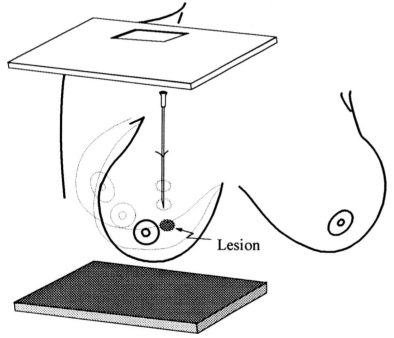

D

Lesion

FIG. 21-20. *Continued.* The radiologist is holding the needle in one hand, and while the technologist slowly uncompresses the breast, he advances the needle further into the breast and pulls the breast up around the needle to be sure to keep the tip beyond the lesion **(C)**. If the needle is not advanced while the breast is being uncompressed, the lesion may pull off of the needle as the breast re-expands to its normal position **(D)**.

Because most patients look immediately down to the breast to see what has been done, it is wise for the radiologist to keep a hand over the needle to prevent the patient from seeing it. Viewing the needle in her breast increases the likelihood that she will experience a vasovagal reaction. She will need to turn her head away, regardless, when she is repositioned in the machine.

With the patient away from the machine, the gantry is rotated 90 degrees in preparation for determining the Z, or depth, coordinate. This final maneuver is facilitated by replacing the large compression paddle with the small spot-compression device. At this point in the procedure it is no longer necessary to compress the entire breast. It is only necessary to be able to visualize the relationship of the needle tip to the targeted lesion so that the tip can be pulled back to establish its appropriate relationship to the lesion. By using the spot compression plate over the area, the lesion is held firmly (Fig. 21-21A), and the relationship of the tip of the needle to the lesion is visible (Fig. 21-21B). By using the spot-compression paddle, there is room for the radiologist to get to the hub of the needle to adjust its depth and engage a wire (Fig. 21-21C, D).

In the initial projection, the needle is passed to a depth that is beyond the lesion. This distance can be measured on the orthogonal mammogram (see Fig. 21-21B). If a simple needle technique is used, this orthogonal projection is the final view required as it gives the surgeon the relationship of the lesion along the shaft of the needle (see Fig. 21-21C). The needle tip should be at least 1 cm beyond the lesion so that the lesion remains along the needle shaft regardless of the position of the breast at surgery (Fig. 21-21D).

The orthogonal view permits withdrawal of the needle so that the tip can be precisely positioned. Cytologic material can be obtained by withdrawing the needle until the tip is in the lesion (although this risks the possibility that the needle will be pulled out of the lesion and the whole procedure will have to be performed again from the beginning). We have done core needle biopsies in this fashion, positioning an introducing needle through which the core needle was passed. If this orthogonal projection

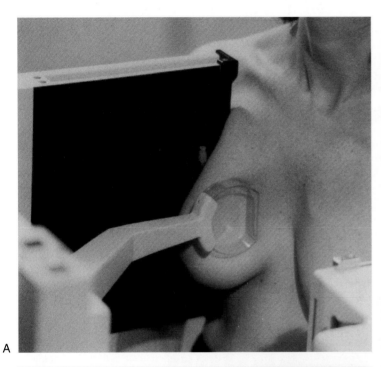

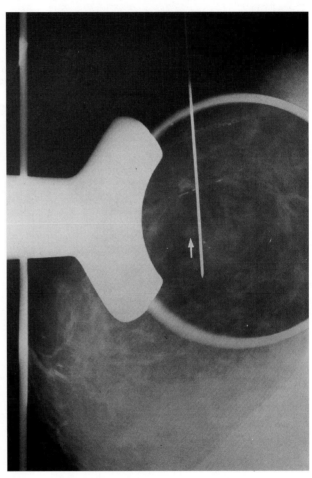

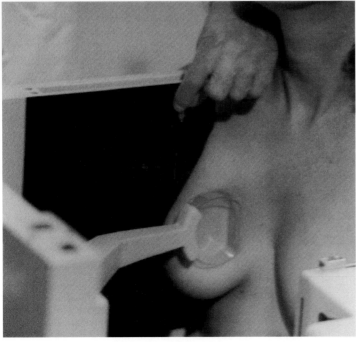

FIG. 21-21. The spot-compression paddle is used to compress perpendicular to the course of the needle **(A)** to image the needle tip and the lesion **(B)**. If a hook-wire is to be introduced, this image is used to determine how far back the needle should be pulled (*arrow*) to position the hook at the appropriate depth. By using the spot-compression paddle, the radiologist can easily reach the needle to pull it back to the desired depth **(C)**. *Continued.*

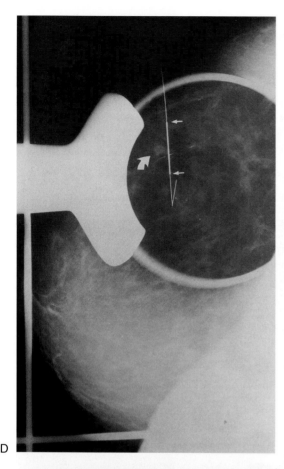

D

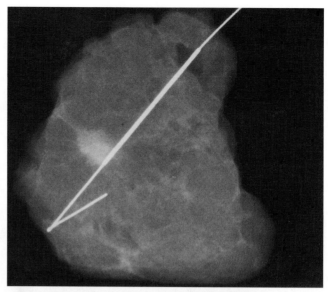

E

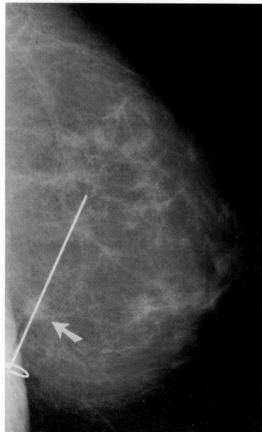

F

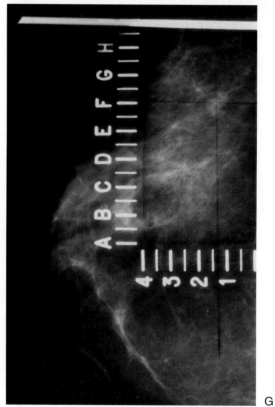

G

FIG. 21-21. *Continued.* A hookwire should be engaged so that the hook is beyond the lesion **(D)** (*curved arrow*), and the lesion is along the thickened segment (*small arrows*). The surgeon should remove a small amount of tissue around the thickened segment, and the excised tissue should be sent for specimen radiography. Specimen radiography confirms that the lesion and wire have been successfully removed **(E)**. In this second patient **(F)** a straight, flat-head needle has been placed from the bottom of the breast using the craniocaudal (CC) projection. This provides only two-dimensional accuracy, and the surgeon must use the image to determine how far along the needle to go to find the lesion (*arrow*). Note that with a straight needle technique the tip should be well beyond the lesion to preclude having the lesion slip off the needle shaft. In this third patient the shortest distance is from the lateral side, so the breast is positioned in the lateromedial projection **(G)** with the window over the lateral skin surface.

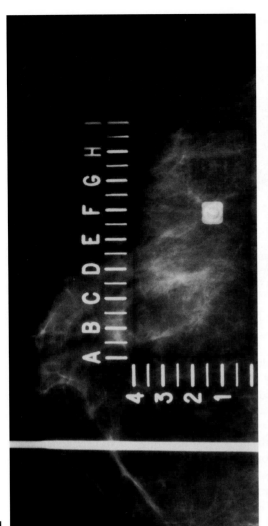

H

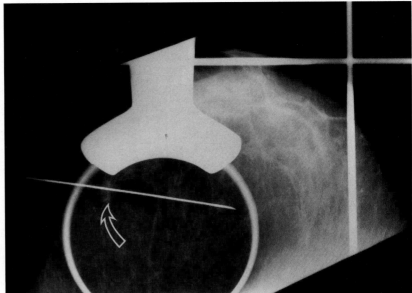

I

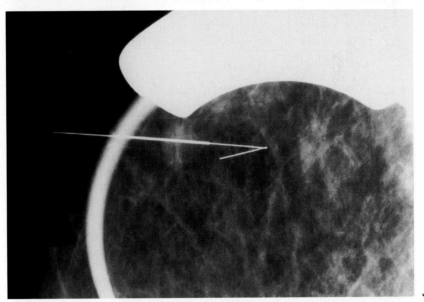

J

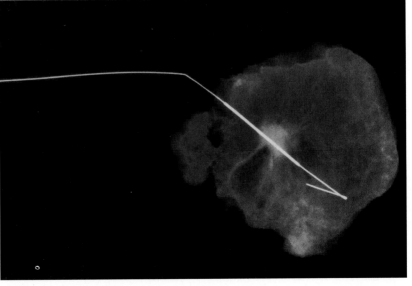

K

FIG. 21-21. *Continued.* The needle is introduced and its position is confirmed **(H)**. The needle is advanced as the compression is released, and the spot-compression device is substituted for the window compression. The gantry is rotated 90 degrees into the CC projection, and the breast is recompressed to show the distance from the lesion (*arrow*) to the needle tip **(I)**. The needle is pulled back and the wire engaged with the lesion ideally located on the thickened segment of wire just proximal to the hook **(J)**. Excision of the invasive ductal carcinoma is confirmed on the specimen radiograph **(K)**.

shows that the lesion has come off the needle shaft and is beyond the tip, accurate localization is lost. The lesion may no longer be in line with the needle and, although readvancing it may give the appearance that it intersects the lesion, the needle may be in a different plane. Accurate localization will be lost, and the surgeon may fail to excise the area of concern. Should the needle be pulled out of the lesion, it is best to start the procedure from the beginning and be certain that the needle remains through the target tissue.

If a hookwire system is used for localization, the needle is withdrawn so that its tip is at the level at which the hook will be placed. In general, it is best to anchor hooks slightly deeper than the lesion so that the wire passes through the lesion. We prefer using wires with a 2-cm thickened segment just proximal to the hook as a guide for the surgeon (see Hookwire Systems, earlier in this chapter). With these wires, the hook is ideally engaged 1.0 to 1.5 cm beyond the lesion so that the lesion is on the thickened segment just proximal to the hook (Fig. 21-21E). This ensures that if there is any movement of the wire with slight traction at surgery the hook will pull into the lesion and not away from it.

The surgeon can use the thickened distal segment of wire as a marker to indicate that the level of the lesion has been reached and that the hook is 2 cm beyond. The surgeon should ideally remove a small cylinder of tissue around the thickened segment that provides a small margin of tissue around the lesion and includes the hook. If the lesion has a high probability of cancer, a wider excision may be desirable to avoid the need for re-excision. Specimen radiography should be obtained to confirm that the lesion has been excised (Fig. 21-21F).

Accurate engagement of hookwires is accomplished by pulling the needle out so that its tip is positioned at the desired location for the end of the wire. The wire is then afterloaded into the needle from the hub. By advancing the wire up the mark on the proximal portion, the hook will be folded just inside the needle tip. The proximal wire should then be held in position while the needle is withdrawn back over it and out of the breast. In this way the hook will engage where the needle tip had been.

On occasion the needle tip may become firmly embedded in fibrous tissue such that when it is withdrawn the tip pulls the tissue with it. Although it appears that the needle is being pulled out of the breast, when the wire is engaged and the tissue elastically returns it to its normal position, the hook may be pulled farther beyond the lesion than is desirable (a hook that is too deep with the lesion along the wire is preferable to one that is too shallow with the lesion beyond the hook). A similar result can occur by inadvertently feeding the wire out the needle tip rather than pulling the needle out while holding the wire stationary. The wire can follow the needle track, or, if the breast is primarily fat, can be pushed through the fat if there is no fibrous tissue to prevent this advance.

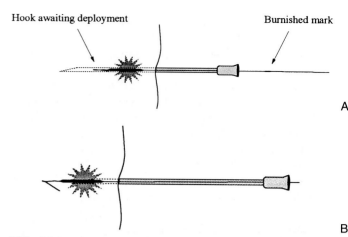

FIG. 21-22. It is occasionally helpful to position the hook within the needle in its desired location in space, as shown on this schematic **(A)**, and then to pull the needle back to release the hook in the appropriate position just beyond the lesion **(B)**.

The problem of the needle tip being fixed in tissue and the wire ending up deeper than desired can be avoided by turning the needle to break it loose from these tissues as it is withdrawn and increasing the pressure of the compression device to prevent the tissues from moving. It is also useful to position the hook in space, while it is still contained in the needle, before pulling the needle back (Fig. 21-22). If the needle tip is to be pulled back 2 cm for proper positioning of the hook, the wire can be inserted so that the burnished mark is 2 cm outside the needle hub. Even though the needle tip is still beyond the appropriate point, the hook is in the desired position relative to the lesion. If the proximal wire is held firmly and the needle is turned and withdrawn, the tip usually frees itself from the deeper tissue by the time the hook is exposed, and the hook engages in the desired tissue.

Some of our surgeons have found it valuable to have a metallic marker placed at the skin insertion site, so that on the final film obtained with the hook engaged they can see how far down the wire the lesion is from the skin (with the understanding that the breast is compressed).

Accuracy and Safety

Virtually all complications of preoperative localization can be avoided if the procedure is carefully thought through and care is exercised in the positioning of guides as well as in the surgical excision of the lesions. In an analysis of 100 consecutive guided wire-directed biopsies performed by radiologists with all levels of expertise (residents, fellows, and staff), we routinely positioned the wire through or within 2 mm of the lesion 96% of the time and were within 5 mm in all 100 procedures. This made it possible for the surgeon to remove a minimum volume (often <5 ml) of tissue without missing the lesion (20).

Completing the Localization Procedure

Once the needle or wire is appropriately placed, the patient is removed from the compression system and the breast is allowed to assume its normal position. In some instances some of the wire is enveloped by the re-expanding breast. This should be anticipated and a long enough wire should be used so that this can be permitted. It is best to not bend or tape the wire to the skin in such a way that it places the hook under tension as this may cause the hook to pull out of the targeted tissue. The exposed wire should be gently looped away from the expected incision site (some surgeons prefer to leave this part of the wire taped to the skin during surgery) and the end taped to the skin (Fig. 21-23). A sterile gauze is placed over the insertion point so that it is protected, but the wire should not be bent or firmly taped at this location because that might put the hook under traction and breast movement might dislodge it. If taped without tension, the wire may slide in and out of the skin with breast movement, but there will be no traction on the hook. By not bending the wire, the surgeon can introduce a needle over the wire in the operating room to provide a stiffer target during surgery.

Discussion with the surgeon or careful diagrammatic portrayal of the relation of the lesion to the wire is suggested so that the surgeon understands the course of the wire and the relationship of the lesion to the hook. We send the localization films with the patient to the operating area.

As noted earlier, once a hookwire is engaged it is not a good idea to compress the breast in the direction of wire insertion. Some surgeons request that an image be obtained looking down the wire. This is not advised and is not necessary. Because the original needle transfixed the lesion, if the needle was not pulled completely out of the lesion before engaging a wire, there is no reason to return to the original projection once a hookwire is engaged because the wire must be where the needle had been (X and Y cannot change). Compressing the breast in the direction of the wire placement could result in advancing the wire farther beyond the lesion and the loss of an accurate Z placement. The surgeon can obtain the X and Y relationship from the original second film with the view looking down the needle shaft and can obtain the Z relationship from the final orthogonal view of the wire and lesion.

SURGICAL EXCISION OF A NONPALPABLE LESION AFTER PLACEMENT OF A GUIDE

Some of the problems with needle localization and biopsy result from the fact that surgeons are reluctant to ask colleagues how to best perform these procedures. Many surgeons remove far more tissue than is required and cause a much larger defect than is needed. Some remove all of the tissue from the skin entry point to the lesions. This is unnecessary.

Two approaches appear to work best. Some surgeons follow the wire from its skin entry site (Fig. 21-24A) down to the thickened segment and then remove a cylinder of tissue around the thickened segment to the hook. This ensures complete removal of the wire as well as the lesion. A second approach is to estimate the location of the lesion and to cut down to the wire from the anterior surface of the breast closer to the lesion than the skin entry site so that there is a shorter distance to dissect along the wire (Fig. 21-24B). Another useful maneuver is to deliver the proximal wire through the incision so that the surgeon can operate looking down the wire (Fig. 21-25). If the wire has been placed so that the lesion is proximal to the hook along the thick segment, a cylinder of tissue around this thick segment is removed to the hook. This will encompass the lesion.

A third approach is to undertake a circumareolar incision, which some surgeons prefer for its cosmetic value, but, as noted above, there is some debate as to the safety of this approach for reaching peripheral lesions that prove to be malignant. Finding a wire when such an approach is used may be difficult. By passing a 20- or 22-gauge needle or specially formed blunt-tipped cannula over the wire, using the wire as a guide, a stiffer target is created to approach a deep lesion (28).

The surgeon should understand that any wire can inadvertently be pulled out of the breast if sufficient traction is placed on it. Furthermore, if the wire is positioned predominantly in fat, there is little tissue for any hook to adhere to and wires can be moved in fat. The wire should be used as a guide and not as a retractor. By placing the

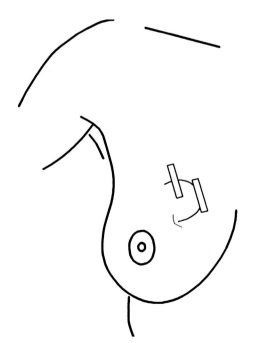

FIG. 21-23. The wire should be taped to the skin in a gentle loop with no tension.

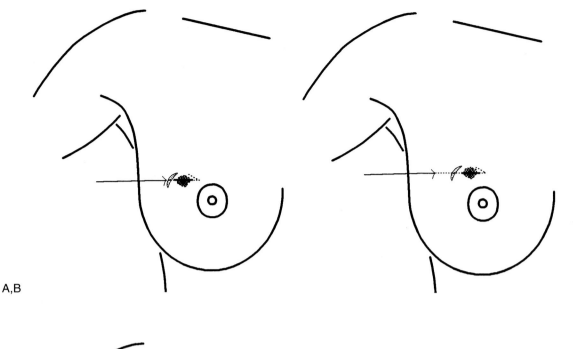

FIG. 21-24. Schematic of the process of **excisional biopsy following the positioning of a hookwire.** The surgeon can dissect straight down the wire from its insertion site **(A)** or anticipate its path and cut down to it and then along its path to the thickened segment **(B).**

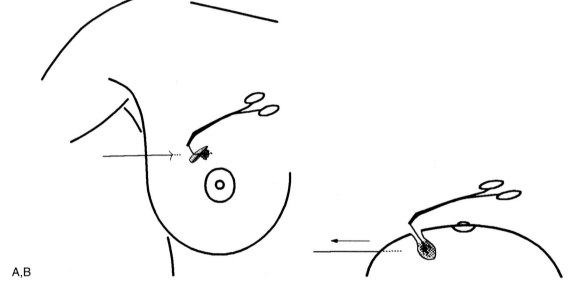

FIG. 21-25. Some surgeons transect the wire and deliver the distal portion through an incision that is remote from the skin entry site **(A).** This permits the surgeon to operate looking down the axis of the wire to facilitate the removal of a small cylinder of tissue around the thick segment and the hook **(B)** and containing the lesion.

lesion along the thickened segment proximal to the hook, any traction applied to the wire pulls the hook back into the lesion rather than away from it. The thick segment acts as an indicator for the surgeon so that the distance to the hook can be anticipated.

If regular needles are used to localize lesions, they should be of sufficient length to transfix and pass beyond the lesion and are advanced flush with the skin. Based on the mammograms the surgeon can estimate the distance down the needle the lesion lies and dissect to this area. Tissue is then taken out in a cylindrical manner around this portion of the needle and sent for specimen radiography to confirm the removal of the lesion.

Dye Injection

If a dye injection technique is used either alone or in conjunction with guide placement, the needle for such injections may be positioned in the same way as described earlier. A vital dye is chosen, and a very small amount is injected into the region of the lesion. The needle may remain in place or be withdrawn slowly, injecting the dye as the needle is withdrawn, staining the track. Although this provides a visible track that can be followed by the surgeon to the tissue in question, it can be difficult to follow and many surgeons who use dye injections leave a needle guide in as well. Although diffusion of dye into a much larger volume than desired has been a problem for some surgeons, proponents argue that this is a rare occurrence.

Some advocate mixing the vital dye with iodinated contrast material to confirm the position of the stained tissue relative to the lesion on the mammogram. This, however, may obscure the lesion in the subsequent specimen radiograph. If these techniques are used, the practitioner must be aware of the potential for contrast reactions as well as possible allergic reactions to the vital dye.

Carbon particles are used in Europe. They are inert and can be positioned weeks in advance because they do not move. Some use these at the time of FNAB so that the surgeon has a guide to the suspicious tissue. Following a thin black line to a lesion, however, can be difficult and may result in the need to remove an excessively large amount of tissue.

Excised Specimen

Except for rare circumstances, all localized biopsies can be performed in the outpatient surgical setting. Most can be done under local anesthetic, often with "conscious sedation." Immediately after the surgical excision, while the biopsy cavity remains open, the specimen should be radiographed to confirm that the targeted abnormality has been removed. Even if the surgeon feels confident that the lesion is out, specimen radiography should be performed for documentation. The specimen should be gen-

tly compressed within the mammographic system or in a special specimen radiography unit so that air interfaces do not obscure the visualization of masses in the specimen (Fig. 21-26).

Specimen radiography is facilitated if the surgeon places the intact specimen in a plastic bag that can be sealed to facilitate handling. If the tissue must be kept cold, this bag can be inserted into a second bag containing ice. The specimen, in its bag, can be placed in the mammography unit and gently compressed using the compression system. If a specimen radiographic unit is used, the specimen can be gently (so as not to crush the tissue) compressed under a piece of Plexiglas.

Magnification radiography of the specimen is preferable because it can improve the visualization of calcifications. Compression of the specimen permits the visualization of masses as well as calcifications in the tissue samples. The radiologist should also analyze the relationship of the lesion to the visible margins on the specimen radiograph to alert the surgeon if the lesion appears to be close or abutting the surgical margin.

Some radiologists advocate performing the specimen radiograph in two projections, but with small compressed specimens it is likely that a good appreciation of the proximity of the lesion to the margin of the specimen can be observed despite the fact that the anterior and posterior margins are not well seen with single-view specimen radiography.

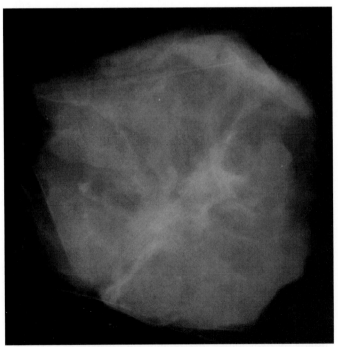
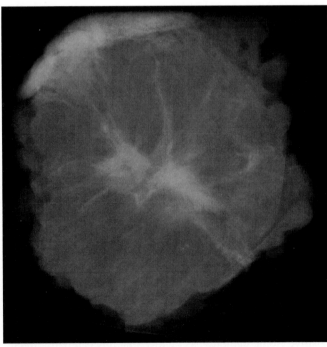

A   B

FIG. 21-26. The specimen should be gently compressed (not crushed) to perform specimen radiography. Detail may be lost if the specimen is not compressed **(A)**. Masses may not be visible at all. With compression and magnification **(B)** excellent detail is seen, and the removal of masses as well as calcifications can be confirmed.

Some have found that marking the location of the lesion within the specimen with additional needles or the use of special specimen containers with grid coordinates aids the pathologist in ensuring that the lesion that was of concern is actually evaluated. Marking the surfaces of the specimen with sutures or colored dyes is used by some surgeons to guide re-excision should cancer be found abutting the margin of the excised tissue.

We routinely obtain two specimen radiographs and retain one for the imaging record; the second accompanies the tissue to the pathology department to alert the pathologist as to the lesion that was targeted.

Ultrasound Specimen Imaging

Lesions that are not visible on the mammogram and are localized using ultrasound may not be visible using specimen radiography. By placing the specimen in a plastic bag the tissue can be evaluated using ultrasound while still in the bag by applying coupling gel to the surface of the bag. The specimen's own moisture provides coupling on the inside, and the lesion can be identified in this way using ultrasound of the specimen.

Margin Analysis

Although the overall prognosis is determined by whether cancer has spread systemically, successful treatment of breast cancer involves preventing recurrences within the breast. Multiple studies have shown that recurrence rates are reduced if a rim of normal tissue is removed around the tumor. Resection to clear margins is the desired goal of an excisional procedure, and analysis of the margins is used to determine whether they are free of tumor, increasing the likelihood (although not guaranteeing) that the tumor has been excised. The specimen radiograph can give a preliminary assessment of part of the margin.

One of the important duties of the pathologist is the assessment of the relationship of cancer to the margins of the excised tissue. If there is tumor present at the margin of the lesion, then a significant amount of residual tumor is likely still in the breast and the recurrence rate in the breast will be higher (58,59). Before sectioning, the pathologist should paint the surface of the specimen with India ink or some similar stain, so that the proximity of cancer to a margin can be assessed after sectioning and during viewing under the microscope (60). Some pathologists use different colored inks to identify the different surfaces of the specimen so that if a margin is positive they can inform the surgeon of its relative position in the breast. If a margin is positive, some pathologists believe that this can help direct the surgeon as to which part of the biopsy cavity wall should be re-excised if re-excision is needed for a positive margin. Unfortunately, although important, margin analysis

is quite crude. The pathologist is viewing only a tiny portion of the specimen.

One specimen radiograph is retained for the patient's record. The second specimen radiograph provides the pathologist with an understanding of the lesion that was excised so that the histologic review can be correlated with the expected pathology to ensure concordance. The volume of the tissue excised may be quite small, but the lesion itself usually occupies a much smaller portion of the sample. Permanent histologic sections are generally approximately 4 μm thick. This, however, is a very small sample of even the smallest biopsy specimen. It would take 2,000 5-μm-thick histologic samples to completely evaluate just a 1-ml volume of breast tissue. Thus, it is possible for the pathologist to inadvertently overlook the actual lesion. Because of this major opportunity for sampling error, even careful margin analysis may fail to reveal that cancer is extending to the margin. It is almost impossible to determine when DCIS has been completely excised because it might extend into a duct that is not included in any of the sections viewed microscopically. With DCIS, even when there are pathologically clear margins, residual in situ cancer is found at re-excision or in the mastectomy at least 40% of the time. Presumably radiation therapy reduces the recurrence rate for DCIS by killing this residual tumor in the breast (61).

If there is any question as to whether the lesion has been seen by the pathologist, radiographs of any remaining unprocessed biopsy tissue or of the paraffin blocks can be obtained and samples of the residual tissue at various levels processed to ensure that complete evaluation has occurred. If there is any question as to where in the specimen the lesion can be found, the sectioned specimen can be radiographed to determine the slices that contain the lesion.

On occasion it may be necessary to radiograph the paraffin blocks containing residual tissue to determine whether the lesion is still deeper in the block, requiring additional histologic sections. Sometimes imaging the block by turning it on its side (Fig. 21-27) (62) can demonstrate that suspicious calcifications are deep in the block and that levels through the block should be obtained.

Some reports have suggested that cancers may occur at a distance from microcalcifications, and this has been used to argue that larger biopsied samples are indicated. This is more than likely a serendipitous occurrence most frequently found with lobular carcinoma in situ. Most calcifications associated with cancer are in the tumor, and in general a small tissue sample is desirable. This is especially true given that the majority of nonpalpable breast lesions prove to be benign, and cosmetic preservation is desirable. If a lesion proves to be malignant and the margins are not free of tumor, re-excision of the biopsy cavity with several centimeters of normal tissue should probably be undertaken, unless the patient chooses mastectomy as the primary course of therapy. Some surgeons "shave" the walls of the cavity at

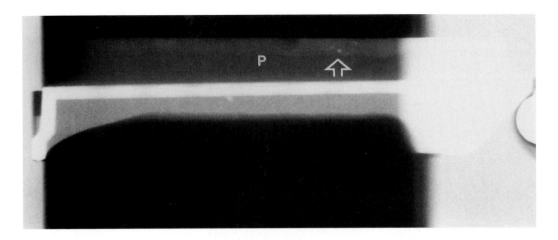

FIG. 21-27. If the pathologist does not find calcifications in the specimen, they may be deeper in the paraffin blocks. Here a paraffin block (P) has been turned on its side so that the radiograph can show the depth location of calcifications (*arrow*) in the block.

the time of excision. If there is tumor in this immediate re-excision, they advise mastectomy.

MAMMOGRAPHICALLY GUIDED CYST ASPIRATION OR FINE-NEEDLE ASPIRATION

Through the use of ultrasound many mammographically detected, clinically occult lesions can be identified as cysts. On occasion, when a lesion is small or when internal echoes are present, the confident diagnosis of a simple cyst cannot be achieved with ultrasound. If the lesion potentially represents a cyst but warrants further intervention, aspiration can be achieved under mammographic or ultrasound guidance. Mammographic guidance is accomplished using the preliminary steps described earlier for the preoperative localization of other occult lesions.

In the case of a potential cyst, but where suspicion is high, the patient can be scheduled for a CNB or for surgical removal to follow the aspiration if it is unsuccessful. If aspiration is unsuccessful, a CNB can be performed or a wire can be afterloaded through the same needle used for aspiration (47) or the needle can be left in place and the patient can undergo surgical excision of the lesion as with any localization.

Cyst Aspiration

Using the fenestrated compression paddle, a needle can be placed into the lesion with the patient in a mammographic position and, using the same procedure described for needle localization, fluid can be aspirated (Fig. 21-28). When the breast is compressed, a cyst is under pressure and

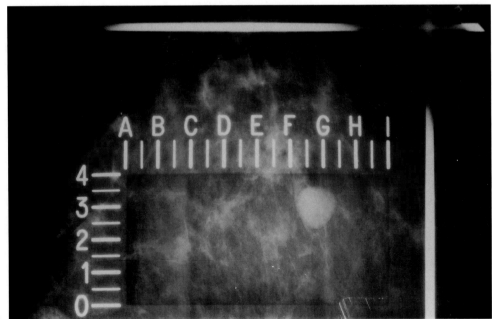

A

FIG. 21-28. When performing **mammographically guided cyst aspiration**, the lesion is positioned in the window of the compression paddle **(A)**. *Continued.*

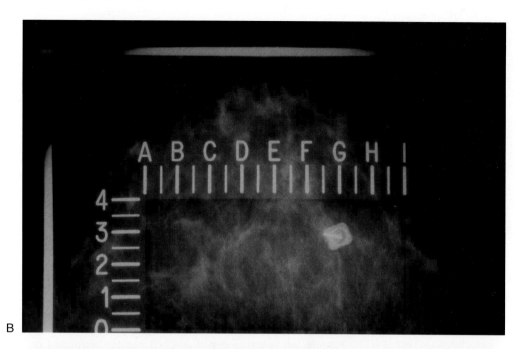

B

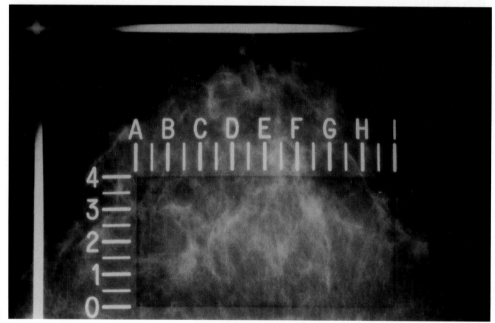

C

FIG. 21-28. *Continued.* The needle is introduced as with a standard needle localization but with connecting tubing attached to a syringe. Once the skin is punctured, an assistant can begin aspirating while the operator advances the needle. The position of the needle can be checked with a mammogram **(B)** to ensure that the lesion has been hit and drained. A final film confirms the resolution of the cyst **(C)**.

fluid may be ejected as soon as the needle passes into the lesion. If a cyst is suspected, it is prudent to attach connecting tubing to the needle so that as it is advanced any fluid forced from the cyst collects in the tubing. The end of the tubing can be connected to a syringe, and an assistant can aspirate as the needle is advanced. The TARGET can be used to guide needle placement by attaching a stopcock to the needle, the TARGET to the top connection, and the connecting tubing to the side port (Fig. 21-29). If there is no intention to follow an aspiration with immediate surgery, we introduce the needle from the CC projection. This allows the needle to reach the most dependent portion of a cyst so that it can be completely aspirated.

If a needle localization is planned but fluid is obtained at aspiration, the needle should be passed through the lesion and the localization should proceed. By viewing the needle in the 90-degree projection, it can be determined whether complete resolution has been achieved. If not, the needle can be pulled back into the lesion and re-aspiration performed (Fig. 21-30A). If the lesion completely disappears and the fluid is turbid yellow, green, or brown, it is safe to terminate the localization and cancel the surgery. If, however, there is no fluid, there is a residual mass, or the fluid appears to contain old blood (thick and maroon in color), it is prudent to proceed with a needle biopsy or localization and excision (Fig. 21-30B).

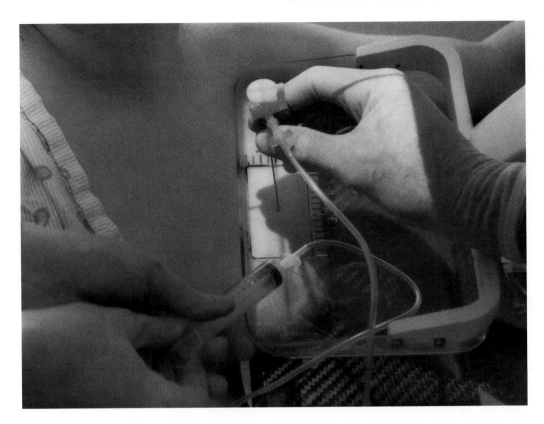

FIG. 21-29. The TARGET can be used for mammographically guided cyst aspiration by placing it on a stopcock in the needle hub. Suction can be applied by an assistant through connecting tubing attached to the side port of the stopcock.

Cytology and Cyst Fluid

Since we began aspirating cysts, we have always sent the fluid for cytologic analysis. Of >500 aspirations, only four have been positive. Two of these were cysts that had an associated mass, and two were large, solitary cysts, one of which contained old blood. Most observers acknowledge that routine cytologic analysis of cysts is very expensive, and, because intracystic cancer is so rare, not cost-effective. Most radiologists advocate discarding fluid that is clear, yellow, milky, brown, or green. The safety of this has been demonstrated by Smith et al. (62a). If the aspirate reveals old blood (maroon in color), then cytologic review may be indicated, although we recommend that the cyst be excised even if the cytology is negative. We often introduce a small amount of air to permit additional evaluation of the cyst, but there is no good scientific evidence that this is of any significant benefit (see Pneumocystography).

Skin Calcification Localization

As noted in Chapter 22, calcifications in the skin can occasionally be mistaken for suspicious intramammary deposits. Virtually all of the skin and calcifications in the skin, project over the breast on two-view mammography (Fig. 21-31). The ability to prove that calcifications are benign deposits in the skin is important to avoid raising unnecessary concern.

The way to confirm that calcifications are in the skin is to obtain a tangential view of the skin and demonstrate the calcifications in the dermis. This can be accomplished by using the fenestrated grid. If indeterminate calcifications are thought to be in the skin (there is no reason to evaluate obvious skin calcifications) (Fig. 21-32A, B), the breast is positioned so that the skin surface thought to contain the calcifications is accessible through the window compression and a marker is taped to them (Fig. 21-32C). The breast is then positioned so that the x-ray beam is tangential to the skin surface at the marker (Fig. 21-32D). The calcifications can be shown to be dermal and, therefore, of no consequence.

Ideally the radiologist will avoid recommending a biopsy for skin deposits, but the biopsy can still be avoided if the needle localization is done using the PCW approach from the shortest distance. Problems will occur, however, if freehand localization is used because there is no way of deducing that the calcifications are actually in the skin if this approach is used.

If the possibility of dermal calcifications is not appreciated and a needle localization is performed, there is still the opportunity to avoid unnecessary surgery. Using the PCW localization technique described previously, a needle introduced from the closest skin surface will pass through the calcifications if they are in the skin. When the patient is removed from the first position in the mammography system and the gantry is rotated and repositioned in the orthogonal projection, dermal

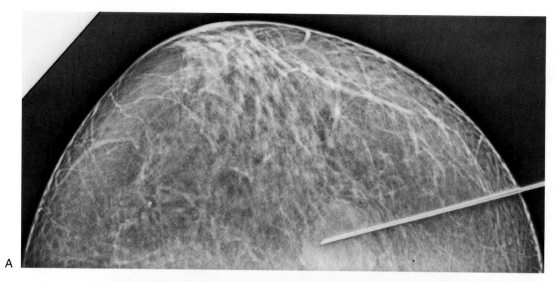

A

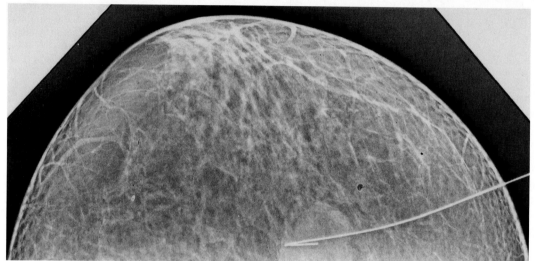

B

FIG. 21-30. If a lesion does not produce fluid, a wire can be afterloaded through the same needle. In this patient the needle has been withdrawn into the mass, as seen on this negative-mode xerogram **(A)**. When no fluid could be withdrawn a hookwire was introduced **(B)**, and surgery revealed an invasive ductal carcinoma.

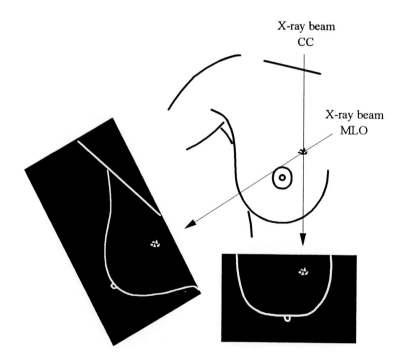

FIG. 21-31. As demonstrated on this schematic, **calcifications that are in the skin of the breast usually project over the breast tissue.**

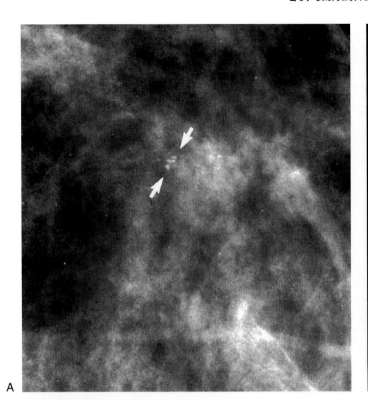

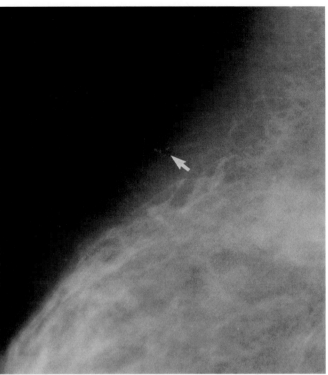

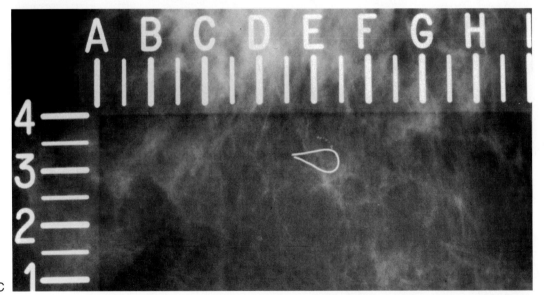

FIG. 21-32. These calcifications (*arrows*) are indeterminate on the craniocaudal **(A)** and lateral **(B)** projections. Using the window compression, a marker is taped to the skin **(C)** overlying the calcifications (or taped to them if they are in the skin). *Continued.*

deposits should be suspected if the calcifications are close to the needle hub (assuming it has been placed flush to the skin) or if the calcifications are close to the skin entry site (Fig. 21-33A). These can be confirmed by obtaining an image with the x-ray beam in tangent to the needle skin entry point (Fig. 21-33B). The localization should be terminated, the patient reassured, and the surgeon notified that a biopsy is not needed.

Parallax Needle Localization

On rare occasions a lesion is visible only on one projection, and the lesion cannot be seen on orthogonal views. Stereotactic devices that can be used to direct needles to such nonpalpable lesions are available, but simple parallax using conventional mammography can be used to position

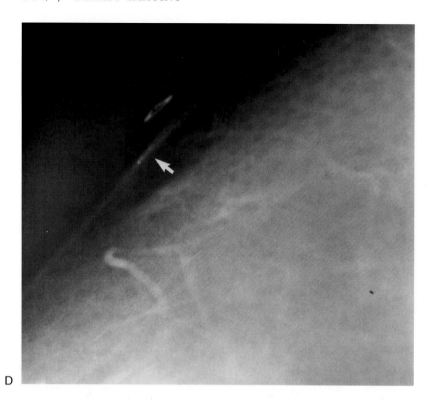

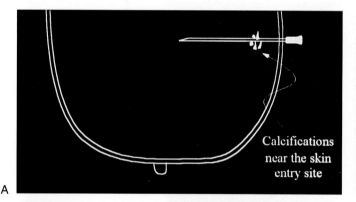

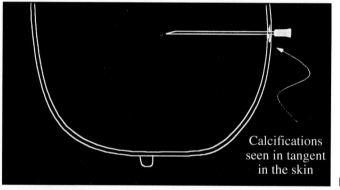

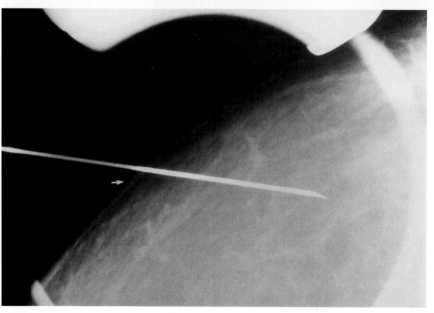

FIG. 21-32. *Continued.* A tangential view **(D)** shows them in the skin *(arrow)* and proves that the calcifications are **dermal deposits** and, therefore, of no consequence.

Calcifications near the skin entry site

Calcifications seen in tangent in the skin

FIG. 21-33. If the calcifications appear to be close to the needle entry site **(A)**, they may be in the skin. **A tangential view to the needle entry site (B) can confirm dermal deposits** so that the needle localization and biopsy can be canceled. In this case surgery was canceled when the radiologist realized that the calcifications were in the skin at the needle entry site **(C)** *(arrow)*.

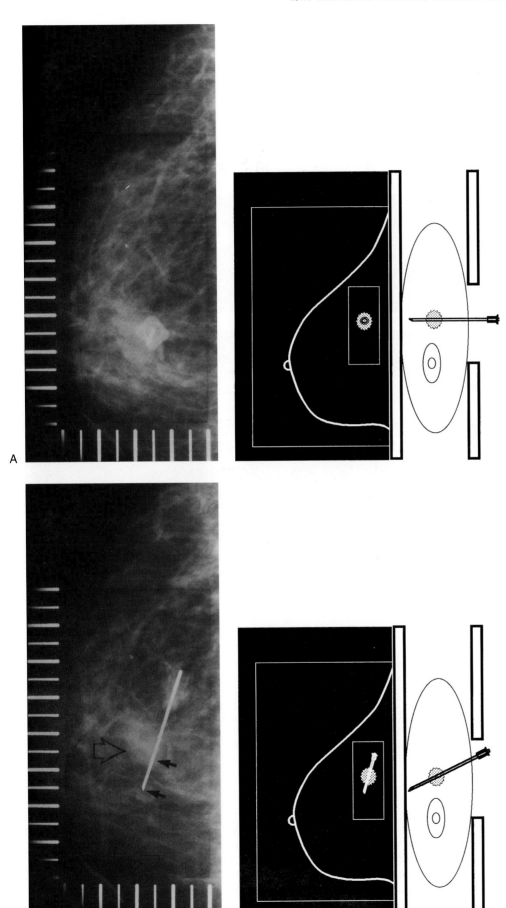

FIG. 21-34. The technique of parallax localization can be seen in the localization of this lesion from the lateromedial approach. The mass has been placed in the window and the needle introduced in the standard fashion and pushed almost to the other side of the breast **(A)**. Compression is reduced slightly and the skin pulled or the breast rolled so that the needle tilts over **(B)**. The needle is now visible at an angle so that its projected length is foreshortened. The open arrow points to the mass. The short arrows define the projected distance that the needle must be pulled back from the lesion (PDL). *Continued.*

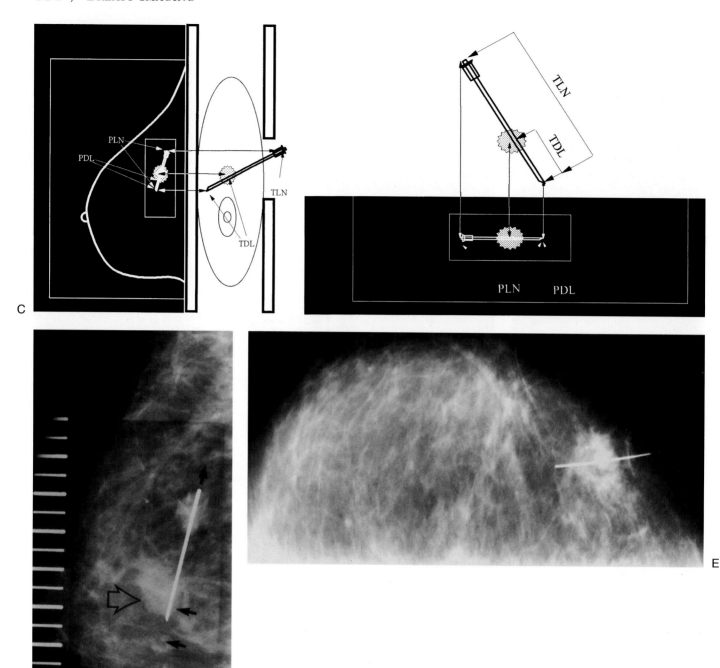

C

D

E

FIG. 21-34. *Continued.* PDL is related to the true distance that the needle must be pulled back (TDL) as the projected length of the needle (PLN) seen on the mammogram **(C)** is to the true length of the metal portion of the needle (TLN). The TDL is calculated, and the needle is pulled back this distance **(D)** and a wire engaged. In this example, the accuracy of the technique can be seen in the relationship of the hooked end to the lesion **(E)**.

needles for aspiration cytology or to guide placement for the surgical excision of these lesions.

This can be accomplished by first noting the shift of the lesion between two slightly different projections. If the lesion is seen on the MLO projection, the straight lateral view can be used to determine its location. Similarly, rolled CC views can be used to triangulate a lesion seen in the CC projection (see Chapter 22). The basic location of the lesion in the medial, middle, lateral, top, or bottom of the breast can be ascertained in this way (41).

A needle longer than the anticipated distance to the lesion from the skin surface is then selected. The breast is positioned in the usual manner, with the lesion in the window of the compression plate. The needle is passed in the direction of the x-ray beam, as in a standard, PCW localization procedure (Fig. 21-34A), so that the tip of the needle is passed beyond the lesion almost to the other side of the breast. The breast is then partially uncompressed. By pulling on the skin or slightly rolling the breast and recompressing, the needle is tilted over (any direction works) and when another image is obtained the needle is seen at an oblique angle (Fig. 21-34B). The targeted lesion can be seen along the needle, and its projected distance along the shaft and projected distance from the tip can be measured from the film.

Simple geometry can be used to determine how far beyond the lesion the tip of the needle actually lies. This actual distance can be calculated by comparing the ratio of the true distance of the lesion from the tip of the needle (*TDL*) to the projected distance of the tip of the needle from the lesion (*PDL*) to the ratio of the true length of the needle (*TLN*) to the projected length of the needle (*PLN*) (Fig. 21-34C) and then solving for the true distance from the lesion.

$$\frac{TDL}{PDL} = \frac{TLN}{PLN}$$

Solve for *TDL*:

$$TDL = PDL \times \frac{TLN}{PLN}$$

The needle can then be withdrawn the true distance that the lesion lies from the tip (TDL), and the tip of the needle will then be at the lesion (Fig. 21-34D). Cytology can be obtained or a hookwire can be introduced and engaged in the tissues, and the lesion will be at the level of the hook (Fig. 21-34E) (24).

This technique has been used successfully to position a guide for the excision of calcifications seen adjacent to a silicone gel implant where the lesion could only be seen in one projection (Fig. 21-35). The implant was in the way so that stereotaxis could not be performed, and the parallax method was used to place a wire for surgical excision. The implant was displaced using a spot-compression device with a window cut out to hold the implant out of the field of view. The needle was passed down the x-ray beam trajectory through the breast almost to the other side. The compression was relaxed slightly so that the skin could be pulled and the needle tipped. The ratios were obtained and the distance to pull back was calculated, permitting accurate localization of the lesion.

The same method can be used to place two needles or a combination of needles and wires at a lesion so that their intersection can be used to guide the surgeon (Fig. 21-36).

If the needle bends, then the calculations will not be accurate so a stiff needle should be used (at least 20 gauge). Because the breast is compressed in the direction of the needle, small distances from the needle tip·to the lesion are amplified when the breast is uncompressed.

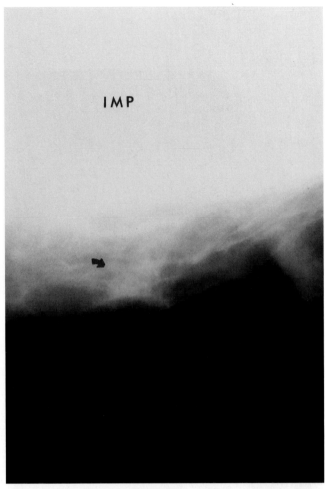

FIG. 21-35. Parallax localization. This patient's implant (IMP) and calcifications were seen at the bottom of the breast (*arrow*) only on the lateral projection **(A)**. *Continued.*

Some Pitfalls

If these localization techniques are followed, there are very few problems that can arise. The accuracy of the localization can be diminished if the needle is pulled out of the lesion (Fig. 21-37). If in the orthogonal position the needle is inadvertently pulled out of the lesion, it cannot be accurately replaced because the lesion and the needle may be at different planes once the lesion comes off the shaft of the needle. Usually the procedure should be started from the beginning to try to ensure accuracy.

Wires can be gently pulled out of the breast (even completely) if the hook has been positioned too far beyond the lesion. This should be done carefully. If resistance is met then an image should be obtained to see if the hook is overbending. Overbending may stress the spring and could result in breaking off the hook. If the hook is in fat, there is little on which it can hold and it can be pulled back. It generally holds tightly in connective tissue.

Wires have been cut at surgery (see Fig. 21-37), and fragments have been left in the breast (Fig. 21-38). The signifi-

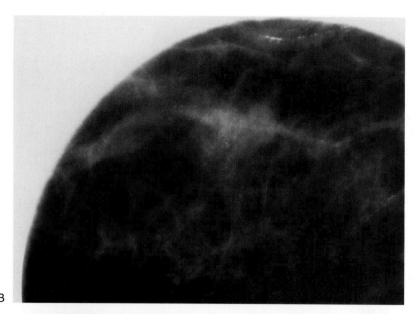

B

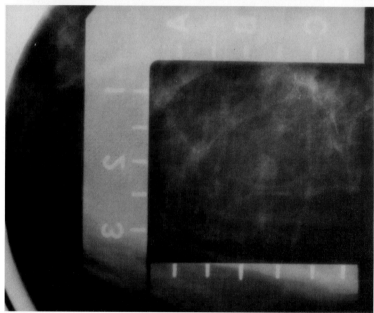

C

FIG. 21-35. *Continued.* The calcifications are more clearly seen on this spot-compression lateral projection with the implant displaced superiorly **(B)**. As a consequence of the implant, the calcifications were not visible on any other projection. They could not be seen on a stereotactic system and had to be localized using the parallax technique. Using a spot-compression paddle with a fenestration, the implant was displaced up and the calcifications were positioned in the window **(C)**. *Continued.*

cance of this varies with the type of wire and the method of positioning it in the breast. Fragments of wires that were positioned parallel to the chest wall have been followed, many for >10 years. They have virtually all remained stable with no significant sequelae. Significant migration of wire fragments, however, has been reported with wires that were positioned freehand and directed back toward the chest wall. One was eventually removed from a cervical neuroforamen (49) and another extruded from behind the knee after traversing the abdomen over several weeks.

Wires are cut when surgeons dissect with scissors. Scalpel dissection avoids the problem. The wire should not be pulled hard because the hook may overbend and break off. Surgeons should be cautioned not to touch wires with electro-

cautery because this may also fragment the wire as well as possibly burning the tissue along the wire's course. In our experience transection of a wire is extremely rare, having occurred only 10 times in >6,000 procedures (0.2%).

It is not a good idea to try to advance a wire once it has been deployed. This could result in bending it at the junction of the thick section and the hook (Fig. 21-39) and could break the wire.

Beware of disappearing masses. On occasion a mass seems to disappear during a localization procedure when the needle is introduced. If morphologically it may represent a cyst and fluid comes out of the *lumen* of the needle, then it is likely a cyst. However, if the lesion seems to have disappeared and there is no fluid to account for its disappearance,

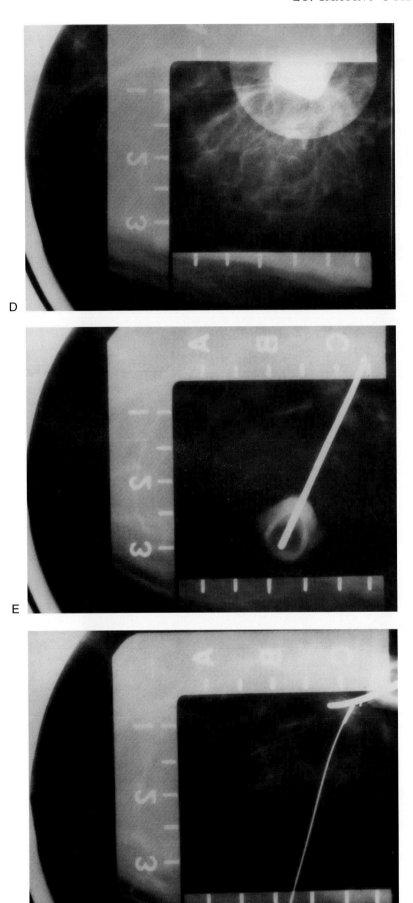

FIG. 21-35. *Continued.* A needle was placed straight through the calcifications **(D)**, and then the needle was tilted by pulling on the skin with the breast in compression **(E)**. By calculating the distance using the parallax formula, the needle was pulled back and a wire was engaged at the calcifications. A second needle was inserted as a precaution. The calcifications are at the intersection of the wire and needle **(F)**.

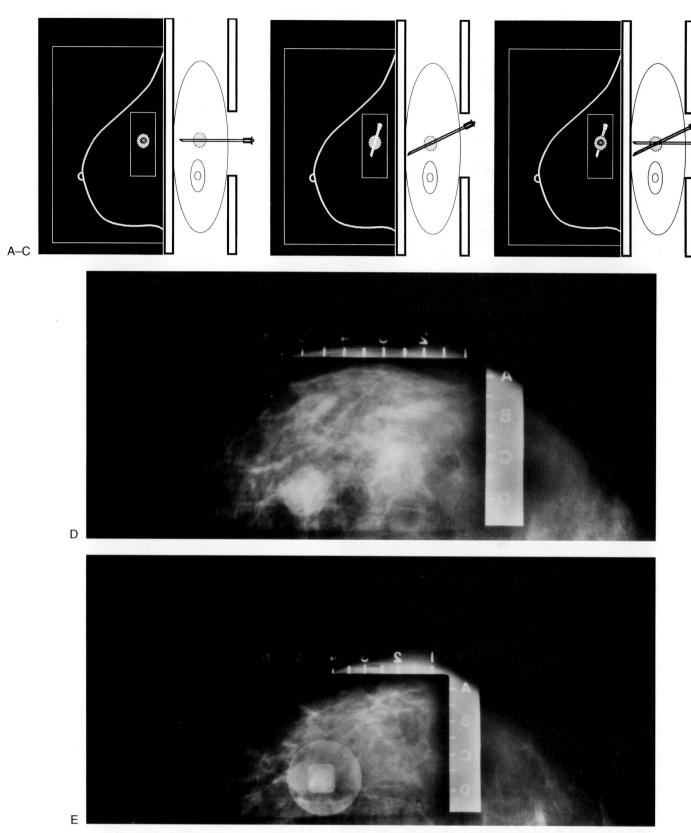

FIG. 21-36. Another aid in needle localization is to use two needles. As shown schematically, and in Figure 21-31, one needle is placed using the standard localization approach **(A)** and then the breast is rolled, tipping the needle **(B)**. A second needle is introduced in the direction of the x-ray beam **(C)**. The lesion will lie at the intersection of the two needles. This approach was used in this case. The mass **(D)** was positioned in the fenestrated compression system. A needle was passed vertically through it. This image looks directly down the needle **(E)**. *Continued.*

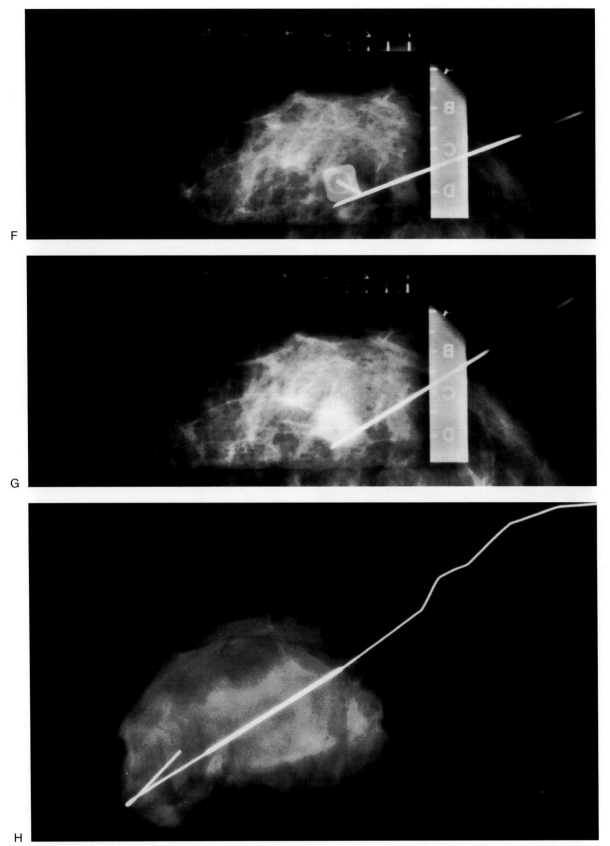

FIG. 21-36. *Continued.* The breast was rolled, showing that the needle tip was just beyond the mass **(F)**, and a second needle was introduced vertically **(G)**. A wire was deployed through the first needle, and the second needle was taped in place. The surgeon removed the tissue at the intersection **(H)**, which proved to be benign focal fibrosis.

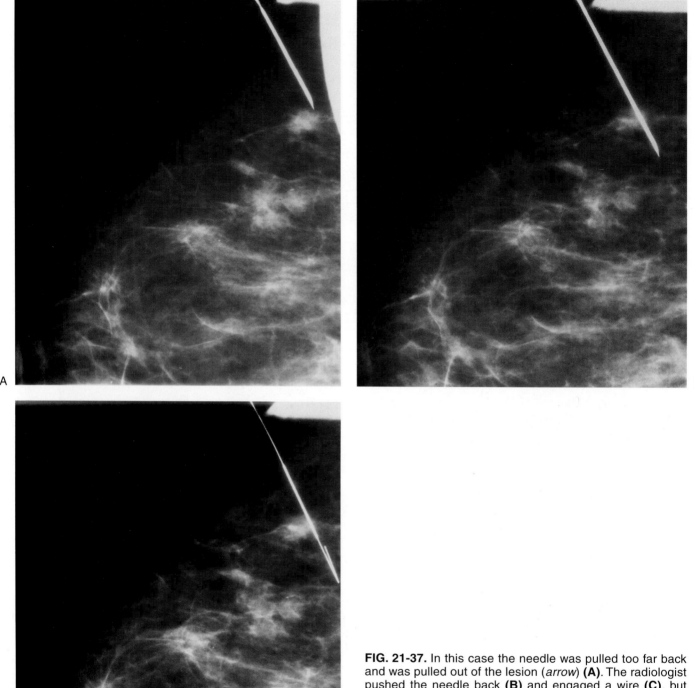

A

B

C

FIG. 21-37. In this case the needle was pulled too far back and was pulled out of the lesion (*arrow*) **(A)**. The radiologist pushed the needle back **(B)** and engaged a wire **(C)**, but the surgeon missed the abnormality. This was likely due to the fact that once the needle has pulled out of the lesion the plane of the needle and the lesion may separate. As a result, the wire ended up at a different level than the lesion, even though it appears to project over it, and the surgeon missed the cancer with his first attempt. The needle cannot be accurately readvanced without starting the localization from the beginning.

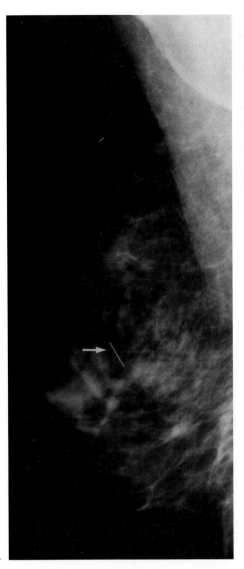

A

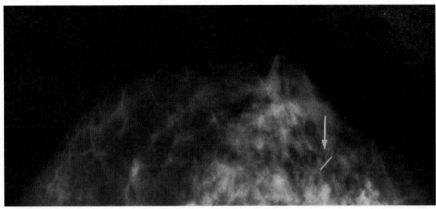

B

FIG. 21-38. The wire fragment (*arrows*), seen here on the mediolateral oblique **(A)** and the craniocaudal **(B)** projections, was left at surgery following a needle localization performed 9 years earlier. It has remained stable with no evidence of movement.

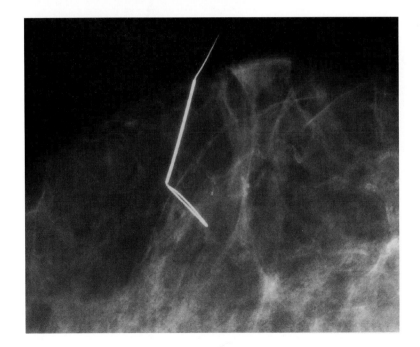

FIG. 21-39. The radiologist tried to advance this wire after it had been deployed from the needle during a freehand localization. This caused a bend at the junction between the thickened segment and the hook.

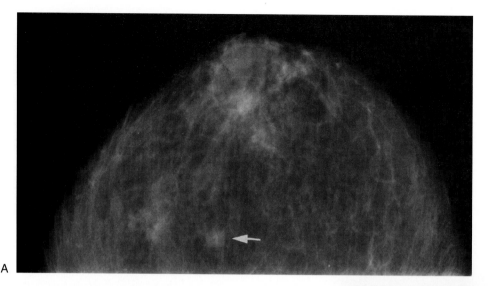

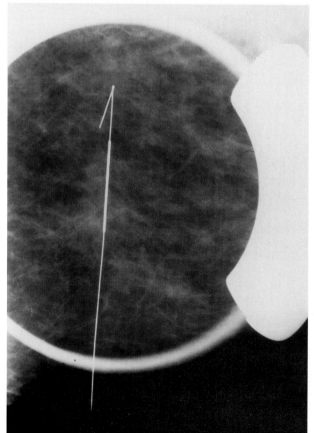

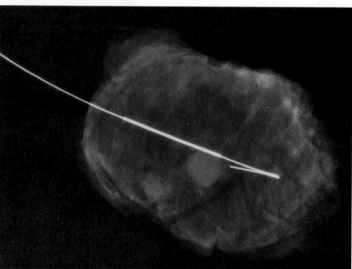

FIG. 21-40. The mass, seen here on the craniocaudal projection **(A)**, seemed to disappear when the needle was placed from the bottom of the breast and the wire was engaged, as seen on this mediolateral projection **(B)**. The excision of the area of concern was completed, however, since no fluid had been expressed through the needle lumen, and the small invasive cancer was clearly evident in the specimen radiograph **(C)**.

the image is likely due to distortion of the tissues or contusion around the mass caused by the needle. It is very unusual to lacerate a cyst and have it decompress without any fluid coming out of the needle lumen. The lesion is likely still there, and the localization should be completed in the area of the "disappeared" lesion and excision carried out (Fig. 21-40). The mass will be seen on the specimen radiograph.

ULTRASOUND-GUIDED NEEDLE PROCEDURES

The most efficacious role for ultrasound is the evaluation of clinically occult, mammographically detected masses to determine whether they are cystic or solid and the occasional evaluation of selected palpable lesions. Ultrasound is also very useful for guiding needle procedures, such as the aspiration of cysts when necessary (43), FNAB for cytology or CNB of nonpalpable masses (37,63), and preoperative localization of masses that need to be excised. A needle can be guided into virtually any lesion that is visible by ultrasound as long as the needle can be imaged with the ultrasound system.

Transducer Selection

High-frequency transducers (7.5 MHz or higher) focused in the near field to a depth of 3 to 5 cm are needed. Linear arrays appear to be the best for guiding needle positioning.

Patient Preparation

Just as with x-ray–guided needle localization, the procedure should be carefully explained to the patient and her questions answered. Because ultrasound-guided procedures are directed back toward the chest wall, it is probably best to discuss the possibility of pneumothorax (extremely rare) as well as the potential need for a chest tube if a pneumothorax occurs. Hematomas are fairly common. The possibility of infection, although also extremely rare, should also be mentioned.

Patient Positioning

Fenestrated compression plates and mammography systems can be used to hold the breast and prevent a lesion from moving during ultrasound-guided procedures (Fig. 21-41). However, most ultrasound-guided procedures can be performed with the patient lying fairly comfortably in the supine position. She should be rolled into whichever oblique position causes the portion of the breast that contains the lesion to be as thin as possible against the chest wall to reduce the amount of tissue that the ultrasound beam and the needle must traverse. A bolster behind the patient can help her maintain the appropriate position. The breast can be further thinned on the chest wall by having the patient extend her arm, placing the palm of her hand behind her head. Tightening the tissues against the chest wall in this fashion also helps to hold the lesion and prevent it from being pushed aside by the needle.

The radiologist should always be aware that with the patient in this position needles are directed back toward the anterior chest wall, and the operator should always avoid the inadvertent placement of a needle into the lung or mediastinum. If there is concern that this might occur, it may be best to consider the use of the mammography compression system to hold the target lesion away from the chest wall.

Aspiration and Localization

Various methods of using ultrasound to guide needle placement have been described in the literature (37,64,65).

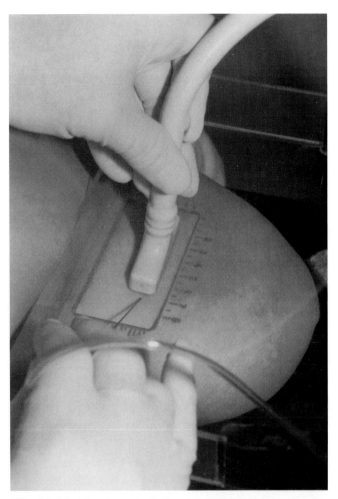

FIG. 21-41. The fenestrated compression plate can be used to hold the breast and lesion **while performing ultrasound-guided procedures.**

With modern ultrasound equipment, the needle and its tip can be followed as it is passed through the breast tissue and into a cyst or tumor. Most cysts can be aspirated, FNAB or CNB of solid masses performed, and wires placed to guide surgical excision under direct ultrasound observation.

After the procedure has been explained to the patient, she should be positioned supine and oblique to flatten the position of the breast, containing the target, against the chest wall to help fix it in position so that the needle traverses a small volume of tissue and the lesion is not able to move out of the way of the introduction of the needle. We prefer to use alcohol or sterile saline as the coupling medium during these procedures so that the breast does not become slippery, making it difficult to maintain the transducer position. A 7.5- or 10.0-MHz linear array transducer is preferred.

The "Third Hand"

We find it very helpful to use a flexible arm and gooseneck to support the transducer and cable. The transducer is clamped to the end of the support, and the cable is held by

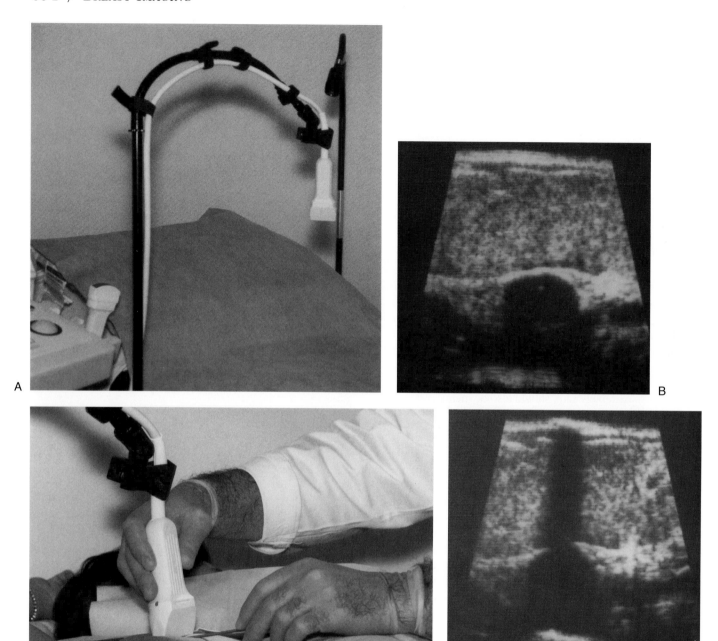

FIG. 21-42. The transducer is fastened to the "third hand" **(A)**. The transducer is then positioned over the lesion **(B)**, and a straw is passed perpendicular to the plane of the section between the skin and transducer **(C)**. When its shadow appears over the lesion **(D)**, its tip is used to mark the skin over the lesion **(E,F)**. A second mark is made at the end of the transducer on the skin where the needle will be inserted.

Velcro straps (Fig. 21-42A). A sterile cover can be placed over the entire assembly so that the transducer is always available, suspended above the patient.

A small straw such as that used to stir coffee can be slipped under the transducer (Fig. 21-42B). When its shadow just becomes visible on the monitor over the lesion,

it is an indication that the tip of the straw is over the lesion. The straw is raised perpendicularly so that the tip can be used to make a mark on the skin using slight pressure (Fig. 21-42C). This impression on the skin is a constant reference so that the location of the lesion is clearly evident on the skin during the procedure. A second mark is placed at the

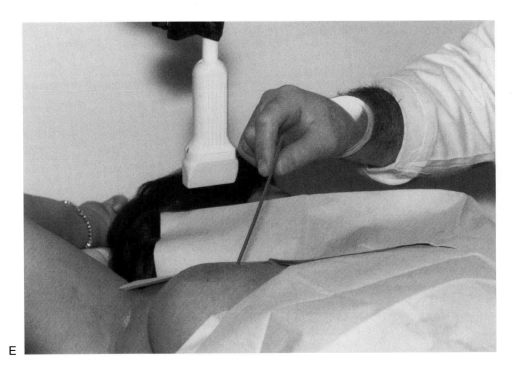

E

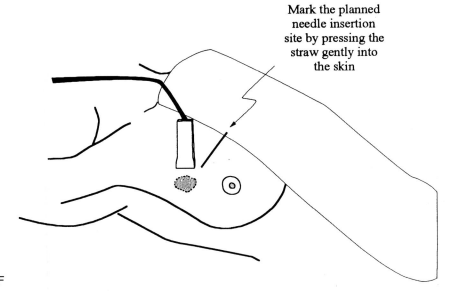

Mark the planned
needle insertion
site by pressing the
straw gently into
the skin

F

end of the transducer to identify the point of needle insertion. The skin is sterilely prepared in the usual manner, and a fenestrated sterile drape is placed over the breast leaving the skin over the lesion and the needle entry point exposed. This provides a sterile field.

As with any procedure in which contact with body fluids is possible, universal precautions should be observed when performing needle procedures in breast tissue.

When a cyst is being aspirated, local anesthesia is frequently not needed, and its use may be more painful than the procedure. The procedure should not be painful. We use anesthesia without hesitation if the patient experiences any discomfort. The anesthetic can be injected through the aspirating needle, and as it leaves the tip of the needle it is fre-

quently visible on ultrasound as it displaces tissue. This can be used to confirm the location of the needle tip.

Breast cyst fluid may be very viscid; therefore, a 19-gauge needle (or a 20-gauge thin-walled needle) is desirable for aspiration of breast lesions. We find it easiest (see Mammographically Guided Cyst Aspiration) if the needle is connected to the syringe with connecting tubing (Fig. 21-43A). This permits the operator to introduce the needle while an assistant provides syringe suction when needed.

Although there have not been any reports of infection, we believe that it is prudent to cover the transducer head with a sterile cover, placing coupling gel inside the cover. Alcohol or sterile saline is dripped over the skin to act as the coupling medium, and the lesion is found once again with the transducer.

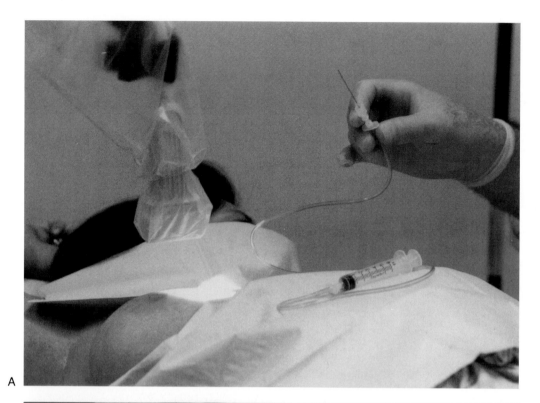

A

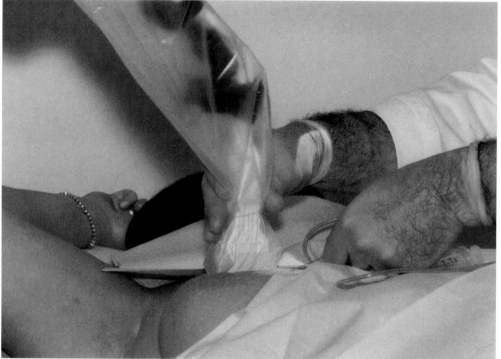

B

FIG. 21-43. We find that there is more sensitive control of the needle if it is connected to a syringe using tubing and the syringe is given to an assistant, who provides suction as needed **(A)**. Following suitable sterile preparation, the needle is introduced at the end of the transducer and directed toward the lesion with its course monitored by ultrasound **(B)**.

The needle is introduced just off the end of the long axis of the transducer so that its tip can be monitored as it is advanced into the field of view of the transducer and is directed toward the lesion (Fig. 21-43B). The operator should be able to monitor the tip of the needle at all times. If it is not visible, the orientation of the transducer or the direction of the needle should be adjusted so that the location of its tip is visible to avoid inadvertent transgression of the chest wall (Fig. 21-44).

At times a more horizontal course for the needle, providing a more perpendicular direction for the sound reflection, may improve the visibility of the needle. On occasion, the wall of a cyst may be painful when punctured, and if the

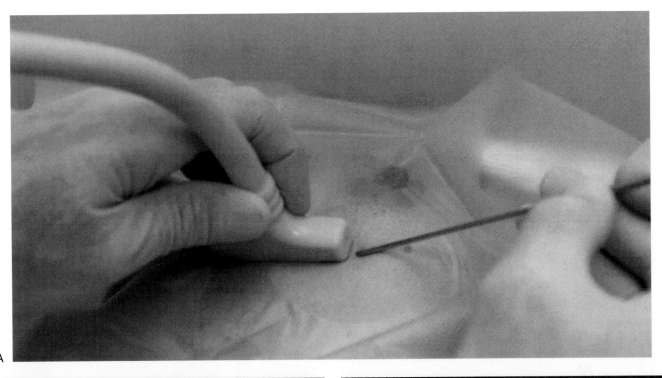

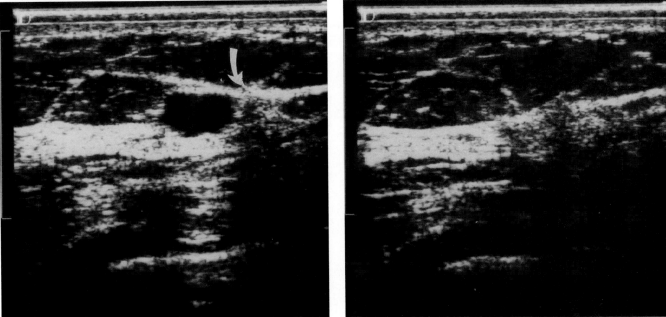

FIG. 21-44. By **introducing the needle along the plane of the section (A)**, its tip can be monitored at all times. The needle is visible entering from the right, and its tip (*arrow*) is just at the margin of the cyst **(B)**. The needle is advanced into the cyst, which is completely drained under real-time observation **(C)**.

patient is experiencing anything more than a feeling of pressure lidocaine should be injected.

Once the needle has penetrated into the cyst, the fluid can be aspirated by an assistant while the operator monitors the withdrawal of fluid and the needle position under ultrasound. If the fluid resists aspiration, the tip can be rotated or repositioned to better drain the cyst's contents. Once the fluid has been removed, a small amount of air (less than the

amount of withdrawn fluid) can be introduced so that the cyst and its wall can be seen easily on postaspiration mammography, which is used as a check (Fig. 21-45) to be certain that the aspirated lesion was what had raised concern on the mammogram. There is, however, no proof that this pneumocystography is of any benefit, and it can be omitted.

If difficulty is encountered in aligning the needle, it is sometimes helpful to have a colleague hold the transducer

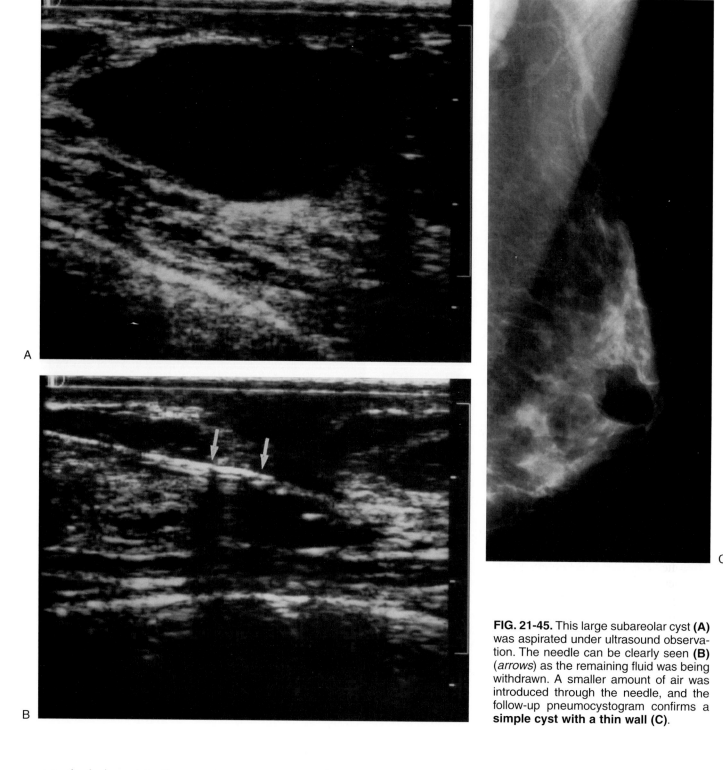

A

B

C

FIG. 21-45. This large subareolar cyst **(A)** was aspirated under ultrasound observation. The needle can be clearly seen **(B)** (*arrows*) as the remaining fluid was being withdrawn. A smaller amount of air was introduced through the needle, and the follow-up pneumocystogram confirms a **simple cyst with a thin wall (C)**.

over the lesion while the operator concentrates on keeping the needle in the plane of section and in view under ultrasound.

When the needle is withdrawn, firm pressure should be placed over the aspiration site and applied back toward the chest wall for several minutes to try to prevent formation of a hematoma. Using this technique, we have rarely had a

hematoma form after a cyst aspiration. If the fluid that is withdrawn does not resemble old blood, then we do not send it for cytologic analysis unless it is from a recurrent cyst.

Betadine ointment or alcohol can provide acoustical coupling if there is any need for postaspiration ultrasound evaluation. The cyst should have completely resolved, or at the most a small slit of residual fluid may persist. If a hypoechoic tissue mass persists, it should be considered suspicious and justification for surgical excision.

Ultrasound can also be used in conjunction with mammographic compression by aligning a cyst in the fenestrated mammographic compression system and positioning the needle while the breast is held away from the chest wall. This has the advantage that the compression holds the cyst, so that it does not move and so that it can be punctured without fear of entering the chest wall. It is also a way to ensure that what is visible by ultrasound corresponds to what was of concern on the mammogram.

Fluid Analysis

Breast cyst fluid is rarely crystal clear. It is usually turbid yellow, cream colored, brown, or green. The viscosity of cyst fluid can vary from that of water to that of thick mucus that is almost impossible to aspirate. These colors are almost always associated with benign processes. When the fluid is thick and maroon or dark brown, suggesting old blood, an intracystic process should be suspected, such as a papilloma or carcinoma. Many argue that if there is no evidence of old blood, it is not cost-effective to send fluid for cytologic analysis. Most merely dispose of typical cyst fluid. It appears that if the fluid shows no evidence of old bleeding (as opposed to blood-tinged new bleeding from the needle), then cytologic analysis is usually fruitless. Not only is intracystic cancer extremely rare, but negative cytology does not eliminate the possibility of malignancy. The vast majority of cysts are benign.

Recurrent Breast Cysts

If patients are followed long enough, a large number of aspirated cysts will recur. We found that 40% recurred by 2 years. Although surgeons are often concerned about cysts that recur after aspiration, there are no data that suggest that further intervention is required if a cyst that had been evaluated by imaging and completely aspirated subsequently recurs.

Although we have seen a single case in which a cyst by ultrasound was aspirated completely, had an abnormal cytology, and recurred having cancer in the wall, this is exceedingly rare and should not dictate usual care. If a cyst is aspirated completely, the fluid does not represent old blood, there is no other reason to suggest malignancy, and it recurs, there are no data to support any additional intervention. There is no scientific reason to reaspirate it. The management of recurrent cysts is subject to local anecdotal practice, and there is no universal standard of care. If the cyst is reaspirated some would argue that its fluid should be sent for cytologic analysis, although the yield of cancer in this setting is undocumented.

Pneumocystography

Some have claimed that inflating a cyst with slightly less air than the amount of fluid withdrawn will prevent its recurrence.

In our experience air does not seem to reduce the rate of recurrence. Introducing air does permit the sharp definition of the cyst wall and is a way of confirming that the aspirated abnormality does correspond to the mammographically imaged finding. It should be considered an optional maneuver.

Ultrasound-Guided Needle Placement Under Direct Real-Time Observation for Surgical Excision

Ultrasound can be used to determine the location of nonpalpable lesions found in the breast by mammography whose three-dimensional position cannot be determined mammographically, and it can be used to direct the positioning of needle guides to permit the surgical removal of nonpalpable masses (49).

Positioning guides for the surgeon under ultrasound observation has the advantage of direct observation of the introduction of the needle. In addition, it permits the surgeon to dissect through the smallest volume of tissue in the direction that many surgeons prefer to operate. High-resolution ultrasound systems with high-frequency transducers (≥ 7.5 MHz) can be used to directly monitor the position of the needle as it is inserted into a mass in the breast in real time.

Many breast lesions are relatively superficial, and, by positioning the patient supine and oblique with the ipsilateral arm behind her head, the breast tissue can be thinned to permit needle placement through a minimum of tissue. This benefits the patient as well as the surgeon. Alcohol or sterile saline is the best coupling materials for these procedures as gels make the breast slippery and difficult to stabilize. The lesion is triangulated and the needle introduced in the same fashion as described for cyst aspiration under direct ultrasound observation. The needle should be passed through or immediately alongside the lesion so that the tip is approximately 0.5 to 1.0 cm beyond the lesion.

The transducer is positioned over the lesion. The needle is inserted in the same fashion as for a cyst aspiration along the long axis of the transducer. It is advanced in the plane of the scan so that its passage through the tissues can be monitored (Fig. 21-46). By using a shallow angle, the needle is more easily visualized because the angle of the incident sound is closer to perpendicular to its surface. This also reduces the chances of entering the muscle or thorax.

The goal is to visualize the tip of the needle as it passes under the transducer to the lesion. On some ultrasound units the needle is not always directly visible, but its passage through the tissue is usually evident as the tissue distorts and moves along its course. The injection of a local anesthetic as the needle is advanced can frequently be seen under ultrasound, indicating the tip of the needle.

Attachments are available that vibrate the needle so that its tip can also be monitored using color Doppler; however, with modern ultrasound transducers, this should not be necessary as the systems permit direct visualization of the needle. On occasion, a lesion cannot be entered because it

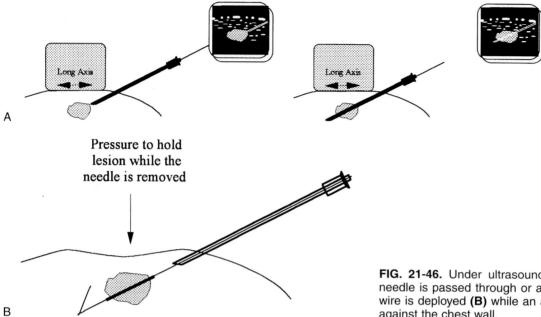

A

Pressure to hold
lesion while the
needle is removed

B

FIG. 21-46. Under ultrasound observation the localizing needle is passed through or alongside the lesion **(A)**. The wire is deployed **(B)** while an assistant presses the breast against the chest wall.

moves out of the way as the needle presses against it. An assistant can help to stabilize the lesion, but the operator should always be cognizant of the other hands to avoid an inadvertent needle stick.

Once the needle is positioned in or alongside the lesion, a springhook wire can be deployed and the needle removed. During removal of the needle and deployment of the hookwire, an assistant should hold the breast around the needle down against the chest wall so that the lesion is not pulled off the needle before engaging the hook. A follow-up mammogram is sometimes useful to confirm the relation of the wire to the lesion (Fig. 21-47). As with computed tomography–guided localizations, the wire must be sufficiently long so that it is not enveloped completely by the breast when the patient sits up.

As with biopsies after mammographically guided localizations, the excised tissue should be placed in a plastic bag and sent for imaging confirmation. If the lesion was visible by ultrasound, ultrasound imaging of the specimen directly through the plastic bag can be used to confirm the removal of the lesion (Fig. 21-48).

COMPUTED TOMOGRAPHY–GUIDED LOCALIZATION

Lesions that are difficult to successfully triangulate by mammographic projections or ultrasound can be located by CT (26). CBT can be used to guide FNAB and even CNB,

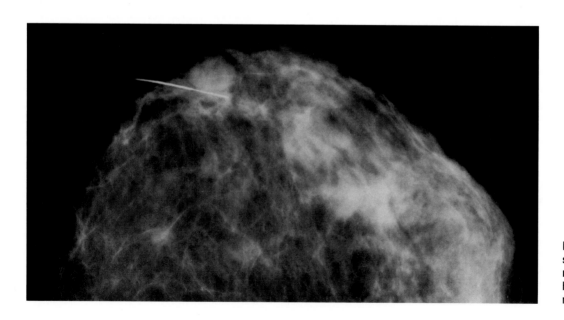

FIG. 21-47. A postultrasound localization mammogram confirms that the hook is just posterior to the margin of the mass.

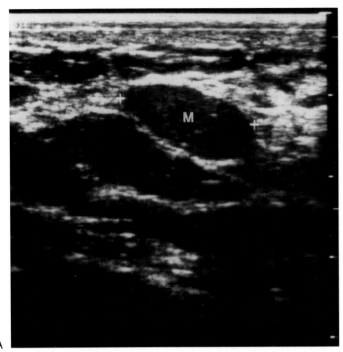

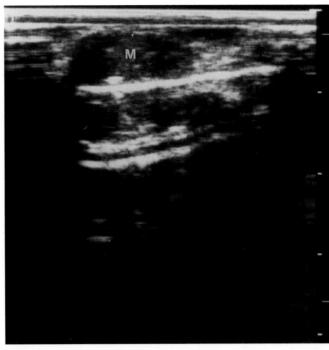

A   B

FIG. 21-48. This mass (M), seen on the prelocalization ultrasound **(A)**, is confirmed in the ultrasound of the excised specimen **(B)**. The bright linear structure is the wire in the specimen.

as well as for placing guides for the surgical excision of suspicious lesions.

The patient is positioned within the scanner so that her breasts are symmetrically positioned and aligned with the plane of scan. This permits the comparison of symmetric areas so that asymmetric areas can be detected. Usually CBT is needed when a lesion is visible only in the lateral projection close to the chest wall. The breast is scanned with 1-cm–thick slices at 1-cm intervals covering the portion of the breast in which the lesion is anticipated based on the mammogram. Once the lesion is located (Fig. 21-49A), a needle for FNAB or a wire guide can be placed preoperatively at the lesion using the scanner.

It is important that the patient remain within the scanner during the localization procedure to avoid shifting the breast on the chest wall with table movement. The skin is sterilely prepared and a sterile piece of wire or a thin needle is taped sagittally over the expected region of the lesion (Fig. 21-49B). This fiducial wire should be visible on the scanner but should not be thick enough to cause artifacts. This wire remains during the procedure as a constant reference.

The patient is then positioned in the gantry with her arm extended and her body rotated so that a minimum amount of breast tissue overlies the lesion. If the lesion is close to the chest wall, it might be preferable to rotate the patient so that the needle passes parallel to the chest wall to avoid entering

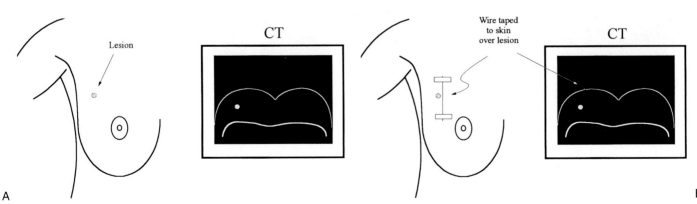

A   B

FIG. 21-49. Computed tomography can be used to guide needle and wire placement. The lesion is identified by CT **(A)**. The skin is prepared, and a sterile wire is taped over the approximate location of the lesion **(B)** as a constant reference mark, so that the patient can remain in the scanner to ensure that her breast does not move. The plane containing the lesion is located, and the patient remains at that table location. *Continued.*

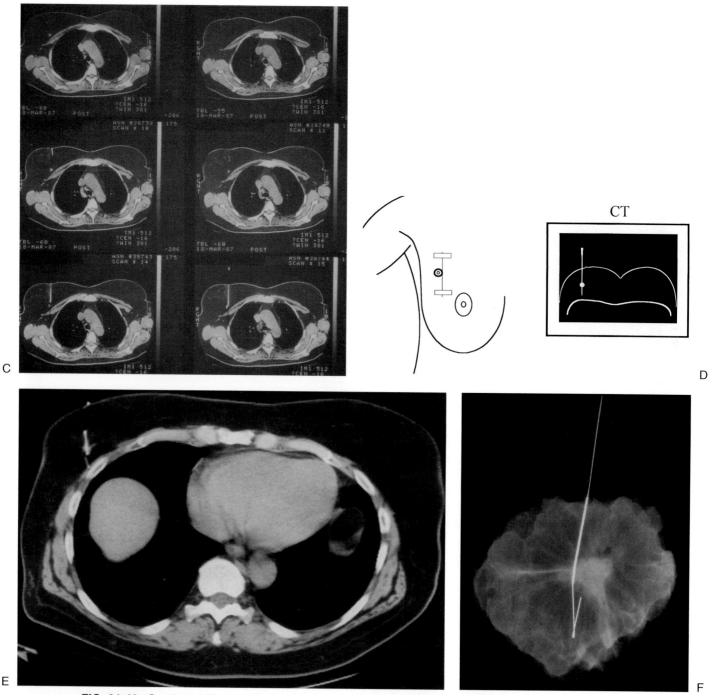

FIG. 21-49. *Continued.* The needle is inserted, being sure to identify the entire length of the needle to avoid going too deep **(C)**. With an assistant holding the breast against the chest wall, a wire is engaged and the needle removed. Ideally the hook will be just beyond the lesion, as in this case where the hook is just deep to the lesion that is on the thickened segment **(D)**. The specimen radiograph **(E)** of this invasive cancer confirms the accuracy of this technique. Another localization sequence **(F)**.

the chest wall with the needle. The lesion is again located by scanning and accurately triangulated using thinner slices. Thin slices (≤5 mm) should be used when positioning needles so that the tip and hub are visible within the scan plane. This avoids the needle's angling through the plane, giving the appearance that the tip is further from the chest wall than it actually is. By measuring the location of the lesion relative to the reference wire on the skin, along with the depth of the lesion on the scan, a needle can be introduced using the laser and the skin wire to triangulate the point of entry and depth of insertion. Care should be taken to avoid entering the pectoralis or thorax. A hookwire can be engaged when the needle tip is satisfactorily positioned just deep to the lesion (Fig. 21-49C, D).

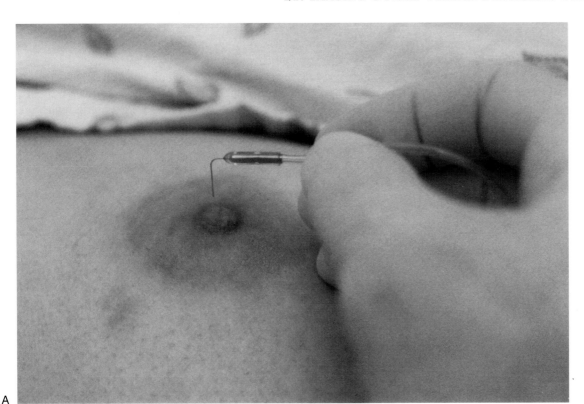

A

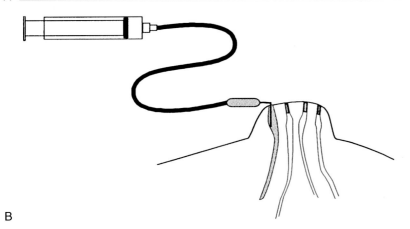

B

FIG. 21-50. A galactogram is performed by producing a small amount of discharge to identify the location of the duct opening. The bent sialogram needle is held by the flexible tubing **(A)** so that excessive pressure is avoided, and the needle is introduced into the duct gently **(B)**.

Because the needle is placed from the front of the breast and the wire is engaged with the patient supine, a long wire should be used as the breast will re-expand when the patient sits up. The wire may be engulfed by the breast and should be sufficiently long to avoid its disappearance completely into the breast. The external wire is then loosely taped to the skin and a sterile gauze placed over the entry site.

GALACTOGRAPHY AND NEEDLE LOCALIZATION

Although the introduction of contrast material into a discharging duct has not proved to be particularly valuable as a diagnostic technique, it can be used to limit the amount of surgical resection needed to diagnose and treat the cause of a nip-

ple discharge. If a focal abnormality is visible on the duct injection, then it can be targeted for needle localization. This is accomplished by first performing the galactogram and then positioning the breast as for a standard needle localization, choosing the shortest distance to the filling defect in the contrast filled duct.

Galactography requires that a single discharging duct be evident. The nipple is sterilely prepared. A 30-gauge blunt-end sialogram needle attached to flexible connecting tubing is filled and flushed with iodinated contrast material (60% for intravenous injection). Care should be taken to avoid air bubbles. A 1- to 3-cc syringe is usually sufficient. We prefer to use a sialogram needle that takes a 90-degree bend.

The patient lies supine for the introduction of the sialogram needle. The face of the nipple looks like a cracked surface criss-crossed by crevices. The duct openings are generally at the bottom of these crevices. Keratin debris frequently fills the crevices and must be picked out gently using the tip of the sialogram needle.

Using a magnifying lens the breast is squeezed to express a small drop of discharge and the tip of the needle is placed in the crevice in which the discharge was expressed (Fig. 21-50). If the needle is held by the flexible tubing, excessive force cannot inadvertently be applied to the needle as the operator wiggles it in the crevice until it falls into the discharging and generally distended duct. The needle is advanced up to the bend, and tape is placed to hold it in the duct.

The patient is moved to the mammography machine, taking care to avoid dislodging the needle. Moderate compression is applied with the patient seated and the breast in the CC projection. Contrast medium is injected. If there is resistance, the needle tip may be against the wall of the duct and should be repositioned (frequently by pulling back slightly and moving it parallel to the axis of the nipple). If resistance continues or contrast refluxes from the duct, it could be due to an obstructive lesion. A mammogram, which can be performed with the sialogram needle remaining in the duct, will answer the question. Contrast should be introduced until there is reflux or the patient experiences a feeling of fullness or pain or burning. The latter may indicate extravasation, and the procedure should be terminated. Extravasation may be due to the needle tearing the duct or to a process, such as cancer, that has disrupted the duct. Generally the breast feels full when the ducts of that network are all opacified and before filling of the lobules. The latter is not desirable, because filled lobules can obscure the detail from the ducts.

Galactography is a nonspecific test. It cannot be used to exclude malignancy. Cancer may present as a filling defect or as a mass associated with the filled duct. The most common reason for a filling defect is an intracystic papilloma. Cancer can cause a single defect or multiple filling defects,

or it can cause an abrupt termination of the duct. If an abnormality is found in this fashion, imaging-guided localization or needle biopsy can be performed in exactly the same way as for any lesion, placing a guide through or alongside the filling defect (Fig. 21-51). Instead of having to dissect out an entire duct network, the surgeon needs only to remove the lesion seen on the galactogram.

If there is a dilated duct but there is no duct discharge, we have done a galactogram by cannulating the duct under ultrasound and introducing contrast directly into the duct.

FINE-NEEDLE ASPIRATION CYTOLOGY AND CORE NEEDLE BIOPSIES

As the number of women being screened has increased, the number of abnormal mammograms has increased, and these have led to an increase in the number of biopsies being performed for diagnosis. Excisional biopsy is extremely safe, but it is physically and psychologically traumatic, as well as expensive. It has been suggested that 30% of the cost of screening is due to the induced costs of tissue diagnosis through an open biopsy. Lindfors and Rosenquist have estimated that if CNB is used for the same indications as surgical biopsy the marginal cost per year of life saved by screening can be reduced by as much as 23%. They estimated that the cost of screening could be reduced from $20,770 per year of life saved to $15,934 (66). For these reasons a reduction in the need for open surgical biopsy is a desirable goal.

Although it would be extremely desirable for an imaging test, such as magnetic resonance imaging, ultrasound, or nuclear medicine, to be able to accurately distinguish benign from malignant lesions without the need for a cytologic or histologic diagnosis, it is unlikely that these will replace cytologic or tissue diagnosis given the safety and low mor-

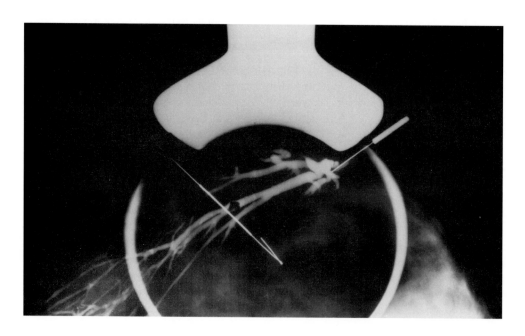

FIG. 21-51. A filling defect was identified by galactography in a woman with a nipple discharge, and using the grid localization system a wire guide was placed into the lesion, which at excision proved to be a **benign, intraductal papilloma.** The galactogram permitted limited tissue removal by identifying the lesion and permitting its localization.

bidity of obtaining cytologic or histologic material. For the foreseeable future there will be the need for the pathologist to evaluate cells or tissue directly. FNA cytology and CNB have been used for years in other parts of the body for diagnosis, and there is no reason to believe that these techniques cannot be successfully applied to the breast.

There is one critical difference between the use of needle biopsy in the breast and its use in other parts of the body. In other organs, a false-negative biopsy does not carry the same significance as in the breast. There are no data that prove that the earlier diagnosis of a lung cancer, pancreatic cancer, or metastatic lesion can result in a life being saved. A false-negative biopsy for these lesions is not as significant as a false-negative biopsy for a breast cancer, where studies have shown conclusively that earlier detection can be lifesaving.

Surgeons have for years used needle biopsy to assist in the management of palpable lesions of the breast. However, because the sampling error (the needle misses the tumor) can be as high as 20%, most surgeons rely on needle biopsy primarily if the results indicate cancer rather than a benign process.

Some surgeons believe that if the lesion has a low probability of malignancy based on the clinical examination and mammography, a negative aspirate or a negative CNB reinforces the certainty of the diagnosis. This has been termed the *triple test* (67). If any of the three analyses (CBE, mammography, or needle biopsy) suggests cancer, then the lesion is excised. This approach has been suggested for needle biopsy of nonpalpable lesions, excluding the clinical evaluation (because the lesions are not palpable). If the needle biopsy results are not concordant with the mammographic expectation, then excision is indicated. The difficulty with this approach is that needle biopsy has been advocated for lesions that are interpreted as BIRADS categories 4 and 5 (see Chapter 24). These are lesions that are "suspicious and biopsy should be considered" and those that are "highly suggestive of malignancy." What has never been defined is when a benign needle biopsy result is concordant with a mammographic interpretation of "suspicious" or "highly suggestive of malignancy."

Replacing imaging-guided excisional biopsy with needle biopsy techniques should be done with caution. The only reason for screening asymptomatic women is to detect breast cancers earlier in their growth, when there is the potential for cure. If cancers that could have been diagnosed earlier through surgical excision after needle localization are missed by needle biopsy techniques and diagnosis is delayed, the benefit of screening may be reduced or lost.

General Considerations

For needle biopsies to be efficacious replacements for needle localization and surgical excisions, they must be performed accurately and their results must be reliable. If this is the case, then considerable savings can be realized. Because needle localization and surgical excisional biopsy are so accurate and safe, needle biopsies must have a false-negative rate that is at least as low as excisional biopsy, or the cancers missed by needle biopsy must be subsequently diagnosed while still at a curable size and stage.

Needle Biopsy and Benign Lesions

If the needle biopsy reveals a benign process and the results are reliable, then an excisional biopsy can be avoided altogether. From a cost perspective, needle biopsy will only lower costs if it is used to evaluate lesions that, in its absence, would be subjected to localization and excisional biopsy for diagnostic purposes.

Some have advocated needle biopsies for lesions classified as probably benign. These are lesions that would ordinarily be followed by mammography at approximately 6-month intervals for 2 to 3 years. Because the vast majority of these prove to be benign (21), it is not cost-effective to add needle biopsy to the standard short-interval follow-up for these lesions. There are potential psychological benefits to providing women with a definitive diagnosis so that they do not have to return at short intervals, but biopsying lesions that have an extremely low likelihood of being malignant (<2%) will lead to increased and not decreased costs (68).

Needle Biopsy and Malignant Lesions

The major benefit from needle biopsy will occur if it can reliably determine that a suspicious finding is, in fact, benign so that no further evaluation is needed. Needle biopsy may also aid in the management of malignant lesions. If a needle biopsy reveals that a lesion is malignant, then the patient and her physician can discuss the options prior to definitive surgery. If the patient elects breast conservation, then the surgeon, already knowing that the lesion is malignant, can perform a lumpectomy (wide excisional biopsy) and an axillary dissection for staging at a single session, exposing the patient to only one excisional procedure and the general anesthesia needed for the axillary dissection. Alternatively, the patient may prefer a mastectomy and having needle-biopsy evidence of a malignant lesion would also require only one operation.

This approach may change in the future. The need for axillary dissection is already being questioned (69). In the past the decision to use chemotherapy or hormonal therapy to treat disseminated disease was determined by the presence of tumor in axillary lymph nodes. Because there appears to be no survival advantage to removing these nodes (70) and there is morbidity associated with their removal, including pain, numbness, and arm edema, and because data have shown that even node-negative women can benefit from systemic therapy, the removal of nodes may become unnecessary in the future.

An intermediate possibility that will permit limited node sampling under local anesthesia has been termed *sentinel-node evaluation*. This involves the injection of technetium 99m sulfur colloid (or a vital dye) around the tumor. These migrate to the axillary nodal chain defining the first lymph nodes draining the area around the tumor. The removal of these first nodes may be sufficient to permit accurate prediction of whether systemic disease is likely present as predicted by nodal involvement (see Chapter 26). If either approach is used, the benefit of needle biopsy may be diminished because there will either be no need for axillary dissection or the removal of the sentinel node can be accomplished using local anesthesia.

Fine-Needle Aspiration for Cytology

FNAB is used in an effort to tear loose cells from an area of concern so that the cytologic features of the cells can be assessed to determine whether they are benign or malignant. The procedure is often called *fine-needle aspiration* biopsy because needles as thin as 25 gauge have been used successfully. The technique takes advantage of the fact that cancer cells tend to be less cohesive and can be broken off more readily than benign cells. The aspiration is accomplished by placing the needle into the tissue to be sampled and moving the needle in and out firmly and rapidly. Some observers advocate the use of suction on the needle, whereas others believe that moving the needle without suction and relying on capillary attraction is preferable. The needle should be moved in the lesion at least 20 times.

If material begins to appear in the hub of the needle, the needle should be withdrawn because it is difficult to retrieve cells once they are in the syringe. The aspirated material is spread on a slide, stained, and interpreted. Blood can make it very difficult to interpret the cytology; therefore the aspiration should be terminated if blood appears in the needle hub.

Aspiration can be performed by inserting a larger introducer needle into the lesion and then performing multiple passes with smaller needles passed through the introducer needle. Generally a needle that is two gauges smaller will fit through the introducer. For example, a 22-gauge needle will fit through a 20-gauge introducer needle. This method has the advantage of requiring only a single pass through the skin (generally the most uncomfortable part of the procedure) but has the disadvantage of directing the aspirating needle into the same part of the lesion each time, potentially reducing the volume of tissue sampled and possibly contributing to a sampling error. One of the advantages of FNAB is that the rapid oscillation of the needle in and out of the lesion causes the tip to deflect and sample larger volumes of tissue.

Once material begins to appear in the hub of the needle (needles with clear hubs are desirable), the needle should be withdrawn and smears made on glass slides. The preparation of the slide is very important. This includes the type of glass slide to be used (clear or frosted), the method of spreading the material, as well as its preservation. Some cytopathologists prefer the slides to air dry, whereas others prefer that the slides be immediately placed in a fixative. Because the accuracy of the diagnosis is dependent on the skill of the interpreter, slide preparation should be performed according to instructions from the cytopathologist.

Advantages

FNAB has a number of advantages. Very thin needles can be used, making it a relatively painless and safe procedure. Even hematomas are uncommon. There is no evidence that cancer cells have been seeded elsewhere in the breast using FNAB techniques. Because the needle is moved in and out of the lesion fairly aggressively, it is likely that the needle deflects in many directions, increasing the volume of the tissue sampled. Cytopathologists tend to be very conservative, and it is extremely rare for a suspicious cytology not to represent true carcinoma. The false-positive rate is generally extremely low. As a result, the false-negative rate may be fairly high. Thus, if the FNAB results are discordant with those expected based on the mammogram or CBE, either the biopsy should be repeated or the lesion should be excised.

Disadvantages

Perhaps the major disadvantage of FNAB is the need for highly trained cytopathologists. The trend in the United States has been toward CNB, due in large part to the lack of trained cytopathologists.

Although deflection of a thin needle may improve the coverage of tissue sampled, thin needles may be difficult to accurately direct at and into the target.

The aspiration technique is highly operator dependent. It is fairly common for the aspirate not to provide satisfactory material. This problem can be obviated by having the cytopathologist or a trained cytotechnologist in the room at the time of the aspiration, often performing the actual biopsy as well as preparing the slides and evaluating them during the procedure. If the cells are not sufficient, additional passes can be made.

The differentiation that can be made by the cytopathologist is frequently only between benign and malignant. Further characterization of a malignant lesion is usually not possible. The cytopathologist is rarely able to make the important therapeutic distinction as to whether malignant cells are from an in situ or an invasive cancer.

Many cytopathologists are very conservative and only diagnose malignancies when the level of certainty is very high. This makes it difficult to rely on a report that suggests that the lesion is benign. There is some advantage to knowing in advance from the cytology that a lesion is likely cancer, but the real benefit would lie in the accurate determination that a lesion is benign and requires no further intervention. It is not clear that FNAB can reliably do the latter.

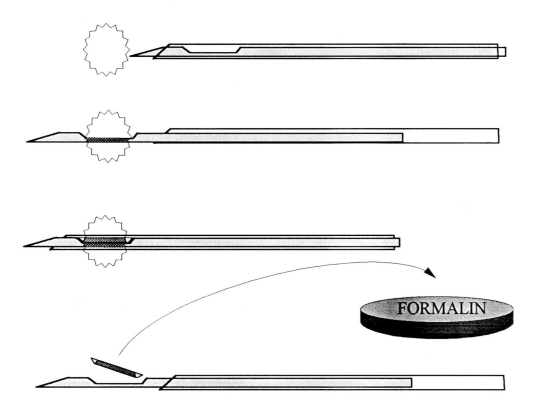

FIG. 21-52. Schematic showing the design of a needle for core biopsy of the breast.

Core Needle Biopsy

Core needle biopsy (CNB) is performed to obtain small slivers of intact tissue. When performed appropriately, the tissue that is obtained is analyzed as histologic material and processed and interpreted in the same fashion as a surgically excised lesion.

The tissue is obtained through large-core needles. Although smaller-core needles are available, most agree that anything smaller than an 18-gauge needle is probably not sufficiently large because the tissue obtained may be insufficient or may fragment. This problem appears to be avoided through the use of 16- or 14-gauge needles. We use 16- or 14-gauge needles for ultrasound-guided biopsies and 14-gauge needles for stereotactically guided biopsies.

Most core needles are variations on the true-cut needle. This is a needle that contains a trocar with a notch just proximal to its tip (Fig. 21-52). The needle and trocar are introduced into a lesion. The outer needle is pulled back so that tissue can fall into the notch. The needle or cannula is pushed back over the trocar, slicing a piece of tissue into the notch.

Spring-Driven Systems

Unfortunately, many lesions cannot be sampled this simply because tissue does not often fall into the notch, and manual biopsies of breast lesions often yield empty notches. Spring-driven systems that automate the process are required. Using high-powered springs in rapid succession, the trocar is driven into the lesion and followed almost instantaneously by the outer needle. These systems take advantage of tissue inertia, making it less likely that the lesion will move out of the way of the needle (like bobbing for apples). Furthermore, the needles are designed to bend and draw the tissue into the notch, producing a higher tissue yield. Most have found that the best combination is a 14-gauge needle with a "long throw" of 2.3 cm and a trocar with a 1.9-cm notch.

When using the spring-driven systems, the operator must remember that the needle will be driven forward and that the notch is behind the needle tip by some distance. The operator must be certain that there is sufficient room behind the lesion so that the lesion can be safely sampled without the tip ending in an undesirable location.

If the lesion is close to surface of the breast adjacent to the film holder (during x-ray–guided procedures), there is the potential that the needle tip may exit the other side of the breast and break or bend against the film holder. If the lesion is close to the chest wall and the needle is directed back in this direction under ultrasound observation, there is the risk of perforating the pectoralis muscle or penetrating into the pleura, mediastinum, or lung. When lesions are close to these structures, needles with stylets that are inserted manually into the lesion followed by assisted-cannula slicing may be preferred so that the needle does not pass uncontrolled beyond the lesion, although our experience with these has resulted in unsatisfactory sampling.

To maximize the amount of tissue removed from the lesion, the needle should be pulled back from the center of the target before firing by the distance of the throw minus the distance from the tip of the needle to the center of the notch in the cocked position (see Stereotactic Biopsy, below). Thus, if the distance from the tip of the stylet to the center of the notch is 1.8 cm and the throw distance of the needle is 2.3 cm, then the needle should be fired 2.3 minus 1.8 cm (0.5 cm) from the center of the target. This places the center of the notch in the center of the lesion at the end of the spring-driven traverse.

Removing the Sample from the Notch

Removing the tissue sliver from the notch can be perplexing. Some "guns" give a "flick" to the trocar when the cannula is pulled back to expose the notch, helping to clear the tissue. The operator must be careful to try not to crush or tear the sample. Some operators use a second needle or a scalpel blade to remove the sample. As always, care should be taken to protect the operator from an inadvertent needle stick. We find that filling a test tube with 2 to 3 cc of normal saline allows the tissue to be washed from the notch by shaking the exposed trocar in the saline (Fig. 21-53). Using a test tube with a screw top permits the samples to be imaged while in the test tube and calcifications confirmed if the target contained calcifications. By using sterile saline the needle can be recocked and used repeatedly. At the end of the procedure, the saline containing the samples is poured into a larger (40 cc) container of formalin. The small amount of saline appears to have no effect on tissue preservation. The system facilitates safe removal of the tissue sample from the notch. The Mueller Tray for interventional procedures, made by Picker International (Highland Heights, OH), contains all of the necessary components needed for these procedures, including a mater-

ial that can hold needles, avoiding the danger of recapping and loose needles during a procedure (Fig. 21-54).

Advantages

Because core samples provide histologic information, they can be interpreted by any pathologist who is trained in breast pathology. Invasive cancers can be distinguished from in situ lesions. Because specific benign histologic diagnoses can be made, it is likely that CNBs will be more practical than cytology from FNAB for reducing the number of open surgical biopsies that will be needed.

Disadvantages

As with any needle biopsy technique, there is always the possibility of sampling error, with the needle obtaining tissue from around the lesion but missing the lesion itself. Because these needles are quite large, the risk of hematoma is greater, and there has been a report of tumor seeding in a needle track (39).

If spring-loaded devices are used, there is an increased risk of unintended trauma from striking the film holder or the thoracic structures.

There has been some concern raised by pathologists that the samples may be too small for diagnostic accuracy. The pathologist frequently uses the relationship of the lesion to its surroundings (context), as well as the extent of the process, for making a diagnosis. Core biopsies force the pathologist to view the lesion through a "key hole." There is some concern that breast cancer may be overdiagnosed.

Spring-assisted core needles, through the force of their traverse through the breast tissue, have been shown to be able to move cells from an intraductal cancer into the normal surrounding tissue so that the pathologist risks misinterpreting an intraductal lesion as an invasive cancer when a core biopsy is followed by an excision. This is not merely hypothetical but has already occurred (Lagios M, personal communication, 1996).

There will be advances made in these needle sampling devices. A modification of the spring-loaded system uses suction to assist in the removal of tissue samples so that the needle does not have to be removed from the targeted tissue. In this Mammotome system, a spring drives the stylet into the tissue. At the bottom of the notch in the stylet is a series of holes. Suction through the holes is applied, pulling tissue into the notch (Fig. 21-55). A rotating cutting cannula is advanced slicing a core of tissue into the cannula. Without withdrawing the needle, the sample can be withdrawn in the cutting cannula out the back of the needle, clearing the notch so that another sample can be obtained without having to remove the needle. Multiple tissue samples can be obtained in this fashion merely by rotating the notch or repositioning the needle without removing it from the targeted area. This increases the size of the samples and facilitates multiple sampling. It should reduce the likelihood of a sampling error.

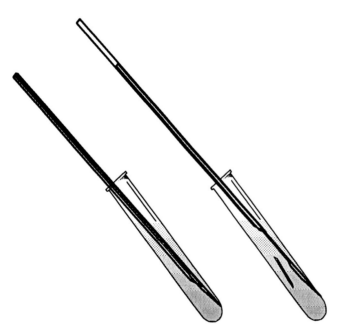

FIG. 21-53. By exposing the notch of the biopsy needle in a test tube with a few cubic centimeters of sterile saline, the tissue can be floated out of the notch and the needle reused.

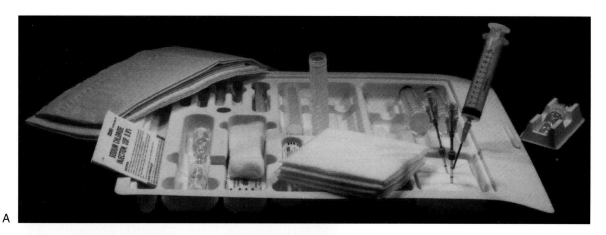

A

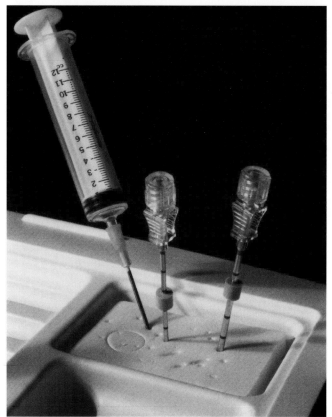

B

FIG. 21-54. The Mueller tray **(A)** contains all of the materials (prep solutions, lidocaine, syringes, hypodermic needles, no. 11 scalpel, sterile saline, glass slides, sterile drapes, and sponges), except the biopsy system, needed for needle biopsy. Of particular value is a pad into which needles can be placed **(B)** and then reused, reducing the risk of an inadvertent needle stick.

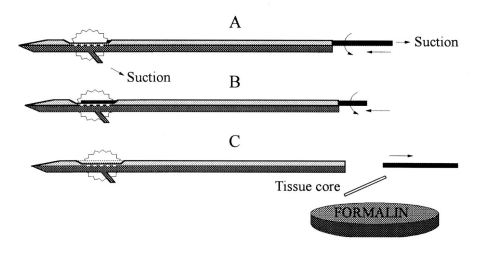

FIG. 21-55. The Mammotome uses suction to pull tissue into the notch **(A)** where a core is cut into a cutting cannula **(B)** so that it can be pulled out the back of the needle **(C)** while the notch remains in place ready for another sample.

Methods of Guiding Fine-Needle Aspiration and Core Needle Biopsy

Two methods are most commonly used to position needles for the biopsy of nonpalpable, imaging-detected lesions: Stereoscopic mammography (stereotactic) and ultrasound can be used to guide these procedures. We have also used conventional needle localization techniques to obtain core samples. Larger percutaneous biopsy systems are being developed. The Advanced Breast Biopsy Instrument (ABBI) is an apple core device that can remove a cylinder of tissue as wide as 2 cm in diameter. Preliminary reports suggest that this is far more complex than core needle biopsy (71).

Stereotactic Guidance

Stereotactic devices have been created to guide needles into lesions from essentially a single projection. This permits the breast and lesion to be held in place while the lesion can be sampled multiple times. The technique relies on the parallax that occurs between the lesion and fiducial marks that are in a fixed location relative to the imaging system (Fig. 21-56). A pair of stereo images is obtained by angling the x-ray tube 15 degrees to one side of the perpendicular to the film plane and then swinging the tube 15 degrees to the other side for a 30-degree difference between the stereo images. Both images contain the projected lesion and fixed reference marks (fiducials). By comparing the

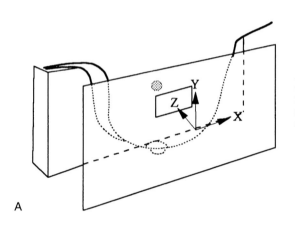

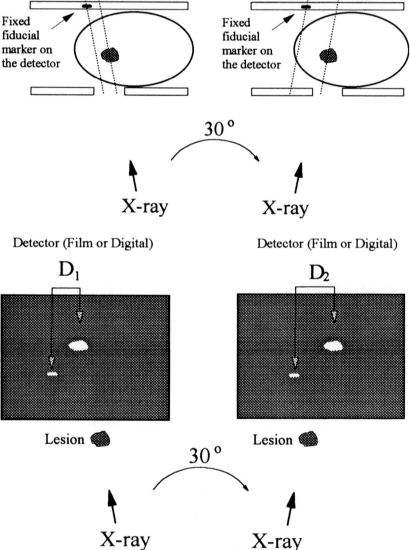

FIG. 21-56. Stereotaxis. This series of schematics demonstrates the basic principles of stereotaxis. **(A)** The breast is positioned in the compression device with the lesion centered in the window. The X and Y coordinates of the location of the lesion in the window are easily seen; all that remains is to calculate its depth. This is done by taking two images 30 degrees apart and measuring how much the lesion appears to shift relative to fixed marks on the detector. The amount of shift is directly related to the height of the lesion above the detector **(B)**. **(C)** shows how the projection of the lesion shifts against the background and in relation to a fixed point on the detector (e.g., film holder) between two mammograms obtained by shifting the direction of the x-ray beam by 30 degrees. The amount of shift ($D_2 - D_1$) is proportionate to the distance of the lesion in front of the film plane and can be used to calculate the depth of the lesion within the breast **(C)**. By providing the X, Y, and Z coordinates, needles can be positioned very accurately.

A

30°

X-ray   X-ray

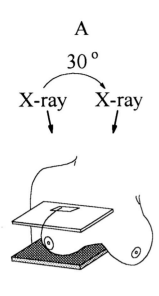

B

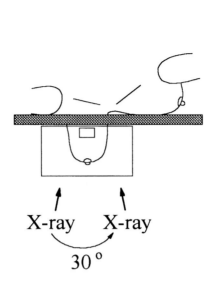

X-ray   X-ray

30°

FIG. 21-57. Stereotactic devices are either additions to conventional mammography equipment with the patient sitting upright **(A)** or dedicated units with the patient lying prone with her breast through an opening in the table **(B)**. A pair of images showing the shift of the lesion relative to the background and the fiducial marks on the film holder is obtained. The amount of movement of the target relative to these marks permits the computer to calculate the depth of the lesion and provides coordinates that permit the accurate positioning of a needle.

amount the lesion appears to move in the two images relative to the fixed marks in the two images (parallax shift), the height of the lesion above the film plane, and consequently the depth (the reciprocal) of the lesion and its distance from the needle holder, can be calculated. Most systems hold the breast in compression so that the lesion is located in the window of a fenestrated compression device.

The patient may be seated with a stereo-mammographic device added on to a conventional mammography system, or the procedure may be performed with the patient prone with her breast in an opening in the table surface and the x-ray device oriented horizontally beneath the table of a dedicated device (Fig. 21-57). The images may be recorded on film or by using a digital detector. The X and Y coordinates are evident from the images (Fig. 21-58), and the Z depth is calculated from the parallax shift. Modern systems use microprocessors to derive all of the lesion's coordinates, permitting a needle guide to be adjusted so that the needle can be precisely introduced into the lesion.

Some units move the needle guide automatically to its appropriate position. By knowing the length of needle that is to be used, the systems can provide coordinates that place the tip of the needle in the center of the targeted tissue with an accuracy that is probably within 1 to 2 mm.

The needle holder and guide can follow polar coordinates so that the needle is angled to target the lesion, or cartesian coordinates can be used so that the needle remains perpendicular to the film plane while it moves in the X and Y planes. Polar coordinates may have a slight advantage by permitting the targeting of lesions closer to the chest wall, although both systems work well.

Once the coordinates of the target are known, the biopsy procedure can begin. Studies suggest that probably at least five tissue samples should be obtained from various portions

of a given lesion (72). Generally the center of the lesion is targeted, as well as locations at 12, 3, 6, and 9 o'clock toward the periphery of the lesion. We generally target tissue between the center and the periphery.

The following sequence is used for stereotactically guided CNB:

1. After discussing the procedure with the patient, including its risks (e.g., missing the lesion, hematoma, infection) and alternatives, informed consent is obtained.

2. The patient is positioned in the compression system so that the lesion is in the biopsy window of the compression plate.

3. A scout image is obtained to confirm that the target is in the window (see Fig. 21-58A).

4. The skin surface is prepared sterilely.

5. A pair of stereo images is obtained, and the needle coordinates are determined (see Fig. 21-58B).

6. A needle is directed at the target using the needle guide to indicate the point where the core biopsy needle will enter the skin.

7. Local anesthesia is injected into the skin at this point and then into the tissues deeper in the breast to include the targeted lesion.

8. Using a no. 11 scalpel blade, a 3- to 5-mm cut is made in the skin into the subcutaneous tissues so that the 14-gauge needle can be introduced.

9. Using the coordinates provided by the stereo pair and computer calculations, the 14-gauge needle, with the spring cocked, is introduced into the breast so that the tip is in the center of the lesion. A stereo pair of x-rays can be obtained to confirm its position (see Fig. 21-58C). Before firing, the needle should be pulled back so that, when the needle or stylet system is fired, the center of the notch is centered in the lesion while the outer cannula slices the tissue into it. Because the notch in

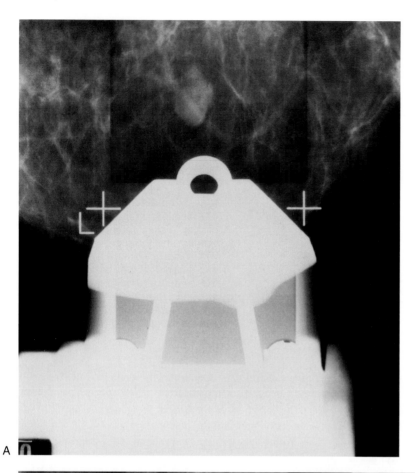

A

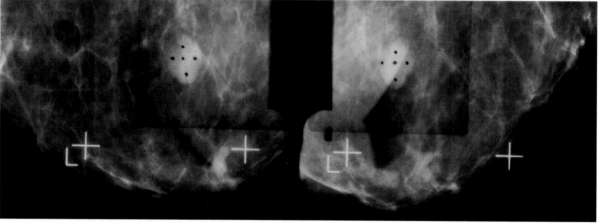

B

FIG. 21-58. The lesion is positioned in the window of the compression system **(A)**. A stereotactic pair of images is obtained, and five points in the lesion are targeted for biopsy **(B)**. Films with the needle in the prefire position can aid in ensuring that the targeted tissue has not moved. *Continued.*

the stylet lies several millimeters back from the tip of the needle, if the system is fired with the tip in the center of the lesion, the center of the notch ends up (for most lesions) partially outside the other side of the lesion and samples only part of the target. The needle should be pulled back prior to sampling, so that when the system is fired the center of the notch ends up in the center of the lesion. The method for calculating this distance is provided below. Films taken after firing (see Fig. 21-58D) can also be used to evaluate the accuracy of the sampling.

The operator should be aware that the lesion may not be far enough from the detector. If, in firing the needle, the

throw will cause it to come out the other side of the breast, the biopsy should not be done (see Fig. 21-58E). This will bend the stylet and could injure the patient.

The distance that the needle must be pulled back before firing can be calculated. It is the difference between the throw distance (how far the spring advances the stylet) and the distance from the stylet tip to the center of the notch (Fig. 21-59). For example, if the center of the notch is 1.8 cm from the tip of the stylet and the spring moves the stylet 2.3 cm, then the needle should be fired from a point that is 5 mm proximal to the center of the lesion. This means that the center of the

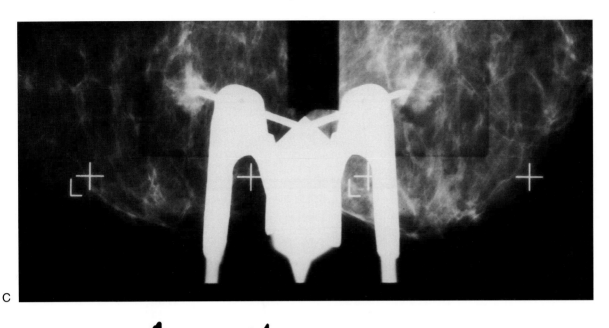

C

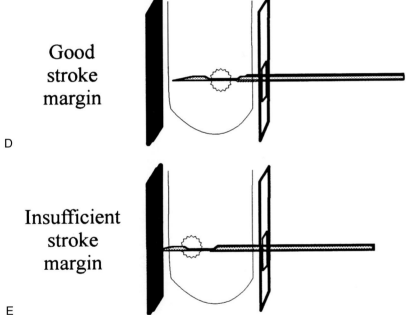

Good
stroke
margin

D

Insufficient
stroke
margin

E

FIG. 21-58. *Continued.* These images **(C)** were obtained prior to obtaining the third specimen. The lesion has become less well defined because of bleeding around it. If the lesion is too close to the back of the detector, a spring-fired cannula may pass through the breast and hit the detector. **(D)** shows the desired relationship to the notch. **(E)** shows that there is insufficient stroke margin to permit a safe biopsy.

notch is positioned 2.3 cm proximal to the center of the lesion so that when the needle is fired the center of the notch moves 2.3 cm and coincides with the center of the lesion.

10. Postfire films can confirm that the needle traversed the lesion (Fig. 21-60).

11. When the needle is withdrawn, an assistant should immediately put pressure over the cut and the lesion to limit hematoma formation.

12. A small test tube is filled with sterile saline, and by moving the stylet with the notch exposed in the saline the sample can be floated out of the notch, avoiding fragmenting or crushing the sample. After all of the samples have been obtained, the samples are poured into formalin. If the amount of saline is small, it will not significantly dilute the

formalin. Samples containing cellular material usually sink. If the samples float, it may indicate that mostly fat has been sampled and additional cores may be needed.

13. If calcifications are targeted, the samples should be x-rayed using magnification mammographic technique to determine whether calcifications are present (see Fig. 21-60E, F) (73). If a plastic test tube has been used, this can be done with the samples in the tube. Otherwise, the samples should be placed in a Petri dish or some other container or on a saline-moistened Telfa pad so that the calcifications in the core will be visible.

14. The sequence is repeated for each targeted portion of the lesion. Taking care to avoid compromising sterility, the skin incision can be moved by traction on the skin so that the

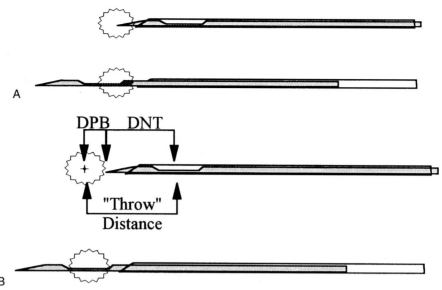

A

DPB DNT

"Throw"
Distance

B

FIG. 21-59. If the maximum possible sample of target tissue is desired, then the lesion must be centered in the notch of the stylet when the cannula slices tissue into the notch. Triggering a spring-loaded stylet with the needle tip in the center of the lesion **(A)** will not center the notch, and some of the tissue sampled will be on the far side of the lesion, increasing the sampling error. Before a spring-loaded needle is fired, the needle should be withdrawn from the center of the target so that when it is fired the center of the notch will coincide with the center of the tissue target. This is accomplished by starting with the center of the notch at the distance back from the center of the tissue **(B)** that is equivalent to the throw distance of the particular needle/gun system being used minus the distance from the tip to the center of the notch. The following formula calculates the pullback distance:

$$DPB = TD - DNT$$

where DPB = the distance to pull back before firing, DNT = the distance from the center of the notch to the tip of the stylet, and TD = the throw distance (distance the spring will drive the stylet). Thus, if the distance from the tip of the stylet to the center of the notch is 1.8 cm and the throw distance of the needle is 2.3 cm, the needle should be fired 2.3 − 1.8 = 0.5 cm from the center of the target.

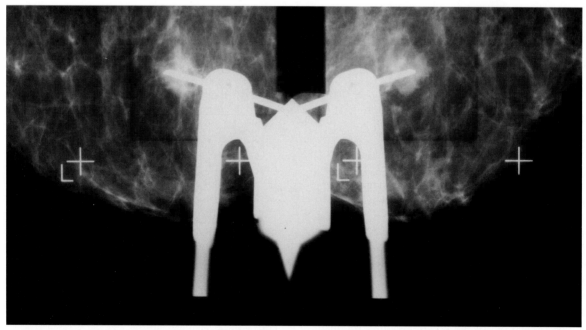

A

FIG. 21-60. Postfire films (A) show that the needle tip is in a slightly different relationship on the two films to the portion of the lesion being targeted (9:00). This may mean that tissue adjacent to the lesion, rather than the lesion itself, was sampled. In this case the mass proved to be a fibroadenoma, but ductal carcinoma in situ was discovered, serendipitously, immediately adjacent to it. *Continued.*

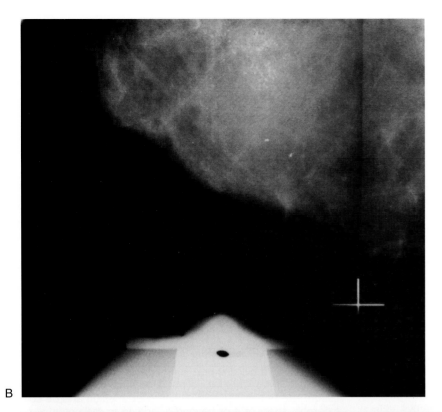

B

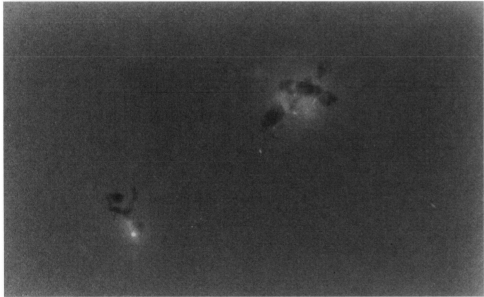

C

FIG. 21-60. *Continued.* In this other patient, calcifications were targeted **(B)** and the samples were x-rayed **(C)**, confirming that there were calcifications in the sample. The radiolucent portions of the tissue represent fat. The calcifications were due to high-grade comedocarcinoma.

sequential needle passes can be made through the same incision without moving the underlying lesion.

15. When the procedure is complete, the patient should be released from compression and firm pressure maintained over the biopsy site for 10 minutes to limit hematoma formation. An ice pack is applied to the biopsy area. Aspirin or other analgesics that slow clotting should be avoided 5 days before the procedure and several days after. A small amount of bleeding is common. Postprocedure orthogonal mammographic images can confirm that the tissue disruption is at the lesion, increasing the likelihood that the lesion has been appropriately sampled.

Because it may be difficult to see a lesion from the two stereo projections 30 degrees apart, some systems permit using the scout image as one projection and a 15-degree stereo to provide the measurement. Depth accuracy can be reduced using this technique.

Another modification permits the needle to be introduced at right angles to the x-ray beam, inserting the needle along the plane at which the computer determines the lesion lies. Because it may be difficult to work between two large plates (the film holder and the compression paddle), a smaller paddle can be substituted in the same way that the spot-compression paddle is used for needle localizations. The accuracy of this method is likely reduced because the needle can deflect out of the plane without the deflection being apparent and the targeted lesion missed without the operator's being aware of the miss.

Contraindications

A prerequisite for stereotactically guided biopsy is that the lesion can be positioned in the compression window. This may prevent access to lesions close to the chest wall and those high in the axilla or close to the sternum.

If the lesion is very superficial, the needle may be outside the skin in the prefire position. The needle must be through the skin before firing or it may merely bounce off the skin.

Because the needle passes through the lesion, if it is too close to the opposite side of the breast or the breast is too thin, the risk of hitting the detector with the needle may preclude needle biopsy.

Any bleeding diathesis may also be a contraindication. We advise patients to avoid ingesting any substance containing aspirin for 5 to 7 days before the procedure.

Sources of Error

Sampling Error. Because a needle biopsy does not remove the entire lesion, it relies on sampling parts of the lesion with the hope that at least one of the samples will be from a portion of the lesion from which an accurate diagnosis can be made. Because these are relatively small samples of even a small lesion, they are subject to missing the significant portion of the lesion. This is termed *sampling error.*

Although in theory stereotactically guided CNB should be very accurate, there are several ways in which the accuracy can be compromised. Movement of the patient, her breast, or the targeted tissue during the procedure can cause the needle to miss the target. The needle biopsies whatever tissue it is directed at. Cancers have been missed because the needle skimmed along the edge of the tumor or missed it altogether. Cancers can be heterogeneous, and the tissue that is sampled may not contain tumor. Although springloading and firing of the stylet/needle combination reduces the risk, the lesion may be pushed out of the needle path or backward away from the needle.

Lesions that are visible on conventional mammograms may be difficult to identify in a pair of stereo images. Targeting the same point in a lesion or the same calcification in a cluster of calcifications may be difficult and is prone to error. The weakest point in a stereotactic procedure is the determination of the targeting points in the pair of stereo images. If the radiologist chooses points on the image that do not truly correspond to the same point in the lesion, the computer may calculate a point in space that is actually not

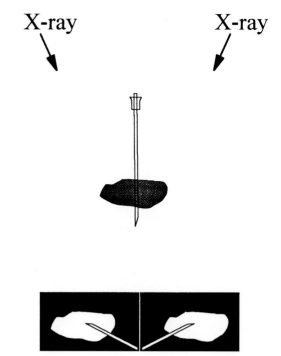

FIG. 21-61. If the same part of a target is not identified for the computer, it can calculate a point in space that is not in the tissue. The needle tip may project over a lesion and be considerably short of it or beyond it, adding to the potential for sampling error.

in the tissue to be sampled. A 5-mm error of this type can lead to a depth error of 1 cm. Because the lesion is being viewed from two angles separated by only 30 degrees, the tip of the needle may appear to be in the lesion when it is in fact short of the target or, worse, beyond it (Fig. 21-61). This can lead to a sampling error removing tissue from in front of or behind the lesion, while mistakenly thinking that the notch of the needle was in the targeted tissue.

The accurate sampling of calcifications can be particularly problematic. Successfully targeting the same portion of a cluster in the two stereo images can be very difficult. Benign calcifications may be associated with malignancies, and the confirmation of calcium in the core samples may be falsely reassuring. Systems that use suction to pull tissue into the needle are likely to reduce the sampling error because they facilitate obtaining multiple large-core samples.

Ultrasound-Guided Needle Biopsy

Ultrasound-guided needle biopsies are performed in the same way that needle aspiration of cysts under direct ultrasound observation is performed (37). The needle is observed using high-frequency ultrasound as it is advanced to the lesion (see above). If spring-assisted CNB is performed, the needle tip should be positioned proximal to the lesion (just as for stereotactic biopsy) so that when the needle is fired the center of the notch ends in the center of the lesion.

The use of an introducing needle (15-gauge for a 16-gauge core needle, 13-gauge for a 14-gauge core) facilitates the process (Fig. 21-62). The introducing needle need only be pushed through the breast tissue to the mass one time (this is the most difficult part of the procedure because the tissues may be extremely fibrous) (see Fig. 21-62 A–C). Once in place just proximal to the lesion, the trocar of the introducing needle is removed and a core biopsy needle is advanced to the lesion (see Fig. 21-62D). A sample is obtained (see Fig. 21-62E), and the core needle is removed through the introducer (see Fig. 21-62F). An assistant should apply pressure over the lesion to reduce hematoma formation while the core sample is removed from the notch. After removing the sample, the spring load can be cocked again and passed back through the introducer to the lesion. By changing the angle of the introducing needle, another sample from a different area of the targeted lesion can be obtained (see Fig. 21-62G, H). Because the introducing needle remains in position, providing easy access through the tissue the process can be repeated numerous times with little trauma to the patient.

It is likely that the spring-loaded needle systems will be replaced by the systems such as the vacuum-assisted Biopsys-Mammotome (Biopsys Medical, Inc., San Juan Capistrano, CA) or systems that remove larger volumes of tissue. These will reduce the sampling error. It is possible to remove the entire lesion through a very small incision or even through a needle.

Advantages

The advantage of ultrasound is that the needle can be monitored throughout the procedure, and its relationship to

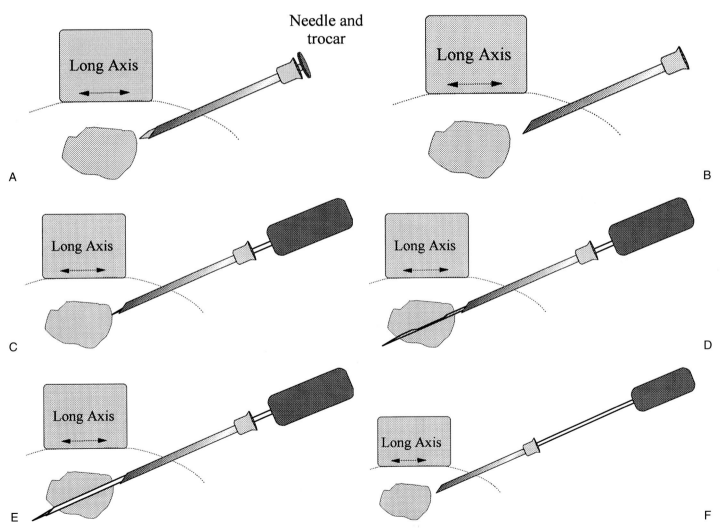

FIG. 21-62. An **introducing needle and coaxial core biopsy system** facilitate needle biopsy. Under imaging guidance (represented here as ultrasound), the introducing needle is advanced to the lesion **(A)**. The trocar is removed **(B)**, and the cocked core needle can be introduced **(C)** through the introducing needle. The core system is fired, and in rapid sequence the notched stylet fires into the mass **(D)**, followed by the cannula, which slices tissue into the notch **(E)**. Then the core needle is removed with the sample **(F)** while pressure is applied over the lesion to reduce bleeding. *Continued.*

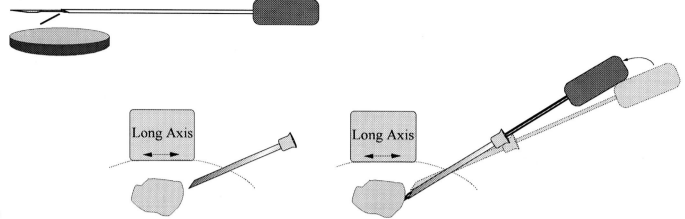

G   H

FIG. 21-62. *Continued.* The tissue is cleared from the core needle and placed into formalin **(G)**. The needle is recocked and introduced back through the introducing needle, which has maintained easy access to the lesion. Another sample can be obtained by changing the angle of the coaxial system **(H)**.

the target can be seen at all times. The equipment is much less expensive than stereotactic guidance equipment. There is no ionizing radiation involved, and the procedure can be performed much faster than stereotactic guided biopsy.

Disadvantages

The procedure is extremely operator dependent. It requires good eye/hand coordination. Many lesions are difficult to see by ultrasound. If the lesion cannot be clearly identified, then an inaccurate biopsy is likely. Microcalcifications are rarely visible. Small lesions (<1 cm) may be difficult to hit. Because the breast is not held, the lesion may be pushed out of the path of the needle as it is introduced into the lesion. Because the needle is directed back toward the chest wall, there is the danger of entering structures of the thorax and causing damage.

Any introduction of a needle into the breast can produce a confusing picture on follow-up ultrasound. Hematomas and edema caused by needle biopsies can produce effects that, when seen by ultrasound, are indistinguishable from cancer (74) and may persist for months.

False-negative biopsies occur.

Ultrasound-Guided Fine-Needle Aspiration Biopsy Versus Core Needle Biopsy

The same arguments that can be used for stereotactically guided biopsies apply to ultrasound-guided procedures. If a trained cytopathologist is available, FNAB is probably more easily performed. The thinner needle is less unwieldy than the spring-driven core needles, and the thinner needles are more easily moved in the unstabilized breast. The thin needles used for FNAB are also less likely to cause any major damage to the breast or the thorax, should it be inadvertently advanced too far. Fornage and colleagues reported ultrasound-guided FNAB of 111 breast lesions (including three

axillary lymph nodes), of which 51 were nonpalpable breast lesions and 60 were palpable masses. They correctly diagnosed 92% of the malignant lesions. The FNAB was positive in 35 of the 38 breast cancers and suspicious in the other three. They had one false-positive result.

Gordon and associates use ultrasound-guided FNAB in conjunction with ultrasound surveys of women with dense breast tissue. Because they could rapidly and with minimum trauma sample suspicious areas found by ultrasound while surveying the breasts of women with dense tissue on mammography, the authors claim that they were able to detect 15 cancers of a total of 213 that were not palpable and not visible by mammography (75). They did FNAB of 123 lesions that were visible by ultrasound alone to find these cancers. They did have 12 false-negative aspirates.

The advantages of needle core biopsy have been discussed previously. The course of the needle can be monitored under real-time ultrasound. Parker and colleagues reported results of 181 procedures. Among these, 49 lesions were excised. They correctly diagnosed the 34 cancers using ultrasound-guided CNB requiring an average of 20 minutes to perform the procedures (76).

SUMMARY

The pressure to reduce the number of excisional biopsies will increase, both from the perspective of cost as well as from the goal of reducing the amount of trauma needed to make a diagnosis. It is likely that the true accuracy of imaging-directed needle biopsies will not be known.

Despite the absence of scientific validation, imaging-guided needle biopsy of the breast has spread rapidly and will likely be applied more frequently. This was in part due to shrewd marketing by manufacturers who placed stereotactic units at a site and got the media to suggest that excisional biopsies were no longer needed. Other practices had to acquire units so that they would not be excluded from caring for patients with breast problems. The dissemination of the procedure is also attractive because a needle biopsy is less traumatic than surgery, and the cost of the procedure is less than the cost of needle localization and surgical excision. Despite the fact that it is inherently less accurate than properly performed needle localization and excision, in an era of cost containment the false-negative rate will be generally accepted although there will undoubtedly be future litigation due to missed cancers. It is hoped that a more scientific analysis will be accomplished, but in its absence women should be informed that the cancer miss rate for CNB is at least 2%, compared to a 0.5% miss rate for properly performed needle localization and excision. Although women should be given the option as to the level of certainty they desire, it is likely that managed care will dictate the lower-cost approach. New biopsy systems are being developed that will allow more tissue to be removed and eventually minimally invasive excision or ablation of lesions.

The Most Suspicious Assessment Should Prevail

It is likely that needle biopsy is not as accurate as excisional biopsy after a properly performed needle localization. Needle biopsy procedures are extremely operator dependent (especially those guided by ultrasound). If needle biopsies are to be used as a substitute for excisional biopsy, the results of the biopsy must be compared with the imaging analysis. Consequently, as with the triple test, benign results from a needle biopsy for a lesion that is very suspicious by imaging should not be reassuring, and the lesion should be excised. If the lesion is suspicious by mammography, then a benign biopsy should not be believed and the lesion should be excised. Lesions revealed to be atypical hyperplasia on needle biopsy should also be excised as many of these prove to be cancer. Needle biopsy is very accurate when invasive cancer is found in the samples, but if only in situ cancer is present in the core samples invasion in another part of the lesion cannot be excluded.

As long as women are informed that needle biopsies are not as accurate as excisional biopsy and they are offered the alternative, the use of imaging-guided needle biopsies, if carefully performed, will likely be a valuable addition to the diagnostic approach to breast lesions.

REFERENCES

1. Van Dijck JAAM, Verbeek ALM, Hendriks JHCL, Holland R. The current detectability of breast cancer in a mammographic screening program. Cancer 1993;72:1933–1938.
2. Kopans DB. Mammography screening for breast cancer. Cancer 1993;72:1809–1812.
3. Moskowitz M. The predictive value of certain mammographic signs in screening for breast cancer. Cancer 1983;51:1007–1011.
4. Swann CA, Kopans DB, McCarthy KA, et al. The halo sign and malignant breast lesions. AJR Am J Roentgenol 1987;149:1145–1147.
5. Cohen MI, Matthies HJ, Mintzer RA, et al. Indurative mastopathy: a cause of false-positive mammograms. Radiology 1985;155:69–71.
6. Bassett LW, Gold RH, Cove HC. Mammographic spectrum of traumatic fat necrosis: the fallibility of "pathognomonic" signs of carcinoma. AJR Am J Roentgenol 1978;130:119–122.
7. Rouanet P, Lamarque JL, Naja A, Pujoi H. Isolated clustered microcalcifications: diagnostic value of mammography—series of 400 cases with surgical verification. Radiology 1994;190:479–483.
8. Meyer JE, Kopans DB, Stomper PC, Lindfors KK. Occult breast abnormalities: percutaneous preoperative needle localization. Radiology 1984;150:335.
9. Gisvold JJ, Martin JK. Prebiopsy localization of nonpalpable breast lesions. AJR Am J Roentgenol 1984;143:477.
10. Rosenberg AL, Schwartz GF, Feig SA, Patchefsky AS. Clinically occult breast lesions: localization and significance. Radiology 1987;162:167.
11. Kopans DB. The positive predictive value of mammography. AJR Am J Roentgenol 1992;158:521–526.
12. D'Orsi CJ. To follow or not to follow, that is the question. Radiology 1992;184:306.
13. Carter CL, Allen C, Henson DE. Relation of tumor size, lymph node status, and survival in 24,740 breast cancer cases. Cancer 1989;63:181–187.
14. Rosen PP, Groshen S, Saigo PE, et al. A long-term follow-up study of survival in stage I (T1 N0 M0) and stage II (T1 N1 M0) breast carcinoma. J Clin Oncol 1989;7:355–366.
15. Tabar L, Fagerberg G, Day N, et al. Breast cancer treatment and natural history: new insights from results of screening. Lancet 1992;339:412–414.
15a. Linver Mn. Mammography outcomes in a practice setting by age: prognostic factors. J Natl Cancer Inst (in press).
16. Baker LH. Breast cancer detection demonstration project: five-year summary report. CA Cancer J Clin 1982;32:194–225.
17. Spivey GH, Perry BW, Clark VA, et al. Predicting the risk of cancer at the time of breast biopsy. Am Surg 1982;48:326.
18. Dupont WD, Page DL. Risk factors for breast cancer in women with proliferative breast disease. N Engl J Med 1985;312:146.
19. Bassett LW, Liu TH, Giuliano AE, Gold RH. The prevalence of carcinoma in palpable vs impalpable mammographically detected lesions. AJR Am J Roentgenol 1991;157:21–24.
20. Smart CR. Highlights of the evidence of benefit for women aged 40–49 years from the 14-year follow-up of the Breast Cancer Detection Demonstration Project. Cancer 1994;74:296–300.
21. Sickles EA. Periodic mammographic follow-up of probably benign lesions: results of 3184 consecutive cases. Radiology 1991;179:463–468.
22. Sickles EA, Herzog KA. Mammography of the postsurgical breast. AJR Am J Roentgenol 1981;136:585–588.
23. Kopans DB. Caution on core. Radiology 1994;193:325–328.
24. Kopans DB, Meyer JE, Lindfors KK, McCarthy KA. Spring-hook-wire breast lesion localizer: use with rigid compression mammographic systems. Radiology 1985;157:537–538.
25. Dowlatshahi K, Yaremko ML, Kluskens LF, Jokich PM. Nonpalpable breast lesions: findings of stereotaxic needle-core biopsy and fine-needle aspiration cytology. Radiology 1991;181:745–750.
26. Parker SH, Lovin JD, Jobe WE, et al. Nonpalpable breast lesions: stereotaxic automated large-core biopsies. Radiology 1991;180:403–407.
27. Elvecrog EL, Lechner MC, Nelson MT. Nonpalpable breast lesions: correlation of stereotaxic large-core-needle biopsy and surgical biopsy results. Radiology 1993;188:453–455.
28. Gisvold JJ, Goeliner JR, Grant CS, et al. Breast biopsy: a comparative study of stereotaxically guided core and excisional techniques. AJR Am J Roentgenol 1994;162:815–820.
29. Gallagher WJ, Cardenosa G, Rubens JR, et al. Minimal-volume excision of nonpalpable breast lesions. AJR Am J Roentgenol 1989;153:957–961.
30. Caines JS, McPhee MD, Konok GP, Wright BA. Stereotaxic needle core biopsy of breast lesions using a regular mammographic table with an adaptable stereotaxic device. AJR Am J Roentgenol 1994;163:317–321.
31. Parker SH, Burbank F, Jackman RJ, et al. Percutaneous large-core breast biopsy: a multi-institutional study. Radiology 1994;193:359–364.
32. Dronkers DJ. Stereotaxic core biopsy of breast lesions. Radiology 1992;183:631–634.
33. Doyle AJ, Murray KA, Nelson EW, Bragg DG. Selective use of image-guided large-core-needle biopsy of the breast: accuracy and cost-effectiveness. AJR Am J Roentgenol 1995;165:281–284.
34. Azavedo E, Svane G, Auer G. Stereotaxic fine-needle biopsy in 2594

mammographically detected non-palpable lesions. Lancet 1989;1: 1033–1036.

35. Layfield LJ, Parkinson B, Wong J, et al. Mammographically guided fine-needle aspiration biopsy of nonpalpable breast lesions. Cancer 1991;68:2007–2011.

36. Franquet T, Cozcolluela R, Miguel C. Stereotaxic fine-needle aspiration of low-suspicion, nonpalpable breast nodules: valid alternative to follow-up mammography. Radiology 1992;183:635–637.

37. Fornage BD, Fariux MJ, Simatos A. Breast masses: US guided fine-needle aspiration biopsy. Radiology 1987;162:409–414.

38. Ciatto S, Del Turco M, Bravetti P. Nonpalpable breast lesions: stereotaxic fine-needle aspiration cytology. Radiology 1989;173:57–59.

39. Harter LP, Curtis JS, Ponto G, Craig PH. Malignant seeding of the needle track during stereotaxic core needle breast biopsy. Radiology 1992; 185:713–714.

40. Berkowitz JE, Gatewood OMB, Gayler BW. Equivocal mammographic findings: evaluation with spot compression. Radiology 1989; 171:369–371.

41. Swann CA, Kopans DB, McCarthy KA, et al. Practical solutions to problems of triangulation and preoperative localization of breast lesions. Radiology 1987;163:577–579.

42. Kopans DB, Waitzkin ED, Linetsky L, et al. Localization of breast lesions identified on only one mammographic view. AJR Am J Roentgenol 1987;149:39–41.

43. Kopans DB, Meyer JE, Lindfors KK, Bucchianeri SS. Breast sonography to guide aspiration of cysts and preoperative localization of occult breast lesions. AJR Am J Roentgenol 1984;143:489–492.

44. Kopans DB, Meyer JE. Computed tomography guided localization of clinically occult breast carcinoma—the "N" skin guide. Radiology 1982;145:211–212.

45. Hall FM, Frank HA. Preoperative localization of nonpalpable breast lesions. AJR Am J Roentgenol 1979;132:101–105.

46. Kopans DB, Deluca S. A modified needle-hookwire technique to simplify the preoperative localization of occult breast lesions. Radiology 1980;134:781.

47. Kopans DB, Meyer JE. The versatile spring-hookwire breast lesion localizer. AJR Am J Roentgenol 1982;138:586–587.

48. Whitman GJ, McCarthy KA, Hall DA, et al. Retained hook-wire fragments in 12 patients: mammography and management. Presented at the meeting of the Radiological Society of North America; 1995; Chicago.

49. Davis PS, Wechsler RJ, Feig SA, March DE. Migration of breast biopsy localization wire. AJR Am J Roentgenol 1988;150:787–788.

50. Homer MJ. Nonpalpable breast lesion localization using a curved-end retractable wire. Radiology 1985;157:259–260

51. Homer MJ, Pile-Spellman ER. Needle localization of occult breast lesions with a curved-end retractable wire: technique and pitfalls. Radiology 1986;161:547–548.

52. Urrutia EJ, Hawkins IF, Hawkins MC, et al. Clinical experience of a new retractable barb needle for breast lesion localization: the first 60 cases. Presented at the 73rd Scientific Assembly of the Radiological Society of North America; December, 1987; Chicago.

53. Czarnecki DJ, Berridge DL, Splittgerber GF, Goell WS. Comparison of the anchoring strengths of the Kopans and Hawkins II needle-hook-wire systems. Radiology 1992;183:573–574.

54. Reynolds HE, Jackson VP, Musnick BS. Preoperative needle localization in the breast: utility of local anesthesia. Radiology 1993;187: 503–505.

55. Feig SA. Localization of clinically occult breast lesions. Radiol Clin North Am 1983;21:155–172.

56. Bristol JB, Jones PA. Transgression of localizing wire into the pleural cavity prior to mammography. Br J Radiol 1981;54:139–140.

57. Kopans DB, Gallagher WJ, Swann CA, et al. Does preoperative needle localization lead to an increase in local breast cancer recurrence? Radiology 1988;167:667–668.

58. Spivack B, Khana MM, Tarafa L, et al. Margin status and local recurrence after breast-conserving surgery. Arch Surg 1994;129:952–957.

59. Gage I, Schnitt SJ, Nixon AJ, et al. Pathologic margin involvement and the risk of recurrence in patients treated with breast conserving therapy. Cancer 1996;78:1921–1928.

60. Lagios MD. Ductal carcinoma in situ: pathology and treatment. Surg Clin North Am 1990;70:853–871.

61. Fisher B, Constantino J, Redmond PHC, et al. Lumpectomy compared with lumpectomy and radiation therapy for the treatment of intraductal breast cancer. N Engl J Med 1993;328:1581–1586.

62. Cardenosa G, Eklund GW. Paraffin block radiography following breast biopsies: use of orthogonal views. Radiology 1991;180:873–874.

62a. Smith DN, Kaelin CM, Korbin CD, et al. Impalpable breast cysts: utility of cytologic examination of fluid obtained with radiographically guided aspiration. Radiology 1997;204:149–151.

63. Rizzatto G, Solbiati L, Croce F, Derchi LE. Aspiration biopsy of superficial lesions: ultrasonic guidance with a linear-array probe. AJR Am J Roentgenol 1987;148:623–625.

64. Davros WJ, Madsen EL, Zagaebski JA. Breast mass detection by US: a phantom study. Radiology 1985;156:773.

65. Parker SH, Jobe WE, Dennis MA, et al. US-guided automated large-core breast biopsy. Radiology 1993;187:507–511.

66. Lindfors KK, Rosenquist CJ. Needle core biopsy guided with mammography: a study of cost-effectiveness. Radiology 1994;190:217–222.

67. Hermansen C, Poulsen HS, Jensen J, et al. Diagnostic reliability of combined physical examination, mammography, and fine-needle puncture ("triple-test") in breast tumors. Cancer 1987;60:1866–1871.

68. Sickles EA, Parker SH. Appropriate role of core biopsy in the management of probably benign lesions. Radiology 1993;188:315.

69. Cady B. Use of primary breast carcinoma characteristics to predict lymph node metastases. Cancer 1997;79:1856–1861.

70. Fisher B, Redmond C, Fisher E, et al. Ten-year result of a randomized clinical trial comparing radical mastectomy and total mastectomy with or without irradiation. N Engl J Med 1985;312:674.

71. Ferzli GS, Hurwitz JB, Puza T, Van Vorst-Bilotti S. Advanced breast biopsy instrumentation: a critique. J Am Coll Surg 1997;185:145–151.

72. Liberman L, Dershaw DD, Rosen PP, et al. Stereotaxic 14-gauge breast biopsy: how many specimens are needed? Radiology 1994; 192:793–795.

73. Meyer JE, Lester SC, Frenna TH, White FV. Occult breast calcifications sampled with large-core biopsy: confirmation with radiography of the specimen. Radiology 1993;188:581–582.

74. Svensson WE, Tohno E, Cosgrove DO, et al. Effects of fine-needle aspiration on the US appearance of the breast. Radiology 1992;185: 709–711.

75. Gordon PB, Goldenberg SL, Chan NHL. Solid breast lesions: diagnosis with US-guided fine-needle aspiration biopsy. Radiology 1993; 189:573–580.

76. Parker SH, Jobe WE, Dennis MA, et al. US-guided automated large-core breast biopsy. Radiology 1993;187:507–511.

Breast Imaging, 2nd ed., by Daniel B. Kopans.
Lippincott–Raven Publishers, Philadelphia © 1998.

CHAPTER 22

Problems and Solutions in Breast Evaluation

As is stressed throughout this text, imaging the breast can be divided into a few major tasks.

1. Find it.
2. Is it real?
3. Where is it?
4. What is it?
5. What should be done about it?

The major objective in breast imaging is the detection of breast cancers at a small size and early stage in an effort to reduce mortality. The screening mammogram (find it) is the most critical study because it is the only opportunity to detect cancers earlier. Once a potential abnormality is found, additional evaluation is frequently needed to determine the significance of the finding (is it real?). If it is determined that a finding is real, then the radiologist must determine its location (where is it?) so that he or she, if needed, can put a needle accurately into the lesion or guide a surgeon to the lesion. The radiologist must decide whether or not the lesion is benign or has the potential of being malignant and then what course of action to pursue to establish the diagnosis.

Finding lesions requires high-quality imaging with proper positioning. Most problems in positioning can be avoided by having well-trained technologists (see Chapter 10) who are compassionate and can work with the patient in an effort to obtain high-quality mammograms (quality control problems are addressed in Chapter 9).

Assuming the images are of good quality, the first clinical problems that the radiologist is likely to encounter can frequently be solved by using techniques that are common to all forms of plain-film radiography. Most problems encountered on a mammogram can be resolved through additional images. These include altering the angle that the x-ray beam takes as it passes through the breast, altering the position of the breast relative to the x-ray beam, the use of spot compression to separate overlapping structures, and the use of magnification mammography to reduce noise and provide sharper images. Ultimately ultrasound, computed tomography, magnetic resonance imaging, and other tests may help resolve specific problems.

MAMMOGRAPHIC FLUOROSCOPY

Mammographic evaluation is similar to fluoroscopy without the fluoroscope. The same principles that are employed in fluoroscopy are used to separate structures by mammography. Just as a compression paddle is used to separate overlapping loops of bowel under fluoroscopic observation, spot compression is used to separate overlapping breast structures. Rolling the breast and viewing it from different projections is the same as the fluoroscopist's rolling the patient to use parallax shifts to distinguish separate structures. The only difference is that fluoroscopy is real time, and with mammography it is the technologist who repositions and compresses the breast during the evaluation.

IS IT REAL?

Once a potential abnormality has been found, determining whether or not it is a real, three-dimensional abnormality can be a complicated process. Not all cancers form a mass, and there is the potential of dismissing an infiltrating process simply because a mass is not evident. The visualization of a finding on more than one additional projection may be required to determine whether or not it is three-dimensionally real or merely a projection artifact of superimposed normal structures. The tendency to rely only on conventional projections may be unnecessarily limiting. Although it is inconvenient, it is better to have the patient return for additional evaluation than to make a management decision based on insufficient information.

The basis of solving problems lies in varying the projections and reorienting the breast structures to provide a better understanding of the three-dimensional relationships (Fig. 22-1).

A Fortuitous Concatenation of Shadows

Many names have been given to the fact that the projection of three-dimensional structures within the breast as a two-dimensional image can result in the superimposition of normal structures, one projected on another, creating the appearance of a worrisome finding. Sickles has termed these

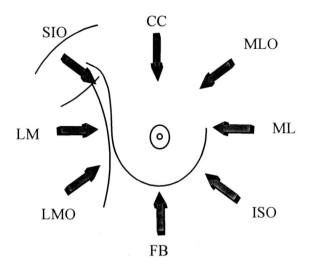

FIG. 22-1. There are an unlimited number of positions that can be used to evaluate the breast. This schematic provides just the standard mammographic projections. (CC, craniocaudal; MLO, mediolateral oblique; ML, mediolateral; ISO, inferosuperior oblique; FB, from below; LMO, lateromedial oblique; LM, lateromedial; SIO, superoinferior oblique.)

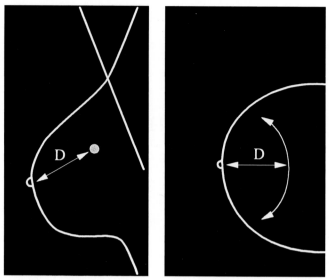

A,B

FIG. 22-2. The **arc method of triangulation** uses the distance from the base of the nipple to the lesion (D) on the view on which the lesion is seen **(A)**. This becomes the radius of an arc that is traced on the second view **(B)**. The lesion should lie close to or on this arc.

summation shadows. Whatever their name, the benign superimposition of normal structures is the most common reason that our screening program recalls women for additional evaluation. This is a bigger problem if single-view mammography is used for screening (1). Not only does single-view screening result in a higher recall rate, but more than 20% of cancer may be missed by using single-view screening (2). The available data suggest that screening should always use two-view mammography to reduce the recall rate and to diminish the chance that a cancer will be overlooked.

Dissecting the Lesion

When an abnormality is suspected in one projection but not evident in another, the radiologist should try to dissect the various components of the finding to determine if it is a true abnormality or merely a concatenation of separate structures. For example, it is not unusual for Cooper's ligaments or small blood vessels to project over one another, forming an image that looks like a spiculated abnormality. True spicules do not pass across a lesion from one side to the other but rather emanate from and blend with its edge. If the abnormality can be made to fall apart as its components are dissected, it is not a real abnormality.

Comparing Projections

Another method of determining whether or not a suspected lesion is real is to determine its location on the projection on which it appears and then to evaluate the corresponding tissues in the other projection. There are two

methods of triangulating a lesion in two projections. One is the arc method and the other is the straight-line method. Neither is perfect, and the accuracy depends on positioning, compression, and the elasticity of the breast tissues.

Arc Method of Triangulating Lesions

One of the methods commonly used for trying to find corresponding areas between mammographic projections involves using the distance from the nipple to the lesion as the radius of an arc with the nipple as its center. This distance is transferred to the other projection, and an arc is swept with the nipple as the center. The tissue along this arc corresponds to the tissues that could contain the suspected lesion (Fig. 22-2). A real lesion should be found somewhere along (close to) this arc in the second image.

Cartesian, Straight-Line Method of Triangulating Lesions

A second method that is used to do the same thing is to measure the distance straight back from the nipple to a point where it is perpendicular to a line dropped from the lesion (Fig. 22-3). This distance is transferred to the other projection. If the lesion is real, it should be somewhere along a line perpendicular to the transferred line at the same distance from the nipple.

There have been two studies that compared these two methods, and they reached opposite conclusions as to which is the more accurate (3). We prefer the arc method. The reader should be aware that these are crude measures. Since the breast is not a uniform shape, neither triangulation

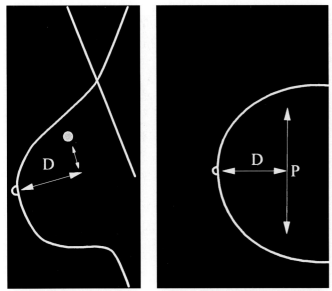

FIG. 22-3. The cartesian, **straight-line method** of triangulation determines the line that is perpendicular to the axis of the nipple that intersects the lesion (D). This is transferred to the other projection, and a perpendicular (P) at this distance is used to try to find the lesion.

method is perfect, and lesions can sometimes seem to be at unexpected distances in the second projection.

Is It Reasonable to Expect That a Finding Is Real?

At times it is fairly obvious that a suspected abnormality is not real. If the breast tissues are predominantly fat and there is no suggestion of an abnormality in the corresponding location on the second view, then it is highly unlikely that the lesion is real. This decision should be made with caution, however, since cancers can be subtle.

Don't Forget the Skin

If a lesion seen on one view is not immediately apparent on the second, the observer should also look carefully at the periphery of the breast at and just under the skin. This is especially true for calcifications seen in only one projection. They are frequently benign deposits in the skin. Methods to prove this are described later in this chapter.

Another possibility when something is seen in one view and not in the other is that it is an artifact. Scratches on the film, dust on the screen, and contaminants on the patient's skin can all cause findings that are only visible on a single view.

BASIC APPROACHES TO POSSIBLE SUPERIMPOSITION OF TISSUES

Tissues that superimpose can be separated in several ways. By changing the path that the x-ray beam takes through the

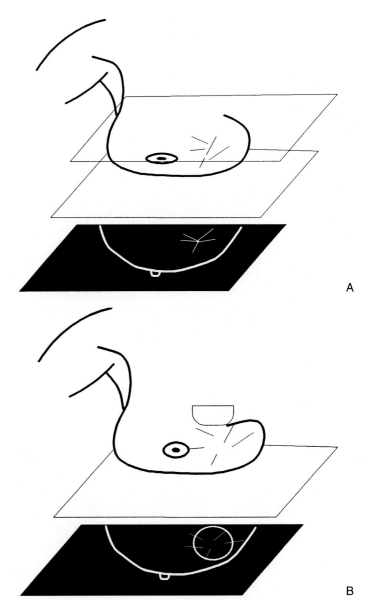

FIG. 22-4. Structures that overlap and cause suspicious shadows on standard compression **(A)** can be spread apart on spot compression **(B)** to eliminate concern. Spot compression can be used to displace tissues that overlap one another, to reduce the amount of overlapping tissue, and to push the tissues closer to the detector, reducing geometric blur.

tissues or by changing the orientation of the tissues relative to the x-ray beam, what at first might appear to be a mass or a spiculated lesion can be shown to come apart when viewed from a different perspective.

Spot Compression

Spot compression can be used to separate overlapping structures. The standard compression paddle presses on the tissues with only as much pressure as the least compressible tissue volume. Spot compression places greater pressure on a

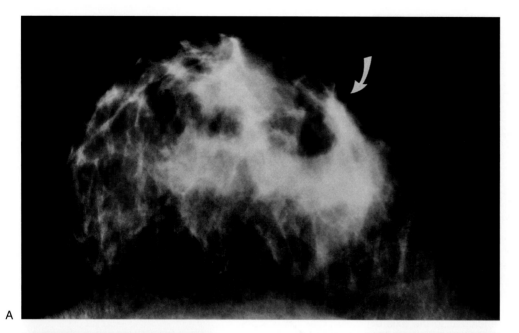

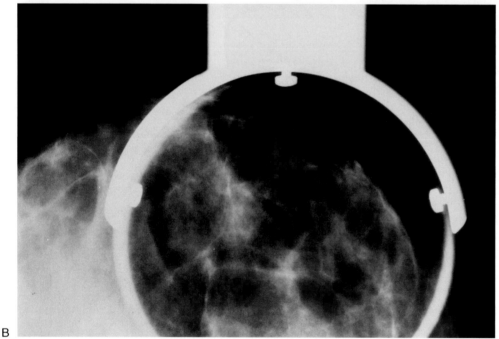

FIG. 22-5. The initial craniocaudal projection **(A)** raised the question of a spiculated mass (*arrow*). On spot compression **(B)**, this was clearly a **superimposition of normal structures.**

smaller volume of tissue. This can displace tissues that overlap one another, reduce the amount of overlapping tissue, and push the tissues closer to the detector, reducing geometric blur (Fig. 22-4). What may initially appear as a significant abnormality can be shown to represent overlapping normal structures using spot compression (Fig. 22-5). It is often useful to use spot compression in addition to changing the position of the breast so that the same structures are not maintained in the same alignment as in the initial image.

Some radiologists like to perform the spot-compression images using magnification. This can be helpful, but it adds another layer of complexity and room for error because any

motion can severely compromise the image sharpness and this is more likely to occur due to the longer exposure times needed for magnification. The benefit of magnification is an improved ability to evaluate the margins of masses and the morphology of calcifications. If it is not certain whether or not a lesion is real, we generally use spot compression without magnification as the first step.

Angulation of the X-Ray System

If the breast is kept in the same position but the gantry is rotated 10 to 20 degrees and then the breast is recompressed,

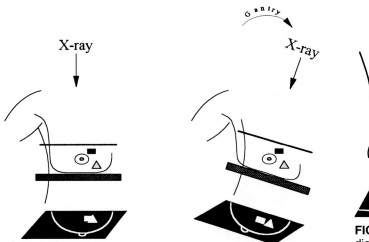

FIG. 22-6. Rotating the gantry and recompressing at a different angle while the breast is kept in the same position can be used to separate normal overlapping structures.

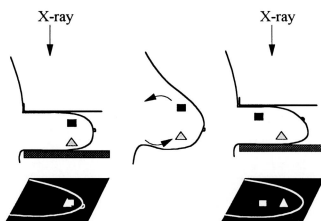

FIG. 22-8. The breast can be rolled front to back, as in this diagram, to accomplish the same results as in the standard rolled views.

the x-ray beam will pass through different tissues and a summation shadow can be made to fall apart into its normal tissue components (Fig. 22-6).

Modified Projections and Rolled Views

Just as the body is rolled under a fluoroscope to reorient overlapping structures, the breast may be rolled to accomplish the same result. The usual maneuver involves rolling the breast around the axis of the nipple (Fig. 22-7). By convention the direction of roll is determined by the movement of the top of the breast (e.g., top rolled laterally). It is occasionally useful to roll tissues from front to back (Fig. 22-8). This will also change the orientation of the various internal structures relative to the x-ray beam so that superimposed structures are not superimposed.

Not only are these maneuvers useful in determining if something is real, but by skillful and thoughtful repositioning, normal tissue that might obscure a lesion can be moved out of the way (Fig. 22-9).

Lesions Seen on Only One Projection

The most common problem occurs when a potential lesion is seen in one projection and not seen in the other view. This often means that the observation is the result of a benign superimposition of normal structures that has formed a summation shadow. The first question to be asked is, "Is it real?" Additional evaluation should begin by determining whether or not the finding is a true abnormality.

Return to the Projection on Which the Lesion Appeared

When a suspected lesion is seen in only one projection, it is best to return to that projection and alter it slightly to determine whether the lesion is real or merely a superimposition of structures. If a potential abnormality is seen on the mediolateral oblique projection (MLO), for example, and not seen on the craniocaudal (CC) projection, it is best to return to the MLO and work from there. If the lesion is not real, then it would be futile and cause unnecessary radiation

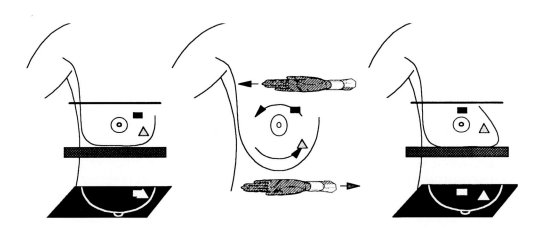

FIG. 22-7. Rolled views. If superimposed tissues are suspected, the breast can be rolled by gently rolling the top in one direction and the bottom in the other and recompressing. Structures that project over one another can be separated using this maneuver.

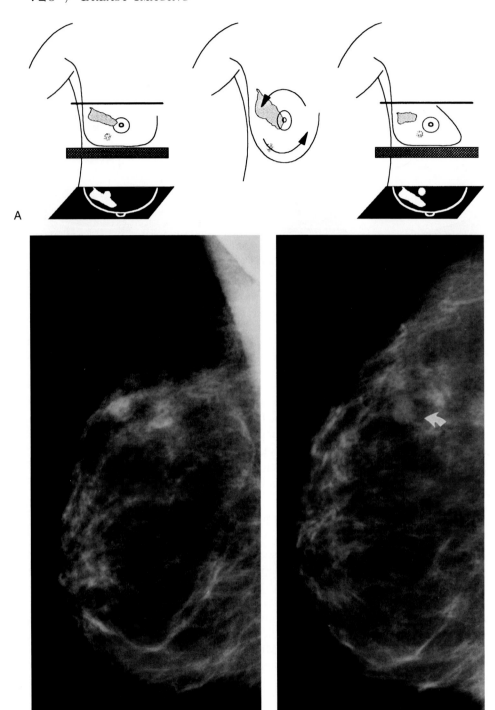

FIG. 22-9. Rolled views or changing the projection may help to eliminate overlapping structures so that a lesion is more clearly visible, as shown in this schematic **(A)**. The dense tissue in the upper outer quadrant is obscuring the visibility of a mass in the lower breast. Rolling the top laterally projects the mass under fat improving its visibility.

In this patient there is the suggestion of a mass on the mediolateral oblique view, but it is obscured by overlapping tissue **(B)**. By obtaining a straight lateral projection **(C)**, the mass, which proved to be a cyst, is more evident (*arrow*).

exposure to search for it by obtaining multiple altered CC projections. If it is not real, then it can never be found on the CC projection! If it is real, by imaging it using a projection that differs slightly from the original, in a predetermined fashion, the lesion can be shown to be real and its location can be determined by its apparent shift against the background of the normal breast structures between the two projections. Once the approximate location of the real abnormality is determined, the orthogonal mammographic

projection can be chosen appropriately to confirm the location and three dimensionality of the lesion.

Problem: A lesion is seen on the MLO projection and not on the CC view. Is it real? The tendency is to obtain multiple projections in the CC position trying to identify the lesion. The fallacy in this approach is that the lesion may not, in fact, be real and thus will not be visible on these projections. It is best to obtain an additional image slightly altering the original position of the breast to determine

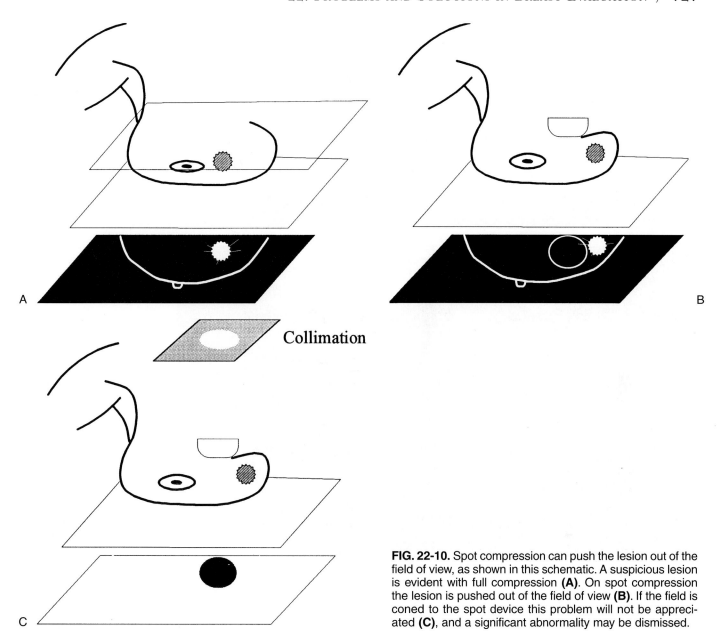

Collimation

FIG. 22-10. Spot compression can push the lesion out of the field of view, as shown in this schematic. A suspicious lesion is evident with full compression **(A)**. On spot compression the lesion is pushed out of the field of view **(B)**. If the field is coned to the spot device this problem will not be appreciated **(C)**, and a significant abnormality may be dismissed.

whether or not the lesion is real. If a superimposition of structures is suspected, a spot compression of the area may be sufficient to exclude a lesion.

Spot compression is a valuable technique, but the radiologist should always be aware that spot compression may squeeze a true lesion out from the field of view, leading to the incorrect impression that it is not real (Fig. 22-10). It is usually best to keep the collimation open on spot-compression views to permit the opportunity to recognize this problem (Fig. 22-11A, B).

The spot-compression view in the same projection may only produce the same superimposition of structures and not differentiate a true lesion from summation shadows. *For lesions seen only on the MLO projection, it is frequently best to go immediately to the straight lateral pro-*

jection. This slight shift in the orientation of the breast structures relative to the x-ray beam is often sufficient to demonstrate that an apparent abnormality is not real but rather a benign superimposition of normal structures (Fig. 22-12 A–G). If the lesion is real, its shift relative to the other structures of the breast between the two projections can help determine its location (see The Triangulation of Breast Lesions), and this information can be used to guide positioning in the CC projection to confirm its three-dimensional location.

Problem: A lesion is seen on the CC view and not on the MLO projection. When a lesion is seen only on the CC projection and not on the MLO, it is best to return to the CC position and alter the orientation of the breast relative to the x-ray beam to determine whether or not the lesion is real.

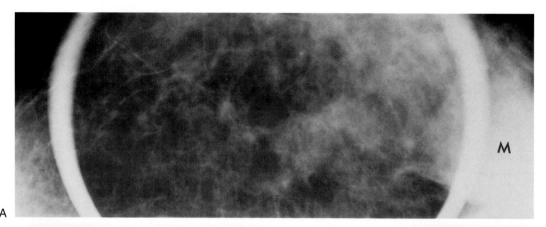

A

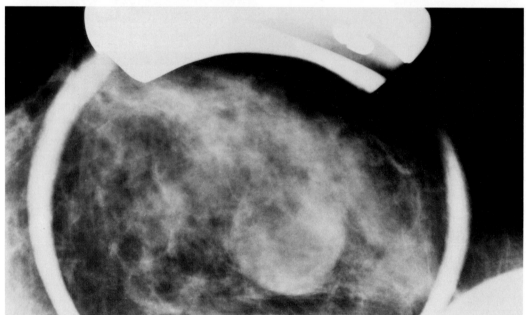

B

FIG. 22-11. In this patient a mass was seen on the craniocaudal projection. On the first spot view **(A)** it appeared that the mass was not real, but rather was superimposed tissue. However, by keeping the cones open the density is visible at the right of the image (M), having been squeezed out from under the paddle. A repeat **(B)** shows the mass, which proved to be a benign cyst.

This may require only spot compression to demonstrate a benign superimposition of structures (Fig. 22-13).

Just as when a radiologist rolls a patient under the fluoroscope, the mammography technologist can gently rotate the breast about the axis of the nipple (rolled view) and recompress in this new orientation. An image obtained in this new orientation may demonstrate that the suspected abnormality was a benign superimposition of normal structures. It may also confirm a true abnormality whose movement relative to the background of the breast may indicate its location in the upper or lower breast and guide positioning in the lateral projection to confirm this location (see Triangulation of Breast Lesions). As noted earlier, rolled views can also be performed by moving the top of the breast back toward the chest wall and pulling the bottom forward. The opposite roll can also be useful.

When obtaining rolled views, it is important for the direction of the roll to be indicated with the top of the breast as a reference. If the top of the breast is rolled laterally and the bottom medially, then the projection is the "top rolled laterally." *The direction of roll is important.* If the lesion is real, then it moves with the breast tissue in which it lies and its location is indicated by knowing which way the top and bottom of the breast were moved. The direction of roll should also be chosen so that, if the lesion is real, following the roll it is projected over fat and not dense tissue so that it is not obscured by dense tissue (see Fig. 22-9).

Use of the Lateromedial Projection

If the lesion is seen in the medial half of the breast on the CC view, positioning the lateral projection as a lateromedial view and placing the medial tissues closer to the detector (Fig. 22-14) may reveal the lesion by reducing geometric blur (Fig. 22-15). Sharpness can be increased by positioning the tissue to be imaged as close to the detector as possible. A caudocranial projection, for example, may provide a clearer image of a lesion in the top of the breast. The film

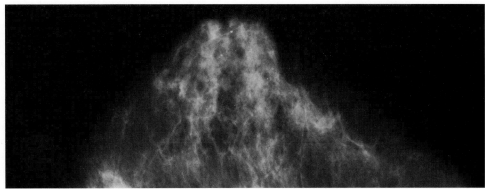

B

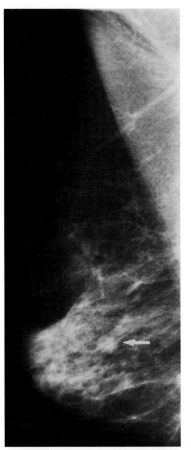

A

FIG. 22-12. There is the suggestion of a mass on the mediolateral oblique (MLO) (*arrow*) **(A)**. There is nothing on the craniocaudal (CC) **(B)** that corresponds. Returning to the view on which it was seen and modifying the projection as a straight mediolateral (ML) **(C)**, there is no abnormality. The original mass was a benign superimposition of normal structures.

In a second patient there appears to be a possible spiculated mass in the upper left breast on the MLO **(D)**. Nothing was visible on the CC projection. A straight lateral ML view **(E)** demonstrates the normal structures that had been projected over one another creating the suspicious, but nonexistent finding.

Simply because an abnormality appears high on the MLO does not mean it is in tail of the breast. *Continued.*

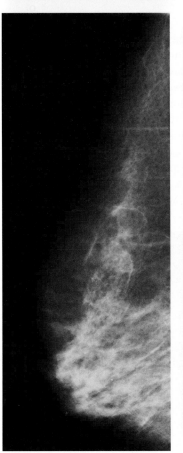

C–E

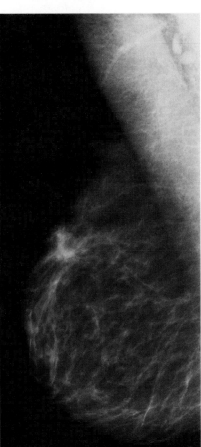

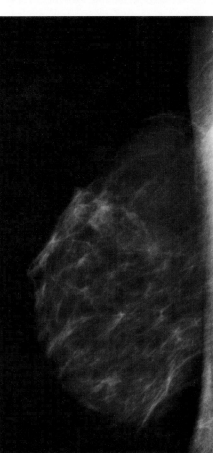

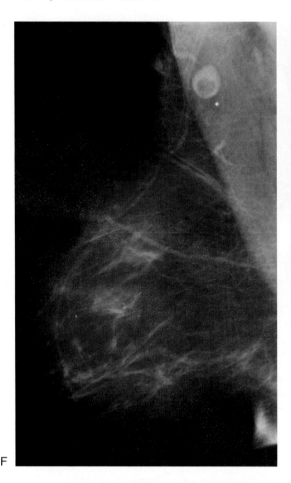

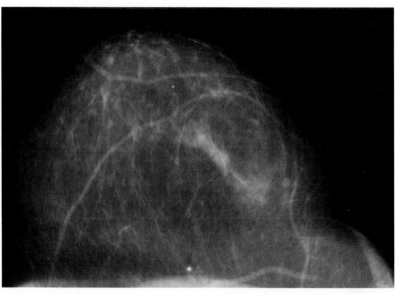

F

G

FIG. 22-12. *Continued.* The metallic marker was placed on a skin lesion and projects high on the MLO **(F)**. Note, however, that it is in the center of the breast on the CC **(G)**. Triangulation is best achieved by obtaining a straight lateral view if a lesion is seen only on the MLO and calculating its location by its movement between the two films.

holder can be placed against any surface of the breast to improve the geometry, and the breast can be rolled or turned to bring the structure in question closer to the film.

TRIANGULATION OF BREAST LESIONS

Whenever possible, any suspicious lesion should be identified in two projections so that its true, three-dimensional location within the breast is known. A good rule of thumb

should be that a biopsy should be never be recommended unless the radiologist is confident of the ability to place a needle tip in the target lesion. Conversely, however, the biopsy of a worrisome lesion should not be deferred by uncertainty as to the location of the lesion.

There are several ways to determine a lesion's location. Triangulation can be accomplished using alterations of conventional mammographic positioning. If this is unsuccessful, ultrasound can be used to find the lesion three dimensionally. If this fails, computed tomography is very

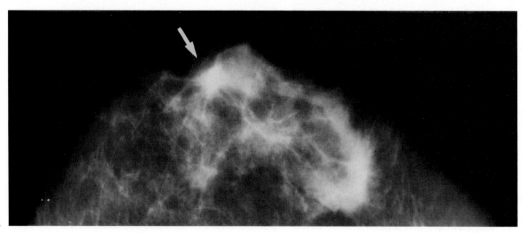

A

FIG. 22-13. For a lesion seen on the craniocaudal (CC) and not on the mediolateral oblique (MLO) projection, return and modify the CC. There is the suggestion of a spiculated lesion on the CC projection **(A)** *(arrow). Continued.*

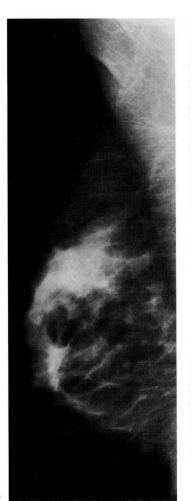

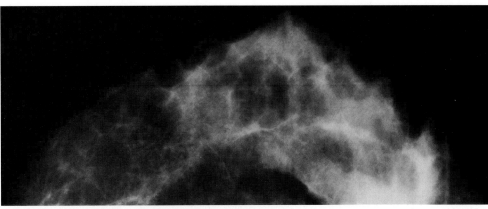

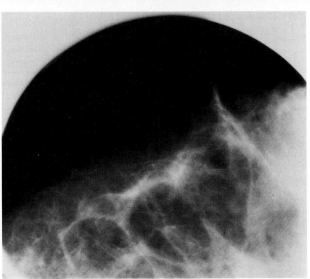

C

B,D

FIG. 22-13. *Continued.* Nothing is evident on the MLO **(B)**. The top of the breast was rolled laterally, and the abnormality fell apart **(C)**. Spot compression, in the CC projection **(D)**, also failed to demonstrate any mass. The original concern had been due to a benign superimposition of normal structures.

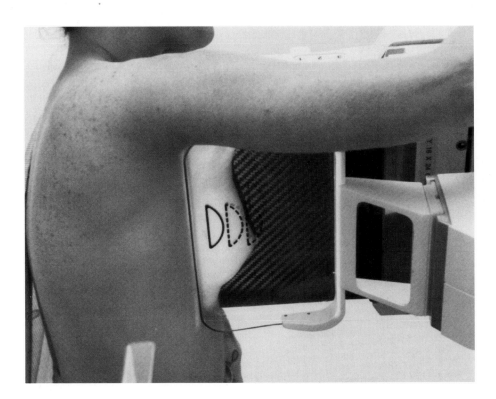

FIG. 22-14. The lateromedial projection, as shown here, is used to place the film close to a lesion that is in the medial breast **to reduce geometric blur**.

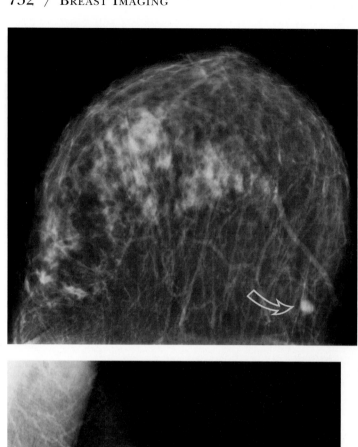

A

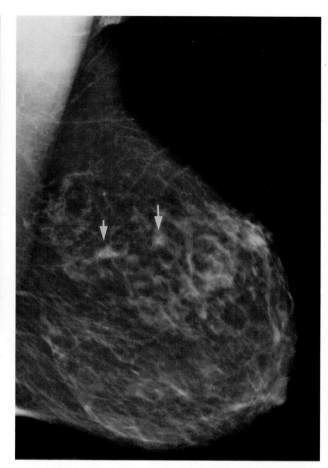

B

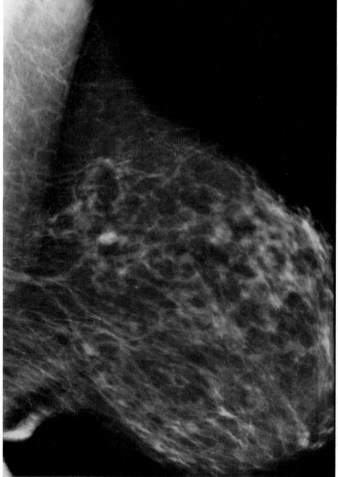

C

FIG. 22-15. The lateromedial projection is useful for imaging the medial tissue with greater sharpness. There is a clearly worrisome mass (*open arrow*) in the medial right breast on the craniocaudal projection **(A)**. It is unclear which of the densities (*arrows*) on the mediolateral oblique **(B)** is the lesion. The lateromedial projection **(C)** clearly demonstrates the lesion.

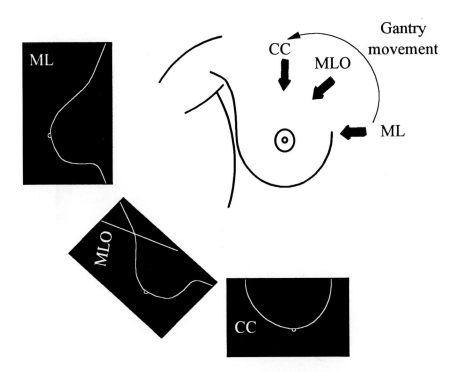

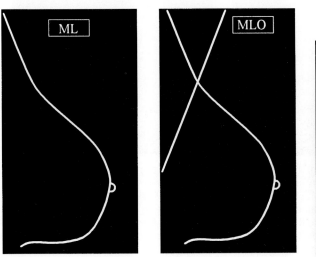

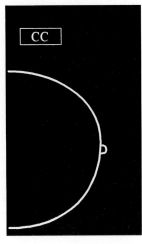

FIG. 22-16. To triangulate lesions seen on the mediolateral oblique (MLO) and not on the craniocaudal (CC), return and obtain the mediolateral (ML). Using the sequence of going from the ML through the MLO to get to the CC, the location of the lesion can be determined.

useful. If the lesion remains visible in only one projection, a needle can be accurately positioned in it using the parallax technique described in the Chapter 21, and some have used stereotactic devices to accomplish this task.

Alteration of Conventional Positioning

Lesions Seen Only on the Mediolateral Oblique Projection

When a real lesion is seen only on the MLO projection, its location can be deduced by altering that projection slightly and obtaining the straight lateral projection. Using the paral-

lax shift of the lesion relative to the background tissues between the two, its location can be determined. There have been several methods devised to assist in this determination (4). The process can be simplified by considering the fact that the straight lateral (90-degree) projection, MLO, and CC views, although obtained in a different sequence, are actually a progression of images. If the mammographic unit were a fluoroscope, the progression would be from the straight lateral through the oblique to get to the CC view (Fig. 22-16). The movement of a lesion relative to the background of the breast from the straight lateral relative to the oblique can be used to predict the lesion's location on the CC projection.

Sickles has devised a simple approach based on geometry (5). The films are placed in line on a view box with the

FIG. 22-17. To determine the location of a lesion seen on the mediolateral oblique (MLO) but not on the craniocaudal (CC), obtain the mediolateral (ML) and align the films on the view box with the nipples at the same level and pointing in the same direction and the axilla at the top of the view box. The films are placed in line on a view box with the straight lateral on one end, the CC view on the other, and the MLO in between.

straight lateral on one end, the CC view on the other, and the MLO in between with the nipple on the same side of each film. The CC view should be positioned with the lateral portion at the top, and the nipples on all three films should be in a line (Fig. 22-17). If the films are arranged in this fashion and in this order, a line drawn from the lesion as it appears on the straight lateral and passing through the lesion on the MLO will point to the portion of the breast in which the lesion can be found on the CC projection. Once the area of the breast is known, the appropriate orthogonal projection can be obtained to confirm the lesion's location.

If a lesion starts in the upper portion of the breast on the straight lateral (Fig. 22-18) *and*

1. It remains high or moves even higher on the MLO, it will be found in the lateral portion of the breast on the CC view (see Fig. 22-18 A–C).
2. It moves down a short distance on the MLO, the lesion is likely in the central portion of the breast.
3. It moves down a large distance on the MLO, then the lesion is likely in the medial portion of the breast on the CC projection (see Fig. 22-18 D–F).

If a lesion starts in the center of the breast on the straight lateral (Fig. 22-19A) *and*

1. It moves higher on the MLO, it will be found in the lateral portion of the breast on the CC view.

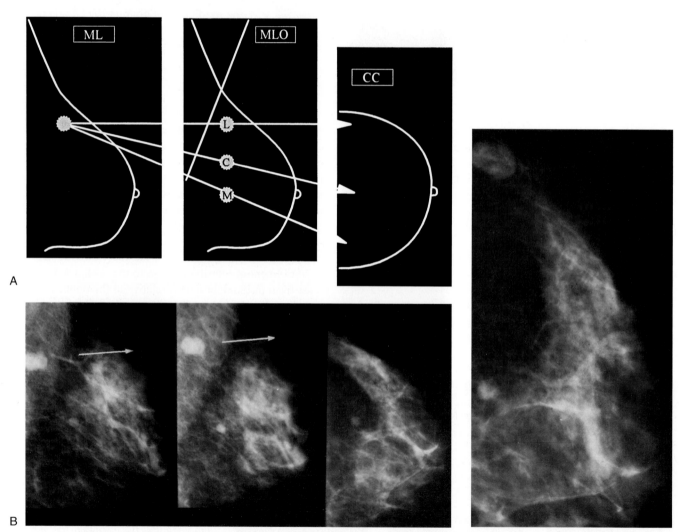

FIG. 22-18. A line drawn from the lesion on the mediolateral (ML) to its location on the mediolateral oblique (MLO) will point to the portion of the breast in which it can be found on the craniocaudal (CC). This diagram **(A)** is for a lesion that is high in the breast on the ML. In this patient a mass was seen on the MLO, but not on the CC, projection. The straight lateral was obtained showing the mass. By lining up the straight lateral followed by the MLO with the CC projection (keeping the nipples in line) **(B)**, a line through the lesion on the two lateral projections points to the lateral portion of the breast on the CC. The location of the lesion in this portion of the breast was confirmed on the CC image exaggerated laterally **(C)**. Note that the second, small mass in the center of the breast is in a line on the three images. *Continued.*

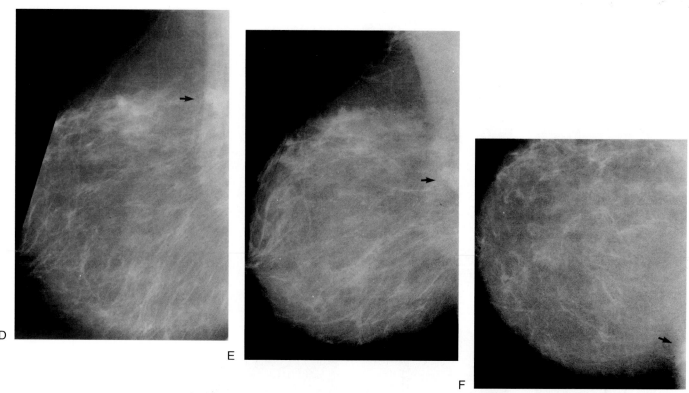

FIG. 22-18. *Continued.* In this second case, lining up the mediolateral (ML) **(D)** with the mediolateral oblique (MLO) **(E)** and the craniocaudal (CC) **(F)** will result in a line connecting the lesion (*arrow*) on the ML and passing through the lesion on the MLO (*arrow*), pointing to the location of the invasive cancer medially (*arrow*) on the CC **(F)**.

2. It remains in the center on the MLO, the lesion is likely in the central portion of the breast.
3. It moves down on the MLO, then the lesion is likely in the medial portion of the breast on the CC projection.

If a lesion starts in the bottom of the breast on the straight lateral (Fig. 22-19B) *and*

1. It stays at the bottom or moves lower on the MLO, it will be found in the medial portion of the breast on the CC view.
2. It moves a short distance up on the MLO, the lesion is likely in the central portion of the breast.
3. It moves a long distance up on the MLO, then the lesion is likely in the lateral portion of the breast on the CC projection.

Lesions Seen Only on the Craniocaudal Projection

The triangulation of lesions seen only on the CC projection can be evaluated using rolled views. By monitoring the direction that the breast is rolled, the location of the lesion is evident. The relationship is simple.

If the top of the breast is rolled laterally and the lesion moves laterally, then it is in the top of the breast (Fig.

22-20A). If it moves medially, then it is in the bottom of the breast (Fig. 22-20B).

Conversely, if the top of the breast is rolled medially and the lesion moves medially, then it is in the top of the breast (Fig. 22-20C). If it moves laterally, then it is in the bottom of the breast (Fig. 22-20D).

If the top of the breast is rolled back toward the chest wall and the lesion moves back, then it is in the top of the breast.

Conversely, if the top of the breast is moved back and the lesion moves forward, then it is in the bottom of the breast.

Use of Ultrasound to Triangulate a Mass

Masses and even some highly calcified lesions can be located by ultrasound. If a lesion is shown to be real but its exact location remains elusive, ultrasound of the expected volume of tissue that contains the lesion can locate it three dimensionally if there are not too many confusing structures nearby (Fig. 22-21). In order to corroborate that what is seen on ultrasound is concordant with what is seen on the mammogram, a needle can be passed through the lesion under ultrasound guidance and then a repeat mammogram should show the needle passing through the lesion.

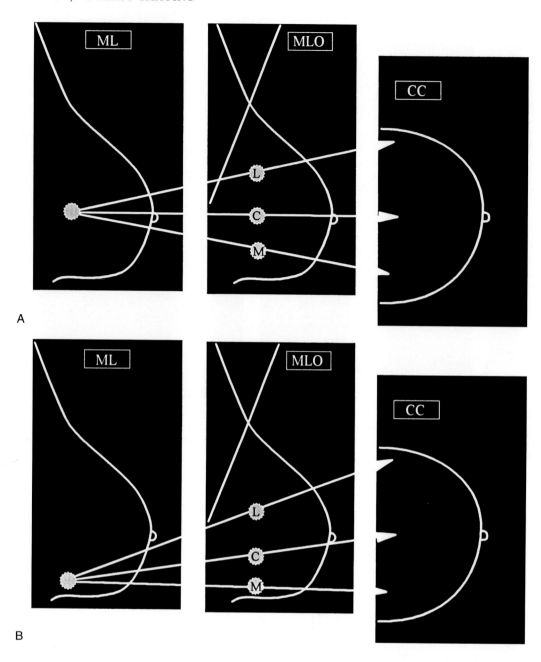

FIG. 22-19. This schematic (A) shows the movement of a lesion that starts in the middle of the breast on the mediolateral (ML). The third schematic (B) shows the location of a lesion that is found in the lower breast on the ML.

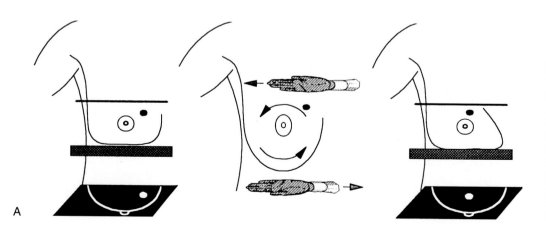

FIG. 22-20. Rolled views can be used to determine the location of a lesion seen only in the craniocaudal (CC) projection. If the **top is rolled laterally** and the lesion moves laterally (A), it is in the top of the breast. This is labeled "CC RL" for craniocaudal projection top rolled laterally. *Continued.*

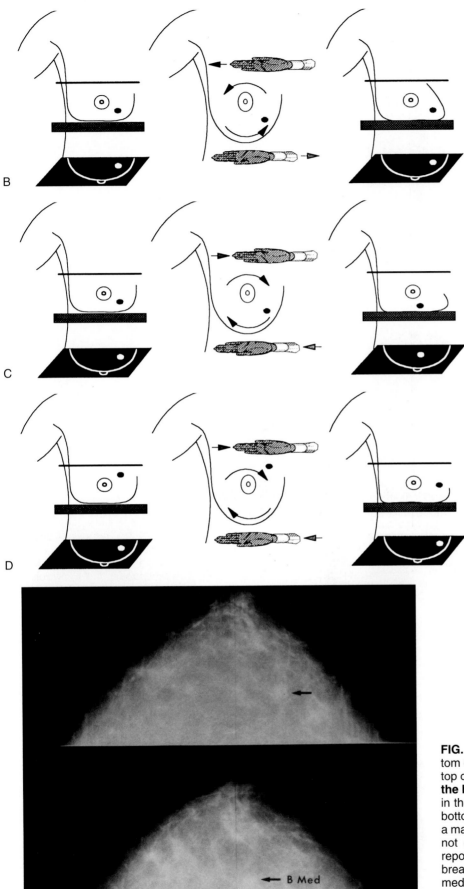

B

C

D

E

FIG. 22-20. *Continued.* If the lesion is in the bottom of the breast, it will move medially when the top of the breast moves laterally **(B)**. If the **top of the breast is rolled medially** (CC RM), a lesion in the top will move medially **(C)**, and one in the bottom will move laterally **(D)**. In this patient **(E)** a mass was seen on the CC view (top image) but not on the mediolateral oblique. The CC was repositioned rolling the top laterally, and the breast was recompressed. The lesion moved medially (bottom image) and consequently was in the bottom of the breast.

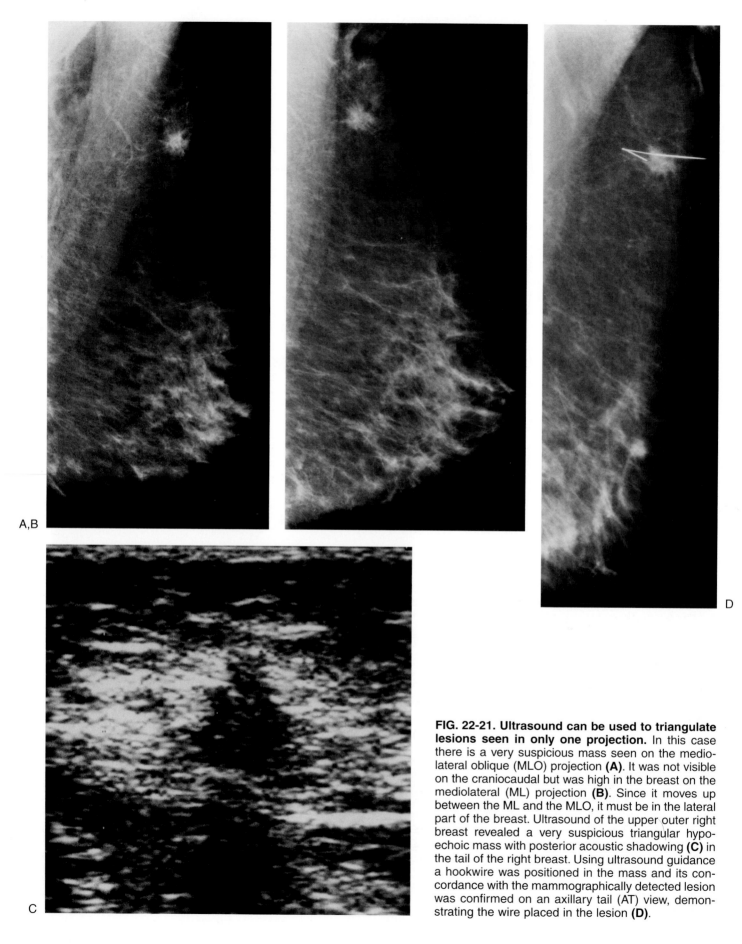

FIG. 22-21. Ultrasound can be used to triangulate lesions seen in only one projection. In this case there is a very suspicious mass seen on the mediolateral oblique (MLO) projection **(A)**. It was not visible on the craniocaudal but was high in the breast on the mediolateral (ML) projection **(B)**. Since it moves up between the ML and the MLO, it must be in the lateral part of the breast. Ultrasound of the upper outer right breast revealed a very suspicious triangular hypoechoic mass with posterior acoustic shadowing **(C)** in the tail of the right breast. Using ultrasound guidance a hookwire was positioned in the mass and its concordance with the mammographically detected lesion was confirmed on an axillary tail (AT) view, demonstrating the wire placed in the lesion **(D)**.

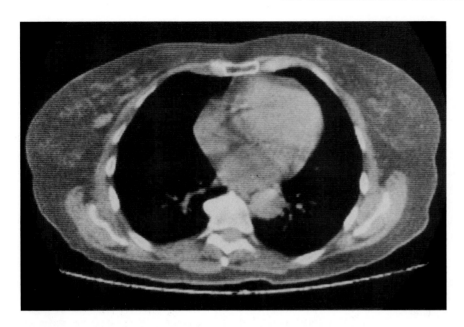

FIG. 22-22. Computed tomography can be used to triangulate a lesion that is difficult to triangulate by mammography or ultrasound. The lesion in the right breast is obvious because it is surrounded by fat.

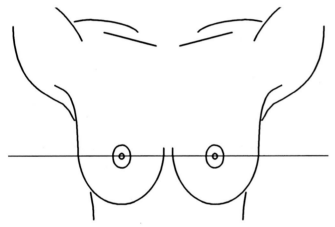

FIG. 22-23. The patient should be positioned so that her breasts are symmetric in the scanner with the nipples in the same scan plane.

Computed Tomography

When additional mammographic views or ultrasound are unable to triangulate the location of a lesion, computed tomography can be very helpful for locating lesions three dimensionally (Fig. 22-22).

The patient is placed in the gantry in the supine position with her arms extended and hands comfortably positioned behind her head. The breasts should be positioned as symmetrically as possible. The patient should be rolled so that nipple areolar complexes are at the same height above the table and in the same scan plane (Fig. 22-23) to try to ensure that the same volumes of tissue are positioned symmetrically. In general, significant lesions are visible as areas of asymmetric attenuation. The appreciation of symmetry and asymmetry necessitates symmetric positioning of the breasts within the gantry, and thus attention to initial positioning facilitates the study.

The patient should be instructed to not take deep breaths. Gentle breathing should be encouraged to avoid shifting the breasts by thoracic movement. In general, the area in question will have been seen mammographically in the upper, middle, or lower portions of the breast, and consequently scans can often be limited to one of these areas.

Initial imaging is performed using 1-cm–thick contiguous slices. The breasts are compared for symmetry on each slice. When the level of concern is identified, thinner slices are useful to refine the image, and are necessary for accurate preoperative localization.

Contrast-Enhanced Computed Tomography

Just as with gadolinium on MRI, cancers enhance with intravenously administered iodinated contrast. This can be helpful in defining the location of a lesion (Fig. 22-24). CT can be used to position needles for localization and biopsy (see Chapter 21).

IMPLANTS

Implants (see Chapter 17) present a problem for breast imaging in that they may prevent optimal visualization of the tissues. If a lesion is suspected, the same maneuvers described previously can be employed in conjunction with implant displacement views. Spot-compression and magnification views are possible. If the lesion is hidden by the implant on all but a single projection, ultrasound may help guide the three-dimensional location, evaluation, needle biopsy localization, and excision of masses.

Conventional, stereotactic, and ultrasound-guided biopsy can be performed by positioning the needle parallel to a tangent to the surface of the implant. By displacing the implant,

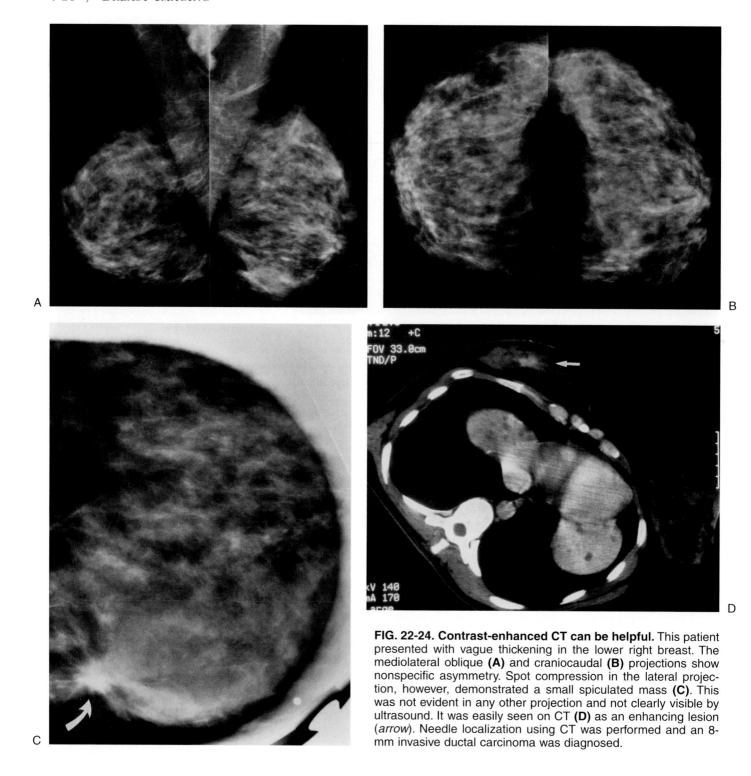

FIG. 22-24. Contrast-enhanced CT can be helpful. This patient presented with vague thickening in the lower right breast. The mediolateral oblique **(A)** and craniocaudal **(B)** projections show nonspecific asymmetry. Spot compression in the lateral projection, however, demonstrated a small spiculated mass **(C)**. This was not evident in any other projection and not clearly visible by ultrasound. It was easily seen on CT **(D)** as an enhancing lesion (*arrow*). Needle localization using CT was performed and an 8-mm invasive ductal carcinoma was diagnosed.

standard needle localization can be performed using a fenestrated compression plate (6) (see Chapter 21). If the implant presents an obstruction, needle positioning can be accomplished using ultrasound or the parallax technique described in Chapter 21. Some radiologists use stereotactic devices to accomplish these procedures with the implant displaced from the field of view.

MAGNIFICATION MAMMOGRAPHY

Magnification mammography theoretically provides an absolute increase in resolution, but in reality the image is improved primarily by the reduction in the noise. Magnification is of value when this will aid diagnosis and management. Magnification is valuable in analyzing the morphology and

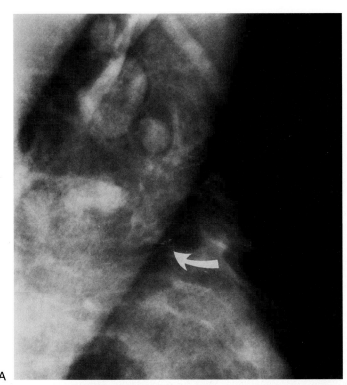
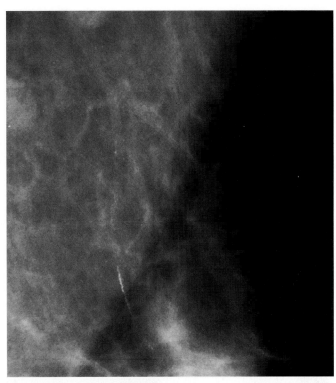

A   B

FIG. 22-25. Magnification is valuable for analyzing the morphology of calcifications. These calcifications (*arrow*) appeared to be heterogeneous, fine, and linear in their distribution **(A)**. Magnification shows that they are in the wall of a tubular structure **(B)** and are benign vascular deposits.

distribution of calcifications (Fig. 22-25) and the margins of lesions. Because of the longer exposures involved, the quality of the magnification image can be compromised by motion. If calcifications seem to disappear on the magnification image, motion is the likely cause.

Problem: The solitary circumscribed mass. Magnification mammography is useful in the evaluation of circumscribed masses to ensure that their margins are indeed well defined. If the lesion is round or oval and has well-defined margins over 75% of its border on magnification in two projections,

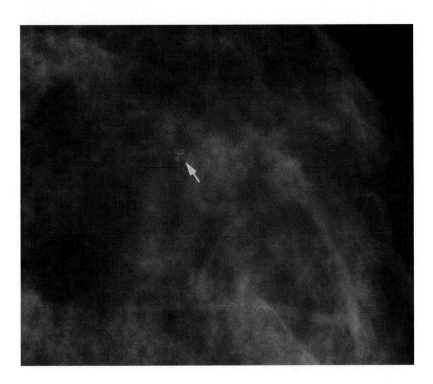

FIG. 22-26. Calcifications in the skin can project as intramammary deposits. These pleomorphic-appearing calcifications (*arrow*) proved to be benign dermal deposits.

it has a <5% probability of malignancy that is independent of its size.

Problem: The focal asymmetric density. A focal asymmetric density may merely represent an island of breast tissue. This can frequently be determined by analyzing the standard mammographic projections. If there is the suggestion that the asymmetry represents a mass, then magnification views may help in the assessment. Generally, if there is truly fat within the lesion, it does not represent cancer (caution: overlapping structures can give the appearance of fat within). There are rare cancers that present as irregular, ill-defined masses that infiltrate in a discontinuous fashion and are interspersed with fat.

Problem: Calcifications may be in the skin. On rare occasions calcifications in the skin can simulate a suspicious intramammary lesion (Fig. 22-26) (7). This can be appreciated if one considers that the breast is a spherical organ, and, because only a very small portion of the skin is seen in tangent, when the breast is compressed in any one projection deposits on its surface can be expected to project as if they lie within the breast itself (Fig. 22-27). Most skin calcifications and skin lesions are easily recognized from their morphology, but if this is not clearly apparent the location of a lesion in the skin can be readily confirmed.

Analyzing the mammogram, the suspected skin surface is determined by the proximity of the lesion to the medial, lateral, inferior, or superior surface of the breast. The patient is positioned in the mammographic system using a fenestrated compression plate in a manner similar to that followed for a needle localization. The window should encompass the area of skin in which the calcifications are expected to lie. It is very important that the proper skin surface is in the window. A small radiopaque marker is taped to the skin at the suspected site of the calcifications (Fig. 22-28). This is confirmed mammographically. The importance of placing the proper surface in the window can be seen, for example, if a marker was placed on the top of the breast. On the mammo-

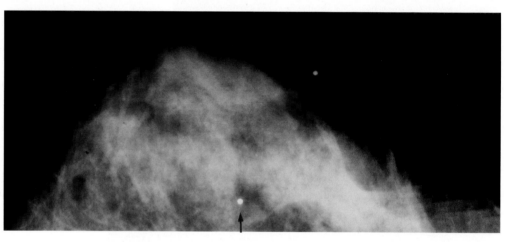

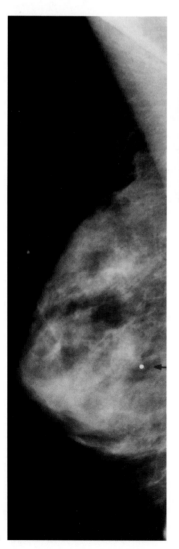

FIG. 22-27. Because only two thin tangents of skin are seen in the two projections, most deposits in (or on) the skin project over the breast. This marker (*arrow*) was placed on a skin lesion. It is clearly on the skin, but it projects over the center of the breast tissues on the mediolateral oblique (**A**) and craniocaudal (**B**) views.

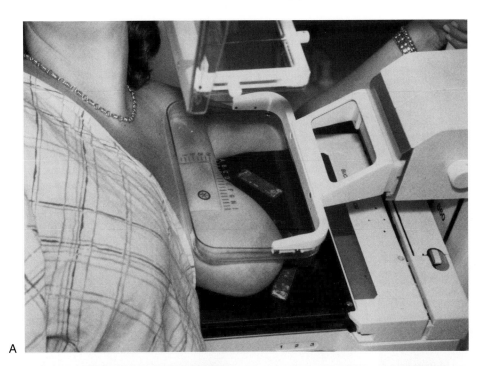

A

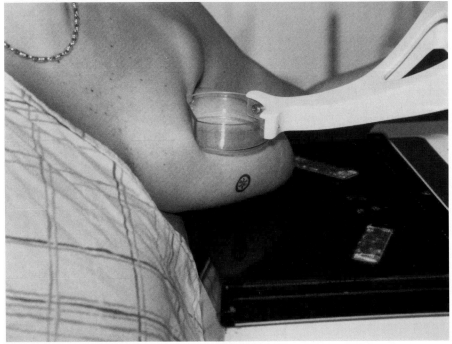

B

FIG. 22-28. Skin localization. To prove that calcifications are in the skin and of no consequence, the breast is positioned in the mammography machine using a window compression system with the skin surface, thought to contain the calcifications, in the window of the compression system **(A)**. A marker is taped to the skin at this location using a scout film and the localization crosshairs to determine the coordinates of the calcifications. The technologist should remember that the marker may appear to be on the calcifications on the mammogram but may actually be on the exact opposite side of the breast. The marker must be taped to the skin surface that contains the calcifications. This marker enables the tangential view **(B)** to confirm that the lesion represents benign dermal deposits. *Continued.*

graphic projection it will look as if it is over calcifications, even if they are actually in the bottom of the breast, and the tangential views will be misleading if the marker is on the wrong skin surface.

Once the marker is in position, the patient is removed from the compression system. The breast is then positioned so that the x-ray beam is tangent to the skin surface under the marker. The skin immediately beneath the marker will be viewed from the side, and if calcifications are present in the skin their

location will be absolutely confirmed or the calcifications will be shown to be in the breast tissue (Fig. 22-29). Dermal deposits are never malignant and need not be biopsied.

Raised skin lesions can project as if they are within the breast. Confusion can be avoided by taping a small radiopaque marker on the skin lesion (Fig. 22-30). Repeat mammography will confirm the correspondence of the marker with the lesion. A tangential view may be obtained to further corroborate this if necessary.

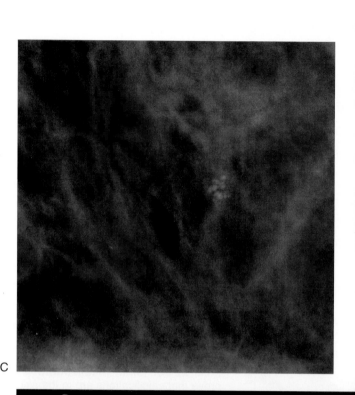

C

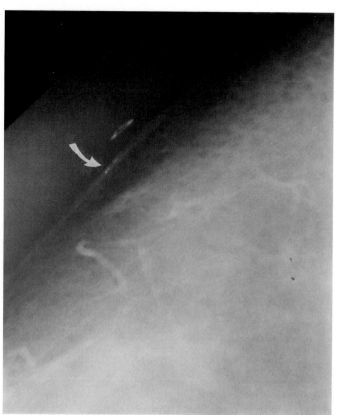

F

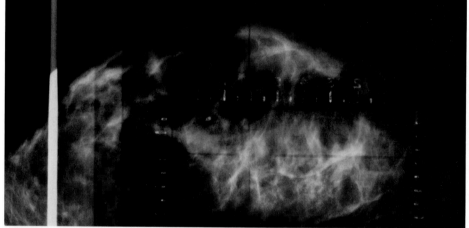

D

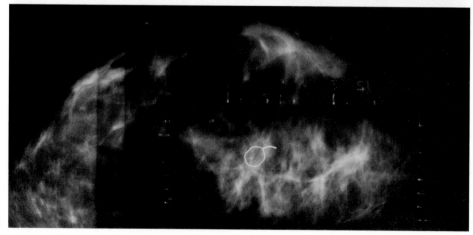

E

FIG. 22-28. *Continued.* In this case calcifications were thought to be worrisome on an outside interpretation **(C)**. The breast was compressed using the window compression paddle, and a marker was placed over the calcifications using the coordinates derived from a scout film **(D)**. The proximity of the marker to the calcifications was confirmed **(E)** and then an image was obtained at low kVp (to image the skin) in tangent to the marker **(F)**. The calcifications are visible in the skin (*arrow*) and of no consequence.

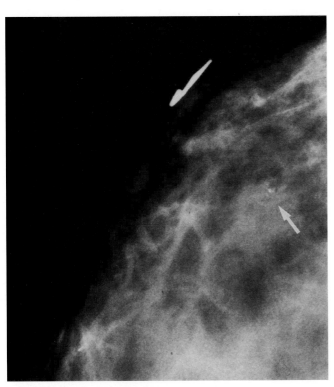

FIG. 22-29. In this case tangential imaging showed that the calcifications were not in the skin. The marker on the skin is distant from the calcifications (*arrow*). A biopsy revealed **ductal carcinoma in situ.**

REFERENCES

1. Sickles EA, Weber WN, Galvin HB, et al. Baseline screening mammography: one vs. two views per breast. AJR Am J Roentgenol 1986;147:1149–1150.
2. Wald NJ, Murphy P, Major P, et al. UKCCCR multicentre randomised controlled trial of one and two view mammography in breast cancer screening. BMJ 1995;311:1189–1193.
3. Folio LR, Bennett CA. Nipple arc localization. Appl Radiol 1994;(December):17–19.
4. Swann CA, Kopans DB, McCarthy KA, et al. Practical solutions to problems of triangulation and preoperative localization of breast lesions. Radiology 1987;163:577–579.
5. Sickles EA. Practical solutions to common mammographic problems: tailoring the examination. AJR Am J Roentgenol 1988;151:31–39.
6. Robertson CL, Kopans DB, McCarthy KA, Hart NE. Nonpalpable lesions in the augmented breast: preoperative localization. Radiology 1989;173:873–874.
7. Kopans DB, Meyer JE, Homer MJ, Grabbe J. Dermal deposits mistaken for breast calcifications. Radiology 1983;149:592.

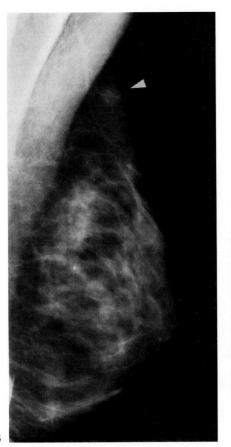
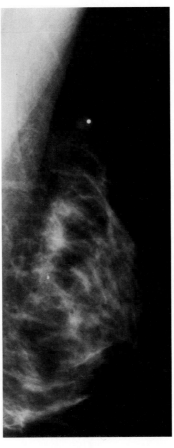

A,B

FIG. 22-30. On the initial study there was the suggestion of a mass in the upper right breast on the mediolateral oblique projection **(A)**. Inspection of the patient's skin revealed a raised skin lesion. A marker was taped to it **(B)**, confirming that the density on the mammogram was the benign skin lesion and no further evaluation was needed.

Breast Imaging, 2nd ed., by Daniel B. Kopans.
Lippincott–Raven Publishers, Philadelphia © 1998.

CHAPTER 23

Palpable Abnormalities and Breast Imaging

Although mammography is used routinely and is a standard of care, it is actually of limited value in the evaluation of clinically evident breast abnormalities. In most cases, by the time a cancer becomes palpable, the potential benefit from mammography has passed. The primary value of mammography is the earlier detection of breast cancer through the screening of asymptomatic women. However, mammography is used routinely to assess the symptomatic individual who has a lump, thickening, discharge, or other sign or symptom that might indicate a possible malignancy.

The efficacy of mammography for symptomatic women is less well defined than its use for screening. Because mammography fails to demonstrate between 5% and 15% of cancers, it cannot be relied on to exclude a malignancy and the ultimate management of a palpable abnormality usually must be determined by the clinical assessment. There is some value from mammography for the symptomatic woman, but its value should not be overestimated.

CLINICAL BREAST EXAMINATION

Clinical breast examination (CBE) is usually a fairly crude evaluation that is compromised by marked variation in the skills of the practitioner and "interperformer" variation. It is often inaccurate due to the heterogeneous texture of normal breast tissues (Fig. 23-1). It is well established, however, that there are breast cancers that can be detected by CBE that are not detected by mammography. The Health Insurance Plan of New York (HIP) demonstrated the efficacy of physical examination screening to reduce the mortality from breast cancer. The women in that trial, who enjoyed a 20% to 30% decrease in mortality, had been screened by both mammography and CBE (1). It has even been suggested that much of the benefit in that trial was due to the CBE because the mammography was not of particularly high quality.

Additional support for screening using CBE was established in the Breast Cancer Detection Demonstration Project (BCDDP), where almost 9% of the cancers were detected only by CBE and were not found by mammography (2).

The benefit from clinical examination is likely to be greatest when the comparison group that is not screened has cancers diagnosed at a late stage, and even clinical examination can lead to a "down-staging" for those screened. This is likely what happened in the HIP study. As more of comparison women have their cancers detected at an earlier stage, it becomes more difficult to demonstrate added benefit.

Although the efficacy of physical examination by itself to reduce mortality has not been tested, it is likely that in a small percentage of women periodic screening by physical examination is efficacious.

It is probable that periodic, properly performed screening with CBE can detect a number of early cancers that might otherwise escape early detection, and CBE should probably be part of a complete screening program. Unfortunately, by the time many cancers are large enough to feel, the patient's course is often already determined and the likelihood that metastatic spread has already occurred is fairly high. Almost 50% of women with cancers that are 2 cm in size or larger have positive axillary lymph nodes (Fig. 23-2) (3) and complete cure is unlikely. Regardless, since a palpable abnormality is apparent to the patient as well as the physician, the care of these patients is of great importance and certainly of medical/legal consequence. The leading cause of malpractice actions in the United States stems from the failure to diagnose palpable cancers.

Who Should Perform Clinical Breast Examination?

Ideally CBE should be performed by well-trained health professionals who take the time to do a thorough examination. In most instances this is the responsibility of the primary care physician. In the National Breast Screening Study of Canada (NBSS) screening trial, highly trained nurses performed high-quality CBE (4). They demonstrated the need for a thorough examination that often took 10 to 15 minutes to perform. Unfortunately, most physicians in the United States do not perform adequate CBEs.

It has been suggested that mammography technologists should be trained to perform breast physical examination. There is no reason not to train technologists, but the primary role of the x-ray technologist is to perform high-quality mammography; she should be highly skilled in mammographic techniques before she takes on any added responsibility. The success of physical examination is as dependent on the care and quality of the examination as the mammo-

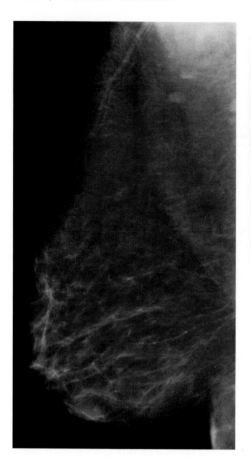

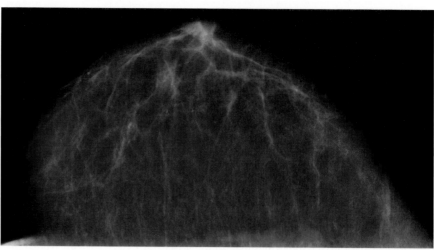

FIG. 23-1. The clinical breast examination (CBE) is often inaccurate. This patient was referred for mammography with the diagnosis of fibrocystic changes and multiple masses on CBE. In fact, the breast tissues are almost all fat. There are no cysts and no masses. The clinician was feeling the lumpy texture of normal breast tissue.

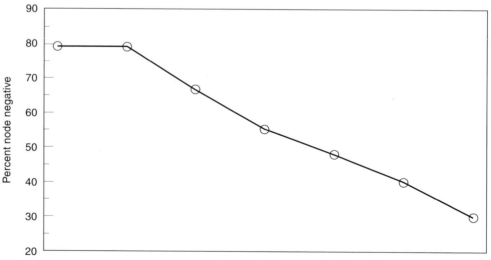

Tumor size in cm.	<0.5	0.5-0.9	1-1.9	2-2.9	3-3.9	4-4.9	>5
Percentage with negative nodes ⊖	79.4	79.4	66.8	55.1	47.9	40.0	29.9

FIG. 23-2. The relationship of tumor size to lymph node involvement. Breast cancer size and nodal status are based on data from the Surveillance, Epidemiology, and End Results program of the National Cancer Institute, 1977–1983. Percentage of woman who are axillary lymph-node negative in relationship to the size of the invasive cancer. (Adapted from Carter CL, Allen C, Henson DE. Relation of tumor size, lymph node status, and survival in 24,740 breast cancer cases. Cancer 1989;63:181–187.)

graphic detection of malignancy is dependent on the care and quality exercised in obtaining and interpreting the mammogram. There are no doubt technologists who are interested in expanding their expertise and responsibility and wish to perform physical examinations as well, but this should not be a requirement and a technologist should not be expected to perform CBE unless properly trained.

Similarly, there are radiologists who extend their expertise and responsibility and perform physical examination. This should be encouraged because it likely enhances interpretive skills in the analysis of breast imaging studies. Physical examination, however, is a separate test from mammography, and the performance of a physical examination should not be a requirement for performing mammography any more than palpation of the abdomen should be a part of the abdominal imaging examination or auscultation of the chest a part of interpreting the chest radiograph.

Physical examination should not be considered a casual function but a technique requiring time, patience, and thoroughness. Only those who are interested in its performance and are willing to be trained and spend the time should be relied on to perform CBEs. The standard of care for the radiologist should be the supervision of the performance of high-quality mammography and careful and thoughtful interpretation of the images.

Correlative Clinical Breast Examination

It has been suggested that the radiologist or technologist perform an exam targeting the area for which the patient was referred. The principal reason for doing this is to ensure that the area of concern is included in the mammogram and to guide spot-compression views if they are to be obtained. One problem with this approach is that there is no way of ensuring that the area palpated by a technologist or radiologist is the same area that concerned the referring physician. At best only the area indicated by the patient can be evaluated.

The basic reason for urging this examination is due to the misinterpretation of data. In 1983 we published a study that suggested that a physical examination by the radiologist was valuable for guiding additional imaging to ensure that a clinically evident abnormality was included in the field of view of the mammogram. At that time, attention to proper positioning was not as rigorous as it is now, and many of the lesions imaged as a result of the additional views prompted by the clinical examination were in regions of the breast that had not been imaged on the initial study. Although we concluded that a correlative physical examination was useful, we did not prove that it had true clinical efficacy (5). Despite our speculation, as far as can be determined these lesions would have been biopsied based on the clinical concern regardless of the mammographic evaluation so that the additional imaging did not actually alter the management of the problem.

A correlative clinical examination by the technologist has also been suggested to help target spot-compression mammography of an area of clinical concern. Technologists are not formally trained to do this, and it should not be considered standard. The reasons for spot compression are discussed later in this chapter, but there are no data confirming that spot compression of an area of clinical concern improves the early detection of breast cancer or alters mortality, which is the basic issue in breast cancer. Spot compression of a palpable area should not be considered a standard of care, although many radiologists may wish to have the additional imaging performed.

DIAGNOSTIC MAMMOGRAPHY

Unfortunately, the success of mammography in detecting early cancers does not mean that it has the truly diagnostic capability of being able to make a diagnosis. In fact, it has been shown repeatedly that there are many cancers that are not even visible by mammography and that mammography lacks diagnostic specificity and cannot reliably differentiate benign lesions from malignant. In our quest to solve the problems of breast cancer, we occasionally imbue the technique with capabilities that it does not possess.

Mammography is best used as a screening technique. By definition, a screening modality is a filter to sift out those most likely to have a given disease from the background of those who are at risk. A Pap test, for example, is useful in determining which women are most likely to have cervical cancer, but additional tests are needed to confirm the diagnosis and false-positives are not uncommon until the definitive biopsy is undertaken. Mammography is the Pap test of the breast. Frequently the mammogram reveals a lesion that is almost certain to be malignant, but because there are rare benign lesions such as radial scars, granular cell tumors, and occasional areas of fat necrosis that can mimic even the classic signs of breast cancer, cytologic or histologic confirmation of malignancy is required.

MAMMOGRAPHY AND THE PALPABLE ABNORMALITY

Numerous articles have shown that in most instances mammography cannot and should not be used to exclude breast cancer (6–8). Even in the most optimistic series, mammography misses at least 5% of breast cancers that are found because they are palpable. If the cancers that reach clinical detectability within a year following a negative screen are included, even more cancers may be undetectable at any given time by mammography. In the BCDDP, 9% of cancers were palpable but not detected by mammography at the time of screening and an additional 20% became clinically evident within one year of a negative screen (2). It is almost certain that these interval cancers were present at the time of screening but were not detectable by mammography.

This false-negative rate for mammography should not be interpreted as a failure of the technique but as rather a reality that must be understood. Mammography does detect the vast majority of cancers and has been shown to be able to detect them 1.5 to 4 years before their clinical detectability (9). Despite the fact that mammography does not detect all cancers, a cancer that is detected by mammography alone is usually at a smaller size and earlier stage than a clinically apparent cancer, and this translates into survival and mortality benefit.

Finally, mammography is not an accurate way to separate benign from malignant lesions. The fact that most lesions detected by mammography that raise concern prove to be benign is evidence of the lack of diagnostic specificity of the test. Even in the Swedish Two County screening trial, which had to keep the false-positive rate as low as possible, 30% of biopsies instigated by mammography revealed benign processes.

These facts emphasize the reality that mammography is a screening technique and not a diagnostic test.

A Negative Mammogram Does Not Exclude Cancer

Because physical examination can detect cancers that are not visible on the mammogram, a negative mammogram does not preclude the possibility of a cancer. The mammogram and physical examination evaluate different tissue characteristics. Two studies have shown that the mammographic appearance of even normal breast tissue cannot predict the characteristics of the tissue that will be found on clinical examination. Conversely, the consistency of the breast on physical examination does not predict its mammographic appearance (10,11). Since the two tests measure different tissue characteristics, concern raised by either test can rarely be negated by the other.

Value of Mammography for Symptomatic Women

One might conclude from the preceding discussion that mammography is not important in the symptomatic patient. This is not the case. There are times when mammography is diagnostic and can aid in the management of a palpable abnormality. Fat-containing lesions such as lipomas, post-traumatic oil cysts, and hamartomas that are seen on mammography need not be biopsied, despite the fact that they are palpable.

In addition, although the absence of suspicious morphologic characteristics on the mammogram does not eliminate the possibility of cancer, on occasion the mammogram shows very suspicious morphologic changes that increase the likelihood that a palpable abnormality is malignant and may prompt earlier intervention when a cancer is present. In most instances, however, the clinician must make a decision based on the clinical evaluation when a palpable abnormality is present.

Even for the symptomatic woman, mammography is primarily a screening test, and if the woman in question can benefit from screening, then mammography is indicated. Since most palpable abnormalities prove to be benign, in the

women with a sign or symptom the mammogram is used to screen the remainder of the ipsilateral breast and the contralateral breast for clinically occult cancer. If the palpable mass is indeed malignant, the prebiopsy mammogram may be useful in assessing the extent of the disease. This becomes important if breast conservation is to be considered as the definitive treatment.

By viewing mammography primarily as a screening test, other questions as to its use can be answered. In women who are not very likely to have breast cancer in the first place (those younger than 35), screening (and, hence, mammography) is not indicated unless they have a genetic predisposition to breast cancer (a mother or sister with bilateral premenopausal breast cancer or a previous high-risk lesion, such as LCIS or ADH, or known BRCA1 or BRCA2 mutations). In women who are not at elevated risk, lumps should probably be evaluated and managed on a clinical basis. From a scientific perspective, mammography is not indicated for these women unless there is a significant likelihood that screening the ipsilateral and contralateral breast will reveal an occult cancer. A mammogram, however, may be useful if the clinical suspicion is not sufficiently high to prompt a biopsy. In the latter case a mammogram revealing suspicious calcifications or a mass might tip the balance toward earlier intervention. Although mammography can demonstrate cancers among these women (12), its value among very young women is based on anecdotal experiences. Williams and colleagues found no clinical benefit from mammography among women younger than age 30 (13). Liberman and colleagues found that among 5,105 asymptomatic women between the ages of 35 and 39 who were screened there were eight cancers (five DCIS and three invasive). The detection rate of 1.6 per 1,000 was the same as their detection rate for women aged 40 to 49 (14). Screening these women may have efficacy. Because women younger than 39 were not included in the screening trials, there are no prospective data supporting the use of mammography before the age of 35. Since there is no universally accepted standard for evaluating these women, in the absence of compelling scientific evidence individual experience should dictate practice.

Mammographic Workup

Many teachers of mammography have become advocates of "the workup." It is suggested that a biopsy should not be advised until additional mammographic views are obtained. Magnification mammography, in particular, with the absolute improvement in sharpness that it provides, may reveal elements that are not apparent on contact imaging. Once again, however, the importance of these extra views is anecdotal and not confirmed by any prospective analysis.

Coned-Down Spot Compression for the Palpable Lesion

The question remains as to whether these additional views have any impact on the proper care of the patient.

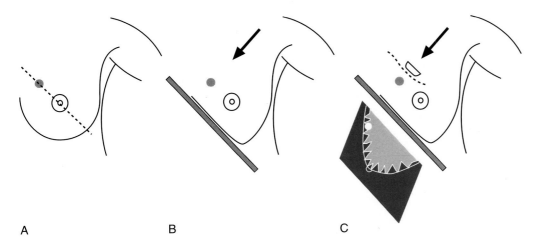

FIG. 23-3. Spot compression to image a palpable mass is best achieved by trying to project the margin of the abnormality against the subcutaneous fat. This is best accomplished by rotating the film holder so that it parallels a plane that passes through the nipple and the lesion **(A, B)** and then using spot compression perpendicular to the plane **(C)**.

Among the approaches promoted is the coned-down spot-compression view of any palpable abnormality. Due to the overlapping structures of the breast, the spot-compression view may reveal details that are not evident on the contact (screening) images. In addition, if the abnormality can be pushed against the subcutaneous fat, its margins may be more clearly evaluated. There is no scientific support, however, for suggesting that the coned-down view can eliminate the possibility of breast cancer so it is of no help in excluding cancer. There are no prospective studies that show that it leads to earlier intervention. There are no data on how many palpable cancers would have the diagnosis delayed as a result of not obtaining the spot-compression view. Faulk and Sickles (15) demonstrated that coned spot compression in conjunction with magnification mammography was often better able to image palpable lesions than the standard screening images. What has not been proved is whether or not these additional views alter patient management. In the Faulk series, among 70 women with palpable masses (76% under the age of 50), 66% of the masses were not visible on the standard two-view projections (86% of the women had dense breast tissue). By adding the spot-compression view, four additional masses were identified. Of the 26 masses visible, eight were reclassified after spot compression and all proved to be benign. All of the malignancies were correctly interpreted before the additional views. Although a few more cancers may become visible using spot compression, there is no evidence that these cancers are not already sufficiently suspicious by clinical examination to warrant intervention, and there are no data proving that the targeted imaging alters patient management.

It has never been shown that this procedure actually influences the course of the patient. There have been no studies that have shown that the patient with a palpable cancer was biopsied solely because of the additional image. Despite the fact that we continue to obtain this image, the advantage of the spot compression is not likely to be statistically significant. Spot compression increases the radiation exposure to the patient as well as the cost of the evaluation. Until a prospective study confirms the validity of the maneuver, it should not be considered a standard of care.

Spot Compression of Palpable Abnormalities

If spot-compression mammography is used to evaluate a palpable mass, the goal is to try to separate it from the surrounding breast tissue and ideally to push it into the subcutaneous fat so that its margins can be better evaluated. Merely compressing it may push it into surrounding breast tissue, obscuring its margins. Spot compression (with or without magnification) of a palpable abnormality is best accomplished by rotating the film holder so that it parallels a plane that passes through the lesion and the nipple (Fig. 23-3). This provides the best geometry to project the lesion as close to the edge of the parenchyma as possible. If it is at the periphery of the parenchyma, as most cancers are (16), this provides the best opportunity to outline at least part of its margin against the subcutaneous fat. This maneuver periodically demonstrates a lesion that is not seen on the conventional images (Fig. 23-4).

Clinical Value of Mammography for Symptomatic Patients

Many physicians fail to understand the role of mammography for the woman who presents with a sign or symptom that could represent breast cancer. Paradoxically some clinicians have expressed a lack of belief in the value of mammography as a screening technique but insist that they would send a patient with a lump, thickening, or other suspicious clinical finding for "diagnostic" mammography. This attitude reveals a lack of understanding of the capability of mammography.

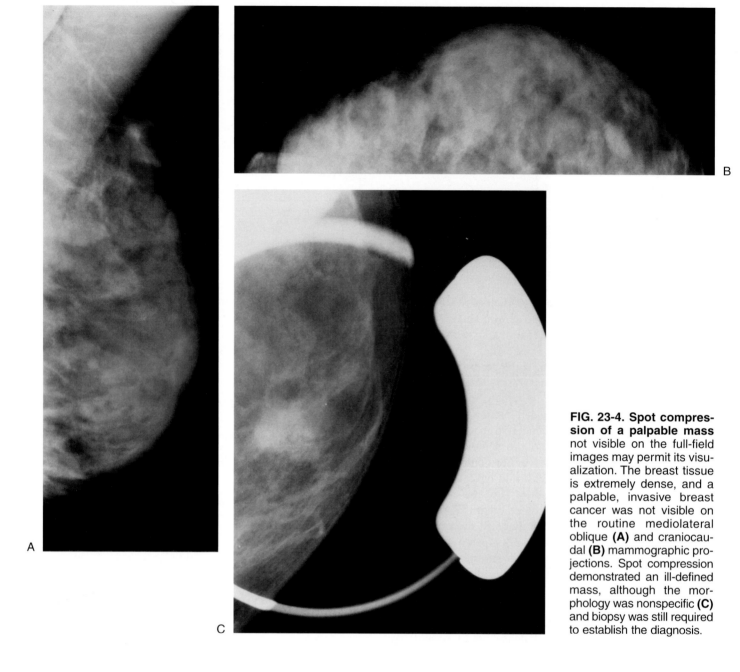

FIG. 23-4. Spot compression of a palpable mass not visible on the full-field images may permit its visualization. The breast tissue is extremely dense, and a palpable, invasive breast cancer was not visible on the routine mediolateral oblique **(A)** and craniocaudal **(B)** mammographic projections. Spot compression demonstrated an ill-defined mass, although the morphology was nonspecific **(C)** and biopsy was still required to establish the diagnosis.

Critical Path and Outcome Analysis

Health planners have begun to focus on aspects of health care that have always been part of medical decision making but have now been provided with new names. The true value of a test is its influence on how the patient does (outcome). An analysis of various interventions and their outcome determines what is now the critical path (the best way to achieve the desired goal). These are not new concepts but merely restate two basic medical questions that should always be asked before a test is ordered: "How will the result of this test alter the care of the patient?" and "How will action based on the result benefit the patient?"

These same questions should be asked when evaluating the use of mammography or any other imaging technique or intervention as a diagnostic modality. The answers for the use of mammography in evaluating a palpable mass can be anticipated by reviewing the range of clinical situations listed below.

Assume that an abnormality is palpated. The clinical examination produces a certain level of concern. The woman then has a mammogram. There are several possible results from the mammogram:

Scenario 1. The lump is visible on the mammogram and has the characteristics of a classically benign lesion, such as a fat-containing mass (lipoma, oil cyst, or harmartoma) or a

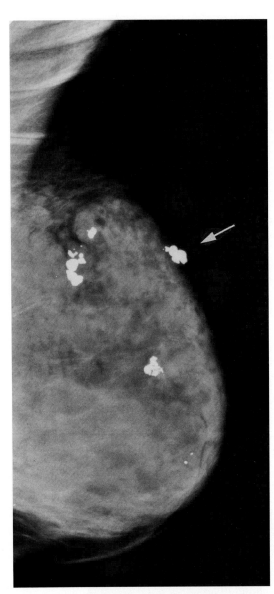

FIG. 23-5. Mammography can occasionally be used to avoid a biopsy of a palpable mass. This patient had a rock-hard mass in the upper outer right breast. The mass corresponded to the densely **calcified fibroadenoma** visible on the mammogram. The mammogram is diagnostic, and a biopsy is not needed.

calcified fibroadenoma (Fig. 23-5). This is one of the few situations in which the mammogram is diagnostic. These lesions have no significant malignant potential. When their mammographic appearance is typical and the mammographic finding corresponds to the clinical abnormality, they do not require biopsy or even further evaluation. In this situation, management is altered by the mammogram, and the patient benefits from the mammogram. This is one of the reasons for obtaining a mammogram to evaluate a palpable abnormality. Unfortunately, this is also an extremely rare occurrence.

Scenario 2. The palpable lump is not visible on the mammogram (see Fig. 23-4). It is well established that there are cancers that are evident on CBE but not visible on the mammogram; therefore, the clinician cannot rely on a negative mammogram to exclude a cancer. Thus, the clinician must still pursue a diagnosis, and management is not altered by the mammogram. This is the most common situation.

Scenario 3. The lump is visible on the mammogram, but its appearance is not specific (Fig. 23-6). The clinician must still pursue the diagnosis, and management is not altered. This is also fairly common.

Scenario 4. The lump is visible on the mammogram, and its morphologic characteristics are very suspicious for malignancy (Fig. 23-7). This often occurs when the lesion felt on clinical examination is actually cancer. Because these lesions are almost always very suspicious on the clinical examination alone, the mammogram rarely alters management. It is possible, however, that without the additional mammographic evidence, the clinician might have decided that his or her clinical suspicion was not sufficiently high to pursue the diagnosis. If this is the case, then the mammogram could have resulted in earlier intervention and management would be altered. The frequency, however, of this particular scenario has never been documented scientifically, and in our experience is very uncommon. Usually when a palpable mass has mammographic features that strongly suggest cancer, the clinical examination is highly suspicious and a biopsy would have been performed on the basis of the clinical findings regardless of the mammographic features. Basic management is not altered by the mammogram.

Finally, it is frequently forgotten that the only efficacious reason for performing mammography is to reduce the death rate from breast cancer. There are no studies that prove that its use in evaluating palpable abnormalities has any influence on mortality, which is the most important measure of outcome.

This review of the basic possibilities makes it evident that the results of the mammogram only rarely alter the management of a clinically evident abnormality. This does not mean that mammography is not valuable in this role but that its value is limited.

The value of the test in the evaluation of the individual with a palpable abnormality is listed below.

Role of Mammographic Evaluation of the Symptomatic Woman

1. For the rare instance in which the mammogram can demonstrate that the palpable abnormality is benign and avoid further intervention (calcified involuting fibroadenoma, lipoma, oil cyst, galactocele, or hamartoma)
2. To reinforce the impression that the palpable abnormality is likely malignant and to support earlier intervention
3. To search the remainder of the ipsilateral breast for an occult cancer
4. To search the contralateral breast to find breast cancer that is not palpable and is clinically occult

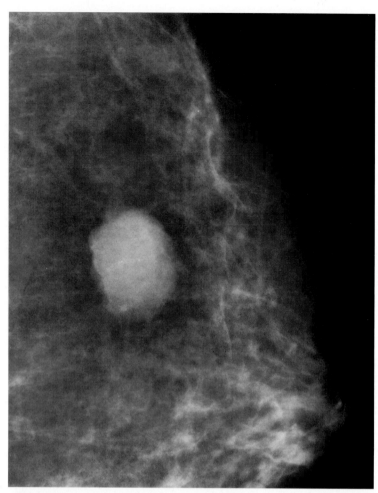

A

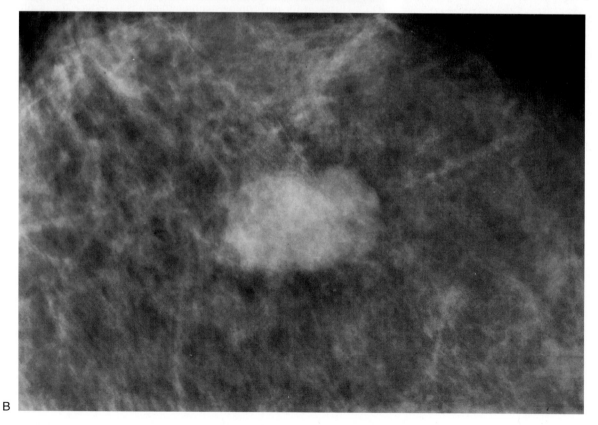

B

FIG. 23-6. The **palpable mass** is visible on the mammogram, but its morphology is nonspecific. This mass is irregular in shape with a microlobulated margin on the mediolateral oblique **(A)** and craniocaudal projections **(B)**. Its morphology was also nonspecific on ultrasound (see Fig. 23-11). It proved to be a cyst.

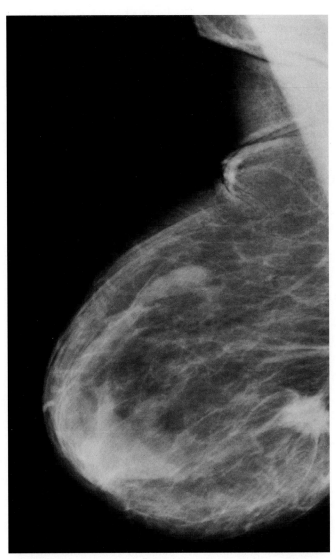

FIG. 23-7. If the mammographic appearance strongly suggests malignancy, malignancy is very likely. This palpable mass is visible on the mammogram. Its irregular shape, spiculated margin, and high x-ray attenuation make it almost certain to be malignant. If the biopsy had proved to be benign, an early repeat mammogram (in 2 to 3 weeks) would have been obtained to ensure that the lesion had been removed. Biopsy of this mass revealed an **invasive breast cancer.**

5. To try to assess the extent of a malignancy and multifocality when cancer is diagnosed

Mammography Is a Screening Test Even for Symptomatic Women

The last three indications listed above for the mammogram are perhaps the most important. Most clinically evident abnormalities are benign. Just as mammography can detect early breast cancer in the asymptomatic woman, early breast cancer can be detected by mammography in the symptomatic woman. The fact is that the major role for mammography in any woman, whether she is asymptomatic or has a clinically evident problem, is screening to detect clinically unsuspected cancer.

Because there are no prospectively obtained data that prove that mammographic evaluation of a palpable abnormality has any impact on mortality, the only efficacious role for mammography is screening to detect breast cancers before they become palpable. It is scientifically inconsistent to suggest that mammography is valuable for the woman who has a lump but not to support its use for screening asymptomatic women.

Evaluation of the Mammographically Detected, Clinically Occult Lesion

An additional role for mammography that has been termed *diagnostic* is its use to further evaluate and characterize abnormalities detected at screening that are not clinically evident. Diagnostic mammography is used to determine if a radiographically detected abnormality is real, its three-dimensional location, and its etiology, if possible, and to guide its management. Additional views, magnification mammography, spot compression, and ultrasound are all techniques that aid the radiologist in determining what to advise the woman and her physician about how to best manage the clinically occult, mammographically detected abnormality.

Clinical Decisions

Mammography can occasionally assist in the management of palpable lesions, but the management of a clinically evident lesion usually requires clinical decisions and a negative mammogram should usually not interfere with earlier intervention if there is sufficient clinical concern. Management of a breast abnormality should usually be guided by the analysis that provides the greatest level of concern. Just as a negative clinical examination does not override a suspicious mammogram, a negative mammogram does not negate a suspicious clinical examination.

Avoiding a False-Negative Breast Biopsy

There is an additional reason for obtaining a mammogram, despite the fact that a palpable abnormality is to be biopsied. As noted previously, one of the important functions of mammography in a woman with a palpable lesion is the demonstration that the lesion has very suspicious morphology on the mammogram. If the mammogram suggests that a palpable lesion is likely to be malignant (Fig. 23-8A) and the biopsy reveals a benign diagnosis, the clinician should question whether the lesion was actually excised. The patient should have a repeat mammogram as soon as possible (Fig. 23-8B), as it is likely that the cancer was missed at surgery (17).

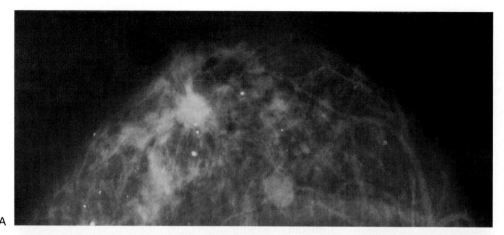

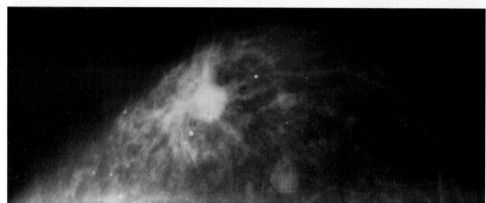

FIG. 23-8. If it looks like cancer, be suspicious if the biopsy results are benign. The surgeon felt the spiculated mass in the lateral right breast, as seen on this craniocaudal projection **(A)** and biopsied the clinical abnormality. The biopsy result was benign tissue. An early repeat mammogram revealed that the lesion was still present **(B)**. The postsurgical change is visible immediately adjacent to the persistent mass. Re-excision following a needle localization established the correct diagnosis of **invasive breast cancer.**

Adjunctive Evaluation

As with all tests, the value of additional imaging should be assessed as to its impact on management. If the results will not alter management, then performing additional imaging is not justified. The reason for using mammography to evaluate women who have signs or symptoms of breast cancer is that occasionally but anecdotally, the mammographic evaluation of the palpable abnormality may be helpful.

ROLE OF ULTRASOUND IN EVALUATION OF A PALPABLE MASS

There is little question that tests are often used for subjective and medical-legal reasons in the absence of scientifically derived efficacy. All physicians are guilty of relying on having "seen a case" where obtaining a study made a difference in the care of the patient. It is likely that better care is rendered because of an individual practitioner's experience, but care (and standards of care) should not be determined based on anecdote.

The use of ultrasound to evaluate the palpable mass is an example of anecdote preceding scientific evaluation. It comes from the reluctance of the radiologist to state that a lesion is indeterminate based on the mammogram. It is

rarely possible to determine whether a noncalcified lesion is cystic or solid by mammography alone. With regard to the nonpalpable mass detected only by mammography, one might argue that it is the radiologist's responsibility to resolve an indeterminate lesion since the clinician has no way of evaluating the nonpalpable lesion. Ultrasound is not yet efficacious for screening asymptomatic women, but ultrasound does provide a useful adjunctive study to mammography when a nonpalpable mass is found, and the radiologist must resolve the nature of the nonpalpable, indeterminate mass detected only by mammography.

The palpable abnormality should be considered the responsibility of the clinician, but it has increasingly become the responsibility of the radiologist. As already shown, mammography is used in this situation primarily to screen the uninvolved breast tissue. If a mass is clinically evident, the vast majority require clinical resolution. Given the cost of ultrasound, it is not economically defensible to use ultrasound to evaluate a palpable mass if the reason is to avoid stating that the palpable abnormality is indeterminate on the mammogram. Since it is rarely possible to determine whether a lesion is cystic or solid by mammography alone, ultrasound can be used to make this clinically important differentiation, but the efficacy of this is not clear.

Most women do not wish to have a palpable lump. For many women they are painful. Clinically guided needle

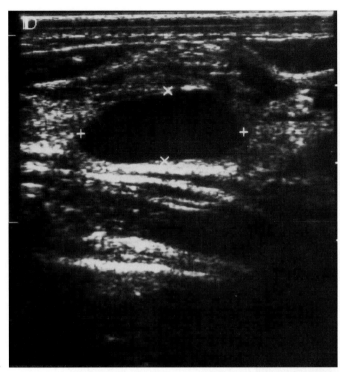
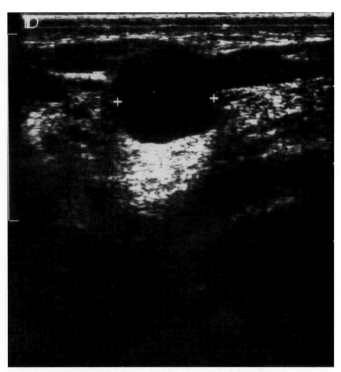

A   B

FIG. 23-9. The ultrasound diagnosis of a cyst is very accurate if all criteria are met. These include a round or oval shape, a sharply defined anterior and posterior wall, no internal echoes, and enhancement through-transmission of sound. These characteristics are seen in the transverse **(A)** and sagittal **(B)** images of this palpable cyst. If these characteristics are present, no further intervention is needed.

aspiration is extremely safe, usually accomplished with little discomfort, and, for the cyst, simultaneously diagnostic and therapeutic. If a lesion is to be aspirated, ultrasound adds an unnecessary test and a layer of health care expense that is wasted. If, however, the demonstration of a cyst avoids an aspiration, then ultrasound of a palpable mass is efficacious.

True intracystic breast cancer is extremely uncommon, so some radiologists argue that intracystic tumors will be missed if ultrasound is not performed. This is a specious argument since the vast majority are in fact benign papillomas.

Once again there are no prospective data from carefully designed trials that show that ultrasound plays any significant management role except cyst/solid differentiation. Because clinically guided cyst aspiration is simple, safe, and often less expensive than ultrasound, it is likely that the ideal sequence for evaluating a palpable mass that is thought to be a cyst is the following:

1. Clinical evaluation and clinically guided aspiration.
2. Mammography in the appropriate age or risk groups to screen the rest of the breast and the contralateral breast (if there has been bruising from the aspiration, then the mammogram should be delayed 2 to 3 weeks).
3. Ultrasound should be used if clinically guided aspiration fails to resolve the mass, since there are some palpable cysts that defy clinically guided aspiration for various reasons.

There are some cysts that for various reasons defy clinically guided aspiration and are presumed to be solid. These lesions will likely be removed surgically unless it can be established that they are truly cysts. In this situation excisional biopsy can be avoided if ultrasound demonstrates a cyst. This can be confirmed by imaging-guided aspiration (18). The use of ultrasound in this sequence of imaging will significantly reduce its use but will make that use appropriate.

Demonstration of a Cyst

When the ultrasound criteria for a cyst are present, the diagnosis is very accurate and further intervention is not required (Fig. 23-9). The only time ultrasound becomes efficacious in the primary analysis of a palpable mass is when the patient and her physician agree that the demonstration of a cyst by ultrasound will be sufficient and will obviate the need for aspiration or surgery (19,20). If this is the case, then ultrasound may be the procedure of choice.

The primary role of ultrasound remains the differentiation of cystic from solid masses and the guidance of needle procedures. Some have suggested that ultrasound can be used to reliably differentiate benign from malignant solid masses, but this is purely a statistical phenomenon (most oval homogeneously solid masses are benign). Given the safety of obtaining a tissue diagnosis (needle biopsy or excisional biopsy) and the importance of early

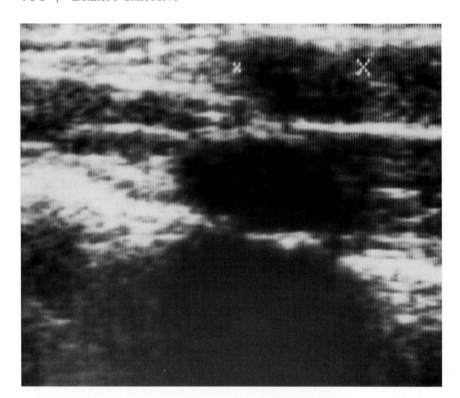

FIG. 23-10. Ultrasound is often nonspecific. This is the ultrasound of the palpable mass in Figure 23-3. Although oval and fairly well defined with a homogeneous echo texture, it still proved to be an **invasive breast cancer.** Note that the hypoechoic mass beneath the cancer is a normal rib.

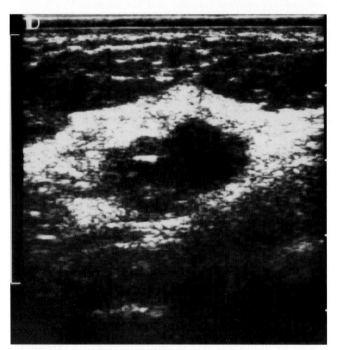

FIG. 23-11. Some cysts appear to be solid by ultrasound. This is the ultrasound of the palpable mass in Figure 23-5. It is irregular in shape and has an irregular echo texture. Biopsy revealed **a benign cyst with a thick wall.**

The fact that a palpable mass should be considered the responsibility of the referring physician does not preclude involvement by the radiologist who is interested in being involved at all levels of breast health care. Many radiologists do physical examinations as well as cyst aspirations, and complete breast care should be encouraged to avoid fragmentation and inefficient service. However, this is not the standard to which all radiologists who provide mammographic services should be held.

Unless the radiologist and referring physician agree otherwise, the palpable abnormality is ultimately the responsibility of the referring physician, just as the mammographically detected, clinically occult lesion requires the radiologist to advise proper management. There will be an increasing reliance on the primary care physician for the care of breast problems. Should the primary care physician wish to avoid a surgical referral for a simple cyst, then ultrasound or imaging-guided aspiration will be used more frequently to evaluate palpable masses.

If the patient is self-referred to the radiologist and the radiologist accepts the referral, then all abnormalities of the breast are the radiologist's responsibility until care has been transferred.

SUMMARY

In general the management of a palpable abnormality should be determined by the clinical evaluation. Mammography is of some use for evaluating the area of concern and may be helpful in limited circumstances where the palpable abnormality has morphologic characteristics that are diag-

cancer detection, reliance on ultrasound carries a risk of a false-negative interpretation that is difficult to justify (Fig. 23-10). Ultrasound is frequently not even specific for the diagnosis of a cyst, and more aggressive intervention may be indicated (Fig. 23-11).

nostic mammographically. Mammography is primarily useful for screening the remaining ipsilateral breast tissue and the contralateral breast to find occult cancer. The demonstration of a morphologically malignant lesion should indicate a high probability of cancer, and if the biopsy indicates a benign result, the accuracy of the biopsy should be reviewed.

Ultrasound is of limited, legitimate value in assessing a palpable lesion unless the demonstration of a cyst avoids aspiration (assuming that the ultrasound is less costly than the aspiration). Ultrasound is not sufficiently diagnostic to rely on it for differentiating benign from malignant solid lesions.

The practitioner should be aware, however, that there has been an increasing emphasis on the use of ultrasound in the evaluation of palpable masses. This emphasis by those who rely heavily on ultrasound has already resulted in the settlement of a lawsuit for the failure to have performed an ultrasound on the breast of a woman who claimed she felt something when nothing was felt by her physician or even the radiologist (beyond the standard of care). There is little question that there are expert witnesses who will testify that ultrasound is the standard of care for the evaluation of palpable abnormalities despite any scientific validation of this role and that position will likely dictate in a malpractice case. It is unfortunate, because this practice will greatly increase the cost of health care.

REFERENCES

1. Shapiro S, Venet W, Strax P, Venet L. Periodic Screening for Breast Cancer: The Health Insurance Plan Project and Its Sequelae, 1963–1986. Baltimore: Johns Hopkins University Press, 1988.
2. Baker LH. Breast Cancer Detection Demonstration Project: five-year summary report. CA Cancer J Clin 1982;32:194–225.
3. Carter CL, Allen C, Henson DE. Relation of tumor size, lymph node status, and survival in 24,740 breast cancer cases. Cancer 1989;63:181–187.
4. Miller AB, Baines CJ, Turnbull C. The role of the nurse-examiner in the National Breast Screening Study. Can J Public Health 1991;82:162–167.
5. Meyer JE, Kopans DB. Breast physical examination by the mammographer; an aid to improved diagnostic accuracy. Appl Radiol 1983;103–106.
6. Mann BD, Giuliano AE, Bassett LW, et al. Delayed diagnosis of breast cancer as a result of normal mammograms. Arch Surg 1983;118:23–24.
7. Burns P, Grace MCA, Lees AW, May C. False negative mammograms causing delay in breast cancer diagnosis. Can Assoc Radiol J 1979;30:74–76.
8. Holland R, Hendriks JHCL, Mravunac M. Mammographically occult breast cancer: a pathologic and radiologic study. Cancer 1983;52:1810–1819.
9. Moskowitz M. Breast cancer: age-specific growth rates and screening strategies. Radiology 1986;161:37–41.
10. Swann CA, Kopans DB, McCarthy KA, et al. Mammographic density and physical assessment of the breast. AJR Am J Roentgenol 1987;148:525–526.
11. Boren WL, Hunter TB, Bjelland JC, Hunt KR. Comparison of breast consistency at palpation with breast density at mammography. Invest Radiol 1990;25:1010–1011.
12. Meyer JE, Kopans DB, Oot R. Mammographic visualization of breast cancer in patients under 35 years of age. Radiology 1983;147:93–94.
13. Williams SM, Kaplan PA, Peterson JC, Lieberman RP. Mammography in women under age 30: is there clinical benefit? Radiology 1986;161:49–51.
14. Liberman L, Dershaw DD, Deutch BM, et al. Screening mammography: value in women 35–39 years old. AJR Am J Roentgenol 1993;161:53–56.
15. Faulk RM, Sickles EA. Efficacy of spot compression—magnification and tangential views in mammographic evaluation of palpable masses. Radiology 1992;185:87–90.
16. Stacey-Clear A, McCarthy KA, Hall DA, et al. Observations on the location of breast cancer in women under fifty. Radiology 1993;186:677–680.
17. Meyer JE, Kopans DB. Analysis of mammographically obvious breast carcinomas with benign results on initial biopsy. Surg Gynecol Obstet 1981;153:570–572.
18. Fornage BD, Faroux MJ, Simatos A. Breast masses: US-guided fine-needle aspiration biopsy. Radiology 1987;162:409–414.
19. Jackson VP. The role of US in breast imaging. Radiology 1990;177:305–311.
20. Bassett LW, Kimme-Smith C. Breast sonography. AJR Am J Roentgenol 1991;156:449–455.

Breast Imaging, 2nd ed., by Daniel B. Kopans.
Lippincott–Raven Publishers, Philadelphia © 1998.

CHAPTER 24

Breast Imaging Report: Data Management, False-Negative Mammography, and the Breast Imaging Audit

The communication of breast imaging results to the patient and her physician has been increasingly analyzed over the past several years. Although the same issues are applicable to all imaging studies, the high visibility and public concern over breast cancer and mammographic screening and the fact that mammography, unlike most other imaging studies, is principally used in asymptomatic, healthy individuals has focused greater attention on these communications.

Although mammography serves the same purpose for the breast that a Pap smear does for the cervix, the psychological issues are clearly different. Unlike the case with cervical testing, women and their physicians are urged to require immediate analysis and communication of the results of their screening mammogram. From a scientific and medical perspective, however, a rushed interpretation of a screening mammogram to provide an immediate report is a mistake. What many women and their physicians fail to understand is that there is no reassurance in a negative mammogram, and, hence, there is no urgency to find out that the mammogram was negative. It is well established that mammography misses 5% to 15% of cancers that are present and palpable at the time of a screening, and as many as 20% of cancers become clinically evident within 1 year of a negative mammogram (1). Mammography cannot tell a woman that she does not have breast cancer. The only benefit from mammography is the potential to detect cancers earlier. The process of mammographic review should be to maximize the detection of small cancers and not to be rushed to provide immediate false reassurance.

Women will be denied access to screening if the costs are not kept low. The best way to keep the cost low and the likelihood of detecting cancer earlier high is to have screening centers where the resources are used to obtain high-quality images in a cost-effective manner. This generally means that the radiologist is off site, where his or her time can be managed more efficiently through batch interpretation of films (see Chapter 11). This may delay the interpretation, but it permits a less hurried review of the images and cost-effective double reading. Regardless of the approach, the analysis of the mammogram should be clear and concise. It should be decision oriented and provide guidance, when appropriate, for the next course of action.

GENERAL PRINCIPLES

Mammography is primarily a screening technique. When a lesion is detected, it is usually no more than an educated guess as to its true histology. The overriding decisions are whether or not it has a significant probability of malignancy and whether or not a biopsy is indicated. Presumably, significant lesions will be biopsied and any decisions that relate to histologic criteria should be based on direct microscopic evaluation.

Speculation concerning true histology that is based on the mammogram contributes little to overall management. Unless pathognomonic signs are present, cysts, fibroadenomas, metastatic lesions, primary breast cancers, and other pathologic processes may have identical mammographic appearances. Thus, the radiologist should use descriptive terminology rather than an attempt to define true histology.

Mammography is an excellent technique for finding small masses or microcalcifications in the breast, many of which prove to be malignant. Mammography is poor at determining which of these is benign and which is malignant, and histologic correlation is inexact. The interpreter should be well aware of this and choose appropriate descriptive terms and summary assessments. It serves no useful purpose and in fact may be misleading to overinterpret mammograms.

Because there is a significant overlap in the appearance of varying histologies in the breast, it is preferable to describe findings in radiographically appropriate terms. The terms fibrocystic disease, fibrocystic changes, fibrocystic tissues, dysplasia, and hyperplasia are inappropriate and should be eliminated from image interpretation. There is no good support for the belief that histology can be accurately inferred from the mammogram, with the exception of benign pathognomonic lesions such as intramammary lymph nodes, cal-

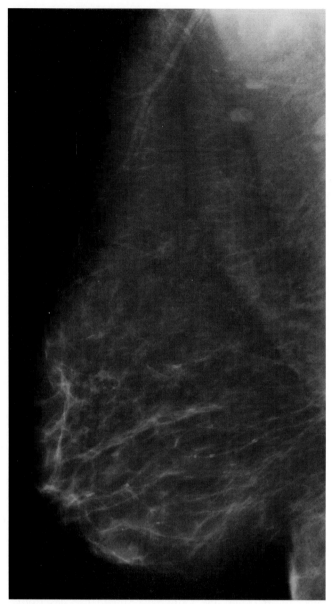

FIG. 24-1. Fibrocystic disease is a meaningless and inaccurate term. This patient was sent for a mammogram with a diagnosis of fibrocystic disease. In fact, her mammogram clearly shows that she has no cysts and very little fibrosis. Her doctor was feeling the **lumpiness caused by locules of fat and Cooper's ligaments.**

cified fibroadenomas, vascular calcifications, and the fat-containing lesions.

Histopathologic terms should be reserved for the pathologist and should be avoided in the clinical evaluation. When a physical examination is performed, the terminology should be appropriate for that test. Stating that a woman with lumpy breasts or mammographically dense tissue has fibrocystic disease does little more than frighten the patient and create the unsubstantiated prejudice that she is more likely to develop breast cancer. This

may unfairly influence recommendations for management and from a practical point of view even affect health insurance premiums. In fact, in breasts that are lumpy there may be little fibrosis and no cysts (Fig. 24-1). The normal breast is a heterogeneous organ with varying tissue composition, and many breasts feel extremely heterogeneous on clinical examination.

Radiographically there is an equally broad spectrum of tissue patterns found on mammograms. In 1976 John Wolfe described four basic breast tissue patterns and his belief that they were associated with varying risks for the development of breast cancer (2). There are some new data to suggest that there is some increased risk for dense patterns (3), although this is not at this time of any clinical value. Wolfe's system was succinct, and a similar system has been adopted by the American College of Radiology (ACR), Breast Imaging Reporting and Data System (BIRADS) (see the following section). As with clinical examination, there is a broad spectrum of radiographic appearances (see Chapter 12), and, based on our current level of knowledge, it is impossible to determine which of these are normal and which represent significant pathologic changes.

The mammographic report should contain only findings that are of significance in patient management and that reflect the level of sensitivity for detecting small cancers that mammography has in a given individual. At the current level of understanding, overall radiographic density is significant only for the fact that small cancers are harder to detect in the dense breast.

AMERICAN COLLEGE OF RADIOLOGY BREAST IMAGING REPORTING AND DATA SYSTEM

The importance of high-quality mammography has been established and federally mandated in the Mammography Quality Standards Act (MQSA). A component of quality is the clear, concise transmission of the results of the interpretation of the mammogram. Recognizing the need to provide clear and accurate reports, the ACR developed BIRADS. BIRADS consists of a lexicon of terminology with definitions to provide standardized language, a reporting structure, and a decision-oriented approach to the assessment of the mammogram. A coding system is provided to facilitate database maintenance. The goal of BIRADS is to standardize mammography reporting so that reports are clear, understandable, and decisive. If data are acquired in a similar fashion, then they can be pooled to permit greater insight into the breast cancer screening effort.

Historical Perspective

A wide variation in mammographic quality in the United States, demonstrated by the Food and Drug Administration's

Nationwide Evaluation of X-Ray Trends (NEXT) study in 1985 (4,5), and an interest on the part of the American Cancer Society (ACS) to designate sites for the ACS National Breast Cancer Awareness Screening Programs led to the development of the ACR's Mammography Accreditation Program (MAP) in 1986 (6). This program established a process for the certification of mammographic equipment; training requirements for radiologists, technologists, and medical physicists; and maintenance of rigorous quality control measures. This process has been adopted by the FDA under the MQSA.

The ACR recognized that part of a strong quality assurance program is the accurate formulation and communication of the mammography interpretation. Concerns had been raised by medical organizations such as the American Medical Association (7) that mammography reports were often ambiguous and interpretation indecisive. Much of the problem was due to the lack of a universally accepted set of descriptive terms and a structured, decision-oriented reporting system.

As a quality assurance measure, the Breast Task Force of the ACR appointed a committee of experts in breast imaging to develop standardized mammographic terminology and an organized reporting system in an effort to reduce confusing breast imaging interpretations.

In addition, although screening services have proliferated, the diversity of health care delivery in the United States and the lack of comprehensive databases have made it difficult to assess the effect of screening nationally and to determine where improvements can be made. Consequently, an additional goal of the ACR committee was to develop a database that would permit pooling of screening results to facilitate outcome monitoring. The overall goal was to improve the quality of breast cancer screening.

Primarily composed of experts in mammography, the committee that developed the ACR's BIRADS was a cooperative effort with assistance and input from several groups, including representatives of the National Cancer Institute, the Centers for Disease Control, the Food and Drug Administration, the American Medical Association, the American College of Surgeons, the College of American Pathologists, and other ACR committees. With such a broad base of support, it is expected that BIRADS will be adopted nationwide.

Contents of BIRADS

BIRADS was conceived as a system that will change with time as new data emerge. The following is our summary of BIRADS. It does not constitute an official copy of the system. The reader is encouraged to contact the ACR to obtain the latest copy of BIRADS.

BIRADS provides a framework for standardizing mammography reports. Clear, succinct reports are encouraged. It is organized into a general framework for breast evaluation, including a dictionary of defined terms and a

reporting structure that is decision oriented. It is hoped that the recommended data collection will permit the pooling of information on a national level. The coding system is designed to facilitate the use of computers to simplify the process.

The system comprises an introduction and five major sections: an introduction, a breast imaging lexicon, the reporting system, a report coding system, a pathology coding system, and a description of follow-up and outcome monitoring.

The introduction to BIRADS provides general principles in breast cancer detection and diagnosis. It establishes the differences between screening (the evaluation of asymptomatic women in the search for unsuspected cancers) and diagnostic evaluation (symptomatic patients or women requiring additional evaluation because of an abnormal screening study). Not only is BIRADS important for radiologists, but the distinctions between these functions and their definitions are important for all physicians to understand. The introduction emphasizes the need for coordinated breast care and defines the role of imaging in that care.

Screening

It is stated that the major role for mammography is the earlier detection of breast cancer in asymptomatic women. Although mammography can detect the majority of breast cancers, there are some that are palpable yet elude mammographic detection (8). BIRADS reinforces that physical examination remains an important component of screening. In addition, although mortality reduction has not been objectively shown, breast self-examination is encouraged in the document.

Breast Evaluation

Although mammography is primarily a screening technology, when it is used in conjunction with other breast imaging techniques, such as sonography, it may be helpful in the evaluation of women who have a sign or symptom that suggests breast cancer. It is stated, however, that breast cancer cannot be excluded on the basis of mammographic evaluation. Just as management decisions must be made on the basis of abnormal mammographic findings, in women with normal findings on clinical examination, there are many decisions that must be based on the clinical evaluation when the mammogram is negative.

As a source of information to the clinician, statements indicating the somewhat lower sensitivity of mammography in the dense breast or the further disposition of a clinical finding with normal mammographic findings may be added. It is well established, however, that mammography does not demonstrate all breast cancers and that the clinician should pursue any significant clinical concern even if the mammogram is negative. As this is now common knowledge,

BIRADS acknowledges that routine general disclaimers are not necessary in mammography reports.

BIRADS acknowledges that screening is appropriately practiced in two major settings. In many centers there is a radiologist on site, and additional imaging is performed immediately when a possible abnormality is detected. In an effort to reduce the cost of screening, so that it can be available for all women, screening is increasingly being performed in high-quality and highly efficient screening centers or using mobile units, where there is no radiologist on site and the mammographic interpretation is not rendered immediately. This means that the patient may be recalled for additional study to evaluate possible abnormalities detected at screening. Regardless of the approach, screening should include two-view mammography incorporating the mediolateral oblique (MLO) and craniocaudal (CC) projections because single-view mammography has been shown to overlook as much as 25% of breast cancers (9).

These two approaches to screening are acknowledged in the reporting system. In the BIRADS report approach, it is required that all mammograms have a final assessment that is decision oriented. The decision that a study is indeterminate is not acceptable. Consequently, women who require additional imaging after a screening mammogram are considered as having an incomplete evaluation. The evaluation is incomplete until a final assessment can be reached.

Breast Imaging Lexicon

The lexicon is a dictionary of terms to be used in mammographic interpretation. The atlas at the end of this chapter provides images to clarify the definitions. The terms chosen in BIRADS are defined and intended to provide a clear and accurate communication of the mammographic findings. These definitions were arrived at by the committee after lengthy discussions and input from radiologists and clinicians across the country. In the interest of clarity, some familiar terms were dropped. The terms that were ultimately included were chosen and carefully defined to provide clear and accurate communication of the findings detected by mammography. Ambiguity is eliminated.

The interpreter of the mammogram should use these terms to provide a description of any significant findings in the body of the report. For masses this includes the size, shape (round, oval, lobular, irregular, or architectural distortion), margin characteristics (circumscribed, microlobulated, obscured, indistinct or ill-defined, and spiculated), and relative x-ray attenuation (high, isodense, low density, or fat-containing) of the abnormality. These are the characteristics that most experts acknowledge as useful for determining the likelihood of a mass being benign or malignant.

The lexicon also includes definitions for the many special situations that are commonly encountered and have a

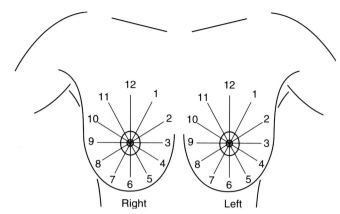

FIG. 24-2. Lesion location should be provided using clinical references that are based on the face of a clock. Note that the same clock description describes a different location depending on which breast is involved. For example, 1:00 on the right breast is in the upper inner breast, whereas on the left it is upper outer.

pathognomonic appearance, such as a tubular density, which may also be called a dilated duct or an intramammary lymph node. These require no further description. Other definitions, such as the difference between a focal asymmetric density and asymmetric breast tissue, are also included.

The various types of calcium deposits are defined. They are divided into those that are typically benign, such as skin deposits and vascular calcifications, and distinguishable as such, as well as the coarse calcifications of an involuting fibroadenoma, the rod-like calcifications of secretory deposits, the lucent-centered calcifications of fat necrosis, and others. These are distinguished from calcifications that are of intermediate concern (amorphous or indistinct) and those with a higher probability of malignancy, such as pleomorphic or heterogeneous calcifications or fine and/or branching calcifications.

These last two categories of calcifications require the use of the distribution modifiers of *grouped* or *clustered*, *linear*, *segmental*, *regional*, or *diffuse/scattered*. The total evaluation of calcifications includes their number, size, morphology, and distribution. All these are defined in the lexicon.

As with masses, the location of significant calcifications should be included in the report. BIRADS has adopted the clinical reference system that uses the face of a clock to define location (Fig. 24-2) and divides the breast into anterior, middle, and deep tissues (Fig. 24-3). This does require the radiologist to convert the location, as determined on the mammogram, into the clinical reference system.

Additional definitions are provided for other associated findings, such as skin or nipple retraction, skin or trabecular thickening, adenopathy, and others so that the descriptive portion of the report is complete.

A thorough discussion of the descriptors can be found in an article by D'Orsi and Kopans (10).

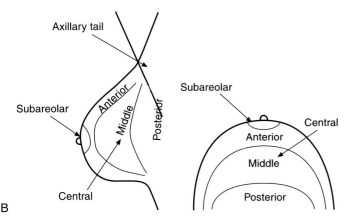

FIG. 24-3. The breast is divided by depth into anterior, middle, and posterior tissues, as seen in the lateral **(A)** and craniocaudal **(B)** projections.

Reporting System

The heart of BIRADS is the reporting system. This defines the report organization and requires the interpreter to decide on the significance of the mammographic findings. A vague report is not permitted. There are five specific categories of assessment other than category 0 (used in the autonomous screening setting, which means that additional evaluation is required), and the interpreting physician must be decisive in determining which category is appropriate. The report should include:

1. Mention of comparison with any pertinent previous studies
2. Brief description of the type of breast tissues being analyzed to provide the referring physician an estimate of the expected sensitivity of the mammogram
3. Description of any significant findings
   a. For masses
      (1) Size (generally the largest dimension; spicules are not included if there is a visible mass)
      (2) Shape
      (3) Margin characteristics
      (4) X-ray attenuation
      (5) Associated calcifications
      (6) Associated findings and location in clinical terms (using the face of a clock)
   b. For calcifications
      (1) Morphology
      (2) Distribution
      (3) Associated findings
      (4) Location (based on the clinical location)
4. One of five decision-oriented assessments outlining a course of action

Breast Imaging Report

In addition to noting any comparison to previous studies, BIRADS requires that the report should include a statement of the general breast tissue type with four categories that are similar to those originally described by Wolfe:

1. The breast is almost entirely fat.
2. There are scattered fibroglandular densities that could obscure a lesion on mammography.
3. The breast tissue is heterogeneously dense. This may lower the sensitivity of mammography.
4. The breast tissue is extremely dense, which lowers the sensitivity of mammography.

If an implant is present, it should be stated in the report (11).

These descriptions of tissue patterns are provided as an indication of the likely sensitivity of the test (12,13), acknowledging that mammography is less sensitive in the dense breast and alerting the referring physician as to the type of breast being evaluated.

The body of the report should include a description of significant findings using the appropriate descriptors, any associated findings, the size of the abnormality, and its location. Any findings should be described in the report using BIRADS terminology provided by the BIRADS lexicon.

The following language is taken from BIRADS. The accompanying figures are our interpretation of those descriptions:

A. Masses are space-occupying lesions seen in two different projections. If a potential mass is seen in only a single projection it should be called a *density* until its three dimensionality is confirmed.
   1. Shape (Fig. 24-4A)
      a. Round (Fig. 24-4B): A mass that is spheric, ball shaped, circular, or globular.
      b. Oval (Fig. 24-4C): A mass that is elliptical or egg shaped.
      c. Lobular (Fig. 24-4D): A mass that has contours with undulations.
      d. Irregular (Fig. 24-4E): The lesion's shape cannot be characterized by any of the above.
      e. Architectural distortion (Fig. 24-4F): The normal architecture is distorted with no definite mass visible. This includes spiculations radiating from a point and focal retraction or distortion of the edge of the parenchyma. Architectural distortion can also be an associated finding.
   2. Special cases
      a. Solitary dilated duct or tubular density (Fig. 24-5) is a tubular or branching structure that likely represents a dilated or otherwise enlarged duct. If unassociated with other suspicious clinical or mammographic findings, it is usually of minor significance.
      b. Intramammary lymph nodes (Fig. 24-6) are typically reniform or have a radiolucent notch due to fat at the hilum and are generally 1 cm or smaller in size. They may be larger than 1 cm and normal when fat replacement is pronounced. They may be multiple, or marked fat replacement may cause a

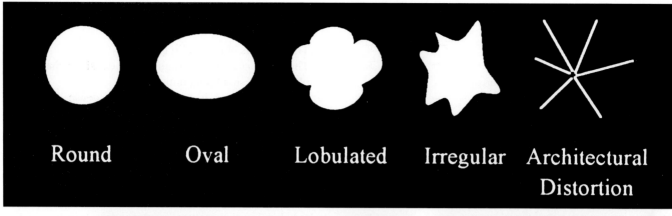

Round   Oval   Lobulated   Irregular   Architectural Distortion

A

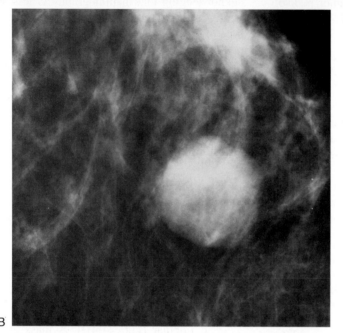

B

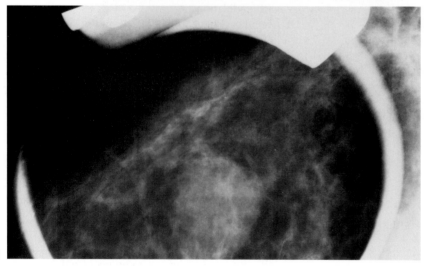

C

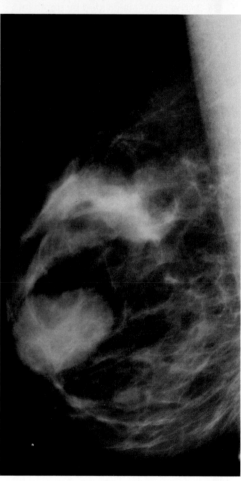

D

FIG. 24-4. (A) Masses should be described according to their shapes: round, oval, lobulated, irregular, and architectural distortion. **(B)** This cyst has a round shape. **(C)** This fibroadenoma has an oval shape. **(D)** This fibroadenoma has a lobulated shape. *Continued.*

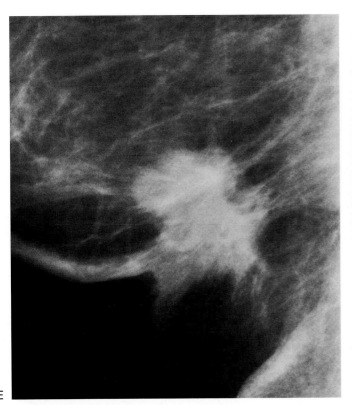

E

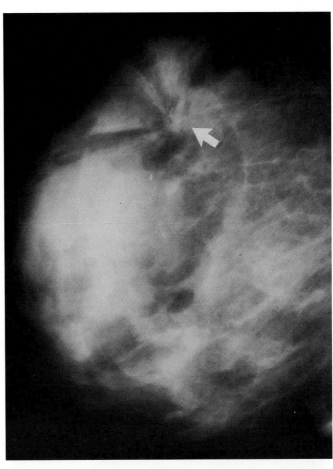

F

FIG. 24-4. *Continued.* **(E)** This **invasive cancer** has an irregular shape. **(F)** This architectural distortion was due to a benign, radial scar.

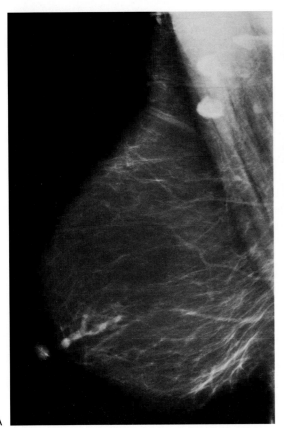

A

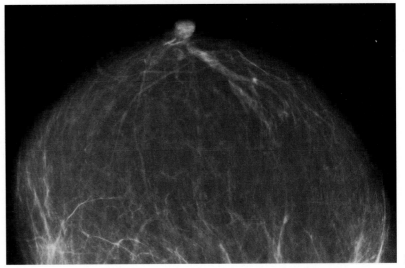

B

FIG. 24-5. The tubular structure in the subareolar region on the mediolateral oblique **(A)** and craniocaudal **(B)** projections is consistent with an ectatic duct, a **solitary dilated duct.**

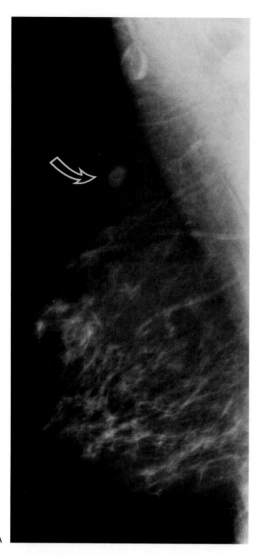

A

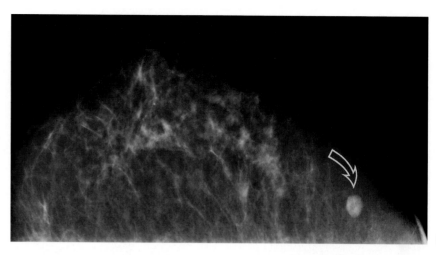

B

FIG. 24-6. A benign intramammary lymph node projects over the upper breast on the mediolateral oblique **(A)** and the outer left breast on the cranio-caudal **(B)** projections (*arrows*).

single lymph node to look like several rounded masses. This specific diagnosis should be made only for masses in the lateral half and usually upper portion of the breast.

c. Asymmetric breast tissue (Fig. 24-7) is judged relative to the corresponding area in the other breast and includes a greater volume of breast tissue, greater density of breast tissue, or more prominent ducts. There is no focal mass formation, no central density, no distorted architecture, and no associated calcifications. Asymmetric breast tissue usually represents a normal variation but may be significant when it corresponds to a palpable asymmetry.

d. Focal asymmetric density (Fig. 24-8) is a density that cannot be accurately described using the other shapes. It is visible as asymmetry of tissue density. It could represent an island of normal breast, but its lack of specific benign characteristics may warrant further evaluation. Additional

imaging may reveal a true mass or significant architectural distortion.

3. Margins (These modify the shape of the mass.) (Fig. 24-9A)

a. Circumscribed (well defined or sharply defined) margins (Fig. 24-9B) are sharply demarcated with an abrupt transition between the lesion and the surrounding tissue. Without additional modifiers there is nothing to suggest infiltration.

b. Microlobulated margins (Fig. 24-9C) undulate with short cycles producing small undulations.

c. Obscured margins (Fig. 24-9D) are hidden by superimposed or adjacent normal tissue and cannot be assessed any further.

d. Indistinct (ill-defined) margins (Fig. 24-9E) are poorly defined and raise concern that there may be infiltration by the lesion that is not likely due to superimposed normal breast tissue.

e. Spiculated margins (Fig. 24-9F). The lesion is characterized by thin lines radiating from the mar-

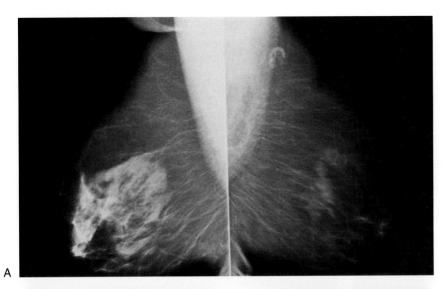

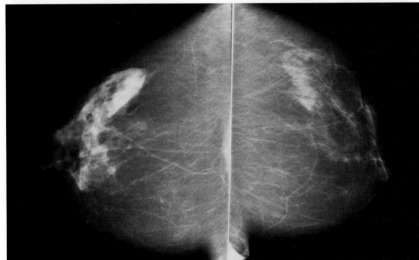

FIG. 24-7. To make the diagnosis of **asymmetric breast tissue,** there should be no mass formation, no significant calcifications, and no architectural distortion. If there is no corresponding palpable asymmetry, this represents a normal variation. In this 45-year-old patient there was no palpable finding, despite the fact that there is prominent asymmetry visible on the mediolateral oblique **(A)** and craniocaudal **(B)** projections. The mammogram had been unchanged for 5 years, and this is a normal variation.

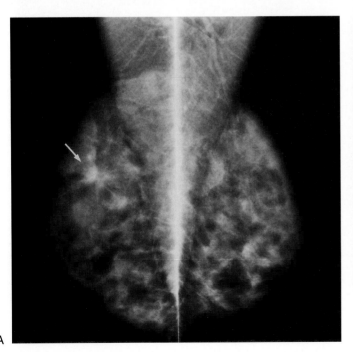

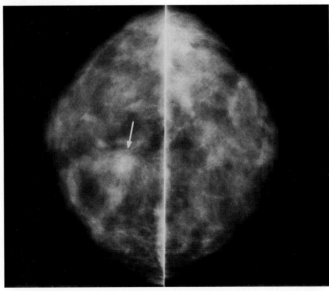

FIG. 24-8. This **focal asymmetric density** on the mediolateral oblique **(A)** (*arrow*) and craniocaudal **(B)** (*arrow*) views **proved to be invasive ductal carcinoma** with an in situ component.

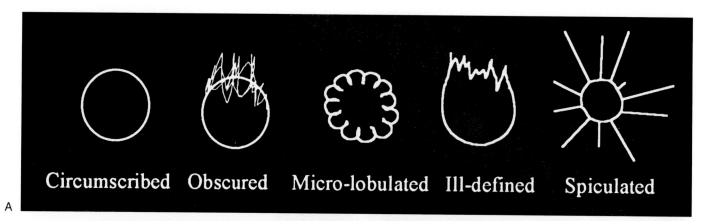

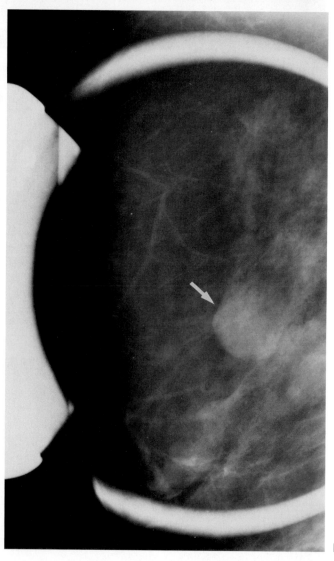

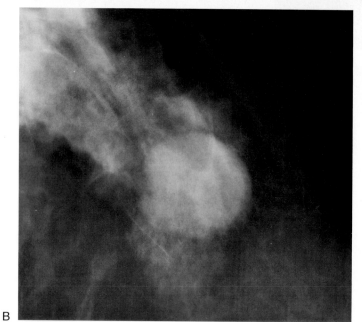

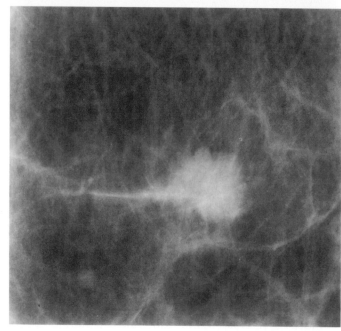

FIG. 24-9. (A) The **margins of a mass** should be described as circumscribed, obscured, microlobulated, ill-defined, or spiculated. **(B)** This cyst has circumscribed margins that can be seen through the overlapping breast tissue. **(C)** This invasive cancer has microlobulated margins. **(D)** Part of the posterior margin of this cyst (*arrow*) is obscured by normal tissue. *Continued.*

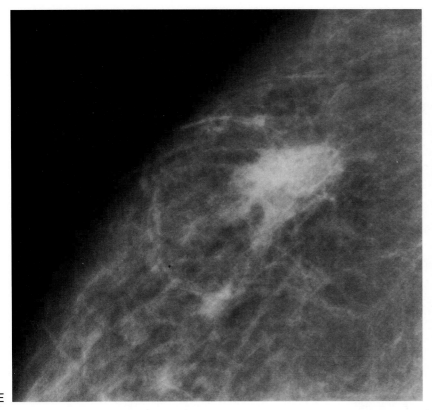

E

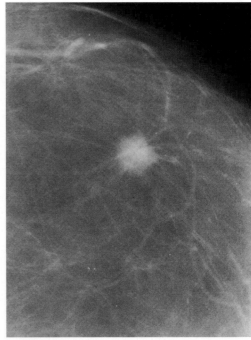

F

FIG. 24-9. *Continued.* **(E)** This **cancer** with an ill-defined margin had **both invasive and intraductal** components. **(F)** This small **invasive cancer** has a spiculated margin.

gins of a mass. If there is no visible mass, the basic description of *architectural distortion* with spiculation as a modifier should be used.

4. Density (attenuation) is used to define the x-ray attenuation of the lesion relative to the expected attenuation of an equal volume of fibroglandular breast tissue. It is important in that most breast cancers that form a visible mass are of equal or higher density than an equal volume of fibroglandular tissue. It is rare (although not impossible) for breast cancer to be lower in density. Breast cancers are never fat containing (radiolucent), although they may trap fat.

   a. High density (Fig. 24-10A)
   b. Equal density (isodense) (Fig. 24-10B)
   c. Low density (lower attenuation but not fat containing) (Fig. 24-10C)
   d. Fat containing (radiolucent) (Fig. 24-10D). This includes all lesions containing fat, such as oil cysts, lipomas, or galactoceles, as well as mixed lesions, such as hamartomas or fibroadenolipomas. (When appropriate, histologic terms may be included.)

B. Calcifications. Benign calcifications are usually larger than calcifications associated with malignancy. They are usually coarser, often round with smooth margins, and

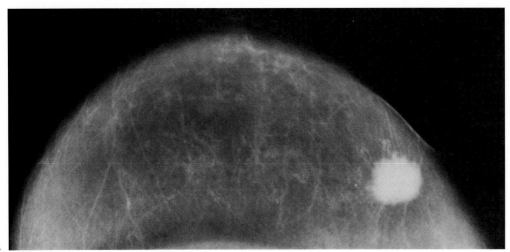

A

FIG. 24-10. Radiographic density can be of some help in analyzing masses. **(A)** This **invasive cancer** is denser than fibroglandular tissue. *Continued.*

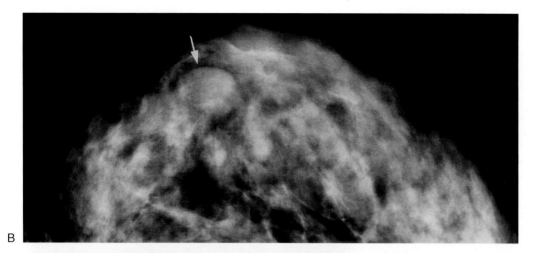

B

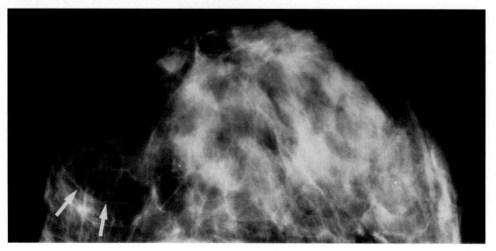

C

D

FIG. 24-10. *Continued.* **(B)** This **fibroadenoma** (*arrow*) is equal or **isodense** with the fibroglandular tissue. It would be indistinguishable from the breast tissue on this craniocaudal projection were it not for the abutting fat and its ovoid shape. **(C)** This **fibroadenoma** is less dense than fibroglandular tissue. **(D) This encapsulated fat-containing lesion** (*arrows*) **is a lipoma.**

are much more easily seen. Calcifications associated with malignancy are usually very small and often require the use of a magnifying glass to see them well.

When a specific etiology cannot be given, a description of calcifications should include the morphology and distribution of the calcifications. Benign calcifications need not always be reported. They should be reported if the interpreting radiologist is concerned that other observers might misinterpret them. Types and distribution of calcifications:

1. Typically benign (Fig. 24-11A)

a. Skin calcifications (Fig. 24-11B) are typical lucent-centered deposits that are pathognomonic. Atypical forms can be confirmed, by tangential views, to be in the skin.
b. Vascular calcifications (Fig. 24-11C): Parallel tracks or linear tubular calcifications that are clearly associated with blood vessels.
c. Coarse or popcorn-like calcifications (Fig. 24-11D) are the classic calcifications produced by an involuting fibroadenoma.

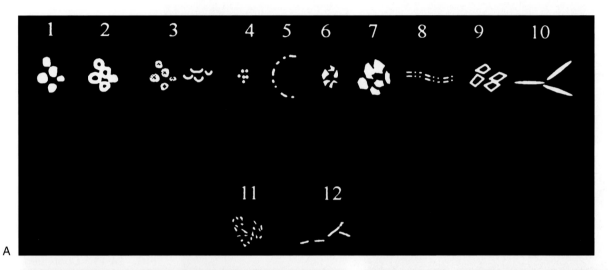

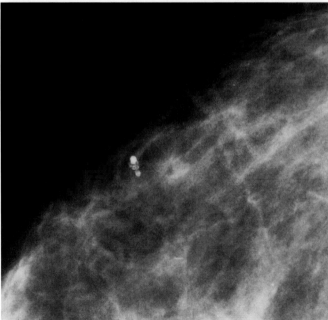

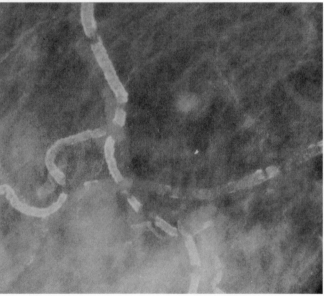

FIG. 24-11. (A) Calcium deposits form numerous shapes, as defined in this schematic. Large, round, solid calcifications (1) are always due to a benign process, as are round, lucent-centered calcifications (2). Milk of calcium (3) layers in the lateral projection. Small, very round calcifications are usually formed in small acinar cysts (4). Rim calcifications (5) form in the wall of cysts or fat necrosis. Coarse calcifications (6, 7) are almost always in involuting fibroadenomas or merely dystrophic. Vascular calcifications (8) form as parallel deposits in the wall (intima) of the vessel. Lucent-centered calcifications (9) with geographic shapes are almost always dermal deposits. Solid rods (10) are due to secretory deposits. Pleomorphic calcifications (11) and fine linear branching calcifications (12) have a high probability of being due to cancer. **(B)** Skin calcifications are usually lucent centered with round or geographic shapes. **(C)** These are vascular calcifications. *Continued.*

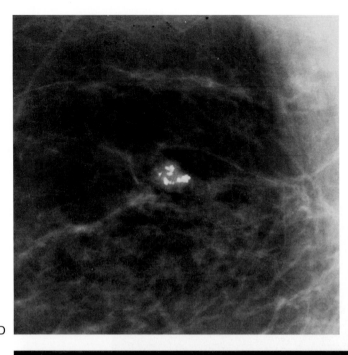

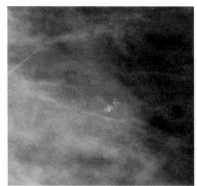

D

F

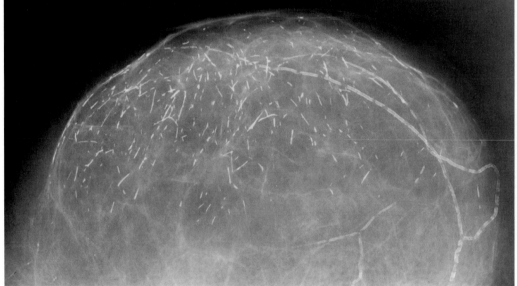

E

FIG. 24-11. *Continued.* **(D)** Large, coarse, "popcorn" calcifications are typical of an **involuting fibroadenoma. (E)** These rod-shaped calcifications are due to **calcified secretory material. (F)** These round calcifications, which are each <0.5 mm in diameter, have been stable for several years and are most likely in dilated acini due to a benign process. *Continued.*

d. Large rod-like calcifications (Fig. 24-11E) are benign calcifications that form continuous rods that may occasionally be branching, are usually >1 mm in diameter, may have lucent centers, and likely fill or surround ectatic ducts. These are the kinds of calcifications found in secretory disease, plasma cell mastitis, and duct ectasia.

e. Round calcifications (Fig. 24-11F), when multiple, may vary in size. They are usually considered benign and when small (<1 mm) frequently are formed in the acini of lobules. When <0.5 mm, the term *punctate* can be used.

f. Spherical or lucent-centered calcifications (Fig. 24-11G) are benign calcifications that range from

<1 mm to >1 cm. These deposits have smooth surfaces, are round or oval, and have a lucent center. The wall that is created is thicker than the rim or eggshell type of calcification. Included are areas of fat necrosis, calcified debris in ducts, and occasional fibroadenomas.

g. Rim or eggshell calcifications (Fig. 24-11H) are very thin benign calcifications that appear as calcium deposited on the surface of a sphere. These deposits are usually <1 mm in thickness when viewed on edge. Although fat necrosis can produce these thin deposits, calcifications in the walls of cysts are the most common rim calcifications.

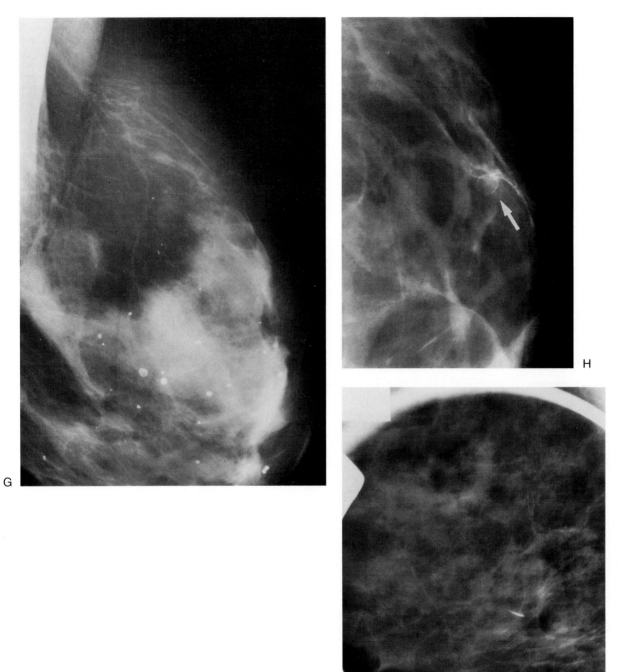

FIG. 24-11. *Continued.* **(G)** These **lucent-centered calcifications** are due to calcification of debris in the ducts or to fat necrosis. **(H) Rim, or eggshell, calcifications** usually are found in the walls of cysts or, as in this case (*arrow*), fat necrosis. **(I) Milk of calcium** has this typical appearance in the magnification lateral projection with the precipitated calcium layering in the dependent portion of a cyst. *Continued.*

h. Milk of calcium calcifications (Fig. 24-11I) are consistent with sedimented calcifications in cysts. On the CC image they are often less evident and appear as fuzzy, round, amorphous deposits while on the horizontal beam lateral image they are sharply defined, semilunar, crescent shaped, curvilinear (concave up), or linear, defining the dependent portion of cysts.

i. Suture calcifications (Fig. 24-11J) represent calcium deposited on suture material. These are rela-

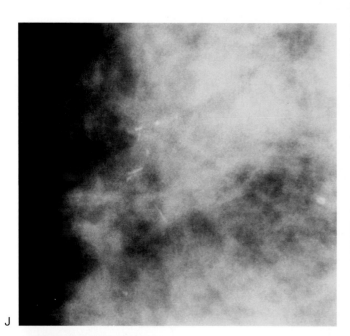

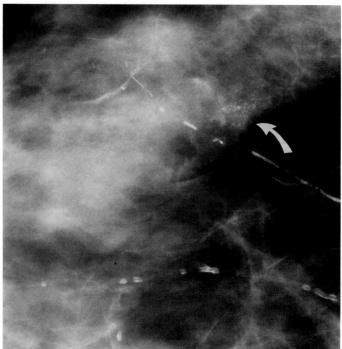

J

L

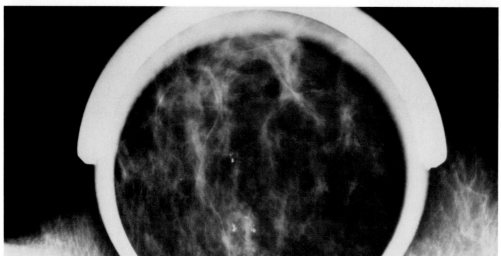

K

FIG. 24-11. *Continued.* **(J) Suture calcifications** do not always have knots. These linear calcifications are at the site of previous surgery in a breast that has been irradiated. **(K) Dystrophic calcifications** are commonly associated with surgery and irradiation as were these. **(L) Punctate calcifications are fairly uncommon.** They are pinpoint particles that are, nevertheless, sharply visible on mammography. These were benign deposits in a microcystically dilated lobule. *Continued.*

tively common in the postirradiated breast. They are typically linear or tubular in appearance and knots are frequently visible.

j. Dystrophic calcifications (Fig. 24-11K) are calcifications that usually form in the irradiated breast or in the breast following trauma. Although irregular in shape, they are usually >0.5 mm in size. They may have lucent centers.

k. Punctate calcifications (Fig. 24-11L) are round or oval, <0.5 mm with well-defined margins.

2. Intermediate concern calcifications are indistinct or amorphous (Fig. 24-11M). They are often round or flake-shaped calcifications that are sufficiently small or hazy in appearance that a more specific morphologic classification cannot be determined.

3. Higher probability of malignancy
   a. Pleomorphic or heterogeneous calcifications (granular) (Fig. 24-11N) are neither typically benign nor typically malignant irregular calcifications with varying sizes and shapes that are usually less than 0.5 mm in diameter.
   b. Fine or branching (casting) calcifications (Fig. 24-11O) are thin, irregular calcifications that appear linear but are discontinuous and <1 mm in width. Their appearance suggests irregular filling of the lumen of a duct involved irregularly by breast cancer.

4. Distribution modifiers (Fig. 24-12) are used as modifiers of the basic morphologic description and describe the arrangement of the calcifications.

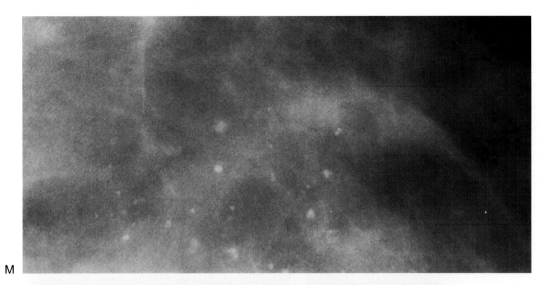

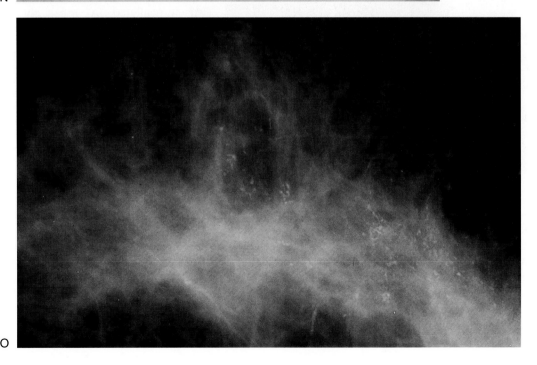

FIG. 24-11. *Continued.* **(M) Amorphous calcifications have fuzzy edges.** These are 1 mm and smaller in diameter and had formed in very small cysts. **(N)** Pleomorphic, heterogeneous calcifications should arouse suspicion. Individually these were <0.5 mm in diameter. They proved to be in a small **involuting fibroadenoma.** **(O)** Fine linear or branching calcifications are almost always due, as in this case, to **high-grade intraductal cancer.**

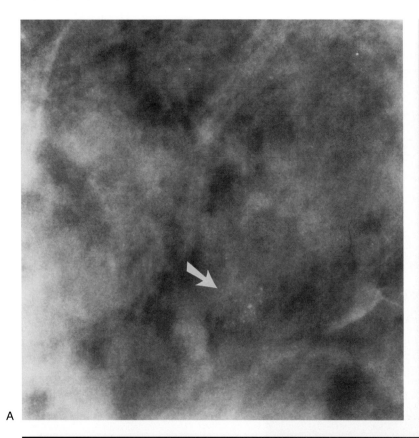

A

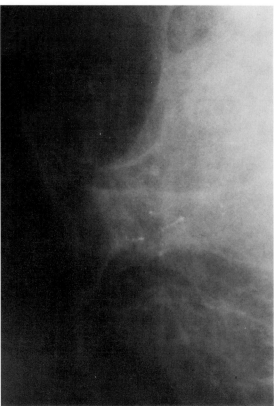

B

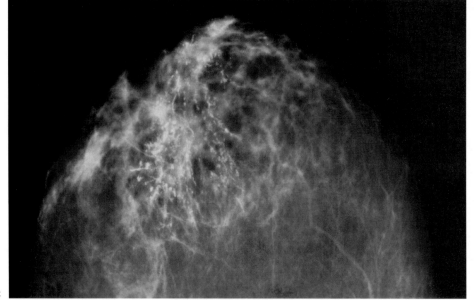

C

FIG. 24-12. The distribution of calcifications ranges from clustered to linear, segmental, regional, and diffusely scattered. **(A)** These **clustered calcifications** (*arrow*) were due to adenosis. **(B)** These calcifications form a **linear distribution** heading toward the nipple. They were due to ductal carcinoma in situ (DCIS), and the patient had Paget's disease of the nipple. **(C) Segmentally aligned calcifications** suggest the distribution of branches in a duct network and are highly suspicious, as in this patient with poorly differentiated DCIS. *Continued.*

a. Grouped or clustered (see Fig. 24-12A) calcifications: Although historically the term *clustered* has connoted suspicion, the term shall now be used as a neutral distribution modifier and may reflect benign or malignant processes. The term should be used when multiple calcifications occupy a small volume (<2 cc) of tissue.

b. Linear (see Fig. 24-12B) calcifications are arrayed in a line that may have branch points.

c. Segmental (see Fig. 24-12C) calcifications are worrisome in that their distribution suggests deposits in a duct and its branches, raising the possibility of multifocal breast cancer in a lobe or segment of the breast. Although benign causes of segmental calcifications such as secretory disease exist, this distribution is of greater concern when the morphology of the calcifications is not specifically benign.

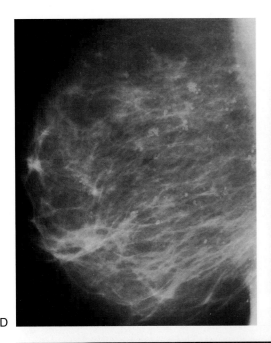

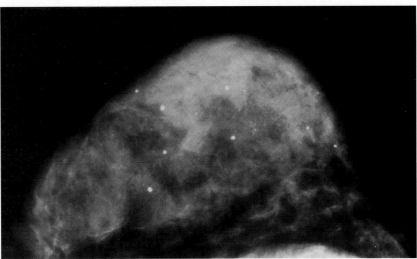

D

E

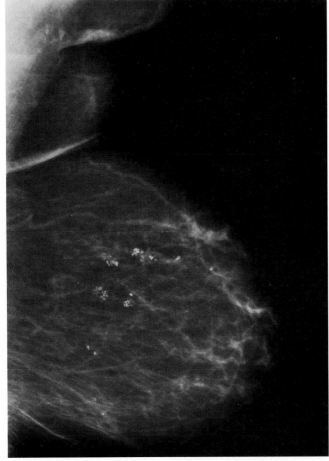

F

FIG. 24-12. *Continued.* **(D)** Regional calcifications are scattered over a large volume of breast tissue. These are usually benign, as with these skin calcifications that spread over the inner half of the left breast on the mediolateral oblique **(D)** and craniocaudal **(E)** projections, but on occasion a large segment can be involved with DCIS producing regionally distributed calcifications. **(E)** These large and small calcifications are diffusely scattered throughout the breast. These are virtually always due to a benign process. **(F)** This is an example of multiple groups of calcifications. These have been stable over many years and are almost certainly benign.

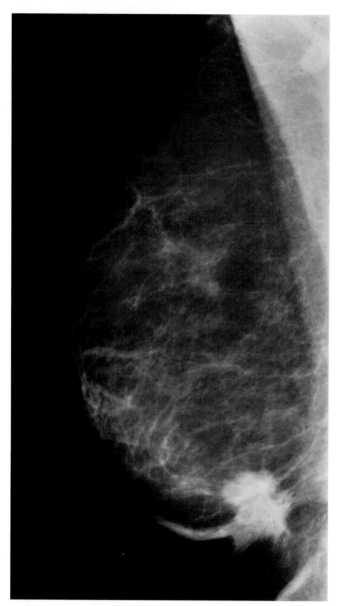

FIG. 24-13. **Skin retraction** is due to the large underlying malignancy.

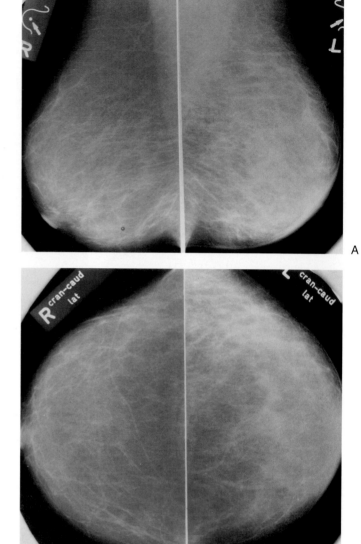

A

B

FIG. 24-15. **Skin thickening** is evident in the left breast on the mediolateral oblique **(A)** and the craniocaudal **(B)** projections due to inflammatory carcinoma.

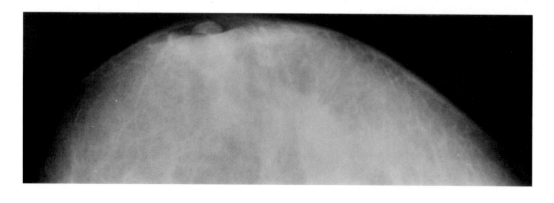

FIG. 24-14. **Nipple retraction** is visible in this under-penetrated craniocaudal projection that also demonstrates **skin thickening associated with a breast cancer** that had been neglected by the patient.

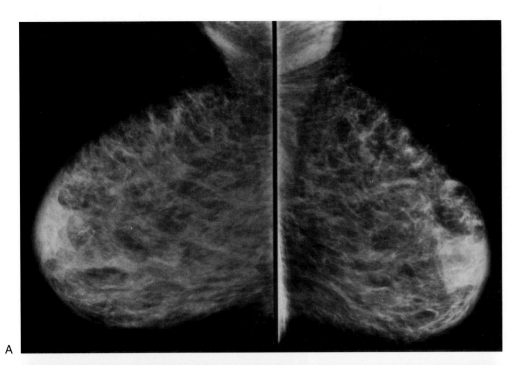

A

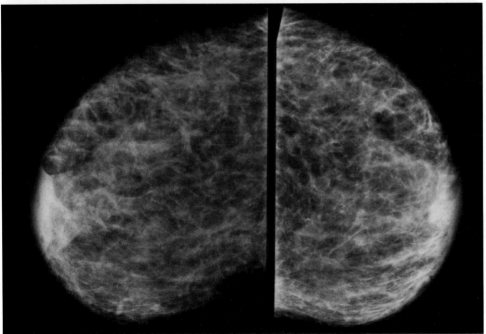

B

FIG. 24-16. There are a number of causes of trabecular thickening. This patient had **superior vena caval obstruction** secondary to lung cancer, causing edema in both breasts, as seen on the mediolateral oblique **(A)** and craniocaudal **(B)** projections. Note that the fine lines of the breasts are markedly thickened.

d. Regional (see Fig. 24-12D) calcifications are scattered in a large volume of breast tissue, not necessarily conforming to a duct distribution, that are likely benign, but they are not everywhere in the breast and do not fit the other more suspicious categories.

e. Scattered or diffuse (see Fig. 24-12E) calcifications are distributed randomly throughout the breast.

f. Multiple groups (see Fig. 24-12F): These modifiers are used when there is more than one group of calcifications that are similar in morphology and distribution.

C. Associated findings: Used with masses or calcifications or may stand alone as findings when no other abnormality is present.

1. Skin retraction (Fig. 24-13): The skin is pulled in abnormally.

2. Nipple retraction (Fig. 24-14): The nipple is pulled in or inverted.

3. Skin thickening (Fig. 24-15): This may be focal or diffuse.

4. Trabecular thickening (Fig. 24-16): This is a thickening of the fibrous septae of the breast.

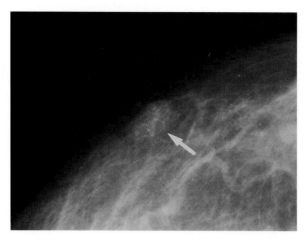

FIG. 24-17. The mass (*arrow*) on this craniocaudal projection is a benign, **raised skin lesion.**

5. Skin lesion (Fig. 24-17): Commented on when it projects over the breast in two views and may be mistaken for an intramammary lesion.
6. Axillary adenopathy (Fig. 24-18): Enlarged, nonfatty, replaced axillary lymph nodes may be commented on. Mammographic assessment of these nodes is unreliable.
7. Architectural distortion: When no mass is present this is used as a finding by itself. As an associated finding it can be used in conjunction with a finding to indicate that the normal tissue structure is distorted or retracted surrounding the finding.

Final Assessment Categories

Once significant findings have been described, a final assessment that summarizes the findings and classifies the study as one of six possible decision categories should be provided.

0. Need additional imaging evaluation. This category should, with rare exception, be used only when there is no radiologist to immediately review the study and the patient must be recalled for additional evaluation (e.g., magnification mammography, rolled views, ultrasound) before a final assessment can be rendered. This category actually means that the study is incomplete until additional imaging is completed and a final assessment can be rendered.

1. Negative. The vast majority of screening mammograms are in this category. There is nothing on the mammogram to suggest the presence of malignancy.

2. "Benign finding"—negative. This category is used when a benign finding that the observer wishes to report appears on the mammogram, but the finding has no likelihood of malignancy and there is no need for further evaluation. This might include a fat-containing lesion, such as a lipoma or an oil cyst, or calcifications, such as secretory or vascular, that

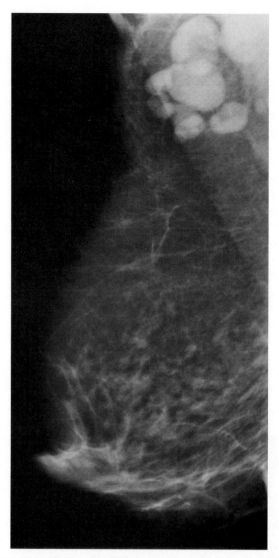

FIG. 24-18. Axillary adenopathy was secondary to **lymphoma.**

might be confusing to the untrained observer or have some implications for the management of a palpable finding.

3. Probably benign—short-interval follow-up suggested. This category will most likely evolve as data that help to refine characteristics that distinguish benign from malignant lesions are accumulated. Individual interpreters may include different findings in this category. Pooling of data should ultimately allow actual and accurate probabilities of a malignant tumor being present to be determined for the various findings.

The category is used for a finding whose characteristics suggest that it is almost certainly benign, but because a very small possibility exists that it is a malignant tumor it is thought to be prudent to follow up at a shorter interval to assess its stability.

Approaches to such lesions have been described (14,15). One of the common lesions that fits into this category is the solitary circumscribed mass. Sickles, who has done the most work in this area, has shown that, if a mass found on a prevalence (first) mammogram is round, oval, or lobulated and has well-defined margins over 75% of its surface in two magnification projections, it can be safely followed at short interval. His follow-up consisted of a mammogram at 6 months and then 3 additional years of annual mammograms, not just as screening mammograms but as highly recommended annual follow-up mammograms. Our own short-interval follow-up is more intensive, with mammography every 6 months but for a total of 2 years (stability of a cancer for more than 2 years is extremely rare).

The principle behind short-interval follow-up is the fact that if a lesion has a low probability of cancer based on its morphology and given that the probability of cancer being stable over time is also very low, then the probability of a lesion with low probability morphology as well as stability being a cancer is extremely low (the probabilities are multiplicative). Follow-up is done to try to detect the few cancers that have benign morphology as early as possible while trying to avoid unnecessary traumatic intervention.

4. Suspicious abnormality—biopsy should be considered. Most impalpable lesions that come to biopsy fall into this category. The range of "suspicious" is determined by the interpreter. It is hoped that as data accumulate it will be possible to provide specific probabilities for a given finding so that the patient and her doctor can determine the appropriate level of intervention. Needle biopsy techniques are evolving that may alter the degree of intervention (16–18).

The phrase *biopsy should be considered* was adopted at the request of the American College of Surgeons. There is no proscription against stating "biopsy is recommended," but BIRADS clearly states that "this is an assessment where the radiologist has sufficient concern that biopsy is warranted unless there are other reasons why the patient and her physician might wish to defer the biopsy." When the statement is used, the referring physician should interpret it as meaning that the radiologist is recommending a biopsy.

5. Highly suggestive of malignancy—appropriate action should be taken. Although mammography cannot provide histologic diagnoses, there are many lesions whose morphology is so characteristic that the diagnosis of malignancy is almost certain. An irregular spiculated mass, for example, is virtually always cancer. It goes without saying that a lesion in this category requires intervention.

It should be noted that these are final assessment categories. As noted earlier, a patient whose screening mammogram suggests the need for additional evaluation because a finding cannot be categorized into one of the five assessment

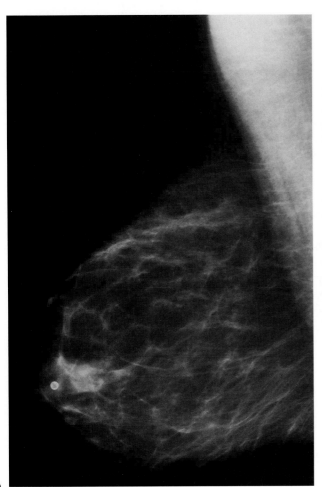

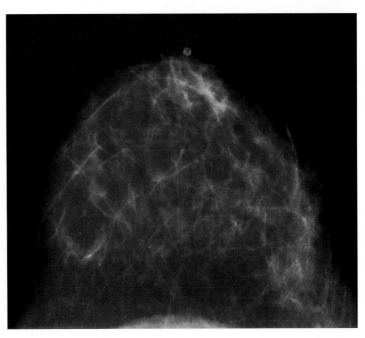

A

B

FIG. 24-19. This is a normal mediolateral oblique **(A)** and craniocaudal **(B)** mammogram of a 39-year-old woman with predominantly fatty breasts.

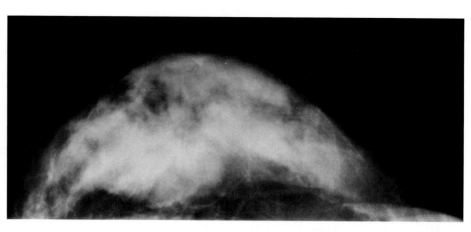

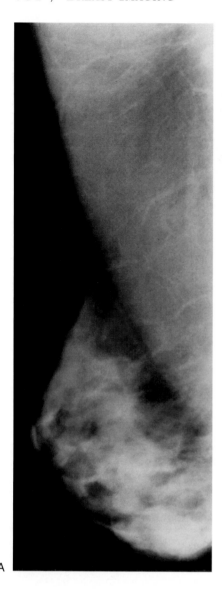

A

FIG. 24-20. The breast tissues are extremely and heterogeneously dense on the mediolateral oblique **(A)** and craniocaudal **(B)** projections. This somewhat lowers the sensitivity of mammography, but the mammogram is normal.

groups is considered to be incompletely assessed until additional imaging is done and the findings assigned to one of the five categories.

The terminology used to define these categories was carefully crafted in consultation with nonradiologists. BIRADS alerts the referring physician to the fact that these are assessments based on the imaging study. They cannot, with rare exception, be used to eliminate concern raised over a clinically suspicious abnormality and do not obviate the need for clinical assessment of the breast as well. The decision to perform a biopsy of most palpable lesions must still be based on the clinical assessment when the mammogram is unrevealing.

Sample Reports

Each radiologist may have a different way of phrasing the ultimate report. Some, for example, may wish to provide direct advice such as "a biopsy is recommended," as opposed to the BIRADS-supported "biopsy should be con-

sidered." This is acceptable as long as the basic BIRADS criteria and content are met and the final assessment provides unambiguous guidance.

Negative Mammogram. Mammograms that are unremarkable fall into two categories. The first is the breast that is predominantly fat and the parenchyma is radiographically lucent. The sensitivity of mammography for small lesions in breasts in this category should be quite high. In this circumstance our report would read as follows:

Example: Fig. 24-19
The breast tissues are predominantly fat. No masses or clustered microcalcifications are visible.
Conclusion: There is no mammographic evidence of malignancy.

When the breast tissues are inhomogeneous or radiographically dense and a lesion could be obscured, we prefer the following:

Example: Fig. 24-20
The breast tissues are heterogeneously dense. This somewhat lowers the sensitivity of mammography. No focal masses or

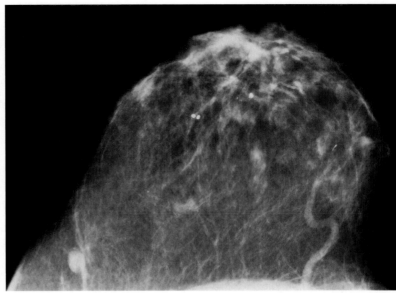

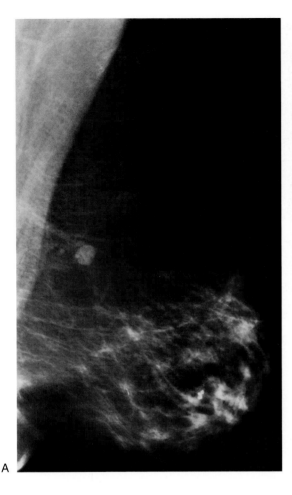

FIG. 24-21. The density that projects over the upper outer right breast on the mediolateral oblique **(A)** and craniocaudal **(B)** projections is a **benign intramammary lymph node.**

clustered microcalcifications are seen, although the dense surrounding tissue could obscure a lesion.
Conclusion: Dense mammary tissues with no mammographic evidence of malignancy.

Such reporting accurately reflects what is seen mammographically and conveys the somewhat diminished sensitivity level in the mammographically dense breast.

For the Patient Who Is Referred for an Area of Clinical Concern. If a patient is referred with a clinically evident abnormality that is not evident or is indeterminate on the mammogram, our report might read:

The breast tissues are heterogeneously dense. This somewhat lowers the sensitivity of mammography. No abnormality is seen in the area indicated by the patient. Any decision to biopsy at this time should be based on the clinical assessment.
Conclusion: There is no mammographic evidence of malignancy.

In the literature and in educational forums it has been clearly conveyed that mammography cannot be used to exclude a malignancy. Just as a mammographically detected abnormality that is not clinically evident must be resolved, so too must a clinically evident abnormality be resolved, even if it is not apparent on the mammogram. Our report in such circumstances merely reminds the clinician that decisions must be made based on a suspicious clinical assessment just as they must be made as a result of a suspicious

mammographic assessment, and the two are frequently mutually exclusive.

We use the terminology "in the area indicated by the patient" because, in reality, unless the clinician were to accompany the patient for her mammogram, there is no way of knowing precisely what area was of concern to the clinician. Even if the radiologist chooses to perform a clinical examination, there is no guarantee that he or she will be concerned about the same area of the breast. The only reliable individual for indicating the area of clinical concern is the patient.

Report When an Abnormality Is Present. The second final assessment category involves the notation of radiographically visible findings that are of no concern but, nevertheless, warrant inclusion in the report. This may be done so that their presence has been noted and if they appear in future studies confusion can be avoided by inexperienced film interpreters. This category may include some benign intramammary lymph nodes, scattered bilateral calcifications, skin calcifications, secretory deposits, and other definitely benign findings.

Example: Fig. 24-21
The breast tissues are predominantly fat.
A benign intramammary lymph node projects over the upper outer right breast. No focal masses or clustered microcalcifications are visible.
Conclusion: There is no mammographic evidence of malignancy.

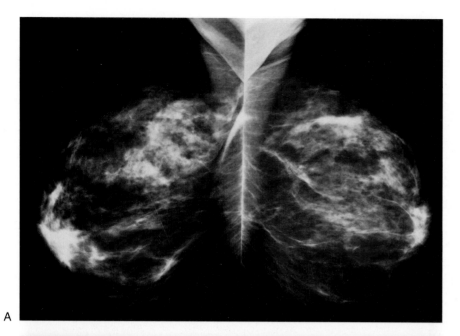

A

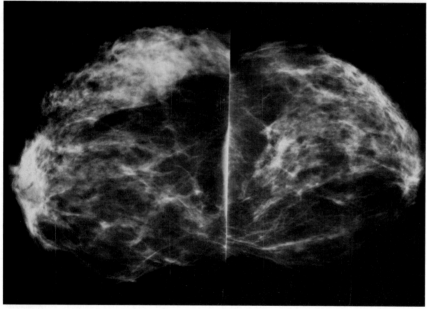

B

FIG. 24-22. There is **asymmetric breast tissue** that projects over the upper outer left breast on the mediolateral oblique **(A)** and craniocaudal **(B)** projections. If this is palpable it should be viewed with suspicion. Otherwise it represents a normal variation.

Short-Interval Follow-Up. BIRADS category 3 is for lesions that are virtually always benign, but because of a slight concern the radiologist prefers an early and closer level of follow-up than the regular screening. This situation is identical to the clinician's requesting that a woman return in a few months for a follow-up when an area has been detected on the clinical examination that the clinician strongly believes to be benign but would prefer to evaluate over time to establish its stability to reinforce confidence that it is benign.

Because we recommend that all women of screening age (≥40 years) have annual mammograms, our short-interval follow-up was chosen as halfway through the interval. This was chosen somewhat arbitrarily but was based on the fact

that the average doubling time for breast cancers is 100 to 180 days. A doubling of the volume increases the diameter by approximately 25%. If the follow-up is too early, then a change may not be apparent. At 6 months (approximately one doubling time) there has been sufficient opportunity for any lesion that might change to do so. The change will be visible, but if the lesion proves to be malignant not so much time has passed that treatment is jeopardized.

Lesions that are placed in a "probably benign" short-interval follow-up category are lesions that are not expected to be cancers. This is not a category, for example, for suspicious lesions that are seen only in one projection. If a lesion is suspicious, it must be dealt with promptly. Lesions for category 3 have a very low probability of malignancy. Although

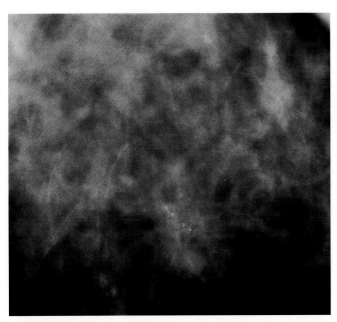

FIG. 24-23. These clustered calcifications proved to be due to **poorly differentiated intraductal carcinoma.**

stability is not a perfect guarantee of a benign process, stability on top of benign morphology reinforces the likelihood of a benign lesion. The stability of a suspicious abnormality such as a spiculated lesion, on the other hand, is not reassuring (19).

There are, in fact, no objective data on which to base follow-up. Some clinicians are replacing the short-interval follow-up with fine-needle aspiration cytology or core biopsy. This increases the cost of screening because most physicians still request the follow-up even when the sampling is benign.

Example: Fig. 24-5
The breast tissues are predominantly fat.
There is a dilated duct in the subareolar region of the left breast. This almost certainly represents a benign process. Nevertheless, careful follow-up is suggested with a repeat study in 6 months.
Conclusion: Probable benign duct dilatation, but follow-up is suggested.

Asymmetric Breast Tissue. Women with asymmetric breast tissue should be evaluated in conjunction with physical examination. It is relatively common to see asymmetric breast tissue in normal women (20). If there is a palpable asymmetry on physical examination that coincides with increased density on the mammogram, the findings should be considered additive and lead to prompter intervention. Thus, asymmetric tissue should be described as a probable normal variation but with the caution that if there is a palpable asymmetry, it should be considered more suspicious.

Example: Fig. 24-22
The breast tissues demonstrate fibronodular densities bilaterally. There is asymmetric breast tissue in the upper outer quadrant of the left breast. If there is a palpable asymmetry in this area, it should be viewed with suspicion. It otherwise represents a normal variation.

Conclusion: Asymmetric breast tissue in the upper outer quadrant of the left breast. Careful clinical assessment is suggested.

Suspicious Abnormality; Biopsy Should Be Considered. Category 4 is quite broad. Different practitioners have different thresholds for intervention. If a low false-negative rate is desired, then the false-positive rate will be higher. If the goal is to have a low false-positive rate, then cancers will be missed and the false-negative rate will be higher.

There are many lesions that have a low but finite probability of malignancy, such as clustered microcalcifications. Although many of these are unlikely to be cancer, they are of sufficient concern that we feel they should be biopsied.

Example: Fig. 24-23
The breast tissues are extremely dense.
There are pleomorphic, microcalcifications in a linear distribution in the 10:00 middle portion of the right breast. These should be viewed with suspicion, and biopsy should be considered. If biopsy is contemplated, imaging-guided core needle biopsy or preoperative radiographically guided localization could be performed.
Conclusion: Suspicious calcifications in the upper outer quadrant of the right breast. Biopsy should be considered.

Highly Suggestive of Malignancy. Lesions in category 5 have a very high probability of being malignant. When a lesion has spiculated margins, it is virtually always malignant and this should be stated in the report.

Example: Fig. 24-24
The breast tissues are heterogeneously dense.
The present study is compared to previous mammograms. A 1.2-cm irregular mass with spiculated margins has developed in the 4:00 middle region of the right breast. On spot-compression imaging, this has the features of a malignant process.
Conclusion: There is a malignant lesion in the lower inner quadrant of the right breast.

The Ultrasound Report. Similar caution should be exercised with ultrasound analysis. The efficacious use of ultrasound involves the differentiation of cysts from solid lesions (and to guide interventional procedures).

Example: Fig. 24-25
Transverse and longitudinal scans of the upper left breast were obtained. The 1.5-cm nonpalpable mass, seen by mammography in the 12:00 region, has the ultrasound appearance of a cyst with sharply defined margins, no internal echoes, and has enhanced through-transmission of sound.
Conclusion: The mass seen by mammography in the upper left breast is a cyst by ultrasound. No further evaluation is needed.

On a statistical basis solid masses that are oval with their long axis parallel to the chest wall or smoothly lobulated with sharply defined margins with a homogeneous internal echo texture by ultrasound are almost always benign. However, if certainty is needed, ultrasound cannot be used to differentiate benign from malignant solid lesions. The degree of concern can be conveyed based on the ultrasound analysis (see Chapter 16). If a solid lesion has a triangular shape with irregular margins and causes shadowing, it is more likely to represent a malignant process. However, the radiol-

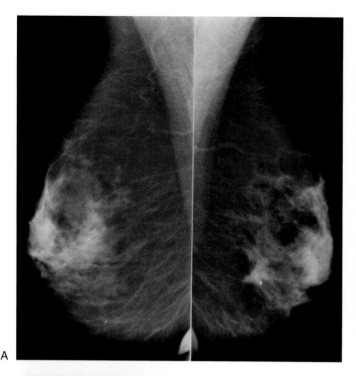

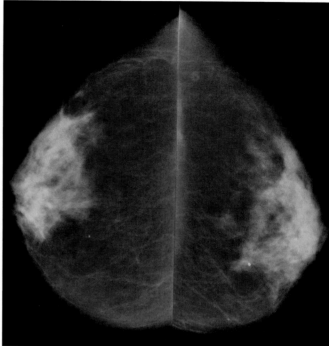

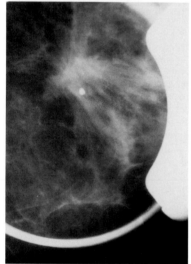

FIG. 24-24. There is an irregular, ill-defined mass in the lower inner aspect of the right breast, as seen on the mediolateral oblique **(A)** and craniocaudal **(B)** projections. On spot-compression imaging **(C)** this represents a spiculated mass that proved to be an **invasive ductal carcinoma.**

ogist should be aware that benign breast structures can have malignant appearances, and malignant lesions can have what is generally considered benign morphology.

Our ultrasound report reflects whether or not the finding of clinical or mammographic concern can be explained on the basis of a macrocyst being present. If the lesion is not clearly a cyst but is a three-dimensionally definable solid lesion with regular ultrasound features, it is so described.

Example: Fig. 24-26
Transverse and longitudinal scans of the upper outer right breast were obtained. The 2.5-cm mass, visible by mammography, in this area is seen by ultrasound. It is ovoid with smooth margins

and a homogeneous internal echo texture. There is enhanced through-transmission of sound. The appearance is consistent with a solid breast mass.
Conclusion: The mass seen by mammography in the upper outer right breast is solid by ultrasound. Although its characteristics are suggestive of a benign process, this cannot be absolutely determined by imaging and biopsy should be considered.

In women under the age of 30, there is an overwhelming statistical likelihood that a mass is a fibroadenoma. It could even be argued that imaging for these women is not warranted. In our report we may suggest that a well-circumscribed solid lesion most likely represents a fibroadenoma but caution the referring physician that this cannot be absolutely determined by imaging techniques.

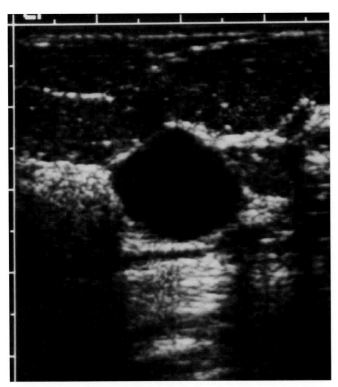

FIG. 24-25. A cyst by ultrasound is round, oval, or lobulated with sharply defined margins, no internal echoes, and enhanced through transmission of sound.

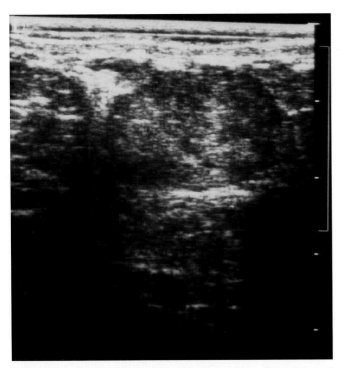

FIG. 24-26. This well-defined, solid mass with uniform internal echoes proved to be a **fibroadenoma** at core needle biopsy.

Transverse and longitudinal scans of the area indicated by the patient in the upper outer right breast reveal a 2-cm ovoid, sharply marginated mass with a homogeneous internal echo texture and good sound transmission. In a patient of this age, this almost certainly represents a fibroadenoma; however, this cannot be absolutely determined by any imaging study. If certainty is required, ultrasound-guided core needle biopsy or surgical excision is suggested.

Conclusion: Solid mass in the right breast.

Report Coding System

A significant goal for BIRADS is to encourage the maintenance of a database that can be used by individuals or groups to monitor the results of their programs (outcomes) in the hope that this will help maintain a high degree of accuracy in breast cancer detection. The collection of similar data may permit the development of a national database as a quality assurance process to assist in the maintenance of high-quality screening. By pooling data, analysis of breast cancer trends can be made. Individuals or groups can compare their own results with the national results and use that information in their quality assurance programs to improve their own performance. Image interpretation can be refined using large data sets.

To simplify the entry of data into a database, BIRADS provides a coding system. This coding system is easily integrated into any computer database system for the maintenance and analysis of the image interpretation and monitoring of results. The codes have been made as simple as possible to facilitate their use and are mnemonic wherever possible.

Pathology Coding System

As with the mammography coding system, the pathology coding system is designed to simplify data entry. Results monitoring is the best way to evaluate the success of screening and to refine a screening program. The pathology coding system permits simple data recording. The old numeric codes that required a complicated dictionary have been replaced by mnemonic codes such as ID for invasive ductal carcinoma, IL for invasive lobular carcinoma, ADH for atypical ductal hyperplasia, and ALH for atypical lobular hyperplasia. Whenever possible, acronyms have been used to simplify coding. This should facilitate the monitoring and recording of results.

Follow-Up and Outcome Monitoring

BIRADS is a quality assurance system. It is not sufficient merely to interpret mammograms in a vacuum. The maintenance of a database is an important element of the ACR system. Without monitoring the results of screening it is impossible to know the success of the program. It is important to know such information as how many studies have been performed, how many women have required evaluation beyond the routine screening, and how many cancers have been detected and their sizes and stages. Each group should maintain the suggested data so that the accuracy of the individual screening programs and their success in diagnosing breast cancers at an earlier stage can be determined. This will also allow each group to adjust its thresholds by comparison with pooled national data.

BIRADS has evolved over several years, and a great deal of thought, effort, and discussion has gone into it. It is not a departure from traditional imaging analysis; rather it simply defines the basic structure of mammographic interpretation. BIRADS merely describes what most radiologists do on a daily basis. It does not eliminate the individual expertise of the radiologist but structures mammographic evaluation in an organized and understandable fashion. BIRADS is not a perfect system. The ACR has planned that BIRADS will evolve with time. The ACR BIRADS committee will evaluate any submitted suggestions for improvement.

Mammography represents the best method available to reduce breast cancer mortality. The use of BIRADS is an important component in the overall delivery of high-quality breast evaluation. Its use will improve the communication of mammography results and permit an ongoing improvement in mammographic quality and interpretation.

DATA MAINTENANCE AND THE SCREENING AUDIT

The only way to determine how well a screening program is functioning is by monitoring the program. BIRADS includes an overview of recommended data to be collected. It is suggested that the following data be maintained by all who provide mammographic services. Some of these data and others may become mandated by law, and the practitioner should be aware of the various state and federal requirements. The goal should be to determine how a program is functioning so that its ability to detect and diagnose early breast cancer can be improved.

Data to Be Monitored

1. Number of women screened
2. Number of women for whom additional evaluation is requested (e.g., extra views, ultrasound)
3. Number of women who actually have extra imaging
4. Number of women recalled who prove to be negative
5. Number of women recommended for short-interval follow-up
6. Number of women for whom a biopsy is recommended
7. Number of women recommended for needle biopsy (fine-needle aspiration or core)
   a. Positive predictive value (number of women diagnosed with cancer divided by the number of women biopsied)
   b. False-negatives

   c. Cyst diagnosed
8. Number of women interpreted as "suspicious—biopsy should be considered." Positive predictive value (the number of women diagnosed with cancer divided by the number of women biopsied)
9. Number of women read as probable cancers. Positive predictive value (the number of women diagnosed with cancer divided by the number of women biopsied)
10. Number of cancers detected (percent palpable in retrospect after mammography)
11. Number of mammographically detected cancers
    a. Number of invasive cancers by size and stage
    b. Number and percent of total cancers that are DCIS
    c. Lobular carcinoma listed separately and not counted as cancer
12. False-positives
13. False-negatives (as can best be ascertained)
14. Interval cancers (diagnosed between screenings) as best determined
15. Pathology data
    a. Benign lesions: size and histology
    b. LCIS and atypical hyperplasias should be tracked separately
    c. Pathologic staging of cancers
       (1) Size (pathologic): gross greatest diameter
       (2) Histology
       (3) Histologic grade
       (4) Margin status
       (5) Nodal status
       (6) Stage
       (7) Other prognostic indicators (e.g., estrogen receptors, progesterone receptors)
    d. Number of deaths (breast cancer and other)
16. Statistical issues: Once the data are acquired, various summary figures can be calculated
    a. True positive: The number of cancers detected by mammography (palpable vs. nonpalpable should be counted separately)
    b. False-positive
       (1) Recall based on the screening study that proves to be benign
       (2) Lesion that is biopsied based on the mammogram that proves to not be cancer
    c. True negative: A negative mammogram in a woman who does not have cancer
    d. False-negative: Negative mammogram in a woman who proves to have cancer; BIRADS includes any cancer that is diagnosed within 1 year of a negative mammogram
    e. Positive predictive value: Number of women diagnosed with cancer divided by the number of women whose study raised the question of cancer
    f. Negative predictive value: Number of women who actually do not have cancer divided by the number of women whose study is interpreted as not showing cancer

Sensitivity and Specificity

Sensitivity and specificity are often cited as the most important measures of a screening program.

Specificity is the number of women whose mammograms are interpreted as negative divided by the number of women who truly do not have breast cancer. Superficially specificity is a measure of how reliable a negative mammogram is in determining there is no cancer present. However, it can be misleading since breast cancer is very uncommon. If a group of 1,000 women is being screened every year, and 1 year the mammograms are all reported as negative without even being looked at, the specificity will be 99.96% to 99.98% because there will be only two to four cancers that become detectable in 1,000 women each year. Even though all of the cancers are missed, the negative predictive value is very high and hence the specificity is high.

Sensitivity is the number of cancers detected by the mammogram divided by the number of actual cancers in the population over a specified time period. It is an important measure of the success of screening. Sensitivity is an overall measure of the cancers detected by screening that are diagnosed over a defined interval. For example, using the Breast Cancer Detection Demonstration Project (BCDDP) rates, if there are actually 100 cancers among a group of women who are screened every year and mammography detects 74 of the 80 cancers that are detected at the time of screening (93% of those detectable by clinical examination together with mammography) and an additional 20 cancers become apparent before the next screening (the woman feels a lump), then the total number of cancers available for detection was 100 (80 detected by the screening and 20 interval cancers). The sensitivity of mammography over the interval was 74/100 = 74%. Because clinical breast examination only detected 58 of the 80 cancers detected at the time of the screening (46%) and another 20 surfaced between screenings, the sensitivity for clinical breast examination would be 58/(80 + 20) = 58%.

Sensitivity is valuable for comparing screening results, but because all clinically relevant cancers eventually are detected (100% sensitivity), the sensitivity figure must be evaluated in conjunction with the size and stage of the cancers detected. A sensitivity of 100% is of little value if all of the cancers are 2 cm or greater in size. A sensitivity of 75% may be very valuable if 50% of the invasive cancers detected are <1 cm and thus highly curable.

Factors That Affect Sensitivity

The accuracy of mammography can appear better or worse than it actually is. The preselection of patients can alter the apparent sensitivity of mammography. For example, assume that a population is screened using mammography and clinical examination and that mammography can detect 85% of the cancers detectable at screening. Further assume that 50% of the cancers are detected only by mam-

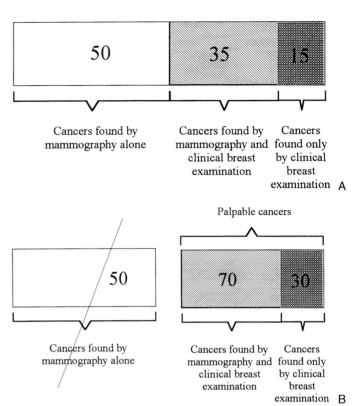

FIG. 24-27. (A) If there are 100 cancers in a population and mammography detects 85% of them, then the sensitivity of mammography is 85%. If 50% of the cancers are only found by mammography and 35% are both clinically evident and visible by mammography while 15% are not found by mammography but are evident by clinical examination, the sensitivity of clinical examination is 50% and the false-negative rate for mammography is 15%. **(B)** If the group studied is made up only of women with palpable masses, then the sensitivity of clinical examination jumps to 100% (by definition) and the sensitivity of mammography falls to 70%. Such a screening, however, would miss the 50% of cancers that could be found earlier that are not palpable.

mography. This means that the sensitivity of mammography is 85%, and the false-negative rate for mammography is 15%. If, on the other hand, the sensitivity of mammography is evaluated for a patient population referred for mammography because of palpable abnormalities, the sensitivity of mammography will appear diminished. Preselection would exclude the asymptomatic women who make up the 50% of the cancers that could be found only by mammography. Thus, the sensitivity of mammography among women who have palpable masses would drop to 70% (Fig. 24-27).

The sensitivity of mammography would be improved in the above example if additional views were performed based on the clinical breast examination. Although it is not clear that management will be affected, obtaining spot compression views that try to push the palpable lesion into the subcutaneous fat will reveal an additional 10% of lesions not evident on routine two-view mammography (21,22). It has

TABLE 24-1. *Screening data analysis*

Mammogram Result	Proven Cancer	No Cancer
Negative	False-negative	True negative
Positive	True positive	False-positive

Sensitivity = TP/(TP + FN)
Specificity = TN/(TN + FP)

also been shown that the detection rate of mammography increases with the number of projections obtained.

In the major screening programs, sensitivities for mammography (screening-detected cancers divided by screening-detected cancers plus interval cancers) have ranged from 45% to 88% (23).

Most analysts view these data as a two-by-two table (Table 24-1).

FALSE-NEGATIVE MAMMOGRAPHY

The ability of mammography to demonstrate abnormalities that are subsequently shown to be malignant varies depending on the patient population and the intensity of the mammographic evaluation. The false-negative rate is difficult to determine accurately because it requires follow-up on all negative screening mammograms. This is impossible for most practices without linkage to state databases, since women shift their health care and the diagnosis of breast cancer may be made in some other facility. Most groups can only develop crude measures for missed cancers, but their analysis may help reduce the rate in the future.

The false-negative rates for a test depend on the standard against which the test is compared and the length of follow-up of the population. For example, in the BCDDP (8) 20% of cancers became apparent within 1 year of screening, having been missed by a combination of mammography and physical examination. Assuming an average doubling time of 100 to 180 days, these interval cancers were present at the time of screening and were not detected. However, the same data indicate that of the cancers detected by screening (clinical examination or mammography) mammography missed fewer than 9% of the total, whereas 42% of the cancers were detected only by mammography and were not palpable (the false-negative rate for clinical breast examination was 42%).

Thus, the false-negative rate for mammography is determined by the number of cancers missed at a screening by mammography divided by the number of cancers that could be detected at that screening (mammographically missed cancers/[mammographically detected cancers + clinically detected cancers]).

The interval cancer rate is the percentage of cancers that surface in the interval between screenings divided by the total number of cancers detected over the entire period (cancers surfacing in the interval between screens/[cancers surfacing in the interval + screen-detected cancers]).

Accuracy

Accuracy is the number of correct study results divided by the total number of patients studied, which equals the true positives plus the true negatives divided by the total patients studied.

For breast cancer screening, this is not that valuable a measure because cancer is so uncommon the accuracy is dominated by negatives.

Audit Results

There are no absolute figures for determining a successful screening program. It depends on the prior probability of cancer in the population (how much breast cancer is actually present to detect). Tabar has shown that it is better to detect invasive cancers before they become >1 cm, although he has suggested that the median size should be 1.5 cm or smaller (24). We believe that the goal should be 1 cm or smaller. In addition to Tabar's data, this goal is reinforced by the data from Memorial Sloan-Kettering, which demonstrated a significant survival benefit among women with stage 1 cancers when the cancer was 1.0 cm or smaller (25).

In our own program we find approximately eight to ten cancers (DCIS + invasive) in the first screening (prevalence) and approximately two to four new cancers in women who have had previous mammograms (incidence). Our interventional policy is quite aggressive, and 60% of the invasive cancers are 1.0 cm or smaller and 30% of the cancers detected are DCIS. These results are at the cost of a positive predictive value for a breast biopsy of approximately 12% for women age 40 and rising steadily to approximately 45% by age 79 for a mammographically instigated biopsy (the positive predictive value increases with the prior probability of cancer). In Sickles' audit (26) with a slightly less aggressive approach such that the positive predictive value ranged from 26% for women in their forties to 56% for women over age 70, 39% of the invasive cancers were 1.0 cm or smaller and 30% of the cancers were DCIS. In Sickles' audit, 79% were stage 0 or stage 1 cancers (negative axillary lymph nodes).

Reasons for False-Negative Mammography

Much has been made of the fact that dense breast tissues may make it more difficult to detect breast cancers; however, there are many false-negatives that occur in women whose tissues are not dense. There are several reasons that cancers are not shown by mammography. Cancers will be missed if the breast is not properly positioned (Fig. 24-28) and if high-quality, high-resolution images are not obtained. Rigorous mammographic technique is important. The importance of

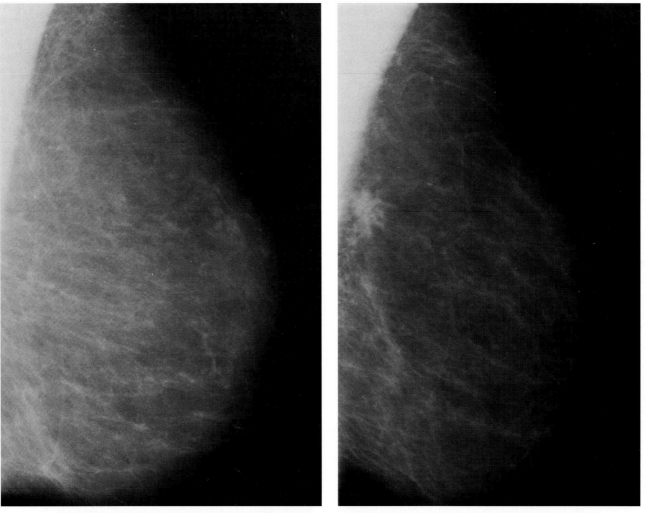

A
B

FIG. 24-28. Cancer can be missed due to poor positioning. This poorly positioned straight lateral mammogram **(A)** (the position used during much of the Canadian screening trial; see Chapter 4) is negative. A repeat mediolateral oblique on the same day **(B)** reveals the cancer, despite the fact that even it is not well positioned.

positioning cannot be overemphasized. Even well-performed mammograms miss some of the breast tissues. Cancers high in the breast and close to the chest wall are difficult to project onto a two-dimensional recording system. It is critical that the breast be pulled away from the chest wall as vigorously as the patient permits to project the deep tissues over the detector system. Mammography should not damage the breast, although on occasion a bruise may result or friable skin, particularly in the intertriginous inframammary fold, may split. Fortunately, most women do not find mammography painful, but some women do find it uncomfortable (27). The technologist must be sensitive and work with the patient to ensure that the breast is drawn as far as possible into the mammographic unit while trying to minimize discomfort. There is a significant danger of missing lesions near the chest wall if this is not done.

Positioning is complicated by the curvature and slope of the chest wall, and in some women the standard two views may not image the entire breast. Blind spots are most common laterally toward the axilla and medially close to the sternum. High upper inner quadrant lesions are especially difficult to project onto conventional detectors.

Between 30% and 50% of the failures to detect cancers on the mammogram are unavoidable (28,29) because the tumors do not produce primary or secondary changes that are visible with current techniques. If the tumor is surrounded by tissue of similar x-ray attenuation and there is no architectural distortion or deposition of calcium, a large cancer may be invisible mammographically.

On approximately one-third of false-negative mammograms, cancers are visible mammographically but are missed by interpreter oversight. Another third have subtle signs of malignancy that may not be appreciated by the inexperienced radiologist. Interpretive errors will always occur, but they can be minimized by proper training. Every radiologist, no matter how skilled, however, cannot avoid overlooking cancers. Because there is a psychovisual threshold below which it does not appear possible to operate, overlooking even an occasional obvious malignancy cannot be avoided. Because observers overlook different things, several studies have now shown that having a second reader review the cases reduces the possibility of oversight by 5% to 15% (30–32). Double reading is desirable, but it can only be effective if it is performed efficiently. This can be accomplished by delaying interpretation and mounting studies on multiviewers. Two or more radiologists can read these very efficiently without increasing the cost. If the process is inefficient, then the cost of screening must go up and women will be denied access.

The importance of high-quality imaging cannot be overemphasized. Mammographic detection of breast cancer is completely image dependent. Proper equipment is essential, and well-trained, motivated technologists are the key to optimizing the study. Experienced interpreters cannot compensate for poor-quality mammography, and strict attention to positioning and quality control should be a constant obligation.

Unfortunately, not only does mammography not detect all cancers, but mammography does not detect all cancers early enough to result in a cure. At this time, breast cancer can only be cured if it is detected and treated before it has successfully spread to other parts of the body. The primary cancer in the breast is not lethal. It is the metastatic disease that eventually kills. Some cancers are likely metastatic very early in their growth. The ability to pass into the circulation, float to other organs, and successfully invade those tissues likely requires DNA changes beyond those that merely decontrol cell proliferation. The fact that many cancers lack the ability to successfully spread to other organs is the likely reason that some cancers can be stopped and that many women can be cured of breast cancer.

Nevertheless, it is very likely that some cancers develop metastatic capability early in their development. It is entirely possible that in some cancers the first malignant clone has the ability to spread. These cancers may have seeded other organs long before the primary is or even can be discovered, and early detection for these women is simply not early enough. Other cancers are not detectable by either mammography or clinical breast exam until they are quite large and have already metastasized, while still other cancers grow to be very large and never metastasize. The latter situation is rare, since metastatic spread is directly associated with the size of the cancer at diagnosis (33).

Assuming the average doubling time of breast cancer is 100 to 180 days, virtually all cancers that eventually become detectable either clinically or mammographically likely have been present at the microscopic level for 5 or more years before their detection. The fact that mortality can be reduced by mammography screening suggests that many cancers grow to large sizes before they successfully metastasize. There is still much room for improvement in detecting cancer earlier. Since prognosis is clearly related to size,

even earlier detection than is now possible may add additional benefit.

Analyzing False-Negative Mammograms

The analysis of false-negative mammography is complicated by its definition. There are at least five types of false-negative mammograms.

1. Truly false-negative (TFN). On the true false-negative mammogram there is no indication of the presence of a cancer even in retrospect.

2. Single-reader false-negative (SRFN) This second category includes the mammograms that are interpreted as negative, but on a second reading the lesion is detected.

3. Retrospectively visible false-negative (RVFN). The third type of false-negative mammogram is the lesion that is visible in retrospect. Lesions that could have been detected should be included here. Some of these are found by the patient or her physician between screenings, while others are found at a subsequent screening.

Lesions that in retrospect showed subtle changes on previous mammograms but would not likely have ever been detected prospectively should be considered TFN because they are unlikely to ever be detected earlier.

4. Interpreted as benign false-negative (IBFN). These are lesions that are detected but, because of their morphologic appearance, are classified as benign and diagnosis is delayed. This category is strongly influenced by the thresholds for intervention. Circumscribed cancers have been detected but passed because of their benign morphology (34).

5. Technical failure false-negative (TFFN). The last category of false-negative mammography includes the cancers that are not detected due to technical shortcomings. Technical factors that may compromise the ability to image the lesion include poor positioning, poor contrast, image blur, and poor penetration of the dense tissues.

Interval Cancers

In screening programs, an indication of the false-negative mammograms can be found in the interval cancer rate. Most investigators categorize cancers that are diagnosed subsequent to a negative screening but before the next screening as interval cancers. Thus, the rate of interval cancers varies with the time between screenings. Interval cancers indicate the false-negative rate for cancers that become palpable between screenings. They do not indicate how many cancers that are detected at a screening could have been detected at an earlier screening. These retrospectively visible false-negatives (RVFN) have been counted in the screening trials as screen detected and not as false-negatives. They should be legitimately considered screening detected because they would not have been detected any earlier in the absence of screening, but they are lesions that offer the opportunity for improved detec-

TABLE 24-2. *Reasons for false-negative mammography*

Misinterpretation	Percent
Classified as benign	18
Seen on previous mammograms and discounted	17
Seen in only one projection	9
Present at the site of previous biopsy	8
Visible in retrospect	43
Missed due to technical failure	5

Source: Bird RE, Wallace TW, Yankaskas BC. Analysis of cancers missed at screening mammography. Radiology 1992;184:613–617.

tion since they are visible on earlier screenings. Those that were detected but interpreted as benign (IBFN) are another category of lesions where earlier detection is possible.

Bird has provided one of the most complete analyses of false-negative mammograms (13), and among 320 cancers diagnosed between 1985 and 1990, 77 (24%) were missed at screening. The authors used a double-reading system. They found that 11 (14%) of the cancers were detected by the second reader. This is similar to the 15% single-reader false-negative (SRFN) reported by Tabar (31). In our practice we found that 7% of cancers detected by screening were detected by the second reader. Among Bird and colleague's false-negatives, only 19 (25%) were truly false-negative (TFN). Forty-seven of 77 (61%) cancers were retrospectively visible (RVFN). Another 14 (18%) were detected, but diagnosis was delayed because they were interpreted as benign (IBFN). Only four (5%) were missed because of technical failures. In all 40 (51%) of the false-negative mammograms were attributed to misinterpretation, offering room for improvement (Table 24-2).

By comparing the patients whose cancers were missed by mammography, the authors concluded that cancers were more likely to be missed in denser breast tissue or if the cancers did not contain calcifications or where the density developed subtly over time.

In the randomized, controlled trial performed in Malmo, Sweden, interval cancers that are reported differ from Bird's false-negatives. In screening programs a lesion that is visible on a previous mammogram and that does not grow to clinical detectability between screenings is not counted as a false negative despite the fact that diagnosis is delayed. Rather it is counted as a screening-detected cancer. In a review of 96 cancers (20% of the total of 470 found in the screened population) that became clinically evident in the interval between screenings in the Malmö screening program, Ikeda and colleagues, probably for this reason, found a lower percentage of cancers that were retrospectively visible than did Bird. The implication for cancers that rise to clinical detectability between screenings may be that they are more aggressive and fast-growing cancers, or, conversely, that the time between screenings is too long (35).

In the Malmö study, 21,000 women between the ages of 45 and 69 were offered screening at intervals of 18 months. The size of the interval cancers was similar to those in the control groups, with a median diameter of 1.9 cm. Lymph nodes were positive in 23% of the screening-detected cancers, 36% of the interval invasive cancers, and 44% of the controls. Among the screening-detected cancers, 19% were stage II or worse. Although among the interval cancers 42% were stage II or worse and among control group cancers 52% of the were stage II or worse, women with interval cancers were twice as likely to die as the controls. The exact reason for this is unclear.

Among the interval cancers, 46% were diagnosed within 12 months of a negative screening and 75% within 18 months. Proportionally more interval cancers were found in younger women. True false-negative (TFN) mammograms that showed no evidence of cancer on previous mammograms accounted for 63% (63/100) of the patients with invasive carcinoma and ductal carcinoma in situ. There were slight mammographic abnormalities evident in retrospect in 21 (21%). Evidence was visible on previous mammograms of a probable malignancy in 10 of 100 (10%) of the women with interval cancer. Only 2% were felt to have been missed for technical reasons.

Methods to Reduce False-Negative Mammograms

Given the demonstrated ability of earlier detection by mammography to reduce the death rate from breast cancer, it is worth improving the technique to increase its advantages. Efforts should be strongly supported to improve conventional mammography through improvements in the patient interface, better focal spots, tubes with greater output to shorten exposure, better automatic exposure control, improved film/screen combinations, more automated film processing to maintain quality, and double reading. The successful development of digital mammography may reduce the false-negative rate and, more important, increase the number of cancers detected at an earlier stage. This will likely occur through exposure optimization and image display as well as through the use of artificial computer intelligence (computer-aided diagnosis) to act as second readers.

THRESHOLDS FOR INTERVENTION

The ability to detect breast cancers earlier is directly related to the aggressiveness with which abnormalities are pursued. In an endeavor such as screening mammography, where the indications of malignancy are fairly well understood and where they may be similar to those of benign processes, an increase in the detection rate of cancers (true-positive rate) can only come at the expense of an increase in the rate of "false alarms" (false-positive rate). In the European trials, where one goal was to keep costs down and minimize the number of women having biopsies, the detection rate for early cancers was likely lower than it could have been had a more aggressive approach been permitted (36).

The time between screenings is an important piece of the interval cancer component of the false-negative rate. The longer the time between screenings, the greater the chance that a cancer will rise to the surface between screenings. These cancers are more likely to be at a later stage and less likely to be cured. A shorter interval between screenings can reduce the interval and false-negative rates. This appears to also influence mortality. The screening trials that had the shorter intervals between screenings for women under the age of 50 had greater reductions in mortality than those with longer intervals for women form ages 40 to 49 (37). The only exception to this was the Canadian screening program, but there were so many other problems with that trial that the results may never be useful (3).

Based on modern screening data, mammography screening programs should be able to detect more than 50% of the invasive cancers in a population that begins screening by age 40 while those cancers are 1 cm or smaller, and more than 20% of the cancers can be expected to be ductal carcinoma in situ. Fewer than 20% of the women should have positive lymph nodes, and the interval cancer rate should be under 20%.

DIAGNOSTIC MAMMOGRAPHY AND FALSE REASSURANCE

Because there are a significant number of breast cancers that are not evident by mammography, a negative mammogram does not preclude the possibility of cancer. False reassurance is a risk of screening. It cannot be overemphasized that, if a finding is clinically suspicious, it must be resolved despite the fact that the mammogram is negative. Furthermore, women must be taught that a negative mammogram does not exclude breast cancer and does not offer any protection for the future. If a woman feels a change in her breast at any time, even if she has had a recent negative screening, she should bring it to her doctor's attention immediately.

REFERENCES

1. Tabar L, Fagerberg G, Day NE, Holmberg L. What is the optimum interval between screening examinations? An analysis based on the latest results of the Swedish two-county breast cancer screening trial. Br J Cancer 1987;55:547–551.
2. Wolfe JN. Breast patterns as an index of risk for developing breast cancer. AJR Am J Roentgenol 1976;126:1130–1139.
3. Boyd NF, Jong RA, Yaffe MJ, et al. A critical appraisal of the Canadian National Breast Cancer Screening Study. Radiology 1993;189:661–663.
4. Reuter FG. Preliminary report—NEXT-85. In Proceedings of the 18th Annual Conference of Radiation Control Program Directors. CRCPD Publication 86-2. 1986;111–120.
5. Conway BJ, McCrohan JL, Reuter FG, et al. Mammography in the eighties. Radiology 1990;177:335–339.
6. McLelland R, Hendrick RE, Wilcox P, Zinninger MD: The American College of Radiology Mammography Accreditation Program. AJR Am J Roentgenol 1991;157:473–479.
7. Scott WC. Establishing mammographic criteria for recommending surgical biopsy. Report of the Council of Scientific Affairs of the American Medical Association. September, 1989.
8. Baker LH. Breast Cancer Detection Demonstration Project: five-year summary report. CA Cancer J Clin 1982;32:194–225.
9. Wald NJ, Murphy P, Major P, et al. UKCCCR multicentre randomised controlled trial of one and two view mammography in breast cancer screening. BMJ 1995;311:1189–1193.
10. D'Orsi CJ, Kopans DB. Mammographic feature analysis. Semin Roentgenol 1993;28:204–230.
11. D'Orsi CJ (ed). The American College of Radiology Breast Imaging Reporting and Data System (2nd ed). Reston, VA: American College of Radiology, 1995.
12. Holland R, Hendriks JHCL, Mravunac M. Mammographically occult breast cancer: a pathologic and radiologic study. Cancer 1983;52:1810–1819.
13. Bird RE, Wallace TW, Yankaskas BC. Analysis of cancers missed at screening mammography. Radiology 1992;184:613–617.
14. Sickles EA. Periodic mammographic follow-up of probably benign lesions: results of 3184 consecutive cases. Radiology 1991;179:463–468.
15. Varas X, Leborgne F, Leborgne JH. Non-palpable, probably benign lesions: role of follow-up mammography. Radiology 1992;184:409–414.
16. Azavedo E, Svane G, Auer G. Stereotactic fine-needle biopsy in 2594 mammographically detected non-palpable lesions. Lancet 1989;1:1033–1036.
17. Parker SH, Lovin JD, Jobe WE, et al. Nonpalpable breast lesions: stereotactic automated large-core biopsies. Radiology 1991;180:403–407.
18. Parker SH, Jobe WE, Dennis MA, et al. US-guided automated large-core breast biopsy. Radiology 1993;187:507–511.
19. Meyer JE, Kopans DB. Stability of a mammographic mass: a false sense of security. AJR Am J Roentgenol 1981;137:595–598.
20. Kopans DB, Swann CA, White G, et al. Asymmetric breast tissue. Radiology 1989;171:639–643.
21. Meyer JE, Kopans DB. Breast physical examination by the mammographer: an aid to improved diagnostic accuracy. Appl Radiol 1983;103–106.
22. Faulk RM, Sickles EA. Efficacy of spot compression—magnification and tangential views in mammographic evaluation of palpable masses. Radiology 1992;185:87–90.
23. Fletcher SW, Black W, Harris R, et al. Report of the International Workshop on Screening for Breast Cancer. J Natl Cancer Inst 1993;85:1644–1656.
24. Tabar L, Fagerberg G, Day N, et al. Breast cancer treatment and natural history: new insights from results of screening. Lancet 1992;339:412–414.
25. Rosen PP, Groshen S, Saigo PE, et al. A long-term follow-up study of survival in stage I (T1 N0 M0) and stage II (T1 N1 M0) breast carcinoma. J Clin Oncol 1989;7:355–366.
26. Sickles EA. Auditing your practice. RSNA Syllabus Categorical Course in Breast Imaging. 1995;81–91.
27. Stomper PC, Kopans DB, Sadowsky NL, et al. Is mammography painful? A multicenter patient survey. Arch Intern Med 1988;148:521–524.
28. Martin J, Moskowitz M, Milbrath JR. Breast cancers missed by mammography. AJR Am J Roentgenol 1979;132:737–739.
29. Feig SA, Shaber GS, Patchefsky A, et al. Analysis of clinically occult and mammographically occult breast tumors. AJR Am J Roentgenol 1977;128:403–408.
30. Bird RE. Professional quality assurance for mammographic screening programs. Radiology 1990;177:587.
31. Tabar L, Fagerberg G, Duffy S, et al. Update of the Swedish two-county program of mammographic screening for breast cancer. Radiol Clin North Am 1992;30:187–210.
32. Thurfjell EL, Lernevall KA, Taube AAS. Benefit of independent double reading in a population-based mammography screening program. Radiology 1994;191:241–244.
33. Carter CL, Allen C, Henson DE. Relation of tumor size, lymph node status, and survival in 24,740 breast cancer cases. Cancer 1989;63:181–187.
34. Peer PG, Holland R, Jan HCL, et al. Age-specific effectiveness of Nijmegen population-based breast cancer screening program: assessment of early indicators of screening effectiveness. J Natl Cancer Inst 1994;86:436–441.
35. Kopans DB. Screening for breast cancer and mortality reduction among women 40–49 years of age. Cancer 1994;74:311–322.
36. Kopans DB. Mammography screening for breast cancer. Cancer 1993;72:1809–1812.
37. Sickles EA, Kopans DB. Deficiencies in the analysis of breast cancer screening data. J Natl Cancer Inst 1993;85:1621–1624.

Breast Imaging, 2nd ed., by Daniel B. Kopans.
Lippincott–Raven Publishers, Philadelphia © 1998.

CHAPTER 25

Medical-Legal Issues and the Standard of Care

In our litigious society, the failure to diagnose breast cancer has become the leading cause of malpractice claims, and this is likely to increase. It is virtually impossible to be protected from a lawsuit, and even if the physician performs at a very high level, a jury may still decide, based on pity for a woman dying of breast cancer, to find for the plaintiff against the physician. The contingency system, in which a lawyer stands to receive 30% of any monetary award, makes it attractive for lawyers to sue if there is any indication of possible success.

TORT OF NEGLIGENCE

Medical malpractice or negligence is covered by tort law. There are four elements that define the tort of negligence (1):

1. Duty: The physician must have established a duty toward the patient. This is generally implied by having rendered a service with an understood level of expectation for care on the part of the patient.
2. Breach of duty: Breach of duty is the act of failing to fulfill the duty appropriately.
3. Causation: Causation means that the action or failure of action by the physician was directly related to the injury to the patient.
4. Damage: This fourth element requires that the causation resulted in damage or loss to the patient.

TODAY'S STANDARD OF CARE

Today's "standard of care" will be decided by juries of the future, and each jury may differ. Many of the questions concerning the duty of the radiologist have yet to be determined through legal challenges. Most questions cannot be answered prospectively, because they are not matters of law; rather, they are ultimately decided by a jury. The jury is generally asked to decide whether the doctor behaved according to the standard of care at the time. The problem lies in the fact that there is no way of knowing what the standard of care actually is today. It will be decided when someone is sued in the future, and it will depend on each jury's decision because one jury's decision is not binding in any other case.

Although the American judicial system is predicated on a trial by a jury of one's peers, most juries are chosen so that their members have little or no medical or scientific training. The decision of one jury as to what a physician should have done in a specific case has no bearing on the next case, even if the facts of the cases are identical. Trials do not set precedents for health care. The only precedents that may evolve have to do with the law itself. If a verdict is appealed, the appeal is generally based on a legal issue and not a medical question, and it is the appellate courts that determine legal precedents.

Failure to Diagnose

The radiologist is under unreasonable pressure to detect all cancers. The majority of lawsuits involving breast imaging are due to a failure to see a cancer on a mammogram that is visible in retrospect. The plaintiff can always find an "expert" who is willing to testify that the radiologist should have seen the lesion. This is remarkable in that there is no radiologist in the world who has not failed to see a significant abnormality at some time that is visible in retrospect, yet these experts are willing to determine that another radiologist was negligent for having made a similar oversight.

Failure to Perceive an Abnormality

The detection of all breast cancers by mammography is impossible given that at least 5% to 15% of cancers are not visible on the mammogram. Furthermore, it is a well-established and unavoidable phenomenon that all observers periodically miss significant findings. Every radiologist, even the most expert in the field, occasionally fails to see an abnormality that, in retrospect, is evident on the film. This is true not only in the perception of cancer on a mammogram but has been documented in the review of chest x-rays for lung nodules (2,3), barium enemas for polyps, and bone films for fractures.

Problem of Perception

The problem lies in the vagaries of perception. The phenomenon is identical to the simple problem of finding one's keys that all of us have encountered. All of us have had the experience of searching for keys and becoming increasingly frustrated at not being able to find them until someone points out that they are right in front of us. We looked right at them but did not see them. There was a perceptual interruption that had nothing to do with negligence but is rather an apparently immutable psychovisual phenomenon. The same phenomenon makes it impossible for a radiologist to perceive all cancers, even some that are obvious in retrospect. If it is not acknowledged that the failure to perceive an abnormality is not negligent, then the radiologist is held to an impossible standard.

Double Reading

Just as the second reader was able to see the keys when they were overlooked by the first, having two or more readers review imaging studies reduces the failure to perceive an abnormality. Double reading, however, is a nonspecific term. It may mean a review by two readers to reduce errors of perception, or it may be considered as double interpretation, where the second reader may decide the concerns raised by the first reader are unwarranted. Double interpretation is a way to reduce false-positive interpretations, although it could lead to an increase in false negatives if the second reader's lack of concern proves to be incorrect.

The interest in double reading depends on the aims of those who review the process. At a meeting held by the National Cancer Institute in January 1996 to review the value of double reading, health planners were more interested in reducing the number of mammograms interpreted as abnormal because they represent added expense than they were in reducing the error rate in cancer detection. Radiologists and those interested in reducing the death rate from breast cancer were more interested in reducing the failure to perceive a significant abnormality. The cost of health care is of major concern, but the best science and medicine should be determined first, and then society can decide what it can afford. Thus, only the latter use of double reading is discussed below.

Double Perception

Since individuals do not fail to perceive the same things (someone else points out your keys), the problem of missing a cancer may be reduced by instituting a system of double reading with two radiologists reviewing the same mammogram. This is impractical in many practices and would lead to an undesirable increase in the cost of screening. If, however, screening cases are read in bulk on a preloaded alternator, double reading can be done without significantly increasing the cost (see Chapter 11).

In a study performed at the Massachusetts General Hospital, double reading was performed on 5,899 cases. The main reader was methodical in reviewing all previous mammograms, while the quick reader was assigned to scan the cases looking for possible abnormalities. The main reader took approximately 2 hours to review 40 to 50 mammograms, while the quick reader accomplished the same task in less than 15 minutes. Together the two readers detected 39 breast cancers. The main reader detected 36 of the 39 breast cancers diagnosed in the group, and the quick reader detected 31 of the 39. Three of the malignant lesions detected by the quick reader were overlooked by the main reader, but eight malignant lesions were overlooked by the quick reader.

Our results suggest that reading more methodically is more accurate than reading quickly, but that two observers are better than a single observer. Bird has reported a similar experience. Using a second reader increased their detection rate by 5% (4). Tabar has quoted a 15% increase in cancer detection (5) with double reading, and Thurfjell and colleagues also found a 15% increase in cancers detected using a second reader (6).

Double reading is not the standard of care. Requiring double reading may, in fact, be counterproductive. Unless an efficient system is used, double reading is expensive (double the radiologist time). It could result in more cancer deaths, because women will be denied access to screening if the cost is too high. However, if the studies are organized efficiently, then the incremental increase in radiologist time is minimal and double reading is easily accomplished at no additional cost. There has been increasing pressure to provide women having a mammogram with an immediate report. Women and physicians need to be educated that the psychological benefit from an immediate report is falsely reassuring (a negative mammogram does not mean that a woman does not have breast cancer) and that it is preferable to permit a delayed and more careful review and double reading to increase the chance of finding a cancer earlier.

The most efficient method of accomplishing double reading is to separate screening from diagnostic procedures. Centers dedicated to high-quality mammography perform screening studies efficiently. A screening mammogram is obtained (MLO and CC projections), the films are processed and checked for quality, and the patient leaves. This can be completed in approximately 15 minutes. The films are then loaded in batches on an alternator and double read. The second reading adds little cost but adds the benefit of greater sensitivity.

Failure to Communicate

Failure to communicate the fact that an abnormality has been detected is a potentially significant problem. The duty of the radiologist has not been defined in an absolute sense and will not likely ever be universally defined (it may vary from state to state) but rather will be decided with each individual case. A written report is clearly indicated. It is also prudent to contact the physician directly when a significant abnormality (one that needs immediate attention) is detected. This is part of the American College of Radiology (ACR) standard. Although there is no consistent determination of the absolute responsibility of the radiologist, it would also be prudent to establish a follow-up system that would permit the timely detection of a patient with a significant abnormality who has not undergone appropriate follow-up. The use of computers can be extremely helpful in this regard.

Monitor Results

It has been suggested that an important defense in a malpractice action will come from having established a group and individual track record. Maintenance of a database such as recommended by the ACR Breast Imaging Reporting and Data System will help establish the standard of practice within a group and by an individual. A well-thought-out approach to the evaluation of problem lesions rather than a haphazard approach to image interpretation is important. Careful maintenance of records and notation of communication with the referring physician (documentation) is strongly recommended.

The following practices would seem prudent.

1. Strive to obtain high-quality mammograms (use well-trained technologists).
2. Require and document continuing education for radiologists and technologists.
3. Develop an organized approach to interpretation.
4. Consider double reading.
5. Be certain that you have a rationale for your recommendations that is logical and backed by scientific support wherever possible. If you choose to recommend follow-up instead of biopsy be sure that your reasoning is clear.
6. Develop a database for your practice to document your results. Knowing your sensitivity and estimating your specificity may be important. Merely quoting the literature is likely insufficient.
7. Communicate important abnormal results by phone and through written reports and document the communication.
8. Develop a tracking system to ensure that patients needing additional evaluation do not fall through the cracks.
9. Avoid extraneous materials in patient records. Only include information for which you are willing to be and should be responsible.
10. If breast diagrams are employed, record only significant information. If you allow anyone to record a mass on a diagram, it is likely that you will be expected to have followed up on that mass to ensure that it was properly evaluated, even if the mammogram was negative.
11. Be sure you and your staff (including receptionists and clerical workers) are courteous, kind, considerate, compassionate, and supportive of patients, who are usually under considerable stress.

REALITY OF MALPRACTICE

There is no way to guarantee that an individual will not be sued and no way of preventing loss in a suit. As noted previously, although the whim of a jury is the ultimate factor, most decisions are supposed to revolve around whether or not the physician performed according to the standard of care. This is defined as a level of performance that would be expected from the average physician in the same circumstance. The problem arises because the standard of care is usually decided by a jury that has no medical or scientific background. This is always a retrospective decision. The jury must decide what the standard of care was at the time of the supposed error.

The legal system does not understand and does not recognize scientific proof. Decisions are based on the testimony of witnesses who claim to be experts, but there are only loose definitions of expertise. Virtually any physician can be accepted as an expert witness. There are no qualifications that are required. As was evident in the famous football star murder trial, opinion is as valid as science. The only check on pseudo-experts is if the opposing attorney can discredit the expert's testimony.

One jury may decide that a certain standard applied at the particular time, while another might decide just the opposite. Neither jury's decision is binding on the other. In fact, two juries, isolated and separately hearing the exact same testimony on closed circuit television, could arrive at exactly opposite decisions, and whichever jury the defendant had would determine the outcome.

Not only is the decision in a jury trial essentially arbitrary, but it is also not binding on future litigation. One jury might decide, for example, that it was not the standard to use ultrasound to evaluate a palpable mass, while 1 week later another jury might decide that it was the standard. One jury's decision does not set a precedent for any other. The only precedents that can be set are precedents that involve particular aspects of the law, and these are set at the appellate level. They have no influence on any decisions of fact or any influence in determining standard of care.

Perhaps even more disconcerting is the fact that it is ultimately the insurance company that is insuring a physician that decides what course of action to follow.

Case Report

Because insurance companies are primarily at risk, they may decide to settle with the plaintiff and not risk a possible greater loss from a jury decision. In one case the plaintiff complained that she felt something in her breast in 1992. Her primary care physician was unable to feel anything but sent her for a mammogram. The radiologist interpreted the mammogram as dense with no evidence of cancer. Retrospective review of the mammogram, even by the plaintiff's attorney, concurred. The radiologist had even gone beyond the standard of care and examined the patient himself and felt nothing.

One year later the patient again complained of a mass in her breast, and this time her doctor felt it. The mammogram revealed a new density and ultrasound showed a solid, 1.5-cm mass. A biopsy removed a 3-cm fibroadenoma. Two months later the patient complained that she still felt a mass, and a second biopsy revealed an invasive breast cancer.

The radiologist was sued for almost $2 million for having not performed an ultrasound study when the patient first complained of an abnormality. Despite the fact that there was nothing on mammography or clinical examination to be evaluated the plaintiff's expert (chosen from a computer list of physicians seeking the high fees paid for consultation as expert witnesses), who read an occasional mammogram but had no other credentials, acknowledged that the mammograms had been interpreted correctly but testified that the ultrasound should have been done. Two nationally recognized experts in breast imaging supported the defendant and testified that the ultrasound was not indicated.

Following deposition of the defendant's experts before trial, the plaintiff agreed to settle for $250,000. Unwilling to risk a jury trial in which they could have lost $1 to 2 million and despite the fact that science and expertise were on the defendant's side, the defendant's insurance company lawyers decided to settle for $250,000 because they feared a much higher loss if the jury ignored the facts and found for the plaintiff.

Since the radiologist had actually performed beyond the standard of care and was certainly not guilty of negligence, this case demonstrates that the system is designed to permit what amounts to legalized extortion. Not only did the plaintiff's lawyers extort money from the insurance company, but, despite the fact that he had done nothing wrong, the radiologist was automatically placed in a national computer database as having lost a malpractice case.

Incentive to Pursue a Suit

In another case in which a radiologist had also done nothing wrong, an expert for the defendant queried the lawyer (off the record) why he was pursuing the suit despite the radiologist's having done nothing wrong. The reply was that if the suit was dropped, then the lawyer, who had already invested a considerable amount of time in the case, would not be compensated because he was to be paid (in the usual fashion) a contingency fee only if he won the case. It was worth his while to pursue the case on the chance that a jury would find for his client. Fortunately, in that case, the jury found for the defendant.

It's to See Who Wins

It is important to realize that the jury system in the United States is not designed to determine the truth but is rather designed to see who wins. It is a contest between opposing lawyers to try to sway the jury. A decision can hinge on the sympathy that a jury has for the plaintiff or its attitude toward the bearing of the plaintiff or defendant or even the lawyers and their experts. As noted earlier, opinion carries the same weight as scientific argument.

Part of the problem with medical malpractice is that a jury of individuals who have little or no familiarity with medicine is frequently asked to interpret complex scientific and medical issues. It is not surprising that juries often decide cases based on which individual they liked or which was more convincing rather than on science and fact. Another problem is that so-called expert witnesses need no specific qualifications, although a judge can exclude one deemed inappropriate. It is usually up to the attorneys to discredit the opposing expert.

Unfortunately, the system encourages litigation and the pursuit of marginal cases and, despite the fact that extortion is illegal, this does not apply to lawyers suing for malpractice. Since the outcome of a jury trial cannot be predicted on the basis of facts, money is often extorted and paid to avoid a potentially larger loss.

TORT REFORM

Unfortunately, those responsible for this system and who benefit the most from it are also in control of the legislation that could change it. Not only is it a profitable system for lawyers, but, because their profession is based on the principle that suit is a routine method for settling grievances, they fail to understand why doctors are concerned about the system.

AN EXPERT OPINION ON THE STANDARD OF CARE IN BREAST IMAGING

Because the standard of care lies at the heart of medical malpractice and the failure to diagnose breast cancer is one of the leading reasons for litigation, the following section is provided as an expert analysis to define the standard of care. It is adapted from an article published in *Radiology* in 1993 (7).

Introduction

There has been an increasing emphasis by some radiologists that in breast imaging, more is better. The frequent use of additional mammographic projections, magnification mammography, ultrasound, and other tests is urged to try to derive a more thorough understanding of an abnormality in order to suggest appropriate management. It is argued by some radiologists that decisions should not be made based on the screening study alone, and, if a questionable finding or abnormality is detected, they insist that the radiologist should work it up. Others urge the increased use of ultrasound to evaluate possible abnormalities. What is lacking in this reflexive exhortation is the importance of determining how the additional evaluation will actually influence the care of the patent and benefit the patient. Ultimately the cost of interventions is a stress in the opposite direction. Doctors may be sued for having not performed a test, while they may lose their jobs in a managed care system if they order tests that are not indicated.

What separates medicine from the "snake oils" of the past is science. It is the careful analysis and objective study of an intervention, using the scientific method, to determine its value and efficacy that raise medically justified procedures above the level of the "copper bracelet." The mere fact that an individual believes in a procedure does not validate that procedure.

Additional imaging and analysis beyond the screening mammogram may be clinically useful if the added information expedites patient care and provides information that influences management decisions to the benefit of the patient. This is particularly true in the setting of screening with mammography, where the care of a clinically asymptomatic woman with a mammographically detected abnormality depends on the radiologist's interpretation. In this situation, sufficient imaging analysis is required to permit the radiologist to advise the patient and her physician as to the appropriate course of action. The mere fact that an additional test adds information, however, does not necessarily justify its use, particularly in light of rising health care costs. There is little doubt that performing every possible test on every patient adds some benefit to a few, but it definitely leads to unjustifiable costs, and, more important, probable harm to many patients from spurious but ultimately insignificant findings.

As with all tests, the value of additional imaging should be assessed for its impact on care. If the results of a test do not have the potential to alter the course of patient care in a beneficial fashion, then its use is not justified and it should not be considered the standard of care. If the use of a test has no scientifically demonstrated efficacy, then it should not be considered a standard.

Clearly every approach to care has not been and cannot be validated scientifically. However, anecdotal experience should not dictate a standard of care for all physicians without supporting scientific validation. For example, there were many radiologists who believed that whole-breast ultrasound could replace mammography in the early detection of breast cancer. Whole-breast ultrasound units proliferated and could have been construed as the standard of care. It was not until the systems were evaluated in a scientific fashion that their lack of efficacy was demonstrated.

A number of experts believed that women who have been treated for breast cancer conservatively should always have magnification views of the tumor site in their follow-up mammograms. This could have been misconstrued as a standard had it not been for a study by DiPiro and colleagues, who showed, in a scientific fashion, that this had no advantage over the standard two views with the addition of magnification views for the small number of women for whom the contact views raised a question (8).

What Is the Standard of Care?

The definition of standard of care, as with all American case law, continues to evolve. In the past, a practitioner's judgment was compared to a local community standard. National standards are now the measure. The terminology is both specific and nebulous. Brenner, citing the 1962 court decision in *Skeffington v. Bradley*, suggests that "liability is imposed only when the mistake results from a failure to comply with recognized standards of medical care exercised by physicians in the same specialty under similar circumstances" (1). Potchen's interpretation described standard of care as "a duty to use that degree of care and skill that is expected of a reasonably competent practitioner of the same specialty" (9).

The definition of standard of care should incorporate the important qualification *care with established efficacy*. For example, in the 1980s many physicians were using diaphanography (transillumination), which was subsequently shown to have no efficacy. Failure to use a technique before its efficacy has been established in prospective analysis should not constitute a violation of the standard of care. Unfortunately, our legal system permits opposite conclusions for identical circumstances. As new approaches to breast problems are developed, their efficacy should be established whenever possible before they are unjustifiably interpreted as standards of care.

Breast cancer remains the leading cause of nonpreventable cancer death among women in the United States. The powerful emotional implications associated with problems of the breast has subjected breast imaging, and mammography in particular, to heightened public awareness and scrutiny. The fact that mammography remains the main weapon in the breast cancer battle has led to greater expectations for the modality than are warranted. In our effort to reduce the devastation from breast cancer, there is the danger of overestimating our capabilities and perhaps suggesting approaches that may not be efficacious.

The Only Demonstrated Efficacy for Mammography Is as a Screening Technology

Although mammography is frequently used for women with clinically evident breast abnormalities, it has only been scientifically validated for use as a screening test. Earlier detection using mammography leads to a reduction in the size and stage of breast cancer at the time of diagnosis (5), and this has been shown to not only prolong survival (10) but to absolutely reduce mortality from breast cancer (11). Unfortunately, mammography is frequently imbued with greater capability than it can provide. Even the term *diagnostic mammography* suggests that the technique can be used to determine the etiology of an abnormality, while in reality this is rarely the case.

Although most medical professionals recognize that the term *diagnostic* is used in a similar fashion to *diagnostic imaging* and actually means *as an aid to diagnosis*, some may take the term literally and this should be clarified. Diagnosis is defined as "the art of distinguishing one disease from another" (12). With the exception of morphologically classic lesions, such as calcified fibroadenomas, lipomas, some forms of fat necrosis, or spiculated cancer, mammography is not diagnostic by this definition. Morphologic criteria can be used to develop probabilities of malignancy, but imaging alone is usually insufficient to determine whether a lesion is benign or malignant.

Mammography as a screening technique acts as a filter to sift out those women most likely to have the disease from the background of those who are at risk. Most screening tests require diagnostic procedures to confirm or exclude the presence of a disease process, and mammography is no exception. Cervical screening using the Pap test, for example, is useful in determining which women are most likely to have cervical cancer. False-positives are fairly common, and a biopsy is often required to establish a diagnosis. Although the psychological implications of a suspicious mammogram may be different from the psychological implications of a suspicious Pap smear, mammography is the Pap test of the breast and histologic confirmation of malignancy is required before definitive therapy is instituted.

It is clear that mammography can never and should never be used to exclude cancer. Frequently, a palpable abnormality is not even visible on the mammogram (13), or if visible its morphologic characteristics are not diagnostic.

Standard of Care for Screening Mammography

The standard of care for the radiologist involved in screening mammography should be to supervise the generation of high-quality mammograms in which the breasts are positioned symmetrically in the mammography system in an effort to image as much tissue as the patient's habitus and level of cooperation permit. The image should be exposed so that the tissues are penetrated sufficiently to see structures through the dense tissues and with sufficient contrast to permit the detection of soft tissue masses and significant calcifications.

The radiologist should be expected to know the various manifestations of malignant lesions and practice a systematic approach to reviewing the mammograms in an effort to find abnormalities that might represent malignancy. The radiologist should not be expected to perceive every cancer but, once an abnormality has been detected, should have an approach and clear rationale for the evaluation and management of that abnormality and should have a system in place to convey the interpretation to the referring physician or, if the patient is self-referred, to the patient.

For radiologists who act as consultants, follow-up care for the patient should ultimately be the responsibility of the patient's primary physician who referred the patient for the consultation. Efforts by the radiologist to track the needed follow-up should not be the standard but should be encouraged. If the radiologist has assumed primary responsibility for the management of the patient's breast problem, follow-up should be pursued until a satisfactory resolution has been achieved.

Standard of Care for Symptomatic Patients

There is no scientific proof that mammography, when used to evaluate women with a palpable abnormality, has any true efficacy. There are no studies that prove that the imaging analysis of women who are already symptomatic can alter the course of cancer and reduce the likelihood of death. Its use in this application is purely anecdotal.

The true importance of mammography in the woman with a clinically evident abnormality is not the evaluation of the abnormality but rather for screening the remainder of the affected breast, as well as the contralateral breast, for clinically occult cancer (14). It is paradoxical and the result of practice based on anecdote that physicians who do not as yet believe in the benefit of screening nevertheless insist that a woman with a sign or symptom of breast cancer have a mammogram. This has caused the courts to find clinicians liable for having not ordered a mammogram in a patient with a symptom, where they have not yet agreed whether the failure to order a screening mammogram for an asymptomatic woman is malpractice (15).

Occasionally, but anecdotally, the mammographic evaluation of the palpable abnormality may be helpful. If the lesion has the classic morphologic characteristics of cancer, then the clinical impression is reinforced and the surgeon should expect a malignant histology. Should the clinically suspicious area prove to be benign in the setting where the mammographic evidence suggests a malignancy, immediate reevaluation and, if necessary, rebiopsy should be undertaken because the cancer may have been missed at the clinically guided biopsy (16).

An additional diagnostic role that has been recently suggested for mammography is its use in treatment planning for the woman with breast cancer who desires breast preservation. Some studies have suggested that radiation therapy has a higher failure rate if a biopsy reveals extensive intraductal carcinoma, possibly indicating an excessive residual tumor burden beyond the margins of the excision (17). It has been proposed that the mammogram, through its use in assessing the extent of a tumor and the likelihood of residual tumor, can be used to reduce the probability of recurrence for women who are to be treated conservatively by lumpectomy and radiation (18). The fact is that it has never been proved that this application reduces the likelihood of recurrence, and, perhaps more important, it has not been shown that this affects overall survival. Since there is not yet proof of either contention, the use of mammography for this purpose, although in my opinion possibly beneficial, should not constitute a standard of care.

Clinical Breast Examination by the Radiologist or Technologist

The Health Insurance Plan of New York (HIP) demonstrated the efficacy of the combined use of physical examination and mammographic screening to reduce the mortality from breast cancer (19). Although the efficacy of physical examination alone to reduce mortality has not been confirmed in other trials, it is likely that for a small percentage of women periodic screening by physical examination is efficacious. It has been suggested that performing a clinical breast examination (CBE) should be a responsibility of the mammography technologist. Technologists certainly can be trained to perform CBEs, but the primary role of the x-ray technologist is to perform high-quality mammography. The value of physical examination is as dependent on the care exercised in its performance as the mammographic detection of malignancy is dependent on the care exercised in obtaining a high-quality mammogram. Training programs for technologists do not include any more than a cursory reference to CBE, if they include any mention at all. There are no formal training programs to teach technologists CBE. No doubt there are technologists who are interested in expanding their expertise and responsibility and wish to perform the CBE as well, but this should not be a requirement and it is certainly not a standard.

Similarly, there are radiologists who would like to extend their expertise and responsibility and perform CBEs. This is quite reasonable for an individual, but physical examination is a separate test from mammography. The performance of a physical examination should not be a requirement for performing mammography any more than palpation of the abdomen should be a part of the abdominal imaging examination or the performance of auscultation by the radiologist a component of chest imaging. The CBE should not be considered a casual function but rather a technique requiring time, patience, and thoroughness. Only those who are interested in its performance and are willing to be trained and to spend the time required to perform it properly should undertake CBEs. No postgraduate courses in breast imaging teach CBE, and it should not be considered a standard of care for radiologists who supervise the performance of mammography and interpret mammograms.

We and others have suggested that a correlative breast examination by the radiologist, nurse, or technologist be performed to ensure that an area of clinical concern is appropriately included on the mammogram (20). In 1983 we published a study that suggested that a physical examination by the radiologist was valuable for ensuring that a clinically evident abnormality was imaged. Our review had been undertaken at a time when attention to proper positioning was not as rigorous as is presently the case, and many of the

lesions imaged as a result of the additional views prompted by the clinical examination were in regions of the breast that had not been imaged on the initial study. Although we concluded that a correlative physical examination was useful, we did not prove that it had true clinical efficacy (21). Despite our speculation, as far as can be determined, these lesions would have been biopsied based on the clinical concern (the patients were referred with palpable abnormalities) regardless of the mammographic evaluation.

Faulk and Sickles reviewed 70 cases of women referred with palpable abnormalities. In 66% the abnormality was not visible on the standard projections. By using spot compression they identified four additional masses and reclassified eight of the masses (31%) based on the spot compression. All of these were benign. All of the cancers were correctly diagnosed before the spot-compression views. Thus, although a few more masses were visible after spot compression, there was no evidence that the spot-compression views had any effect on the earlier detection of cancer (13).

Most cancers that are palpable and visible by spot compression are very suspicious on clinical examination and should be biopsied regardless of the mammogram. There are no prospectively derived data that prove that spot-compression imaging leads to earlier and beneficial intervention. Despite the fact that some enthusiasts espouse its use, there are no prospective data confirming the efficacy of the correlative breast examination and there are no data to support requiring it as a standard of care.

Role of Mammography in the Evaluation of a Woman with a Palpable Breast Mass

It has been shown repeatedly and emphasized in numerous articles that mammography cannot be used to exclude breast cancer (22,23). Even in the most optimistic series, mammography fails to reveal at least 5% to 15% of breast cancers that are palpable, and if cancers that reach clinical detectability within 1 year following a negative screen are included an additional 20% may be undetectable by mammography at the time of screening (24). This false-negative rate for mammography should not be considered a failure of the technique, but rather a reality that must be acknowledged. Mammography permits the detection of the majority of cancers 1.5 to 4 years before their clinical detectability (25), but a negative mammogram does not preclude the possibility of breast cancer. The mammogram and physical examination evaluate different tissue characteristics. Two studies have shown that the textural consistency of the breast on physical examination does not predict the mammographic appearance (26,27). Consequently, concern raised by either test can rarely be negated by the other. There are exceptions such as fat-containing, encapsulated lesions, which are benign and have a characteristic appearance on the mammogram and need not be biopsied despite the fact that they are palpable, but the majority are not characteristic. Often the mammogram shows very suspicious morphologic changes that increase the likelihood that a palpable abnormality is malignant, but the absence of such elements does not eliminate the possibility of cancer. In most instances, the clinician must make a decision based on the clinical evaluation when a palpable abnormality is present.

Role of Ultrasound in the Evaluation of a Palpable Mass

The use of ultrasound to evaluate the breast is an example of anecdote preceding scientific evaluation and incorrectly guiding practice. In the 1970s ultrasound was advocated for screening before any efficacy testing merely because it could be used to show cancer that was already known to exist. Once the appropriate prospective studies were performed, it became evident that ultrasound could not be used to reliably find cancer and, in fact, was not efficacious for screening.

Ultrasound does provide a useful adjunctive study to mammography when a nonpalpable mass is found on the mammogram. It is the radiologist's responsibility to resolve the nature of the nonpalpable, indeterminate mass detected only by mammography, because the clinician has no way of evaluating these lesions. On the other hand, the palpable abnormality should be considered primarily the responsibility of the clinician, unless by agreement with the referring physician the radiologist shares or assumes responsibility.

The use of ultrasound in the evaluation of palpable masses is derived from the reluctance of the radiologist to state that the character of a lesion is indeterminate based on the mammogram. It is rarely possible to determine whether a lesion is cystic or solid by mammography alone, and ultrasound can be used to make this clinically important differentiation. The question is, is this efficacious for palpable masses? As has been previously discussed, mammography should be used in the woman with a palpable mass primarily to screen uninvolved breast tissue. If a mass is clinically evident, it will likely require clinical resolution. Most women do not want to have a palpable lump. For many women a lump is painful or psychologically disturbing. Clinically guided needle aspiration is extremely safe, usually accomplished with little discomfort, and often less expensive than ultrasound. If the mass proves to be a cyst, aspiration is simultaneously diagnostic and therapeutic.

If a lesion is to be aspirated regardless of the ultrasound results, then ultrasound adds an unnecessary test and a layer of expense that is wasted. There are some cysts that for various reasons defy clinically guided aspiration. In this situation, excisional biopsy can be avoided if a subsequent ultrasound demonstrates a cyst that is confirmed by imaging-guided aspiration (28). The use of ultrasound in this sequence will significantly reduce its utilization. The

use of ultrasound in the primary analysis of a palpable mass becomes efficacious only if the patient and her physician agree that the demonstration of a cyst by ultrasound will be sufficient and will obviate the need for aspiration or surgery (29,30).

It will be argued that intracystic cancer will be missed if ultrasound is not performed. The majority of intracystic tumors are in fact benign papillomas. True intracystic breast cancer is extremely rare, and there are no prospective data (other than anecdotal) that show that ultrasound plays any significant management role except for cyst/solid differentiation or as a guide for interventional procedures.

The fact that a palpable mass should be considered the responsibility of the referring physician does not preclude participation by the radiologist who is interested in involvement at all levels of breast health care. Many radiologists already perform physical examinations, cyst aspirations, fine-needle aspiration, and core biopsy. Complete breast care should be encouraged to avoid fragmentation of services; however, this is not the standard to which all radiologists who provide mammographic evaluation should be held. If, however, the radiologist accepts self-referred patients, then all abnormalities of the breast are the radiologist's responsibility until care has been transferred (1).

There are no data supporting the use of ultrasound to evaluate a breast in which there is not already an abnormality evident by either mammography or clinical breast examination. Gordon and colleagues reported a series of cases in which they claim to have found nonpalpable, mammographically occult cancers using ultrasound alone (31). Their patient selection, imaging parameters, and cancer stages were not provided, and, until their results can be reproduced, their approach is not the standard of care (32).

Breast Imaging and the Woman Under 40 with a Sign or Symptom of Breast Cancer

Despite a recent article advocating the use of mammography in women who are under the ages commonly suggested for screening (younger than 35 to 40) (33), there are no commonly agreed on guidelines for its use in these women. The risk of radiation induction of breast cancer is related to the age at which the radiation is sustained (34). The younger the woman, the higher the potential risk. For women older than 40, the risk is extremely low and may no longer exist at any level of exposure (35), but in younger women there is likely a finite (although small) risk. In these women one must balance the exposure to the radiation against the benefit to be derived from the study.

Because mammography is not sufficiently accurate to be able to safely distinguish most benign from malignant palpable masses and because mammography is primarily useful for screening, its use at any age should be guided by the probability of detecting clinically occult breast cancer. The major screening studies have only tested the efficacy of screening mammography in women age 40 and older. Guidelines suggesting a baseline study at age 35 were not actually based on data but on the belief that it was desirable to have a baseline exam for future comparison obtained at a time when breast cancer is unlikely. As a result, obtaining a baseline study before age 40 is no longer supported by any major organization.

Among teenage women and women in their early 20s, breast cancer is extremely rare. Fewer than 0.3% of breast cancers occur in women under the age of 30. In these very young women, even the very low radiation risk may outweigh any benefit. This does not mean that mammography is not useful in caring for younger women with breast problems; it only means that there are no prospective data that support the use of mammography for screening younger women (under 40).

Because mammography cannot exclude breast cancer and a palpable mass must be dealt with clinically and there are no data to support screening women under 40, the value of mammography in these women is only anecdotal. Anecdotal experience may be reasonable to follow for an individual practice if there are no objective, prospective studies on which to rely. Nevertheless, anecdotes are not sufficient to determine a national standard of care, and until such objective data are available mammography in younger women should not be considered a standard but should be dictated by individual experience. Any decision to biopsy a palpable mass in the breast of a woman in this age group, as in older women, remains a clinical decision.

Conclusion

This commentary may be viewed as being overly negative toward the application of breast imaging techniques in the care of breast problems. This could not be further from the truth. Any test or maneuver that can improve the quality of care should be explored, but intuitive approaches are not always correct, as evidenced by the legitimate controversies that surround the issue of screening. Any approach that is considered the standard of care should require validation. This does not mean that individuals and practices should be prevented from going beyond the standard to explore new approaches. Tests are often legitimately used based on anecdotal experience when scientifically derived proof of efficacy is unavailable. In some circumstances care must rely on the art of medicine. All radiologists, at one time or another, have relied on having seen a case where performing a particular maneuver or obtaining an additional study made a difference in caring for a patient.

It is likely that better care is rendered because of an individual practitioner's experience, but the standard of care—that to which all should adhere—should, whenever possible, be derived from scientifically proved techniques and should not be based on intuitive assumptions and anecdotal observations.

REFERENCES

1. Brenner RJ. Medicolegal aspects of screening mammography. AJR Am J Roentgenol 1989;153:53–56.
2. Kundel HL, Nodine CF, Thickman D, et al. Nodule detection with and without a chest image. Invest Radiol 1985;20:94–99.
3. Kundel HL. Predictive value and threshold detectability of lung tumors. Radiology 1981;139:25–29.
4. Bird RE. Professional quality assurance for mammographic screening programs. Radiology 1990;177:587.
5. Tabar L, Fagerberg G, Duffy SW, et al. Update of the Swedish two-county program of mammographic screening for breast cancer. Radiol Clin North Am 1992;30:187–210.
6. Thurfjell EL, Lernevall KA, Taube AAS. Benefit of independent double reading in a population-based mammography screening program. Radiology 1994;191:241–244.
7. Kopans DB. Breast imaging and the "standard of care" for the "symptomatic" patient. Radiology 1993;187:608–611.
8. DiPiro PJ, Meyer JE, Shaffer K, et al. Usefulness of the routine magnification view after breast conservation therapy for carcinoma. Radiology 1996;198:341–343.
9. Potchen EJ, Bisesi MA, Sierra AE, Potchen JE. Mammography and malpractice. AJR Am J Roentgenol 1991;156:475–480.
10. Seidman H, Gelb SK, Silverberg E, et al. Survival experience in the Breast Cancer Detection Demonstration Project. CA Cancer J Clin 1987;37:258–290.
11. Tabar L, Fagerberg CJG, Gad A, et al. Reduction in mortality from breast cancer after mass screening with mammography. Lancet 1985;1:829–832.
12. Dorland's Medical Dictionary (26th ed). Philadelphia: Saunders, 1981.
13. Faulk RM, Sickles EA. Efficacy of spot compression—magnification and tangential views in mammographic evaluation of palpable masses. Radiology 1992;185:87–90.
14. Kopans DB, Meyer JE, Cohen AM, Wood WC. Palpable breast masses: the importance of preoperative mammography. JAMA 1981; 246:2819–2822.
15. Brenner RJ. Medicolegal aspects of breast imaging: variable standards of care relating to different types of practice. AJR Am J Roentgenol 1991;156:719–723.
16. Meyer JE, Kopans DB. Analysis of mammographically obvious breast carcinomas with benign results on initial biopsy. Surg Gynecol Obstet 1981;153:570–572.
17. Harris JR, Lippman ME, Veronesi U, Willett W. Breast cancer (three parts). N Engl J Med 1992;327:319–328, 390–398, 473–480.
18. Sadowsky NL, Semine A, Harris JR. Breast imaging: a critical aspect of breast conserving treatment. Cancer 1990;65:2113–2118.
19. Shapiro S, Venet W, Strax P, Venet L. Periodic Screening for Breast Cancer: The Health Insurance Plan Project and Its Sequelae, 1963–1986. Baltimore: Johns Hopkins University Press, 1988.
20. Kopans DB. Breast Imaging. Philadelphia: Lippincott, 1989.
21. Meyer JE, Kopans DB. Breast physical examination by the mammographer: an aid to improved diagnostic accuracy. Appl Radiol March/April 1983;103–106.
22. Burns P, Grace MCA, Lees AW, May C. False negative mammograms causing delay in breast cancer diagnosis. Can Assoc Radiol J 1979;30:74–76.
23. Mann BD, Giuliano AE, Bassett LW, et al. Delayed diagnosis of breast cancer as a result of normal mammograms. Arch Surg 1983; 118:23–24.
24. Baker LH. Breast Cancer Detection Demonstration Project: five-year summary report. CA Cancer J Clin 1982;32(4):194–225.
25. Moskowitz M. Breast cancer: age-specific growth rates and screening strategies. Radiology 1986;161:37–41.
26. Swann CA, Kopans DB, McCarthy KA, et al. Mammographic density and physical assessment of the breast. AJR Am J Roentgenol 1987; 148:525–526.
27. Boren WL, Hunter TB, Bjelland JC, Hunt KR. Comparison of breast consistency at palpation with breast density at mammography. Invest Radiol 1990;25:1010–1011.
28. Fornage BD, Faroux MJ, Simatos A. Breast masses: US-guided fine-needle aspiration biopsy. Radiology 1987;162:409–414.
29. Jackson VP. The role of US in breast imaging. Radiology 1990; 177:305–311.

30. Bassett LW, Kimme-Smith C. Breast sonography. AJR Am J Roentgenol 156;1991:449–455.
31. Gordon PB, Goldenberg SL. Malignant breast masses detected only by ultrasound: a retrospective review. Cancer 1995;76:626–630.
32. Kopans DB, Sickles EA, Feig SA. Malignant breast masses detected only by ultrasound: a retrospective review. Cancer 1996;77: 208–209.
33. Donegan WL. Evaluation of a palpable breast mass. N Engl J Med 1992;327:937–942.
34. Feig SA, Ehrlich SM. Estimation of radiation risk from screening mammography: recent trends and comparison of expected benefits. Radiology 1990;174:638–647.
35. Boice JD, Harvey EB, Blettner M, et al. Cancer in the contralateral breast after radiotherapy for breast cancer. N Engl J Med 1992;326:781–785.

Breast Imaging, 2nd ed., by Daniel B. Kopans.
Lippincott–Raven Publishers, Philadelphia © 1998.

CHAPTER **26**

Future Advances in Breast Imaging

Conventional x-ray mammography using film/screen detectors continues to be the only imaging technique with the proven capability to detect clinically occult breast cancer at an earlier size and stage than clinical examination. Conventional film/screen mammography is the only imaging technique that has been shown to decrease mortality through screening asymptomatic women (1,2). This is likely to remain so until film/screen detectors are gradually replaced by digital detectors.

Although x-ray mammography provides significant benefit, it is not the complete solution to the increasing breast cancer problem, and research into better methods of detecting early stage breast cancer is critical. Nevertheless, using conventional imaging, a 30% to 50% reduction in mortality can be expected from mammographic screening (3,4). Preventive measures are being explored, but until these can be demonstrated to be effective or a universal cure is discovered, earlier detection remains the best hope for reducing the death rate from breast cancer.

SCREENING AND DIAGNOSIS

Imaging techniques can be applied as screening tests or for diagnostic purposes.

Screening for breast cancer involves the evaluation of apparently healthy, asymptomatic women (no sign or symptom of cancer) on a periodic basis in an effort to detect breast cancer earlier in its development to prevent or defer death.

New screening techniques should be compared to conventional mammography, which represents the "gold standard."

Diagnostic evaluation of the breast is the process of differentiating benign from malignant lesions.

New diagnostic techniques should be compared to the gold standard, which is the removal of cells or tissue for microscopic evaluation.

The major benefit from any breast imaging technique is saving lives through the earlier detection of breast cancer by screening. The ability to define noninvasively whether a detected lesion is benign or malignant is of secondary benefit, although potentially of great value. A new technology should not be expected or required to do both, and it is likely that a single technology will not be the solution to either problem.

X-ray mammography is today, and likely will remain for the foreseeable future, the only method that has proven efficacy for breast cancer screening. It has been clearly shown to be able to detect breast cancer at an earlier size and stage than clinical examination (2), and randomized, controlled trials have provided proof that mortality can be reduced by periodic mammographic screening (5) (see Chapter 4).

There are ongoing efforts to improve the ability to find cancers earlier using mammography. It is hoped that the development of digital mammography systems will permit improved detection and diagnosis. Investigators are searching for other techniques that will be even more successful in finding early cancer and permit a greater opportunity for cure as well as less invasive methods of diagnosis.

OTHER REASONS FOR BREAST EVALUATION

In addition to detection and diagnosis, imaging techniques are being evaluated to determine their value in the assessment of other factors involved in breast cancer management. These include refining the determination of tumor extent, staging and prognostication, response to treatment, and detection of recurrence following treatment.

Assessing the Extent of Cancer

Surgery is currently performed with the goal of reducing the tumor burden by removing the bulk of the malignancy. If the breast is to be preserved, it must be irradiated to destroy any tumor that remains and thereby prevent local recurrence. The entire breast must be treated because there is no way at the present time to determine the true limits of a tumor's border. Even with the removal of large volumes of breast tissue, it is not possible to ensure that all tumor has been excised. Tumor spreads along the duct network (6,7) (Fig. 26-1). This is often not visible and is frequently not appreciated by the surgeon, who may leave behind significant amounts of cancer. Since the pathologist is able to evaluate less than 1/10,000 of the tissue removed, it is not surprising that, even if the margins of the excised tissue appear to be free of tumor, there is as much as a 40% chance that there is residual tumor in the breast. Whole-breast irradiation is used to destroy any remaining cancer cells.

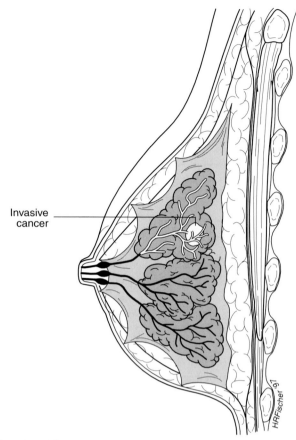

Invasive
cancer

FIG. 26-1. This diagram demonstrates how **tumor can spread within the duct network,** making it impossible to determine the absolute margins of the lesion. The white ducts represent intraductal spread.

Radiation therapy destroys cancer cells logarithmically, killing a percentage of the remaining cells with each course of therapy. Unfortunately, it kills indiscriminately, and normal cells are killed along with cancer cells. The total dose applied must balance the ablation of cancer cells relative to the killing of normal cells. Recurrences following conservation therapy likely occur when the residual tumor burden, following the primary extirpation, is too great to be eliminated by radiation. Techniques that could provide more accurate assessment of cancer extent, multifocality (tumor within the same duct segment) and multicentricity (noncontiguous, separate primary lesions in different duct systems) would greatly facilitate more appropriate tailoring of treatment to the individual situation. Until better methods are developed to define the true extent of a malignancy, the entire breast must be treated.

A number of investigators are studying the possibility of treating cancers without surgical removal. It is possible to insert a probe and freeze the primary tumor using cryotherapeutic techniques. High-frequency ultrasound can be applied to heat the tumor sufficiently to kill it, and lasers can be introduced through fiber-optic guides to ablate cancer in vivo. All of these techniques are limited by the same problem—the lack of definition of the tumor's extent. The abil-

ity to accurately define the microscopic extent of the cancer could prove to be of great value for tailoring the level of treatment needed for a given individual. It would permit targeting the cancer while sparing normal tissues.

Staging

Despite the major efforts applied to finding methods to treat cancer in the breast, the overall survival of the individual is not dependent on the treatment of cancer in the breast. Cancer that is confined to the breast is not lethal. It is the metastatic spread to other organs that makes breast cancer deadly, and it is the prevention of this spread or its eradication that determines the individual's ultimate survival. In an effort to eradicate any occult sites of metastatic disease, many women are now treated with systemic chemotherapy to try to eliminate putative disease outside the breast. A significant percentage of women who are treated systemically do not have systemic cancer, and the treatment is unnecessary. Because for many cancers it is not yet possible to determine which have spread, many women are subjected to the morbidity and (small) mortality risk from these toxic agents in order to improve survival among a few. The ability to more accurately predict who can benefit from systemic treatment would have significant importance, and efforts continue to develop more accurate prognostic measures.

The best predictor of likely spread is the presence of tumor in the axillary lymph nodes. To assess risk of systemic disease, the axilla is dissected to remove and analyze lymph nodes. If cancer is found in these nodes, it is an indication that the tumor has developed a metastatic capability and must be presumed to have spread elsewhere. The absence of cancer in the nodes suggests a better prognosis, although it is not a guarantee that there has been no spread since approximately 30% of women whose axillary lymph nodes are negative still recur with distant metastases. Less invasive, or noninvasive, methods of assessing the axillary lymph nodes or the discovery of other indicators of systemic spread would be very valuable.

Assessment of the axillary lymph nodes remains one of the best methods for predicting outcome. Although the role of axillary dissection is evolving, therapeutic decisions, such as the choice of adjuvant chemotherapy or hormonal (Tamoxifen) treatment, are influenced by the results of the axillary analysis. Axillary staging requires surgery under general anesthesia and is not without morbidity. Among other problems, it can lead to long-term arm edema. Less invasive methods of staging and more accurate methods of prognostication are desirable.

Treatment Monitoring and the Detection of Recurrent Breast Cancer

New approaches to treatment, such as the application of neoadjuvant chemotherapy (systemic treatment before

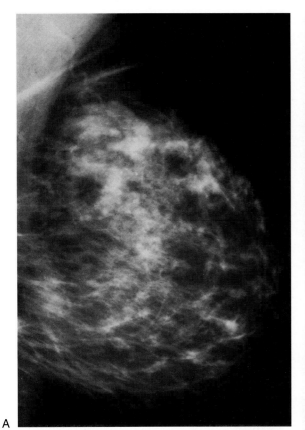

FIG. 26-2. With standard mammography systems, the deep tissues are often not imaged. This patient had metastatic disease and had this mammogram of her right breast to search for the primary tumor. The mediolateral oblique **(A)** and craniocaudal **(B)** images were interpreted as negative. A chest CT scan performed to evaluate the lungs revealed the cancer deep in the breast **(C)**. The mass was barely visible on repeat mammography, despite the fact that the CT revealed a significant amount of tissue even deeper than the cancer.

removal of the primary lesion), could benefit from accurate methods of in vivo monitoring of the response of the tumor.

Although there is no proof that early detection of breast cancer recurrence following therapy alters the ultimate course of the cancer, there is some evidence suggesting a possible benefit (8). The development of techniques that are more sensitive to recurrence than clinical examination and mammography might be of value.

The following sections discuss areas in which development is likely to produce an immediate benefit in the early detection of breast cancer.

CONVENTIONAL FILM/SCREEN MAMMOGRAPHY

Although some of the goals for the improvement of conventional mammography will be superseded with the devel-

opment of digital detectors, many can also be implemented with digital detectors and will enhance the technique.

Patient Interface and Breast Compression

Conventional mammography, using film/screen combinations, and dedicated mammographic equipment has developed into a very efficient technology for the early detection of breast cancer (9). Although research into better methods of detection and diagnosis is critical, conventional mammography is likely to remain the primary screening technology for the next several years. Although a fairly mature technology, improvements can be made in conventional mammographic systems. Several of these improvements would also be of use when digital detectors are substituted for film/screen combinations.

At the present time, proper positioning of the breast in the mammographic unit is extremely operator dependent (10).

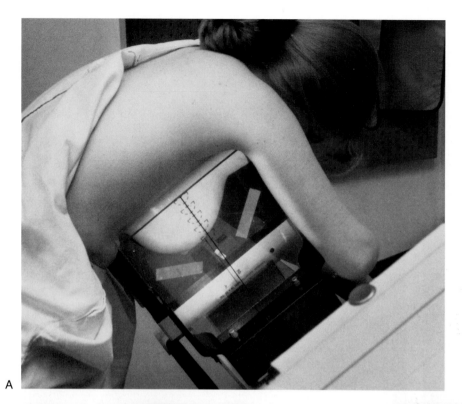

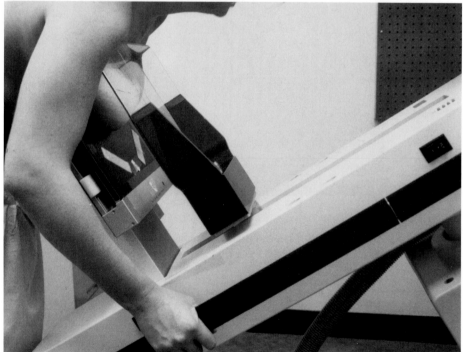

FIG. 26-3. Pendent positioning permits the use of gravity to pull the breast away from the chest wall on the lateral **(A)** and craniocaudal **(B)** projections.

Better human engineering might improve the interface between the patient and the mammographic system and reduce reliance on the "artistry" of the technologist to ensure proper position and reduce false-negative examinations from positioning errors. Even with high-quality mammography, deep tissues are not always completely imaged (Fig. 26-2).

Pendent Positioning

Pendent positioning with the patient leaning forward or almost prone with the pectoralis musculature relaxed results in more efficiently obtained, more complete, and more reproducible images. This technique permits the breast to align itself under the influence of gravity in the

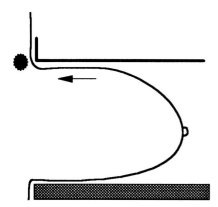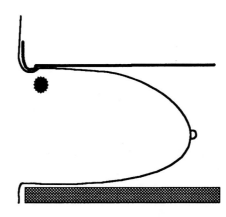

FIG. 26-4. A ridged compression plate traps the tissue in the field of view so that the deep tissues are not squeezed out.

mammographic system. Although primarily suspended by the skin, attachments of the breast to the pectoralis musculature through fascial penetrating vascular and lymphatic elements require that the axillary tail of the breast be viewed in two-dimensional imaging through the pectoralis musculature. By relaxing this muscle with the arm extended forward while the patient is in a prone position with the back humped, the breast and muscle fall away from the chest wall into the field of view of the imaging system (Fig. 26-3). Systems that can be angled to better suit the habitus of the individual are already available. Further refinements of pendent positioning will likely have additional benefits.

Tailored Compression

Compression of the breast is needed to spread structures apart and improve the projection of the internal structures of the breast (see Chapter 10). Applying breast compression first along the chest wall, either with an angled variable compression plate or ridged compression system, will prevent the breast from being pushed by the parallel compression plates out of the mammographic device and out of the field of view (Fig. 26-4).

Tilting Compression Paddles

Although the current recommendations suggest that the compression plates remain parallel, better compression and separation of tissue structures (particularly at the front of the breast) can be achieved by angling the compression system at the front of the breast to better conform to its conical shape (Fig. 26-5). These modifications will likely result in more reproducible and complete imaging of the breast tissue.

A Separate Compression System

The use of compression plates on either side of the breast, separated from the detector, might permit better imaging of the deeper structures by allowing the detector to be moved around the curve of the chest wall, eliminating loss from the dead space at the edge of the detector (Fig. 26-6).

Traction

Other techniques are being developed to assist in drawing the breast over the detector to reduce the volume of tissue

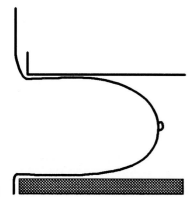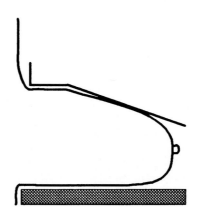

A,B

FIG. 26-5. A standard compression paddle **(A)** only compresses the thickest part of the breast (usually the back). A **tilting paddle** is hinged at the chest wall. Its chest wall surface is flat, while the surface toward the front of the breast is angled **(B)**. It can bring compression to bear on the front of the breast, permitting better separation of the anterior structures. *Continued.*

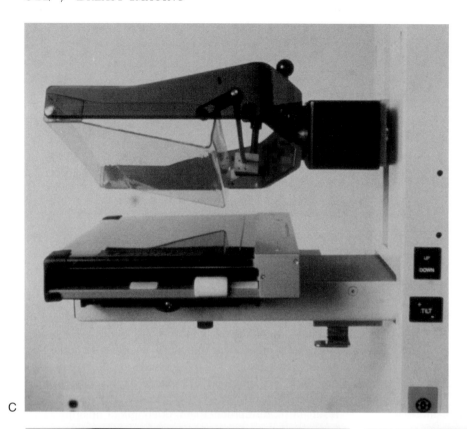

C

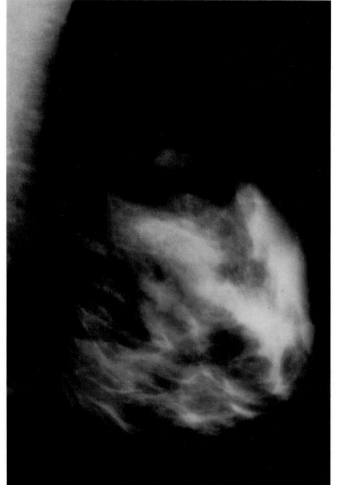

D

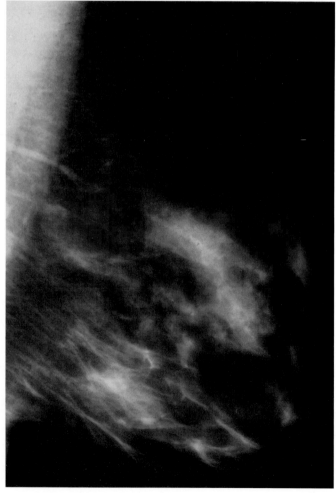

E

FIG. 26-5. *Continued.* This is an example of a tilting paddle **(C)**. This mediolateral oblique projection **(D)** was obtained using standard compression. Note that with the tilt compression **(E)** the anterior tissues are spread apart.

Compression system
independent from the detector

X-ray

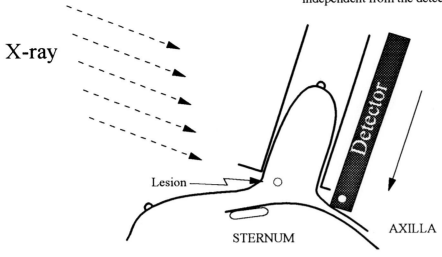

Lesion

STERNUM

AXILLA

FIG. 26-6. If the entire breast **compression system is separate from the detector,** the detector can be moved around the chest wall so that the deep tissues can be imaged.

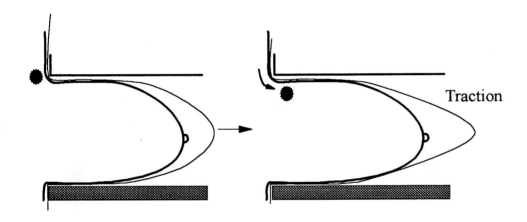

Traction

FIG. 26-7. Moving radiolucent sheets placed between the breast and the compression system can permit **traction on the breast** while in compression, pulling it deeper into the machine to image the deeper tissues.

that is not imaged. Movable sheets of material can be placed between the detector and the breast and between the compression paddle and the breast. These can be used to pull the breast further into the field of view, even after compression has been applied (Fig. 26-7).

Scatter Reduction

Oscillating Grids

Stationary grids are not appropriate for imaging the breast since the grid lines may interfere with the visualization of fine details. Although the present oscillating grid systems are extremely effective in reducing the effect of scatter, there is room for improvement in scatter reduction. Standard grids not only absorb scatter photons, but they also block the primary beam (Fig. 26-8). This requires additional exposure to fill in these areas when the grid oscillates, resulting in more than doubling the dose to the patient.

One new grid design is a honeycomb that reduces scatter in all directions.

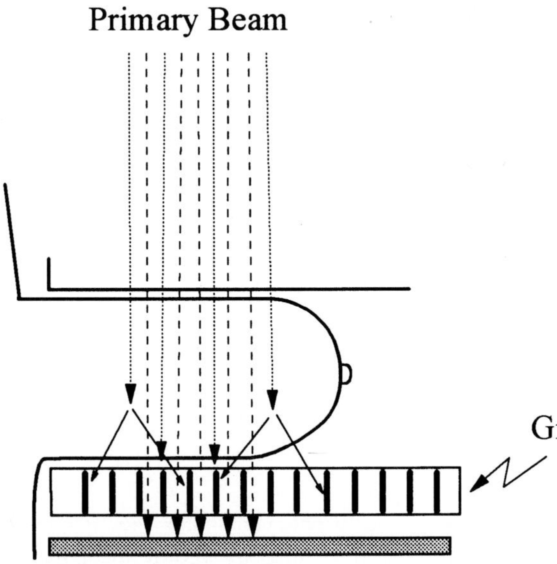

Primary Beam

Grid

FIG. 26-8. A standard grid blocks not only scattered photons (*small arrows*) but also some of the primary beam (*long dashed arrows*). Because half of the primary beam is also blocked by the grid (*long dotted arrows*), an increase in dose is needed to complete the image.

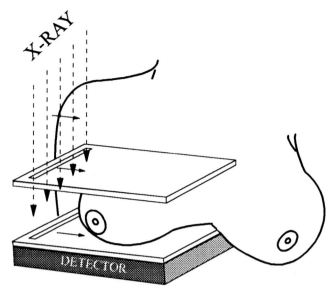

FIG. 26-9. A **moving slot** between the breast and the detector efficiently eliminates most scatter. If it is coupled with a pre-breast slot, then the tissues are protected from unused exposure.

Grazing Incidence

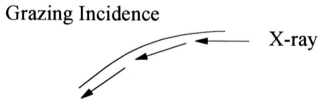

FIG. 26-10. A **grazing incidence system** might one day be used to focus x-rays. If glass or plastic tubes are formed with the proper curvature, they can alter the course of the x-rays and permit them to be "focused."

Slot Systems

Scatter reduction can be made even more efficient using various slot configurations. A slit in a metal plate that is positioned between the breast and the detector permits only the directly transmitted x-rays to pass through to the detector (Fig. 26-9). This is among the most efficient methods for reducing the amount of scatter reaching the x-ray detector. Various forms of aligned slit technology can virtually eliminate scatter (11). By coupling pre- and post-breast slot devices, scatter can be reduced and a slot in front of the breast will protect it from wasted exposure (see Fig. 26-9).

Focusing X-Rays

Although it is generally believed that x-rays cannot be focused, carefully bent glass tubes as well as specially fabricated metal have been shown to be able to alter the course of x-rays using the principle of grazing incidence (Fig. 26-10). The development of "lenses" for focusing x-rays could have a major impact on breast cancer detection and

diagnosis. Not only might this permit the selection of mono-energetic beams, but such a system could virtually eliminate scatter by permitting precise alignment of the incident x-ray beam with a corresponding post-breast lens system so that only perpendicularly incident x-rays passing directly through the breast would be conducted into the detector and off-angle photons would be rejected.

Magnification

Magnification has been shown to improve the visibility of masses and calcifications. It is presently used to evaluate areas that have raised concern on contact imaging. The routine use of whole-breast magnification to improve the signal-to-noise ratio and the spatial resolution of mammography might permit an increase in the early detection of breast cancer. This would require either a further reduction in the size of the x-ray focal spot or a truly microfocal spot that was small over a large area of the detector. Magnification mammography can provide a true increase in the resolution of intramammary structures (12,13). This improved resolution can be used to better evaluate the morphologic characteristics of breast lesions and to improve the detectability of early-stage breast cancer. If magnification could be applied to the entire breast routinely, it would likely result in the ability to detect an increased number of breast cancers at an earlier stage. More powerful x-ray tubes that are able to handle the heat generated by small focal spots are needed to provide high-resolution images with short exposure times to avoid blur due to motion.

Stereomammography and Tomography

Stereomammography and tomography of the breast (see Digital Mammography) are presently being evaluated using digital detectors. Stereotactic guidance of needles is already helpful in the diagnosis of various breast lesions. Stereomammography has been tried in the past but has not become standard. It would likely be helpful in the assessment of suspected abnormalities detected at screening. Stereotactic imaging would be useful to confirm that a finding is a true mass rather than a summation shadow from the superimposition of normal structures. Overlapping normal structures in the breast are a constant problem in the detection and diagnosis of breast cancers.

Investigation into the development of tomographic methods of mammographic evaluation should be encouraged. Conventional blurred-image tomograms of the breast would be extremely valuable. Digital tomosynthesis (see Digital Tomosynthesis later in this chapter) or other computer-aided methods of tomography would be extremely valuable. Some preliminary reports suggest that a better appreciation of the three-dimensional distribution of calcifications in a suspicious cluster may provide greater differentiation of benign from malignant lesions.

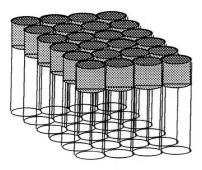

FIG. 26-11. Optical fibers with the phosphor integrated in the fiber could permit a thicker phosphor layer while reducing light spread in the screen.

Screen Design

Improving screen phosphors and devising screens with greater quantum detection efficiency without increasing imaging blur are potential improvements. This may be accomplished by etching screens or bundling extremely small optical fibers containing appropriate phosphors such that light is conducted directly back at the film with minimum light spread in the phosphor (Fig. 26-11). Improved film emulsions with greater resolution (spatial and contrast) and less noise will improve the ability to detect breast cancer.

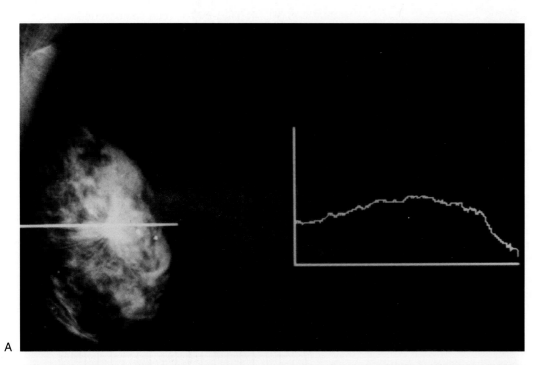

A

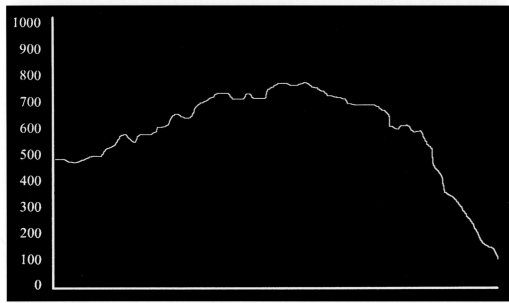

B

FIG. 26-12. Digitization converts an analog signal into a digital signal. If the density of the film (assume completely black is zero and pure white is the highest signal) is measured across a line of the image **(A)**, it appears as a continuous line **(B)**, depending on the whiteness or blackness of the image at each point along the line. *Continued.*

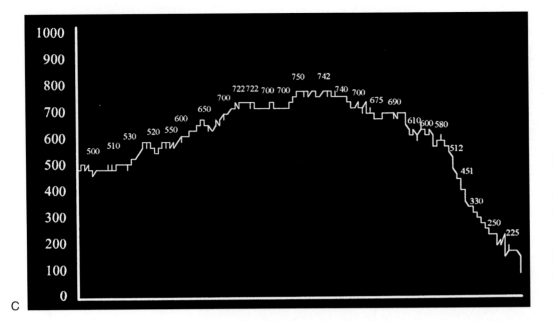

FIG. 26-12. *Continued.* The height of the line can be represented by numbers at any specified points **(C)** (digital conversion), and this produces a digital measure. Every point on the image can be converted to a number. The size of the point determines the fineness or coarseness of the digital representation.

Automatic Exposure Control

Consistency in imaging is important to maintain quality. Automatic exposure-control (AEC) devices should be linear over all breast thickness and composition. This reduces the dose requirements by eliminating repeat exposures and enhances throughput. Underexposure of dense breast tissues remains a problem. Some systems permit greater flexibility in the positioning of the AEC. Devices to sample the exposure under the entire breast to optimize the penetration of dense tissues will likely further improve the ability to produce high-quality mammograms.

Film Processing

Until digital mammography becomes a practical reality, quality control in film processing is of critical importance and should be automated to eliminate human error. Assessment of optimum processing should be built into film processors, and operating parameters should be constantly and automatically monitored by the processor to detect problems and take corrective action.

DIGITAL MAMMOGRAPHY

A Digital Image

Conventional mammography using film/screen detectors to record the x-ray photons that pass through the breast produces an analog image. Although limited by the grain size of the film emulsion, the components of a film image are fairly continuous. If the density of the film along a line across the image was measured, the transition from white through gray to black would appear to be fairly uninterrupted (Fig.

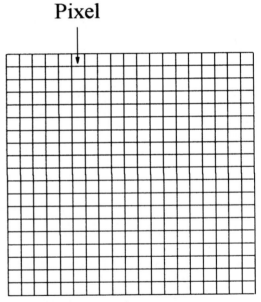

FIG. 26-13. A digital image is made of a series of picture elements (pixels). Any image can be made into a grid of rows and columns. Each block of the grid is called a pixel. By assigning a level of gray (black to white) to each pixel, the image can be created. Because the location of each pixel is represented by a row and column number and each level of gray can be translated into a number, the image can be represented as rows and columns of numbers with a gray scale figure and the image becomes digital.

26-12A, B). A digital image can be thought of as sampling this continuous signal at fixed points and assigning numbers (digits) to represent each point depending on its level of gray (Fig. 26-12C). The closer the sampling, the finer the image; the coarser the sampling, the lower the quality of the image.

Most people are now familiar with digital images because they have become ubiquitous in the computer age. The idea is

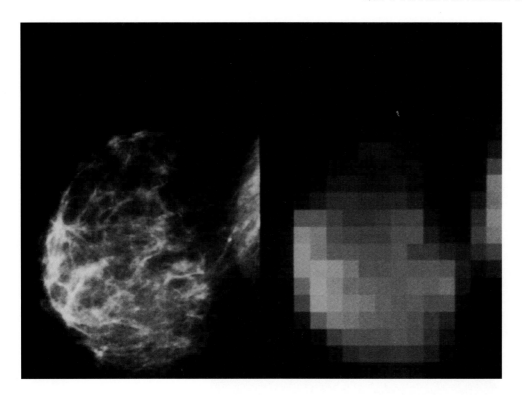

FIG. 26-14. An image with small pixels contains more detail than an image with large pixels that covers the same area. These images exaggerate the point. The data on the left represent an image digitized with a pixel size of 42 μm. The same data were used to form the right image but are averaged to a pixel size of 1 cm per pixel.

fairly straightforward. A picture can be thought of as a two-dimensional grid of rows and columns (Fig. 26-13). Each block defined by the grid is a pixel (for picture element). By filling the pixels with colors or levels of black, gray, or white a picture can be recreated. The smaller the pixels, the sharper the detail (Fig. 26-14). Once the image is created as pixels, a number can be assigned to each shade of gray in the image. Since the coordinates of the pixel (its row and column) and its level of gray can be defined in terms of numbers, the image can be defined as a digital image. By knowing the corresponding levels of gray that are represented by the numbers of the gray scale and by knowing the organization of the rows and columns, the image can be reproduced perfectly, an unlimited number of times, just from the numbers. Because numbers can be sent over wires by satellite or fiber optics, manipulated, saved electronically, and carefully checked for accuracy, the exact image can be sent anywhere in the world and perfectly reproduced as many times as needed.

Since the image is represented by numbers, the various scales and ranges that include these numbers can be altered electronically to enhance the image and improve the visibility of structures. Windows (the range of the gray scale) and levels (the center of the gray scale) can be altered, and various electronic filters can be applied to enhance the image. One simple maneuver, for example, is inversion of the gray scale. Since the image is electronic, it can easily be reversed so that blacks become white and whites become black (Fig. 26-15). At times this makes some structures more easily appreciated. On a conventional mammogram the only way to see structures in the dark portions of the film is to use a

bright light. A digital image, however, can be adjusted so that all areas of the image are visible by using such techniques as histogram equalization or unsharp masking, in which the darker areas are lightened without altering the visibility of structures in the lighter portions of the image. With a digital image computers can be used to analyze the image, and the image can be securely stored. Digital images offer enormous advantages over analog images.

From Film to Digital

It is the ability of x-ray imaging to demonstrate the internal structures of the breast at high resolution and the concomitant detection of breast cancer at a smaller size and earlier stage than any other method that has been shown to reduce the death rate from breast cancer. The x-ray image is created from the variable absorption of x-rays by normal and abnormal tissues that results in varying numbers of x-ray photons that pass through the breast and out the other side. It is this variable absorption and transmission of these photons by the breast tissues (normal and abnormal) that results in the shadows of the x-ray image. The detection of these photons when they exit the breast and their conversion into a viewable image was first accomplished by exposing film alone to the x-rays. Plain film was the detector. Subsequently, fluorescent screens were developed that converted the x-ray photons into light. The light from the screen was more efficient in exposing the film. The efficiency gained by coupling a screen with the film permitted a major reduction in the dose required to image the breast.

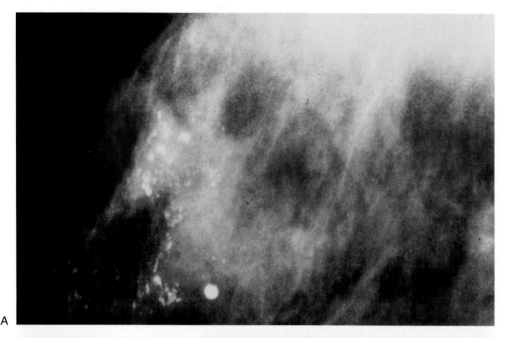

A

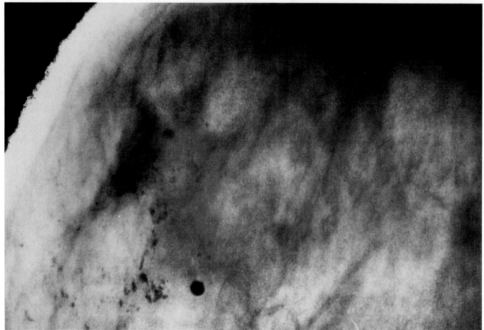

B

FIG. 26-15. Positive or negative image presentation. A simple manipulation, easily performed with a digital image, is the reversal of the image so that white on black **(A)** becomes black on white **(B)**.

Advantages of Film

Film has significant advantages. It is relatively inexpensive and, when coupled with a screen, it is quite efficient in producing an image. Mammographic film has the theoretic ability to resolve 17 to 20 line-pairs per millimeter, permitting the evaluation of very fine details. The amount of information contained on a piece of film is enormous, making it an excellent storage medium. Film permits the storage of a great deal of information in a very small space, and the information can be displayed very inexpensively.

Disadvantages of Film

There are several important disadvantages of film/screen combinations, however. As a consequence of the fact that the film is both the detector and the display medium, the actual exposure requirements are dictated by the need to form a viewable image. Film does not respond linearly to incident photons. It is not very sensitive to the early photons striking it so that areas of high x-ray absorption in the breast (low transmission of photons to the film) all appear similarly white on the image (the toe of the Hunter and Driffield

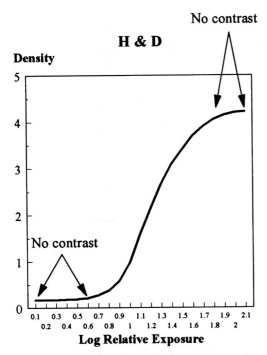

FIG. 26-16. If there is no contrast between two structures, they cannot be distinguished. At both ends of the Hunter and Driffield (H&D) curve where it flattens out (the very white areas of the film and the very dark areas), there is no contrast between structures of both high and low attenuation.

curve) (Fig. 26-16), and it is only over a fairly narrow range of exposure that small changes in attenuation result in differences in film blackening (contrast). Since the normal structures of the breast and cancers of the breast have similar x-ray attenuation, this limitation can make it difficult to visualize and separate normal from abnormal structures. Contrast is extremely important. Although film has high spatial resolution, if there is insufficient contrast between two small structures then they will not be separately visible.

Another limitation of film is that once the image is developed it is immutable. The information is displayed in only a single presentation, and if the exposure has not been optimal then the image will be suboptimal. The film is the only record of the image, and if it is lost or damaged the loss is irretrievable. Storage of x-ray films requires large amounts of space, and studies are not infrequently lost. If a consultation with another physician or expert is desired, the images must be physically provided to the consultant.

Advantages of Digital Mammography

As in other areas of imaging, digital mammography overcomes many of the limitations of conventional mammography and will provide the opportunity to improve on the basic technique. It is hoped that this will further improve our ability to find early breast cancer. Interest in digital mammography has paralleled the interest in digital imaging of other organ systems, but development has been delayed because of the need for higher spatial resolution than required by other x-ray studies.

Numerous approaches are being considered. These range from digitization of conventional mammograms to digitization of information obtained using an intermediate receptor, such as photostimulable phosphor, to direct acquisition of photon fluxes through the breast by solid state detectors, producing direct digital data acquisition.

One of the fundamental benefits of digital images results from the fact that the parameters involved in acquiring the digital image are not dependent on displaying the image. This permits a wide dynamic range for digital systems and improved contrast between tissues. Multiple presentations of the same data can be obtained from this system for each image acquired (Fig. 26-17 A–C). It is likely that this will enhance cancer detection, particularly in the radiographically dense breast where inherent contrast is low. Other benefits include the ability to use the computer to manipulate the image information (Fig. 26-17D, E). The major impediments to digital imaging at the present are the limitations of display technology. High-resolution monitors are still unable to provide the amount of information needed for mammographic assessment simultaneously. As improved displays are developed, however, the benefits of digital imaging will accrue to mammography. Image manipulation and the application of computer-aided diagnosis will be facilitated (14). Telemammography and teleconsultation will become possible.

With primary digital acquisition the potential exists to perform dual energy-subtraction studies. By subtracting breast tissue and improving the perspicuity of calcifications, the detection of early stage breast cancer will likely be enhanced.

Cancers have been shown to enhance following the intravenous infusion of iodinated contrast material under computed tomographic observation (15) as well as digital subtraction angiography (16). This is likely a function of the increased concentration of vessels due to tumor neovascularity (17) or increased permeability of the tumor vessels. The use of contrast material in the breast will be limited by individual reactions to the contrast material, but digital contrast subtraction may be valuable in the high-risk woman whose mammary parenchyma is radiographically extremely and heterogeneously dense.

True digital acquisition will permit improved utilization of artificial intelligence systems to enhance the image and assist the radiologist in detection and diagnosis. Algorithms are being devised to evaluate digitized conventional images, but this approach is not likely to be particularly useful because there are no more data available in the digitized image than on the original film. Primary digital acquisition, on the other hand, offers a greater depth of information, but the challenge will be to determine the best way to present it to the observer since the combinations will be essentially limitless.

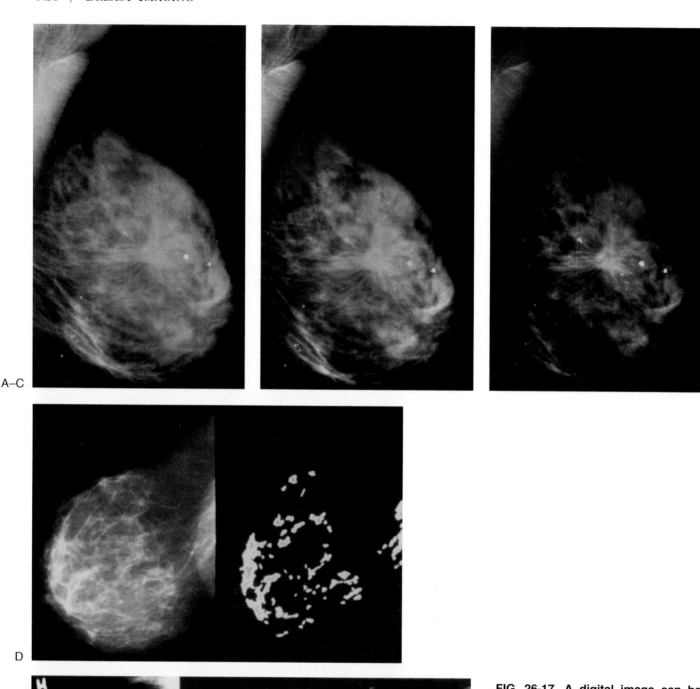

FIG. 26-17. A digital image can be manipulated in an infinite number of ways to enhance the visibility of structures. These images were all derived from a single exposure. The computer was used to enhance different features using a wide gray scale **(A)**, an intermediate scale **(B)**, and high contrast **(C)**. Computer enhancements can be applied to digital images. The image on the right **(D)** used a thresholding technique to highlight the densest portions of the image for parenchymal pattern analysis. Electronic magnification is demonstrated on this digital image **(E)** at three levels of enlargement, revealing segmentally distributed calcifications.

In the near future computers will assist in the identification of suspicious groups of calcifications. As algorithms improve and computer power increases, assistance in detecting and diagnosing noncalcified lesions of the breast may become possible (18).

Digitized Mammograms versus Primary Digital Acquisition

Digitization of Film

Devices that allow the conversion of a conventional film mammogram into a digital representation continue to improve (19). An evaluation of an early system was performed by Smathers and colleagues (20), using a laser scanner that permitted the production of a 2048 × 2048 matrix with a 12-bit (4096) range of pixel intensity (20). Digitizers work by passing light through the radiograph and recording the intensity of the transmitted light at each point in the picture and assigning a number to that light intensity. In their study the image was scanned to record the light passing through each 0.10- × 0.18-mm area of the film. In this way a numeric value can be assigned to the densities of the film. Thus copied into a digital form, the window center and width can be varied, permitting computer manipulation and greater range in display of the data acquired by the film/screen system. Electronic filtering techniques were used to enhance the visibility of structures in the original image. Simulated microcalcifications were evaluated, and based on the ability to discriminate 50% of the microcalcifications of a given size, the authors found that in a review of the digitized conventional film/screen images their ability to detect simulated microcalcifications improved.

Although there are some advantages to digitizing film, there are significant disadvantages. A major advantage of a digital system derives from contrast manipulation and electronic filtering techniques. Although a digitized image permits the use of computer assistance in detection and diagnosis, the digitized image has somewhat less information than the original image (information is lost and noise is added whenever an image is copied). Spatial and contrast resolution of images digitized from another medium are limited by the spatial and contrast resolution of the initial image. Digitization of conventionally obtained mammograms does not add information, although it may permit the improvement in the observer's ability to appreciate information that may not be obvious owing to the narrow exposure latitude of film and its compressed dynamic range. Digitization merely permits manipulation of the image to enhance the visibility of the structures.

Once digitized, an image can be enlarged. Optical magnification, in addition to image manipulation, probably contributes to the ability to discern subtle structures. Techniques such as unsharp masking (21) to enhance the high-frequency signal, and hence the fine detail, by blurring the low-frequency broad-area structures make it easier to see microcalcifications. Electronic magnifying glasses do not add information but may make it easier to perceive important detail.

Direct Digital Imaging

Advantages of Direct Digital Acquisition for X-Ray Mammography

To maximize the information contained in an x-ray "shadowgram" of the breast, direct measurement of the x-ray photons passing through the breast is desirable. To collect the most information, the goal of digital imaging is literally to count the number of photons that pass through the breast. A digital detector should have no threshold (it should detect the first and last photons through) and should be able to count a wide range of photons reaching it (photon flux). This provides the truest representation of the varying attenuation of the tissues through which the photons passed. If there is a difference in x-ray absorption between these tissues, a photon counter offers the best opportunity of displaying those differences.

Contrast versus Spatial Resolution

X-ray film has very high spatial resolution. Some film has the ability to resolve 17 to 20 line-pairs per millimeter. This means that it can demonstrate structures that are as small as 25 μm in size. This is much greater resolution than what is actually obtained using conventional film/screen mammography. Without magnification, mammography generally cannot resolve calcifications that are smaller than 200 μm. Theoretical spatial resolution is determined under ideal circumstances and where the structures being resolved differ significantly in contrast. Spatial resolution may appear to be very high when the study object (phantom) consists of metal lines alternating with empty spaces so that the contrast between the two is almost 100% (the metal blocks all the photons, while the spaces permit them all to pass through).

The ability to resolve structures may diminish rapidly if the objects are similar in contrast. If, for example, there are two masses that are side by side and they are imaged with a technique that has insufficient spatial resolution, then they will appear as a single structure (Fig. 26-18). If the system can display them at different contrast (contrast resolution), however, then they may be visible as separate entities to the observer even if the spatial resolution is not optimal. Spatial resolution cannot be evaluated without measuring contrast resolution.

Modulation Transfer Function

Generally a good measure of the performance of a system is determined by its modulation transfer function (MTF).

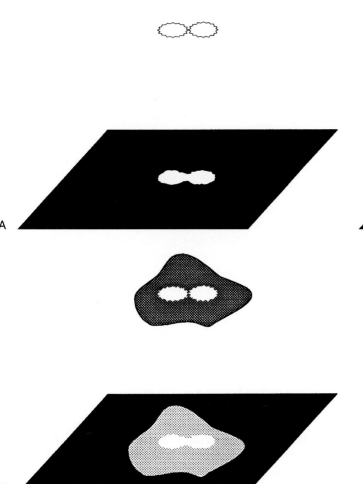

FIG. 26-18. Spatial resolution versus contrast resolution. If two structures are too close together for the system to resolve, then they appear as one structure. These simulated calcifications appear as one if there is insufficient spatial resolution **(A)**. Even if the system has high spatial resolution, if there is insufficient contrast resolution then the calcifications and the tissue in which they lie appear as a single structure and the calcifications are not visible **(B)**. Even if the spatial resolution is not high, the structures may be seen if they can be resolved by differences in contrast. These simulated calcification are visible in the dense tissue due to high contrast, although their morphology is indistinct due to low spatial resolution **(C)**.

The MTF gauges the percentage of the signal strength entering the system relative to the signal coming out of the system at varying frequencies (Fig. 26-19). The smaller the structure being imaged, the higher the frequency of the signal that represents it and the higher the frequency that must be recorded to display it. For most imaging systems the MTF decreases as the spatial frequency increases. It is the rate of decrease and its level that influences the effectiveness of the system. A system may be able to display high-frequency structures, but the signal may be so low that it cannot be seen because it is lost in the noise of the system.

Signal-to-Noise Ratio

The MTF is not the only measure of a system's potential. The signal-to-noise ratio (SNR) is a major factor. An image can be thought of as combination of desirable information (signal) and undesirable information that clouds the image (noise) (Fig. 26-20). Film has a fairly high MTF at high spa-

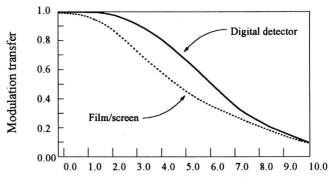

Spatial frequency in line pairs per mm.

FIG. 26-19. These are **the modulation transfer functions** for a high-resolution film/screen system and a full-field digital system. Note that the digital system has high-contrast resolution for the lower spatial frequencies. The film/screen system will have greater contrast transfer at the higher frequencies, but this better spatial resolution may not be visible because the contrast will be very low and the structures will be invisible to the observer.

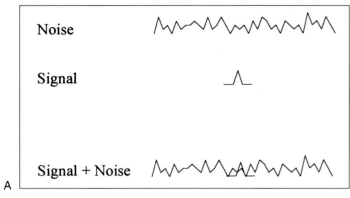

A

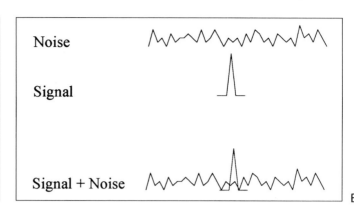

B

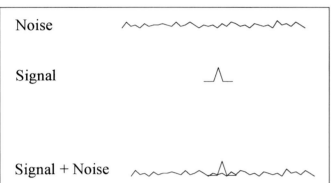

C

FIG. 26-20. Signal-to-noise ratio. When the signal is low relative to the noise, the structure (signal) cannot be seen **(A)**. By increasing the signal **(B)** or decreasing the noise, the structure becomes more evident **(C)**.

tial frequencies, but the film image is composed of discrete grains spaced randomly through the emulsion of the film. At high spatial frequencies very small structures are close to the size of the film grains. The grains produce a random background of white and black dots, and the structure to be imaged may not be separable from the random noise. Blur caused by the screens that are coupled with the film in conventional mammography also degrades the spatial resolution of film/screen combinations (see Chapter 8). At high frequencies (small details), the SNR ratio usually becomes very low, and the image signal is lost in the noise of the film/screen detector. As a consequence the potential spatial resolution of film is not realized in day-to-day mammographic imaging.

One method of improving the SNR for film is radiographic magnification. This spreads the signal over a larger area. Since the noise remains the same regardless of the magnification, enlarging the signal area increases the ratio of the signal to the noise. Digital detectors can be made that produce a higher SNR than film/screen combinations, and this is one of their advantages. Although they may not have the same absolute spatial resolution and high-frequency capture as a film detector, the MTF and SNR of some digital systems is greater than film/screen for the display of moderately high-frequency information. A crude demonstration of this is seen in imaging the ACR breast phantom. There are no film/screen systems presently in use that can image all of the objects in the American College of Radiology (ACR)

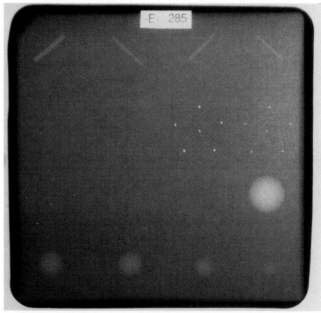

FIG. 26-21. Digital mammography and a test phantom. All of the test objects in the ACR phantom are visible using the General Electric flat-panel imager due to its wide dynamic range.

phantom. The General Electric full-field imager can demonstrate all of the objects in the ACR phantom, despite having lower spatial resolution than film/screen systems (Fig. 26-21), because it has higher contrast resolution.

Dynamic Range

The ability to differentiate structures of similar but not identical x-ray attenuation is the contrast resolution of a system. This is described in terms of dynamic range. For example, a system that can represent the x-ray attenuation of the tissues through which the x-ray beam passed using only 8 shades of gray (from white to black) has a much lower dynamic range than one with 4,096 shades of gray. Film/screen systems have a very narrow dynamic range, and the exposure must be made to fit that narrow range; otherwise, the image will be underexposed or overexposed. Because a digital system is not limited in this way, it can record a much larger range of photon flux and can record and differentiate much more subtle differences in contrast (its dynamic range is greater). This longer scale means that tissues of similar but slightly different contrast that would not be differentiated using film can be differentiated with a digital system. Digital systems offer the opportunity for much higher contrast resolution.

Possible Configurations for a Digital Imager

Numerous methods of collecting x-ray photons to form a digital image have been proposed. Spatial resolution is important for a digital mammography system. In order to be able to resolve 5 line-pairs per millimeter, the pixel size of the detector must be 100 μm (0.1 mm). If the goal is 10 line-pairs per millimeter, then the pixel size must be 50 μm (0.05 mm). The large conventional mammographic film size is 24 × 30 cm. If the digital imager has a pixel size of 100 μm, it would have 10 pixels for every millimeter, which means there would be 100 pixels for every centimeter, and it would take 2,400 × 3,000 pixels for a total of 7,200,000 pixels to cover the same area as a piece of film. Thus, without any attention to the brightness (gray levels) of the image, each image is 7.2 megabytes in size. If the imager is to have a 50-μm pixel size to provide 10 line-pairs of resolution, then the area covered must be 4,800 pixels wide by 6,000 pixels long for a total of 28,800,000 pixels (28.8 megabytes).

This is an underestimate of the amount of memory required for digital mammography because the image is defined not only by the pixel size and number but also by the shades of gray (brightness) that can be represented at each pixel. Brightness is determined by the dynamic range (the scale of gray between no photons recorded [pure white] to complete transmission of x-rays [totally black]). If the pixel were to be only black or white, then an additional bit of computer memory would be required. If 2 bits are available, the imager could display four shades of gray, 3 bits provide eight shades, 4 bits 16, 5 bits 32, 6 bits 64, 7 bits 128, 8 bits 256, 9 bits 512, 10 bits 1,024, 11 bits 2,048, 12 bits 4,096, 13 bits 8,192, and 14 bits 16,384 shades of gray. Most interpreters believe that at least 12

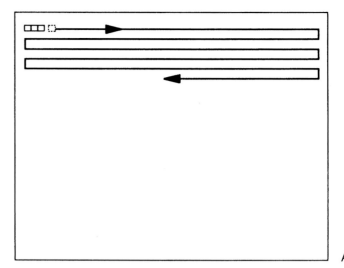

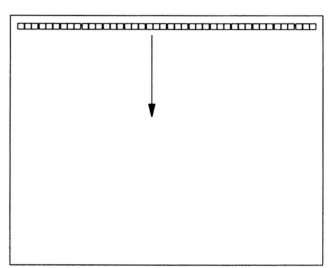

FIG. 26-22. There are several approaches to forming a digital mammogram. **(A)** Sweeping **a point of x-rays** across the breast and detecting the transmitted photons at each point is the simplest way to make a digital image, but it is extremely slow. **(B) A line-scanning system** with detectors following a fan beam of x-rays that sweep across the breast is feasible but very slow. *Continued.*

bits are needed for contrast. Most images in fact have 16 bits available (2 bytes of computer memory). This means that the amount of data included in each image must multiply the number of pixels by 2 bytes. An imager with 5 line-pairs per millimeter (100-μm pixel size) will require 7.2 megabytes × 2 bytes = 14.2 megabytes of memory for each image. At 10 line-pairs per millimeter (50-μm pixel size), the image will be 28.8 × 2 = 57.6 megabytes. These extremely large image files have been part of the reason for the slow evolution of digital mammography, but recent improvements in memory capacity now make digital mammograms feasible.

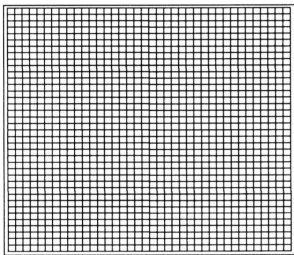

C

D

FIG. 26-22. *Continued.* **(C) A pixel array** (several rows of detectors) can be scanned under the breast and exposed by a fan beam in a fairly efficient fashion. **(D) An area detector** that records all points of the image simultaneously is desirable.

Approaches to Digital Acquisition

Spot Scanning

The simplest method of forming a digital image is to have a single detector behind the breast and to sweep a very small pencil beam of x-rays across the breast. The x-rays recorded at each point would create the image (Fig. 26-22A). Unfortunately this is an extremely slow way to make an image. If, for example, the goal is to have an imager with 50-µm pixel size and the beam must stop at each point for 1 second to ensure that sufficient x-ray photons pass through each point to make an image, it would take 32,640,000 seconds, or 378 days to make an image. Needless to say this would compromise throughput.

Line Scanning

Efficiency can be increased by making a row of detectors and sweeping a line of x-rays aligned with the detector across the breast (Fig. 26-22B). This requires only 100 minutes to make an image if the line is 50 µm wide. If higher-energy photons are used, then it takes less time at each position to reach sufficient flux to create the image and an image can be made in a reasonable time period. Line-scanning systems have been made. One such system, described in the following section, uses a higher-energy spectrum beam and can sweep the breast in approximately 22 seconds. More recently a variation has been built that takes a detector that is made up of with several 256×256 (or 512×512) pixel arrays mounted in a line that moves along with the fan beam of x-rays to make the image (Fig. 26-22C). By sweeping a wider beam across the breast and integrating the results for each line, an image can be made in several seconds. If it takes a number of seconds to make an image motion could be a theoretical problem. However, the image for any portion of the breast is recorded in a fraction of the total time, so that overall motion should not be a problem for a scanning system. A slot that moves with the detector is fairly efficient at removing scatter.

Area Detector

Film is an area detector. The entire area of the breast is exposed simultaneously. If scatter reduction is not an issue, then a digital area detector, in which all of the image is collected simultaneously, is the most desirable system (Fig. 26-22D).

Digital Mammographic Systems

Scatter and Digital Mammography

Area detectors are subject to the same scatter degradation that occurs with conventional mammographic techniques. Point scanning (22) produces the least scatter, but because a fraction of the x-ray beam is used insufficient photon flux is available. Line-scanning systems with slit collimation provide the best compromise (23). The reduced contrast that occurs due to scatter can be compensated for by electronic filtering, but this can be complex, and our preliminary results suggest that for dense breasts or those that do not compress to <4 to 5 cm, a grid can improve the image.

Dose and Digital Mammography

One of the original goals of digital mammography was to reduce the amount of radiation needed to image the breast and detect early breast cancer. Conventional film/screen mammography does not efficiently use all the x-ray photons passing through the breast. This contributes to the need for additional exposure of the patient. As stated by physicists, conventional mammographic images are not "quantum limited." Dose can be reduced by improving the efficiency of the system to account for all the photons reaching the detector. Increasing quantum detection efficiency (QDE) and the translation of those quanta to imaging information as detective quantum efficiency (DQE) by using systems that use detectors that record photon flux over a broad area simultaneously usually results in decreased resolution. DQE may be improved by making a thicker medium that is more likely to absorb the x-ray photon, but if the absorber works by converting the x-ray photons to light, a thicker medium will permit spread of the light generated by the interaction. Spread of light in the detector produces blurred images.

Early Digital Mammography Systems

Line Scanning

Systems have been developed that use solid state detectors that virtually count the photons passing through the breast. One of the earliest digital mammography systems was invented by American Science and Engineering. They oriented the scintillator material on edge so that the x-ray photons enter the edge of the detector and have a long photon path in which to be absorbed and generate light. A photodiode array was aligned alongside the scintillator with 1,024 detectors per inch with the capability of 40 pixels per millimeter. This detector array was then coupled with a pre- and post-breast slit collimation system that protected the

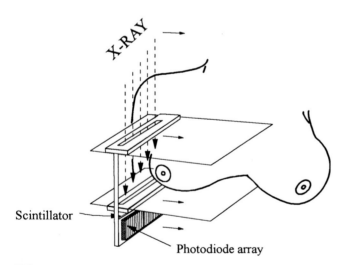

FIG. 26-23. The American Science and Engineering line-scanning, digital mammography system used pre- and post-breast slits to virtually eliminate scatter. The x-rays entered the scintillator along its edge, and the light emitted was converted to electricity by the photodiode array aligned along the scintillator. This provided high x-ray photon detection efficiency with a short light path to reduce spread in the scintillator.

breast from unused radiation and significantly reduced image degrading scatter (Fig. 26-23). The system demonstrated 8- to 9-line-pairs-per-millimeter resolution with the possibility of even higher resolution, but its development was never completed. Greater resolution can be achieved, but it is limited by the capacity of the x-ray tube to generate sufficient photon flux through the breast.

Storage Phosphor Systems

The storage phosphor systems are digital area detectors that have been in use for many years for plain radiography. They continue to be explored and improved so that they might be useful for breast imaging. These involve a hybrid technology using europium-activated barium fluorohalide (24). When this material is exposed to radiation, it stores the incident photon energy in the media by producing a quasi-stable energized state that is in proportion to the radiation striking the medium. The plate is exposed by a conventional mammographic system and then introduced into a special processing system. The stored-energy latent image is read by scanning the media with a helium-neon laser, which releases the stored energy in the form of light that can be electronically recorded in a digital format, once again permitting computer manipulation.

This system has been studied for use as a digital mammography detector. It has been shown to suffer from relatively low resolution. The reusable media theoretically has approximately 5-line-pairs-per-millimeter resolution, although it probably does not come close to achieving this based on its MTF. This may not be a limitation of the media itself but of the capacity of the system to digitize, store, and display the large amounts of data that are required with these techniques, and improvements are likely.

Charge-Coupled Devices

Another way of recording mammographic images digitally is through the use of charge-coupled devices (CCDs). These are essentially chips that have rows and columns of electronic "wells" that collect electrons that are generated by the interaction of light in a photocathode (material that uses light energy to release electrons). The electrons are generated in direct proportion to the light impinging on the photocathode. The charge in each well can be read and expressed digitally. Thus far, mammographic systems that use CCDs have used fluorescent screens to convert the x-ray photons to light. Lens systems have been used to focus the light onto the CCDs, but these proved inefficient. Fiber optics have been used to guide the light from the screen to the CCDs.

Since CCDs have only been made in fairly small sizes, they were initially used as single, limited field-of-view detectors in stereotactic devices. A single CCD allowed imaging an area of approximately 4 to 5 cm on a side.

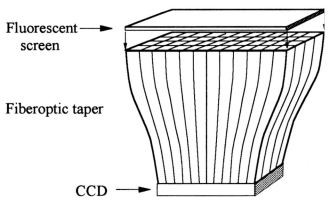

Fluorescent screen →

Fiberoptic taper

CCD →

FIG. 26-24. A fiber-optic taper can be used to channel the light emitted from the fluorescent screen down to the smaller area of the charge-coupled device (CCD).

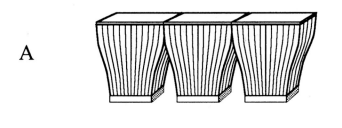

A

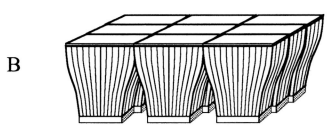

B

FIG. 26-25. Multiple fiber-optic tapers coupled to charge-coupled devices can be joined to form a scanning detector **(A)** or butted together to form a full-field detector **(B)**.

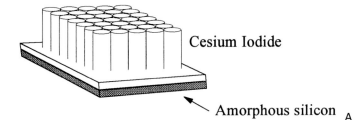

Cesium Iodide

Amorphous silicon A

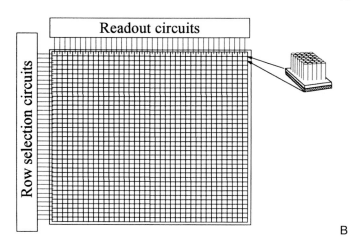

Readout circuits

Row selection circuits

B

FIG. 26-26. The General Electric full-field, amorphous silicon detector system is based on a thin film of amorphous silicon with an X and Y grid of electronics bonded to it using lithographic techniques. The phosphor is grown on the film epitaxially so that the cesium iodide crystals form columns at each pixel **(A)** that conduct the light emitted by that crystal to the silicon photodiode so that there is little image-degrading light spread in the detector. Microcapacitors (each pixel) are discharged in proportion to the light reaching the photodiode, producing an electronic signal. Each pixel's charge can be read out individually from the entire matrix **(B)** into a computer to form the digital image.

The actual area of the CCD was much smaller than this. The larger area could be covered by using a fiber-optic taper to channel the light from the screen to the CCD. The taper is formed by taking a bundle of millions of glass fibers aligned in parallel and then drawing out the fibers so that they taper down from an area of 4 to 5 cm on a side to the smaller size of the CCD (Fig. 26-24). One solution to making a full-field digital detector has been to join these together to form an array of multiple fiber-optic tapers and CCDs (Fig. 26-25). This requires careful engineering to avoid gaps where the detectors are butted together. Detectors have been constructed using arrays of 12 CCD elements (3 × 4) to produce a full image of the breast at 10-line-pairs-per-millimeter spatial resolution (50-μm pixels).

Thin-Film Transistor Array

Another approach to forming a full-field digital detector has taken advantage of the development of thin-film transistor technology. These have been used to make active matrix computer displays, and the technique has been used in reverse to produce digital x-ray detectors. As with CCD technology, the x-ray photon is converted into light either by a phosphor that is mated to the electronics or by crystals grown directly onto the thin film of amorphous silicon. Using techniques that were developed for the manufacture of computer chips, small transistors are printed on the amorphous silicon with each transistor connected to an X and Y grid array of wires (Fig. 26-26). Light photons are converted to electrons and are detected by the transistor array. The charge that develops at each transistor can be read using the wire grid that connects each point in the array to the edge of the detector.

Selenium as a Detector

One technology that may well represent a trip "back to the future" is a selenium-based x-ray detector. In the mid-1970s an article by Bailar (25) heightened concern for the potential carcinogenic effect of mammography. This adverse assessment spurred the development of imaging techniques, such as ultrasound and transillumination, that did not involve the use of ionizing radiation. Simultaneously film/screen combinations were developed to reduce the radiation exposure to the patient. The xeroradiographic technique was developed and was used successfully for many years. Xeroradiography (26) was a detector system in which an aluminum plate was coated with selenium, forming a semiconductor. Approximately 2,000 volts was applied to the surface of the plate, which was then introduced into an insulating cassette. X-rays passing through the breast caused a discharge that was in proportion to the amount of radiation reaching the plate. The plate was then extracted from the cassette, and in a special processor a cloud of charged powder was blown across the surface. The powder was attracted like iron filings to a magnet and accumulated in proportion to the amount of charge at each point on the plate. This produced an image of the x-ray transmission through the breast. A plastic-coated paper was placed against the powder image, and the powder was transferred to the paper. Heat was applied, which melted the powder into the plastic surface, forming the Xerox image. This is the same type of technology used in copying machines. Toward the end of the use of xeroradiography liquid toner was substituted for the powder.

Although there were claims that xeroradiography was superior to film/screen technology, no trial was ever performed to objectively compare the two, and the perceived lower dose from film/screen imaging and the switch to this technology by most health care providers involved in breast imaging resulted in the discontinuation of the xeroradiographic system.

Selenium-based digital detectors are being developed. They have the advantage that selenium converts x-ray photons directly to electronic charge without the interposition of a fluorescing screen. Because of light spread in a screen, the image can be blurred. There is no spread of the charge formed in the selenium detector. It is sharply confined to the portion of the detector that absorbs the x-ray photon. This offers the opportunity for very sharp, high-resolution x-ray imaging. Methods to read out the charge directly from the plate are needed before this will become a practical approach to digital mammography.

Limitations of Digital Mammography

As the technical hurdles involved in developing a digital x-ray mammographic imager are surmounted and the storage of these large images becomes less costly, the major limita-

tion to the use of digital mammography will be in the display of the images. Low-cost image displays are not capable of displaying such large amounts of information. Even 2K × 2K monitors cannot display an entire digital mammogram if it is acquired at 50-μm pixel size. Initial studies have required viewing of the entire breast at low-information density and then focusing in on areas of interest that are then displayed, providing all of the data. Progressively more detail is displayed, but the area covered is smaller. The only way to display a full digital mammogram for the foreseeable future is to print the images on film. Although this defeats one of the principal near-term benefits of a digital mammogram, it permits research to move forward to maximize the other benefits from digital mammography.

Other Benefits of Digital Mammography

Digital mammography will permit the development of additional methods of evaluating the tissues.

Dual Energy Subtraction

Dual energy subtraction will permit the direct demonstration of calcifications. At low x-ray energies, calcifications absorb a higher percentage of the incident photons than soft tissue does. At higher energy, the differences in attenuation

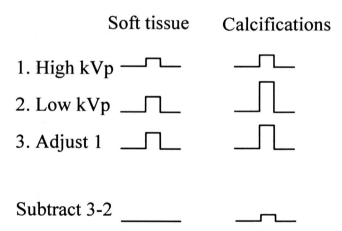

FIG. 26-27. Dual energy subtraction takes advantage of the fact that the change in attenuation is greater for calcifications than for soft tissues when the kVp is altered from high energies to low energies. If the resulting images are adjusted so that the soft tissues in the two images have identical digital representations, then when one is subtracted from the other the soft tissues completely subtract and the only residual signal is from the calcifications, permitting an image of only the calcifications in the breast. This is shown schematically where the signals from a soft-tissue object and calcifications are represented by the curves for the high- (line 1) and low-energy (line 2) exposures. By raising the peaks (line 3) so that the soft tissue curves completely subtract, there is still some signal from the subtracted calcification signals and this difference is the signal for the calcifications only.

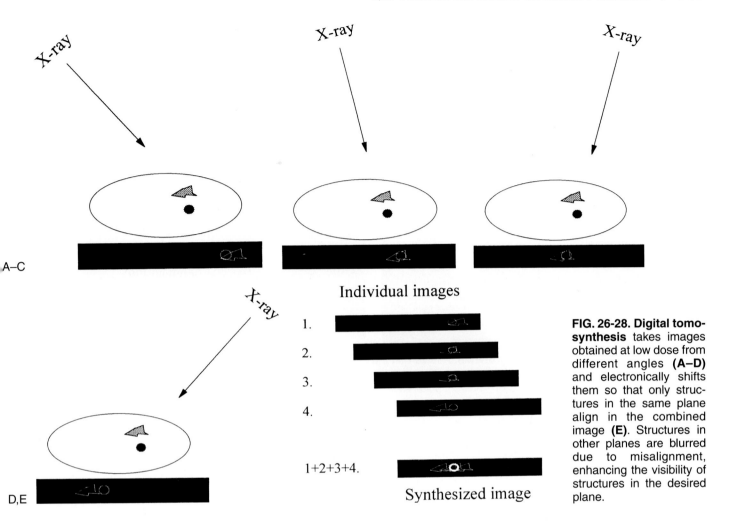

X-ray   X-ray   X-ray

A–C

Individual images

X-ray

1.

2.

3.

4.

1+2+3+4.

Synthesized image

D,E

FIG. 26-28. Digital tomosynthesis takes images obtained at low dose from different angles **(A–D)** and electronically shifts them so that only structures in the same plane align in the combined image **(E)**. Structures in other planes are blurred due to misalignment, enhancing the visibility of structures in the desired plane.

between soft tissues and calcifications are not as wide. By obtaining an image at high kVp and another at low kVp, one of the images can be adjusted so that if the two images are subtracted the soft tissue signal can be made to completely cancel out, leaving only the resultant calcium signal (Fig. 26-27). The only limitation of this approach is that when two images are subtracted the amount of noise is doubled. An increase in photon flux can help improve the SNR, and by also applying computer analysis to the image it is likely that calcifications will be more easily detected, reducing the chance of overlooking an early cancer and facilitating image review and radiologist viewing.

Digital Tomosynthesis

A major impediment to the detection of small cancers comes from the overlap of the normal tissues of the breast. This "structure noise" makes it difficult to perceive lesions and to evaluate them once they have been detected. The reduction in structure noise is one of the main advantages of tomography. CT lacks the spatial resolution of flat-field imaging, although with significantly higher dose a high-resolution CT scanner might have value in breast evaluation.

The geometry of such a scanner, however, would be problematic if the goal was to include the axillary tail. Conventional linear, or polycycloidal, tomography would be difficult in the breast because the patient's head and body would interfere with the required movement of the detector and x-ray tube. Conventional tomography would also involve significantly more dose.

Tomography can, however, be achieved with the breast held in the standard mammography system and with the detector stationary. Digital tomosynthesis is a method that was described many years ago (27) but could not be easily applied until the development of a digital detector that can be read directly without moving the breast in the system. We have developed a modification of the method of digital tomosynthesis that works by combining images taken from several angles with the x-ray tube following an arc above the breast while the detector remains stationary (28). The images can be electronically reconstructed so that planar sections throughout the breast can be viewed. By accurately knowing the location of the x-ray tube relative to the breast, the multiple images are aligned and superimposed so that only structures in the plane of interest are aligned (Fig. 26-28). By obtaining each individual image at lower dose

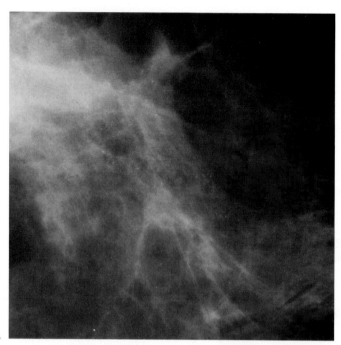
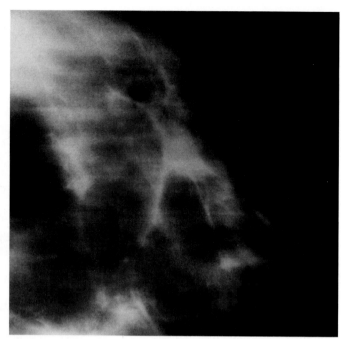

FIG. 26-29. Digital tomosynthesis. A lesion on the standard mammogram of a mastectomy specimen is barely visible **(A)**. It is obvious on the tomosynthesis image **(B)** when the plane in which it resides is in focus.

than a standard mammographic image, the unaligned planes have low contrast and SNR and are effectively blurred, while the signal from the portions that are aligned are added and the structures in the chosen plane become more visible (Fig. 26-29). A series of eight to ten images obtained over a 20- to 30-degree arc permit movement through the breast, developing slices that are effectively only a few millimeters in thickness. Using reconstruction algorithms a three-dimensional model of the breast can be developed. This will likely improve the ability to detect cancers that are presently being overlooked due to the interference of structured noise.

Contrast Subtraction Angiography of the Breast

Numerous studies have now demonstrated that cancers develop an increased blood supply to permit their growth. These vessels are often more numerous than in an equal volume of normal tissue. Furthermore, they are less well formed than normal vessels, and are "leaky." Intravenous contrast material has been used to enhance the visibility of cancers by demonstrating these tumor vessels with computed tomography, angiography, and most recently magnetic resonance imaging. Digital detectors, with their increased ability to resolve low-contrast structures, will permit the ability to demonstrate tumors using intravenous iodinated contrast infusion at much lower cost than computed tomography or magnetic resonance imaging. This will offer additional opportunity to determine the importance of an abnormality found by mammography, as well as the potential to find cancers earlier in selected populations.

It remains to be proved that digital imaging can provide as much information as conventional mammography, but our initial experience suggests that the wider dynamic range of these systems and the ability to manipulate the image will provide more information than conventional mammography. Furthermore, contrast subtraction or temporal subtraction studies with such systems will allow further study of the properties of malignant lesions when contrast material is infused. Chang and colleagues (15), using computerized body tomography of the breast, and Watt and associates (16), using digital subtraction angiographic techniques, have demonstrated that not only does contrast material produce a blush from the neovascularity recruited by the tumor, but enhancement persists in significant quantities in breast cancer for relatively long periods of time, presumably due to leakage of the contrast out of tumor vessels that are known to be poorly formed and leaky (Fig. 26-30). Watt and co-workers demonstrated that after iodinated contrast infusion, the peak contrast flow through the tumor's neovascular structure occurred within 10 seconds. However, 0.3 mg/cm of iodine remained within a 36-cc tumor, and this persisted for more than 3 minutes. Higher-resolution digital techniques may permit utilization of this phenomenon to aid in the diagnosis of breast cancer. Because overlap between benign and malignant lesions is likely, contrast subtraction studies will more than likely have their greatest impact in the radiographically dense breast, in which they may be used to improve the sensitivity of mammography by enhancing lesions that are obscured by the surrounding tissue on the conventional study.

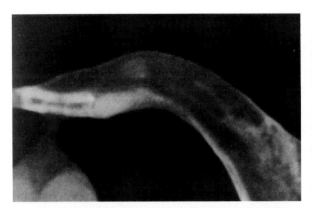 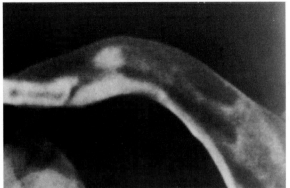

FIG. 26-30. Cancers enhance with iodinated contrast. The cancer is seen on the unenhanced image on the left as a vague area of attenuation in the medial left breast. Following the intravenous administration of iodinated contrast there is marked enhancement, as is evident on the right image.

Clinical Impact

Digital mammography will offer the opportunity to revolutionize x-ray imaging of the breast. In addition to the already proved efficacy of x-ray mammography in the earlier detection of breast cancer and the resulting decrease in deaths, digital imaging will enhance the ability of mammography to save lives. Since the image will no longer be constrained by the narrow limitations of a film picture and since the image can be adjusted after the exposure, unsatisfactory images will be eliminated. This will reduce the overall exposure of the population and the time and cost involved in repeating technically unsatisfactory images. The increased contrast resolution of a digital image will make cancers that are presently overlooked using conventional mammography become more visible. Computer analysis of the images will reduce the likelihood that a cancer will be overlooked by the human reader. Storage will be more secure, reducing the likelihood that images will be lost, and consultation anywhere in the world will be facilitated through the use of telemammography.

Computer-Aided Detection and Diagnosis

Once an image is in digital form it can be analyzed by a computer. Features can be extracted, and the computer can learn to recognize calcifications, masses, and architectural distortion. This can be done directly or using neural networks that let the computer select the features that help it to most accurately detect a specific abnormality. Computer-aided detection and design (CAD) will not likely replace the radiologist, but numerous studies have shown that all radiologists, regardless of skill level, fail to see a significant abnormality at some time or other. Have a second reader (double reading) has been shown to increase the detection rate of cancers by 5% to 15% (1,29–31). A computer can function as a second reader and indicate areas of concern on the film that might have been overlooked by the radiologist.

Systems to assist in the detection of breast cancer are already being evaluated. One of the challenges is to have the computer's threshold be sufficiently low so that it detects cancers overlooked by the radiologist but not so low that it generates a large number of false positives so that the radiologist ceases to use it.

Telemammography

Enormous advances continue to be made in telecommunications. These have resulted in the ability to transmit information virtually instantaneously anywhere in the world. Remote medical evaluation using standard television video images (telemedicine) has been used for many years and continues to improve and expand so that patients may be evaluated and even have treatment instituted by physicians hundreds or thousands of miles away.

Television images, however, have significant limitations. They are based on analog signals. Because they are relatively low in resolution, they are not useful for sending images that must be high in detail. In addition, analog signals cannot be perfectly reproduced. An image that is in digital form becomes a fixed record that can be transmitted as an electrical signal over telephone lines, dedicated telecommunication lines, or by satellite. The transmitted image is a perfect reproduction of the original when it is sent as a string of numbers. Furthermore, by using numbers to send an image, carefully devised techniques are available to correct any mistakes that may occur in the transmission so that the image that is received is identical to the image that was transmitted.

The development of digital mammography will permit more widespread use of the ability to send mammographic images anywhere in the world. One of the limitations that prevented the transmission of high-quality mammograms until recently was the enormous size of the digital file that was needed to encode a complete mammogram. Over the last few years the ability to transmit the file size needed for mammography has improved significantly. In a program funded by the National Cancer Institute that allied an industrial group with an academic medical center, we demonstrated that a digitized mammogram can be sent from one part of the country to another using a satellite relay in less than 4 minutes without an error.

The development of telemammography will permit experts in breast imaging to evaluate images from anywhere in the country or even the world. Women in rural areas who do not have access to high-quality breast cancer screening could be visited by a mobile mammography unit. A digital mammogram could be obtained and immediately transmitted by satellite to a breast screening center, where a radiologist could immediately interpret the images and relay any need for additional evaluation back to the mobile unit so that the additional evaluation could be undertaken while the patient was still at the screening vehicle. This would not only permit underserved women access to high-quality screening, but it would facilitate the evaluation of lesions found at screening and reduce the likelihood that if a significant problem was identified the individual might not be properly evaluated because she would not avail herself of follow-up services because they were too far away.

OTHER IMAGING TECHNIQUES

Ultrasound

Ultrasound has been discussed in detail. Ultrasound has demonstrated efficacy in the differentiation of cysts from solid lesions and is useful in guiding interventional procedures, but it is unreliable for the differentiation of benign solid lesions from those that are malignant (32,33). Although in the past ultrasound has been shown to have no role in screening, there have been several reports that modern technology may offer the possibility of detecting early cancers that are not visible on mammography or evident on clinical examination. Gordon and Goldberg reported on anecdotal cases of cancers detected by ultrasound alone (34,35). Kolb and associates reported on 2,300 women who had radiographically dense breasts on whom they performed screening ultrasound studies. They found 10 cancers among these women after a negative mammogram and clinical breast examination (36). They reported that the cancers that were detected were similar in size (11.3 mm) to those detected by mammography (10.9 mm) as well as similar in stage (83.3% vs. 90.2% stage I). This is a significant detection rate (4/1,000) and suggests the need to reevaluate ultrasound as a second-level screening technique. This needs to be done prospectively in a triple-blind evaluation of clinical breast examination, mammography, and ultrasound with the investigators initially blinded to the mammogram and then with the knowledge of the mammogram. The technique of scanning needs to be defined and reproducible, and the criteria for intervention carefully defined since by ultrasound there are many findings in any breast that could represent cancer. Given the improvements in the technology that have taken place over the past 10 years, ultrasound should be reevaluated as a screening technique. Until efficacy has been demonstrated, however, ultrasound should not be considered as a screening technique.

Ultrasound is the primary breast diagnostic technique for differentiating benign cysts from solid masses. Ultrasound is also valuable for guiding the accurate placement of needles under direct observation into masses to obtain fluid, cytologic material, or core-needle samples. Ultrasound is also useful for monitoring the placement of guides to direct surgeons in the excision of nonpalpable lesions.

The technique has improved significantly since the early 1980s when whole-breast ultrasound was found to be unsatisfactory for screening (37). It is possible that in the not too distant future three-dimensional whole-breast ultrasound evaluation will be possible. Microbubbles will be injected intravenously and provide sonographically visible contrast. The neovascularity that can indicate a cancer on CT, MRI, or nuclear medicine studies may reveal itself using ultrasound.

Magnetic Resonance Imaging

MRI *without contrast enhancement* has not proved useful in the detection or diagnosis of breast cancer. Data suggest that *contrast-enhanced* scans may be helpful in determining the extent of breast cancer as a management aid (38), detecting unsuspected foci of multifocal or multicentric tumors and perhaps aiding in differentiation of benign from malignant lesions (39). MRI may one day aid in primary detection. MRI has demonstrated efficacy in the evaluation of women with silicone implants to demonstrate rupture of the implant. Pulse sequences that suppress fat and water tissue signals make it possible to differentiate silicone (40) (see Chapter 20).

MRI without contrast has thus far failed to demonstrate sufficient sensitivity and specificity to justify the great expense and time needed to perform these studies. Just as has been seen with iodinated contrast and x-ray imaging, breast cancer demonstrates useful signal intensity change on MRI following the infusion of contrast agents such as gadolinium DTPA (38,41–43). The earliest, most likely clinically efficacious role for MRI will be the evaluation of women with known breast cancer in whom MRI will be used to assess the extent of the tumor and assist in treatment decisions. If the cost can be reduced significantly and the throughput increased, MRI of the breast offers promise for the earlier detection of breast cancer, as a screening technique, particularly in the radiographically dense breast.

Computed Tomography

CT of the breast has shown some promise in the past for the definition of cancers through the use of intravenously administered iodinated contrast enhancement. This phenomenon has been confirmed using digital subtraction angiographic techniques. CT's only practical application in breast imaging at this time, however, is to triangulate some lesions and guide needle localization in difficult situations (44,45). Nevertheless, the advantage of cross-sectional images in permitting the separation of a significant lesion from the structure noise of the surrounding breast tissue should not be ignored. High-resolution CT scanning with the use of intravenously administered iodinated contrast reflects the same phenomena as gadolinium-enhanced MRI and should be investigated as a possible lower-cost alternative. CT may permit more accurate detection and evaluation of lesions in dense breast tissues.

Transillumination

Transillumination, light scanning, and diaphanography (46) are all synonymous with the passage of far red (R) and near infrared (IR) light through the breast. Proponents believe that breast cancers absorb these wavelengths owing to blood in their neovascular networks. Most systems attempt to evaluate the total light transmission through regions of the breast as well as compare the ratio of infrared to red light transmitted. Severely compromising this technique is the fact that it uses a broad, diffuse light source, and virtually all of the light transmitted is scattered and diffused, reducing resolution in a similar manner to scatter radiation and geometric unsharpness in x-ray imaging.

Early favorable assessments were anecdotal reports of unscientific evaluations. Bartrum and Crow (47) were the first to critically assess the technique. They were optimistic in their preliminary assessment, despite the fact that in their blind reading, 24% of cancers were not detected by light scanning, while mammography detected 94% of the cancers. Sickles reported a prospective series of 1,239 women with 83 proven cancers studied with both light scanning and mammography (48). Once again mammography detected 96% of the cancers, whereas transillumination was able to reveal only 53%. More discouraging is the fact that the technique missed 67% of the cancers in women with negative axillary nodes and 81% of the cancers <1 cm in size. Marshall and colleagues (49) were somewhat more encouraged in their study of 1,000 women, but the 26 of 29 cancers they demonstrated on light scanning were clinically evident lesions. Furthermore, in their series, light scanning failed to demonstrate three of eight cancers <1 cm.

Geslien and coworkers (50) studied 1,265 women in whom they found 33 cancers. Light scanning missed 42% of the cancers and 45% of the nonpalpable cancers as well as 70% of the 10 tumors less than 1 cm in size. They also assessed the technique as a diagnostic procedure and found that it was not as sensitive as ultrasound for differentiating cysts from solid lesions.

Further evidence that light scanning is not useful in breast evaluation was added by Gisvold and associates (51) in a study of 822 women and 67 cancers. Although 96% of the cancers were found by mammography, only 67% were evident by light scanning.

The poor results from light scanning are due to the poor depth resolution of the technique. Simulating light transmission through the breast in a phantom study, Drexler and coworkers showed that under ideal conditions, a lesion could not be detected at a depth greater than twice its diameter (46). The geometry of the light source and the virtually complete scattering of the light by the breast severely compromise the technique.

Laser Imaging

Visible light and light in the near infrared portion of the spectrum can pass through human tissues. Just as with x-rays, this can be used to form shadows of the internal structures of the breast. Unfortunately, an extremely small amount of light, if any, passes directly through the breast. The vast majority is scattered and diffused, reducing or eliminating the signal relative to the noise.

It is theoretically possible to eliminate the scatter and collect only the directly transmitted light to gain information about the internal structures of the breast. This will most likely be accomplished using low-energy lasers. Laser breast imaging has only begun to be studied. Multispectral diffuse transillumination (diaphanography) of the breast has been shown to have no value in the detection or diagnosis of breast cancers (52). It is possible, however, that laser transillumination techniques may one day be useful. One method of eliminating scatter is through the use of range gating. In this method, using picosecond switches, only the "fast light" (the directly transmitted light) is collected before the scatter reaches the detector. Other scatter elimination methods may one day make laser transillumination useful in breast evaluation.

One company is developing a CT scanner that uses a laser instead of x-rays. The efficacy of these systems has yet to be demonstrated. It is more likely that lasers will be applied toward tissue diagnosis through the use of fiber-optically guided light pulses that raise electrons surrounding atoms into higher energy levels. When these electrons return to a lower energy state, they give off light that is a spectral signature of the atoms, molecules, and possibly the tissue that were excited by the light. The acquisition of spectral information from relaxation energies may be used to characterize the tissues. Lasers may also ultimately have application in the in vivo treatment of breast cancers by heating or even vaporizing tumors in situ. Unless, however, precise definition of the extent of a cancer can be determined in vivo it will be difficult to utilize closed ablation techniques such as lasers, high-frequency ultrasound, microwaves, or cryotherapy.

DIAGNOSTIC TECHNIQUES

Although there are no better screening techniques than mammography on the horizon, other techniques may have significant value when applied to the problems listed in this chapter, and some may ultimately be shown to be efficacious for earlier detection of breast cancer. Even if a test is not efficacious as a primary screening technique for the entire population, it may be useful as a secondary screening in a selected segment of the population. For example, the subset of women with dense breast tissue, in whom mammography is less sensitive, might benefit from a secondary screening technique if that test can be shown to detect earlier-stage cancer that is not revealed by mammography.

The breast is one of the safest organs from which to obtain a tissue diagnosis, and a less invasive procedure must be very accurate to avoid a needle biopsy or even a guided excision. There is, nevertheless, great interest in trying to reduce the amount of trauma (and cost) required for the successful diagnosis and treatment of breast cancer.

Scintigraphic Imaging

Thallium and Technetium 99m Sestamibi

Preliminary studies have raised recent interest in the use of radionuclides for evaluating breast lesions. Tracers that were originally developed for myocardial imaging have been found to concentrate in breast malignancies. Thallium 201 has been used to image some breast malignancies. In one series of 81 women with palpable breast masses, thallium identified 45 of the 47 malignancies (sensitivity of 96%). Only three false positives were identified among the 13 patients who were found to have fibroadenomas. There were no additional false positives in the 21 women with other benign masses. The cancers in this study, however, were all palpable and the smallest was 1.3 cm in greatest dimension (53).

Technetium 99m sestamibi has similar properties to thallium, having its origin as a cardiac agent. It is undergoing an extensive trial to evaluate its ability to differentiate benign lesions from malignant lesions detected by mammography or clinical examination (Fig. 26-31). Early data with a small number of patients reported a sensitivity of 96% and a specificity of 85% (54). An updated review included 387 women and 3 men (55), who were evaluated for mammographically or who had clinically detected abnormalities. There were 182 palpable abnormalities, 222 nonpalpable lesions, and 20 normal volunteers. The smallest mass was 8 mm. The patients received 20 mCi of technetium 99m sestamibi (MIBI) intravenously by hand injection. The breasts were imaged sequentially from the lateral side while the patient lay prone with the breast being imaged while pendent and as close to the camera as possible. Five minutes after the injection, the breast was imaged for 10 minutes. Several patients

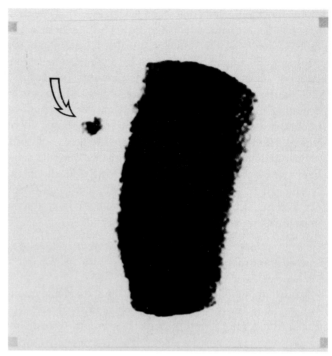

FIG. 26-31. The large cancer in this breast enhanced with **technetium 99m sestamibi** (*arrow*).

were also evaluated using single photon emission CT (SPECT). The investigators considered a focal area of uptake as significant. Mild diffuse uptake or none at all was negative. The agent appeared to concentrate in the lesions with a ratio of target-to-background activity that ranged from 1.3 to 5.8. The authors reported that the scans correctly identified 90% of the cancers with a 3% false-negative rate and a 7% false-positive rate.

Our own evaluation of sestamibi was less encouraging (56). We evaluated a group of 31 patients with lesions detected only by mammography (nonpalpable). The lesions consisted of 14 groups of calcifications, 12 masses, and five areas of architectural distortion. There were seven malignancies and 24 benign lesions. The sensitivity of the sestamibi was only 29%, with a specificity of 83%. Three invasive cancers and two cases of ductal carcinoma in situ were false-negative, and there were four false-positive scans (Fig. 26-32). These results raise serious doubts concerning the efficacy of the tracer for evaluating nonpalpable lesions.

The agent appears to delineate cancers in two ways. Circulating in the blood it is likely more concentrated where there is a high density of blood vessels, such as in the neovascularity that develops in many cancers. This is similar to the early enhancement of cancers that is seen following the intravenous administration of iodinated contrast and the enhancement by gadolinium on MRI. It also appears that there is some active uptake by the mitochondria of the cells.

The initial sestamibi studies are trying to determine whether scintigraphy of the breast can aid in reducing the

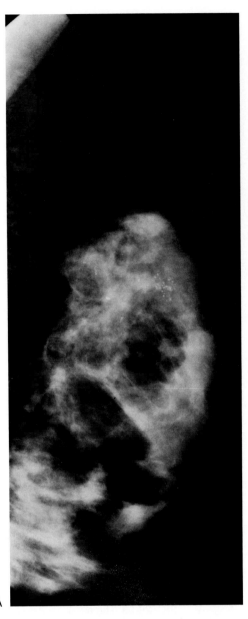

A

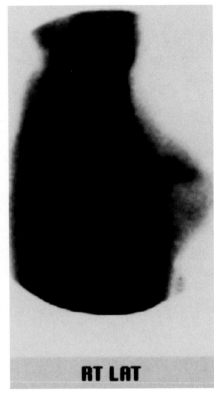

RT LAT

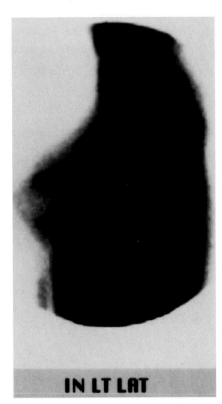

IN LT LAT

B,C

FIG. 26-32. Technetium 99m sestamibi. The calcifications seen on this mediolateral oblique mammogram **(A)** delineate a nonpalpable intraductal cancer with microscopic areas of invasion in a 44-year-old woman. The sestamibi study was positive for this lesion **(B)** but was also falsely positive on the contralateral side **(C)**.

need for intervention for lesions detected by mammography by the noninvasive differentiation of benign from malignant lesions. There are as yet no data to support its use for screening. Use of the agent for axillary staging has not been studied in any rigorous fashion. The development of other labeled molecules may permit greater refinement in breast cancer detection and diagnosis.

Positron Emission Tomography

Positron emission tomography (PET) requires highly specialized equipment. Early results suggest that breast cancers have elevated metabolic activity. This can be detected through the use of fluorine 18–labeled glucose (FDG) (57) (Fig. 26-33). Preliminary information suggests that PET may be a method for staging breast cancers by assessing the

axillary nodal status and possible distant metastatic spread. PET may also be valuable in assessing the possibility of recurrence following breast cancer treatment. Large trials are necessary to establish any efficacy in the screening of asymptomatic women for breast cancer. This application for PET will likely be limited by the requirement for the injection of radioactive material that is difficult to produce since it must be made using a cyclotron. Investigators are considering the possibility of using FDG with SPECT scanning to take advantage of the metabolism of FDG without the need for an expensive PET scanner.

The risk from present-day tracers is greatest for the bladder due to clearance in the urine, and this will likely limit its usefulness to older women.

PET scanning offers the opportunity not only to determine whether a lesion is benign or malignant but to assess

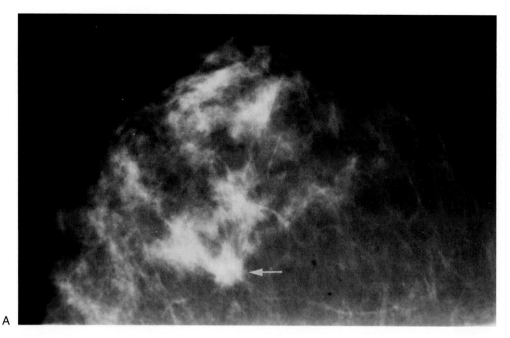

A

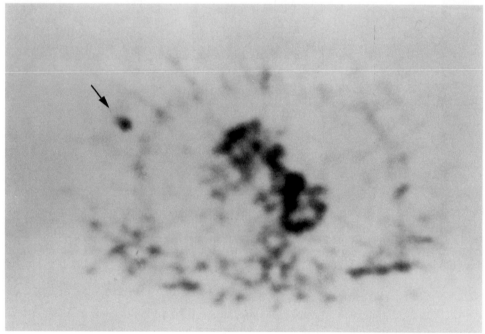

B

FIG. 26-33. The small cancer **(A)** seen on this mammogram (*arrow*) was visible on this positron emission tomography scan **(B)** because it was glucose avid.

some metabolic parameters that might be of prognostic value by their utilization or incorporation of the labeled molecule. The isotopes that are used, however, are very short lived and must be produced by an on-site accelerator, increasing the cost of performing PET studies.

Glucose labeled with fluorine 18 to form 2-[fluorine 18]-fluoro-2-deoxy-D-glucose (FDG) is one of the most widely studied molecules. This agent has been used to demonstrate lesions that are metabolically active and have an increased utilization of glucose. Early results suggest that many breast cancers have elevated metabolic activity that can be detected

through the use of FDG. Wahl and associates found increased uptake in 10 of 10 primary breast cancers (57). Adler and coworkers studied 28 women with 35 masses that were larger than 1 cm and found increased uptake in 26 of the 27 malignant lesions (sensitivity of 96%) with no false-positive scans (specificity of 100%) (58). These authors were also able to identify increased activity in the axillae in 9 of the 10 of the women who were shown to have positive axillary nodes.

Nieweg and associates had similar preliminary results in their study of 20 women. Fluorine 18–labeled glucose accumulated in 10 of the 11 lesions in women with cancer. These authors had one case in which there was some uptake in a woman whose biopsy revealed only fibrocystic tissue (false-positive). All five of the women who had axillary uptake demonstrated tumor in their axillary lymph nodes (59).

These are all preliminary findings, and the evaluation of PET for breast imaging has thus far been limited. This is in part due to limited access to scanners and the need for agents with short half-lives that must be generated by a nearby cyclotron. It remains to be seen whether PET will be accepted as a diagnostic technique to differentiate benign from malignant lesions to obviate the need for needle or open biopsy.

Large trials would be necessary to establish any efficacy in the screening of asymptomatic women for breast cancer. This application will be unlikely due to the cost of the procedure and the requirement for the injection of radioactive material although the radiation risk is very low. The critical organ for FDG, which is cleared in the urine, is the bladder, which receives approximately 0.32 rad/mCi of injected activity (60). In most studies the patients were injected with 10 to 20 mCi. This will likely limit its usefulness to older women.

The few studies that have been published have used PET to image large cancers. Its ability to evaluate small cancers is questionable. Although our own experience is very limited, we have already had a 7-mm invasive breast cancer that was not evident on the PET scan. Adler and colleagues compared the normalized activity of the lesions with the nuclear grade of the cancers, and their data suggest that higher grade (poorly differentiated) lesions exhibited greater activity (58). This suggests that PET may be useful as a prognostic test.

All of these preliminary results are encouraging, but the studies are very limited. The patients were highly selected, and the results must be analyzed accordingly. At this time, PET of the breast should be considered experimental with no as yet proven clinical efficacy.

Axillary Node Assessment

Sentinel Node

It has been shown in patients with melanoma that technetium sulfur colloid, injected at the periphery of the melanoma, will concentrate in the first lymph node that drains the area of the tumor, making it identifiable using a gamma probe (61,62). Removal and examination of this node is predictive for the presence or absence of metastatic disease, reducing the need for more complex nodal dissection and its associated morbidity and expense.

There appear to be sentinel nodes for breast cancer. A preliminary report is encouraging (63). In this study, following the injection of 0.4 mCi of technetium 99m sulfur colloid mixed in 0.5 ml of saline into the tissue in a 180-degree arc around the tumor along its axillary perimeter, a probe was held over the axilla. The sentinel node was found where there were at least 30 counts in 10 seconds. The node was removed and evaluated for the presence of metastatic disease and compared to the results of the full axillary dissection. In a study of 22 women, a sentinel node was identified in 18 women who had full axillary dissections (all three levels) following radionuclide injections 1 to 9 hours prior to surgery. Among the 18 women, 62 radioactive and 170 nonradioactive nodes were removed. In all seven of the women who had positive nodes, the sentinel node contained tumor. In three of the patients, only this node contained tumor.

If the predictive value of the sentinel node can be validated in other trials, then the need for a full axillary dissection can be avoided. This would greatly facilitate the surgical approach to breast cancer and permit all surgery for women who elect breast preservation to be performed using only local anesthesia. This would have implications for imaging-guided needle biopsy since it would permit diagnosis, staging, and local treatment (lumpectomy) with a single operative procedure using local anesthesia.

INTERVENTIONAL TECHNIQUES

The gold standard for diagnosis is the evaluation of tissue under a microscope. Methods for improving the ability to obtain tissue, ranging from traditional fine-needle aspiration to large histologic samples, will continue to be developed. Investigators should consider that it may be possible to improve on histologic diagnosis. It is conceivable that the diagnosis of a significant breast lesion (one with lethal potential) may be more accurately determined using in vivo imaging technologies rather than in vitro histologic techniques. Such a shift in prognostication, however, would require very large trials.

Increased attention is focusing on the ability to diagnose a lesion once it has been detected by mammography. Efforts to develop noninvasive imaging methods to differentiate benign from malignant lesions should continue, but these have rarely been able to replace direct tissue acquisition in other organs. In settings with access to skilled cytopathology, fine-needle aspiration cytology is valuable (64). However, core-needle biopsy has the advantage of providing histologic information such as whether the tumor is invasive. Core-needle biopsy is likely to become the primary diagnostic technique for mammographically detected, clinically occult breast lesions (65,66). This technique offers the greatest promise because core material is obtained in a less operator-dependent fashion than fine-needle aspiration, and the core material can be interpreted by any pathologist skilled in breast histology and pathology. Although the accuracy of core-needle biopsy of the breast has never been fully validated (67), the pressure to reduce cost and surgical trauma will result in its increasing application. Because of the sampling error involved in any needle procedure, the process will be improved by permitting larger amounts of tissue to be removed through small skin entry points in a minimally invasive approach.

The development of minimal excision surgical breast biopsies in which cubic centimeter or greater volumes of tissue are removed through very small incisions will eliminate the likelihood of a sampling error that compromises the accuracy of needle techniques. Reduced trauma to the patient and diminished expense to society are valuable goals. These should be achieved, however, without reducing the accuracy of diagnosis presently afforded by needle, dye, and wire localization followed by excisional breast biopsy.

PREDICTING THE FUTURE

Film/screen mammography will likely remain the primary method of breast cancer detection over the next several years. As digital detectors improve, they will likely supersede film-based systems and permit the increased use of computer-aided detection and diagnosis. If the cost of MRI can be reduced, it may become a second-level screening technology for individuals with dense or complex breast tissues. Radionuclide scintigrams may have a role as a second-level screening, but sensitivity and the fact that the patient is exposed to radioactivity may limit the application of these techniques.

The application of imaging to the differentiation of benign lesions from malignant (diagnosis) will have limited value. Needle biopsy techniques and other forms of minimally invasive methods of tissue sampling will become more accurate and so safe and cost effective that it will be difficult to avoid obtaining tissue from questionable lesions unless an imaging test is almost 100% specific (i.e., can exclude cancer).

The role of needle biopsy in lesions that have a high probability of cancer will likely diminish, as will the need for extensive lymph node evaluation. There are some who already are foregoing axillary dissection, arguing that it does not truly influence long-term survival, and systemic treatment is determined based on tumor size and the histology and grade of the lesion. In the National Surgical Adjuvant Breast Project Trial B-04, in women with stage II cancer, there was no difference in survival between women whose axillae were irradiated or who had lymph nodes surgically resected. For women with stage I cancer, there was no difference in survival among women who had their lymph nodes surgically removed, treated by irradiation, or not treated at all (68). If axillary node evaluation is no longer necessary, then the diagnostic excisional biopsy for many lesions will be all that is required.

A second possibility is that sentinel node evaluation will be all that is required, and the identification of the primary drainage node will permit evaluation under local anesthesia, eliminating the need for an axillary dissection under general anesthesia.

Efforts to accurately define the extent of breast cancer have thus far been inaccurate. A percentage of intraductal cancers are not detectable by MRI, and thus it will be difficult to treat tumors in vivo using high-energy sound or lasers or even progressive tissue removal without additional treatment to the entire breast. Neoadjuvant chemotherapy may reduce the need for extensive excisional biopsy, but it is likely that some form of overall breast treatment will be required to eliminate any residual disease. More accurate prognostication such as the emerging newer classifications of intraductal cancer (69,70) may help select individuals for tailored or less or more intense therapy.

Efficacy Must Be Established Before a Technique Is Widely Adopted

The evaluation of a new technique must ask critical questions concerning the device and its capabilities. The primary role for an imaging technique is the *detection* of breast cancer at a time when its natural history can be interrupted and death from breast cancer avoided or deferred. Many of the structures found by screening may prove to be benign, but as long as the group as a whole contains small, early stage, clinically occult cancers, then the technique may be useful.

The requirements for a *diagnostic* technique differ. Because a surgical excision is almost 100% accurate and is very safe, a less invasive technique must be almost perfect to replace excisional biopsy (some women may be willing to accept a lower specificity). It is likely that the same technique cannot perform both functions well. Mammography can detect a significant number of earlier-stage cancers, but it frequently cannot differentiate them from other lesions it detects. Ultrasound is useful diagnostically to differentiate benign cysts from solid breast lesions, but it is not useful as a screening technique to detect breast cancer. As new technology emerges, its capabilities in these two separate areas must be evaluated. Screening devices should fulfill the criteria outlined by Moskowitz and associates (71) before they can be accepted as efficacious. Diagnostic techniques are only useful if they can be shown to alter the course of patient management. The scientific method should be applied. New tests should be evaluated in blinded studies, without the knowledge of the other test results. The new test can then be reread using other information, but its contribution can only be assessed without the results of the established test biasing the assessment. Science is tedious, but adding layers of tests that may add information but do nothing to improve the care of the patient will only add to the cost of health care and not to the benefit.

REFERENCES

1. Tabar L, Fagerberg G, Duffy SW, et al. Update of the Swedish two-county program of mammographic screening for breast cancer. Radiol Clin North Am 1992;30:187–210.

2. Bassett LW, Liu TH, Giuliano AE, Gold RH. The prevalence of carcinoma in palpable vs impalpable mammographically detected lesions. AJR Am J Roentgenol 1991;157:21–24.
3. Fletcher SW, Black W, Harris R, et al. Report of the International Workshop on Screening for Breast Cancer. J Natl Cancer Inst 1993;85:1644–1656.
4. Smart CR, Hendrick RE, Rutledge JH, Smith RA. Benefit of mammography screening in women ages 40–49: current evidence from randomized, controlled trials. Cancer 1995;75:1619–1626.
5. Shapiro S. Screening: assessment of current studies. Cancer 1994;74:231–238.
6. Ohuchi N, Furuta A, Mori S. Management of ductal carcinoma in situ with nipple discharge. Intraductal spreading of carcinoma is an unfavorable pathologic factor for breast-conserving surgery. Cancer 1994;74:1294–1302.
7. Ohtake T, Abe R, Izoh K, et al. Intraductal extension of primary invasive breast carcinoma treated by breast conservative surgery. Cancer 1995;76:32–45.
8. Orel SG, Fowble BL, Solin LJ, et al. Breast cancer recurrence after lumpectomy and radiation therapy for early-stage disease: prognostic significance of detection method. Radiology 1993;188:189–194.
9. Kimme-Smith C. New and future developments in screen-film mammography equipment and techniques. Radiol Clin North Am 1992;30:55–66.
10. Eklund GW, Cardenosa G. The art of mammographic positioning. Radiol Clin North Am 1992;30:21–53.
11. Kopans DB. Nonmammographic breast imaging techniques: current status and future developments. Radiol Clin North Am 1987;25:961–971.
12. Sickles EA, Doi K, Genant HK. Magnification film mammography: image quality and clinical studies. Radiology 1977;125:69–76.
13. Sickles EA. Further experience with microfocal spot magnification mammography in the assessment of clustered microcalcifications. Radiology 1980;137:9–14.
14. Vyborny C. Can computers help radiologists read mammograms? Radiology 1994;191:315–317.
15. Chang CHJ, Nesbit DE, Fisher DR, et al. Computed tomographic mammography using a conventional body scanner. AJR Am J Roentgenol 1982;138:553–558.
16. Watt CA, Ackerman LV, Windham JP, et al. Breast lesions: differential diagnosis using digital subtraction angiography. Radiology 1986;159:39–42.
17. Weidner N, Semple JP, Welch WR, Folkman J. Tumor angiogenesis and metastasis—correlation in invasive breast carcinoma. N Engl J Med 1991;324:1–8.
18. Kegelmeyer WP, Pruneda JM, Bourland PD, et al. Computer-aided mammographic screening for spiculated lesions. Radiology 1994;191:331–337.
19. Sommer FG, Smathers RL, Wheat RL, et al. Digital processing of film radiographs. AJR Am J Roentgenol 1985;144:191.
20. Smathers RL, Bush E, Drace J, et al. Mammographic microcalcifications: detection with xerography, screen-film, and digitized film display. Radiology 1986;159:673.
21. McSweeney MB, Sprawls P, Egan RL. Enhanced image mammography. AJR Am J Roentgenol 1983;140:9.
22. Kushner D, Cleveland R, Herman TE, et al. Detection and evaluation of chest abnormalities with low-dose scanning beam digital radiography: comparison with standard radiographs. Presented at the 69th Scientific Assembly of the Radiological Society of North America, November 1983, Chicago.
23. Tesic MM, Sones RA, Morgan DR. Single-slit digital radiography: some practical considerations. AJR Am J Roentgenol 1984;142:697.
24. Sonoda M, Takano M, Miyahara J, Kato H. Computed radiography utilizing scanning laser stimulated luminescence. Radiology 1983;148:833.
25. Bailar JC. Mammography: a contrary view. Ann Intern Med 1976;84:77.
26. Kopans DB. Breast Imaging. Philadelphia: Lippincott, 1989.
27. Miller ER, McCurry EM, Hruska B. An infinite number of laminograms from a finite number of radiographs. Radiology 1971;98:249–255.
28. Niklason LT, Christian BT, Whitman GJ, et al. Improved visualization of breast lesions with digital tomosynthesis imaging. Presented at the 82nd Scientific Assembly of the Radiological Society of North America, December 1996, Chicago.
29. Bird RE. Professional quality assurance for mammographic screening programs. Radiology 1990;177:587.
30. Thurfjell EL, Lernevall KA, Taube AAS. Benefit of independent double reading in a population-based mammography screening program. Radiology 1994;191:241–244.
31. Hulka CA, Mrose H, McCarthy K, et al. The value of double reading in screening mammography. Presented at the 80th Scientific Assembly and Annual Meeting of the Radiological Society of North America, November 27–December 2, 1995, Chicago.
32. Jackson VP. The role of US in breast imaging. Radiology 1990;177:305–311.
33. Kopans DB. Recent issues in breast cancer and the pre-market approval by the Food and Drug Administration of a U.S. system for breast lesion evaluation. What happened to science? Radiology 1997;202:315–318.
34. Gordon PB, Goldenberg SL, Chan NHL. Solid breast lesions: diagnosis with US-guided fine-needle aspiration biopsy. Radiology 1993;189:573–580.
35. Gordon PB, Goldenberg SL. Malignant breast masses detected only by ultrasound: a retrospective review. Cancer 1995;76:626–630.
36. Kolb TM, Lichy J, Newhouse JH. Detection of otherwise occult cancer with ultrasound in dense breasts: diagnostic yield and tumor characteristics. Presented at the 82nd Scientific Assembly of the Radiological Society of North America; December 4, 1996, Chicago.
37. Kopans DB, Meyer JE, Lindfors KK. Whole breast ultrasound imaging—four-year follow-up. Radiology 1985;157:505–507.
38. Pierce WB, Harms SE, Flamig DP, et al. Three-dimensional gadolinium-enhanced MR imaging of the breast: pulse sequence with fat suppression and magnetization transfer contrast. Radiology 1991;181:757–763.
39. Orel SG, Schnall MD, LiVolsi VA, Troupin RH. Suspicious breast lesions: MR imaging with radiologic-pathologic correlation. Radiology 1994;190:485–493.
40. Gorczya DP, Sinha S, Ahn CY, et al. Silicone breast implants in vivo: MR imaging. Radiology 1992;185:407–410.
41. Kaiser WA, Zeitler E. MR imaging of the breast: fast imaging sequences with and without Gd-DTPA. Radiology 1989;170:681–686.
42. Heywang SH, Wolf A, Pruss E, et al. Imaging of the breast with Gd-DTPA: use and limitations. Radiology 1989;171:95–103.
43. Stack JP, Redmond OM, Codd MB, et al. Breast disease: tissue characterization with Gd-DTPA enhancement profiles. Radiology 1990;174:491–494.
44. Kopans DB, Meyer JE. Computed tomography guided localization of clinically occult breast carcinoma—the "N" skin guide. Radiology 1982;145:211–212.
45. Spillane RM, Whitman GJ, McCarthy KA, et al. Computed tomography-guided needle localization of nonpalpable breast lesions: review of 24 cases. Acad Radiol 1996;3:115–120.
46. Drexler B, Davis JL, Schofield G. Diaphanography in the diagnosis of breast cancer. Radiology 1985;157:41.
47. Bartrum RJ, Crow HC. Transillumination light scanning to diagnose breast cancer: a feasibility study. AJR Am J Roentgenol 1984;142:409.
48. Sickles EA. Breast cancer detection with transillumination and mammography. AJR Am J Roentgenol 1984;142:841.
49. Marshall V, Williams DC, Smith KD. Diaphanography as a means of detecting breast cancer. Radiology 1984;150:339.
50. Geslien GE, Fisher JR, DeLaney C. Transillumination in breast cancer detection: screening failure and potential. AJR Am J Roentgenol 1985;144:619.
51. Gisvold JJ, Brown LR, Swee RG, et al. Comparison of mammography and transillumination light scanning in the detection of breast lesions. AJR Am J Roentgenol 1986;147:191.
52. Alveryd A, Balldin G, Fagerberg G, et al. Lightscanning versus mammography for the detection of breast cancer in screening and clinical practice: a Swedish multicenter study. Cancer 1990;65:1671–1677.
53. Waxman AD, Ramanna L, Memsie LD, et al. Thallium scintigraphy in the evaluation of mass abnormalities of the breast. J Nucl Med 1993;34:18–23.
54. Khalkhali I, Mena I, Jouanne E, et al. Prone scintimammography in patients with suspicion of breast cancer. J Am Coll Surg 1994;178:491–497.
55. Diggles L, Mena I, Khalkhali I. Technical aspects of prone dependent-breast scintimammography. J Nucl Med 1994;22:165–170.
56. Whitman GJ, Fischman AJ, Lee JM, et al. Sestamibi breast imaging with histopathologic findings in 31 nonpalpable breast lesions. Pre-

sented at the 82nd Scientific Assembly of the Radiological Society of North America; December 2, 1996, Chicago.

57. Wahl RL, Cody RL, Hutchins GD, Mudgett EE. Primary and metastatic breast carcinoma: initial clinical evaluation with PET with the radiolabeled glucose analogue 2-[F-18]-fluoro-2-deoxy-D-glucose. Radiology 1991;179:765–770.

58. Adler LE, Crowe JP, Al-Kaisi NK, Sunshine JL. Evaluation of breast masses and axillary lymph nodes with [F-18] 2-deoxy-2-fluoro-D-glucose PET. Radiology 1993;187:743–750.

59. Nieweg OE, Kim EE, Wong W, et al. Positron emission tomography with fluorine-18-deoxyglucose in the detection and staging of breast cancer. Cancer 1993;71:3920–3925.

60. Dowd MT, Chen CT, Wendel MJ, et al. Radiation dose to the bladder wall from 2-[18F]fluoro-2-deoxy-D-glucose in adult humans. J Nucl Med 1991;32:707–712.

61. Alex JC, Krag DN. Gamma-probe guided localization of lymph nodes. Surg Oncol 1993;2:137–143.

62. Alex JC, Weaver DL, Fairbank JT, Krag DN. Gamma-probe guided lymph node localization in malignant melanoma. Surg Oncol 1992;2:303–308.

63. Krag DN, Weaver DL, Alex JC, Fairbank JT. Surgical resection and radiolocalization of the sentinel lymph node in breast cancer using a gamma probe. Surg Oncol 1993;2:335–340.

64. Azevado E, Svane G, Auer G. Stereotactic fine-needle biopsy in 2594 mammographically detected non-palpable lesions. Lancet 1989;1:1033–1036.

65. Parker SH, Lovin JD, Jobe WE, et al. Nonpalpable breast lesions: stereotactic automated large-core biopsies. Radiology 1991;180:403–407.

66. Dowlatshahi K, Yaremko ML, Kluskens LF, Jokich PM. Nonpalpable breast lesions: findings of stereotaxic needle-core biopsy and fine-needle aspiration cytology. Radiology 1991;181:745–750.

67. Kopans DB. Caution on core. Radiology 1994;193:325–328.

68. Fisher B, Redman C, Fisher E. Ten-year results of a randomized clinical trial comparing radical mastectomy and total mastectomy with or without radiation. N Engl J Med 1985;312:674–681.

69. Holland R, Peterse JL, Millis RR, et al. Ductal carcinoma in situ: a proposal for a new classification. Semin Diagn Pathol 1994;11:167–180.

70. Silverstein MJ, Poller DN, Waisman JR, et al. Prognostic classification of breast ductal carcinoma-in-situ. Lancet 1995;345:1154–1157.

71. Moskowitz M, Feig SA, Cole-Beuglet C. Evaluation of new imaging procedures for breast cancer: proper process. AJR Am J Roentgenol 1984;140:591.

Subject Index

A

Abscesses
  acoustic shadowing on ultrasound and,
    439
  diagnosis of, 430–431
  hematoma compared with, 430
  implants and, 474
  in male breast, 502
  mammogram, not demonstrated on, 298
  nursing and, 287
  ultrasound instance of, 430, 435
Accessory breast tissue, 6
  in axilla, 231
  breast development and, 4–5, 231
  ectopic breast and, 6
  formations of, 6
  location of, 4–5
  mammographic instance of, 230
  milk line and, 5, 231
  nipple(s), 4, 6
    breast development and, 4
    formation of, 6
    xerographic instance of, 231
Acini
  adenosis and, 25
  appearance of, 232
  calcifications and, 325–326
    mammographic instance of, 362
  cysts and, 429
  lobular, calcifications in
    benign nature of, 361–362
    mammographic instance of, 362
  menstrual cycle, influence on mitotic
    rate, 19
  microcyst formation and, 24
Acoustic shadowing, lesions that produce,
  438
Adenoid cystic sarcoma, 601, 602–603
Adenoma, nipple, 516
Adenopathy. *See also* Axilla
  axillary lymph nodes and, 347
  benign, 347
  free silicone and, 475
  gel bleed and, 475
  malignant, 347
  mammography and, 347
Adenosis, 515–516, 546, 548–551
  acinar structures and, 25

diffusely scattered calcifications and, 367
mammographic appearance of, 550–551
radial scars and, 305
and relative risk for invasive breast cancer, 512, 548, 550
sclerosing, 25, 546, 548, 549
ultrasound appearance of, 551
Adjuvant chemotherapy. *See* Chemotherapy, adjuvant
Adjuvant radiation therapy. *See* Radiation
  therapy, adjuvant
Adolescent breast, masses in, 231
Age 50
  biological irrelevance of, 79–81, 98
  and breast tissue, no dramatic change at,
    235
  as surrogate for menopause, 79–80
Age
  at exposure, radiation risk, varies with,
    103
  and mammography, woman under 40
    with a sign or symptom of
    breast cancer, 804–805
Aging
  arterial calcifications and, 362
  breast cancer risk and, 30–31, 45, 46
  breast tissue, changes in, 20–21,
    511–512
  involution of breast and, 20–21
  lesions, cancer probability increasing
    with, 376
American Cancer Society (ACS)
  breast cancer screening, baseline study,
    recommendations regard-
    ing, 441
  and randomized controlled trials, 97–98
  recommendations of, 97–98, 98
American College of Radiology (ACR)
  accreditation requirements, 169
  Breast Imaging Committee, mammogra-
    phy guidelines and, 77
  Breast Imaging Reporting and Data
    System (BIRADS),
    762–790
  analyzing masses, approach to,
    267–279
  and clock face method of location,
    274

contents of, 763–764
  breast evaluation, 763–764
    two major settings for, 764
  lexicon, 764
  screening, 763
data maintenance and screening
  audit, 790–792
  data to be monitored in, 790
  sensitivity and specificity, 791–792
final assessments and, 222
goal of, 762
historical perspective, 762–763
mammogram assessment, categories
  for, 254
Mammography Accreditation Program, 763
mammography outcome monitoring
  and, 218
mammography reporting and, 218
  assessment categories for,
    225–227
  standardized language for, 157
mass
  margins defined by, 275
  shape defined by, 275
microlobulated term used by, 384
patterns
  of breast tissue, 238–239
  calcification distribution, 334–337
  parenchymal, 238–239
  seen on ultrasound, 423–424
reporting system of, 765–789
  breast imaging report, 765–782
  calcifications, classification of,
    771, 773–781. *See also* Cal-
    cifications, classification of
  masses, classification of,
    765–771. *See also* Masses,
    classification of
  description of significant find-
    ings, 765–782
  description of tissue pattern, 765
  sample reports, 784–78
    asymmetric breast tissue,
      787
    highly suggestive of malig-
      nancy, 787
    negative mammogram, 784–785

American College of Radiology (ACR),
Breast Imaging Reporting
and Data System (*contd.*)
for patient referred for area of
clinical concern, 785
short-interval follow-up,
786–787
suspicious abnormality, 787
ultrasound, 787–789
coding system, 789
for pathology, 789
follow-up and outcome monitoring,
789–790
terminology, microlobulated margins,
274–279, 295
Committee on Quality Assurance in Mammography, manuals of, 165
guidelines to quality control procedures.
See Breast Imaging Report-
ing and Data System
(BIRADS), quality control
and
mammographic dose, recommendations
of, 153
mammography equipment, specifications for, 135
National Mammography Accreditation
Program, and quality assurance compliance, 168
phantom, 823
baseline optimized by, 166
criteria for, 166
resolution and, 142
to establish optimized baseline, 166
quality control and
Committee on Quality Assurance in
Mammography, manuals of,
165
guidelines for procedures, 158
Standard for Diagnostic Mammography,
screening programs and, 470
American Joint Committee on Cancer
(AJCC)
classification of breast cancer, 108–109
prognostic factors, and criteria for, 112
staging
confirmation of diagnosis, microscopic required, 109
system of, 107
TNM definitions, 108–109
Angiosarcoma, 596, 598, 599
occurrence of, 26
Anodes, screen-film mammography and,
138–139
Apocrine carcinoma, 590–591
Apocrine metaplasia
and cyst formation, 537, 538
and relative risk for invasive breast cancer, 512
Apoptosis
arbitrariness of juries and, 799, 800

and breast cancer, 19
in development of, 32–33
telomeres, cell cycle and, 38
Arc method of triangulation, 722
Architectural distortion
adjunctive assessment of
rolling the breast for, 348
spot compression for, 348
after biopsy, mammographic instance
of, 449
benign causes of, 299, 384–385
biopsy and, 278–279, 384, 449
breast cancer and, 298–302
evaluation of
rolled views and, 299
spot compression and, 299
fat necrosis, benign, 384–385
hamartoma and, mammographic
instance of, 307
hematoma and, 290–291
mammographic instance of, 243, 276,
300, 301, 302
normal flow of structures and, 384
parenchymal edge, 301–302, 385–386
mammographic instance of, 385–387
parenchymal fat interface, mammographic instance of, 384
persistent after surgery, 450
as postsurgical change, 278–279,
379–380, 466
common change, 457–458
mammography efficacy and, 471
markers on skin scar, 451, 453
postsurgical scarring, 299, 304
benign, 384–385
mammographic instance of, 385
radial scars and, 299, 305, 385
reduction mammaplasty and, mammographic instance of, 450
sclerosing adenosis and, 25
spiculated, 301–302
mammographic instance of, 279
stable, invasive ductal carcinoma, mammographic instance of, 311
tumors indicated by, radiographically
dense breasts and, 242
Areola
anatomy of, 3, 14–15
calcifications in, 14–15
Artifacts
mammographic instance of, 369
misinterpretation of, 367
Asian women, age at menarche of, and
breast cancer risk among, 44
Aspiration of cysts
cytologic analysis after, 679, 680
for diagnosis and elimination, 283–284
mammographically guided, 677–680
Asymmetric breast tissue, 768, 769.
benign
characteristics of, 262

mammographic instance of, 263
biopsy, when needed, 312
breast development and, surgery
avoided for, 231
cancer, invasive, and 401–403
causes of, 401, 402
clinical breast examination and, 264,
403
biopsy and, 402
mammogram correlated with biopsy
need and, 312
dense
cancer associated with, 265
invasive ductal carcinoma, mammographic instance of, 265
vs. focal asymmetric density, 260, 262,
313, 315
mammographic instance of, 260, 261
distinguished from focal asymmetric
density, 387–388
magnification views and, 388
iatrogenically created, 265
mammographic instance of, 265
invasive, mammographic instance of,
314
location of, 264–265
lump, before puberty, 6
malignancy and, 312–313
mammographic instance of, 313
normal architecture preserved in, 383
normal variation, 401
origin of, 264–265
palpable
biopsy recommended for, 264, 313
risk and, 264
presenting as prominent ducts, mammographic instance of,
264
risk, unfounded implication of, 263–264
sample report for, 787
significant, mammographic instance of,
314
term defined, 260–261
ultrasound and, 417
Asymmetric ducts, 403
Asymmetric gynecomastia
bilateral nature of, 502
in contralateral breast, evident by mammography, 497
in male breast, 497
imaging of, 501
mammographic instance of, 498, 502
Asymmetric tissue density
assessment of, 221–222
increasing, mammographic instance of,
382
preliminary assessment of, 387
Asymmetric vasculature. *See* Vascular
asymmetry
Asymmetries
as developmental phenomenon, 7

focal
  further evaluation needed for, 256–257
  mammographic instance of, 256, 257–267
  mirror images and, 220
  palpable and mammographic, suspicion of, 383
Ataxia-telangiectasia gene, radiation risk and, 102
Atypical hyperplasia
  cancer risk and, 1
  ductal, 526
    risk associated with, 230
  ductal epithelial, intraductal carcinoma and, 22
  epithelial
    development of carcinoma in situ and, 117
    increased risk for breast cancer, 48
    risk factors, histologic, 18–19
  excisional biopsy warranted in, 226
  explanation for, 7
  as a field phenomenon, 123–124
  gynecomastia and, 497
  lobular, 526–527
    risk associated with, 230
  mammographically defined indications of, no, 230
  phenotypic changes and, visibility of, 41
  possible explanation for, 7
  risk for breast cancer, 30
  role in breast cancer, continuum theory and, 123
Atypical proliferative changes, as risk factor for breast cancer, 47
Augmentation mammaplasty, silicone implant and, 472. See also Implants, breast
Automatic exposure control (AEC)
  cleavage view and, 198–199
  failure to position under dense tissue, underexposed mammogram and, 150
  future of, 816
  in mammography
    breast thickness and, 150
    purpose of, 150
  Mammography Quality Standards Act, requirement of, 150–151
  quality assurance and, 157
  selection, 151
Axilla
  accessory breast tissue and, 4, 5, 231
  mediolateral oblique projection and, 176, 179
Axillary dissection
  conservation therapy and, 467
  radionuclide injections and, 12
Axillary lymph node(s). See also Lymph node(s)
  adenopathy and, 347

anatomy, cancer staging and, 109
assessment of
  positron emission tomography, 345
  surgical sampling, 345
breast cancer staging and, 12
calcified, gold deposits in, 347–348
  mammographic instance of, 347–348
cancer staging and, 107
enlarged
  causes of, 407–408
  mammographic instance of, 406–407
  tumor in, prognosis and, 406–407
evaluation of, 4–7
fat infiltration and, 407
imaging
  computed tomography, 345
  lymphoscintigraphy, 345
involvement
  diagnosis of intraductal carcinoma and, 122
  metastases and, 132
  number of involved, prognosis and, 108
  positive, adjuvant chemotherapy and, 108
  predictors of, 107
  prognosis and, 108, 112, 117
  systemic treatment and, 132
  tumor in
    prognostication and, 108
    therapeutic decisions and, 108
involvement in tumor, treatment selection and, 107
location, 333, 345
lymphatic drainage through, 345
lymphoma and, 347
mammographic instance of, 345, 346, 347
mammography and, 4–7
metastases, prognosis and, 132
negative, thresholds for intervention and, 218
negative for tumor involvement, treatment and, 107
nonmalignant causes of, 406–407
prognosis and, 131
size of, 345, 440–441
  of normal, 407
spread of tumor to, 808
  magnetic resonance imaging and, 345
  prognosis and, 345
Axillary node levels, location, 465
Axillary tail view, mammographic projection, 196, 197, 198

B

Bacterial infections, of breast, 568
BEIR V, radiation risk, calculations of, 102, 104
Benign breast disease, as risk factor for breast cancer, 47–48

Benign breast lesions, 516–569. See also Adenosis; Cysts; Duct ectasia; Duct network, and pathologic processes; Extralobular terminal ducts, benign lesions of; Fat necrosis and scarring; Galactoceles; Lipomas
  histologic types of, relative risks of, 48
  morphologically indistinguishable from cancers, 62
  nipple adenomas, 516
  secretory deposits, 523–524, 525
  unusual, 558–569
    from bacterial infections, 568
    diabetic mastopathy, 562–563
    extra-abdominal desmoid tumor, 563–565
    focal fibrosis, 561–562, 563
    granular cell tumors, 560–561
    hamartoma
      mammary (fibroadenolipoma), 558–560
      myoid, 567, 568
    from parasitic infections, 568–569
    pseudoangiomatous stromal hyperplasia, 563
    radial scars, 565–566
    superficial thrombophlebitis (Mondor's disease), 566–567
Benign dermal deposits, mammographic findings and, 207
Benign fibrosis, shadowing and, ultrasound instance of, 438
Benign hyperplasia
  axillary lymph node enlargement and, 407–408
  of epithelium of distal duct and lobular ductules, 513
Benign secretory calcifications, rod, shape of, 393
Biochemical markers, prognostic factors, TNM staging and, 112
Biopsy. See also Excision, surgical, after guide placement
  and abnormal mammogram, recall rates and, 81
  architectural distortion and, mammographic instance of, 449
  benign abnormality and, 81
  of benign lesions and, 56
    scarring after, 81, 456–457
  and breast buds, inadvertent removal of, 6–7
  cosmetic results after, 458–459
  costs associated with, 411
  diagnostic capability of, 211
  ductal carcinoma in situ, diagnostic for, 118
  false-negative, 375
  false-positive, 81, 375

Biopsy (contd.)
  guide placement for, 459
  and mammogram, effect on, 447
  margins of excised tissue and, 129
  morbidity with, 375, 411
  mortality with, 411
  and need for clinical breast examina-
      tion, correlated with mam-
      mogram and, 312
  needle, 637–720
    controversy over, 641–644
      early studies on core needle biopsy,
          642
      error rate, 643–644
    core. See Core needle biopsy
    false-negative, avoiding, 755
    fine-needle aspiration. See Fine-
        needle aspiration biopsy
    general considerations, 705–706
      with benign lesions, 705
      with malignant lesions, 705–706
        sentinel-node evaluation, 705
    imaging-guided, 645
      positioning of needles and guides
          for, 653–673
        accuracy and safety of, 646, 672
        anteroposterior approach,
            654–656
          caution with, 656
          circumareolar incision for,
              656
          freehand localization from
              front of breast, 654–655
          advantages of, 655
          disadvantages of, 655
          wire migration with, 656
        completing procedure, 673
        guides introduced parallel to
            chest wall, 657–673
          alignment of centering light,
              658, 659
          fenestrated compression plates
              for, 658, 663–664
          introduction from skin surface
              closest to lesion, 658, 660,
              661, 664–672
          breast positioning, 664
          embedding of needle tip in
              fibrous tissue, 672
          TARGET for, 665–666
        preparation of patient, 653–654
          anesthesia, 654
          support of the patient, 654
    indications for, 645–646
    positive predictive value of, 637–640
      early intervention, 640
      interval cancers and detection tar-
          gets, 640
      sensitivity, 640
  positive predictive value and, 81
  safety of, 375

  screening and, 56
  signs that warrant, 312
  surgical, 641
  suspicions prompting, 375
  suspicious lesion and, 226
  thresholds for intervention and, 90
  ultrasound and, 411
BIRADS. See American College of Radiol-
      ogy (ACR) Breast Imaging
      Reporting and Data System
Blastomycosis, of breast, 568
Blood clot, in breast cyst, 564, 548
Blue-domed cyst, 540
Blur
  breast compression and, 145
    focal spot and, 140–141
  heel effect and, 140
  in screen-film imaging, 135, 136–137
Bone, as metastatic site, cancer staging
      and, 109
Bone marrow transplantation, treatment,
      selection of based on stag-
      ing, 107
Brain, as metastatic site, cancer staging
      and, 109
BRCA1 gene
  age for screening of women with, 46
  breast cancer, heredity and, 2
  DNA abnormality, radiation risk and,
      102
  heritable genes, breast cancer and, 40
  inherited, 127
  predisposition to breast cancer and, 126
  risk of breast cancer and, 46, 47
  risk of ovarian cancer and, 47
BRCA2 gene
  breast cancer, heredity and, 2
  DNA abnormality, radiation risk and,
      102
  heritable genes, breast cancer and, 40
  inherited, 127
  predisposition to breast cancer and, 126
  risk of breast cancer and, 47
  risk of ovarian cancer and, 47
Breast anatomy
  Cooper's ligaments in, 13
  enervation and, 11
  epithelial elements, 13
  glandular elements, 13
  lymphatics, tumor spread and, 11
  stromal elements, 13
  supporting structures, 13–14
    fibrous tissues, 13
  vascular supply, 10–11
Breast augmentation. See Implants
Breast biopsy. See Biopsy
Breast bud(s)
  development of, 6
    asymmetric, 610
  removal of, 231
    inadvertent, 6–7

Breast Cancer Detection Demonstration
      Project (BCDDP), 749
  and mammography, detection ability
      demonstrated in, 72
  and minimal cancer, definition of, 133
  screening and, 101
    age for, 77
      lead time gained and, 93
    negative, false reassurance and, 90
  survival rate data, 86–87
  Surveillance, Epidemiology, and End
      Results (SEER) data and,
      mortality compared in, 72
Breast cancer screening. See Screening
Breast cancer(s). Ductal carcinoma in situ
      (DCIS); Lobular carci-
      noma; Lobular carcinoma
      in situ (LCIS); Multicentric
      breast cancer; Multifocal
      breast cancer
  advanced, skin thickening due to, 341
  age and, 130–131
    at diagnosis, 79–80
    at onset, 117
  assessment, systematic approach to,
      223–224
  apoptosis and, 19, 32–33
  axillary lymph nodes, breast cancer
      staging and, 107
  baseline risk of developing, 1
  benign lesions, morphologically indis-
      tinguishable from, 62
  characteristics of, as predictors of axil-
      lary nodal involvement, 107
  chromosomal damage, and ability to
      infiltrate and, 107
  circumscribed, 291–292
  clonal nature of, 40–41
  colloid subtypes, attenuation of, 383
  compared with cancer of cervix, 96
  compared with prostate cancer, 117
  compared with thyroid cancer, 117
  complexity of, 1
  contralateral axillary lymph nodes and,
      408
  death and, 1, 55
  definition of, 117
  detection of
    imaging quality and, 227
    incidence screening and, 91–92
    interpretation, 227
    mammography and, 55
    myths, 78–79
    psychological aspects of, 212
    rates, age and, 80–81
    requirements for, 227
    systematic approach to, 219–227
    women with implants and, 492, 494
  determining extent of tumor and, 469
  development of, 124
    alcohol and, 125

autopsy studies and, 124–125
as continuum, 117
continuum theory of, 124
DNA sequences involved in, 122
dual theory of, 124–125
as duality of growth, 117
epithelial transition to cancer, 117
hormones and, 43
initiation phase, 36
more than one, 470
    survival determined by worst
        lesion, 470
in parenchyma, 14
progression phase, 36
promotion phase, 36
schools of thought on, 117
variation of, 107
various courses of, 117–118
diagnosis of
    myths and, 78–79
    psychological aspects of, 212
differences in, due to age of women,
    86
DNA alterations and, 1
duct network and, 15
early detection and, 43
    survival and, 32
early stage, defined, 133
etiologies, 1, 52
extensive intraductal component and,
    255
    adjuvant radiation therapy and, 255
fat and, 262, 383
genetics and, 34–36
growth
    patterns of, 64
        periodic screening and, 64–65
    rate
        doubling time, 129
        prognosis and, 85–86, 131
    screening and, 93
    unlikely within 1 year of surgery, 304
    variation of, 107
heredity, genetic components of, 2
histologic grade
    prognosis and, 117, 131
    Surveillance, Epidemiology, and End
        Results (SEER) study,
        131–132
history of, as risk factor for breast can-
    cer, 47
hormone receptors and, prognosis and,
    131
hormones, factor in development of,
    32
host responses to, varying, 133
hypoechoic quality of, 409, 439
identification, systematic approach to,
    219
implants. See also Implants, breast
    no increased risk with, 483

reduced risk with, 483
in situ, significance of, 117. See also
        Ductal carcinoma in situ
        (DCIS)
inherited susceptibility to, 127
initiation, 133
    during breast development, 104
invasive capability of, reasons for, 42
invasive
    as only true cancer, 117
    with in situ carcinoma, 23–24
    model, 42
investigation of
    size implications for, 440–441
Klinefelter's syndrome
    increased incidence with, 498
large, primary chemotherapy and, 471
lead time, survival and, 32
lesions that mimic, 378–380
lethal potential, effect on treatment, 117
level of incurability of, 63
local tumor control
    radiation with, 464
    surgical treatment, 464
location of
    along milk line, 269
    epithelial elements, 272
    mammographic blinds spots and,
        271–272
    most common, 269, 271
    parenchymal cone periphery, 240, 271
        mammographic instance of, 240
    parenchymal periphery, 301–302
in male breast, 497, 506–509
    age of patient with, 498
    appearance of, 506
    distinguishing from gynecomastia,
        506
    gynecomastia, no increased risk with,
        498
    histologically indistinguishable from
        female breast cancers, 501
    infiltrating ductal tumors, 500–501
    ionizing radiation exposure and, 498
    location of, 506
    mammographic instance of, 507,
        508
    mammography and, 506
    palpable, 500
    prognosis for, 497, 498, 500
    ultrasound instance of, 507
    uncommon, 497, 498
    xerographic instance of, 499, 505,
        506, 509
malignant, epithelial origin of most, 17
mammographic detection
    growth rate and, 129–130
    lead times for, 85
    prognosis of, 95
mammographic projections, similar on
        both, 453–454

management, systematic approach to,
    219, 224–227
margins of
    ill-defined, 295
        on ultrasound, 439
margins of excised tissue and, 128, 129
metastasis, 133
    cellular requirements for, 42
    changes necessary for, 130
    lethal, 42
    lymph nodes and, 12
    model, 42
    potential
        lymph node involvement and, 11
    potential for, 12
    requirements for, 127
    sites of, 127–128
    staging and, 107
metastatic to breast, characteristics of,
        432, 434
model of, 42
morphologic characteristics of, 375
    densities, similar to benign lesions,
        375
    margins, similar to benign lesions,
        375
    shapes, similar to benign lesions, 375
mortality, 130
    aging and, 55
    lifetime risk from mammographic
        radiation, 104, 105
mortality reduction and, 85
    age at diagnosis and, 51, 52
multiplicity of findings, usual indica-
        tion of benign processes,
        311
mutation, ability to infiltrate and, 107
natural history, 1, 123, 133
    calcifications showing, xerographic
        instance of, 398–399
    continuum theory of, 123
    epithelial lining of duct and, 123
    interruption of, 43, 63–64, 91, 117
        early detection and, 77
    interruption of possible, 76
    long, 85
    neglected, skin thickening due to, 341
    neovascularity of, prognosis and, 133
    old film review, mammographic
        instance of, 252–254
origin of. See Precursor lesions
palpability of, 107
postmenopausal form of, 31–32
pre-pubertal females and, 7
pregnancy
    diagnosed during, 446
    risk reduced with, 446
premenopausal form of, 31–32
presence in lymphatics, prognostic sig-
        nificance of, 12
presentation, in augmented breast, 494

Breast cancer(s) (*contd.*)
  presenting as asymmetry, mammo-
      graphic instance of, 258
  prevention
    as goal for, 52
    at early age, exposure to carcinogens
        and, 8
    in older women and, 8
    Tamoxifen and, 52
  prognosis
    axillary lymph node involvement and,
        117
    factors, 130–131
      TNM staging and, 112–114
    histology of tumor and, 131
    size of lesion and, 32, 63–64, 117
    stage of lesion and, 32
  progression, 133
  proliferation, model, 42
  promotion, 133
  recurrence
    after conservation therapy, 467–470
    detection of, 471
    mammography efficacy and, 471
    mechanism of, 15
    microcalcifications and, 471
    new mass and, 471
    new microcalcifications and, 471
    signs of, 471
  residual, adjuvant radiation therapy and,
      15
  risk factors, 52
    of new, from radiation therapy, 471
    screening and, 98
    tissue density and, 239–240
  screening
    defined, 56
    frequency, 91–93
    lead time gained by, 91–93
    size of primary cancer, 55–56
  second lesion, morphology of, different
      from first lesion, 470–471
  site of origin of, 1
  size of, 81–82
    at diagnosis, mortality reduction and,
        229
    Breast Cancer Detection Demonstra-
        tion Project (BCDDP)
        study, 131
    importance of, 129–130
    prognosis and, 112, 117, 131–132,
        133
      primary cancer, 55–56
    staging schemes and, 131
  skin thickening and, 341
  spiculations pathognomonic of, 302
  spread of, lymphatic system as route
      for, 11
  stages, 133
    at diagnosis, mortality reduction and,
        229

  cell proliferation, 42
  initiation, 41–42
  progression, 41
  promotion, 41
    treatment decisions based on, 107
  staging, 107. *See* Cancer staging
  survival, and age at diagnosis, 51, 84,
      130–131
  susceptibility, influences on, 39
  systemic treatment. *See also*
      Chemotherapy
    evolving use of, 464
    hormonal manipulation, with Tamox-
        ifen, 464
    surgical, 131
    survival advantage of, 464
  treatments for
    local tumor control of, 464
    primary concerns of, 464
    systemic treatment, 464
  triangulation. *See* Triangulation
  types of, 31–32, 279
  ultrasound and, 412–413, 439–440. *See
      also* Ultrasound
    ultrasound instance of, 413
  variations of, 118
  verification, systematic approach to,
      219, 222–223
  viral etiologies suggested, 45
  x-ray attenuation of, 307–308
    mammographic instance of, 307, 308
Breast compression. *See also* Compression
  advantages of, 145
  chest wall and, 177, 178
  discomfort from, 145–146
  fear of damage unwarranted, 145
  goals of, 174–175
  importance of, 145–146
  mammographic image quality and, 171
  mammographic screening, noncompli-
      ance and, 145
  pain and, 175
  pounds per square inch, 145–146
  pressure applied, 175
  proper, 175
  reasons for, 145–146
  scatter radiation, effect on, 148
  system, detector separated from, 147
  traction system and, 147
  with implants, 485
Breast conservation. *See* Conservation
      therapy
Breast development
  asymmetric, 231–232
    normal, 312
    surgery avoided for, 231
  asymmetry resolved in ultimate, 7
  damage from carcinogens during, 49–50
  involution and, 386–387
  lobular development and, 8
  phases of, 386

  pregnancy and, 446
  radiation carcinogenesis and, 49
  radiation exposure, age of sensitivity to, 8
  radiation risk, puberty and, 104
  reversal, age of, 386
  stem cells and, 37
  symmetry of normal, 231
  terminal buds and, 49
Breast elevation, craniocaudal projection
      and, 184–185
Breast imaging. *See also* Computed
      tomography; Magnetic res-
      onance imaging; Mammo-
      grams; Mammography
  after explantation, 492
  after irradiation, mammographic
      instance of, 466
  after mastectomy
    computed tomography and, 484
    magnetic resonance imaging and, 484
  assessment
    Breast Imaging Reporting and Data
        System (BIRADS) and, 222
    computerized reporting system and, 222
  detection and diagnosis, organized
      approach to, 212
  detection defined, 211
  diagnosis defined, 211
  lactation, ultrasound and, 446
  magnetic resonance imaging
  of male breast, reasons for, 497
  menstrual cycle, influence on, 19
  mirror images
    architecture and, 221–222
    density distribution and, 221–222
    subareolar regions, 221
  quality of images and, 219
  radiology, 1
  results, communication of, 227
  screening defined, 211
  systematic approach to, 219
    principles of, 211
  two-view examination for, 219
  with implants, 485. *See also* Implants,
      breast
Breast Imaging Reporting and Data Sys-
      tem (BIRADS). *See* Ameri-
      can College of Radiology
      (ACR) Breast Imaging
      Reporting and Data System
Breast involution. *See* Involution, of breast
Breast irradiation, purpose of, 465
Breast lesion evaluation, defined, 222
Breast pain, 11
Breast parenchyma, chest wall imaging
      and, 146
Breast patterns, American College of
      Radiology (ACR) Breast
      Imaging Reporting and
      Data System (BIRADS),
      description of, 245

Breast self-examination
  among Chinese women, 96
  biopsy and, 82
  efficacy of, 77
  randomized controlled trials, none
      shown to reduce mortality,
      91
Breast size, cancer risk unrelated to, 7
Breast stem cell, evidence for, 124
Breast tissue patterns
  age and, 51
  mammographic instance of, American
      College of Radiology
      (ACR) patterns, 239
  mammographically determined, risk
      indicators, 50
Breast tissue(s)
  abnormal, 230
  acoustic properties of, 421–422
    ultrasound instance of, 422
  after irradiation
    clinically soft, 466
    radiographically dense, 466
  age and, variation with, 232–236
  aging and, 20–21
  anterior
    imaging, positioning and, 171
    tilting compression paddles and, 181
  architectural distortion and, 298–299
  asymmetric. See Asymmetric breast tissue
  changes to, 305
  connective tissue, breast development
      and, 7
  deep, imaging, positioning and, 171
  dense
    cancer risk and, 232
    limitations on contrast between vari-
      ous tissues and, 144
    mammogram of, properly exposed,
      150
    risk for cancer and, 238, 239–240
    tungsten anodes and, 144
  dense patterns, mammograms and, 230
  density of
    age and, 80
    assessment of symmetry of, 221–222
    changes to, 233–237
    during lactation, 20, 446
    hormone replacement therapy and,
      240–242, 387
      mammographic instance of, 241
    increase in, 402
      reasons for, 240–242
      weight changes and, 240
    increasing over time, 386, 387
    mammographic instance of, 235, 236
    pregnancy and, 235
    radiographic, 237
    weight loss and, 387
  density increased from radiation, mam-
      mography efficacy and, 471

diffuse density, parenchymal patterns
    and, 239
distribution of high attenuation, auto-
    matic exposure control,
    reduced accuracy in mam-
    mograms with, 150
dramatic changes to, weight change
    and, 237
    mammographic instance of, 236,
      237, 238
elasticity of, compression and, 186
fat
  carcinoma visible in, mammographic
      instance of, 243
  content, increase in, 237–238
  parenchymal pattern and, 238
fatty patterns of, 233–234
  mammographic instance of, 235, 236,
    237
fibrous structures, attenuation of, 243
fibrous tissues, 13
firmness of, radiographic density not
    related to, 237
interlobular, 13
involution, aging and, 19–20
lactation and, 20
  changes to, 446
location of, 173
mammography of, not projected onto
    detector, 195
medial, craniocaudal projection and,
    185
medial tissues, mammographic imaging,
    cleavage view, 198–199
muscles and, 8
neodensity in, 305
nodular densities in, parenchymal pat-
    tern and, 238
normal, echo texture of, 422
normally symmetric flow of, 298–299
on mammogram
  asymmetric distribution of, further
      evaluation needed, 256–257
  symmetric distribution of, 256–257
patterns, 238–239
  age and, 80
  Breast Imaging Reporting and Data
      System (BIRADS), seen on
      ultrasound, 423–424
pectoralis major muscle and, pendent
    positioning in CT scan,
    174
pregnancy and, 19–20
reduction mammaplasty, appearance
    after, mammographic
    instance of, 461–463
spread apart, during compression, 145
stability of, 305
stromal, 13
stromal fibrosis, parenchymal patterns
    and, 239

subareolar, tilting compression paddles
    and, 181
subcutaneous adipose tissues, breast
    development and, 7
types, on ultrasound, 423
upper, lumpogram for, 201
weight change and, dramatic changes
    to, 237
Breast(s)
  anatomy of, 1, 3–4, 4, 8–10, 8–12
  architecture, asymmetric differences,
      assessment of, 221
  as dynamic organ, 19
  asymmetric, 231–232
    mammographic instance of, 231
    psychological difficulties with,
      231–232
    reason for, 231–232
  composition of, variable, 232
  development of, 1, 4
    cell proliferation during, 43
  ductal elements of, location, 172
  fatty tissue, cancer detection in,
      244–245
    mammographic instance of, 243
  glandular elements of, location, 172
  histology of, 3
  immature
    carcinogen and, 8
    stem cells vulnerable in, 8
  large, imaging as a mosaic and, 181,
      182
  lobule, 4
  mammographic appearance, 251
  mammographic changes on, 1–2
    menstrual cycle and, 1–2
  margins of, mammographic positioning
      and, 177
  maturation of, 8
  normal, 1–2
    aging and, 229
    cyclic hormonal fluctuations and, 18
    histologic information concerning,
      229
    involution of, age and, 18
    lack of definition of, 21
    variation in, 229
    wide range of, 18
  pathology of, 3
  radiographically dense, tumors borders
      invisible in, 242
  size, cancer risk and, 7, 232
  skin of, anatomy of, 3
  stability of, 376
  symmetry of, 221–222

C

Calcifications. See also Microcalcifica-
    tions
  in acini, adenosis and, 25
  adenosis and, 332

Calcifications *(contd.)*
  after breast biopsy
    benign results and, 460
    suture material and, 460
  after radiation therapy
    analysis of, 467
    benign, 467
  associated with cancer
    removal of suggested, 470
    types of, 391
  and associated findings, 780–782
    architectural distortion, 782
    axillary adenopathy, 782
    nipple retraction, 780, 781
    skin lesion, 782
    skin retraction, 780, 781
    skin thickening, 780, 781
    trabecular thickening, 781
  associated with implant capsule, 494
  in axillary nodes
    fine irregular, metastasis suspected
        with, 347–348
    large
        mammographic instance of, 348
        no significance to, 347
  benign, reabsorption of, 397
  benign and malignant, mammographic
        instance of, 396
  benign processes
    association and, 324–332
    mammographic instance of, 396, 397
    requiring no intervention, 351–370
  Breast Imaging Reporting and Data
        System (BIRADS) lexicon
        for, 764
  branching, 334
  cancer-associated, 323
    excision of, 468–469
    location of, intraductal portion of the
        cancer, 322
    postoperative mammography and,
        469
  casting, tissue necrosis within cancer
        and, 323
  categorization of, 322–323
  central lucent zones in, benign process,
        395–396
    mammographic instance of, 396
  classification of, 771–782
    coarse or popcorn-like, 774
    dystrophic, 776
    fine or branching (casting), 776, 778
    grouped or clustered, 778
    indistinct or amorphous, 776, 777
    large rod-like, 774
    linear, 778
    milk of calcium, 775
    multiple groups, 779, 781
    pleomorphic or heterogeneous, 776,
        777
    punctate, 776

  regional, 779, 781
  rim or eggshell, 774, 775
  round, 774
  scattered or diffuse, 779, 781
  segmental, 778
  skin, 773
  spherical or lucent-centered, 774, 775
  suture, 775–776
  typically benign, 773
  vascular, 773
clustered, 334–335
  mammographic instance of, 372
  number of, significance of, 388
  significance of, 318–319, 388–390
clusters, new, probability of malignancy
    with, 377
coarse deposits, involuting fibroadeno-
    mas and, 325
comedo, 551
and cysts, 541, 544, 545
determining risk of malignancy,
    321–322
and diffuse breast cancer, 551
diffusely scattered, 334, 335, 337
  benign nature of, 366–367
  bilateral, benign process and, 391
  etiology unclear, 367
  mammographic instance of, 367, 392
  shape of, 367
distribution of, 317–318, 391
  significance of, 393
ductal carcinoma in situ and, 118,
    119–120
  indications of, 122
  mammographic instance of, 400
dystrophic, benign process, 329–332
evaluation of, 393–394
  mammographic views for, 199–200
extensive, caution exercised with, 365
extensive intraductal component and,
    317
extent of cancer and, 393
in fibroadenoma, diagnostic, 282
final assessment categories for,
    782–784
  "benign finding"—negative, 782
  highly suggestive of malignancy, 783
  need additional imaging evaluation,
    782
  negative, 782
  probably benign, 782
  suspicious abnormality, 7834
follow-up of, 338
granular, term for pleomorphic, 332
heterogeneous, significance of, 332–333
and implants
  computed tomographic instance of,
    487
  mammographic instance of, 487
and involuting fibroadenomas, charac-
    teristics of, 358–359

irregular linear, segmental distribution,
        mammographic instance of,
        381
line linear, 334
lobular carcinoma in situ associated
        with, 230–231
location of, major determination, 319
lost in noise, 149
lucent-centered, mammographic
        instance of, 452
lucent-centered skin, evaluating
    magnification mammography using,
        324
    tangential views using, 324
magnification mammography for ana-
        lyzing, 741, 742–743
morphology clearer with, 255
in male breast, mammographic instance
        of, 499
malignant
    morphologic characteristics associ-
        ated with, 393
    shapes of, 393–394
mammographic instance of, 318–338,
        348
mammographic interpretation and, 251
masses associated with, 315–316
milk of calcium, 328
morphology of, 317–319, 322–323
    benign, 319
    breast cancer and, 332
    judged by worst, 321
multiple groups of, 337–338
no associated mass, analysis of,
        317–319
number of, 321–32
    and pattern, risk of malignancy,
        321–322
    threshold, 321–322
of nipple, Paget's disease and, 320
patterns of
    breast cancer associated with,
        389–390
    malignancy and, 381
    of deposits, 321–322, 323
    of distribution, 334
        American College of Radiology
            (ACR) Breast Imaging
            Reporting and Data System
            (BIRADS) definition of,
            334
peripheral, benign masses and,
        359–360
pleomorphic, significance of, 332–333
postsurgical and irradiation, mammo-
        graphic instance of, 467
punctate, fibrous stroma and, 332
and radiation therapy and, 397
radiopaque, composition of, 390
recurrent cancer and, mammographic
        instance of, 469

regional, 334, 335, 337
residual
   radiation therapy after surgery, 255
   significance of, 255
rim calcifications, cyst wall and, 326,
   328
risk of malignancy, determining,
   321–322
rod-shaped
   plasma cell mastitis term, 365
   secretory disease and, 325
round
   acinar, 325–326
   regular
      mammographic instance of, 400
      significance of, 400
secretory, pattern produced by, 337
secretory disease and, 365
segmentally distributed, 334, 335–336
   ductal, mammographic instance of,
      394, 395
shape of, 391
   biopsy required due to, 318
   significance of, 393
silicone injection and, 471
size of, 321, 391
of skin, 723, 741, 742–745, 773
   benign nature of, 365
   etiology of, 365–366
   localization of with mammography,
      679–681, 682
   typical appearance of, 320–321
spherical lucent-centered, result of
      benign processes, associa-
      tion with breast cancer,
      326–327
stability of, 397
   for indeterminate or suspicious mor-
      phology, 338
   with benign processes, 338
suspicious, 393
and suture material, mammographic
      instance of, 368
sutures and, 329, 330, 367
types of, 317
   in lesions, mammographic instance
      of, 395
ultrasound, usually not seen on, 425
vascular
   distinctive appearance of, 362
   magnification mammography and,
      324, 362
   mammographic instance of, 318, 363
visibility of
   magnification mammography and,
      319
   x-ray mammography requirements
      for, 139
without masses, benign, 360–367
   lucent-centered, 360–361
   morphologies characteristic, 360–361

Calcified fibroadenoma, mammographic
      demonstration and evalua-
      tion of, 215
Calcium deposits
   causes of, 391
   composition of, 317
   mammography, not visible by, 390
   in skin, mammographic findings and,
      207
Cancer detection, lead-time bias and, 65
Cancer foci. *See* Multicentric breast
      cancer; Multifocal breast
      cancer
Cancer formation, epithelial cells and, 16
Cancer growth, screening intervals and, 58
   sojourn time and, 58–59
Cancer initiation and progression, natural
      history and, 123
Cancer promotion
   natural history and, 123
   stromal-epithelial interactions and, 17
Cancer staging, 107, 808
   axillary node involvement and, 12, 108
   basis of, 108
   at clinical level, 108
   data form for, 115–116
   distant site involvement and, 108
   future of, 108
   MRI and, 631
   pathologic staging, 108
   size of tumor and, 108
   thresholds for intervention and,
      218–219
   and tumor involvement, levels of, 107
Cancer(s). *See* Breast cancer(s)
Capsular contracture
   implants and, 474
   problems caused by, 475
   reducing likelihood of, 475
   time of occurrence, 475
Carcinogenesis
   age and, 49
   radiation and, 49
Carcinogens
   as initiators of cancer, 36
   DNA damage and, 39
   effective during breast development,
      104
   environmental, increased exposure to,
      breast cancer risk and, 34
   exposure to
      age at, 124
      stem cell, cancer development and, 8
Carcinoma in situ, gynecomastia and, 497
Carcinomas, breast
   multiple simultaneous ipsilateral pri-
      mary, TNM classification
      criteria, 110
   simultaneous bilateral, staging of, 110
Cartesian, straight-line method of triangu-
      lation, 722–723

Casting, calcifications with cancer and,
      323
Caudocranial projection
   gantry rotation for, 201
   use of, 201
CC projection. *See* Craniocaudal projec-
      tion
Cell growth. *See also* Stem cells
   breast cancer development and, 43
   carcinogenesis component of, 42
   chromosomal DNA and, 36
   DNA damage and, 37–38
   growth factors, protein category, 36
   proto-oncogenes and, 38–39
   stages of, 37–38
Cell pleomorphism, histologic grading
      systems and, 131
Cell ploidy
   abnormal cells and, 38
   normal cells, 38
Cells in S phase, flow cytometry to mea-
      sure percent of, 132
Cellular tumors, on ultrasound, 425
Cervical screening, acceptance of, 97
Chemotherapy, 131, 464. *See also* Primary
      chemotherapy
   adjuvant
      axillary lymph node involvement and,
         108
      selection of based on staging, 107,
         108
   determinant for use, menopause and,
      79–80
   primary
      hormone-receptor negative tumors,
         response of, 471
      large breast cancers and, 471
      tumor reduction and, mammographic
         instance of, 471
      uses of, 471
   systemic treatment
      lymph node involvement and, 132
      use of evolving, 464
Chest wall
   anatomy of, 110
   imaging
      breast parenchyma not necessarily
         imaged with, 146
      focal spot and, 139–140
      heel effect and, 139–140
      mammography for, after mastectomy,
         465
   ultrasound and, 409
Chinese women, breast self-examination
      among, 96
Choriocarcinoma, gynecomastia and, 497
Chromosomal abnormalities, risk for can-
      cer and, 29
Chromosome 17, tumor suppressor genes
      and, 47
   breast cancer and, 127

Chromosomes, damage to, cancer initiation and, 42
Circumscribed margins
   defined, 275, 277
   mammographic instance of, 277
Circumscribed masses, halo sign surrounding, 279
Classification rules, staging and
   clinical, 109
   pathologic, 109–110
Cleavage view
   automatic exposure control and, 199
   mammographic projection, 198–199
   medial breast tissues and, 198–199
   positioning for, technologist and, 198–199
Clemmesen's hook, breast cancer incidence and, 32
Cleopatra view. See Axillary tail view
Clinical breast examination (CBE), 747–749. See also Physical examination
   asymmetric breast tissue, palpable, significance of, 264
   benefit from, National Breast Screening Study of Canada (NBSS) and, 91
   biopsy and, 82, 96
   breast compression and, 145
   cancers detected by, 61
   compared with mammography
      Health Insurance Plan (HIP) of New York trial, 71–72
      screening trials and, 75–76
   correlative, 749
   correlated with mammogram, biopsy, signs for, 312
   false-positive mammography and, 96
   focused, mammographic positioning and, 193, 195
   lesions, fat-containing lucent, 355
   mammography and, 77
      referrals and, 192
   oil cyst presentation of, 355
   pressure applied during, 175
   and radiologists, not required to perform, 192
   randomized controlled trials and, 91
   screening
      importance of, 60
      mammography and, 98
   systematic performance of, 192
   tissue characteristics evaluated, 77, 403
   who should perform, 747, 749
Clinical staging, elements of, 109
   imaging, 109
   pathologic examination of tissue, 109
   physical examination, 109
Clinically detected abnormality
   and mammography, screening remainder of breast(s) using, 215

resolution by clinical evaluation, 215
Clock face method of location, Breast Imaging Reporting and Data System (BIRADS) and, 274
Collagen
   in breast, age and, 21
   focal fibrosis and, 287, 289
Collagen, imaging of, 513
College of American Pathologists (CAP), prognostic factors and, 112
Colloid carcinoma, 587, 588
   margins of, 279
Comedo calcifications, 551
Comedocarcinoma, poorly differentiated (high-grade), 572–575. See also Ductal carcinoma in situ (DCIS)
   mammographic appearance of, 575
   ultrasound appearance of, 575
   vs. well-differentiated ductal carcinoma in situ, 575–576
Comedo-necrosis
   calcification pattern associated with, 381
   calcifications due to, 323
Committee on the Biological Effects of Ionizing Radiation, radiation risk
   model developed by, 103
   varies with age at exposure, 103
Complex sclerosing lesions, radial scars, 26
Compression paddles
   craniocaudal projection and, 185–186, 272
   disadvantages of, 147
   mediolateral oblique projection and, 179
   screen-film mammography and, 147
   tilting, axillary tissue thickness and, 181
   use of, 147
Compression plates, fenestrated, for introducing guides parallel to chest wall, 657
Compression. See Breast compression
Compton scattering, x-ray image and, 148
Computed tomography
   cost-effective approach to, 212
   future role in breast imaging, 832–833
   imaging cancers with
      intravenous contrast agents and, 414
      neovascularity and, 414
   implants and
      detecting rupture in, 492
      evaluation and, 486
   lesion location and, 223
   needle biopsy and, 447
   for triangulation, 739

Computed tomography–guided needle localization, 700–703
Coned-down spot compression. See Spot compression
Congestive heart failure, skin thickening and, 341
Connective tissues, breast development and, 7
Connective-tissue disorders, silicone implants and, 473
Conservation therapy
   axillary dissection and, 467
   completeness of primary excision, recurrence rate and, 468
   defined, 467
   excision and radiation, advanced cancers treated with, 128
   follow-up, extensive intraductal component and, 470
   gross malignancy elimination for, 464
   indications for, 464
   lumpectomy, clear margins and, 467
   magnification mammography and, 254–255
   radiation therapy and, 464
      compared with mastectomy, 465–466
   recurrent cancer after, 469–470
   surgical incisions for, 468
Contralateral cancer risk, radiation therapy and, 471
Contrast
   in screen-film imaging, 135–136
   resolution, human eye and, 142
Contrast subtraction angiography of the breast, 830, 831
Contusion. See also Trauma
   distinguished from hematoma, 289–290, 296, 298
   mammographic instance of, 288
Cooper's ligaments, 3
   anatomy of, 342
   architectural distortion and, 298–299
   breast anatomy and, 3, 13
   normal margins to parenchyma and, 302
   parenchymal edge distortion and, 385–386
   role in breast, 342
   shadowing and, 438
   shadows from, ultrasound instance of, 438
   skin and, 339
   skin changes and, 340, 405
   ultrasound and, 413, 423, 425
   ultrasound instance of, 425
Core needle biopsy, 644, 707–709. See also Needle biopsy
   accuracy in diagnosis, 448
   as adjunctive technique, 217
   advantages of, 708
   cost-effective approach to, 212

disadvantages of, 708
hematomas and, 449
of indeterminate lesion, 226
Mammotome for, 709
Mueller tray for, 708, 709
radial scar, insufficient for, 299
removing sample from notch, 708
spring-driven systems, 707–708
stereotactic guidance for, 710–716
  contraindications, 716
  sources of error, 716
ultrasound-guided, 716–718
  advantages of, 717–718
  disadvantages of, 718
  vs. ultrasound-guided fine-needle
    aspiration biopsy, 718
use of, 2
Craniocaudal projection
breast elevation for, technologist and,
    184–185
ideal positioning for, 184–186
inframammary fold, elevation of, 184
lesions seen only on, 735, 736–737
maximizing tissue imaged on,
    187–189
medial tissues and, 185–187
missed lesions in, 272
nipple axis and, 184
opposite breast, positioned symmetri-
    cally, 187
second mammographic view, 184
standard view, 184
Cribriform cancers, ductal carcinoma in
    situ and, 120, 121
Cyst(s), 515, 537–546
and apocrine metaplasia, 537, 538
blue-domed, 540
and cancer, 538, 540
fluid of, 540
  characteristics of 286–287
halo around, due to Mach effect, 541,
    542
mammographic appearance of, 541
and menopause, 540
and relative risk for invasive breast can-
    cer, 512
role of duct obstruction in formation of,
    537–538
septated, 544, 546, 547
spontaneous resorption of, 541, 543
ultrasound appearance of, 544, 545,
    546
aspiration of, 283, 540, 544
  confirmation by, 359
  eliminated by, 281
  fluid produced by, 427–429
  mammographic guidance of, 421
  recurrence after, 540–541
  ultrasound guidance and, 421
benign, ultrasound instance of, 414
blood in, 546, 548

calcifications and, 541, 544, 545
  mammographic instance of, 360
calcified wall, mammographic instance
    of, 315
cancers abutting, 287
  ultrasound instance of, 419
cancers associated with, 285
  mammographic instance of, 285
characteristics of, 429
common, 282
consequence of, 18–19
debris suspended in fluid, imaging, 427
demonstration by ultrasound, aspiration
    and, 441
diagnosis of
  aspiration, 283
    therapeutic, 284
  ultrasound and, 247, 283–284
    criteria for, 283–284
diffusely scattered calcifications and,
    367
family history of breast cancer and,
    18–19
formation, risk factor for breast cancer,
    48
hyperplasia and, 22
in lobule, benign, 24
in male breast, 502
  mammographic instance of, 498
location of, lobules, 273–274
mammographic instance of, 282–287,
    293, 295
management of, 283, 348
margins of, 295–296
multiplicity of, 311
no internal echoes in, 427
obscured margins and, 294–295
pericystic fibrosis and, ultrasound
    instance of, 438
peripheral calcifications and, 359
pneumocystography for, 699
reaspiration, no longer recommended,
    286
recurrent, 699
round mass, mammographic instance of,
    275
spontaneous resolution of, 286, 287
traumatic, x-ray attenuation of, 355
ultrasound appearance, 225
ultrasound assessment and, 224
ultrasound criteria for, 415
ultrasound demonstration of, manage-
    ment implications of, 348
ultrasound diagnosis and, 18, 281, 305
ultrasound instance of, 284, 285, 287,
    349, 420–421, 427–428
Cyst, aspiration of. See Aspiration of
    cysts
Cystic mastitis
normal breast physiology and, 18
poor term, 18

Cystosarcoma phylloides. See Phylloides
    tumors
Cytologic analysis
fine-needle aspiration and, 448

D
DCIS. See Ductal carcinoma in situ
    (DCIS)
Dense breasts. See also Breast tissue(s);
    Normal breast; Parenchy-
    mal pattern
cancer detection in, 243–244
dense tissue
  architectural distortions detected in,
    51
  microcalcifications detected in, 51
  radiographic density and, 237,
    242–243
  ultrasound used to image, 414
Dense fibroglandular tissue, cancer hidden
    in, mammographic instance
    of, 378
Densitometry, halo effect and, 280
Dermis, breast anatomy and, 13–14
Desmoid tumor, extra-abdominal, 563–565
Desmoplasia, spiculations, cancers with-
    out, 382
Detection
distinguished from diagnosis, 229
mammography as technique for, 211
Diabetes, arterial calcifications and, 362
Diabetic mastopathy, 562–563
Diagnosis
distinguished from detection, 229
techniques of, 247
ultrasound and, 247
Diagnostic mammography, as poor term,
    214, 222
Diagnostic tests, ultrasound, uses of,
    211
Diet, risk for breast cancer and, 33, 44
alcohol consumption, 50
Diffuse adenosis
as a field phenomenon, 124
explanation for, 7
possible explanation for, 7
Diffuse breast cancer, 551
Digital angiography, imaging cancers with
    intravenous contrast agents and, 414
  neovascularity and, 414
Digital mammography. See also Mam-
    mography, digital
clustered calcifications and, 390
compression, less firm necessary, 145
digital detectors
  ACR phantom and, 142
  screen thickness and, 153–154
input requirements for, 135
principles of, 135
reciprocity law failure, not relevant to,
    143

Digital mammography (contd.)
  systems
    future requirements of, 155
      phantom and, 142
      spatial resolution and, 142
    with contrast enhancement, uses of, 53
    with dual energy subtraction, uses of, 53
Digitization of film, 821
Dissecting the lesion, 722
DNA
  alterations
    altered genotype, cells with, 36
    breast cancer development, patterns of, 40
    breast stem cell and, 124
    cancer initiation and, 123
    chromosomal, mechanism for breast cancer development, 44
    hereditary breast cancer and, 46–47
    malignant transformation and, 36
    tumor aggression and, 128
  content, in cancer cells, flow cytometry to measure, 132
  damage
    aging and, 31
      increasing incidence of breast cancer and, 34–35
    breast cancer, ovulatory cycle and, 32–33
    cell cycle and, 33, 37–38
    environmental carcinogens, breast cancer and, 34–35
    spontaneous mutation, breast cancer and, 34–35, 35–36
  protein synthesis and, 35
  repair, BRCA1 and BRCA2 genes and, 126
  replication, cancer development, terminal ducts and, 7
Doppler ultrasound
  indeterminate lesions, confirmation needed for, 414
  rationale for, 413–414
Double reading
  mammogram interpretation, accuracy and, 212, 213–214
  mammography, high-quality and, 247
  as standard of care issue, 798
Dual-energy subtraction studies, clustered calcifications and, 390
Duct ectasia, 513, 521–523
  as cause of plasma cell mastitis, 522
  diagnosis of, 429
  nonspecific, 21
  and relative risk for invasive breast cancer, 512
  ultrasound instance of, 429
Duct(s)
  anatomy of, 15

appearance of, contrast enhancement and, 232, 233
breast cancer
  confined to single, 15
  metastasizing within, 15
connective tissue elements and, 13
network, pathologic processes of, 513–516. See also Benign breast lesions
Ductal carcinoma, distinctive, 581, 583–591
  apocrine, 590–591
  colloid or mucinous, 587, 588
  inflammatory, 590, 591, 592
  medullary, 588–590
  Paget's disease, 583–584, 585
  papillary, 586–587
  tubular cancer, 584, 586
Ductal carcinoma in situ (DCIS), 125, 514, 570–572. See also Comedocarcinoma, poorly differentiated (high-grade); Intraductal carcinoma in situ; Invasive ductal carcinoma NOS
  architectural features in, 393
  as earliest manifestation of breast cancer, 118
  calcifications and, 118, 119–120
    mammographic instance of, 392, 394, 395
    screening and, 122
  categories of, 118
  classification system, Lagios, 120–121
  comedo-necrosis, calcifications with, 391
  cytologic differentiation
    intermediate, 391, 393
    pleomorphic cells and, 391
    poorly differentiated, 391, 393
    well differentiated, 391, 393
  detection by mammography demonstrated, 72
  ducts, confined to, 118
  extent of, difficulties of determining, 128
  forms of, 22
  histologic grading, 121
    systems, 118, 120–121
    uses for, 122
  histologic review, 121
  histopathology of, 393
  in male breast, 506
  and calcifications, 572, 585
  characteristics of, 570
  earliest stage of, 570
  high-grade, 574
  histologic types of, 570–571
  incidence of, 29, 571
  invasions overlooked in, 122
  and invasive breast cancer, 1, 125
    development of, 571

related to, 118
risk of, compared with LCIS risk, 26
lesion excision, sufficiency of, 118
long-term follow-up, importance of, 121–122
mammographic appearance, 119–120
mammographic instance of, 294
management of, grading systems used in, 121
margins of excised tissue and, 129
minimal breast cancer, size of, 133
mortality from, 117
on MRI, 630–631
natural history, interruption of, 122
necrosis in, 393
nuclear morphology, prognostic indicator, 391
patterns of, 23
prognosis of, 571
recurrence, prediction of, 120–121
residual cancer, after tumor excision, 464
role in breast cancer, continuum theory and, 123
significance of, 23, 128
  age at development of, 125
subclassification of, 118, 391
treatment studies (National Surgical Adjuvant Breast Project), 572
Van Nuys Prognostic Index for, 570
well-differentiated (macropapillary and cribriform lesions), 575–576
Ductal epithelium
  aging, atrophy and, 20
  breast anatomy and, 14
  breast cancer and, development of, 107
  cancer of. See Ductal carcinoma in situ (DCIS)
  invasive cancer, development of, 40–41
  invasive ductal carcinoma and, 23–24
  male breast and, 497
Ductal hyperplasia. See Extralobular terminal ducts, benign lesions of, hyperplasia
Ductography, to evaluate nipple discharge, 520
Ducts(s)
  anatomy of, 15–16
  asymmetric, 403
  breast cancer origin and, 1
  cancer in situ in, reasons for, 42
  contrast material injected into, 14
  cross section of, 16
  development of, 6
    DNA alteration of stem cell, breast cancer and, 7
  DNA alteration and
    cancer and, 7

stem cells and, 7
cancer and, 37
lesions of, 21–24
Dysplasia
normal breast physiology and, 18
as poor term, 18
Dystrophic calcifications
in irradiated breast, 366
mammographic instance of, 366
significance of, 366

E

Echogenic noise, of free silicone, ultrasound and, 489
Ectasia, dilated ducts due to
mammographic instance of, 309–310
ultrasound instance of, 310
Ectatic ducts, ultrasound instance of, 429
Ectopic breast tissue, development of, 231
Edinburgh trial
analysis of data, 86
clinical breast examination used in, 96
randomized controlled trials, 74–75
effect of insurance companies on, 799–800
Embryonal cell carcinoma, gynecomastia and, 497
Encapsulation, of implants, cause uncertain, 475
Endogenous hormonal imbalance, gynecomastia and, 497
Environmental factors, breast cancer risk and, 44
Epidermal growth factor, prognosis and, 133
Epidermal inclusion cysts
benign, no intervention needed, 351
in male breast, mammographic instance of, 504
inframammary fold and, 351
ultrasound and, 351
Epithelial elements
breast cancer(s)
location of, 272
natural history of, 123
cancer formation and, 16
pregnancy and, 19–20
Epithelial hyperplasia
in male breast, 497
radial scars and, 305
Epitheliosis. See Extratubular terminal
ducts, benign lesions of, hyperplasia
Epithelium
and breast cancer development, theories of, 124–125
radiation and, 445
Estrogen
breast cancer development and, 43
receptors
detected in tumors, 43

prognosis and, 132
Tamoxifen use and, 132
unopposed, carcinogenic effect of, 43
Estrogen receptor
activity, prognosis and, 112
cancers, Tamoxifen treatment and, 52
Exaggerated craniocaudal view laterally,
mammographic projection,
196–197
Excessive residual tumor burden, adjuvant
radiation therapy and,
255
Excision, surgical, after guide placement,
673–677
with dye injection, 674–675
margin analysis after, 676–677
specimen from, 675–676
ultrasound of, 676
Excisional biopsy
architectural distortion after, mammographic instance of, 453
cost-effective approach to, 212
masses, solitary, with margins circumscribed, 281
Exogenous hormones. See also Hormone
replacement therapy (HRT)
estrogens, gynecomastia and, 498, 501
tissue density increase, diffuse nature
of, 241–242
Explantation
imaging after, 492
scarring after, 492
Exposure time, focal spot size and, 143
Exposure values, of film, automatic exposure control, purpose of,
150
Extensive intraductal component (EIC)
as risk for recurrence, 470
tumor type, 255
Extent of tumor, assessing, 807–808
Extra-abdominal desmoid lesions, spiculated margins of, mimic of
malignancy, 378
Extra-abdominal desmoid tumor, 563–565
Extralobular terminal ducts
anatomy of, 16
benign lesions of, hyperplasia, 524–527
atypical
ductal, 526
lobular, 526–527
mammographic appearance of,
527
incidence of, 524, 526
multiple peripheral papillomas, 527

F

"Fallen envelope sign," with ruptured
breast implants, 626
False-negative mammography. See Mammography, false-negative
False-negative rate, acceptable, 217–218

Familial breast cancer, distinguished from
hereditary breast cancer, 46
Family history, and risk factor for breast
cancer, 30, 46
fibroadenoma, 25
Fascia
breast anatomy and, 13
retromammary, 3
breast anatomy and, 13–14
retromammary fat and, 14
superficial layer of, 3
Fat
in breast
age and, 21
normal, 18
hypoechoic quality of, 409, 423
ultrasound instance of, 424
magnetic resonance imaging of, signal
intensity, 492
ultrasound and, 412–413, 424–425
Fat necrosis
architectural distortion and, 384–385
calcifications and, 361
mammographic instance of, 362
peripheral, 359
post-traumatic oil cysts, 430
mammographic instance of, 306
postsurgical, 450
calcifications and, 279
common change, 457–458
mammographic instance of, 450, 456
and scarring, 554–557
calcium deposition with, 555–556
causing post-traumatic oil cysts, 554,
555–556
differentiation of postbiopsy change
from cancer, 555
mammographic spectrum, 554–556
ultrasound appearance of, 556–557
spiculated
lucent structure within is diagnostic,
380
mammographic instance of, 379
mimic of malignancy, 378
ultrasound instance of, 435, 436
Fatty enlargement
bilateral, in male breast, 497
distinguished from gynecomastia, 497
Female, as risk factor for breast cancer,
45–46
Fetus, radiation exposure to
background radiation and, 445
mammography and, 105, 445
scatter radiation and, 445
Fibroadenolipoma, 558–560. See also
Hamartoma
Fibroadenoma(s), 527–537
acini and, 24–25
acoustic shadowing on ultrasound and,
439
benign, ultrasound instance of, 433

Fibroadenoma(s) *(contd.)*
  calcifications of, 530, 531, 532, 533, 534
    dystrophic, 366
    typical, 282
  calcifying
    mammographic instance of, 359
    types of, 359
  cancer alongside, 532, 534
  cancers in, 24–25
  change over time to, 305
  classic, 529
  complex
    family history of breast cancer, risk and, 25
    and increased risk of future development of breast cancer, 528
  giant, 528
  halo around, due to Mach effect, 530
  hypoechoic quality of, 431
  and invasive breast cancer, relative risk for, 512
  involution of, 528, 530, 531, 532
  juvenile, 528, 532, 534
  lobulation of, 530
  in lobule, benign, 24–25
  location of, lobules, 273–274
  mammographic appearance of, 528–534
  mammographic instance of, 282, 294
  margins of, 281–282
    ill-defined, mammographic instance of, 296
  multiple, 311
    mammographic instance of, 358
    metastases considered with, 434
  obscured margins and, 294–295
  phylloides tumor and, 291, 528
  physiology of, 24–25
  radiographic characteristics
    indistinguishable from carcinoma, 281
    indistinguishable from cyst, 281
  sensitivity to hormones, 528
  shadowing caused by, ultrasound instance of, 438
  signs of malignancy with, 359
  ultrasound appearance of, 534–537
    echoes, 534
    for differentiation from cancer, 534, 536
  ultrasound instance of, 430, 432, 435
Fibrocystic disease
  breast cancer risk and, 19
  as confusing pathologic terminology, 18, 19, 47–48, 229, 512–513
  normal breast physiology and, 18–19
  and relative risk of invasive breast cancer, 512–513
Fibroglandular densities
  mammograms and, 4

multiple rounded, 356
Fibroglandular elements, normal breast and, 18
Fibrosarcoma, 596
  occurrence of, 26
Fibrosis
  acoustic shadowing and, 438
  focal, 561–562, 563
  and relative risk for invasive breast cancer, 512
Fibrous capsule, after explantation of implants, 492
  mammographic instance of, 493
Fibrous contracture, implant problems and, 478
Fibrous encapsulation, implants and, 475
Fibrous histiocytoma, malignant, 599, 601, 602
Fibrous tissue, ultrasound and, 412–413
Field phenomena
  cells abnormality and, 7
  DNA changes, cells at risk and, 123
  possible explanation for, 7
  stem cells and, 37
Film
  characteristics of, x-ray attenuation and, 135
  developer, processor quality control tests, 151
  exposure, intensity and time, reciprocal parameters, 143
  processing of mammographic, 151–152
Film-screen mammography. *See* Mammography, film-screen
Filters, mammographic, 144
  artifacts and, 144
Fine-needle aspiration biopsy, 644, 706.
    See also Aspiration of cysts
  breast enervation and, 11
  cysts and, 2
    management of, 348
  cytology
    accuracy in diagnosis, 448
    as adjunctive technique, 217
    cost-effective approach to, 212
    criteria for using, 410
    ultrasound as guide for, 409, 410
  masses
    palpable, 441
    solitary with circumscribed margins, 281
  stereotactic guidance for, 710–716
    contraindications, 716
    sources of error, 716
  ultrasound-guided, 415, 716–718
    advantages of, 717–718
    disadvantages of, 718
    vs. ultrasound-guided core needle biopsy, 718
  use of, 2

Flow cytometry
  DNA content, measured in cancer cells, 132
  ploidy of cells and, 132
Focal asymmetric density
  annual screening and, 388
  asymmetric dense breast tissue, distinguished from, 313, 315
  benign, mammographic instance of, 262
  characteristics of that warrant biopsy, 257, 260
  magnification mammography of, 257
  mammographic instance of, 388, 389
  normal asymmetric breast tissue, distinguished from, mammographic instance of, 260
  perception of, 257
  significant distinguished, 387–388
  spot compression of, 257
  ultrasound and, 417
Focal asymmetries, distinguished from asymmetric breast tissue, 400
  mammographic instance of, 401, 402
Focal fibrosis, 561–562, 563
  as islands of density, 287, 289
  ill-defined margins of, 298
  mammographic instance of, 288
Focal spots
  blur and, 141
  design of, 139
  geometric blur and, 140–141
  heel effect and, 139–140
  location on breast and, 139–140
  magnification requirements and, 154
  mammographic system and, 139
  shape of, resolution and, 143
  size, spatial resolution and, in screen-film mammography, 138
Food and Drug Administration (FDA)
  ATL ultrasound unit approval, 412
  screening programs and, 227
  silicone gel prohibited by, 485
  silicone implants banned by, 472
Foreign bodies, in breast
  calcium deposition and, 367
  four sections of, 513
  mammographic instance of, 369, 370, 371

G
Galactoceles, 557–558
  benign, 306
  characteristics of, 436
  mammographic appearance of, 356, 557–558
  ultrasound appearance of, 558
  x-ray attenuation of, 306, 355
Galactography, 703
  limitations of, 345
  performing, 344–345
Gantry, rotation of, 196
Gel bleed, implants and, 475

Gene(s)
  abnormal, blood testing to screen for, 126–127
  alterations
    amplification, 36
    breast cancer and, 133
      clonal nature of, 41
      development of, 117–118
      invasive, development of, 125
    breast stem cell and, 124
    cancer natural history and, 123, 124
    deletions, 36
    methods of, 36
    prognosis and, 112
    reasons for, 133
    translocation, 36
  BRCA1, blood testing for, 126–127
  cell growth and, 36
  defects of, loss of heterozygosity, breast cancer cells and, 7
  histologic aberration and, 127
  oncogenes, cell growth and, 38–39
  p53, 42
    as tumor suppressor, 127
  proto-oncogenes, cell growth and, 38–39
  tumor suppressor genes, 39
Genetic abnormalities
  blood testing to screen for, 126–127
  heredity of breast cancer and, 38
Genetic controls, telomeres, DNA sequences and, 38
Genetic repair, DNA damage and, 38
Genotype, DNA alterations and, 36
Germ cell abnormalities, heredity breast cancers and, 35, 40
Giant fibroadenoma
  asymmetric breast and, 232
  mammographic instance of, 276
Glandular acini, terminal duct lobular unit and, 16
Gothenburg trial
  analysis of data, 86
  randomized controlled trials, 74
Granular cell tumors, 560–561
  spiculated margins of, mimic of malignancy, 378
Granular tumors, in male breast, 505, 506
Granulomas
  after explantation of implants, 492
  free silicone and, 475
  gel bleed and, 475
  silicone injection and, 471
Gynecomastia
  asymmetric. See Asymmetric gynecomastia
  bilateral, in male breast, 497
  bilateral nature of, mammographic instance of, 504
  breast development and, ultrasound findings, 502, 506

clinical presentation, 497
  defined, 497
  discoid density formed, xerographic instance of, 501
  drugs associated with, 497
  hypoechoic nature of, ultrasound instance of, 505
  indistinguishable from female breast
    mammographic instance of, 503
    xerographic instance of, 503
  mammographic appearances, 501–504
  nipple retraction and, xerographic instance of, 504
  skin thickening and, xerographic instance of, 504
  symmetric, mammographic instance of, 499
  ultrasound findings, 502
  unilateral, in male breast, 497

H

Halo, due to Mach effect, 280
  solitary circumscribed mass and, 397
  xerographic instance of, 280
Hamartoma
  benign
    characteristics of, 436
    mammographic instance of, 307
  mammary, 558–560
  mammogram, characterized as benign from, 307
  mammographic instance of, 215, 356
  mixed-density lesion
    appearance of, 355–356
    fat content of, 307
Health Insurance Plan of New York trial
  age for screening and, 77, 82
  analysis of data, 86
  Breast Cancer Detection Demonstration Project, development of, 72
  clinical breast examination used in, 96
  evaluation of results of, 77
  mortality rates, 133
    concerns regarding screening and, 95
  randomized controlled trials, 73
    clinical breast examination in, 71
    mammogram in, 71
    screening efficacy proved in, 71
  screening
    benefits demonstrated by, 101
    death rate and, 71
    earlier detection of cancers in, 128
    noncompliance in, 70
  statistical significance of, 76
Heel effect, focal spot in mammography and, 140
Hematomas
  abscess compared with, 430
  diagnosis of, 430–431

distinguished from contusion, 289–290, 296, 298
  due to core needle biopsy, mammographic instance of, 448
  implants and, 474
  mammographic instance of, 289
  margins of postsurgical, 455–456
  oval mass, mammographic instance of, 275
  postsurgical, 455–456, 470
    architectural distortion and, 289–290
    resolution of, 289–290
    ultrasound instance of, 430
    seromas indistinguishable from, 455–456
Hepatic disease, chronic, gynecomastia and, 497–498
Hereditary breast cancer(s)
  abnormal genes and, 40
  age at occurrence of, 47
  distinguished from familial breast cancer, 46
  genetic abnormalities and, 38
  germ cells and, 40
    abnormalities of, 35
  screening, age for, 47
  tumor suppressor genes and, 40
Hereditary relationships, breast cancer risk and, 44
Hiroshima, radiation, high-dose exposure, breast cancer risk increased from, 101, 103–104
Histologic grading
  systems, cell pleomorphism and, 131
  thresholds for intervention and, 218–219
Histology, not determinable by ultrasound, 432
Hodgkin's disease, risk for breast cancer, after irradiation, 49
Hookwire systems, for localization and excisional biopsy, 651–653, 672
  advantages of, 651–652
  disadvantages of, 652
  length of, 652
  side-port protruding, 653
  thickened distal segment of, 652–653, 672
Hormonal fluctuations
  in adolescent males, gynecomastia and, 7
  due to menstrual cycle, influence on breast of, 19
Hormonal manipulation, systemic treatment, with Tamoxifen, use of evolving, 464
Hormone receptors, absence or presence of, prognosis and, 132

Hormone replacement therapy (HRT)
  breast cancer risk and, 34, 50
  breast tissue density and, 241, 387
    increase in, mammographic instance
        of, 286
    mammographic instance of, 241, 242
  cyst development and, 242, 287
  fibroglandular density increase and,
        287
  neodensity and, 376
Hormone therapy
  axillary lymph node involvement and,
        108
  determinant for use, menopause and,
        79–80
  treatment, selection of based on staging,
        107, 108
Hormone-independent cancers
  epidermal growth factor, prognosis and,
        133
  transforming growth factor alpha, prog-
        nosis and, 133
Hormone-receptor negative tumors, pri-
        mary chemotherapy,
        response to, 471
Hormones, role in development of breast
        cancer, 32
Hyperplasia, 514. See also Extralobular
        terminal ducts, benign
        lesions of, hyperplasia
  atypical. See Atypical hyperplasia
  benign, of epithelium of distal duct and
        lobular ductules, 513
  mild, and relative risk for invasive
        breast cancer, 512
  of terminal duct, 22
  and relative risk for invasive breast can-
        cer, 512
  risk factor for breast cancer, 48
  role in breast cancer, continuum theory
        and, 123
Hysterectomy
  breast cancer risk reduction and, 46
  with oophorectomy, risk for breast can-
        cer reduced, 33

I
Ill-defined margins
  defined, 277
  mammographic instance of, 278
Ill-defined mass, mammographic instance
        of, 295, 297, 298
Imaging-guided aspiration, cysts and, 283,
        284
Imaging-guided needle biopsy
  cost-effective approach to, 212
  sentinel node, predictive value of, 12
IMF. See Inframammary fold (IMF)
Immunohistochemical stains, DNA syn-
        thetic activity, measurement
        of, 132

Implants, breast. See also Linguine sign;
        Magnetic resonance imag-
        ing, and breast implants
  after subcutaneous mastectomy, 462
  autoimmune reactions and, 472–473
  breast cancer detection and, 483
  breast compression and, 483
  cancer and, risk of developing, 483
  cancer detected with
    mammographic instance of, 479
    ultrasound instance of, 480
  capsular contracture and, 474
  changes to, 480–482
  collapsing envelope, 492
    magnetic resonance imaging of, 492
    rupture indicator, 492
    ultrasound visualization of, 492
  concern over, 474–475
  contents of, 622
  deformity of, 481
    intact, 620
    types, 480
  double-lumen, mammographic instance
        of, 474
  envelopes of, 622
    torn, 621
  explantation, 492
    imaging after, 492
    scarring after, 492
  extracapsular rupture of, 480
    imaging, 417
    stepladder appearance
        on magnetic resonance imaging, 417
        on ultrasound, 417
  fibrous contracture, mammography and,
        478
  fibrous encapsulation, 481, 619
    xerographic instance of, 487
  herniated, 481, 620
  high attenuation of, 481
  imaging, mammography and, 485
  intracapsular rupture and, 480, 482
    imaging of, 417
  iridium, radiation therapy and, 466
  mammographic instance of, 490
  mammography and, 475, 483
    positioning, 483
  needle biopsy, guided to avoid ruptur-
        ing, 483
  placement
    locations of, 475
    mammography and, 475
  polyurethane foam applied to surface of,
        475
  postsurgical complications with
    bleeding, 473
    infection, 473
    rupture of, 473
    toleration of, 473
  as problems in optimal visualization,
        739–740

radial folds due to, 621
regulations concerning, 472
retroglandular placement, 475, 476, 619
    mammographic instance of, 476
retropectoral placement, 475, 477, 619
    mammographic instance of, 477, 485
rheumatoid syndromes and, 472
rupture, 619–620, 621
    concern over, 474–475, 478
    detection of, 485–486, 492
        by mammography, 620, 621, 622
    extracapsular, 619
    extruded silicone in, 478, 480
    forms of, 480–482
    indistinguishable from herniation,
        mammographic instance
        of, 487
    intracapsular, 619
    mammograms and, 485–486, 487
    mammographic diagnosis of, 478
    mammographic instance of, 479, 488
    mammographic pressure as cause of,
        486
    of saline implants, 478–480
    silicone outside as proof of, 484
    silicone rubber envelope and, 478
    ultrasound instance of, 489
    ultrasound to determine, 416
    xerographic instance of, 487
silicone
    connective-tissue disorders and,
        472–473
    in livers of women with, 474
silicone envelope, collapse of, ultra-
        sound instance of, 417
silicone exposure and, 474
silicone gel for, 472
silicone "snowstorm" and, ultrasound
        instance of, 488
surgery related to, 474
texturing of, 475
types, 472, 475
ultrasound and, 484
    evaluation of palpable lesions with, 416
    to screen for breast cancer, no data
        supporting, 416
ultrasound instance of, 416
with polyurethane, hepatic cancer risk
        and, 480
In situ cancer. See also Ductal carcinoma
        in situ (DCIS); Lobular car-
        cinoma in situ (LCIS)
  significance of, 118
  within invasive cancers, reasons not
        often found, 125
  incentives to pursue suits, 800
Incidence, of breast cancer(s), 29
  age and, 30–31, 42, 80–81
  implants and, 483
  increasing, 29, 34, 78, 130–131
  young women and, 441

Incidence screen
    sojourn time and, 61
    successive breast cancer screens, 61
Indeterminate lesions, mammographic category, possibilities within, 255–256
Infection
    in treated breast, 471
    mammogram, not demonstrated on, 298
Infiltrating (invasive) ductal carcinoma, 576–581
    collagen production and calcium deposition of, 577, 580
    irregular shape of, 577
    mammographic appearance of, 577–580, 581
    mammographic instance of, 292, 295
    not otherwise specified, 577
        as circumscribed mass, 279
    subclassification of, 577
    ultrasound appearance of, 580, 582, 583, 584
Infiltrating (invasive) lobular carcinoma, 593–594.
    asymmetric density and, 261
    lobular carcinoma in situ and, 26
Infiltrating ductal tumors, in male breast, 500–501
Inflammatory carcinoma, 590, 591, 592
    characterization of, 110
    skin thickening and, 341, 406
    TNM classification of, 110
Inframammary fold (IMF)
    elevation of, craniocaudal projection and, 184
    mediolateral oblique projection and, 177, 178, 179, 183, 187–188
    visibility on mammogram and, 249–250
Interlobular stroma, lesions arising in, 21
Interval cancer rate, 792, 794–795
Interventional techniques, future of, 837–838
Intracystic bleeding, x-ray attenuation of, 308
Intracystic cancer
    bleeding and, 285
        mammographic instance of, 285, 308
    in male breast, 506
    mammographic instance of, 428–429
    rarity of, 285–286
    ultrasound instance of, 428–429
Intracystic papillary carcinoma, in male breast, ultrasound instance of, 507
Intracystic papillomas, 517–518
Intraductal calcifications, distinguished from vascular calcifications, 362
Intraductal cancer
    calcification pattern associated with, diagnostic, 381

ductal carcinoma in situ, tumor stage, treatment decisions based on, 107
Intraductal carcinoma in situ, 514. See also Ductal carcinoma in situ (DCIS)
    axillary lymph node involvement and, 122
    calcifications of, 393
        mammographic instance of, 394
    diagnosis, by biopsy, 118
Intraductal clones, breast cancer growth and, 41
Intraductal disease, diffuse, risk for recurrence, after radiation therapy, 470
Intraductal papilloma. See also Papillomas, large duct (intraductal)
    benign, risk for breast cancer and, 48
    calcified, presentation of, 360
    duct dilatation and, 308–309
    histologic cross section of, 22
    location of, 287, 310
    mammograms, not evident on conventional, 287
Intralobular connective tissue, characteristics of, 13
Intralobular terminal duct, anatomy of, 16
Intramammary lymph node(s). See also Lymph node(s)
    appearance of, classic, 352
    benign, 272–273
        location of, 351–352
        mammographic instance of, 354
    diagnosis of, 273, 352
    enlarged, causes of, 352–353
    lucent hilum in, 352
    mammographic instance of, 273
    mammography
        characteristic appearance of, 273
        routinely seen on, 273
    morphology unclear, magnification mammography and, 273
    psoriatic dermatopathic, xerographic instance of, 354
Intrauterine growth, breast development and, 4
Intravenous contrast agents
    imaging cancers with, technologies for, 414
    ultrasound evaluation and, 414
Invasive breast cancer(s)
    continuum theory and, 124–125
    denser than surrounding tissue, mammographic instance of, 382, 383
    detection by mammography demonstrated, 72
    development of, from single cell, 125
    growth of, screening intervals and, 94
    in situ cancer, associated with, 125

mortality from, 117
    tumor stage, treatment decisions based on, 107
    ultrasound instance of, 433
    upper outer quadrant, mammographic instance of, 274
Invasive carcinoma, minimal breast cancer, size of, 133
Invasive ductal cancers
    appearance on ultrasound, 439
    distinguished from invasive lobular cancer, 26
    not otherwise specified, cytologic features of tumor, 23–24
    ultrasound instance of, 439
Invasive ductal carcinoma. See also Infiltrating (invasive) ductal carcinoma
    focal asymmetry presentation of, mammographic instance of, 259
    in male breast, xerographic instance of, 505, 506, 509
    ultrasound instance of, 433, 434, 435, 437
    varying manifestations of differentiation in, prognosis, 131
Invasive lobular cancer, distinguished from invasive ductal cancer, 26
Invasive lobular carcinoma. See Infiltrating (invasive) lobular carcinoma
Involuting fibroadenomas, calcifications, 315
    characteristic of, 358–359
    mammographic instance of, 315
Involutional changes in breast, 511–512
    age and, 233
    before menopause, 20–21
    menopause and, 20–21
Irradiation
    male breast, breast cancer risk and, 498–499
    scarring and, 278–279
Irregular mass, mammographic instance of, 276

J
Jewish women, risk for breast cancer and, 47, 127

K
Kidney cancer, metastatic to breast, characteristics of, 432, 434
Klinefelter's syndrome
    breast cancer development and, 497
    breast cancer incidence and, in male breast, 498
    gynecomastia and, 497
Kopparberg trial
    analysis of data, 86

Kopparberg trial *(contd.)*
  randomized controlled trials, 73–74
  survival rate data, 86
Kyphotic women, mammography for, cau-
      docranial projection and,
      201

L

L/AP ratio. *See* Length-to-height ratio
Labels
  mammograms and, 220–221
  lack of recognition for scientific proof,
      799, 800
Lactation
  breast maturation and, 8
  breast tissues
    changes during, 445, 446
    density of, 20
    return to baseline after, 447
    x-ray attenuation of, 446
  ducts and, 16
  long duration of, breast cancer risk and,
      44
  mammography during, 445, 446
    problems with, 446
  pregnancy and, 19–20
  radiographic density of breast during, 20
  risk for breast cancer and, 33, 50
    reduced during long periods of, 33
Lactiferous ducts, anatomy of, 15
Lactiferous sinuses, 3
  nipple and. *See* Montgomery's glands
Laplace's law, duct dilatation and, 309
Large duct papillomas. *See* Papillomas,
      large duct (intraductal)
Laser imaging of breast, future role of,
      833
Lateromedial projection
  medial breast tissues and, 200–201
  positioning for, 200–201
  to reduce geometric blur, 728–730, 731,
      732
Latissimus dorsi, used for breast recon-
      struction after mastectomy,
      484
Length-to-height ratio
  of benign and malignant lesions, differ-
      entiating between, 431–432
  schematic of, 432
  use of, questionable, 432
Lesion(s). *See also* Mass(es); Precursor
      lesions
  analyzing, approach to, 251
  assessment of
    adjunctive, 348–349
    benign findings, 223
    lucent centers and, 223
    magnification and, 222–223
    mammographic interpretation and,
      223
    morphologic analysis of, 223

  ultrasound as adjunctive study, 224
benign
  categorization of, 21
  Doppler ultrasound and, 414
  following, 224
  intramammary lymph nodes and,
      272–273
  location of, 272–274
  mammographic instance of, 352–359
  mammography and, 376
  pathology review of, 456
  radiolucent, 306
  x-ray attenuation of, 306–307
biopsy criteria, 224–227
calcifications in
  more than one type, 393, 395
  significance of, 317
circumscribed, evaluation of, 292
classification of, by ultrasound,
      411–412
determining reality of, 207–209
diagnosis, biopsy needed for, 211
ductal carcinoma in situ, classification
      of, 118, 120–121
extent of, defined with magnification
      mammography, 254–255
fat-containing lucent, x-ray attenuation
      of, 355
ill-defined margins, 295–296
  biopsy needed for, 296
  malignancy and, 382, 437
internal echoes of, aspiration of, 429
intramammary lymph nodes, mammo-
      graphic appearance of, 224
length-to-height ratio, differentiating
      benign and malignant,
      431–432
location, 251
  computed tomography and, 274
  importance of, 274
  rolled views and, 223
  triangulation and, 204–207, 223
  ultrasound and, 274
lucent-centered calcifications, mammo-
      graphic appearance of, 224
malignant
  categorization of, 21
  gross cancer removal and, 226–227
  margins of excised tissue, 226–227
  postsurgical mammography with
      magnification, to assess
      extent of, 226
  x-ray attenuation not increased, 383
    mammographic instance of, 383
mammographic detection
  more extensive than calcifications
      indicate, 128
  ultrasound evaluation of, 419–420
mammography, diagnosis of malig-
      nancy, not possible with,
      376

margins of, significance of, 223–225,
      275, 277, 296, 377, 382,
      384, 437
  microlobulated, 295, malignancy
      probable, 384
  obscured
    differentiating, 294–295
    ultrasound and, 294–295
missed in surgery, 455
mixed density, benign nature of,
      355–356
morphology of, biopsy determined by,
      309, 311
nonpalpable, only detected by mammo-
      gram, and radiologist's
      responsibility, 284
of major ducts
  duct ectasia, etiology of unknown, 21
  large duct papilloma, 22
  Paget's disease, 22
  and periductal inflammation, 21
of minor and terminal ducts, 22–24
  ductal carcinoma
    in situ, 23
    invasive, 23–24
  hyperplasia, 22
  papillomas, multiple peripheral, 22–23
on ultrasound, 425
palpable, ultrasound in management of,
      441
probably benign
  classification of, 370–371
  definition of, 371
  evaluation of, with magnification
      mammography, 371
  mammographic instance of, 371
  management of, 370–373, 372–373
  short-interval follow-up for, 371,
      372–373, 375–376
  threshold for intervention of, 373
    cost determining, 373
radiolucent, benign, 306–307
raised skin, seborrheic keratosis, no
      intervention needed, 351
reality of
  morphology and, 254
  parallax used to determine, 204–205
short-interval follow-up for, 227
  doubling times of breast cancer and,
      227
size of
  at time of diagnosis, prognosis and,
      274–275
  ductal carcinoma in situ (DCIS), 122
skin, mammographic findings and, 207
solid, characteristics of cyst
  aspiration of questionable, 420–421
  internal echoes only differentiating
      factor, 420–421
solitary dilated duct, as indicator of can-
      cer, 308

spiculated margins
    breast cancer(s) with, 302–304
    dense irregular mass with, malig-
        nancy and, 377
    intervention needed for, 224–225
    malignancy and, 377
    mammographic instance of, 378, 379
    specimen radiography instance of,
        390
    stability possible, 377
    uncommon, 305
    stability over time and, 226
staging, 107
subareolar region, evaluation of, 440
summation shadows, distinguished
        from, 222
suspicious, tissue diagnosis, 349
thresholds for intervention and,
        224–227
triangulation. See Triangulation
ultrasound analysis of, 425–427. See
        also Ultrasound
    benign masses, 426
    cancers, 427
    cysts, 426
    malignant lesions, 426
    pericystic fibrosis, 426
    systems for, 425–427
unusual, 305
verification of, 222–223
    magnification and, 222–223
    noise reduction and, 222–223
visibility of, x-ray mammography
        requirements for, 139
visualization improvement, scatter radi-
        ation elimination and, 148
well-circumscribed, 434
x-ray attenuation of, low, 306
Leukemia
    bilateral adenopathy and, 347
    risk from radiation therapy, 471
Light scanning, future role in breast evalu-
        ation, 833
Linguine sign
    computed tomographic instance of,
        491
    magnetic resonance imaging instance
        of, 491
    significance of, 489
    ultrasound instance of, 490
    with ruptured breast implants, 626,
        627
Lipomas, 551–554
    benign, 306
    characteristics of, 434–436
    in male breast, 497, 502
    mammographic demonstration of, 215
    mammographic instance of, 306, 355,
        552, 553
    mammographic view of, 216
    ultrasound instance of, 436, 553–554

vs. liposarcoma, 553
x-ray attenuation of, 306, 355
Liposarcoma, 596
    occurrence of, 26
Liver, as metastatic site, cancer staging
        and, 109
Liver cancer, polyurethane and, 475
Lobe(s), anatomy of, 15
    lactiferous ducts, 15
Lobular acini. See Lobule(s)
Lobular carcinoma (neoplasia), 516
Lobular carcinoma in situ (LCIS), 516,
        592–593
    appearance of, 26
    as field phenomenon, 122, 123
    breasts at risk, both, therapy ramifica-
        tions of, 122
    calcifications and, risk for invasive car-
        cinoma and, 48
    cancer risk and, 1
    cluster of calcifications, found in biopsy
        for, 391
    diagnosis of, coincidental, 122
    vs. ductal carcinoma in situ, 122
    explanation for, 7
    high risk lesion, 26
    incidence of, 29
    invasive cancer
        bilateral risk for, 26
        indicator of increased risk for, 122
    mammographically defined indications
        of, no, 230–231
    mammography and, 48
    minimal breast cancer, size of, 133
    risk associated with, 230
Lobular epithelium
    breast cancer and
        development of, 107
Lobular neoplasia. See Atypical lobular
        hyperplasia; Lobular carci-
        noma in situ (LCIS)
Lobule(s)
    anatomy of, 3–4
    appearance of, 232
    DNA alteration and
        cancer, 7
        stem cells and, 7
    lactation and, 445
    lesions of
        benign, 24, 514–516, 527–551. See
            also Fibroadenoma
        malignant, 592–596
            infiltrating (invasive) lobular carci-
                noma, 593–594, 595–596
            lobular carcinoma in situ,
                592–593
    pregnancy and, 20
    stem cell, DNA alteration of, cancer
        and, 37
Localization, cost-effective approach to,
        212

Localization techniques. See also Aspira-
        tion of cysts; Calcifications,
        of skin, localization of with
        mammography; Parallax
        needle localization
    computed-tomography–guided,
        700–703
    galactography, 703–704
    needle, for excisional biopsy, 646–653
        estimating lesion location, 646–647
        guides for, 648, 649
            anchored needles, 653
            conventional hypodermic needles,
                648, 649–650
            curved wires protruding from nee-
                dle tip, 653
            hookwire systems, 651–653. See
                also Hookwire systems, for
                localization and excisional
                biopsy
            side-port portruding hookwire,
                653
        locating occult lesions three dimen-
            sionally, 647–649
        preoperative, 646
            general considerations for, 649
    pitfalls of, 685, 690–692
    ultrasound-guided. See Ultrasound-
        guided needle procedures
Lumpectomy. See also Surgical breast
        biopsy
    as conservation therapy, 467
    clear margins, radiation therapy and,
        464
    ductal carcinoma in situ, with radiation
        therapy, recurrence rate
        and, 118
    goal of, 448–449
    imaging-guided needle biopsy and, 12
    magnification mammography and,
        254–255
    recurrence of cancers after, 118,
        448–449
    residual tumor after, 464
    tissue removed in, 464
    tumor margins and, 448–449
Lumpogram, use of, 201
Lung, as metastatic site, cancer staging
        and, 109
Lung cancer
    gynecomastia and, 498
    metastatic to breast
        characteristics of, 432, 434
        ultrasound instance of, 434
Lung diseases, gynecomastia and, 498
Lymph node positivity, prognosis and, 132
Lymph node(s). See also Axillary lymph
        node(s)
    anatomy of, 12
    cancer staging and, 109
    axillary dissection for analysis, 467

Lymph node(s) *(contd.)*
  intramammary
    location of, 12–13
    visible by mammography, 13
  location of, 12–13
  mammography and, 12
  staging and, 107
  tumor in
    excised, 12
    metastatic potential indicated by, 11
    radiation treatment and, 12
Lymphatic drainage, breast anatomy and, 12
Lymphatic system, tumor access to, 130
Lymphatics, 107
Lymphoma
  axillary lymph nodes and, 347
    enlargement of, 407–408
  bilateral adenopathy and, 347
  of the breast, 604–606, 607–608
  characteristic appearance of, 434
  in male breast, 506
  intramammary lymph node, enlargement of, 353
  mammographic instance of, 291, 292
  margins of, 279
  metastasizing to breast, 292
  morphological characteristics of, 291
  ultrasound instance of, 435

M

Mach effect
  halo, 280
    around cysts on mammography, 541, 542
    around fibroadenoma, 520
  solitary circumscribed mass and, 397
Magnetic resonance imaging, 617–636
  appearance of silicone implants, 624–626
    after rupture, 625, 626
    "linguine" or "fallen envelope" sign, 626, 627
    postoperatively, 625
    preference for sagittal images, 625
    with T1- and T2-weighted images, 625
  cost-effective approach to, 212
  costs of, 52–53
  of ductal carcinoma in situ, 630–631
  fast spin-echo and, 489
  future of, 633–634, 832
  gadolinium enhancement with, uses of, 470
  imaging cancers with
    intravenous contrast agents and, 414
    neovascularity and, 414
  implants and, 489
    detecting rupture in, 492
    evaluation of, 486, 489, 491–492
    extracapsular rupture of, 417
    suppression techniques, 489–491

techniques for. *See also* Implants, breast
    artifact from cardiac motion, 624
    limitations of, 623–624
    pulse sequences for, 623
    silicone-selective imaging, 623
  of lesions, 626, 628–634
    background, 626, 628
    detecting chest wall recurrences after reconstruction with implant or TRAM flap, 632
    in differentiating benign from malignant, 628, 629, 630
    in differentiating scar tissue from cancer recurrence, 631–632
    with Gd-DTPA contrast enhancement, 626, 629–630
    techniques for, 628–629
      dose of Gd-DTPA, 628
      double coil for, 628
      echoplanar imaging, 628–629
      eliminating fat from, 628
      pulse sequences for, 628
      standard radiofrequency spoiled gradient echo or FLASH imaging, 628
    for tumor staging, 631, 632
  needle biopsy and, 447
  resonance frequencies
    of fat, 489–491
    of silicone, 489–491
    of water, 489–491
  signal intensities, 491
  surface coils and, 489
  T1-weighted images, and cancers with surrounding fat, 617, 618
  T2-weighted images, and cysts, 617, 618
Magnetic resonance spectroscopy in women with implants, to detect silicone in livers of, 474
Magnification mammography, 740–745
  approaches to, 154–155, 212
  calcifications, 741, 742–745
    morphology clearer with, 255
    vascular, 362
    visibility of, 319
      improvement of, 209
  clarification of problem and, 171
  degree of magnification, formula for, 154
  disadvantage of, 154
  dual spot, 209
  focal asymmetric density, used to determine, 388, 742
  focal spot, 348
    size and, 209
  ill-defined mass, evaluation of, 298
  lesions
    adjunctive assessment of, 348

    indeterminate, 255–256
    probably benign, evaluation of, 371
    verification of, 222–223
  longer exposure required for, 154
  mammographic resolution, 141
    noise reduction and, 141, 209, 255
  margins of masses, clearer, 255
  of palpable finding, 193, 195
  performance of, 209
  radiation dose and, 209
  scatter reduction and, 209
  for solitary circumscribed mass, 741–742
  subareolar tissues and, 344
  uses of, 209, 254–255
Male breast. *See also* Breast cancer(s), in male breast
  adolescent, transient changes in, 497
  benign lesions in, 502
  cysts in, 497
  development in, ultrasound findings, 502, 506
  ductal epithelium in, 497
  imaging
    asymmetric gynecomastia and, 501
    reason for, 501
    unilateral lump found during, 501
  lobule formation in, 497
  mammography for
    caudocranial projection and, 201
    positioning for, 201, 202
  normal, 501
    histology of, 497
    mammographic instance of, 500
Malignancy
  development of, different courses for, 123
  diagnosis of, spiculated lesions and, 377
Malignant breast lesions, 569–612. *See also* Ductal carcinoma, distinctive; Ductal carcinoma in situ; Infiltrating (invasive) ductal carcinoma; Lobule, malignant lesions of; Metastatic lesions to the breast; Tumor masses, in preadolescent females
  distribution of types, 569
  histologic categories of, 569
  lymphoma of the breast, 604–606
  unusual, 594, 596–604. *See also* Sarcomas of the breast
Malignant fibrous histiocytoma, 599, 601, 602
  imaging of, no distinguishing features by, 292
Malmö trial
  analysis of data, 86
  mortality rates, concerns regarding screening and, 95
  randomized controlled trials, 74
Malpractice, 799–800. *See also* Standard of care issues

Mammary dysplasia
    as confusing pathologic terminology,
        19, 512–513
    normal breast physiology and, 18–19
    and relative risk of invasive breast can-
        cer, 512–513
Mammary gland, cancer staging and, 109
Mammary hamartoma, 558–560
Mammary ridges, breast development and,
    4
Mammogram(s). *See also* Mammographic
        terms; Mammography
    after biopsy, care with, 450
    artifacts visible on, 250
    assessment categories, Breast Imaging
        Reporting and Data System
        (BIRADS) and, 254
    baseline
        guidelines for, 87
        new 6 months after radiation treat-
            ment, 470
        new after biopsy, 450
        new with questionable finding, short-
            term follow-up for, 470
    benign findings
        no further evaluation needed, 254
        reporting for, 225
    blur, causes of, 250
    breast cancer mortality reduced by,
        105
    breasts symmetrically positioned for,
        mammographic instance of,
        249
    compression for, Cooper's ligaments
        and, 343
    craniocaudal projection, breast anatomy
        and, 9
    data, American College of Radiology
        (ACR) recommendations
        for, 220–221
    detection and, 247
    diagnosis, not suited for, 247
    diagnostic mammography, as mislead-
        ing term, 87
    double reading and, 213–214, 247
    early repeat, missed lesion revealed dur-
        ing, 455
    example of need for two views, 173
    false-positive screening and, biopsy rec-
        ommendation and, 81
    film for, 219
    film positioning
        as mirror images, 248
        conventions of, 248
    findings, intervention required for vari-
        ous, 225–227
    follow-up, after surgery, 450
    high probability of malignancy finding,
        reporting for, 225
    identification of, 191–192
        conventions regarding, 192

image evaluation and, 248–249
indeterminate lesion
    characteristics of, 226
    interventions for, 226
    reporting for, 226
    short-interval follow-up for, 226
interpretation of, 219–222, 247
    accuracy of, 212
    associated findings and, 338–348
    asymmetry appreciation and, 251
    double reading and, 212, 213–214,
        247
    elements to consider during, 250–251
    human perception, psychovisual
        threshold and, 213–214
    old film review and, 251
        mammographic instance of,
            252–254
    organization needed for, 247
    positioning film for viewing and,
        220–221
    psychovisual phenomenon and, 247
    radiologists', 247
        reading rate for, 212
    systematic review of, 251, 349
    viewing techniques for, 250–251
labeling of, 191–192
lactation and, 445
lesion features of, receiver operating
        characteristic curve and,
        218
mediolateral oblique projection (MLO)
    breast anatomy and, 9
    ideal positioning for, 175–181
menstrual cycle and, 230
mirror images
    interpretation and, 221
    viewing as, 187
negative, reporting for, 225
nipple in profile on, 249
normal, variation in, 230–231
positioning of patient for
    optimal, 249–250
        proper penetration and, 250
            mammographic instance of, 250
        tissue maximization, 250
postbiopsy, reason for, 454–455
pregnancy and, 445
radiographic density determined by, 243
radiopaque markers, conventions
        regarding, 220–221
suspicious lesion seen during
    intervention for, 226
    reporting for, 226
thresholds for intervention, guidelines
        for, 254
two-view film-screen, radiation risk
        from, 104–105
view box analysis of, 248
viewing conditions for, 248
    quality control and, 248

Mammographic equipment, quality of, 219
Mammographic findings
    architectural distortion, probability of
        malignancy with, 376
    focal asymmetries, 256–267
        mammographic instance of, 256–267
    neodensity and, probability of malig-
        nancy with, 376
    new calcifications, cluster of, probabil-
        ity of malignancy with, 376
    new mass, probability of malignancy
        with, 376
    possibility of malignancy with, 376
    probably benign, 397
    spiculated lesions
        mammographic instance of, 378
        probability of malignancy with, 377
    suspicion aroused by, 382
Mammographic positioning
    standard views, 171
    with implants, 483
Mammographic screening. *See also*
        Screening
    of asymptomatic women, efficacy of, 52
    benefit-to-risk ratio, at age of beginning
        screening, 104
    cost of, 211–212
    efficacy of, debate over, 55
    technologists, well-trained, importance
        of, 212
Mammographic systems, compression
        and, 145
Mammography. *See also* Blur; Contrast;
        Digital mammography;
        Mammograms; Mammog-
        raphy terms; X-ray mam-
        mography
    additional evaluation
        multifocality and, 255
        reasons for, 255–267
        residual cancer and, 255
    after mastectomy, 484
    artifacts
        recurrent, 144
        sources of, 137
    as screening technology, 105–106
    of axilla, after mastectomy, 465
    baseline, two views for, 171
    benefit from, 215
    benign mass, used to avoid biopsy of,
        214
    and biopsy
        after screening, and thresholds for
            intervention, 90
        needle, 447
        resulting from, positive predictive
            value of, 96
    breast compression
        coned-down spot compression, clari-
            fication of problem and,
            171

Mammography *(contd.)*
  discomfort and, 175
  implants and, 485
  need for, 174–175
  breast imaging team roles
    physicist, 163
    radiologist, 163
    technologist, 163
  breast traction device and, 174
  bremsstrahlung photons in, 138
  calcification evaluation, and straight
      lateral projection,
      199–200
  cancer detection and, 244–245
  categories of lesions in, 255–256
  chest wall, after mastectomy, 465
  clinically evident abnormality and, 193
    resolution by clinical evaluation and,
        215
  compared with clinical breast examina-
      tion, screening trials and,
      75–76
    Health Insurance Plan of New York
        trial, 71–72
  correlated with ultrasound, 414–415
  cost reduction of, 229
  craniocaudal projection, exaggerated,
      196–197
  detection ability demonstrated in, Breast
      Cancer Detection Demon-
      stration Project, 72
  detection and, 211
    threshold of, 63–64
  diagnostic intervention and, effective-
      ness of screening and, 90
  digital, 816–832. *See also* Digital mam-
      mography
    advantages of, 819–821, 828–830
      contrast subtraction angiography,
          830, 831
      digital tomosynthesis, 829–830
      dual-energy subtraction, 828–829
    clinical impact of, 831–832
      computer-aided detection and diag-
          nosis, 831
      telemammography, 831–832
    image, composition of, 816–817
    direct, 821–832
      advantages of for x-ray mammog-
          raphy, 821
      contrast vs. spatial resolution, 821
      dynamic range, 824
      modulation transfer function,
          821–822
      possible configurations for imager,
          824
      signal-to-noise ratio, 822–823
    dose and, 825–826
    from film to, 817–818, 821
    image acquisition, approaches to, 825
    limitations of, 828

  scatter, 825
  systems for, 825–828
    early, 827–828
      charge-coupled devices, 826
      line scanning, 826
      selenium as a detector, 828
      storage phosphor systems, 826
      thin-film transistor array, 827
  dual screen/dual emulsion systems,
      153–154
    parallax and, 153–154
  ductal carcinoma in situ, detection of, 72
  during lactation, and reduced sensitivity,
      446
  during pregnancy, efficacy of, 446
  early detection and, 81–82, 247
  efficacy of, 77, 106
  equipment, 157
    artifacts and, 159
    beryllium windows in tubes, 144–145
    dedicated, radiation exposure to fetus
        and, 445
    detector, 158
    film processing, 158–159
    film processor, maintenance of, 159
    film-screen contact, 158
    gantry, 196
    grid, 158, 159
    image quality and, 171
    processing chemistry, 159–160
    quality control program and, 155
  equipment acceptance testing
    quality control and, 158
  exaggerated views, 195–201
    compression paddles and, 196–197
  exposure for, 157
  false-negative, 792–795
    accuracy measure, 792
    analyzing, 794
    audit results, 792
    and interval cancer rate, 794–795
    methods to reduce, 795
    reasons for, 792–794, 795
      positioning, 793
  film
    developer chemicals for, 151
    processing of, 151, 157
      artifacts and, 151
      chemical agitation and, 161
      chemical replenishment rates,
          160–161
      darkroom requirements, 163
      extended, 151–152
      film drying and, 161
      optimum, 152
      temperature requirements, 161
      time requirements, 161
      wash cycle and, 161
  processor
    problems, 152
    procedure for optimizing, 161–163

  quality control tests and, 151
  underprocessing, effect of, 152
  used as detector in, 137
  film viewing, 163
  film-screen
    combinations, extended processing
        not needed for new, 152
    conventional, advantages and disad-
        vantages of, 818–819
    radiation risk and, 104
  focused, 193, 195
  future improvements in, 809–816
    automatic exposure control, 816
    film processing, 816
    magnification, 814
    patient interface and breast compres-
        sion, 809–813
      pendent positioning, 810–811
      tailored compression, 811–813
        separate compression system,
            811
        with tilting compression pad-
            dles, 811, 812
        traction, 811, 813
    scatter reduction, 813–814
      focusing x-rays, 814
      oscillating grids, 813
      slot systems, 814
    screen design, 815
    stereomammography and tomogra-
        phy, 814
  goal of, 157
  guidelines for, 77
  high-quality, 247
    double reading and, 247
    high-contrast resolution and, 135
    positioning of patient and, 247
  image sharpness
    on different parts of breast,
        139–140
    magnification and, 154
  and implants, 480–481, 485
    evaluation and, 486–487
    polyurethane-coated, 486–487
    rupture of, 485–486, 492
    standard view for, 494
  in male breast, does not exclude cancer,
      506
  and intervention, parameters for, 218
  involutional changes to breast, micro-
      scopic study of, 233–234
  kilovolt peak and, 138
  lactation, effect of, mammographic
      instance of, 447
  lateral breast tissues
    axillary tail view, 196, 197–198
    craniocaudal view, exaggerated,
        196–197
  magnification. *See* Magnification mam-
      mography
  of mastectomy site, 465

of medial tissues, using cleavage view, 198–199
and medical physicist, responsibilities of, 158
missed cancers and, 99
modified projections, clarification of problem and, 171
and mortality rate, reducing, 99
National Breast Screening Study of Canada (NBSS) and, poor quality, 87–88
negative, intervention for clinically significant abnormality and, 99
noise in
quantum mottle and, 137
sources of, 137
outcome monitoring, American College of Radiology (ACR), Breast Imaging Reporting and Data System (BIRADS), 218
of palpable lesions. See Palpable lesions, mammographic workup for
pectoral major muscle and, 8–9
physical examination as complementary to, 215, 216
and physicians, responsibility of, 157
poor image, positioning and, 172
positioning of patient, 157, 271–272
focused, clinical breast examination and, 193, 195
implants and, 485
importance of, 171, 172
incapacitated patient accommodation and, 172
quality control and, 186–189
pendent, 172, 173, 174
seated, 172
standing, 172
postaspiration, mammographic instance of, 421
and pregnancy, avoid routine screening during, 445
pressure from
increased growth of metastatic lesions from, 95
safety of, 95
principles of imaging, 135–136
quality of, 62
effectiveness of screening and, 90
maintained and monitored throughout, 157
radiation for Hodgkin's disease, following, 49
radiation risk and, 101
radiographic density of breast and, 62
and radiologist
responsibilities of, 158
training for, 88
recurrent breast cancers and, 471

regulations for
Mammography Quality Standards Act (MQSA) and, 168
state, 168
reporting standardization. See Reporting, of breast imaging
resolution of
formula for, 141
increase of, 141
magnification and, 141
variation in actual spatial, 142
role of, 229
rolled views and, 206–207
scatter radiation, fetal radiation exposure and, 445
scatter-reduction grids, high-quality images and, 148–149
screen-film combinations, 135
primary detector, 143
resolution capability of, 142
screen thickness and, 153–154
screening
after subcutaneous mastectomy, 462
age to begin, 441–442
detection of cancers and, 60
efficacy of, 375
elements for success of, 62–63
findings of, 351
importance of, 171
not diagnostic technique, 82
not excluding, 442
randomized controlled trials and, 55
results of, 76
younger women and, 441–442
sensitivity of, 62
signal-to-noise ratio and, magnification and, 154
spatial resolution and, measurement of, 142
spot compression and, 193
standard views, 171
implants and, 485, 486
subcutaneous mastectomy and, 494
for symptomatic women, value of, 750, 751–755
critical path and outcome analysis, 752–753
as technically demanding procedure, 157
technologists, highly skilled needed, 155
thresholds for intervention, prognostic measurements and, 218
tissue characteristics evaluated by, 403
clinical breast examination (CBE) and, 77
value of, 222
x-ray tube design for, 138
younger women and, 441–442
Mammography aid to positioning (MAP)
axilla and, 190

craniocaudal projection, evaluation of, 191
pectoralis major muscles in, 189–191
positioning, importance of, 189
training technologists, aid to, 189–191
use of, 189–191
Mammography Quality Standards Act (MQSA), 762
quality assurance, required by, 157
quality control, required by, 157
regulations, automatic exposure control (AEC) required by, 150–151
requirements of, 168
Mammography terms
false-positive results defined, 217
incidence defined, 216
interval cancers defined, 217
lead time defined, 216
positive predictive value defined, 216–217
prevalence defined, 216
prior probability of cancer defined, 216
sensitivity defined, 217
specificity defined, 217
true-negative results defined, 217
true-positive results defined, 217
Mammotome, for needle biopasy, 708, 709
Margins, lesion
analysis of excised tissue, 676
importance of, 464
brush border, mammographic instance of, 378
clear, conservation therapy and, 467
defined, American College of Radiology (ACR), Breast Imaging Reporting and Data System (BIRADS), 275
halo effect, xerographic instance of, 280
ill-defined
invasive cancer, photomicrograph appearance of, 280
malignancy and, 382, 437–438
interface of mass with surrounding tissue, 275, 277
magnification to evaluate, mammographic instance of, 298
in male breast, 506
of masses, magnification mammography and, 255
microlobulated, malignancy probable, 384, mammographic instance of, 384
obscured
defined, 277
dense normal fibroglandular tissue and, 382
significance of, 275, 277
on ultrasound, 423

Mass(es)
  analysis of
    American College of Radiology
        (ACR), Breast Imaging
        Reporting and Data System
        (BIRADS) approach,
        267–279
    location of, 267–269
  benign
    calcifications characteristic of,
        358–360
    mammogram finding, and no inter-
        vention needed, 351–352
    peripheral calcifications and, types
        of, 359–360
  calcifications and, 315–316, 358–360
  circumscribed
    hypoechoic, significance of, 431
    mammographic instance of, 291, 292,
        293
    management of, 279
    probability of malignancy and,
        280–281
    rare, 292
    size, risk of malignancy and, 281
    solitary
      biopsy indicated in, 399
      interventions for, 281
      mammographic instance of, 399
      management of, 397, 399–400
      ultrasound used with, 399
  classification of, 765–771
    by density, 771, 772
    by margins, 768, 770
    by shape, 766
  ill-defined
    biopsy for, 298
    evaluation of, 298
  in region of previous biopsy, follow-up
      reasonable for, 304–305
  location of, 267–269
  margins, stability over time and, 309
  shape
    defined by American College of
        Radiology (ACR) Breast
        Imaging Reporting and
        Data System (BIRADS),
        275
    malignancy, probability and, 275
    mammographic instance of, 275,
        276
    stability over time and, 309
  size, factor when lesion is cancer, prog-
      nosis and, 281
  solid, acoustic enhancement and, ultra-
      sound instance of, 422
  spiculated, mammographic instance of,
      381
  stability over time
    as indication of benign nature of, 309
    margins of, 309

shape and, 309
  ultrasound instance of, 416
Massachusetts General Hospital, double-
    reading system, mammo-
    gram interpretation and,
    214
Mastectomy
  as curative procedure, 128
  compared with breast conservation with
      radiation, 465–466
  ducts and, 14
  imaging after, 484
  for in situ disease, 128
  primary chemotherapy and, 471
  radical, pectoralis major muscle and,
      14, 465
  radical modified
    standard incision for, 465
    when indicated, 464–465
  reconstruction after
    implants, 483
    silicone implants for, 472
    tissue expanders, 483
    transverse rectus abdominis myo-
        cutaneous flap and,
        483–484
  reduction mammaplasty after, 461
  residual tumor extension, ducts and, 14
  subcutaneous
    cancer risk reduction and, 462
    epithelial elements remain, 462
    implant and, 462
    mammography screening indicated
        after, 462
    residual breast tissue after, 462
Mastitis
  plasma cell, 522, 523
  radiation treatment for, radiation risk for
      breast cancer and, 103
  and relative risk for invasive breast can-
      cer, 512
  skin thickening and, 340
Mastopathy
  normal breast physiology and, 18
  as poor term, 18
Medial mass, imaging of, craniocaudal
    projections and, 9
Medial tissues, mammographic imaging of
    craniocaudal projection and, 185–187
    lateromedial projection and, 200–201
    cleavage view, 198–199
    mediolateral oblique projection, 185
      missed cancers in, 271–272
Medical physicist, role in mammography,
    163–165, 166
Medicare, screening intervals permitted
    by, effect on detection, 93
Mediolateral oblique positioning. See also
    Mediolateral oblique pro-
    jection (MLO)
  compression and, 183

nipple, as reference point in, 183, 184
  proper, pectoralis muscle in, 183
Mediolateral oblique projection (MLO).
    See also Mediolateral
    oblique positioning
  maximizing tissue imaged on, 187
  medial tissues and, 185
  missed lesions on, 271–272
  opposite breast, positioned symmetri-
      cally, 187
  positioning films of, as mirror images,
      248
  positioning for, 175–181
    how to gauge, 181, 183
  triangulation for lesions seen only on,
      733–735
Medullary cancers
  carcinoma, 588–590
  margins of, 279
  prognosis and, 131
Melanoma
  lymph node involvement and, 12
    technetium 99m sulfur colloid injec-
        tion and, 12
  metastatic to breast, 292
    characteristics of, 432, 434
    mammographic instance of, 293
Menarche
  breast development and, 6
  early onset
    annual incidence of breast cancer
        and, 33
    as risk factor for breast cancer, 33,
        45, 46
    late onset, as risk factor for breast can-
        cer, 43
Menopause
  age 50 as surrogate for, 79–80
  age of, risk for breast cancer and, 33,
      34, 43, 45, 46
  and breast cysts, 540
  and breast tissue, no dramatic change
      in, 235
  relationship to involution and, 20–21
Menstrual cycle
  acinar cells
    follicular phase, 19
    luteal phase, 19
    mitotic rate of, estrogen-stimulated,
        19
  changes in, and breast imaging, 511
  mammogram and, 230
    histologic evaluation and, 230
Metaplastic bone formation, 607, 610
Metastatic breast cancer, 127–130
  negative mode xerographic instance of,
      355
Metastatic lesions
  to the breast, 607, 609
  major sites of involvement, 109
  model for, 130

primary cancer of, 292
tumor size and, 129–130
Metastatic potential
breast cancer and, natural history of, 123
lymph nodes and, presence of tumor in,
11
Metastatic spread
cell changes required for, 42
intramammary lymph node and,
enlargement of, 353
Microcalcifications. *See also* Calcifications
benign, 389–390
clustered, mammography capable of
detecting, 388
definition of, 389
malignancy and, varied, 395–396
malignant, 389–390
mammographic findings and, 207
mammographic interpretation of, 220
mammography, magnifying lens and, 222
new, recurrent breast cancer and, 471
size of, 389
threshold number for biopsy, 388–389
Microlobulated margins
defined, 277
malignancy and, 295
mammographic instance of, 278, 294,
295
Microscopic invasion, ductal carcinoma in
situ and, 122
Milk line, 4
accessory breast tissue and, 5, 231
breast development and, 4
Milk of calcium
benign process, 328
diagnosis of, 362
lobular acini and, 361–362
mammographic instance of, 363
Milroy's disease, skin thickening and, 341
Minimal cancer
Breast Cancer Detection Demonstration
Project (BCDDP), defini-
tion of, 133
early-stage, definition of, 133
as poor term, 133
Minority women, and lack of inclusion in
screening trials, 69
Mirror images
film positioning of mammograms and,
248
mammogram viewing, asymmetry and,
221
MLO projection. *See* Mediolateral oblique
projection (MLO)
Mole markers, radiopaque, for skin
lesions, 351
Molybdenum anodes
contrast of mammography and, 144
screen-film mammography and, characteristic radiation and,
138–139

Mondor's disease, 566–567
Montgomery's glands
anatomy of, 3
breast anatomy and, 3
Morgagni's tubercles
anatomy of, 3
breast anatomy and, 3
Mortality, breast cancer
and benefit from screening, 65
Breast Cancer Detection Demonstration
Project (BCDDP) data, Surveillance, Epidemiology,
and End Results (SEER)
data and, 72
cancer detection and, 65
screening, 66
compared with other causes, 66
randomized controlled trials, surrogate
end points to predict, 57
MRI. *See* Magnetic resonance imaging
Mucinous carcinoma, 587, 588
Mueller tray, for needle biopsy, 708, 709
Multicentric breast cancer, defined, 125
Multifocal breast cancer
defined, 125
lesions of, connections between,
125–126
Multiple rounded densities
causes of, 356
cysts and, 356
defined, 311
fibroglandular tissue and, 356
follow-up for, 311–312
mammographic instance of, 312, 357,
358, 359
metastatic lesions and, 356
morphology suspicious, biopsy for,
311–312
ultrasound
not recommended for, 311
to evaluate, not standard of care, 356,
358
Multiple vague densities, follow-up for, 312
Muscles. *See also specific muscles*
orientation of, 5
Myocutaneous flaps. *See* Transverse rectus
abdominis myocutaneous flap
Myoepithelial cells
lactation and, 16
pregnancy, changes during, 20
Myoid hamartomas, imaging, no distinguishing features by, 292

N

Nagasaki, and high-dose radiation exposure, breast cancer risk
increased from, 101,
103–104
National Breast Screening Study of
Canada (NBSS) trial
age for screening, 77, 82

efficacy of, 87
breast tissue patterns, dense, breast cancer risk and, 50
clinical breast examination used in, 96
contamination and, 87
design of, 75–76, 82
diagnostic intervention, effectiveness of
screening and, 90
lymph node–positive participants,
88–90
population with, 75–76
mammographic screening, compared
with physical examination,
67
mammography, quality
effectiveness of screening and, 90
poor in, 87–88
mortality rates, concerns regarding
screening and, 95
negative screening, false reassurance
and, 90
randomized controlled trials, 75–76
need for, 66
populations for study and, 68
results of
complications with, 91
summary, 90
risk for breast cancer, tissue density
and, 240
statistical significance of, 88–89
thresholds for intervention, 90
validity of, 88–90
volunteers for, 75, 88
screening trial design and, 69
National Cancer Advisory Board (NCAB),
screening guidelines and, 78
National Cancer Institute (NCI). *See also*
Surveillance, Epidemiol-
ogy, and End Results
(SEER)
lifetime risk and, Surveillance, Epidemiology, and End Results
(SEER) data, 30
position on screening efficacy, 97–98
randomized controlled trial data and,
97–98
screening
denied to women in their 40s, inappropriate data analysis and,
68
guidelines and, 78, 87
National Institutes of Health Consensus
Development Conference
(CDC)
conflicts of interest and, 97–98
organization of, 97–98
recommendation of, 97–98
National Surgical Adjuvant Breast Project
(NSABP), ductal carcinoma
in situ, study of treatments,
118

Necrosis
  calcifications with, 317
  prognostic feature, ductal carcinoma in
    situ and, 121
Needle biopsy. *See also* Core needle
    biopsy; Biopsy, needle
  clinical guidance with, 447
  imaging guidance with, 447
    implants and, 483
  implants and, 494
  increasing use of, 375
  of indeterminate lesion, 226
  mammogram and
    changes on, after, 449
    effect on, 447
  radial scars, unreliable for, 380
  ultrasound-guided, reliability of, 412
Needle localization
  fenestrated compression plates and, 494
  for lesion in implanted breast, 494
  ultrasound with, 495
Needle positioning
  accurate methods of, 226–227
  computed tomography and, 226
  magnetic resonance imaging and, 226
  mammographic unit and, 226
  ultrasound and, 226
Needles, hypodermic, for localization and
    excisional biopsy, 648–650
Neo-adjuvant chemotherapy. *See also*
    Chemotherapy, primary
  tumor reduction and, mammographic
    instance of, 472
Neodensities
  cysts, 305
  fibroadenomas, 305
  mammographic instance of, 377
  mammographic interpretation of, 251
Nijmegen, the Netherlands, and screening
    programs, cancers over-
    looked in, 245
Nipple(s). *See also* Nipple axis line
    (NAL); Nipple discharge
  adenoma of, 516
  anatomy of, 3, 14–15
  areolar complex, imaging positions,
    ultrasound instance of, 418
  areolar contraction, mammographic
    instance of, 342
  as axis
    craniocaudal projection, 184
    rotation and, 205
  breast anatomy and, 3
  breast disease in, 513. *See also* Papillo-
    mas
  calcifications in, 14–15
  cancers immediately beneath, 16
  changes to, asymmetric gynecomastia
    and, 502
  deviation of, secondary sign of malig-
    nancy, 406

hypoechoic, ultrasound and, 422
inversion of
  benign processes and, 342–343
  malignancy, secondary sign of, 406
  mammographic instance of, 405
keratin plugs in, 308
male, breast cancer and, 500
mammographic imaging of
  craniocaudal projection and, 186
  positioning for, 249
  secondary to breast imaging, 339
muscle in, 14
Paget's disease and, 22, 343
reference point and, mediolateral
    oblique projections and,
    183, 184
retraction of, 780, 781
  benign processes and, 342–343
  clinical examination of, 342
  gynecomastia and, xerographic
    instance of, 504
  in male breast, breast cancer and, 500
  malignancy, as secondary sign of,
    342–343, 406
sebaceous glands in, 14
surface of, 3
  ducts and, 16
tissue eccentric from, architectural dis-
    tortion, 384
Nipple axis line (NAL)
  craniocaudal projection and, 188–189
  mammogram positioning and, 248–249,
    249–250
  mediolateral oblique projection and,
    188–189
Nipple discharge
  bilateral, hormonal cause and, 343
  bloody or serous. *See* Papillomas, large
    duct (intraductal)
  breast cancer associated with, 343
  characteristics of, 343
  clinical examination, trigger point and,
    344
  duct dilatation and, 308
    in association with cancer, 309
  galactography to evaluate, 344
  in male breast, breast cancer and, 500
  mammography obtained with, 344
  management of, 343–344
  and nipple lesions, 513
  papillomas and, intraductal, 360
  unilateral
    benign duct ectasia and, 343
    benign processes causing, 343
Nodular densities, breast tissue patterns
    and, 239
Noise
  calcifications lost in, 149
  magnification to reduce, 209
  reduction of
    lesion verification and, 222–223

magnification mammography, 255
mammographic resolution and, 141
Nulliparity. *See also* Pregnancy
  breast cancer risk and, 47, 446
Nutrition and maturation, breast cancer
    risk and, 44

O

Obesity, as risk for breast cancer, 44, 50
Occult lesion, clinically, evaluation of
    mammographically
    detected, 755
Oil cyst(s)
  acoustic shadowing on ultrasound and,
    439
  calcified, mammographic instance of, 360
  mammographic demonstration of, 215
  postsurgical, as common change,
    457–458
  post-traumatic, 554, 555–556
Oncogenes
  activation sequence of, breast cancer
    and, 127
  cell growth and, 38–39
  tissue assay and, 132
Oral contraceptives, breast cancer risk and,
    34, 50
Osteogenic sarcoma, 599, 600
Ostergotland trial
  mortality rates, concerns regarding
    screening and, 95
  randomized controlled trials, 73–74
Ovarian cancer, metastatic to breast, 292
  mammographic instance of, 293
Ovulatory cycles
  breast cancer development and, 43
  earlier onset of, annual incidence of
    breast cancer and, 33
  risk for breast cancer, reduction and, 33
  suspension of, breast cancer risk
    reduced with, 47

P

p53 gene, tumor suppressor, breast cancer
    and, 127
p53 protein, cell cycle regulation, 38
Paget's disease, 513, 583–584
  calcifications of nipple and, 320
  characterization of, 22
  intraductal cancer and, 343
  TNM classification of, 110
Palladium, filters used in mammography
    and, 144
Palpable abnormalities, mammographic
    visibility and, 215
Palpable lesions
  clinical value of mammography for,
    751–755
    critical path and outcome analysis,
    752–753
  diagnosis of, 441

mammographic workup for, 750–751
  spot compression, 750–751
treatment of, 441
use of ultrasound to assess, 348,
    756–758
  demonstration of cyst, 757–758
Papillary cancers
  intracystic nature of, 279
  carcinoma, 586–587
    margins of, 279
  papilloma. *See* Papillomas
Papillomas, 513, 516–521
  calcifications and, 315, 361
  large duct (intraductal), 516–521
    intracystic, 517–518
    location of, subareolar region,
      273
    mammographic appearance of,
      518–521
    mammography, not visible by, 273
    producing shell-like calcific deposits,
      519–520
    relationship to nipple, 518–519
    solitary, 22
    ultrasound appearance of, 520, 521
    vs. papillomatosis, 516
  multiple peripheral, 22–23, 527
  and relative risk for invasive breast can-
    cer, 512
Papillomatosis
  in distal ducts, 514
    vs. intraductal papilloma, 516
  radial scars and, 305
Paraffin injection, illegal status of, 471
Parallax, lesion location and, 204–206
  needle localization, 681, 683–685,
    686–688, 690
Parenchyma
  density of, male breast mammographic
    finding, 501
  and implant obscuring, 494
  magnetic resonance imaging of, signal
    intensity, 492
  normal, variations in, on ultrasound,
    423
  ultrasound and, 409
  ultrasound instance of, 424
  variations in, automatic exposure con-
    trol, reduced accuracy in
    mammograms with, 150
Parenchymal cone
  breast anatomy and, 14
  periphery of
    architectural distortion of, 385–386
      common type of, 301–302
      mammographic instance of, 301,
        385–387
    cancer development, frequency of, 240
    cancer location, 271
    intramammary lymph nodes, location
      of, 351

subcutaneous fat interface
  Cooper's ligaments and, 385–386
  retinacula cutis and, 385–386
Parenchymal pattern. *See also* Dense
    breast
  breast tissue types and, 238–239
  mammographic, 21
Pathologic staging
  clinical staging data as part of, 109–110
  elements of, 108, 109–110
  gross assessment of tumor, 108
  histologic evaluation, 108
  pathologic examination of primary car-
    cinoma as part of, 109–110
  surgical exploration and resection as
    part of, 109–110
Peau d'orange
  inflammatory carcinoma and, 590, 591,
    592
  skin thickening and, 341, 406
Pectoralis muscle(s), 3
  breast anatomy and, 5, 8, 13–14
  cancer staging and, 107–108
  craniocaudal projection and, 189
  density of, 8
  hypoechoic quality, ultrasound instance
    of, 424
  implant placement and, 475–477
  location of, 3
    mammography and, 8–9
  mammogram positioning and,
    249–250
  mammogram visibility and, 11
  mammography aid to positioning
    (MAP) and, 189–191
  mediolateral oblique projection and, 10,
    175–176, 188–189
  modified radical mastectomy and, 465
  orientation of, 5
  pendent positioning, mammographic
    image and, 172, 173, 174
  structure of, 3, 5
    importance for breast imaging, 3
  ultrasound and, 409
Pendent positioning, 172, 173, 174
Perception, psychovisual threshold
  double reading and, 213–214
  mammogram interpretation and,
    213–214
Pericystic fibrosis, margin appearance and,
    295–296
Pericystic inflammation, margin appear-
    ance and, 295–296
Periductal mastitis, and relative risk for
    invasive breast cancer, 512
Periductal stroma, tumor infiltration and,
    107
Phantom images. *See* American College of
    Radiology (ACR), phantom
Phenotype, DNA alterations, malignancy
    and, 36

Phylloides tumor(s), 594, 596, 597–598,
    599
  benign, 436
  dense, 356
  fibroadenoma and, 25–26, 528
  growth of, 25–26, 291
  malignant potential of, 25–26
  mammographic instance of, 290
  natural history of, 291
  ultrasound instance of, 434
Physical examination. *See also* Breast self-
    examination; Clinical breast
    examination (CBE)
  negative, mammogram and, 215
  palpable lesions found on, 192
  radiographic density and, no relation-
    ship between, 242–243
  screening mammography as comple-
    mentary to, 215, 216
  screening, detection of cancers and, 60
Physicians, ultrasound, responsibilities
    with, 419
Plasma cell mastitis, 522, 523
  mammographic instance of, 364
  rod-shaped calcifications and, 365
Pleomorphic calcifications
  as indicators of cancer, 315–316
  in lymph node, metastatic breast cancer
    and, 347
  mammographic instance of, 316, 318,
    394
  significance of, 332–333
Ploidy of cells, flow cytometry to mea-
    sure, 132
Pneumocystography, 699
Poland's syndrome, 611–612
Polyurethane
  exposure to, implants and, 475
  hepatic cancer risk and, 483
  on implants, ingrowth of tissue and,
    475
Positioning, for mammography
  and false-negative mammography, 793
  importance of, 171
  for mediolateral oblique projection
    proper, 175
    technologist and, 177, 179
  pendent, 172, 173, 174
Positive predictive value
  age, increasing with, 376
  biopsy, seen as recommendation for, 217
  and breast cancer presentation, variabil-
    ity of, 217
  context of, 217
  threshold for intervention and, 211
  variation in, 217
Positron emission tomography
  axillary lymph nodes assessment and,
    345
  future role in evaluating breast lesions,
    835–837

Post-traumatic oil cyst
  after reduction mammaplasty
    mammographic instance of, 450–451,
      462
  characteristics of, 436
  diagnosis of, 436
  mammographic instance of, 355
  postsurgical, mammographic instance
    of, 456
  x-ray attenuation of, 306
Post-treatment changes
  long-term follow-up, screening treated
    breast, 470
  magnetic resonance imaging, recurrence
    distinguished from, 470
  new baseline, 6 months after radiation,
    470
Post-treatment follow-up, clinical exami-
    nation and, 471
Postsurgical changes. See also Scarring
  architectural distortion, mammographic
    instance of, 379
    persistent, 460
  asymmetric tissue, mammographic
    instance of, 460
  biopsy technique and, 458–459
  calcifications and, 329, 330
  diagnosis of, 304
  fat necrosis, 456
  healing of, 379
  hematoma and, 449, 451
    mammographic instance of, 304
  mammogram projections, difference
    between, 379–380,
    453–454
  mammograms and, 449
  markers for cutaneous scar and, 380
  missed cancer, biopsy for, 380
  pathology review for questions, 380
  persistent, 457–458
    short-interval follow-up of, 466–467
  prominence on different projections,
    453–454
    mammographic instance of, 453
  radiation therapy, 466
    healing delayed after, 449
  resolution of, 455, 456–457, 459
    mammographic instance of, 454,
    457–458
    ultrasound instance of, 458
  scarring and, 304
  stability of, 456–457
  tissue distortion, reducing, 459–460
Precursor lesions, field abnormalities and,
    230
Pregnancy. See also Nulliparity
  age at, risk for breast cancer and,
    33, 34
  breast cancer(s) and, 104
    development and, 43
    diagnosed during, 446

prognosis of, 446
  risk reduced for, 446
  survival and, 446
breast changes during, 8, 445
breast density and, 235
breast development and, 104
early and repeated, risk for breast can-
    cer and, 33
effect on breast, 19–20
epithelial cells and, 19–20
lactation and, 8
Premalignant lesion, breast cancer model
    and, 42
Prevalence screen, first breast cancer
    screen, 61
Primary care physicians, breast evalua-
    tions and, 441
Primary excision
  size of, risk of recurrence and,
    468–469
  staining of, for histologic evaluation,
    469
Progesterone
  breast cancer development and, 43
  receptors, detected in tumors, 43
    activity, prognosis and, 112
Progestins, hormone replacement therapy
    and, breast cancer risk and,
    34
Prognosis
  size of lesion and, 281
  thresholds for intervention and,
    218–219
Prognostic factors
  anatomic, 114
  cellular, 114
  College of American Pathologists
    (CAP) and, 112–114
Projections. See also Superimposition of
    tissues, basic approaches
    to; Triangulation
  comparison of, 722–723
    arc method, 722
    cartesian, straight-line method,
    722–723
  craniocaudal. See Craniocaudal projec-
    tion
  dissecting the lesion, 722
  importance of varying, 721–723
  lateromedial. See Lateromedial projec-
    tion, to reduce geometric
    blur
  mediolateral oblique. See Mediolateral
    oblique projection
  rolled views, 725–726, 728
Proliferative changes, atypical, as risk fac-
    tor for breast cancer, 47
Proteins, growth factors, tumors and, 36
Proteolytic enzymes
  breast cancer model and, 42
  cathepsin D, measurements of, 132–133

tumor metastasis and, 127
Proto-oncogenes
  activation of, breast cancer mechanism,
    126
  cell growth and, 38–39
Pseudoangiomatous stromal hyperplasia,
    563
  lesions categorized as, 289
Pseudogynecomastia, and fat deposition,
    501
Psoriasis, skin thickening and, 341
Psychovisual threshold, mammogram
    interpretation and, 213–214

Q

Quadrant section
  reconstruction after, 464
  residual tumor after, 464
  tissue removed in, 464
Quality assurance
  compliance programs
    American College of Radiology
      (ACR) National Mammog-
      raphy Accreditation Pro-
      gram, 168
    Mammography Quality Standards Act
      (MQSA), 168
    mammography, management program
      of, 157
    mammography unit, equipment accep-
      tance testing and, 158
Quality assurance program
  manual, contents of, 164
  responsible person for program,
    163–164
Quality control
  compromised images, examples of
    artifact, 165
    between film and screen, 168
    developer chemistry and, 160
    grid lines on mammographic image,
    159
    motion blur, 167
  mammography and, 157–158
  quality maintenance through, 157–158
  testing, image quality and, 158
  tests
    American College of Radiology
      (ACR) recommendations
      of, 164–165
    objectives for
      compression force appropriate, 168
      darkroom cleanliness, 165
      darkroom fog checked, 168
      fixer retention, 168
      mammography technique chart
        and, 168
      phantom images and, 166
      processor quality control and, 165
      repeat analysis tracked, 168
      screen cleanliness, 166

screen-film contact and, 168
view box cleanliness, 166
visual checklist, 168
scheduling of, 164–165
Quantum mottle, mammography noise
and, 137

R

Radial scars, 565–566
adenosis and, 305
architectural distortion and, 305
benign lesion, spiculation of, mammographic instance of, 380
biopsy for, 299, 380
epithelial hyperplasia and, 305
etiology of, 26–27
idiopathic lesion, 305
etiology unknown, 380
indistinguishable from cancer, mammographic instance of, 385
mammographic appearance of, 26–27
mammographic instance of, 300, 305
other terms for, 299
papillomatosis and, 305
spiculated margins of, mimic of malignancy, 378
spicules produced by, 279
biopsy required for diagnosis, 279
Radiation carcinogenesis, of developing
breast, 49
Radiation risk
age and, 103, 104
at exposure and, 103–104, 105,
441–442
assessment, screening and, 95
carcinogenesis of the breast, 103
doses and, 102–103
effect of radiation, latency period for,
103
fetus and, 105
low-dose risk estimates, age at exposure
and, 103–104
mammographic dose limit and, 152
mammography, 105
high quality and, 104
safety of, 101
screening and, 98
significance of, 102–103
tuberculosis patients and, 103
Radiation therapy. *See also* Radiation
adjuvant treatment
after surgical removal of tumor, 465
excessive residual tumor burden and,
255
intentions of, 15
breast conservation and, 464
calcifications and, 397
contralateral cancer risk and, 471
ductal carcinoma in situ, with lumpectomy, recurrence rate and,
118

excision of tumor, 464
and future cancer, no protection from,
471
iridium implants with, 466
leukemia risk, 471
and lumpectomy, 118, 464
magnification mammography and,
254–255
new breast cancer risk, 471
postsurgical change and, 466
protocols, 466
residual tumor burden and, 465
sarcoma risk, 471
skin thickening and, 405
Radiation. *See also* Radiation therapy
breast carcinogenesis and, 101
carcinogenic effects of, 445
on epithelium, pregnancy and, 445
chest fluoroscopies, for tuberculosis, 101
DNA damage and, risk for breast cancer
and, 48
doses used in mammography
detective quantum efficiency and,
153
determination of, 152–153
and dose limit, image quality not
compromised for, 152
dose reduction and, 153
glandular dose and, 152–153
half-value layer and, 152–153
measurement of, 152–153
midbreast dose and, 153
National Council on Radiation Protection and Measurements,
manual published by,
152–153
reduced with xeroradiographic technique, 101
signal-to-noise ratio, 153
detective quantum efficiency formula, 153
skin entrance dose and, 153
high-dose exposure, breast cancer risk
increased from, 101–102
ionizing
carcinogen, 101
exposure to, breast cancer risk in
male breast, 498
irradiation, for Hodgkin's disease,
101–102
organs sensitive to, 101
residual disease and, 255
risk
age at exposure and, 48–49
DNA damage and, 48–49
therapeutic doses of, for mastitis, 101
Radioactive thymidine, DNA synthetic activity, measurement of, 132
Radiographic density
concern over, 242
firmness distinct from, 242–243

predictors of, 243
Radiologists
clinical breast examination
consequences of performing, 193
not required to perform, 192
training for, 192
mammogram interpretation and, 212,
247
double reading and, 213–214
responsibilities of, and lesions detected
by mammogram only,
284
role in mammography, 163–165
ultrasound, responsibilities of, 418
untrained, National Breast Screening
Study of Canada (NBSS)
and, 88
Radionuclide imaging, needle biopsy and,
447
Radiopaque markers
conventions regarding, 192
mammogram labeling and, 191–192
Randomized controlled trials
analysis of results, 82–83, 84, 85
cancer interruption possible, 117
deaths odds ratio for, 76
design of, 67–68, 82–83
earlier diagnosis, mortality reduced
from, 128
Edinburgh trial, 74–75
efficacy of, size and, 86
efficacy of an intervention, proof of,
66–67
factors that influence, 67, 70
follow-up for, 68
Gothenburg trial, 74
Health Insurance Plan of New York
trial, 73
age of screening and, 82
background survival among controls
and, 84
Kopparberg trial, 73–47
Malmö trial, 74
analysis of results, 83
mammography and, 55
mortality reduction, demonstration of,
83–85
National Breast Screening Study of
Canada (NBSS), 75–76
age of screening and, 82
lymph node–positive breast cancer in,
69
populations for study, 68
treatment bias and, 69
validity of, 88–89
Ostergotland trial, 73–74
populations for study, selection of, 68
results summarizing, statistically significant benefits and, 98
screening and, 56–57
efficacy of, 56–57

Randomized controlled trials *(contd.)*
   intervals, 85
   quality, 70
   proof of efficacy and, 66
   statistical power of, sample size, 67
   Stockholm trial, 74
   surrogate end points in, 57
   Swedish trials, 73–74
   threshold for intervention, 70
   treatment bias and, 69
   Two County trial, 73–74
   validity of, 88–89
RCTs. *See* Randomized controlled trials
Reactive hyperplasia, axillary lymph
       nodes and, 345
Recall rates, biopsy recommendation and,
       81
Receiver operating characteristic curve,
       lesion features, recognized
       by mammogram readers,
       218
Reciprocity law failure, film exposure in
       mammography and, 143
Recurrence
   after irradiation, mammographic
       instance of, 469
   and conservation therapy, completeness
       of primary excision, 468
   detection of, 467, 808–809
   rates of
      after lumpectomy and radiation, 470
      screening and, 131
Reduction mammaplasty
   architectural distortion
      mammographic instance of, 450
      persistent after, 450
   breast tissue appearance after, mammo-
      graphic instance of, 461–463
   calcification of suture material and, 367
   incisions of, 461
   mammography after, 460–462
   reasons for, 461
Regional lymph nodes
   anatomy, cancer staging and, 109
   relative risk of cancer based on patho-
      logic examination of benign
      tissue, 512–513
Renal cell carcinoma, metastasizing to
       breast, 292
Reporting, of breast imaging, 761–796
   Breast Imaging Reporting and Data
      System (BIRADS) and,
      225–227. *See also* Ameri-
      can College of Radiology
      Breast Imaging Reporting
      and Data System
      (BIRADS)
   general principles, 761–762
   histology terminology, 761–762
   similarity to fluoroscopy, 721
   Wolfe's breast tissue patterns, 762

Residual tumor burden
   after surgery, radiation efficacy and, 465
   survival rate and, 465–466
Resolution
   contrast and, 142
   elements of, mammography and, 142
   focal spot, shape and, 143
   improving with magnification, 154
   variation in actual spatial, mammogra-
      phy and, 142–143
Retinacula cutis
   breast anatomy and, 13
   location of, 14
   parenchymal edge distortion and,
      385–386
   skin and, 339
Retromammary fascia. *See* Fascia, retro-
      mammary
Retromammary fat
   breast cancer found in, 34
   hypoechoic quality, 425
      ultrasound instance of, 424
   ultrasound and, 409
Rhodium
   anodes used in mammography and, 144
      characteristic radiation and, 138–139
   filters used in mammography and, 144
Ribs
   as hypoechoic structures, 425
   ultrasound and, 409
   ultrasound instance of, 424
Risk factors for breast cancer
   annual incidence and, 30
   assessing, 44–45
   atypical hyperplasia, 30
   atypical proliferative change and, 45
   complexity of, 45
   dietary, 44–45
   family history of breast cancer, 45
   for invasive breast cancer, hormones, 29
   height, 45
   hormones, 43–33
   lactation, 44
   lifetime defined, 30
   mammographic screening and, 45
   obesity, 44
   ovulatory cycles and, 43–44
      total number of, 43–45
   pregnancy, 44
   significance of, 29
RODEO pulse sequence, for fat suppres-
      sion on MRI of breast
      lesions, 628
Rolled views, 725–726, 728
   lesion location and, 223
   positioning for, 205, 206–207

S
Saline, as implant type, 475
Sarcomas
   angiosarcomas, rarity of, 26

   of the breast, 594, 596–604
      adenoid cystic, 601, 602–603
      angiosarcoma, 596, 598, 599
      fibrosarcoma and liposarcoma, 596
      malignant fibrous histiocytoma, 599,
       601, 602
      mucoepidermoid carcinoma,
       603–604
      osteogenic, 599, 600
      phylloides tumor, 594, 596, 597–598,
       599
   fibrosarcomas, rarity of, 26
   imaging, no distinguishing features by,
      292
   liposarcomas, rarity of, 26
   risk from radiation therapy, 471
Scarring. *See also* Fat necrosis and scar-
      ring; Postsurgical changes
   after explantation, 492
   architectural distortion and, 384–385
   healing of, 378–380
   postsurgical
      biopsy of benign lesion and, 456–457
      hematoma and, 457
      mammographic instance of, 303
      spiculated margins of, mimic of malig-
       nancy, 378
Scatter radiation
   breast compression effect on, 148
   breast thickness effect on, 148
   Compton scattering and, 148
   grid use and, 148
      types of grids, 148–149
   magnification mammography and, 154
   radiation dose and, 148
   scatter reduction, contrast and, 148
Schistosomiasis, 568–569
Scintigraphic imaging, future role in evalu-
      ating breast lesions, 834–835
Scleroderma, silicone implants and, 472
Sclerosing adenosis. *See also* Adenosis
   architectural distortion and, 25
Screen-film mammography
   beam filtration type, 137
   blur in, 135
   contrast in, 135–136
   focal spot size, spatial resolution and,
      138
   image quality
      quantum mottle and, 149
      radiation dose and, 149
   industrial film mammography, original
      type, 149
   modern type, 149
   molybdenum anodes, characteristic
      emission of, 138–139
   photon energy, importance of uniform,
      139
   positioning and, 149
   radiographic sharpness of, 135
   resolution limitations of, 138

rhodium anodes, characteristic emission of, 138–139
screen-film combination
    choice of, 149
    image quality and, 149
systems of, 137
techniques and, 149
tungsten anodes, characteristic emission of, 138–139
x-ray generators and, 139
Screening. *See also* Screening programs
age to begin, 1, 51, 78, 85–86
    genetic risk and, 47
    National Breast Screening Study of Canada (NBSS) trial and, 75
age to stop, 96
benefits of, 56, 72
    determining, 57–58
    statistically significant, in women aged 40 to 49, 97
breast cancer, compared with cervical cancer, 97
cancer detection, early intervention and, 71
cancer growth rate and, 63
compared with cervical screening, 97
contamination and, 76
cost-benefit analyses of, 96–97
costs of, 56, 57
    relationship to intervals of, 94, 95
defined, 56, 71, 211
detection threshold for, 70
diagnosis separated from, 219
earlier detection of cancers, mammography and, 29
early detection and, 133
    mortality reduction, 51–52
efficacy of, 1, 56, 76, 133, 211
    National Cancer Institute, position of, 97
frequency of, 1, 91, 133, 388, 470
guidelines
    baseline mammogram, 77
    mammography intervals, 77
health planners and, 96
incidence rate of cancers diagnosed and, 61
increased incidence and, 34
intervals between, 62
    cancer growth rate and, 64–65
    importance of, 58, 59–60
intervention results and, 96–97
interventions from compared, 96
lead time and, 62
    gained by, 91–93
length-biased sampling, cancer growth rate and, 65
Malmö, Sweden, report of mortality reduction, 55
mammographic study and, 171

mammography and
    clinical breast examination and, 98
    costs and benefits of, 98
    detection of cancers and, 60, 229
    efficacy of, 2
Massachusetts General Hospital, tumor size and, 133
methods, efficacy of, 2
mortality rate reduction, 52, 133
negative, false reassurance and, 90
noncompliance and, 76
physical examination, detection of cancers and, 60
problems with, and cancers morphologically indistinguishable from benign lesions, 62
procedure
    technical quality of, randomized controlled trials and, 67
    thresholds for intervention and, 67
public health issues and, 57
purpose of
    false-negative rate and, 218
    false-positive rate and, 218
radiation risk and, 95
randomized controlled trials
    analysis of data from, 57
    proof of benefit and, 56–57
    proof of efficacy and, 56–57, 66
recommendations for, American Cancer Society, 98
risk factors and, 52
risks of, 56
single-view mammography, missed cancers and, 70, 91
statistical significance and, 57
survival time and, 65–66
Swedish results, 29
Swedish Two County trial, 32
terminology of, 216–217
thresholds for intervention, importance of, 58
two-view mammography, detection and, 91
Screening programs. *See also* Screening
abnormalities, tracking of, 227
cancers detected and, 217
detection of early-stage cancers and, 87
for women treated for breast cancer, American College of Radiology (ACR) Standard for Diagnostic Mammography position, 470
Nijmegen, the Netherlands, cancers overlooked in, 245
successful
    goals for, 217
    measures of, 217
UCSF, intervals between screening, 94
Screening trials. *See also* Randomized controlled trials
contamination and, 69, 70

design of, 68–69
earlier detection, mortality reduction and, 130
Edinburgh trial, 70
follow-up, length needed for, 70
Health Insurance Plan of New York, 70
    death rate and, 71
Malmö trial, 70
National Breast Screening Study of Canada (NBSS), 70
noncompliance and, 69, 70
Ostergotland trial, 70
Two County trial, 70
Sebaceous cysts, mammographic projection ability, 267
Sebaceous glands. *See* Montgomery's glands
Seborrheic keratosis
    benign skin lesion, 351
    characteristics of, 269
    mammographic findings and, 207
    mammographic instance of, 268, 269, 270
    mammographic projection ability, 267
Secretions, produced in male breast, 497
Secretory calcifications
    benign, 361
    coincidental cancer with, mammographic instance of, 365
    mammographic instance of, 364
Secretory carcinoma, 611
Secretory deposits, 523–524, 525
Seminoma, gynecomastia and, 497
Sensitivity, of mammographic screening program, 791–792
Sentinel node
    for breast cancer, radionuclide injections and, 12
    evaluation, 705
Seromas
    hematomas indistinguishable from, 455–456
    postsurgical development of, 470
Short-interval follow-up, lesion(s), classification determining, 227
Silicone
    antigenic properties of, 472
    breast implants. *See* Implants, breast
    collections outside implant, as indication of implant rupture, 487, 489
    exposure to
        implant rupture and, 478
        with implants, 475
    gel
        anechoic character of, normal, 489
        composition of, 475
        implant type, 475
        implant evaluation and, on ultrasound, 489

Silicone *(contd.)*
  injections
    calcified granulomas from, xerographic instance of, 473
    illegal status of, 471
  and magnetic resonance imaging, signal intensity, 492
  residual, after explantation of implants, 492
    mammographic instance of, 492
Silicosis, silicone implants and, 472
Single-view mammography
  detection and, 91
  missed cancers and, 91, 171, 172
  recall rates, 171, 172
  screening trials and, 73–74
Single-view screening, problem of, 721–722
Skin
  after irradiation, susceptible to trauma, 466
  anatomy of, 339
  benign deposits in, 723
  breast reconstruction after mastectomy and, 483–484
  calcifications, 773
    differentiated from intramammary lesions, 223
    etiology of, 365–366
    lucent-centered, benign nature of, 365
    mammographic instance of, 361, 365
    mole markers used with imaging, 366
    when to suspect, 366
  changes
    asymmetric gynecomastia and, 502
    clinically evident, 339
    Cooper's ligaments and, 405
    differential diagnosis for, 340
    evaluation of, 403–406
    mammographic abnormalities and, 338–339
  Cooper's ligaments and, 339, 405
  contamination
    mammographic instance of, 368
    on mammogram, 367
  cyst
    mammographic instance of, 353
    ultrasound instance of, 353
  dimpling, xerographic instance of, 404
  focal changes, clinical examination and, 339
  lesions
    air interface and, 267
    benign, no intervention needed, 351
    differentiated from intramammary lesions, 223
    mammographic findings and, 207
    mammographic instance of, 268–270
    mammographic projection of, 267

  mole marker use, 267, 269
    mammographic instance of, 269
  line
    mammographic view of, 219
    visible on mammogram, reasons for, 152
  mammographic findings on, 207
  mammographic imaging of, secondary to breast tissues, 339
  normal
    hypoechoic structure, ultrasound instance of, 423
    on ultrasound, 423
    thickness of, 3, 339
  retraction
    clinical examination of, 339, 342
    desmoplastic reaction to cancer, 339
    mammographic instance of, 339, 404
  thickening of. *See* Skin thickening
  TNM classification of, 110
  ultrasound and, 409
Skin thickening
  associated with cancer, advanced disease and, 405
  breast cancer and, 341
  causes of, 339–340
    benign, mammographic instance of, 341
    breast cancer and, 341
  clinical findings, 406
  congestive heart failure, xerographic instance of, 340
  diffuse, causes, 340–341
  focal, causes, 340
  gynecomastia and, 497
    xerographic instance of, 504
  inflammatory carcinoma and, 406
  irradiation of breast and, 340–341, 466
  in male breast, 497
  mammographic instance of, 340
  and peau d'orange, 341
  radiation therapy and, 471
    mammographic instance of, 466
  tumor invasion of dermal lymphatics, poor prognosis and, 405
  on ultrasound, 423
  used to demonstrate, 339
Sojourn time
  cancer growth and, 58–59
  detection of cancers, screening and during, 60
  early, 58–59
  incidence screen and, 61–62
  synchronized cancers, detection of, 59–60
Solitary circumscribed mass. *See also* Mass(es)
  management of, 397
  probably benign, 397, 399–400
Solitary dilated duct
  biopsy and, 400
  duct dilatation and, 308

  malignancy, secondary sign of, 400
  mammographic finding, 400
  mammographic instance of, 309, 373
  management of, 400
Spatial resolution, magnification mammography and, 154
Specificity, of mammographic screening program, 791
Spiculated margins
  defined, 277
  mammographic instance of, 278
Spiculated masses
  biopsy of, 278–279
    repeat mammogram for benign, 215
  extension of, 377
  mammographic instance of, 301, 302
  mammographic view of, 215
  postsurgical, 278–279
  superimposed normal structures and, mammographic instance of, 258
Spiculations
  desmoplastic, 302, 304
  fibrosis interspersed with tumor, 302
  postsurgical change, mammographic instance of, 303, 455
  significance of, 302
  spot compression for, mammographic instance of, 257
Spot compression, 723–724
  ability to push lesion out of field of view, 727
  accurate placement for, measuring techniques, 207–209
  area of concern, suggested by patient, 193, 195
  clinical breast examination and, 193, 195
  clinically evident abnormality and, 193, 195
  coned-down techniques and, 207–209
    circumscribed lesions, evaluation of, 292
    focal fibrosis and, 289
  goal of, 193
  ill-defined mass, evaluation of, 298
  lesions, adjunctive assessment of, 348
  magnification and, 193, 724
  nonpalpable lesions, compression paddles and, 207–209
  palpable finding, 193, 195, 750–751
    image improvement and, 194
    not standard of care, 195
    role in altering management of, rare, 193, 195
  summation shadow demonstrated by, 207
Squamous metaplasia, and relative risk for invasive breast cancer, 512
Staging, of breast cancer. *See* Cancer staging
Standard of care issues, 797–799, 800–805
  care with established efficacy, 801

careful documentation, 799
clinical breast examination with screening mammography, 803
double reading, 798
double perception, 798
in evaluation of woman with palpable breast mass
with mammography, 803–804
with ultrasound, 804
evolution of definition of, 801
failure to communicate, 798–799
failure to diagnose, 797
failure to perceive an abnormality, 797
problem of perception, 797–798
proven efficacy of mammography as screening technique only, 749, 750, 755, 801–802
for screening mammography, 802
for symptomatic patients, 802–803
for women under 40 with signs and symptoms of breast cancer, 804–805
Staphylococcus, causing breast infections, 568
Stem cells
alteration in immature breast, carcinogen exposure and, 8
breast cancer origins and, 124
field phenomena and, 124
for mammary ducts, 37
role of, 37
Stereomammography, 814
Sternalis muscle, location, mammography and, 9
Stockholm trial, randomized controlled trials, 74
Straight lateral projection
calcification evaluation and, 199–200
lesion location and, 223
positioning for, 199–200
Stromal fibrosis, parenchymal patterns and, 239
Stromal-epithelial interactions, cell transformation and, 17
Subareolar cancers, surgery for, 464
Subareolar mass, mammogram positioning and, 249
Subcutaneous adipose tissues, breast development and, 7
Subcutaneous fat
breast anatomy and, 3, 14
breast cancer found in, 34
male breast, normal, mammographic instance of, 500
ultrasound and, 409, 423
Subcutaneous mastectomy, mammography and, 494
Summation shadow, 721–722
overlap of structures, benign, spot compression used to demonstrate, 207

Superficial fascia, breast anatomy and, 13
Superimposition of tissues, basic approaches to, 723–730
angulation of x-ray system, 724–725
modified projections and rolled views, 725
with lesion seen on only one projection, 725–730
return to projection in which lesion was seen, 725–728
spot compression, 723–724. *See also* Spot compression
Supraclavicular nodes, tumors in, cancer staging and, 108
Surgical breast biopsy
accuracy in diagnosis, 448
excisional biopsy, 448
incisional biopsy, 448
lumpectomy, and excision of malignant process, 448
Surrogate end points, used in randomized controlled trials, 57
Surveillance, Epidemiology, and End Results (SEER) program
data from, 78–79
histologic grade of tumor, prognosis and, 131–132
incidence rates for breast cancer, 29
tumor registries of, 29
increase in breast cancer incidence, 30
Survival rates
and age at diagnosis, 84
staging classification and, 113
Survival time, cancer detection and, 65–66
Suture calcifications, 467
after breast biopsy, 460
after radiation therapy
characteristics of, 467
mammographic instance of, 468
after reduction mammaplasty, 462
mammographic instance of, 462
Swedish trials
mortality benefit shown from, 94
mortality rate, 133
randomized controlled trials, 73–74
Systemic treatment, survival advantage of, 464

T
Tamoxifen
breast cancer treatment, 52
endometrial cancer risk and, 52
estrogen inhibitor, inhibiting lesion growth and, 43
women eligible for, 52
TDLU. *See* Terminal duct lobular unit (TDLU)
Technologists. *See also* X-ray technologists
clinical breast examination and, consequences of performing, 193

mammographic screening, importance of training for, 212
proficiency of, 219
role in mammography, 163–165
role in positioning patient, 171
Telemammography, 831–832
Telomeres, cell division and, 38
Terminal duct lobular unit (TDLU), 4, 513, 514, 515. *See also* Lobule(s)
anatomy of, 4, 16–17
appearance of, 17
benign lesion development in, 17
cancer development in, 14, 17, 18
importance of, 16
stem cells in, 7
Testes, gynecomastia and, 497
Testicular tumors, gynecomastia and, 497
Tests. *See also* Mammogram; Ultrasound
acceptability of, 375
accuracy of, 411–412
avoiding biopsy with, 411–412
efficacy of, 411–412
management of patient, alteration due to, 411–412
Thelarche, breast development and, 6
Thresholds for intervention
benefit of screening and, 63
false-negative rate determining, 375
importance of, 58, 59–60
National Breast Screening Study of Canada (NBSS) and, 90
positive predictive value and, 211
survival advantages to, 218
Thrombophlebitis, superficial, 566–567
Tilt paddles. *See* Compression paddles
Tissue resection, size of, risk of recurrence and, 468–469
Tissue sampling, differentiating benign and malignant lesions with, 432
TNM classification
cancer staging, 107
distant metastasis, 111
histopathologic grade, 112
histopathologic type, 111–112
microinvasion of breast carcinoma, 110
pathologic classification, 111
primary tumor, 110–111
prognostic factors and, 112
regional lymph nodes, 111
stage grouping, 111
Tomography, 814
Tort of negligence, 797
Tort reform, 800
Trabecular thickening, 403
after irradiation, 466
mammographic instance of, 466
causes of, 342
mammographic instance of, 405

Trabecular thickening *(cont.)*
TRAM flap. *See* Transverse rectus abdominis myocutaneous (TRAM) flap
Transillumination, future role in breast evaluation, 833
Transverse rectus abdominis myocutaneous (TRAM) flap
  mammographic instance of, 484
  reconstruction after mastectomy and, 483–484
  schematic of, 484
Trauma. *See also* Contusion
  fat necrosis and, 290–291
  post-traumatic oil cyst and, 290–291
Triangulation, 204–207, 223, 274, 730–739. *See also* Projections; Superimposition of tissues, basic approaches to
  alteration of conventional positioning, 733–735
    lesions seen only on craniocaudal projection, 735
    lesions seen only on mediolateral oblique, 733–735
  arc method, 722
  cartesian, straight-line method, 722–723
  computed tomography for, 739
  mammographic tricks of, 204–207
  parallax and lesions in the mediolateral oblique projection, 204–206
  orthogonal x-ray imaging and, 274
  rolled views and lesions in the craniocaudal projection, 206–207
  systematic approach to, 219, 223
  ultrasound for, 735
Triple test, 705
Tubular cancer, 584, 586
Tumor aggression, theories of, 128
Tumor angiogenesis, prognosis and, 133
Tumor burden. *See* Residual tumor burden
Tumor masses, in preadolescent females, 610, 611
  secretory carcinoma, 611
Tumor neovascularity, metastasis and, 127
Tumor phenotype, evaluation of, prognostic factors and, 114
Tumor suppressor genes
  chromosome 17 and, 47
  deactivation of, breast cancer mechanism, 126
  DNA damage and repair, p53, 39
  gene function and, 40
  p53, 39, 40
    prognosis and, 112
Tumor(s). *See* Breast cancer(s)
Tungsten anodes
  dense breast tissue and, 144

screen-film mammography and, characteristic radiation and, 138–139
Two County trial
  mammography screening, radiation risk and, 104
  mortality rates, concerns regarding screening and, 95
  randomized controlled trials, 73–74
  screening, lead time gained by, 93–94
  statistical significance of, 76
  tumor size, 131
    prognosis and, 133
Two-view mammography
  detection and, 91
  radiation risk and, 104
  screening studies, preferred for all, 171
  screening trials and, 74

U

Ultrasound. *See also* Doppler ultrasound
  advances in, 409
  aspiration of cysts and, 415
  asymmetric breast tissue and, 417
  ATL unit, 412
  cancer detection rate of, 410
  cancer lesion, shadowing and, ultrasound instance of, 419
  characteristics of findings, 411
  correlated with mammography, 414–415
  cost-effective approach to, 212
  costs of, 440
  of cysts
    criteria for diagnosis, 348–349, 415
    diagnosis of, 283–284, 412, 429
    differentiated from solid masses, 409, 440
    in male breast, 508
  demonstrated lesion as a cyst, management implications, 414–415
  Doppler. *See* Doppler ultrasound
  during pregnancy, uses of, 446
  echoes, differentiated from noise and, 418
  efficacy of, 440, 442
  equipment
    gray scale adjustment algorithms and, 418–419
    hand-held, high-resolution systems
      patient positioning, 417
      preferred, 417
    high-frequency transducers for, 417
    whole-breast ultrasound units, patient position in, 417
  focal zone, transducer and, 419
  follow-up with, 413
  future role in breast imaging, 442, 832
  gain settings
    importance of, 418
    improper, ultrasound instance of, 418

ultrasound instance of, 420
guide for aspiration and, 409
histology, not determined by, 432
ill-defined mass, evaluation of, 298
implants, 416–417, 483
  detecting rupture in, 492
  evaluation of, 486
    free silicone and, 489
internal echoes, importance of correct scan factors for, 420–421
lactation and, 446
lesions
  adjunctive assessment of, 348
  detection of
    clinically occult, 413
    mammographically occult, 413
  location and, 223
  with obscured margins and, 294–295
linguine sign, implants and, 490
of male breast, 502
  hypoechoic lesions and, 508
  spiculated lesions and, 508
malignant mass, differentiated from benign mass, reliability of, 411
mammographic confirmation of, mammographic instance of, 420
multiple rounded densities
  avoided for, 312
  evaluation by not standard of care, 356, 358
needle biopsy and, 447
normal breast physiology and, 18–19
of normal breast structures
  findings of, 412–413
  hypoechoic qualities of, 412–413
operator-dependency of, 417
of palpable mass, in evaluation of, 2, 756–758
  demonstration of cyst, 757–758
patient positioning for, 409, 419
performance of, 409
physical assessment during scanning, 419
physicians, responsibilities with, 417, 419
post-treatment breast, evaluation of, 470
primary use of, 440
reliability, biopsy avoidance and, 411
sample report for, 787–789
scanning technique, need for definition of, 411
scans, standard planes of, 419
screening, 409, 442
  efficacy of, 410–411
silicone, hypoechoic nature of, 416
skin thickening, demonstrated using, 339
solid focal area by, biopsy considered for, 383

solitary circumscribed masses, evaluation of, 281
standard of care issues for, 804
survey technique, 412–413
system
  problems with, 418
  requirements of, 418
tissue diagnosis and, 412
tissues evaluated by, 409
transducer, variable compression with, 436
  ultrasound instance of, 437
transducer-skin interface, specular reflection at, 423
triangulation of lesions and, 415, 735, 738
unable to avoid biopsy with, 442
use of, appropriate, 414–415
and viewing all contiguous tissue, 419
whole-breast systems of, 442
Ultrasound-guided aspiration, of cyst, ultrasound instance of, 415
Ultrasound-guided biopsies, reliability of, 415–416
Ultrasound-guided FNA cytology. See Fine-needle aspiration
Ultrasound-guided needle procedures, 692–700
  aspiration and localization, 693–699
  "third hand," 693–699
  fluid analysis, 699
  patient positioning, 693
  patient preparation, 693
  transducer selection, 693
  under direct real-time observation for surgical excision, 699–700

Union Internationale Contre Le Cancer (UICC), staging system of, 107

V
Van Nuys Prognostic Index for ductal carcinoma in situ, 570
Vascular asymmetry
  benign, mammographic instance of, 266
  causes of, 403
  mammographic instance of, 403
  as normal variation, 265–266
  origin of, 265
  palpable breast cancer and lateral xerographic instance of, 266
  secondary to thyroid cancer, mammographic instance of, 267
Vascular calcifications. See Calcifications, vascular
Vascular system, tumor access to, 130
Viruses, etiologies for breast cancer and, 45

W
Weight change, breast tissue change and, 376
Wens. See Epidermal inclusion cysts
Whole-breast ultrasound, ultrasound instance of, 410
Wolfe, John, breast tissue patterns described by, 762

X
X-ray anode
  bremsstrahlung and, 143
  composition of, 143
  molybdenum anode, filters and, 143
  molybdenum filters and, 144
  tungsten anode, characteristics of, 143

X-ray attenuation
  breast tissue patterns and, 243–244
  high, little contrast between areas of, 135
  of lesion, measure of significance of, 306
  of radiolucent lesions, 355
X-ray film
  composition of, 149–150
  image mechanism of, 149–150
X-ray image
  digital acquisition of, 135
  formation of, 148
  scatter radiation and, 148
X-ray imaging, patient interface, improvements possible to, 146–147
X-ray mammography
  goal of, 135
  radiation doses for, 101
  visibiiity of calcifications, high resolution required for, 139
  visibility of lesions, high resolution required for, 139
X-ray technologists. See also Technologists, and clinical breast examination (CBE)
  not required to perform, 192
  training for, 192
X-ray tube, composition of window, importance of, 144–145
X-rays
  anode composition, importance of, 138
  energy characteristics of, 138
  spectra, 137, 138
Xeroradiographic technique, radiation doses, mammography and, 101